A MEDICAL BIBLIOGRAPHY

A MEDICAL BIBLIOGRAPHY

(Garrison and Morton)

AN ANNOTATED CHECK-LIST OF TEXTS ILLUSTRATING THE HISTORY OF MEDICINE

Leslie T. Morton FLA

LIBRARIAN, NATIONAL INSTITUTE
FOR MEDICAL RESEARCH, LONDON

THIRD EDITION

A GRAFTON BOOK

ANDRE DEUTSCH

FIRST PUBLISHED 1943
SECOND EDITION 1954

REPRINTED 1961 BY ANDRE DEUTSCH
SECOND EDITION REVISED 1965
THIRD EDITION COMPLETELY RESET AND PRINTED 1970 BY
ANDRE DEUTSCH LIMITED
105 GREAT RUSSELL STREET
LONDON WC1
SECOND IMPRESSION OF THIRD EDITION SEPTEMBER 1976

PRINTED PHOTOLITHO IN GREAT BRITAIN BY
EBENEZER BAYLIS AND SON LTD
THE TRINITY PRESS, WORCESTER, AND LONDON
ISBN 0 233 96130 5

INTRODUCTION TO THIRD EDITION

"Every discovery, however important and apparently epoch-making, is but the natural and inevitable outcome of a vast mass of work, involving many failures, by a host of different observers."—STARLING.

The need for a third edition of this bibliography has provided an opportunity for a thorough revision and for the addition of references to recent discoveries and advances in medicine, although no attempt has been made to approach too close to the present.

The previous edition contained 6,808 items; 744 have been added and 118 removed in the present edition. The total number of entries (7,534) includes some 3,700 from Garrison's original *Check-List*. The insertion of new entries has been made in such a way as not to disturb the original numbers. Numbers for deleted items have not been used for new entries except in the sections devoted to the histories of subjects.

I am greatly indebted to the librarians of the Royal Society of Medicine and the Wellcome Institute of the History of Medicine for permission to use their libraries and for much help while doing so. I have found much information in the Wellcome Institute's *Current Work in the History of Medicine*. I have drawn heavily on Miss Joan Emmerson's extremely useful *Translations of medical classics*, 1965 (No. 6786.6). Mr. S. Watkins has again given assistance in the revision of the historical sections and in verifying references, Miss Sheila Mayo has helped in the preparation of the manuscript and my wife has assisted in the compilation of the indexes. I am grateful to Mr. Eric Gaskell for reading the proofs and for drawing my attention to some errors and omissions, and to several other friends and colleagues for information and advice.

The kind reception given to previous editions leads me to hope that the present revision will prove just as useful to those interested in the past achievement and future progress of medicine.

L. T. MORTON

EXTRACT FROM INTRODUCTION TO THE FIRST EDITION

This bibliography is an attempt to bring together in convenient form references to the most important contributions to the literature of medicine and its ancillary sciences, and, by means of annotations, to show the significance of individual contributions in the history and development of the medical sciences. In its construction I have endeavoured to take into account the special needs of research workers, librarians, bibliographers, and students of the history of medicine. The work has been arranged in a manner considered most convenient for the user, while full details of names and dates of authors, important medical eponymic terms, translations and reprints are given wherever possible. Under each subject the important works showing the development of that subject are arranged in chronological order. While such an arrangement makes necessary the occasional duplication of certain details, it has the advantage that each subject, and each entry, are self-contained units, which can be utilized without reference elsewhere. In a comparatively small book such as this only the most important references can be included, but further information can be obtained from the histories of special subjects, which will usually be found at the end of each section.

To Sir William Osler belongs the credit for first suggesting such a work as this. The late Fielding H. Garrison carried his suggestion into effect, and the list compiled by him appeared in the *Index-Catalogue of the Library of the Surgeon-General's Office*, Washington, 1912, 2nd Series, xvii, 89–178. Garrison himself wrote that he used the list "as a convenient scaffolding for a book on the history of medicine." Those familiar with his great *Introduction to the History of Medicine* will appreciate the value of the material in that list. Later Garrison revised the list and republished it in the *Bulletin of the Institute of the History of Medicine*, Baltimore, 1933; i, 333–434, entitling it "A Revised Students' Check-List of Texts Illustrating the History of Medicine," and it is this later Check-List which forms the basis of the present work. Much has been added and a little deleted. The Check-List of 1933 contained 4,186 entries, of which 3,826 have been retained, and to which 1,680 new entries have been added. Discarded entries consist principally of references to subjects not directly concerned with medicine, and histories which have since been superseded. The addition of annotations to most entries will, it is hoped, explain more clearly the significance of these entries. Another addition is the provision of author and subject indexes.

Much has been omitted which might have been included; it is hoped that nothing has been included which ought to have been omitted. Every effort has been made to check the accuracy of the references and other data, but this has not been possible in every case. Some of the books and journals mentioned here are not to be found in British libraries, while others have been stored in safe but inaccessible places or have recently been destroyed. The book has benefited from the help and advice of several friends, but responsibility for the accuracy and completeness of the information given in it rests solely with the present compiler, who will be grateful for details of errors and omissions.

I can but hope that this book will in some measure fulfil its object of assisting those who are interested in the record of past achievement and in the further development of medical science. Perhaps it may be considered worthy to serve as a starting-point for something better, to the construction of which both the specialized knowledge of the medical historian and the bibliographical skill of the librarian can at some future date be devoted.

L. T. M.

CONTENTS

1–86.4 COLLECTED WORKS; OPERA OMNIA

See also 2189–2238, MEDICINE, general works; 5547–5632, SURGERY, general works.

1 HAMMURABI, *King of Babylon.*
The code of Hammurabi, King of Babylon about 2250 B.C. Autographed text, transliteration, translation, glossary, index of subjects, lists of proper names, signs, numerals, corrections, and erasures, with map, frontispiece and photograph of text, by ROBERT FRANCIS HARPER. Chicago, *Callaghan & Co.*, 1904.

The Code of Hammurabi was found among the clay tablets of the library of Ashurbanipal. It was first published in Scheil: *Mémoires de la Délégation en Perse*, Paris, 1902, 4, 4–162. The Code mentions the fees payable to a physician following successful treatment; these varied according to the station of the patient. Similarly, the punishment for the failure of an operation is set out. At least this shows that in Babylon 4,000 years ago the medical profession had advanced far enough in public esteem to warrant the payment of adequate fees.

2 EBERS PAPYRUS.
Papyros Ebers. Das älteste Buch über Heilkunde. Aus dem Aegyptischen zum erstenmal vollständig übersetzt von H. Joachim. Berlin, *G. Reimer*, 1890.

The Ebers Papyrus dates from about 1552 B.C. The original, now at Leipzig, was discovered about 1862 and was purchased by Georg Ebers in 1873. The papyrus measures 20.23 m. in length and 30 cm. in height. It is the most important medical papyrus yet recovered; it is written in hieratic script and contains the most complete record of Egyptian medicine known. Ebers published a facsimile of the papyrus, with a partial translation, in 1875.

3 ——. The papyrus Ebers. The greatest Egyptian medical document. Translated by B. EBBELL. Copenhagen, *Levin & Munksgaard*, 1937.

Best English translation so far published.

4 WRESZINSKI, WALTER. 1880–
Der grosse medizinische Papyrus des Berliner Museums (Pap. Berl. 3038) in Facsimile und Umschrift mit Uebersetzung, Kommentar und Glossar. Herausg. von W. WRESZINSKI. Leipzig, *J. C. Hinrichs*, 1909.

The Greater German Papyrus (Brugsch Papyrus) dates from about 1300 B.C. The above facsimile reproduction and translation forms vol. 1 of the *Medizin der alten Aegypter* series.

5 CHESTER BEATTY PAPYRUS.
Le papyrus médical Chester Beatty. Par le Dr. FRANS JONCKHEERE. Bruxelles, *Fondation Égyptologique Reine Elisabeth*, 1947. *La Médecine Égyptienne*, No. 2.

A hieratic papyrus of the 13th-12th century B.C. It is a fragment of a monograph on diseases of the anus. It was reproduced with hieroglyphic transcription by A. H. Gardiner in 1935.

6 KÜCHLER, Friedrich.

Beiträge zur Kenntnis der assyrisch-babylonischen Medizin. Texte mit Umschrift, Uebersetzung und Kommentar. Leipzig, *J. C. Hinrich*, 1904.

Medical texts from the library of Ashurbanipal, together with German translations. A valuable paper on this subject is M. Jastrow's "The medicine of the Babylonians and Assyrians", *Proc. roy. Soc. Med.* 1913–14, **7**, Sect. Hist. Med., 109–76.

7 THOMPSON, Reginald Campbell. 1876–1941

Assyrian medical texts. From the originals in the British Museum. London, *Oxford Univ. Press*, 1923

Facsimiles of the texts of 660 cuneiform medical tablets, many of which were hitherto unpublished, from the library of Ashurbanipal. The tablets date back to the seventh century B.C. No translations are included, but Thompson has interpreted and systematized many of the texts in a later work (*Proc. roy. Soc. Med.*, 1924, **17**, Sect. Hist. Med., 1–34; 1926, **19**, Sect. Hist. Med., 29–78.)

8 AYURVEDA.

The Ayurvedic system of medicine. By Nagendra Nath Sen Gupta. 3 vols. Calcutta, *K. R. Chatterjee*, 1901–07.

Ayurveda is the most ancient system of Hindu medicine; only fragments of the original remain. The early Hindus believed it to be of divine origin and ascribed it to Brahma. It dates from *circa* 1400–1200 B.C.

9 CHARAKA SAMHITA.

[Charakasamhita. Edited by Jibananda Vidyasagara.] Calcutta, *Sarasvati Press*, 1877.

Sanskrit text. Authorities vary as to the date of Charaka. He is said to have lived at times varying between 800 B.C. and A.D. 78. The Samhita, or Sanhita, is one of the most ancient and complete systems of Hindu medicine to have survived. It is arranged in the form of dialogues between master and pupil and is divided into eight books. Charaka's writing is superior to that of Suśruta in the accuracy of his descriptions. What Suśruta is to surgery Charaka is to medicine.

10 ——. The Caraka Samhita. Edited and published with translations in Hindi, Gujerati and English, by Shree Gulabkunverba Ayurvedic Society. 6 vols. Jamnagar, 1949.

11 SUŚRUTA SAMHITA.

[Susruta Samita. The system of Hindu medicine taught by Dhanwantari. Compiled by Susruta. Edited and published by Pandit-kulapati Jibananda Vidyasagara]. 5th ed. Calcutta, 1909.

Sanskrit text. The Suśruta Samhita required a good educational foundation of a student of medicine. The writings of Suśruta and Charaka formed the groundwork of all the Hindu medical and surgical systems which followed. The Suśruta is divided into six books and contains a fairly accurate description of the human body, besides some surgery.

12 ——. An English translation of the Sushruta Samhita . . . translated and edited by K. K. Bhishagratna. 2nd ed. Varanasi, *Chowkhamba Sanskrit Series Office*, 1963.

13 HIPPOCRATES. 460–375 B.C.
Œuvres complètes d'Hippocrate. Traduction nouvelle avec le texte grec en regard . . . Par E. LITTRÉ. 10 vols. Paris, *J. B. Baillière*, 1839–61.

Classical philologists consider that many of the writings attributed to Hippocrates were in fact written by members of the Hippocratic School, of which he was one. Hippocrates himself is, by common consent, the greatest physician of all time, the "Father of Medicine". The first complete edition of his works to be printed in Latin was issued from Rome by Fabius Calvus in 1525. Aldus printed a Greek edition in 1526. The above Greek-French bilingual represented 22 years of continuous labour, is one of the most important editions of Hippocrates extant, and is a permanent memorial to Littré's industry and scholarship.

14 ——. The genuine works of Hippocrates. Translated from the Greek, with a preliminary discourse and annotations by FRANCIS ADAMS. 2 vols. London, *Sydenham Society*, 1849.

This is a valuable translation of Hippocrates, although limited to the so-called "genuine works". A reprint, edited by E. C. Kelly, was published in 1939 and reprinted in 1946.

15 ——. Opera. Edidit H. KUEHLEWEIN. 2 vols. Lipsiae, *B. G. Teubner*, 1894–1902.

Garrison considers this the most authoritative edition of Hippocrates in respect of collations and emendations of readings from the known manuscripts.

16 ——. Works. With English translation. Edited by W. H. S. JONES and E. T. WITHINGTON. 4 vols. London, *Heinemann*, 1923–31.

The most important English translation of Hippocrates was that published by Francis Adams (No. 14), containing only the so-called "genuine" works. The above bilingual edition, in the *Loeb Classical Library*, supersedes it in usefulness to the English reader.

16.1 ——. The medical works of Hippocrates. A new translation by J. CHADWICK and W. N. MANN. Oxford, *Blackwell*, [1950].

17 ARISTOTLE. 384–322 B.C.
Opera. Edidit Academia Regia Borussica. 5 vols. Berolini, *Reimer*, 1831–70.

Greek-Latin bilingual text. Aristotle, at one time tutor to Alexander the Great, was the founder of comparative anatomy. He made many dissections of animals. His views had a profound influence in determining the direction of medical and biological thought; perhaps no other man has so dominated and advanced science as a whole than Aristotle.

18 ——. The works of Aristotle translated into English. Edited by J. A. SMITH and W. D. ROSS. 11 vols. Oxford, *Clarendon Press*, 1908–31.

19 ASCLEPIADES *of Bithynia*. 124–56 B.C.
Fragmenta. Digessit et curavit C. G. GUMPERT. Vinariae, *Industrie-Comptoir*, 1794.

After the fall of Corinth (146 B.C.), Greek physicians migrated to Rome. There, before the advent of Asclepiades, the Greek physicians were despised and distrusted. Asclepiades may be said to have established Greek medicine in Rome on a respectable footing. Gumpert has preserved what is left of his writings in the above Greek edition. See R. M. Green, *Asclepiades, his life and writings*, New Haven, 1955, which includes a translation of Gumpert's *Fragmenta*.

20 CELSUS, AULUS AURELIUS CORNELIUS. 25 B.C.–A.D. 50
De medicina. Florentiae, *Nicolaus* [*Laurentius*], 1478.

The *De Medicina* is the oldest medical document after the Hippocratic writings. It was written about A.D. 30. After the invention of printing it was still considered important, being one of the first medical books to be set in type. Celsus has left the best account of Roman medicine; he was the first important medical historian. The manuscript of the *De medicina* was lost during the Middle Ages and re-discovered in Milan in 1443. The above edition was edited by Bartholomaeus Fontius. See Osler, *Incunabula medica*, 147.

21 ——. De medicina. With an English translation by W. G. SPENCER. 3 vols. London, *Heinemann*, 1935–38.

Loeb Classical Library. Text in Latin and English.

22 ARETAEUS *the Cappadocian*. A.D. 81–?138
Τά Σωδομένα. The extant works of Aretaeus, the Cappadocian. Edited and translated by FRANCIS ADAMS. London, *Sydenham Society*, 1856.

Aretaeus left many fine descriptions of disease; in fact Garrison ranks him second only to Hippocrates in this respect. He was a follower of the "Pneumatic School". His works were first printed in 1554; the valuable edition by Adams includes the Greek text with an English translation.

23 RUFUS *of Ephesus*. *circa* A.D. 98–117
De vesicae renumque morbis. De purgantibus medicamentis. De partibus corporis humani . . . Nunc iterum typis mandavit GULIELMUS CLINCH. Londini, *J. Clarke*, 1726.

The name of Rufus of Ephesus was known to all mediaeval physicians. In his day he stood out among his contemporaries as a great surgeon. He is particularly remembered for his work on haemostasis; he also wrote a treatise on gout. Rufus is mentioned by Chaucer's Doctor. Of his 36 works only 12 survive. The first Greek edition was printed in 1554. The above is a Greek-Latin bilingual text.

24 ——. Œuvres, texte collationné sur les MSS., traduit pour la première fois en français avec une introduction. Publication commencée par CH. DAREMBERG, continuée et terminée par CH. ÉMILE RUELLE. Paris, *Baillière*, 1879.

With Greek and Latin texts. First French edition.

25 ANONYMUS LONDINENSIS.
Anonymus Londinensis. Auszüge eines unbekannten aus Aristoteles-Menons Handbuch der Medizin und aus Werken anderer älterer Aerzte. Berlin, *G. Reimer*, 1896.

The important B. M. Papyrus 137, found in 1891, was deciphered by Sir Frederick Kenyon; a Greek text edited by Hermann Diels was published in 1893, and the above German translation (by H. Beckh and F. Spät) appeared in 1896. The work is a treatise on medicine, written about A.D. 150. It contains extracts from a lost collection of the opinions of the earlier Greek physicians, and throws some light on early Greek medicine.

26 ——. The medical writings of Anonymus Londinensis. By W. H. S. JONES. Cambridge, *University Press*, 1947.

Greek and English text on opposite pages.

27 GALEN. A.D. 130–200
Opera omnia. Ediderunt Andreas Asulanus et J. B. OPIZO. 5 vols. Venetiis, *in aedibus Aldi, et Andreae Asulani soceri*, 1525.

Greek text. First printed edition of Galen's *Opera omnia*.

28 ——. Opera omnia. Editionem curavit C. G. KÜHN. 20 vols. [in 22]. Lipsiae, *C. Cnobloch*, 1821–33.

The founder of experimental physiology, Galen stands second only to Hippocrates in importance in classical Greek medicine. He was the most voluminous of the ancient writers; his writings dominated medicine until the time of Vesalius. The above most useful edition of his works contains both Latin and Greek texts.

29 ——. Opera omnia. 4 vols. Lipsiae, *B. G. Teubner*, 1914–22.

Greek text.

30 ANTYLLUS. *fl.* A.D. 250

Antylli veteris chirurgi quae apud Oribasium libro xliv, xlv et 1 leguntur fragmenta. Dissertatio . . . publice defendet F. C. F. WOLZ. Jenae, *typ. Schreiberi*, [1842].

One of the most daring and accomplished of surgeons, Antyllus is particularly remembered for his work on the surgery of aneurysm. He was first to recognize two forms of aneurysm—one caused by dilatation and the other following wounding of an artery. Much of his writing is available to us only through the industry of Oribasius who included it in his compilations. A German version of Antyllus is in *Janus*, 1847, **2**, 298–329, 744–71; 1848, **3**, 166–84.

31 ORIBASIUS. A.D. 325–403

Œuvres d'Oribase, texte grec, en grande partie inédit . . . traduit pour la première fois en français; par les Drs. BUSSEMAKER et DAREMBERG. 6 vols. Paris, *Imp. nationale*, 1851–76.

Oribasius was a compiler of existing knowledge rather than an original writer. His output was immense; he compiled the *Synagoge*, an encyclopaedic digest of medicine, hygiene, therapeutics and surgery from Hippocrates to his own times, in 70 volumes. The unwieldiness of the work was probably the reason why he also wrote a synopsis of it. Only 17 volumes have survived. It was first printed by Aldus Manutius in Venice, in 1554 or 1555.

32 ——. Collectionum medicarum reliquiae. 4 vols. Lipsiae, *Teubner*, 1928–31.

Contains selections from the writings of medical men the originals of some of whose works no longer exist, and who would have been forgotten but for the compilations of Oribasius. Writers included are Agathinus, Antyllus, Apollonius, Archigenes, Athenaeus, Ctesias, Dieuches, Diocles, Dioscorides, Herodotus, Justus, Lycus, Menemachus, Mnesitheus Atheniensis, Mnesitheus Cyzicenus, Oribasius, Philagrius, Philotimus, Philumenus, Sabinus, Xenocrates, Zopyrus.

33 AETIUS *of Amida*. A.D. 502–575

Βιβλίων, ἰατρικῶν τόμος ά. Librorum medicinalium tomus primus, primi scilicet libri octo nunc primum in ludem editi. [Venetiis, *in aed. haeredum A. Manutii et A. Asulani*], 1534.

In his *Tetrabiblion*, the first printed edition of which is given above, Aetius collected together works of other men which might have been forgotten but for him. Among them may be mentioned Rufus of Ephesus, Antyllus, Leonides, Soranus, Philumenus. In this work is also to be found Aetius's own original work on the treatment of aneurysm by ligation of the brachial artery above the sac. Above work has Greek text; no second volume published.

34 ALEXANDER *of Tralles*. A.D. 525–605

Practica. [Lugduni, *per F. Fradin*, 1504].

35 ——. Alexander von Tralles. Original-Text und Uebersetzung . . . von THEODOR PUSCHMANN. 2 vols. Wien, *W. Braumüller*, 1878–79.

In the main Alexander Trallianus was a compiler, but some of the work in his *Practica* appears to be his own. His original description of worms and vermifuges make him the first parasitologist. The above Greek-German text is the best so far published, and includes a biography. Reprinted, Amsterdam, 1963.

36 PAUL *of Aegina*. A.D. 625–690
The seven books of Paulus Aegineta. Translated from the Greek . . . by FRANCIS ADAMS. 3 vols. London, *Sydenham Society*, 1844–47.

Paulus Aegineta was the most important physician of his day and a skilful surgeon. He gave original descriptions of lithotomy, trephining, tonsillectomy, paracentesis and amputation of the breast; the first clear description of the effects of lead poisoning also comes from him. His work first appeared in Greek from the famous Aldine Press in Venice in 1528. Above is the first English translation.

37 ——. Paulus Aegineta. Ed. J. L. HEIBERG. 2 vols. Lipsiae, *Teubner*, 1921–24.

Greek text.

38 BUDGE, *Sir* ERNEST ALFRED THOMPSON WALLIS. 1857–1934
Syrian anatomy, pathology and therapeutics or "The Book of Medicines." The Syriac text . . . with an English translation, *etc.* 2 vols. London, *H. Milford*, 1913.

Text and translation of a Syrian manuscript which throws some light on Syrian medicine.

39 RHAZES [ABŪ BAKR MUHAMMAD IBN ZAKARĪYA AL-RĀZĪ]. ?850–?923
Liber nonus ad Almansorem, cum commentario SILLANI DE NIGRIS. [Padua, *B. Valdezochius*], 1476.

The *Almansor*, so named after the prince to whom it was addressed, was a popular textbook and one of the first to be printed. Rhazes ranks with Hippocrates and Galen as one of the founders of clinical medicine. Only one copy of the above edition of his work is known to exist; it was bought by Sir William Osler in 1915 and bequeathed by him to the British Museum. For its full collation see the *Bibliotheca Osleriana*, No. 451. Choulant gives the date of Rhazes' birth as 860.

40 ——. Liber Elhavi seu totum continentis Bubikir Zacharie Errasis filii, traducti ex arabice in latinum per MAG. FERRAGIUM. [Brescia, *J. Britannicus*], 1486.

The *Al-Hawi*, or *Continens*. It is a great encyclopaedia of medicine. The above first Latin translation by Ferragut is the largest and heaviest of the medical incunabula. The original manuscript was in Arabic.

41 ——. Opera parva. Luguni, *V. de Portonariis*, 1510.

Contains: Almansor; De aegritudinibus iuncturarum; De morbis puerorum; Aphorismi; Parvum antidotarum; De praeservatione ab aegritudine lapidis; Liber introductorius parvus in medicinam; De sectionibus et cauteriis ac ventosis; Synonyma; Liber divisionum cum novem capitibus in fine additus, et ab aliis impressoribus semper obmissis.

42 HALY ABBAS ['ALI IBN-AL-'ABBĀS AL MAJŪSI]. 930–994
Liber artis medicine, qui dicitur regalis. Venetiis, *B. Ricius*, 1492.

The *Almaleki*, or *Liber regius*, of Haly Ben Abbas was the leading treatise of medicine for a hundred years, when it was displaced by Avicenna's *Canon* (see No. 43).

43 AVICENNA [ABU-'ALI AL-HUSAYN IBN-SINA]. 980–1037
Liber canonis. Mediolani, *P. de Lavagna*, 1473.

Avicenna is said to have written more than 100 books, most of which have perished. He was an experienced physician; he wrote on the aetiology of epilepsy and described diabetes, noticing the sweetish taste of the urine. His *Canon* is the most famous medical text ever written; it is a complete exposition of Galenism. Of it Neuburger says: "It stands for the epitome of all precedent development, the final codification of all Graeco-Arabic medicine." It dominated the medical schools of Europe and Asia for five centuries. The above is a Latin translation by Gerard of Cremona. Choulant mentions two other undated, and probably earlier, editions.

44 ——. Libri V Canonis medicinae. Romae, *typ. Medicae*, 1593.

Arabic text.

45 ——. A treatise on the Canon of Medicine incorporating a translation of the First Book. By O. C. GRUNER. London, *Luzac & Co.*, 1930.

This translation of Book I of the *Canon* is accompanied by a large number of valuable notes and comments on the text, which bring out the close connection between Arabic and Chinese medicine, and the influence which Avicenna had upon many medieval scholars. See also *The general principles of Avicenna's Canon of Medicine* by Mazhar H. Shar, Karachi, 1966.

46 CONSTANTINE *of Africa*. 1015–1087

Opera. 2 vols. Basileae, *H. Petrus*. 1536–39.

Many of the writings of Constantine were merely translations into Latin of Greek Arabic and Jewish writers. His importance lies in the fact that by such latinizing he placed Mohammedan thought and culture at the disposal of European medicine from the 12th to 17th centuries. For a time he taught at the School of Salerno.

47 AVENZOAR [ABUMERON]. ?1092–1162

Liber Teisir, sive rectificatio medicationis et regiminis. Venetiis, *J. & G. de Gregoriis*, 1490.

This is a Latin translation from the Hebrew version of 1280. Avenzoar, the greatest Moslem physician of the Western Caliphate, described the itch-mite, *Sarcoptes scabiei*, serous pericarditis, mediastinal abscess, pharyngeal paralysis and otitis media. He was the first to attempt total extirpation of the uterus. He anticipated the modern stomach tube and advocated rectal feeding. He carefully described, but did not perform, lithotomy, and is apparently the first to mention a lithotrite.

48 AVERROES [ABU'L WELID MUHAMMAD IBN AHMED IBN RUSHD AL MALIKI]. 1126–1198

Colliget. Ferrarae, *L. de Valentia de Rubeis*, 1482.

The *Kitab-al-Kullyat* or *Colliget* (Book of Universals) was an "attempt to found a system of medicine upon the neo-Platonic modification of Aristotle's philosophy" (Garrison, p. 132). Averroes was the best commentator upon Aristotle, and scholars still turn to him for the interpretation of obscure passages in the great philosopher's writings. He was the last of the great Arab physicians.

49 SCHOOL OF SALERNO.

Collectio Salernitana . . . raccolti ed illustrati da G.E.T. [*i.e.*, A.W.E.T. HENSCHEL, C. DAREMBERG ed E. S. DE RENZI. 5 vols. Napoli, *Filiatre-Sebezio*, 1852–9.

The School of Medicine at Salerno dispelled the stagnation of medicine which had persisted throughout the Dark Ages. Its masters were the first medieval physicians to cultivate medicine as an independent science. Many of the documents compiled at the School are included in the above work, having been found in the Breslau Codex of the mid-twelfth century, discovered in 1837. The *Regimen Sanitatis Salernitanum* was among the earlier medical works printed. The School at Salerno was eclipsed by the rise of Montpellier and Bologna to the front rank; it was suppressed by Napoleon in 1811.

50 ——. Magistri Salernitani nondum editi. Ed. PIERO GIACOSA. 1 vol. and atlas. Torino, *frat. Bocca*, 1901.

Reproduction of some of the texts produced at the School of Salerno. In all, it is believed that the total output from the School numbered 100 texts, including the famous poem *Regimen Sanitatis Salernitanum*, or *Flos Medicae*.

51 SCHOOL OF SALERNO.

The school of Salernum. Regimen sanitatis Salernitanum, the English version by Sir JOHN HARINGTON. History of the School of Salernum by FRANCIS R. PACKARD, and a note on the prehistory of the Regimen Sanitatis by FIELDING H. GARRISON. London, *Oxford Univ. Press*, 1922.

New edition, Salerno, 1953.

52 ARTICELLA.

Articella. [Padua, *N. Petri*, *circa* 1476.]

A collection of classical texts on medicine, written in Latin. Includes works of Hippocrates, Galen, Theophilus, and Johannitius.

53 IN HOC VOLUMINE.

In hoc volumine hec continentur. Aphorismi Rabi Moysi. Aphorismi Jo. Damasceni. Liber secretorum Hypocratis, *etc.* Venetiis, *J. Pencium de Leucho*, 1508.

54 MEDICI ANTIQUI OMNES.

Medici antiqui omnes, qui latinis literis diversorum morborum genera et remedia persecuti sunt. Venetiis, *apud Aldi filios*, 1547.

Contains selections from the writings of Celsus, Pliny, Soranus, Apuleius, Musa, Priscianus, Trotula, Macer, Caelius Aurelianus, Marcellus Empiricus, Scribonius Largus, Serenus Samonicus, Strabus Gallus.

55 MEDICAE ARTIS PRINCIPES.

Medicae artis principes post Hippocratum et Galenum. Graeci Latinitate donati. Excudebat H. STEPHANUS. 2 vols. [Paris], *typ. H. Stephanus*, 1567.

Contains works of Aretaeus, Rufus of Ephesus, Alexander of Tralles, Paul of Aegina, Oribasius, Sextus Philosophicus, Aetius, Philaretius, Theophilus, Actuarius Zach. fil., Nicholaus Myrepsus Alexandrinus, Celsus, Scribonius Largus, Marcellus Empiricus, Quintus Serenus Samonicus.

56 MEDICI ANTIQUI GRAECI.

Medici antiqui graeci . . . omnes a JUNIO PAULO CRASSO latio donati. Basileae, *et. off. P. Pernae*, 1581.

Contains works of Aretaeus, Palladius, Rufus of Ephesus, Theophilus.

57 PARACELSUS [BOMBASTUS AB HOHENHEIM (AUREOLUS PHILIPPUS THEOPHRASTUS)]. 1493–1541

Sämtliche Werke . . . Herausg. von K. SUDHOFF und W. MATHIESSEN. 14 vols. München, Berlin, *O. W. Barth*, *R. Oldenbourg*, 1922–33.

Paracelsus, a much-travelled man, was one of the most remarkable figures in medicine. He was first to write on miners' diseases, to establish the relationship between cretinism and endemic goitre and to note the geographic differences in diseases. Karl Sudhoff, perhaps the greatest of all medical historians, has studied Paracelsus exhaustively and is responsible for the above definitive edition of his works. A selection of his writings was edited by J. Jacobi and translated by N. Guterman, 1951; J. Hargrave published a biography in 1951.

58 ——. Theophrastus Paracelsus Werke. Besorgt von W. E. PEUCKERT. Bd. 1–3. Basel, *Schwabe*, 1965–67.

Osler said that Paracelsus was "the Luther of medicine, for when authority was paramount he stood out for independent study".

59 PARÉ, Ambroise. 1510–1590

Œuvres complètes d'Ambroise Paré. 3 vols. Paris, *Baillière*, 1840–41.

The best edition of Paré's works, edited by J. F. Malgaigne. An English translation by Thomas Johnson appeared as early as 1634. See also No. 5565. Janet Doe has published *A bibliography of the works of Ambroise Paré*, Chicago, 1943.

60 BAILLOU, Guillaume de [Ballonius]. 1538–1616

Opera medica omnia. 4 vols. Venetiis, *apud A. Jeremiam*, 1734–36.

De Baillou, "the first epidemiologist of modern times", foreshadowed much that was afterwards taught by Sydenham. He first described whooping-cough and introduced the term "rheumatism". He was Court physician during the reign of Henri IV of France. See the article on Baillou by E. W. Goodall in *Ann. med. Hist.*, 1935 **7**, 409–27.

61 SENNERT, Daniel. 1572–1637

Opera. 6 vols. Lugduni, *J. A. Huguetan*, 1676.

Besides giving early accounts of scarlatina and rubella, Sennert added to the knowledge of scurvy, dysentery and alcoholism. He was an able clinician but a believer in witchcraft. His *Opera* was first published in 1641; the edition given above is regarded as the best.

61.1 HARVEY, William. 1578–1657

The works of William Harvey. Translated from the Latin, with a life of the author, by Robert Willis. London, *Sydenham Society*, 1847.

62 WILLIS, Thomas. 1621–1675

Opera omnia. 2 vols. Genevae, *apud Samuelem de Tournes*, 1676–80.

Willis was remarkable for his careful clinical observation. He was second only to Sydenham in his day. To him we owe the original descriptions of several conditions.

63 SYDENHAM, Thomas. 1624–1689

Opera omnia. Ed. Gulielmus Alexander Greenhill. London, *Sydenham Society*, 1844.

Sydenham is one of the greatest figures in internal medicine, and has been called the "Father of English Medicine". His reputation rests on his first-hand accounts of such conditions as the malarial fevers of his times, gout, scarlatina, measles, etc. A better edition of the above (editio altera) appeared in 1846. The original work, printed in 1685, is called *editio altera*: although no earlier edition is known to exist, it is said that one was published in 1683.

64 ——. The works of Thomas Sydenham. Translated from the Latin edition of Dr. Greenhill with a life of the author by R. G. Latham. 2 vols. London, *Sydenham Society*, 1848–50.

Best English translation of Sydenham's works.

65 REDI, Francesco. 1626–1697

Opere. 7 vols. Venezia, *Remondini*, 1762.

Redi was a leading physician in Italy. He is best remembered for his experiments discrediting the theory of spontaneous generation and for his pioneer work in the field of parasitology (see No. 2448); see also the article on Redi by R. Cole in *Ann. med. Hist.*, 1926, **8**, 347–59.

66 MALPIGHI, Marcello. 1628–1694

Opera omnia. 2 vols. Londini, *R. Scott*, 1686.

Malpighi was the founder of histology and the greatest of the microscopists. In 1660 he was the first to see the capillary anastomosis between the arteries and the veins, thus helping the completion of Harvey's work on the circulation. He was a great embryologist; his name is perpetuated in the "Malpighian bodies", "Malpighi's layer" of the epidermis, "Malpighi's (splenic) corpuscles". Malpighi was an excellent draughtsman but a poor writer.

67 LEEUWENHOEK, ANTONJ VAN. 1632–1723

Ontledingen en ontdekkingen. 6 vols. Leiden, 1693–1718.

Leeuwenhoek was one of the first and greatest of the microbiologists. Many of his discoveries were communicated by him to the Royal Society in London. He discovered protozoa and bacteria. He is said to have had 250 microscopes and 419 lenses, many of them ground by himself. (See also Nos. 98, 265, 860). An English translation of his works appeared in 2 vols. in 1798–1807. Clifford Dobell's study, *Anthony van Leeuwenhoek and his little animals*, London, 1932, reveals many new facts about the man. In 1939 a committee of Dutch scientists began publication of his collected letters (Amsterdam, Swets & Zeitlinger).

68 BAGLIVI, GIORGIO. 1668–1707

Opera omnia medico-practica et anatomica. Lugduni, *Anisson & J. Posuel*, 1704.

Baglivi, Professor of Anatomy at Rome, had a short but brilliant career. He wrote *Praxis medica* and *De fibra motrice*, and originated the so-called "solidar" pathology; he also devoted much time to experimental physiology. He was the first to distinguish between smooth and striped muscle. Baglivi was a strong advocate of specialism.

69 STAHL, GEORG ERNST. 1660–1734

Theoria medica vera. Halae, *lit. Orphanotrophiei*, 1708 [1707].

See 70. A three-volume German translation of the above was published in Berlin in 1831–33.

70 ——. Œuvres médico-philosophiques et pratiques. 6 vols. Paris, *J. B. Baillière*, 1859–64.

Stahl was responsible for the re-introduction of the idea of a "sensitive soul", propounded by van Helmont. The Stahlian "animism" considered the body to be composed of passive or "dead" substance, which became animated by the soul during life, returning to passivity or "death" on the departure of the soul from the body.

71 LANCISI, GIOVANNI MARIA. 1654–1720

Opera quae hactenus prodierunt omnia. 2 vols. Genevae, *J. A. Cramer et fil.*, 1718.

Lancisi, great Italian clinician, was the first to describe cardiac syphilis; he was also notable as an epidemiologist, with a clear insight into the theory of contagion. He was physician to Pope Clement XI, who turned over to him the forgotten copper plates executed by Eustachius in 1552. Lancisi published these with his own notes in 1714. (See No. 391.)

72 HOFFMANN, FRIEDRICH. 1660–1742

Opera omnia physico-medica. (Supplementum, *etc.*) 9 vols. Genevae, *fratres de Tournes*, 1740–53.

Hoffmann of Halle was the most important of the Iatromechanists. He believed an ether-like "vital fluid" to be present in the nervous system and to act upon the muscles, giving them "tonus".

73 BOERHAAVE, HERMAN. 1668–1738

Opera omnia medica. Venetiis, *apud L. Basilium*, 1742.

Boerhaave had a great reputation as a clinician; he was, in fact, the creator of the modern method of clinical teaching. His writings had an enormous influence during his lifetime. Haller, Cullen, Pringle, van Swieten and de Haen were among his pupils. His greatest work was his *Elementa chemiae*, published in 2 vols. at Leiden, 1732. Biography by G. A. Lindeboom, London, 1968.

74 HUXHAM, John. 1692–1768

Opera physico-medica. Lipsiae, *J. P. Kraus*, 1764.

Huxham, a Devonshire man, was a pupil of Boerhaave. His most important contributions to medicine were in connexion with fevers and infectious diseases. Huxham practised at Plymouth; it is related of him that in order to attract attention he used to arrange to be called from church during service. He would then gallop through the town accompanied by a footman and affecting extreme gravity of demeanour.

75 WERLHOF, Paul Gottlieb. 1699–1767

Opera medica. 3 vols. Hannoverae, *imp. frat. Helwingiorum*, 1775–76.

Werlhof, a contemporary and friend of Haller, is remembered for his classical description of purpura haemorrhagica (see No. 3052). He was Court physician at Hanover.

76 CULLEN, William. 1710–1790

The works. 2 vols. Edinburgh, *W. Blackwood*, 1827.

Cullen was the most conspicuous figure in the history of the Edinburgh Medical School during the eighteenth century. He was an inspiring teacher and was instrumental in founding the Glasgow Medical School in 1744. His clinical lectures were notable as being the first given in the vernacular instead of in Latin.

77 CAMPER, Pieter. 1722–1789

Sämmtliche kleinere Schriften. 3 vols. Leipzig, *S. L. Crusius*, 1784–90.

Camper, an artist of skill, made his mark as an anthropologist and craniologist. He discovered the processus vaginalis of the peritoneum and the fibrous structure of the eye, and made several other important contributions to medical science. An English translation of the above appeared in 1794.

78 HUNTER, John. 1728–1793

The works of John Hunter. With notes. Edited by J. F. Palmer. 4 vols. and atlas. London, *Longman*, [1835]–37.

Hunter gave a great impetus to the study of morbid anatomy; he was the veritable founder of experimental and surgical pathology and one of the three greatest surgeons of all time. He was responsible for the commencement of some of the greatest medical museums; the Hunterian museum of the Royal College of Surgeons of England was based on his own private collection; much of it was destroyed during an air raid in May, 1941. Vol. I of the above work includes Drewry Ottley's Life of Hunter. A list of the books written by Hunter, and their location in British libraries, was published by W. R. LeFanu in 1946. Short biographies of Hunter were published by S. R. Gloyne (1950) and E. A. Gray (1952).

79 HEWSON, William. 1739–1774

The works. Edited with an introduction and notes by G. Gulliver. London, *Sydenham Society*, 1846.

Hewson was a pupil of the Hunters. In 1769 his memoir on the lymphatics in fishes won for him the Copley Medal of the Royal Society. His most important work is probably his "Experimental inquiry into the properties of the blood," 1771. See also Nos. 863, 1102.

80 RUSH, Benjamin. 1745–1813

Medical inquiries and observations. 2 vols. Philadelphia, *Prichard & Hall*, 1879–93.

Rush was considered the ablest American clinician of his time. He was a friend of Benjamin Franklin and one of the signatories of the Declaration of Independence. His many writings are distinguished for their classical style; several are dealt with elsewhere in this bibliography. Rush probably had more influence on American medicine than any other single man.

81 RUSH, BENJAMIN. 1745–1813.
The selected writings of Benjamin Rush. Edited by DAGOBERT D. RUNES. New York, *Philosophical Library*, 1947.

82 PURKINJE, JOHANN EVANGELISTA [PURKYNE]. 1787–1869
Sebrané spisy. Opera omnia. Tom. 1– . v Praze, *Purkyňova Spolestnost*, 1918–

In progress. Purkinje was professor of physiology at Breslau and Prague. Eminent as physiologist and microscopist, he was first to use the microtome. His discovery of the ganglionic cells in the cerebellum led them to be called "Purkinje cells" (see No. 1396).

83 PASTEUR, LOUIS. 1822–1895
Œuvres de Pasteur, réunies par Pasteur VALLERY-RADOT. 7 vols. Paris, *Masson*, 1922–39.

One of the founders of bacteriology, Pasteur is at the same time one of the greatest figures in the history of medicine. His work on fermentation, the doctrine of spontaneous generation (which he exploded), virus diseases and preventive vaccinations, was fundamental. René Vallery-Radot's *Life of Pasteur* appeared in 1911.

84 CHARCOT, JEAN MARTIN. 1825–1893
Œuvres complètes. 9 vols. Paris, 1888–94.

Charcot, famous teacher at La Salpêtrière, created there the greatest neurological clinic of modern times. He was a pioneer of psychotherapy and left many memorable descriptions of nervous disorders. Pierre Marie, who died in 1940, was a pupil of Charcot.

85 LISTER, JOSEPH, 1*st Baron Lister*. 1827–1912
Collected papers. 2 vols. Oxford, *Clarendon Press*, 1909.

Lister, a pupil of Sharpey, became Professor of Surgery successively at Glasgow, Edinburgh and King's College, London. He was England's greatest surgeon and the first medical man to be raised to the peerage. The founder of the antiseptic principle, his work had a profound effect upon modern surgery and obstetrics. It is to be remembered that Oliver Wendell Holmes and Ignaz Semmelweis had both, before Lister, striven without success to obtain the adoption of antisepsis in obstetrics. Sir Rickman Godlee's biography of Lister appeared (2nd ed.) in 1918. A shorter biography was published by H. C. Cameron in 1948, and another by D. Guthrie in 1949.

86 KOCH, ROBERT. 1843–1910
Gesammelte Werke. 2 vols. [in 3]. Leipzig, *G. Thieme*, 1912.

By his demonstration of the life-cycle of the anthrax bacillus, Koch in 1877 was the first to show a specific micro-organism to be the cause of a definite disease. For his work on tuberculosis, he received the Nobel Prize in 1905. Koch ranks as the greatest bacteriologist of his day.

86.1 PAVLOV, IVAN PETROVITCH. 1849–1936
Sämtliche Werke. 6 vols. Berlin, *Akademie-Verlag*, 1956.

86.2 EHRLICH, PAUL. 1854–1915
Collected papers of Paul Ehrlich. Compiled and edited by F. HIMMELWEIT. 3 vols. London, *Pergamon Press*, 1956–60.

86.3 CORPUS MEDICORUM GRAECORUM.
Ediderunt Academiae Berolinensis Hauniensis Lipsiensis. 1– , Leipzig, *B. G. Teubner*, 1908–

Reprints of works by classical Greek medical writers.

86.4 CORPUS MEDICORUM LATINORUM.
Editum consilio et auctoritate Instituti Puschmanniani Lipsiensis. 1– , Leipzig, *B. G. Teubner*, 1915–
Reprints of classical Latin medical texts.

87–273.1 BIOLOGY

87 EMPEDOCLES. *circa* 490–430 B.C.
The fragments of Empedocles. Translated by W. E. LEONARD. *Monist*, 1907, **17**, 451–74.
Empedocles was a Greek philosopher, statesman, physician and reformer. His poem on Nature originally ran to 5,000 lines, of which only 400 are now left. He believed in four ultimate elements—fire, air, water and earth, these being brought into union and parted by the two powers, love and hate. His name has been honoured even in modern times in Sicily.

88 LUCRETIUS *Carus*, TITUS. 98–55 B.C.
De rerum natura. Edited by CYRIL BAILEY. 3 vols. London, *Oxford Univ. Press*, 1947.
The first printed edition of the *De rerum natura* was published in Brescia in 1473. The work is a reasoned system of philosophy written in verse. Book V attempts an explanation of the origin of the universe and life, and the gradual advance of man from the savage state. All these topics are treated from the viewpoint that the world is not itself divine nor directed by a divine agency. The above definitive edition includes a translation, commentary, *apparatus criticus* and prolegomena.

89 PLINIUS *Secundus*, GAIUS. A.D. 23–79
Histoire naturelle de Pline. 20 vols. [in 10]. Paris, *C. L. F. Panckoucke*, 1829–40.
Latin-French bilingual. The most ancient encyclopaedia extant, Pliny's *Historia* contained all that was known in his time of geography, mineralogy, anthropology, botany, zoology and meterology. Books XX–XXXII deal with medicine. This was the one work of classical antiquity which, despite the low quality of its material, was read steadily throughout the Dark Ages. The botanical errors were not corrected until 1492 (Leonicenus, see No. 1798). Pliny's work was first printed in 1469 by Johannes de Spira, of Venice. It is one of the finest of the incunabula, a perfect example of ancient typography.

90 ——. Natural history. English translations by W. H. S. JONES and H. RACKHAM. 10 vols. London, *W. Heinemann*, 1938–63.
Loeb edition; Latin and English on facing pages.

91 BARTHOLOMAEUS *Anglicus* [DE GLANVILLA (BARTHOLOMAEUS)] *fl.* 1250
De proprietatibus rerum. [Bazel, *B. Ruppel, circa* 1470.]
A condensed encyclopaedia of what was then understood by natural science. The work was probably written about the middle of the 13th century. It was one of the most widely read scientific works of the Middle Ages. Caxton is said to have learned to print from this book.

92 ——. De proprietatibus rerum. [London, *Wynkyn de Worde*, 1495.]
This English translation of Bartholomaeus Anglicus was made by John of Trevisa in 1398. Bibliographically it is of interest as being one of the earliest books printed in London, one of the finest of the 15th century, and the first book printed on paper made in England.

93 LEONARDO DA VINCI. 1452–1519

Codice sul volo degli uccelli. Pubblicato da T. SABACHNIKOFF; transcrizione e note di G. PIUMATI, con traduzione francese di C. RAVAISSON-MOLLIEN. Paris, *E. Rouveyre*, 1893.

The scientific study of the mechanics of flight begins with Leonardo's investigations on birds, undertaken during his attempts to build a flying machine. The original manuscript of this work is now in Rome; the work first appeared in print in 1492.

94 ——. Leonardo da Vinci's notebooks; arranged and rendered into English, with introductions, by EDWARD MCCURDY. New York, *Empire State Book Co.*, 1923.

95 HERBAL.

Herbarius zu Teutsch. [Mainz, *P. Schoeffer*], 1485.

A compilation of earlier writers. The popularity of this book stimulated Brunfels, Fuchs, Valerius Cordus and others and it is therefore of importance.

96 ——. Ortus sanitatis. Moguntiae, *J. Meydenbach*, 1491.

First edition of a herbal which became very popular. Despite its quaint and often fanciful woodcuts of animals and plants, it stimulated other more scientific treatises on botany and zoology. Available in facsimile in W. L. Schreiber's *Die Krauterbücher des XV und XVI Jahrhunderts*, Munich 1924. An English translation of c. 1521 (S.T.C. 22367) was reprinted London, *Quaritsch*, 1954, edited by N. Hudson.

97 REDI, FRANCESCO. 1626–1697

Esperienze intorno alla generazione degl'insetti. Firenze, *all'Insegna della Stella*, 1668.

Redi's experiments, recorded in the above work, dealt the first real blow to the doctrine of spontaneous generation. In these experiments Redi made use of what we now term "controls".

98 LEEUWENHOEK, ANTONJ VAN. 1632–1723

Arcana naturae. 4 vols. Delphis Batavorum, *H. a. Krooneveld*, 1695–1719.

Leeuwenhoek is one of the greatest microbiologists of all time. Above is a collection of his most important writings. He saw protozoa and, later, bacteria. He was probably also the first clearly to observe the red blood cells.

99 LINNÉ, CARL VON [LINNAEUS]. 1707–1778

Systema naturae. Lugduni Batavorum, *apud Theodorum Haak*, 1735.

In this work Linnaeus developed the first logical and modern classifications of plants, animals and minerals. Its most valuable feature, the binomial nomenclature (genus and species) was probably devised in the first place by Joachim Jung, about 1640. The most important edition of the *Systema naturae* is the tenth, published in 1758.

100 SPALLANZANI, LAZARO. 1729–1799

Saggio di osservazioni microscopiche relative al sistema della generazione. Modena, 1767.

Spallanzani was one of the first to dispute the doctrine of spontaneous generation, making important experiments in support of his views. He was a believer in the "preformation" theory.

101 ——. Prodromi sulla riproduzione animali. Riproduzione della coda del girino. Modena, 1768.

Spallanzani first advanced the doctrine of the regeneration of the spinal cord. By decapitation of the frog he also showed that certain postures may be maintained by a reflex action of the spinal cord.

102 ——. Opusculi di fisica animale e vegetabile. 2 vols. Modena, *Soc. tipografica*, 1776.

Later confutation of the theory of spontaneous generation. Spallanzani's conclusions were similar to those expressed by Pasteur nearly a century later. This work also contains Spallanzani's important investigations upon the gastric juice. His collected works were published in Milan, 2 vols., 1932–33.

103 INGEN-HOUSZ, JAN. 1730–1799

Experiments on vegetables, discovering their great power of purifying the common air in the sun-shine, and of injuring it in the shade at night. To which is joined, a new method of examining the accurate degree of salubrity of the atmosphere. London, *P. Elmsley and H. Payne*, 1779.

Ingen-Housz showed that the green parts of plants, when exposed to light, fix the free carbon dioxide of the atmosphere, but that in darkness plants have no such power. Thus he proved that animal life is dependent ultimately on plant life, a discovery of fundamental importance in the economy of the world of living things. Reprinted, with biography, by H. S. Reed in *Chronica Botanica*, Waltham, Mass., 1949, **11**, No. 5–6.

104 BLUMENBACH, JOHANN FRIEDRICH. 1752–1840

Ueber den Bildungstrieb und das Zeugungsgeschäft. Göttingen, *J. C. Dieterich*, 1781.

Blumenbach, Professor of Medicine at Göttingen, was the founder of modern anthropology. In the above work he advanced a theory of reproduction and embryonic development. He rejected the "preformation" theory and advanced the theory of epigenesis as the true explanation of the phenomenon of evolution.

105 DARWIN, ERASMUS. 1731–1802

Zoonomia; or the laws of organic life. 2 vols. London, *J. Johnson*, 1794–96.

Grandfather of Charles Darwin. The *Zoonomia* contains a system of pathology and a treatise on generation. Darwin believed that "one and the same kind of living filaments is and has been the cause of life".

106 OKEN, LORENZ. 1779–1851

Die Zeugung. Bamberg, Würzburg, *J. A. Goebhardt*, 1805.

Oken maintained that all organic beings originate from, and consist of, cells, and that organisms are produced by an agglomeration of these cells.

107 ISIS.

Isis, oder encyclopädische Zeitung (verzüglich für Naturgeschichte, vergleichende Anatomie und Physiologie), von OKEN. 41 vols. Jena, *etc.*, 1817–48.

Oken, a leading light in the Nature-Philosophical School in Germany, produced important work in the field of biology. He founded the journal *Isis*, which published articles of great value; its incursion into the field of German politics led to a demand for the resignation of Oken from his professorship or the suppression of his journal. Oken resigned and continued to publish *Isis*.

108 DUTROCHET, RENÉ JOACHIM HENRI. 1776–1847

Recherches anatomiques et physiologiques sur la structure intime des animaux et des végétaux. Paris, *J. B. Baillière*, 1824.

109 BROWN, ROBERT. 1773–1858

Observations on the organs and mode of fecundation in Orchideae and Asclepiadeae. *Trans. Linn. Soc.*, 1829–32, **16**, 685–746.

Discovery, in 1831, of the cell nucleus.

109.1 WAGNER, Rudolph. 1805–1864

Einige Bemerkungen und Fragen über das Keimbläschen (vesicula germinativa). *Arch. Anat. Physiol. wiss. Med.*, 1835, 373–7.

Wagner saw and described the nucleolus.

110 DUTROCHET, René Joachim Henri. 1776–1847

Mémoires pour servir à l'histoire anatomique et physiologique des végétaux et des animaux. 2 vols. Paris, *J. B. Baillière*, 1837.

An advance in the knowledge of the chlorophyll system of plants was made when Dutrochet recognized that only those plant cells which contain green matter are capable of absorbing carbon dioxide. The *Mémoires* are a collection of all his more important biological papers.

111 EHRENBERG, Christian Gottfried. 1795–1876

Die Infusionsthierchen als vollkommene Organismen. 1 vol. and atlas. Leipzig, *L. Voss*, 1838.

In this monumental work Ehrenberg extended Müller's bacteriological classification. Like Müller, he made no distinction between protozoa and bacteria, classing them both as infusoria. His classification included *Vibrio, Spirillum* and *Spirochaeta*. The fine plates in this book were drawn by Ehrenberg himself.

112 SCHLEIDEN, Matthias Jakob. 1804–1881

Beiträge zur Phytogenesis. *Arch. Anat. Physiol. wiss. Med.*, 1838, 137–76.

Schleiden demonstrated that plant tissues are made up of and developed from groups of cells, of which he recognized the "cytoblast" or cell-nucleus. He observed with great accuracy certain other activities of the cell, and is an important figure in the development of the cell theory. Unfortunately he held that young cells develop spontaneously from the cytoblast, an acceptance of the theory of spontaneous generation. English translation (Sydenham Society) 1847.

113 SCHWANN, Theodor. 1810–1882

Mikroskopische Untersuchungen über die Uebereinstimmung in der Struktur und dem Wachsthum der Thiere und Pflanzen. Berlin, *Sander*, 1839.

Mainly devoted to the investigation of the elementary structure of animal tissues, Schwann's *Untersuchungen* had an important bearing on the development of the doctrine of the cell structure of animal tissue. In the same work he described the neurilemma, the "sheath of Schwann". Schwann was professor of anatomy and physiology at Liége. English translation (Sydenham Society), 1847. See *The cell of Schwann*, by G. Causey, Edinburgh, 1960.

114 MOHL, Hugo von. 1805–1872

Grundzüge der Anatomie und Physiologie der vegetabilischen Zelle. Braunschweig, *F. Vieweg und Sohn*, 1851.

Von Mohl saw and described cell division. English translation 1852.

115 MOLESCHOTT, Jacob. 1822–1893

Der Kreislauf des Lebens. Mainz, *V. von Zabern*, 1852.

This work attacked Liebig's theories, although courteously. Moleschott, a Dutch physiologist, evolved a purely materialistic conception of the world. He considered life a magnificent metabolic process, and thought a product of the activities of the brain.

116 REMAK, Robert. 1815–1865
Ueber extracelluläre Entstehung thierischer Zellen und über die Vermehrung derselben durch Theilung. *Arch. Anat. Physiol. wiss. Med.*, 1852, 47–57.

Remak was the first to point out that growth of new tissues was accomplished by the division of pre-existing cells. He was the first Jew to be given an academic appointment at a German university.

117 SCHULTZE, Maximilian Johann Sigismund. 1825–1874
Ueber Muskelkörperchen und das, was man eine Zelle zu nennen habe. *Arch. Anat. Physiol. wiss. Med.*, 1861, 1–27.

Schultze showed the cell to be a clump of nucleated protoplasm, stating that each muscle fibre or primitive muscle bundle was developed from a single myoblast by successive divisions of its cell or nucleus. His work settled the controversy with regard to the place of the cell in muscle tissue and stimulated the histologists to investigate the nature of intercellular tissue.

118 BATES, Henry Walter. 1825–1892
Contributions to an insect fauna of the Amazon valley. *Trans. Linn. Soc.*, 1862, **23,** 495–566.

Bates visited the Amazon and there collected 8,000 species of insects new to science. In the above paper he clearly stated and solved the problem of protective mimicry, the superficial resemblances between different species and the likeness between animals and their surroundings for evasion or concealment from their enemies. (See also No. 341).

119 SPENCER, Herbert. 1820–1903
The principles of biology. 2 vols. London, *Williams & Norgate*, 1864–67.

Spencer conceived that every species is endowed with its own type of physiological unit, each unit being capable, under certain circumstances, of reproducing the whole organism. Spencer set forth doctrines of evolution some years before the appearance of the *Origin of species*.

120 HAECKEL, Ernst Heinrich Philipp August. 1834–1919
Die Gastraea-Theorie, die phylogenetische Classification des Thierreichs und die Homologie der Keimblätter. *Jena. Z. Naturw.*, 1874, **8,** 1–55.

Haeckel's gastraea theory, which considers the two-layered gastrula as the ancestral form of multicellular animals.

121 BUTLER, Samuel. 1835–1902
Life and habit. London, *Trübner & Co.*, 1877.

Samuel Butler translated the work of Hering on the psychophysical theory of heredity (No. 227) and used it as a basis for his attacks on Darwinism.

122 FLEMMING, Walther. 1843–1905
Beiträge zur Kenntniss der Zelle und ihrer Lebenserscheinungen. *Arch. mikr. Anat.*, 1879, **16,** 302–436; 1880, **18,** 151–259.

Classical account of cell division and karyokinesis. Translation of Part II in *J. Cell Biol.*, 1965, **25**, No. 1, pt. 2, 3–69.

123 STRASBURGER, Eduard Adolf. 1844–1912
Ueber Zellbildung und Zelltheilung. 3te. Aufl. Jena, *G. Fischer*, 1880.

A pioneer work on the formation and division of cells. In this third edition Strasburger established one of the principles of modern cytology, i.e., that independent cell formation does not occur but that fresh nuclei invariably arise through the division of older ones. The first edition of this book appeared in 1875.

125 LOEB, Jacques. 1859–1924
Der Heliotropismus der Thiere und seine Uebereinstimmung mit dem Heliotropismus der Pflanzen. Würzburg, *G. Hertz*, 1890.
Loeb founded the theory of "tropisms" as the basis of the psychology of the lower forms of life.

127 DAVENPORT, Charles Benedict. 1866–1944
Experimental morphology. 2 pts. New York, *Macmillan*, 1897–99.
Second edition, 1908.

128 MORGAN, Thomas Hunt. 1866–1945
Regeneration. New York, *Macmillan*, 1901.

129 DRIESCH, Hans Adolf Eduard. 1867–1941
Die organischen Regulationen. Leipzig, *W. Engelmann*, 1901.

132 MINOT, Charles Sedgwick. 1852–1914
The problem of age, growth and death. New York, *G. P. Putnam*, 1908.
Minot's theory of ageing, based on cytomorphosis and the rate of growth. This work first appeared as a paper in vol. 7 of the *Popular Science Monthly*, 1907.

133 LOEB, Jacques. 1859–1924
Ueber das Wesen der formativen Reizung. Berlin, *J. Springer*, 1909.

134 KEEBLE, *Sir* Frederick William. 1870–1952
Plant animals. Cambridge, *University Press*, 1910.

135 LOEB, Jacques. 1859–1924
The mechanistic conception of life. Chicago, *University Press*, (1912).
Loeb's mechanistic theory of life.

136 ABDERHALDEN, Emil. 1877–1950
Handbuch der biologischen Arbeitsmethoden. Herausgegeben von E. Abderhalden. Vol. 1–107. Berlin, Wien, *Urban & Schwarzenburg*, 1920–39.

137 PEARL, Raymond. 1879–1940
The biology of death. Philadelphia, *Lippincott Co.*, 1922.
Raymond Pearl, of John Hopkins University, did important work on the subject of vital statistics.

138 ROBERTSON, Thorburn Brailsford. 1884–1930
The chemical basis of growth and senescence. Philadelphia, *J. B. Lippincott*, (1923).

139 LOEB, Jacques. 1859–1924
Regeneration from a physico-chemical viewpoint. New York, *McGraw Hill Book Co.*, 1924.

139.1 BAKER, John Randal. 1900–
The cell-theory: a restatement, history, and critique. *Q. J. micr. Sci.*, 1948, **89,** 103–25; 1949, **90,** 87–108; 1952, **93,** 157–90.

139.2 Lewis, Warren Harmon. 1870–1964
Pinocytosis. *Bull. Johns Hopk. Hosp.*, 1931, **49,** 17–27.
Discovery of pinocytosis.

140 BARR, MURRAY LLEWELLYN. 1908– , & BERTRAM, EWART GEORGE. 1923–
A morphological distinction between neurones of the male and female, and the behaviour of the nucleolar satellite during accelerated nucleoprotein synthesis. *Nature* (*Lond.*), 1949, **163,** 676–7.

Barr and Bertram showed that it is possible to determine the genetic sex of an individual according as to whether there is a chromatin mass present on the inner surface of the nuclear membrane of cells with resting or intermittent nuclei. See also *Anat. Rec.*, 1952, 112, 709–12. and *Surg. Gynec. Obstet.*, 1953, **96,** 641–8.

History of Biology

141 RÁDL, EMMANUEL. 1873–1942
Geschichte der biologischen Theorien. 2 pts. Leipzig, *Engelmann*, 1905–09.

English translation, London, 1930.

142 NORDENSKIÖLD, NILS ERIK. 1872–1933
The history of biology: a survey. Translated by L. B. EYRE. New York, *Knopf*, 1928.

Previously published in Swedish and German editions. Reprinted 1935 and 1960.

143 KROGMAN, WILTON MARION. 1903–
A bibliography of human morphology, 1914–1939. Chicago, *University Press*, 1941.

144 SINGER, CHARLES JOSEPH. 1876–1960
A history of biology. A general introduction to the study of living things. 3rd ed. London & New York, *Abelard-Schuman*, 1959

145 BODENHEIMER, FREDERICK SIMON. 1897–1959
The history of biology. London, *Dawsons*, [1958].

145.1 HUGHES, ARTHUR. 1908–
A history of cytology. New York, *Abelard-Schuman*, 1959.

146–197 ANTHROPOLOGY

See also 198–215, CRANIOLOGY

146 HERODOTUS. *circa* 484–425 B.C.
The History of Herodotus. New version. With notes, etc. By G. RAWLINSON. 4th ed. 4 vols. London, 1880.

George Rawlinson's edition of Herodotus is probably the most useful, the notes being of particular value.

147 ——. Works of Herodotus. Translated by A. D. GODLEY. 4 vols. London, *Heinemann*, 1920–24.

Greek and English text, Loeb Classics series. Herodotus travelled much in Greece. Asia Minor and North Africa, before settling in Italy. His *History* includes careful observations on the nature and habits of various peoples, and may be regarded as the first work on anthropology.

148 GALEN. A.D. 130–200
De temperamentis. *In his* Opera, ed. C. G. KUHN. Lipsiae, 1821, **1,** 509–694.

149 DÜRER, Albrecht. 1471–1528
Vier Bücher von menschlicher Proportion. (Nürnberg, *J. Formschneyder*), 1528.

Dürer's greatest work. The first two books deal with the proper proportions of the human form; the third changes the proportions according to mathematical rules, giving examples of extremely fat and thin figures, while the last book depicts the human figure in motion and treats of foreshortenings. Dürer's work is the first attempt to apply anthropometry to aesthetics. The woodcuts represent the first attempt to employ cross-hatching to depict shades and shadows in wood engraving.

150 PORTA, Giovanni Battista della. 1536–1605
De humana physiognomonia libri IIII. Vici Æquensis, *apud I. Cacchium*, 1586.

Della Porta preceded Lavater in attempting to estimate human character by the features. He was the founder of physiognomy, and this is one of the earliest works on the subject.

151 ELSHOLTZ, Johann Sigmund. 1623–1688
Anthropometria. Patavii, *typ. M. Cadorini*, 1654.

152 CARDANO, Girolamo [Cardanus]. 1501–1576
Metoposcopia libris tredecim et octingentis faciei humanae eiconibus complexa. Paris, *T. Jolly*, 1658.

Contains 800 illustrations of the human face. Cardan, the most celebrated physician of Europe in his time, and professor of medicine at Padua, claimed to be able to draw horoscopes from the appearance of the face. This book was written in 1550; a French translation was published in 1658.

153 TYSON, Edward. 1650–1708
Orang-outang, sive homo sylvestris: or, the anatomy of a pygmie compared with that of a monkey, an ape, and a man. London, *T. Bennet & D. Brown*, 1699.

The first really important work on comparative morphology. Tyson originated the "missing link" idea. He was a prominent comparative anatomist in the 17th century and wrote several classical monographs. Facsimile reprint, 1966.

154 LAVATER, Johann Caspar. 1741–1801
Von der Physiognomik. Leipzig, *Weidmanns Erben*, 1772.

Although not of fundamental importance, this book was popular for many years. Lavater was the last of the descriptive physiognomists.

155 RUBENS, Pierre Paul. 1577–1640
Théorie de la figure humaine. Paris, *C. A. Jombert*, 1773.

This work on the human figure, published more than 100 years after the death of Rubens is notable for its exquisite copper-plate engravings.

156 BLUMENBACH, Johann Friedrich. 1752–1840
De generis humani varietate nativa. Gottingae, *A. Vandenhoeck*, 1775.

Blumenbach was the founder of anthropology. He classified the various subdivisions of the human race according to colour of skin and geographical habitat. His classification, with little modification, has survived to the present day.

157 ——. Beyträge zur Naturgeschichte. 2 pts. Göttingen, 1790–1811.

158 CAMPER, Pieter. 1722–1789
Ueber den natürlichen Unterschied der Gesichtszüge in Menschen verschiedener Gegenden und verschiedenen Alters. Berlin, *Vossische Buchhandlung*, 1792.

This work on physiognomy includes Camper's description of his craniometrical methods the foundation of all subsequent work. Camper is chiefly remembered for the "facial angle" of his own invention. The book first appeared in Dutch in 1791.

159 PRICHARD, James Cowles. 1786–1848
Researches into the physical history of man. London, *J. & A. Arch*, 1813.

Prichard, a Bristol physician, classified and systematized facts relating to the races of men better than any previous writer. The second edition of his book, 1826, contains a remarkable anticipation of modern views on evolution, views which were suppressed in later editions. An atlas of illustrations to the above work appeared in 1844.

160 PURKINJE, Johann Evangelista [Purkyně]. 1787–1869
Commentatio de examine physiologico organi visus et systematis cutanei. Vratislavae, *typis Universitatis*, [1823].

Purkinje was the first to classify fingerprints.

161 KNOX, Robert. 1791–1862
The races of men. London, *H. Renshaw*, 1850.

Knox, anatomist at Edinburgh, and notorious for his association with the resurrectionists, made important researches in the field of ethnology while serving as an army surgeon at the Cape of Good Hope.

164 QUATREFAGES DE BRÉAU, Jean Armand de. 1810–1892
Unité de l'espèce humaine. Paris, *L. Hachette*, 1861.

De Quatrefages was one of France's most eminent anthropologists.

165 HUXLEY, Thomas Henry. 1825–1895
Evidence as to man's place in nature. London, *Williams & Norgate*, 1863.

Huxley showed that in the visible characters man differs less from the higher apes than do the latter from lower members of the same order of primates.

167 ——. On the methods and results of ethnology. London, 1865.

Includes Huxley's classification of mankind by means of the hair.

168 PRUNER-BEY, Franz. 1808–1882
De la chevelure comme caractéristique des races humaines. *Mém. Soc. Anthrop. Paris*, 1865, **2**, 1–35; 1872, **3**, 77–92.

Pruner-Bey did the first important work on the classification of races according to texture and shape in section of hair.

169 BROCA, Pierre Paul. 1824–1880.
Mémoires d'anthropologie. 3 vols. Paris, *C. Reinwald*, 1871–77.

Broca was among the greatest of the French anthropologists. He originated modern craniometry and in that connexion devised many craniometric and cranioscopic instruments.

170 DARWIN, Charles Robert. 1809–1882
The descent of man, and selection in relation to sex. 2 vols. London, *J. Murray*, 1871.

This is really two works. The first demolished the theory that the universe was created for Man, while in the second Darwin presented a mass of evidence in support of his earlier hypothesis regarding sexual selection.

171 QUETELET, Lambert Adolphe Jacques. 1796–1874
Anthropométrie, ou mesure des différentes facultés de l'homme. Paris, *J. B. Baillière*, 1871.

In his classification of various populations Quetelet adopted the plan of determining the standard or typical "mean man" as a basis, using stature, weight, or complexion, etc., as a measure in each particular race or population.

173 SPENCER, Herbert. 1820–1903
Descriptive sociology: a cyclopaedia of facts; representing the constitution of every type and grade of human society, *etc.* London, 1873– .

Spencer founded and edited this great series, which still continues to be published.

174 LOMBROSO, Cesare. 1836–1909
L'uomo delinquente, studiato in rapporto alla antropologia, alla medicina legale ed alle discipline carcerarie. Milano, *U. Hoepli*, 1876.

Lombroso inaugurated the doctrine of a "criminal type". His systematic studies showed that in general the criminal population exhibits a higher percentage of physical, nervous and mental anomalies than the normal population; this he attributed partly to degeneration and partly to atavism.

175 TOPINARD, Paul. 1830–1912
L'anthropologie. Paris, *C. Reinwald*, 1876.

Topinard was curator of the museum of the Société d'Anthropologie de Paris. "Topinard's angle" and "line", both described in this book, are landmarks employed in anthropometry.

176 VIRCHOW, Rudolf Ludwig Karl. 1821–1902
Beiträge zur physischen Anthropologie der Deutschen. *Abh. k. preuss. Akad. Wiss. Berl.* 1876, Phys.-math. Klasse, Abt. 1, 1–390.

Virchow made an important survey of the physical characters of the German people. Outside pathology of which he was the Master, Virchow's greatest scientific interest was anthropology.

177 FAULDS, Henry. 1844–1930
On the skin-furrows of the hand. *Nature* (*Lond.*), 1880, **22,** 605.

Faulds's fingerprint method of identification.

179 PLOSS, Hermann Heinrich. 1819–1885
Das Weib in der Natur- und Völkerkunde. 2 vols. Leipzig, *T. Grieben*, 1885.

A vast amount of data concerning every aspect of woman is collected into these volumes. Anthropology, psychology, aesthetics, physiology are all treated at length in what has become a standard and authoritative work. Subsequent editions were edited by Max and Paul Bartels and by von Reitzenstein. An English translation by E. J. Dingwall was published in London in 1935 (3 volumes); the translator has added much to the value of both text and plates.

180 RATZEL, Friedrich. 1844–1904
Völkerkunde. 2 vols. Leipzig, Wien, *Bibliographisches Inst.*, 1885–88.

One of the greatest books on ethnology. Ratzel emphasized the importance of the investigation of the history of primitive peoples in the study of ethnology.

181 BERTILLON, Alphonse. 1853–1914
Les signalements anthropométriques. Paris, *G. Masson*, 1886.

Bertillon invented a method ("Bertillonage") of identifying persons by means of selected measurements, the five following measurements being used as the basis of his system: head length, head breadth, length of middle finger, length of left foot, and length of forearm from elbow to extremity of middle finger. His method was used particularly for the identification of criminals.

182 QUATREFAGES DE BRÉAU, Jean Louis Armand de. 1810–1892
Les pygmées. Paris, *J. B. Baillière*, 1887.

De Quatrefages showed that pygmies are descended from ancient races and are not, as was believed by many, a retrograde or degenerate type of negro of comparatively recent growth.

183 WIEDERSHEIM, ROBERT ERNST EDUARD. 1848–1923
Der Bau des Menschen als Zeugniss für seine Vergangenheit. Freiburg i.B., *J. C. B. Mohr*, 1887.

184 FRAZER, *Sir* JAMES GEORGE. 1854–1941
The golden bough. 2 vols. London, *Macmillan & Co.*, 1890.
3rd edition, 12 vols., 1911–15. New abridgement, 1959.

185 BRÜCKE, ERNST WILHELM VON, *Ritter*. 1819–1892
Schönheit und Fehler der menschlichen Gestalt. Wien, *W. Braumüller*, 1891.

186 GALTON, *Sir* FRANCIS. 1822–1911
Finger prints. London, *Macmillan*, 1892.
The use of fingerprints as identification marks was known to the Chinese, but Galton was among the first to explain their possibilities in the identification of criminals. "Galton's delta" is a triangular area of papillary ridges on the distal pads of the digits.

187 ELLIS, HENRY HAVELOCK. 1859–1939
Man and woman. London, *W. Scott*, 1894.
A study of the constitutional differences between man and woman.

188 STRATZ, CARL HEINRICH. 1858–1924
Die Schönheit des weiblichen Körpers. Stuttgart, *F. Enke*, 1899.

189 HENRY, *Sir* EDWARD RICHARD, *Bart*. 1850–1931
Classification and uses of finger prints. London, 1900.
In 1901 Henry's system of fingerprint identification of humans was officially adopted in England.

190 MARTIN, RUDOLF. 1864–1925
Lehrbuch der Anthropologie. Jena, *G. Fischer*, 1914.
Exhaustive bibliography. 2nd ed., 1928.

191 KEITH, *Sir* ARTHUR. 1866–1955
The antiquity of man. London, *Williams & Norgate*, 1915.
New edition, 2 vols., 1925.

192 BOULE, PIERRE MARCELLIN. 1861–1942
Fossil men. Elements of human palaeontology. Translated from the French . . . 2nd ed. Edinburgh, *Oliver & Boyd*, 1923.
New edition, London, 1957.

193 SCHEIDT, WALTER. 1895–
Einführung in die naturwissenschaftliche Familienkunde. München. *J. F. Lehmann*, 1923.

194 ——. Allgemeine Rassenkunde. Vol. 1. München, *J. F. Lehmann*, 1925.

195 MOURANT, ARTHUR ERNEST.
The use of blood groups in anthropology. *J. roy. anthrop. Inst.*, 1947, **77**, 139–44.

History of Anthropology

196 HADDON, ALFRED CORT. 1855–1940
History of anthropology. With the help of A. Hingston Quiggin. London, *Watts & Co.*, 1910.
Revised edition, 1934.

197 PENNIMAN, THOMAS KENNETH.
A hundred years of anthropology. London, *Duckworth*, 1952.
Includes a useful chronological table and a valuable bibliography. First published 1935.

198–215 CRANIOLOGY

198 BLUMENBACH, JOHANN FRIEDRICH. 1752–1840
Decas collectionis suae craniorum diversarum gentium illustrata. 6 pts. Gottingae, *J. C. (H.) Dieterich*, 1790–1820.
Blumenbach's most important anthropological work, containing his classical description of 60 human crania. It includes a description of the uncinate ("Blumenbach's") process.

199 OKEN, LORENZ. 1779–1851
Ueber die Bedeutung der Schädelknochen. Jena, *J. C. G. Göpferdt*, 1807.
Oken's vertebral theory of the skull.

200 GOETHE, JOHANN WOLFGANG VON. 1749–1832
Ueber den Zwischenkiefer des Menschen und der Thiere. *Nova Acta Acad. Leopold.-Carol. (Halle)*, 1831, **15**, 1–48.
Goethe discovered the intermaxillary bone; he was one of the pioneers of evolution and the first to use the term "morphology."

201 MORTON, SAMUEL GEORGE. 1799–1851
Crania Americana. Philadelphia, *J. Dobson*, 1839.
In his day Morton was the most eminent craniologist in the United States. He had a collection of nearly 1,000 skulls.

202 RETZIUS, ANDERS ADOLF. 1796–1860
Om formen af nordboernes cranier. *Förhandl. skand. Naturforsch.*, 1842, **3**, 157–201.
Retzius introduced the method of classifying races according to the cranial or cephalic index. A German translation of his paper is available in the *Arch. Anat. Physiol. wiss. Med.*, 1845, 84–129.

203 DAVIS, JOSEPH BARNARD. 1801–1881, & THURNHAM, JOHN. 1810–1873.
Crania Britannica. 6 pts. London, *printed for the subscribers*, 1856–65.

204 SCHAAFHAUSEN, HERMANN. 1816–1893
Zur Kenntniss der ältesten Rassenschädel. *Arch. Anat. Physiol. wiss. Med.*, 1858, 453–78.
First description of the Neanderthal skull. English translation in *Nat. Hist. Rev.*, 1861, **1**, 155–76.

205 RÜTIMEYER, LUDWIG. 1825–1895, & HIS, WILHELM, *Snr*. 1831–1904.
Crania Helvetica. Basel, Genf, *H. Georg*, 1864.

206 QUATREFAGES DE BRÉAU, JEAN LOUIS ARMAND DE. 1810–1892, & HAMY, ERNEST THEODORE JULES. 1842–1908.
Crania ethnica. 2 pts. Paris, *J. B. Baillère*, 1872–82.

207 RETZIUS, MAGNUS GUSTAF. 1842–1919.
Finska kranier. Stockholm, *Central-Tryckeriet*, 1878.

208 TÖRÖK, AUREL VON.
Grundzüge einer systematischen Kraniometrie. Stuttgart, *F. Enke*, 1890.

Török made an exhaustive study of craniometry and proposed 5,000 different measurements of a single skull.

209 VIRCHOW, RUDOLF LUDWIG KARL. 1821–1902
Crania ethnica Americana. Berlin, *A. Asker*, 1892.

Virchow was an expert craniologist.

210 DUBOIS, EUGÈNE. 1858–1940
Pithecanthropus erectus. Eine menschenähnliche Uebergangsform aus Java. Batavia, *Landesdruckerei*, 1894.

The skull-cap of *Pithecanthropus erectus* (Java man), the earliest type of ape-like man known, was discovered by Dubois at Trinil, Java, in 1891. It is here described for the first time.

211 KEITH, *Sir* ARTHUR. 1866–1955
The Piltdown skull and brain cast. *Nature* (*Lond.*), 1913–14, **92,** 197–9, 345–6.

Description of a skull discovered by Charles Dawson at Piltdown, Sussex, in 1912. It was at one time considered to represent one type of human living at the beginning of Pleistocene times but detailed examination by new methods in 1953–54 showed it to be a forgery. See J. S. Weiner, *The Piltdown forgery*, 1955.

212 SMITH, *Sir* GRAFTON ELLIOT. 1871–1937
The Rhodesian skull. *Brit. med. J.*, 1922, **1,** 197–8.

Description of the skull found at Broken Hill, Rhodesia, in 1921.

213 ——. Sinanthropus—Peking Man; its discovery and significance. *Sci. Monthly*, 1931, **33,** 193–212.

Elliot Smith visited Peking to view the skull of *Sinanthropus pekinensis*, discovered by W. C. Pei on December 2, 1929. A preliminary description by Pei is to be found in *Bull. geol. Soc. China*, 1929, **8,** 3.

214 BUXTON, L. H. DUDLEY, & MORANT, GEOFFREY MCKAY.
The essential craniological technique. *J. roy. anthrop. Inst.*, 1933, **63,** 19–47.

215 WEIDENREICH, FRANZ. 1873–1948
The skull of Sinanthropus pekinensis. *Geological Survey of China*, New series D, No. 10, 1943.

216–258.2 EVOLUTION. HEREDITY. GENETICS

216 LAMARCK, JEAN BAPTISTE PIERRE ANTOINE DE MONET DE. 1744–1829
Philosophie zoologique. 2 vols. Paris, *J. B. Baillière*, 1809

Lamarck was one of the greatest of the comparative anatomists. In the above work he showed himself a pioneer in the idea of evolution. He advanced the theory that it occurred by the inheritance of characters acquired by animals as a result of the use or disuse of organs in response to external stimuli. English translation by H. Elliot, 1914.

216.1 ADAMS, JOSEPH. 1756–1818
A treatise on the supposed hereditary properties of diseases. London, *J. Callow*, 1814.

Adams was a pioneer in medical genetics. He distinguished between familial and hereditary diseases, saw that an increase in hereditary disease frequency in isolated areas could be caused by inbreeding, and suggested the establishment of hereditary disease registers.

217 STEENSTRUP, JOHANNES JAPETUS SMITH. 1813–1897
Om Fortplantning og Udvikling gjennem vexlende Generationsraekker. Kjøbenhavn, *C. A. Reitzel*, 1842.

Steenstrup is responsible for the theory of the "alternation of generation". He showed that certain animals produce offspring which never resemble them but which, on the other hand, bring forth progeny which return in form and nature to their grandparents or move distant ancestors. An English translation of the book was published by the Ray Society of London in 1845.

218 CHAMBERS, ROBERT. 1802–1871
Vestiges of the natural history of creation. 2 vols. London, *J. Churchill*, 1844.

This outspoken statement of a belief in evolution, published anonymously but attributed to Chambers, anticipated Darwin's *Origin* by 16 years and generally prepared the public for the latter. Chambers, with his brother William, founded the well-known *Chambers' Journal.*

219 WALLACE, ALFRED RUSSEL. 1823–1913
On the tendency of varieties to depart indefinitely from the original type. *J. Proc. Linn. Soc.* (1858), 1859, **3,** Zool., 53–62.

Wallace, friend of Darwin, independently arrived at conclusions similar in the main to those expressed by Darwin. This paper, read before the Linnean Society on 1 July, 1858, includes an abstract of Darwin's own views, contributed by the latter, and thus becomes a preliminary note to the *Origin of species.*

220 DARWIN, CHARLES ROBERT. 1809–1882
On the origin of species by means of natural selection. London, *J. Murray*, 1859.

Prepared under the advice of Lyell and Hooker, this was Darwin's greatest work and one of the most important books ever published. The whole edition of 1250 copies was sold on the day of publication. The evidence for the existence of evolution and that it resulted from the survival of the fittest by natural selection is marshalled and set out as never before. Garrison considered this "the most wonderful piece of synthesis in the history of science". Darwin's influence on biology was fundamental, its full implications being by no means yet exhausted. An expert critical analysis of the work is in Singer's *History of biology*, 1959. Facsimile reproduction, Cambridge, Mass., 1964.

221 MÜLLER, JOHANN FRIEDRICH THEODOR. 1821–1897
Für Darwin. Leipzig, *Engelmann*, 1864.

Müller, the first German to support Darwin, studied the development of the Crustacea in Brazil and published some of his results in the above little book, which contains much original information. He realized the bearing of individual development on the theory of evolution.

222 MENDEL, GREGOR JOHANN. 1822–1884
Versuche über Pflanzen-Hybriden. *Verh. naturf. Vereines Brünn* (1865), 1866, **4,** 3–47.

The experiments of Mendel led to the formulation of the Mendelian laws of inheritance. These laws are the basis of the science of genetics. An English translation of this paper on pp. 317–361 of Bateson's *Mendel's principles of heredity*, 1909 (No. 244) was republished with an introduction by R. A. Fisher, Edinburgh 1965.

223 HAECKEL, ERNST HEINRICH PHILIPP AUGUST. 1834–1919
Generelle Morphologie der Organismen. 2 vols. Berlin, *G. Reimer*, 1866.

Haeckel, the great morphologist, accepted the general principles of Darwinism, disagreeing on some points.

224 ——. Natürliche Schöpfungsgeschichte. Berlin, *G. Reimer*, 1868.

Haeckel carried Darwinism into Germany, to face the opposition of Virchow. He is among the greatest morphologists of the nineteenth century. His Phyletic Museum at Jena is probably the finest collection of serial illustrations of evolution and development in the world.

224.1 DARWIN, CHARLES ROBERT. 1809–1882
The variation of animals and plants under domestication. 2 vols. London, *J. Murray*, 1868.

Darwin carried out numerous investigations with pigeons and various plants. He recognized continuous and discontinuous variation; he concluded that crossing tends to keep populations uniform.

225 HUXLEY, THOMAS HENRY. 1825–1895
On the physical basis of life. London, 1868.

Huxley has been called the ablest modern interpreter of the ideas of Darwin, whose work he popularized.

226 GALTON, *Sir* FRANCIS. 1822–1911
Hereditary genius. London, *Macmillan & Co.*, 1869.

Galton investigated the families of great men and suggested that genius was hereditary, and thus founded the science of Eugenics, although he did not coin the word until 1883 (*see* No. 230).

227 HERING, KARL EWALD KONSTANTIN. 1834–1918
Ueber das Gedächtnis als eine allgemeine Funktion der organisierten Materie. *Abh. k. Akad. Wiss. Wien*, 1870, **20**, 253–78.

Hering was responsible for the "psycho-physical theory" of heredity, "that facultative memory, the automatic power of protoplasm to do what it has done before, is the distinctive property of all living matter" (Garrison). His belief that the transmission and reproduction of parental characters are the result of the organism's preconscious memory of the past was an idea subsequently reiterated by Samuel Butler (No. 121).

228 WALLACE, ALFRED RUSSEL. 1823–1913
Contributions to the theory of natural selection. London, *Macmillan*, 1870.

A collection of important essays by Wallace.

229 ROUX, WILHELM. 1850–1924
Über die Bedeutung der Kerntheilungsfiguren. Leipzig, *F. Engelmann*, 1883.

Roux identified the chromosomes as the bearers of the units of heredity.

230 GALTON, *Sir* FRANCIS. 1822–1911
Inquiries into human faculty and its development. London, *Macmillan & Co.*, 1883.

Galton, cousin of Charles Darwin, founded the science of Eugenics. In his important *Inquiries* he showed mathematically "the results of his experiments on the relations between the powers of visual imagery and of abstract thought, of the associations between the elements of different sense departments, of the correlation of mental traits, the associations of words, and the times taken in making the associations" (T. K. Penniman). The word "eugenics" first appears in the above book.

231 KÖLLIKER, Rudolph Albert von. 1817–1905
Die Bedeutung der Zellenkerne für die Vorgänge der Vererbung. *Z. wiss. Zool.*, 1885, **42,** 1–46.

Kölliker stated that hereditary characters were transmitted by the cell nucleus.

231.1 BOVERI, Theodor. 1862–1915
Zellen-Studien. *Jena Z. Naturw.*, 1888, **22,** 685–882.

Boveri gave decisive proof of the maintenance of chromosomal individuality.

232 EIMER, Gustav Heinrich Theodor. 1843–1898
Die Entstehung der Arten auf Grund Vererbung erworbener Eigenschaften nach den Gesetzen organischen Wachsens. 3 vols. Leipzig, Jena, *G. Fischer*, 1888–1901.

"Eimer believed that lines of evolution were not miscellaneous and haphazard but were confined to a few definite directions, determined at their initial stages not by natural selection but by the laws of organic growth" (Newman).

233 GALTON, *Sir* Francis. 1822–1911
Natural inheritance. London, *Macmillan & Co.*, 1889.

By the employment of statistical methods Galton propounded a "law of filial regression". This book represents the first statistical study of biological variation and inheritance.

234 WEISMANN, August Friedrich Leopold. 1834–1914
Amphimixis, oder die Vermischung der Individuen. Jena, *G. Fischer*, 1891.

By "amphimixis" Weismann meant the union of the two parent germs, which he considered the principal agent in evolution.

235 ——. Aufsätze über Vererbung und verwandte biologische Fragen. Jena, *G. Fischer*, 1892.

Weismann produced experimental evidence that acquired characters are not directly transmitted.

236 ——. Das Keimplasma. Jena, *G. Fischer*, 1892.

Weismann elaborated the theory of the immortality of the germ plasm.

237 BATESON, William. 1861–1926
Materials for the study of variation treated with especial regard to discontinuity in the origin of species. London, *Macmillan & Co.*, 1894.

Bateson stressed the importance of the study of discontinuance of variation in species, and suggested that variation resulted from Mendelian segregation rather than from evolution by natural selection. He showed that Darwin's concept of variation needed modification in the light of the new knowledge of genetics.

238 WILSON, Edmund Beecher. 1856–1939
The cell in development and inheritance. New York, *Macmillan & Co.*, 1896.

Wilson studied the influence of the reproductive chromosomes on heredity.

239 GALTON, *Sir* Francis. 1822–1911
The average contribution of each several ancestor to the total heritage of the offspring. *Proc. roy. Soc. Lond.*, 1897, **61,** 401–13.

Galton's "law of ancestral heredity".

240 VRIES, Hugo Marie de. 1848–1935
Die Mutationstheorie. 2 vols. Leipzig, *Veit & Co.*, 1901–3.

Mendel's fundamental work was overlooked until 1900, when de Vries and others brought it into prominence and confirmed it in every respect. The theory of mutation was first advanced by de Vries. An English translation of the above is available, published in Chicago in 1909.

241 ——. Befruchtung und Bastardierung. Leipzig, *Veit & Co.*, 1903.

De Vries was the head of the Mutationist School, which considered that new species arise by sudden marked changes in the offspring of a normal parent.

241.1 BOVERI, THEODOR. 1862–1915

Über mehrpolige Mitosen als Mittel zur Analyse des Zellkerns. *Verh. phys.-med. Ges. Wurzburg*, 1903, **35,** 67–90.

Boveri's theory concerning the role of the chromosomes in heredity was similar to that of Sutton. Their views became known as the Sutton-Boveri hypothesis.

242 JOHANNSEN, WILHELM LUDWIG. 1857–1927

Ueber Erblichkeit in Populationen und in reinen Linien. Jena, *G. Fischer*, 1903.

More support for the Mendelian law of inheritance was provided by Johannsen, a Danish botanist, who showed that in certain self-fertilizing plants a pure line of descendants can be maintained indefinitely, in which case natural selection is not effective, selection depending upon genetic variability. He introduced the term "gene" in 1911.

242.1 SUTTON, WALTER STANBOROUGH. 1877–1916

The chromosomes in heredity. *Biol. Bull.*, 1903, **4,** 231–51.

Sutton advanced the theory that the hereditary particles (genes) in the cell are borne by the chromosomes, a view also shared by Boveri.

242.2 BATESON, WILLIAM. 1861–1926, *et al.*

Further experiments on inheritance in sweet peas and stocks; preliminary account. *Proc. roy. Soc. B*, 1906, **77,** 236–8.

W. Bateson, E. R. Saunders and R. C. Punnett noted the phenomena of linkage of chromosomes.

243 GASKELL, WALTER HOLBROOK. 1847–1914

The origin of vertebrates. London, *Longmans, Green*, 1908.

Gaskell was probably the most brilliant of Michael Foster's pupils. His theory of the origin of vertebrates from invertebrate ancestors is not universally accepted.

244 BATESON, WILLIAM. 1861–1926

Mendel's principles of heredity. Cambridge, *Univ. Press*, 1909.

An account of Mendelism and the results which have followed from the application of its principles to later research on heredity. Pre-Mendelian work is considered, and the book includes an English translation of Mendel's classical paper, *Versuche über Pflanzen-Hybriden* (see No. 222.) Bateson was Professor of Biology at Cambridge. Third impression, with additions, 1913.

245 NILSSON-EHLE, NILS HERMAN. 1873–1949

Kreuzungsuntersuchungen an Hafer und Weizen. *Lunds Univ. Årsskr.*, 1909, N.F. Afd.2, **5,** Nr. 2, 1–122; 1911, N.F. Afd.2, **7,** Nr. 6, 1–84.

The "multiple factor" theory advanced by Nilsson-Ehle brought under the Mendelian law cases which, by their extreme variability of inheritance, might be considered exceptions to it.

245.1 MORGAN, THOMAS HUNT. 1866–1945

Sex-linked inheritance in *Drosophila*. *Science*, 1910, **32,** 120–22.

Demonstration of sex-linked inheritance.

245.2 STURTEVANT, ALFRED HENRY. 1891–

The linear arrangement of six sex-linked factors in *Drosophila*, as shown by their mode of association. *J. exp. Zool.*, 1913, **14,** 43–59.

Proof that the genes are arranged in a linear sequence along the chromosome. The work paved the way for the construction of chromosome maps for other species besides *Drosophila*.

246 MORGAN, Thomas Hunt. 1866–1945, *et al.*
The mechanism of Mendelian heredity. New York, *H. Holt*, 1915.

Morgan made great advances in the science of genetics by an intensive study of the mechanism of inheritance in the fruit fly *Drosophila melanogaster*. By the study of cross-over frequencies he was able to map the position of many of the Mendelian factors in the fly along the chromosomes. He was awarded the Nobel Prize for physiology in 1933.

247 PEARL, Raymond. 1879–1940
Modes of research in genetics. New York, *Macmillan & Co.*, 1915.

Raymond Pearl did much to advance the knowledge concerning the part played by the individual human constitution in disease.

248 CASTLE, William Ernest. 1867–
Genetics and eugenics. Cambridge (Mass.), *Harvard Univ. Press*, 1916.

250 MacCURDY, George Grant. 1863–1947
Human origins. New York, *Appleton*, 1924.

251 MORGAN, Thomas Hunt. 1866–1945
The theory of the gene. New Haven, *Yale Univ. Press*, 1926.

251.1 MULLER, Hermann Joseph. 1890–1967
Artificial transmutation of the gene. *Science*, 1927, **66,** 84–7.

Muller was awarded the Nobel Prize in 1946 for his work on the genetic effects of radiation. His paper records the first successful attempt at genetic mutation.

251.2 GRIFFITH, Frederick. ?1879–1941
The significance of pneumococcal types. *J. Hyg.* (*Camb.*), 1928, **27,** 113–59.

Griffith's experiments on transforming type II pneumococci into type III were repeated by Avery who was able sixteen years later (No. 255.1) to demonstrate that DNA was the transforming material.

252 LULL, Richard Swan. 1867–
Organic evolution. New York, *Macmillan & Co.*, 1929.

Third edition, 1945.

253 COWDRY, Edmund Vincent. 1888–
Human biology and racial welfare. Edited by E. V. Cowdry, New York, *P. B. Hoeber*, 1930.

Several authorities collaborated in writing this book.

253.1 FISHER, *Sir* Ronald Aylmer. 1890–1962
The genetical theory of natural selection. Oxford, *Clarendon Press*, 1930.

254 CLARK, *Sir* Wilfrid Edward Le Gros. 1895–
Early forerunners of man. London, *Baillière, Tindall & Cox*, 1934.

254.1 BEADLE, George Wells. 1903– , & TATUM, Edward Lawrie 1909–
Genetic control of biochemical reactions in *Neurospora*. *Proc. nat. Acad. Sci.* (*Wash.*), 1941, **27,** 499–506.

The work of Beadle and Tatum on mutations induced with *Neurospora crassa* opened up a new field, biochemical genetics. They shared the Nobel Prize in 1958 with J. Lederberg (No. 255.2) for their researches on the mechanism by which the chromosomes in the cell nucleus transmit inherited characters.

255 HUXLEY, *Sir* JULIAN SORELL. 1887–
Evolution: the modern synthesis. London, *Allen & Unwin*, 1942.

255.1 AVERY, OSWALD THEODORE. 1877–1955, *et al.*
Studies on the chemical nature of the substance inducing transformation of pneumococcal types. Induction of transformation by a desoxyribonucleic acid fraction isolated from pneumococcus type III. *J. exp. Med.*, 1944, **79**, 137–58.

Demonstration that deoxyribonucleic acid is a primary hereditary material. With C. M. MacLeod and M. McCarty.

255.2 LEDERBERG, JOSHUA. 1925– , & TATUM, EDWARD LAWRIE. 1909–
Gene recombination in *Escherichia coli*. *Nature* (*Lond.*), 1946, **158,** 558.

Discovery of sexual processes in the reproduction of bacteria. Lederberg shared the Nobel Prize with Tatum and Beadle (No. 254.1) in 1958.

256 HERSHEY, ALFRED DAY. 1908– , & CHASE, MARTHA COWLES. 1927–
Independent functions of viral protein and nucleic acid in growth of bacteriophage. *J. gen. Physiol.*, 1952, **36,** 39–56.

DNA shown to be the carrier of genetic information in virus reproduction.

256.1 ZINDER, NORTON DAVID. 1928– , & LEDERBERG, JOSHUA. 1925–
Genetic exchange in Salmonella. *J. Bact.*, 1952, **64,** 679–99.

Description of a new mechanism ("transduction") for the transfer of genetic characters from one bacterial strain to another.

256.2 TJIO, JOE HIN, & LEVAN, ALBERT.
The chromosome number of man. *Hereditas* (*Lund*), 1956, **42,** 1–6.

Proof that the normal chromosome number of man is 46.

257 HOLMES, SAMUEL JACKSON. 1868–1964
A bibliography of eugenics. *Univ. Calif. Publ. Zool.*, 1924, **25,** 1–514.

258 COOK, ROBERT CARTER. 1898–
The chronology of genetics. *Yearb. Agric. U.S. Dep. Agric.*, 1937, 1457–77.

258.1 PETERS, JAMES ARTHUR. 1922–
Classic papers in genetics. Edited by JAMES A. PETERS. Englewood Cliffs, N.J., *Prentice-Hall Inc.*, 1959.

258.2 STURTEVANT, ALFRED HENRY. 1891–
A history of genetics. New York, *Harper & Row*, 1965.

259–273.1 MICROSCOPY

259 STELLUTI, FRANCESCO. 1577–1653
Persio tradotto. Roma, *G. Mascardi*, 1630.

First book to contain illustrations of natural objects as seen through the microscope. The work includes the Latin text of the Satyrae VI of Aulus Persius Flaccus together with an Italian translation and notes by Stelluti.

260 BOREL, Pierre [Borellus.] 1620–1689
Historiarum, et observationum medico-physicaram, centuria. Castris, *apud A. Colomerium*, 1653.

The first work to apply microscopy to medicine. Borel probably saw the blood corpuscles and *Sarcoptes scabiei.*

261 ——. De vero telescopii inventore. Hagae-Comitum, *A. Vlacq*, 1655.

Borel collected evidence to show that Zacharias (sometimes called Zacharias Janssen) invented the compound microscope about 1590. Zacharias was a spectacle-maker of Middelburg, Holland.

262 HOOKE, Robert. 1635–1703
Micrographia, or some physiological descriptions of minutes bodies made by magnifying glasses; with observations and inquiries thereupon. London, *J. Martyn & J. Allestry*, 1665.

Hooke, at one time research assistant to Robert Boyle, constructed one of the most famous of the early compound microscopes. His *Micrographia* is the earliest work devoted entirely to an account of microscopical observations and the first book on the subject in English. It contains many accurate illustrations, beautifully engraved by Hooke himself. It includes also the first reference to cells, which were revealed by the microscope. Facsimile reprint, Oxford, 1938.

263 ZAHN, Johann.
Oculus artificialis teledioptricus sive telescopium. 3 pts. Herbipoli, *Q Heyl*, 1685–86.

Includes the first complete history of ea.ly microscopes.

264 BONANNI, Filippo [Buonanni]. 1638–1725
Observationes circa viventia, . . . cum micrographia curiosa. Romae, *typ. D. A. Herculis*, 1691.

Illustrates several early microscopes, including the famous microscopes of the Bolognese Joseph Campani.

265 LEEUWENHOEK, Antonj van. 1632–1723
Ontledingen en ontdekkingen, *etc.* 6 vols. Leiden, Delft, 1693–1718.

A collection in Dutch of many contributions sent by van Leeuwenhoek to the Royal Society of London. He is one of the greatest figures in the history of microscopy. He was first to describe spermatozoa, and the red blood corpuscles, discovered the crystalline lens, and was the first to see protozoa under the microscope. He introduced staining in histology in 1719 (saffron for muscle fibres). The *Ontledingen* appeared in a two-volume English translation, London, 1798–1807. See No. 67.

265.1 DEIJL, Harmanus van. 1738–1809
Kort bericht der trapsgewijze verbeteringen aan achromatische verrekijkers. *Natuurk. Verh. Maatsch. Wetensch. Haarlem*, 1807, **3**, 133–52.

Van Deijl introduced an achromatic objective.

266 AMICI, Giovanni Battista. 1784–1863
De microscopi catadiottrici memoria. Modena, 1818.

Amici constructed the first microscope with achromatic lenses and suggested water-immersion for improved achromatic lenses of the compound microscope. A translation in French of the above appears in *Ann. Chim. Phys. (Paris)*, 1820, **13**, 384–410.

266.1 GORING, C. R. 1792–1840

On Mr. Tulley's thick aplanatic object-glasses, for diverging rays; with an account of a few microscopic test objects. *Quart. J. Sci.*, 1827, **22,** 265–84.

Goring was an Edinburgh medical practitioner. He commissioned Tulley and others to make various modifications to the microscope. The above paper reports the first effective achromatic object-glass.

267 LISTER, JOSEPH JACKSON. 1786–1869

On some properties in achromatic object-glasses applicable to the improvement of the microscope. *Phil. Trans.*, 1830, **120,** 187–200.

The principle of the modern microscope was worked out by J. J. Lister, father of Lord Lister. His important improvements in achromatic lenses make him one of the most prominent figures in the history of modern microscopy.

267.1 DONNÉ, ALFRED. 1801–1878

Cours de microscopie. 1 vol. and atlas. Paris, *J. B. Baillière*, 1844–45.

The atlas includes the first engravings from photomicrographs. One is reproduced by A. Hughes, *J. roy. micr. Soc.*, 1955, **75,** 1–22 (pl. IV).

268 HIS, WILHELM, *Sr.* 1831–1904

Beschreibung eines Mikrotoms. *Arch. mikr. Anat.*, 1870, **6,** 229–32.

His was more than any other man responsible for the introduction of the microtome, although Ranvier and other Frenchmen had earlier employed microtomes of simpler types.

268.1 STEPHENSON, JOHN WARE.

On a large-angled immersion objective, without adjustment collar; with some observations on "numerical aperture." *J. roy. micr. Soc.*, 1878, **1,** 51–6.

Stephenson suggested the oil immersion lens system to Abbe, who developed it.

269 ABBE, ERNST. 1840–1905

Ueber neue Mikroskope. *S. B. Jena. Ges. Med.*, 1886, **2,** 107–28 (suppl. to *Jena Z. Naturw.*, 1887, **20**).

Fundamental improvements in the microscope were made by Abbe, who was a mathematician. In 1878 he introduced the oil immersion lens; in 1886 he made an apochromatic objective corrected for three colours in which the secondary spectrum was not noticeable, while he is also remembered for the sub-stage condenser which bears his name. A translation of the above article is in *J. roy. micr. Soc.*, 1887 20–34.

269.1 KÖHLER, AUGUST. 1866–1948

Mikrophotographische Untersuchungen mit ultraviolettem Licht. *Z. wiss. Mikr.*, 1904, **21,** 129–65, 273–304.

The ultraviolet light microscope was conceived and designed by Köhler.

269.2 HEIMSTÄDT, OSKAR.

Das Fluoreszenzmikroskop. *Z. wiss. Mikr.*, 1911, **28,** 330–37.

Fluorescence microscopy.

269.3 KNOLL, MAX, & RUSKA, ERNST.

Beitrag zur geometrischen Elektronenoptik. *Ann. Physik*, 1932, **12,** 607–61.

Electron microscope. See also their later paper in *Z. Physik.*, 1932, **78,** 318.

269.4 HAITINGER, Max. 1868–1946
Die Methoden der Fluoreszenzmikroskopie. In E. Abderhalden: *Handbuch der biologischen Arbeitsmethoden*, Berlin, Abt. II, Teil 3, pp. 3307–37, 1934.
Modern methods of fluorescence microscopy were developed by Haitinger.

269.5 ZERNIKE, Frits. 1888–1966
Das Phasenkontrastverfahren b.d. mikroskopischen Beobachtung. *Phys. Z.*, 1935, **36,** 848–51.
Phase contrast microscopy was invented by Zernike. He was awarded the Nobel Prize for physics in 1953.

269.6 BARNARD, Joseph Edwin. 1869–1949, & WELCH, Frank V.
Microscopy with ultra-violet light. A simplification of method. *J. roy. micr. Soc.*, 1936, **56,** 365–71.

269.7 COSSLETT, Vernon Ellis, & NIXON, W. C.
X-ray shadow microscope. *Nature (Lond.)*, 1951, **168,** 24–5.

269.8 EHRENBERG, Werner. 1901– , & SPEAR, W. E.
An electrostatic focussing system and its application to a fine focus x-ray tube. *Proc. phys. Soc.* (*Lond.*) *B*, 1951, **64,** 67–75.
X-ray microscopy.

History of Microscopy

270 HARTING, Pieter. 1812–1885
Het mikroskoop. 4 vols. Utrecht, 1848–54.
Exhaustive history of the microscope. The work was translated into German appearing (second edition) in 1866.

271 CLAY, Reginald Stanley, & COURT, Thomas H.
The history of the microscope. London, *Griffin*, 1932.

272 CONN, Harold Joel. 1886– , *et al.*
History of staining. 2nd ed. Geneva, N.Y., *Biotech Publications*, 1948.

273 FREUND, Hugo, & BERG, Alexander.
Geschichte der Mikroskopie. 3 vols. Frankfurt, *Umschau*, 1963–66.
A biographical history.

273.1 BRADBURY, Savile.
The evolution of the microscope. Oxford, *Pergamon Press*, 1967.

274–358.1 ZOOLOGY AND COMPARATIVE ANATOMY

274 ARISTOTLE. 384–322 B.C.
Historia animalium. *In his* Works . . . edited by J. A. Smith and W. D. Ross, Oxford, 1910, **4,** 486a–633a.
By his careful observations and excellent accounts of the natural history of those living creatures which he was able to investigate, Aristotle may be considered the first and greatest of all naturalists. For an evaluation of the biological work of Aristotle, *see* Singer's *History of biology*, 1950, pp. 9–44.

275 ——. De partibus animalium. *In his* Works . . . edited by J. A. SMITH and W. D. ROSS, Oxford, 1912, **5**, 639a–697b.

This and the preceding entry are English translations.

276 ALBERTUS MAGNUS [ALBERT VON BOLLSTADT.] ?1193–1280
De animalibus libri xxxi. Nach der Cölner Urschrift herausgegeben von H. STADLER. 2 vols. Münster, 1916–21.

Albertus slavishly followed Aristotle, although sometimes criticising him. He was a Dominican monk and the most eminent naturalist of the 13th century; his work on animals contained a good deal of personal observation.

277 TURNER, WILLIAM. 1510–1568
Avium praecipuarum . . . historia. Coloniae, *J. Gymnicus*, 1544.

The first ornithological work in the modern sense. Turner attempted to determine those birds named by Aristotle and Pliny; he added notes from his own observations on birds.

278 BELON, PIERRE [BELLONIUS]. 1517–1564
L'histoire naturelle des estranges poissons marins. Paris, *R. Chaudiere*, 1551.

This, Belon's first biological work, is regarded as the earliest modern scientific work in the field of comparative anatomy.

279 ——. De aquatilibus. Parisiis, *C. Stephanus*, 1553.

280 GESNER, CONRAD. 1516–1565
Historia animalium. 5 vols. Tiguri, *apud C. Froschouerum*, 1551–1587.

Gesner was a man of great industry. His *Historia animalium* is considered one of the starting points of modern zoology; it contains 4,500 pages and nearly 1,000 woodcuts, some being by Albrecht Dürer. It includes the names of all the known animals in the ancient and modern languages, together with a mass of information regarding them.

281 WOTTON, EDWARD. 1492–1555
De differentiis animalium. Lutetiae Parisiorum, *M. Vascosanus*, 1552.

Wotton is considered the founder of modern zoology. Basing his work on Aristotle, he rejected the fantastic additions which had accrued to the writings of the latter during the Middle Ages.

282 RONDELET, GUILLAUME [RONDELETIUS]. 1507–1566
Libri de piscibus marinis. (Universae aquatilium pars altera.) 2 vols. Lugduni, *apud Matthiam Bonhomme*, 1554–55.

Rondelet wrote this book with the idea of verifying Aristotle, but in it he described many forms of fishes for the first time. The book is an accurate account of his investigation of Mediterranean fishes and marine animals, and Singer says that Fig. 51, illustrating the structure of a sea urchin, is the earliest figure we have of a dissected vertebrate. Rondelet also observed the relationship between embryo and mother in the placental dogfish.

283 BELON, PIERRE [BELLONIUS]. 1517–1564
L'histoire de la nature des oyseaux. Paris, *B. Preuost, G. Cauellat*, 1555.

Belon's book on birds is well illustrated, including plates of the skeletons of man and bird side by side and in the same posture, to compare them bone for bone.

284 COITER, VOLCHER. 1534–1576
Diversorum animalium sceletorum explicationes. Noribergae, *in off. T. Gerlachii*, 1575.

Coiter was a pupil of Fallopius and Eustachius, and became town physician of Nuremberg. His book on comparative osteology is the most important of the early works on that subject. Biography by B. T. W. Nuyens and A. Schierbeck, Haarlem, 1956.

285 RUINI, CARLO. ?1530–1598
Dell'anotomia, et dell'infermità del cavallo. Bologna, *G. Rossi*, 1598.

First book devoted exclusively to the structure of a single species other than man. Besides being one of the foundation-stones of modern veterinary medicine, it contains a description of the lesser circulation. The admirable plates are by some authorities attributed to Leonardo.

286 CASSERIO, GIULIO [JULIUS CASSERIUS *Placentinus*]. 1561?–1616
De vocis auditusque organis historia anatomica. 2 pts. Ferrariae, *exc. V. Baldinus, typ. Cameralis*, 1600–01.

Casserius investigated the structure of the auditory and vocal organs in most of the domestic animals. The book includes a description of the larynx more accurate than that of any previous author, and is also notable for its fine illustrations.

287 JONSTON, JOHN [JOHNSTONE]. 1603–1675
Thaumatographia naturalis. Amsterdami, *G. Blaeu*, 1632.

A compilation of all the contemporary zoological knowledge. Jonston, born in Scotland, spent most of his life on the Continent.

288 MOFFET, THOMAS [MOUFET, MUFFETUS]. 1553–1604
Insectorum sive minimorum animalium theatrum. Londoni, *ex off. typ. Thom. Cotes*, 1634.

Moffet travelled extensively in Europe and kept copious notes of his observations on insects. These he published in the above folio, together with many excellent illustrations. To date, this was the best work of its kind and it set a new standard of accuracy in the study of the invertebrates. An English translation, *Theater of Insects*, appeared in 1658.

289 SEVERINO, MARCO AURELIO [SEVERINUS]. 1580–1656
Zootomia Democritaea: id est, anatome generalis totius animantium opificii. Noribergae, *lit. Endterianis*, 1645.

One of the most important of the early works on comparative anatomy. It includes the *Anatomia porci*, attributed to Copho of Salerno. Severinus dissected many animals and was convinced that the microscope would throw light on comparative anatomy.

290 ALDROVANDUS, ULYSSES [ALDROVANDI]. 1522–1607
Opera omnia. 13 vols. Bononiae, *J. B. Bellagamba (and others)*, 1599–1667

Aldrovandi, first director of the botanical garden at Bologna, was a prolific writer. Some of his writings made their first appearance in print after his death. He designed them as a whole to form an enormous encyclopaedia of biology.

291 GOEDAERT, JAN [GOEDARTIUS]. 1620–1668
Metamorphosis et historia naturalis insectorum. 3 pts. Medioburgi, *Jacobum Fierensium*, 1662–67.

English translation, 1682.

292 CHARLETON, Walter. 1619–1707
Onomasticon zoicon, plerorumque animalium differentias et nomina propria pluribus linguis exponens. Cui accedunt mantissa anatomica, et quaedam de variis fossilium generibus. Londoni, *apud. J. Allestry*, 1668.

Gives a list of the English, Latin, and Greek names of all the then known animals.

293 MALPIGHI, Marcello. 1628–1694
Dissertatio epistolica de bombyce. Londini, *J. Martyn & J. Allestry*, 1669.

Malpighi's work on the silkworm represents the first monograph on an invertebrate and records one of the most striking pieces of research work on his part. He dissected the silkworm under the microscope with great skill and observed its intricate structure; before the appearance of this work the silkworm was believed to have no internal organs.

294 SWAMMERDAM, Jan. 1637–1680
Historica insectorum generalis. 2 pts. Utrrecht [*sic*], *M. van Dreunen*, 1669.

Swammerdam, one of the greatest of the early microscopists, spent much time on the study of insects, and mapped out a natural classification of them.

295 PERRAULT, Claude. 1613–1688
Mémoires pour servir à l'histoire des animaux. Paris, *Acad. d. Sci.*, 1671–76.

The early biological work of the French Académie des Sciences was issued chiefly as anatomical descriptions of various animals, and is mostly the work of Perrault. Singer considered this important text on comparative anatomy to be the most sumptuously produced of all biological works.

296 BLAES, Gerard [Blasius]. 1626–1682
Anatome animalium. Amstelodami, *J. a Someren*, 1681.

This work, the result of many years spent on a comparative study of the structure of vertebrates, is a compendium of previous writings on the subject, with some original observations of Blaes. It is the first general systematic treatise on comparative anatomy.

297 GREW, Nehemiah. 1641–1712
Musaeum Regalis Societatis, or a catalogue and description of the natural and artificial rarities belonging to the Royal Society and preserved at Gresham College. Whereunto is subjoyned the comparative anatomy of stomachs and guts. London, *H. Newman*, 1681.

Grew, secretary to the Royal Society, compiled this great illustrated catalogue of its museum, then housed at Gresham College. The second part of the book is a collection of lectures delivered by Grew before the Society in 1676. It is one of the best comparative studies undertaken in the 17th century; Grew himself introduced the term "comparative anatomy".

298 SNAPE, Andrew, *Jnr.*
The anatomy of an horse. London, *M. Flesher*, 1683.

First book in English on equine anatomy.

299 RAY, John. 1628–1705
Synopsis methodica animalium quadrupedum et serpentini generis Londini, *S. Smith, & B. Walford*, 1693.

This work contains the first really systematic classification of animals. Much of its general arrangement of animals survives in modern systems of classification.

300 TYSON, Edward. 1650–1708
Orang-outang, sive homo sylvestris: or, the anatomy of a pygmie compared with that of a monkey, an ape, and a man. London, *T. Bennet & D. Brown*, 1699.

The earliest work of importance in comparative morphology. Tyson compared the anatomy of man and monkeys and between the two he placed the chimpanzee, which he regarded as the typical pygmy. This was the origin of the idea of a "missing link" in the ascent of man from the apes. See also No. 153.

301 RÉAUMUR, René Antoine Ferchault de. 1683–1757
Sur les diverses reproductions qui se font dans les écrevisses, les omars, les crabes, etc. *Mém. Acad. roy. Sci.* (*Paris*), 1712, 226–45.

Réaumur showed that crustaceans replace their lost limbs, a fact until then disputed.

302 VALLISNIERI, Antonio [Vallisneri]. 1661–1730
Istoria del camaleonte Affricano e di varj animali d'Italia. Venezia, *G. G. Ertz*, 1715.

303 VALENTINI, Michael Bernhard. 1657–1729
Amphitheatrum zootomicum. Francofurti ad Moenum, *sumpt. haered. Zunnerianorum*, 1720.

"First extensive work on the comparative anatomy of vertebrates" (Casey Wood).

304 RÉAUMUR, René Antoine Ferchault de. 1683–1757.
Memoires pour servir à l'histoire des insectes. 6 vols. Paris, *Mortier*, 1734–42.

Réaumur's greatest work. It describes the appearance, habits and locality of all the known insects except the beetles, and includes 267 plates.

305 LYONET, Pieter. 1707–1789
Traité anatomique de la chénille. La Haye, 1740.

Lyonet's great monograph on the goat moth caterpillar remains today among the greatest examples of anatomical examination.

306 BAKER, Henry. 1698–1774
An attempt towards a natural history of the polype. London, *R. Dodsley*, 1743.

307 TREMBLEY, Abraham. 1710–1784
Mémoires, pour servir à l'histoire d'un genre de polypes d'eau douce, à bras en forme de cornes. Leyden, *J. & H. Verbeek*, 1744.

Trembley was one of the pioneers of experimental morphology. The above work records how he cut hydras into several pieces, producing new individuals, and how, by cutting up the latter, he obtained a third generation. His experiments were of great importance in the study of regeneration of lost parts, he was first to make permanent grafts and to witness cell-division. A biography of Trembley was published by J. R. Baker, London, 1952.

308 BONNET, Charles. 1720–1793
Traité d'insectologie. 2 pts. Paris, *Durand*, 1745.

Bonnet was a precursor of the *Naturphilosophie* school, and believed in the "performation" theory—that the organism is already formed in the ovum or in the spermatozoon.

309 HUNTER, John. 1728–1793
Observations on certain parts of the animal oeconomy. London, 1786.

Includes John Hunter's observations on the secondary sexual characteristics in birds, on the descent of the testis, on the air sac in birds, on the structure of the placenta, etc., together with the original description of the olfactory nerves.

310 RUSSELL, Patrick. 1727–1805
An account of Indian serpents. 4 vols. London, *G. Nicol*, 1796–1809.
First attempt at a description of Indian serpents and serpent venoms. Includes the original description of Russell's viper, *Daboia russellii.*

311 CUVIER, Georges Léopold Chrétien Frédéric Dagobert, *Baron.* 1769–1832
Leçons d'anatomie comparée. 5 vols. Paris, *Baudouin*, an VIII [1800]–1805.
Cuvier ranks with von Baer as one of the founders of modern morphology.

312 BLUMENBACH, Johann Friedrich. 1752–1840
Handbuch der vergleichenden Anatomie. Göttingen, *H. Dieterich*, 1805.
Blumenbach, physiologist and anthropologist, was Professor of Medicine at Göttingen. He was the first to show the value of comparative anatomy in the study of anthropology; his classical text went through many editions; it was translated into English in 1807.

313 VICQ D'AZYR, Felix. 1748–1794
Œuvres. 6 vols. and atlas. Paris, *L. Duprat-Duverger*, 1805.
Vicq d'Azyr was the greatest comparative anatomist of the eighteenth century. The mammillo-thalamic tract is named the "bundle of Vicq d'Azyr".

314 MECKEL, Johann Friedrich, *the younger*. 1781–1833
Beyträge zur vergleichenden Anatomie. 2 vols. Leipzig, *C. H. Reclam*, 1808–11.
See No. 318.

315 HOME, *Sir* Everard. 1756–1832
Lectures on comparative anatomy, in which are explained the preparations in the Hunterian collection. 6 vols. London, *G. & W. Nicol, etc.*, 1814–28.

316 LAMARCK, Jean Baptiste Pierre Antoine de Monet de. 1744–1829
Histoire naturelle des animaux sans vertèbres. 7 vols. Paris, *Verdière*, 1815–22.
An expansion of Lamarck's *Philosophie zoologique* (see No. 216). As a systematist Lamarck made important contributions to biology. He separated spiders and crustaceans from insects, made advances in the classification of worms and echinoderms, and introduced the classification of animals into vertebrates and invertebrates.

317 CHAMISSO, Ludwig Adalbert von. 1781–1838
De salpa. Berolini, *apud F. Dümmlerum*, 1819.
In this monograph on certain *Vermes* is included the first description of several of the Tunicates and the earliest use of the expression "alternation of generations".

318 MECKEL, Johann Friedrich, *the younger*. 1781–1833
System der vergleichenden Anatomie. 5 vols. [in 6]. Halle, *Renger*, 1821–31.
Meckel is considered the greatest comparative anatomist before Johannes Müller.

319 GEOFFROY SAINT-HILAIRE, Étienne. 1772–1844, & CUVIER, Frédéric. 1773–1838
Histoire naturelle des mammifères. 4 vols. Paris, *Belin & Blaise*, 1824–42.

322 AUDUBON, John James Laforest. 1785–1851
The birds of America. 4 vols. London, *The Author*, 1827–38.

Contains 435 plates. This is the first of the great modern atlases of ornithology. With the assistance of William Macgillivray, Audubon wrote a five-volume text for this atlas, entitled *Ornithological biography*, Edinburgh, 1831–39.

324 BUFFON, Georges Louis Leclerc, *Comte*. 1707–1788
Œuvres complètes. 20 vols. Bruxelles, *T. Lejeune*, 1828–33.

Buffon's great *Histoire naturalle*, published in 44 vols., Paris, 1749–1804, was the first modern attempt to embrace all scientific knowledge. His works influenced Erasmus Darwin, Lamarck, Goethe, Cuvier and others. Buffon believed in the possibility of spontaneous generation.

325 OWEN, *Sir* Richard. 1804–1892
Memoir on the pearly nautilus (Nautilus pompilius, Linn.). London, *W. Wood*, 1832.

326 ROYAL COLLEGE OF SURGEONS OF ENGLAND.
Descriptive and illustrated catalogue of the physiological series of comparative anatomy contained in the Museum. 5 vols. [in 6]. London, *R. & J. E. Taylor*, 1833–40.

When Hunter died his museum was cared for by his faithful assistant William Clift, who persuaded the Government to purchase it. Owen later became curator and his monumental catalogue is still of value to-day. A history of the museum from its foundation to its destruction by a high-explosive bomb in May, 1941, is given in G. Grey Turner's *Hunterian Museum*, 1946. See also No. 2295.

327 CUVIER, Georges Léopold Chrétien Frédéric Dagobert, *Baron*. 1769–1832
Le règne animal. 3me édition. 20 vols. Paris, *Fortin, Masson & Cie.*, 1836–49.

Cuvier's most comprehensive work represented the fruits of a lifetime's study of living and fossil animals. In his day Cuvier exerted an enormous influence on science. He played a leading part in the development of the science of palaeontology and stimulated the study of comparative anatomy. First edition, 1817. Several English translations are available.

328 MÜLLER, Johannes. 1801–1858
Ueber die Lymphherzen der Schildkröten. Berlin, *Druckerei d. k. Akad.*, 1840.

329 OWEN, *Sir* Richard. 1804–1892
Odontography, or, a treatise on the comparative anatomy of the teeth. 2 vols. and atlas. London, *H. Baillière*, 1840–45.

Owen's comprehensive investigation of the morphology of mammalian teeth led him into palaeontology, of which he soon became one of the masters. Owen was from 1836–56 Hunterian professor at the Royal College of Surgeons. For a time he was an opponent of Darwinism.

330 ——. On the archetype and homologies of the vertebrate skeleton. London, *J. Van Voorst*, 1848.

Owen's vertebrate theory of the origin of the skull, later refuted by Huxley and others.

331 SIEBOLD, Carl Theodor Ernst von. 1804–1885, & STANNIUS, Hermann Friedrich. 1808–1883
Lehrbuch der vergleichenden Anatomie. 2 vols. Berlin, *Veit & Co.*, 1846–48.

333 AGASSIZ, LOUIS JEAN RODOLPHE. 1807–1873
Contributions to the natural history of the United States. 4 vols. Boston, *Little, Brown & Co.*, 1857–62.

Agassiz was the leading comparative anatomist in America and an opponent of Darwinism.

334 BRONN, HEINRICH GEORG. 1800–1862
Die Klassen und Ordnungen des Thier-Reichs. Vol. 1– . Leipzig, *C. F. Winter*, 1859–

This great systematic work, begun by Bronn, is being continued by other naturalists. It deals with both recent and fossil zoology.

335 COUCH, JONATHAN. 1789–1870
A history of the fishes of the British Isles. 4 vols. London, *Groombridge and Sons*, [1860]–1865.

Couch, a general practitioner at Polperro, Cornwall, became one of the greatest authorities on British fishes. The work, a monument of industry and patience, includes some fine plates, also by Couch.

336 OWEN, *Sir* RICHARD. 1804–1892
On the anatomy and physiology of the vertebrates. 3 vols. London, *Longmans, Green*, 1866–68.

1. Fishes and reptiles; 2. Birds; 3. Mammals. The most important work on the subject since Cuvier. It is based entirely on personal observations.

337 GEGENBAUR, CARL. 1826–1903
Grundzüge der vergleichenden Anatomie der Wirbelthiere. 2te. Aufl. Leipzig, *W. Engelmann*, 1870.

Gegenbaur's best work. He stressed the value of comparative anatomy as the basis of the study of descent, considering that knowledge of the relations of corresponding parts in different animals was more important even than comparative embryology in this respect.

338 HUXLEY, THOMAS HENRY. 1825–1895
A manual of the anatomy of vertebrated animals. London, *J. & A. Churchill*, 1871.

Huxley was among those who refuted Owen's theory of the vertebrate skull.

339 DOHRN, ANTON. 1840–1909
Der Ursprung der Wirbelthiere und das Princip des Functionswechsels. Leipzig, *W. Engelmann*, 1875.

340 WALLACE, ALFRED RUSSEL. 1823–1913
The geographical distribution of animals. 2 vols. London, 1876.

Wallace studied the fauna of the Malay peninsula and was struck both with its resemblances to and differences from that of S. America. His studies resulted in the above work, still the most important on the subject.

341 MÜLLER, JOHANN FRIEDRICH THEODOR. 1821–1897
Ueber die Vortheile der Mimicry bei Schmetterlingen. *Zool. Anz.*, 1878, **1**, 54–55.

Bates (No. 118) based his explanation of mimicry on the theory of natural selection; this did not explain the "warning colours" of certain animals, for the purpose of holding off their attackers. Müller suggested that life is saved by this mimicry, as it warned others of the danger or inedible nature of these animals, and further that it protected the young and inexperienced of the would-be enemies.

343 WIEDERSHEIM, ROBERT ERNST EDUARD. 1848–1923
Lehrbuch der vergleichenden Anatomie der Wirbelthiere. Jena, *G. Fischer*, 1883.

344 BROCA, PIERRE PAUL. 1824–1880
Mémoires sur le cerveau de l'homme et des primates. Paris, *C. Reinwald*, 1888.

345 LANKESTER, *Sir* EDWIN RAY. 1847–1929
A treatise on zoology. Edited by E. RAY LANKESTER. 9 vols. London, *Black*, 1900–9.

346 THEOBALD, FREDERICK VINCENT. 1868–1930
A monograph of the Culicidae, or mosquitoes. 4 vols. and atlas. London, *Longmans & Co.*, 1901–10.

347 DUCKWORTH, WYNFRID LAURENCE HENRY. 1870–1956
Morphology and anthropology. Cambridge, *Univ. Press*, 1904.

348 MORGAN, THOMAS HUNT. 1866–1945
Experimental zoology. New York, *Macmillan & Co.*, 1907.

349 PATTON, WALTER SCOTT. 1876–1960, & CRAGG, FRANCIS WILLIAM. 1882–1924
A textbook of medical entomology. London, Madras, and Calcutta, *Christian Literature Society for India*, 1913.

350 TILNEY, FREDERICK. 1875–1938
The brain from ape to man. With chapters on the reconstruction of the grey matter in the primate brainstem by HENRY ALSOP RILEY. 2 vols. New York, *P. B. Hoeber*, 1928.

Classical study of the evolution of the central nervous system in the higher mammals.

351 ZUCKERMAN, *Sir* SOLLY. 1904–
The social life of monkeys and apes. London, *Kegan Paul*, 1932.

A study of the relationship of Man to the other primates, from the physiological and biochemical standpoint. Zuckerman's work is considered the first adequate interpretation of simian society.

352 CLARK, *Sir* WILFRID EDWARD LE GROS. 1895–
History of the primates. London, *British Museum (Natural History)*, 1949.

History of Zoology

353 CARUS, JULIUS VICTOR. 1823–1903
Geschichte der Zoologie. München, *R. Oldenbourg*, 1872.

French edition, 1880.

354 BROOKS, WILLIAM KEITH. 1848–1908
The foundations of zoology. London, *Macmillan & Co.*, 1899.

355 ESSIG, EDWARD OLIVER. 1884–
A history of entomology. New York, *Macmillan & Co.*, 1931.

356 WOOD, CASEY ALBERT. 1856–1942
An introduction to the literature of vertebrate zoology. London, *Oxford Univ. Press*, 1931.
A comprehensive summary of the literature on vertebrate zoology.

357 HASSALL, ALBERT. 1862–1942, *et al.*
Index-catalogue of medical and veterinary zoology. Pt. 1– . Washington, *Govt. Printing Off.*, 1932–
In progress.

358 COLE, FRANCIS JOSEPH. 1872–1959
A history of comparative anatomy. From Aristotle to the eighteenth century. London, *Macmillan & Co.*, 1944.

358.1 PETIT, GEORGES, & THÉODORIDES, JEAN.
Histoire de la zoologie des origines à Linné. Paris, *Hermann*, 1962.

359–1588.5 ANATOMY AND PHYSIOLOGY

359–461.1 ANATOMY

359 GALEN. A.D. 130–200
De anatomicis administrationibus, libri i–ix. *In his* Opera, ed. C. G. KÜHN, Lipsiae, 1821, **2**, 215–731.
Galen's anatomical writings are a repository of all contemporary knowledge, together with some of his own views and discoveries. He had a good knowledge of osteology and myology, some knowledge of angiology and less of zoology. Although not to be regarded as the founder of the science of anatomy, he is nevertheless its first important figure. English translations by C. Singer (1956) and W. H. L. Duckworth (1962).

360 ——. Sieben Bücher Anatomie des Galen. 2 vols. Leipzig, *J. C. Hinrichs*, 1906.
Greek text with German translation.

361 MONDINO DE' LUZZI [MUNDINUS]. ?1275–1326
Anothomia. Papiae, *A. de Carchano*, 1487.
The first book devoted solely to anatomy; it was written for his students in 1316. Mundinus re-introduced human dissection, which had been neglected for 1500 years before him; he was the most noted dissector of his period. The mediaeval anatomical vocabulary, well set forth by Mundinus, was derived mainly from Arabic; Singer, in his translation of the work, 1925, has added an ample glossary of terms of Arabic origin. Facsimile reproduction, Bologna, 1930.

362 MONDEVILLE, HENRI DE. ?1260–1320
Die Anatomie des Heinrich von Mondeville. Nach einer Handschrift der Königlichen Bibliothek zu Berlin von Jahre 1304 zum ersten Male herausgegeben von J. PAGEL. Berlin, *G. Reimer*, 1889.
Mondeville was the first teacher known to have lectured with the aid of illustrations, using 13 charts of human anatomy. He lectured at Montpellier.

363 KETHAM, JOHANNES DE. *d. circa* 1490
Fasciculus medicinae. Venetiis, *per Johannem & Gregorius fratres de Forlivio*, 1491.
A collection of short medical treatises. Its great importance is that it includes the first anatomic illustrations of any kind. Singer, who considers the woodcuts the best of the time, edited an English translation of the work which includes notes by Sudhoff and which was published at Milan, 1924.

364 LEONARDO DA VINCI. 1452–1519
I manoscritti de Leonardo da Vinci della Reale Biblioteca di Windsor. Pubblicata da TEODORO SABACHNIKOFF. Transcritti e annotati da GIOVANNI PIUMATI. 2 vols. Parigi, *E. Rouveyre*, 1898–1901.
Includes ff. A-B of his anatomical MSS. Text in French and Italian.

365 ——. Quaderni d'anatomia. I–VI. Fogli della Royal Library di Windsor, pubblicati da C. L. VANGENSTEN, A. FONAHN, H. HOPSTOCK. 6 vols. Christiania, *J. Dybwad*, 1911–16.
Leonardo "the greatest artist and scientist of the Italian Renaissance, was the founder of iconographic and physiologic anatomy" (Garrison). He made over 750 sketches of all the principal organs of the body, drawings which were adequately reproduced only in recent times. His notes accompanying the drawings are in mirror-writing. Text in Italian, English, and German.

366 ——. Leonardo da Vinci on the human body. The anatomical, physiological, and embryological drawings of Leonardo da Vinci. With translations, emendations, and biographical introduction by CHARLES D. O'MALLEY and J. B. DE C. M. SAUNDERS. New York, *Henry Schuman*, 1952.
Includes 215 plates, reproduced by photography.

367 BERENGARIO DA CARPI, GIACOMO. 1470–1550
Commentaria cum amplissimis additionibus super anatomia Mundini una cum textu ejusdem in pristinum et verum nitorem redacto. Bononiae, *imp. per H. de Benedictis*, 1521.
Berengario corrected Mondino and was himself an eminent anatomist. He first mentioned the vermiform appendix and the larger pelvic capacity of the female. He gave the first good description of the thymus.

368 ——. Isagogae breves perlucide ac uberime in anatomiam humani corporis a communi medicorum academia usitatam. Bononiae, *per B. Hectoris*, 1522.
A better work than the preceding, which it was intended to replace. Includes a description of the valves of the heart. English translation by L. R. Lind, Chicago, 1959.

368.1 EDWARDES, DAVID. 1502–1542
De indiciis et praecognitionibus, opus apprime utile medicis. Eiusdem in anatomicen introductio luculenta et brevis. Londini, *R. Redmanus*, 1532.
First anatomical text by an Englishman. The only known copy is in the British Museum. Edwardes made the first dissection in England (1531). Reproduced in facsimile with an English translation by C. D. O'Malley and K. F. Russell, London, 1961.

369 LAGUNA, ANDRÉS [LACUNA]. 1499–1560
Anatomica methodus, seu de sectione humani corporis contemplatio. Parisiis, *apud J. Kerver*, 1535.
Includes the first description of the ileo-caecal valve. Laguna, a Spanish anatomist, travelled much in Europe and became physician to Charles V.

370 DRYANDER, JOHANN [EICHMANN]. 1500–1560
Anatomia capitis humani. Marpurgi, *E. Cervicorni*, 1536.

371 ——. Anatomiae, hoc est, corporis humani dissectionis pars prior. Marpurgi, *apud E. Cervicornum*, 1537.

Dryander was among the first to make illustrations after his own dissections. His unfinished *Anatomiae* is one of the most important of the pre-Vesalian atlases. Choulant ascribes the woodcuts to the school of Hans Brosamer. This book includes Copho's *Anatomia porci.*

372 VESALIUS, ANDREAS. 1514–1564
Tabulae anatomicae sex. Venetiis, *sumpt. J. S. Calcarensis*, 1538.

Only two copies of the original edition of this atlas are known to exist. The book was reprinted privately for Sir William Stirling-Maxwell, London, 1874. The *Tabulae* are also reproduced half-size in *A prelude to modern science*, by C. Singer and C. Rabin, Cambridge, 1946.

373 CANANO, GIOVANNI BATTISTA. 1515–1579
Musculorum humani corporis picturata dissectio. [Ferrara, 1541?].

Contains copper-plates of the bones and muscles of the upper limb, from drawings by Girolamo da Carpi, which "in realism and exactitude surpassed anything between Leonardo and Vesalius; but having seen the woodcuts of [Vesalius's] *Fabrica*, the high-minded Ferrarese deliberately suppressed his own book, and only 11 copies are now extant" (A. C. Klebs). The first book in which each muscle was illustrated separately. This fine work was reprinted in facsimile in Florence, 1925, edited by Harvey Cushing and E. C. Streeter.

374 LOBERA DE AVILA, LUIS. *fl.* 1551
Libro de anatomia. [Alcalá de Henares, *Juan de Brocar*, 1542].

375 VESALIUS, ANDREAS. 1514–1564
De humani corporis fabrica libri septem. Basileae (*ex off. Ioannis Oporini*, 1543).

By this epoch-making work Vesalius, the "Father of Modern Anatomy", prepared the way for the rebirth of physiology by Harvey. More important still, he undermined the widespread reverence for authority in science and prepared the way for independent observation in anatomy and clinical medicine. The publication of this book was the greatest event in medical history since the work of Galen. J. B. de C. M. Saunders and C. D. O'Malley published *The illustrations from the works of Andreas Vesalius*, with a biographical sketch in 1950, O'Malley published a biography in 1964, and Harvey Cushing's *Biobibliography of Andreas Vesalius* appeared in a second edition, Hamden, Conn., 1962.

376 ——. Suorum de humani corporis fabrica librorum epitome. Basileae (*ex off. J. Oporini*, 1543).

The very rare *Epitome* appeared in the same month (June) as the *Fabrica*, and probably after it, although authorities vary in their opinions as to this point. Facsimile reproduction, with translation, New York, 1949.

377 ——. De humani corporis fabrica libri septem. Basileae, *J. Oporinus*, 1555.

A better edition of the *Fabrica*. *See* the remarks of Garrison on page 219 of his *Introduction*, 1929.

378 ESTIENNE, CHARLES [STEPHANUS]. 1504–1564
De dissectione partium corporis humani. Parisiis, *apud S. Colinaeum*, 1545.

First published work to include illustrations of the whole external venous and nervous systems. A French translation appeared from the same press in 1546.

378.1 COLOMBO, MATTEO REALDO [COLUMBUS]. 1516–1559
De re anatomica libri xv. Venetiis, *ex typ. Nicolai Beuilacquae*, 1559.

Colombo was a pupil of Vesalius and succeeded him in the chair of anatomy a Padua before proceeding to chairs first at Pisa and later Rome. His book, which was published posthumously, rectified a number of anatomical errors but he plagiarized and disparaged his predecessors. He described the pulmonary circulation but may have read the account of Servetus published six years previously. He gave a clear description of the mode of action of the pulmonary, cardiac, and aortic valves.

378.2 FALLOPPIO, GABRIELE [FALLOPIUS]. 1523–1562
Observationes anatomicae. Venetiis, *apud M.A. Ulmum*, 1561.

Fallopius studied under Vesalius and became professor of anatomy at Ferrara (1547), Pisa (1548), and Padua (1551). He was a careful dissector, a great observer, and an accurate recorder. He discovered and first described the chorda tympani and semicircular canals, correctly described the structure and course of the cerebral vessels, knew the circular folds of the small intestines. He enumerated all the nerves of the eye, and introduced a number of anatomical names. He is eponymously remembered by the Fallopian tube and the Fallopian aqueduct.

379 BAUHIN, CASPAR [BAUHINUS]. 1560–1624
Theatrum anatomicum. Basileae, *S. Henricpeti*, 1590.

Includes valuable historical data.

380 GUIDI, GUIDO [VIDIUS]. 1508–1569
De anatome corporis humani libri vii. Venetiis, *apud Juntas*, 1611.

Guidi, professor of philosophy and medicine at Pisa, discovered the Vidian nerve the Vidian canal, and the Vidian artery. The above was edited by his nephew.

381 CASSERIO, GIULIO [JULIUS CASSERIUS *Placentinus*]. 1561?–1616
Tabulae anatomicae lxxiix. Venetiis, *apud E. Deuchinum*, 1627.

Includes some of the finest copper-plates produced in the 17th century. Daniel Bucretius (or Rindfleisch) obtained the plates, intending to use them to illustrate the work of Spigelius, but first published them separately. Actually there are 97 plates Bucretius added 20 and destroyed one of the originals.

382 HIGHMORE, NATHANIEL. 1613–1685
Corporis humani disquisitio anatomica. Hagae-Comitis, *S. Broun*, 1651.

Highmore is remembered for his description of the "antrum of Highmore" (already noticed by Casserius and figured by Leonardo da Vinci), the seminal ducts and the epididymis.

383 KERCKRING, THOMAS THEODOR. 1640–1693
Spicilegium anatomicum. Amstelodami, *sumpt. A. Frisii*, 1670.

Kerckring made important investigations on the development of the foetal bones. He was the first to describe the large ossicle sometimes present at the lambdoidal suture; his name is remembered in the *valvulae conniventes* of the small intestine, previously described by Fallopius.

384 GENGA, BERNARDINO. 1655–1734
Anatomia chirurgica. Roma, *A. Ercole*, 1672.

First book devoted entirely to surgical anatomy.

385 BIDLOO, Govert. 1649–1713
Anatomia humani corporis, centum et quinque tabulis, per artificiosiss. G. de Lairesse ad vivum delineatis. Amstelodami, *vid. J. à Someren,* 1685.

The value of Bidloo's *Anatomia* lies chiefly in the 105 fine copperplate engravings drawn by G. de Lairesse. When William of Orange came to England in 1688, Bidloo was chosen to accompany him as his physician. English translation by W. Cowper, 1698. Facsimile reprint, Paris, 1972.

386 GENGA, Bernardino. 1655–1734
Anatomia per uso et intelligenza del disegno ricercata non solo su gl'ossi, e muscoli del corpo humano. Roma, *G. J. de Rossi,* 1691.

Contains 56 copper-plates, excellent anatomically and artistically. This book was the best of its time, in fact one of the finest of all books on anatomy for artists

387 HAVERS, Clopton. ?–1702
Osteologia nova, or some new observations of the bones. London, *S. Smith,* 1691.

Havers discovered the Haversian canals and made important observations on the physiology of bone growth and repair. The Haversian lamellae, glands, and folds, are also named after him. The Haversian canals were observed by van Leeuwenhoek in 1686.

388 VERHEYEN, Philippe. 1648–1710
Anatomia corporis humani. Lovanii, 1693.

This work was widely used for some years after publication, superseding Bartholin in popularity. The second edition, 1710, with supplement, 1731, published at Brussels and Amsterdam, is much better.

389 RUYSCH, Frederik. 1638–1731
Thesaurus anatomicus. i-x. Amstelaedami, *J. Wolters,* 1701–16.

Ruysch, professor of anatomy at Leyden and Amsterdam, is notable for his method of injecting the vessels. The recipe for the material used by Ruysch has remained a secret. He gave the first description of bronchial blood vessels and vascular plexuses of the heart, demonstrated the valves of the lymphatics, and made a great number of other important discoveries in anatomy.

390 CHESELDEN, William. 1688–1752
The anatomy of the humane body. London, *N. Cliff & D. Jackson,* 1713.

Although Cheselden is best known for his accomplishments in the field of surgery, he wrote two important books on anatomy. The above was for many years a text-book of the English medical schools and ran through 13 editions.

391 EUSTACHI, Bartolommeo [Eustachius]. 1520–1574
Tabulae anatomicae. Romae, *ex off. F. Gonzagae,* 1714.

A romantic history attaches to this fine collection of plates, drawn by Eustachius himself and completed in 1552. They remained unprinted and forgotten in the Vatican Library until discovered in the early 18th century, and were then presented by Pope Clement XI to his physician, the famous Lancisi. The latter published them in 1714 together with his own notes. These plates are more accurate than the work of Vesalius; Singer was of the opinion that had they appeared in 1552 Eustachius would have ranked with Vesalius as one of the founders of modern anatomy. He discovered the Eustachian tube, the thoracic duct, the adrenals and the abducens nerve, and gave the first accurate description of the uterus. He also described the cochlea, the muscles of the throat and the origin of the optic nerves.

392 SANTORINI, GIOVANNI DOMENICO. 1681–1737
Observationes anatomicae. Venetiis, *apud J. B. Recurti*, 1724.

Santorini was one of the ablest dissectors of his day. In the above work many new discoveries of anatomical details are set forth, together with corrections of some of the errors of earlier anatomists.

393 CHOVET, ABRAHAM. 1704–1799
A syllabus or index, of all the parts that enter the composition of the human body . . . For the use of those that go through courses of anatomy. London, 1732.

Chovet was born in England and died in Philadelphia. He made many beautiful wax models to illustrate his lectures, and was among the first to popularize the use of wax and natural preparations in the teaching of anatomy, devices which he advocated in his *Syllabus*. The book gives an interesting picture of the methods employed in the teaching of anatomy in the mid-18th century. Chovet's famous collection of models went to Philadelphia University, where it later perished in a fire.

394 WINSLOW, JACOBUS BENIGNUS. 1669–1760
Exposition anatomique de la structure du corps humain. 4 vols. Paris, *G. Desprez et J. Dessesartz*, 1732.

The foramen between the greater and lesser sacs of the peritoneum (described on pages 352–65), is named after Winslow. His *Exposition* is distinguished as being the first book on descriptive anatomy to discard physiological details and hypothetical explanations foreign to the subject. He did much to condense and systematize the anatomical knowledge of his time. English translation, 1733–34.

395 CHESELDEN, WILLIAM. 1688–1752
Osteographia, or the anatomy of the bones. London, 1733.

Considered the best production of the 18th century anatomists. It contained full and accurate descriptions of all the human bones, as well as many of animals. Cheselden is the first person known to have used the camera obscura to gain precision in his illustrations. These are beautifully executed by Van der Gucht, and the whole is a work of permanent value. In 1720 Cheselden inaugurated lectures on anatomy and surgery at St. Thomas's Hospital. See the paper by K. F. Russell, *Bull. Hist. Med.*, 1954, **28**, 32–49, which mentions a trial issue of the book, dated 1728. Facsimile reprint 1968.

396 LIEUTAUD, JOSEPH. 1703–1780
Essais anatomiques. Paris, *P. M. Huart*, 1742.

Lieutaud rectified many anatomical errors, described carefully the structure and relations of the heart and its cavities, and added to the contemporary knowledge concerning the bladder. The trigonum vesicae is named "Lieutaud's trigone."

397 HALLER, ALBRECHT VON. 1708–1777
Icones anatomicae. 8 pts. Gottingae, *A. Vandenhoeck*, 1743–56.

Accurate and beautiful engravings of the diaphragm, uterus, ovaries, vagina, arteries, with explanatory observations.

398 GAUTIER D'AGOTY, JACQUES FABIAN. 1717–1786
Essai d'anatomie en tableaux imprimés. Paris, *chez Gautier*, 1745.

Remarkable for its striking coloured mezzotints.

399 ALBINUS, BERNHARD SIEGFRIED. 1697–1770
Tabulae sceleti et musculorum corporis humani. Lugduni Batavorum, *J. & H. Verbeek*, 1747.

Albinus was one of the greatest anatomical illustrators of the 18th century; his illustrations of the bones and muscles were noted for their beauty and accuracy and his work established a new standard in anatomical illustration. He is said to have spent 24,000 Dutch florins on the production of the illustrations for the above work. English translation, Edinburgh, 1777.

400 SOEMMERRING, Samuel Thomas. 1755–1830
Vom Baue des menschlichen Körpers. 5 pts. Frankfurt a.M., *Varrentrapp u. Wenner*, 1791–96.

Soemmerring's text-book contained only facts actually observed by himself. He departed from the usual practice of including physiology with anatomy. The book was very popular in German medical schools, and Meckel considered it Soemmerring's best work.

401 ——. Tabula sceleti feminini juncta descriptione. Trajecti ad Moenum, *Varrentrapp et Wenner*, 1797.

Soemmerring was noted for his accuracy in anatomical illustration, and the above work is a fine example of his artistic sense. For it he selected the skeleton of a well-built girl of 20 years. Great care was taken in selecting the most appropriate posture and the contour of an ideally perfect female body in which the skeleton might be drawn in order properly to observe its proportions.

402 BELL, *Sir* Charles. 1774–1842
A system of dissections. 2 vols. Edinburgh, *Mundell & Son*, 1799–1801.

Published while Bell was still a student. The anatomical work of Bell was the most important in the British Isles during the early part of the 19th century.

403 BICHAT, Marie François Xavier. 1771–1802
Anatomie générale, appliquée à la physiologie et à la médecine. 2 vols. [in 4]. Paris, *Brosson, Gabon & Cie.*, an X [1801].

One of Medicine's most important books. Bichat revolutionized descriptive anatomy. Where Morgagni and others had conceived of whole organs being diseased, Bichat showed how individual tissues could be separately affected. English translation, Boston, 1822.

404 ——. Traité d'anatomie descriptive. 5 vols. Paris, *Gabon & Cie.*, an X–XII [1801–03].

Bichat's last work, unfinished at his death.

405 BURNS, Allan. 1781–1813
Observations on the surgical anatomy of the head and neck. Edinburgh, *T. Bryce*, 1811.

See also Nos. 2889, 3055. Burns was first to suggest (p. 31) ligature of the innominate artery. His book describes "Burns' space," the fascial space at the suprasternal notch.

406 MEDICO, Giuseppe del.
Anatomia per uso de' pittori e scultori. Roma, *V. Poggioli*, 1811.

Contains 38 good copper-plates in black and red.

407 MECKEL, Johann Friedrich, *the younger*. 1781–1833
Handbuch der menschlichen Anatomie. 4 vols. Halle & Berlin, 1815–20.

408 RIEMER, Pieter de. 1760–1831
Afbeeldingen van de juiste plaatsing der inwendige deelen van het menschelijk ligchaam. 's-Gravenhage, *J. Allart*, 1818.

First use of frozen sections for anatomical illustration. De Riemer appears to have been the first to freeze tissues in order to permit of fine sectioning.

409 CLOQUET, Jules Germain. 1790–1883
Anatomie de l'homme. 5 vols. Paris, *C. de Lasteyrie*, 1821–31.

This fine atlas includes 300 plates. Cloquet was professor of clinical surgery, Paris.

410 QUAIN, Jones. 1796–1865
Elements of descriptive and practical anatomy. London, *W. Simpkin & R. Marshall*, 1828.

Among the most important of the English text-books on anatomy. An eleventh edition was published in 1908–29.

411 FLAXMAN, John. 1755–1826
Anatomical studies of the bones and muscles, for the use of artists. London, *M. A. Nattali*, 1833.

Plates engraved by Henry Landseer from Flaxman's drawings.

412 HUXLEY, Thomas Henry. 1825–1895
On a hitherto undescribed structure in the human hair sheath. *Lond. med. Gaz.*, 1845, **36,** 1340–41.

"Huxley's layer" and "membrane" of the root sheath of hair follicles.

413 HYRTL, Jośzef. 1810–1894
Lehrbuch der Anatomie des Menschen. Prag, *F. Ehrlich*, 1846.

Hyrtl's *Lehrbuch* passed through 22 editions and was translated into the principal modern languages.

414 ——. Handbuch der topographischen Anatomie. 2 vols. Wien, *W. Braumüller*, 1847.

Hyrtl, professor of anatomy at Vienna, published the first text on topographical anatomy in German. He was for 30 years the most popular lecturer on the subject in Europe, and ranks as one of the greatest of medical scholars.

415 KNOX, Robert. 1791–1862
A manual of artistic anatomy. London, *H. Renshaw*, 1852.

Knox, remembered because of his indiscreet association with the Edinburgh "resurrectionists," was one of the best teachers of anatomy during the 19th century.

416 PIROGOV, Nikolai Ivanovich. 1810–1881
Anatome topographica sectionibus per corpus humanum congelatum triplici directione ductis illustrata. 8 pts. Petropoli, *J. Trey*, 1852–59.

Pirogov was the greatest of all Russian surgeons. In Russian medicine he is approached only by Pavlov. He introduced the teaching of applied topographical anatomy in Russia. His great atlas of 220 plates represents the first use on a grand scale of frozen sections in anatomical illustration, an idea first carried out by de Riemer (No. 408).

417 HENLE, Friedrich Gustav Jakob. 1809–1885
Handbuch der systematischen Anatomie des Menschen. 3 vols. Braunschweig, *F. Vieweg u. Sohn*, 1855–71.

Considered by many authorities to be the greatest of the modern systems of anatomy. Many structures are named after him, including the looped portion of the uriniferous tubules of the kidney, the layer of cells in the root sheath of a hair, and the ampulla of the uterine tube.

418 GRAY, Henry. 1825–1861
Anatomy, descriptive and surgical. London, *J. W. Parker & Son*, 1858.

Gray's text-book of anatomy remains to-day a standard work on the subject in the English-speaking world. The 33rd edition appeared in 1962; the first American edition was published at Philadelphia, 1859.

419 HUMPHRY, *Sir* GEORGE MURRAY. 1820–1896
A treatise on the human skeleton, including the joints. Cambridge, *Macmillan & Co.*, 1858.

Humphry was professor of anatomy at Cambridge and became the first professor of surgery there. He founded the *Journal of Anatomy and Physiology* in 1867. "Humphry's ligament" of the knee-joint is described on p. 546 of the above book and pictured on plate 53, fig. 1.

420 OLLIER, LOUIS XAVIER EDOUARD LÉOPOLD. 1830–1900
Des moyens chirurgicaux de favoriser la reproduction des os après les résections. *Gaz. hebd. Méd. Chir.*, 1858, **5**, 572–7, 651–3, 733–6, 769–70, 853–7, 890, 899–905.

"Ollier's layer," the osteogenetic layer of the periosteum.

421 LEIDY, JOSEPH. 1823–1891
An elementary treatise on human anatomy. Philadelphia, *J. B. Lippincott*, 1861.

Leidy himself illustrated this book. He was professor of anatomy at Philadelphia and the leading American anatomist of his time.

422 SIBSON, FRANCIS. 1814–1876
Medical anatomy. 7 pts. London, *J. Churchill*, [1855]–69.

Sibson was professor of medicine at St. Mary's Hospital. "Sibson's fascia" and "muscle" are named after him.

423 HEITZMANN, CARL. 1836–1896
Die descriptive und topographische Anatomie des Menschen. Wien, *W. Braumüller*, 1870.

424 BRAUNE, CHRISTIAN WILHELM. 1831–1892
Topographisch-anatomischer Atlas. Nach Durchschnitten angefrornen Cadavern. Leipzig, *Veit & Co.*, 1872.

Fine illustrations of frozen sections.

425 HYRTL, JOŠZEF. 1810–1894
Die Corrosions-Anatomie und ihre Ergebnisse. Wien, *W. Braumüller*, 1873.

Hyrtl, skilled in making anatomical preparations, built up a collection which was unsurpassed in Europe. In the above work he described a method of his own invention, in which he injected the blood supplies of the different organs, the adjacent parts being eaten away by acids, in order to show the finest ramifications. The technique of wax impregnation and later corrosion was of course known to the Hunters.

426 REID, ROBERT WILLIAM. 1851–1939
Observations on the relation of the principal fissures and convolutions of the cerebrum to the outer surface of the scalp. *Lancet*, 1884, **2**, 539–40.

Reid's base line – the anthropometric base line on the skull.

427 KOLLMANN, JULIUS KONSTANTIN ERNST. 1834–1918
Plastische Anatomie des menschlichen Körpers. Leipzig, *Veit & Co.*, 1886.

"Illustrated with lithographs from hand-drawings, photographs from the nude, ethnic studies of facial features . . . The text . . . is of unusual historic interest, and includes special chapters on the anatomy of the infant, human proportions, and ethnic morphology" (Choulant, transl. Frank.)

428 TESTUT, Jean Léo. 1849–1925
Traité d'anatomie humaine. 3 vols. Paris, *O. Doin*, 1889–92.
7th edition, 1921–23.

429 BRODIE, Charles Gordon. 1860–1933
Dissections illustrated. London, *Whittaker & Co.*, 1892–95.
"Brodie's ligament," the transverse humoral ligament, described.

430 SPALTEHOLZ, Karl Werner. 1861–1940
Handatlas der Anatomie des Menschen. 3 vols. Leipzig, *S. Hirzel*, 1895–1903.
16th edition in English, 1967.

431 MACEWEN, *Sir* William. 1848–1924
Atlas of head sections. Glasgow, *J. Maclehose*, 1893.

432 HIS, Wilhelm, *Snr*. 1831–1904
Die anatomische Nomenclatur. Leipzig, *Veit & Co.*, 1895.
His was largely responsible for the Basle Nomina Anatomica, the first attempt to produce a standard anatomical nomenclature. English translation by L. F. Barker, 1907.

433 BARDELEBEN, Karl von. 1849–1918
Handbuch der Anatomie des Menschen. Herausgegeben von K. von Bardeleben. 32 parts. Jena, *G. Fischer*, 1896–1934.
An important collective work.

434 ——. Lehrbuch der systematischen Anatomie des Menschen. Berlin, Wien, *Urban & Schwarzenberg*, 1906.

435 MERKEL, Friedrich Sigmund. 1845–1919
Die Anatomie des Menschen. 3 pts. Wiesbaden, *J. F. Bergmann*, 1913–14.

436 TANDLER, Julius. 1869–1936
Lehrbuch der systematischen Anatomie. 2te. Aufl. 4 vols. Leipzig, *F. C. W. Vogel*, 1923–29.

436.1 WOERDEMANN, Martinus Willem. 1892–
Nomina anatomica Parisiensia (1955) and B.N.A. (1895). Utrecht, *Oosthoek*, 1957.
Includes historical sketch of the systems of anatomical nomenclature.

History of Anatomy

437 BAUHIN, Caspar [Bauhinus]. 1560–1624
Anatomica corporis virilis et muliebris historia. Lugduni, *J. le Preux*, 1597.

437.1 PORTAL, Antoine. 1742–1832
Histoire de l'anatomie et de la chirurgie. 6 vols. [in 7]. Paris, *P. F. Didot le jeune*, 1770–73.
A biobibliographical survey to 1755.

438 HALLER, ALBRECHT VON. 1708–1777
Bibliotheca anatomica. 2 vols. Tiguri, *apud Orell, Gessner*, etc., 1774–77.

Haller is one of the greatest names in medical bibliography. He compiled bibliographies of botany, anatomy, medicine and surgery which together form the most exhaustive summary of previous writings on these subjects.

439 HYRTL, JOŠZEF. 1810–1894
Antiquitates anatomicae rariores. Vindobonae, *typ. Congregationis Mechitaristicae*, 1835.

440 CHOULANT, JOHANN LUDWIG. 1791–1861
Geschichte und Bibliographie der anatomischen Abbildung. Leipzig, *R. Weigel*, 1852.

In this classical work Choulant traced the evolution of anatomical illustration from the early schematic plates up to his own time, including a valuable bibliography. An English translation of the work by Mortimer Frank appeared in 1920 (Chicago, University Press) and this is enriched by a chapter on anatomical illustration since Choulant, written by F. H. Garrison. A reprint of the translation appeared in 1945 with additional essays by Garrison and others.

442 KEEN, WILLIAM WILLIAMS. 1837–1932
A sketch of the early history of practical anatomy. Philadelphia, *J. B. Lippincott*, 1874.

443 HYRTL, JOŠZEF. 1810–1894
Das Arabische und Hebräische in der Anatomie. Wien, *W. Braumuller*, 1879.

Hyrtl, professor of anatomy at Prague and Vienna, retired in 1874 and devoted his leisure to the writing of this and the following work. He ranks with Littré as one of the greatest medical scholars.

444 ——. Onomatologia anatomica. Geschichte und Kritik der anatomischen Sprache der Gegenwart. Wien, *W. Braumüller*, 1880.

A classical work on anatomical terminology.

446 DUVAL, MATHIAS MARIE. 1844–1907, & CUYER, EDOUARD. 1852–?
Histoire d'anatomie plastique. Paris, *Picard & Kaan*, 1898.

447 TÖPLY, ROBERT, *Ritter* VON. 1856–1947
Studien zur Geschichte der Anatomie im Mittelalter. Leipzig, Wien, *F. Deuticke*, 1898.

448 ——. Geschichte der Anatomie. In Puschmann's *Handbuch der Geschichte der Medizin*, Jena, 1903, **2,** 155–326.

449 HOPF, LUDWIG. 1838–
Die Anfänge der Anatomie bei den alten Kulturvölkern. Breslau, *J. U. Kern*, 1904.

Abhandlungen zur Geschichte der Medizin, Breslau, Heft 9.

450 BARDEEN, CHARLES RUSSELL. 1871–1935
Anatomy in America. *Bull. Univ. Wisconsin*, 1905, No. 115, 85–208.

451 SUDHOFF, KARL FRIEDRICH JAKOB. 1853–1938.
Tradition und Naturbeobachtung in den Illustrationen medicinischer Handschriften und Frühdrucke vornehmlich des 15. Jahrhunderts. Leipzig, *J. A. Barth*, 1907.

452 SUDHOFF, Karl Friedrich Jakob. 1853–1938.
Ein Beitrag zur Geschichte der Anatomie im Mittelalter, speziell der anatomischen Graphik nach Handschriften des 9. bis 15. Jahrhunderts. Leipzig, *J. A. Barth*, 1908.

Studien zur Geschichte der Medizin, Leipzig, Heft 4.

453 CRAIGIE, David. 1793–1866
History of anatomy. *Encyclopaedia Britannica*, Cambridge, 11th ed., 1910, **1**, 921–937.

This excellent short history of anatomy, written for an earlier edition of the *Encyclopaedia Britannica*, was brought up to date by F. G. Parsons.

454 SINGER, Charles Joseph. 1876–1960
The evolution of anatomy. A short history of anatomical and physiological discovery to Harvey. London, *Kegan Paul*, 1925.

This invaluable reference book, by the outstanding British authority on the subject, is an expansion of the FitzPatrick Lectures, 1923–24. Reprinted under the title *A short history of anatomy from the Greeks to Harvey* (Dover reprint, 1957).

456 CORNER, George Washington. 1889–
Anatomical texts of the earlier Middle Ages. Washington, 1927.

Carnegie Inst. Publication No. 364. A valuable study of the history of mediaeval anatomy.

457 ——. Anatomy. New York, *P. B. Hoeber*, 1930.

Clio Medica series.

458 HUNTER, Richard Henry.
A short history of anatomy. 2nd ed. London, *John Bale*, 1931.

459 WEGNER, Richard Nikolaus. 1884–
Das Anatomenbildnis. Seine Entwicklung im Zusammenhang mit der anatomischen Abbildung. Basel, *Schwabe*, 1939.

460 DOBSON, Jessie.
Anatomical eponyms: being a biographical dictionary of those anatomists whose names have become incorporated into anatomical nomenclature, with definitions of the structures to which their names have been attached and references to the works in which they are described. 2nd ed. Edinburgh, *E. & S. Livingstone*, 1962.

461 RUSSELL, Kenneth Fitzpatrick. 1911–
British anatomy 1525–1800: a bibliography. Parkville, *Melbourne Univ. Press*, 1963.

Full descriptions of 901 items.

461.1 WOLF-HEIDEGGER, Gerhard, & CETTO, Anna Maria.
Die anatomische Sektion in bildlicher Darstellung. Basel, *Karger*, 1967.

462–534.1

EMBRYOLOGY

462 ARISTOTLE. 384–322 B.C.
De generatione animalium. *In his* Works . . . edited by J. A. Smith and W. D. Ross. Oxford, 1912, **5**, 715a–789b.

The first great text-book of embryology. Aristotle classified animals according to their embryological characters, wrote at length on generation and the theories concerning it which were current in his day, and dealt exhaustively with the whole subject of embryology. He believed the menstrual blood to be responsible for embryogenesis. "The depth of Aristotle's insight into the generation of animals has not been surpassed" (Needham). Also translated by A. L. Peck (Loeb Classics), 1953.

463 RUEFF, Jacob [Ruff; Ruoff]. 1500–1558
De conceptu et generatione hominis. Tiguri, *C. Froschoverus*, 1554.

This is an improved version of Rösslin's *Der swangern frawen*. Its importance to the embryologist lies in Rueff's illustrations, which show contemporary ideas about mammalian embryology.

464 ARANZI, Giulio Cesare [Aranzio; Arantius]. 1530–1589
De humano foetu. Bononiae, *J. Rubrius*, 1564.

Aranzi believed the maternal and foetal circulations to be separate. He described the ductus arteriosus and ductus venosus of the foetus, and the corpora Arantii in the heart valves. Incidentally, he was the first to record a pelvic deformity.

465 FABRIZZI, Girolamo [Fabricius ab Aquapendente]. 1533–1619
De formato foetu. Venetiis, *per F. Bolzettam*, 1600.

Fabricius wrote at great length on embryology, inventing many theories, some of which were false. His illustrations marked a great advance on previous work. Fabricius recorded for the first time the dissection of several embryos. Facsimile reprint with translation by H. B. Adelmann, 1942.

466 ——. De formatione ovi et pulli. Patavii, *ex off. A. Bencÿ*, 1621.

467 HARVEY, William. 1578–1657
Exercitationes de generatione animalium. Londini, *O. Pulleyn*, 1651.

The most important book on the subject to appear during the 17th century. Harvey was among the first to disbelieve the erroneous doctrine of the "preformation" of the foetus; he maintained that the organism derives from the ovum by the gradual building up and aggregation of its parts. The chapter on midwifery in this book is the first work on that subject to be written by an Englishman. This book also demonstrates Harvey's intimate knowledge of the existing literature on the subject. He corrected many of the errors of Fabricius. See *The analysis of the De generatione animalium of William Harvey* by A. W. Meyer, Stanford Univ. Press, 1936.

468 MALPIGHI, Marcello. 1628–1694
De ovo incubato observationes. Londini, *J. Martyn*, 1673.

First description, from the microscopical point of view, of the chick embryo.

469 ——. Dissertatio epistolica de formatione pulli in ovo. Londini, *J. Martyn*, 1673.

This and the *De ovo incubato* (No. 468) placed the study of embryology on a sound basis, surpassing in accuracy all other contemporary work on the subject and foreshadowing some of the more important general lines of research in embryology.

470 WOLFF, Caspar Friedrich. 1733–1794
Theoria generationis. Halae ad Salam, *lit. Hendelianis*, 1759.

Wolff observed in great detail the early processes of embryonic differentiation. He disposed of the "preformation" theory, substituting his view that the organs are formed from leaf-like (blastodermic) layers. He thus laid the foundation of the "germ-layer" theory of Baer and Pander. His book includes descriptions of the "Wolffian bodies" and "ducts". Reprinted 1966.

471 ——. De formatione intestinorum praecipue. *Novi Comment. Acad. Sci. Petropol.*, 1768, **12,** 43–7, 403–507; 1769, **13,** 478–530.

One of the acknowledged classics of embryology. Wolff's description of the formation of the chick's intestine by the rolling inwards of a leaf-like layer of the blastoderm was important as proving his theory of epigenesis. A German translation of the book by J. F. Meckel was published in 1812.

472 BONNET, Charles. 1720–1793
Considérations sur les corps organisés. 2 vols. Amsterdam, *M. M. Rey*, 1762.

Bonnet believed in the preformation of the embryo. He used many of Haller's arguments to support his own opinions. J. Needham (No. 533) calls him an organicistic preformationist, for his objection to epigenesis lay in the fact that it apparently did not allow for the integration of the organism as a whole.

473 SOEMMERRING, Samuel Thomas. 1755–1830
Icones embryonum humanorum. Francofurti ad Moenum, *Varrentrapp u. Wenner*, 1799.

Soemmerring met William Hunter during a visit to London in 1778. The latter's classical work on the pregnant uterus (No. 6157) dealt only with the latter half of pregnancy. Soemmerring therefore decided in a supplementary volume, to deal with the appearance of the embryo during the first half of pregnancy. This book is one of the best illustrated of Soemmerring's works.

474 PANDER, Heinrich Christian. 1794–1865
Dissertatio sistens historiam metamorphoseos, quam ovum incubatum prioribus quinque diebus subit. Wirceburgi, *T. E. Nitribitt*, 1817.

A well-illustrated monograph on the development of the chick. Pander, with von Baer, developed the germ-layer theory. He recognized three germ layers. The book appeared in German, also in 1817.

475 MÜLLER, Johannes. 1801–1858
Ueber die Entwickelung der Eier im Eierstock bei den Gespenstheuschrecken. *Nova Acta phys.-med. Acad. Caes. Leopold nat. curios.*, Bonn, 1825, **12,** 553–672.

Discovery of the Müllerian duct.

476 PURKINJE, Johann Evangelista [Purkyně]. 1787–1869
Subjectae sunt symbolae ad ovi avium historiam ante incubationem. Vratislaviae, *typ. Universitatis*, [1825].

First description of the germinal vesicle in the embryo, "Purkinje's vesicle."

477 BAER, Carl Ernst von. 1792–1876
De ovi mammalium et hominis genesi. Lipsiae, *L. Vossius*, 1827.

Announces Baer's discovery of the mammalian ovum. The book was reprinted in facsimile in *Isis*, 1931, **16,** 315–30. English translation by C. D. O'Malley, *Isis*, 1956, **47,** 117–53.

478 PRÉVOST, Jean Louis. 1790–1850, & DUMAS, Jean Baptiste André. 1800–1884.
Mémoire sur le développement du poulet dans l'oeuf. *Ann. Sci. nat. (Paris)*, 1827, **12,** 415–43.

First description of the segmentation of the frog's egg.

479 BAER, Carl Ernst von. 1792–1876
Ueber Entwicklungsgeschichte der Thiere. 3 vols. Königsberg, *Bornträger*, 1828–88.

Baer, the father of modern embryology, definitely established the "germ-layer theory," discovered the notochord and the human ovum, and postulated the law of corresponding stages in embryonic development. With Cuvier he is the founder of modern morphology. Later in his life he devoted much time to the study of anthropology.

480 RATHKE, Martin Heinrich. 1793–1860
Abhandlungen zur Bildungs- und Entwicklungs-Geschichte der Menschen und der Thiere. 2 pts. Leipzig, *F. C. W. Vogel*, 1832–33.
Rathke's most notable discovery was of structures homologous with gill slits in bird and mammalian embryos. He discredited the vertebral theory of the skull.

481 SCHWANN, Theodor. 1810–1882
De necessitate aëris atmosphaerici ad evolutionem pulli in ovo incubito. Berolini, *typ. Nietackianis*, 1834.
Proof that air is necessary in the development of the embryo.

482 REICHERT, Karl Bogislaus. 1811–1883
Ueber die Visceralbogen der Wirbelthiere. Berlin, *Sittenfeld*, 1837.
First description of the visceral arches in vertebrates.

483 RATHKE, Martin Heinrich. 1793–1860
Entwicklungsgeschichte der Natter (Coluber natrix). Koenigsberg, *Börntrager*, 1839.
"Rathke's pouch," a diverticulum from the embryonic buccal cavity.

484 BISCHOFF, Theodor Ludwig Wilhelm. 1807–1882
Entwickelungsgeschichte des Kaninchen-Eies. Braunschweig, *F. Vieweg u. Sohn*, 1842.
Bischoff contributed important original work on the development of the rabbit.

485 REMAK, Robert. 1815–1865
Untersuchungen über die Entwickelung der Wirbelthiere. Berlin, *G. Reimer*, 1855.
Simplification of von Baer's classification of the germ-layers.

486 GEGENBAUR, Carl. 1826–1903
Ueber den Bau und die Entwickelung der Wirbelthier-Eier mit partieller Dottertheilung. *Arch. Anat. Physiol. wiss. Med.*, 1861, 491–529.
Proof that the ovum is unicellular in all vertebrates.

487 KÖLLIKER, Rudolph Albert von. 1871–1905
Entwicklungsgeschichte des Menschen und der höheren Thiere. Leipzig, *W. Engelmann*, 1861.
First book on comparative embryology.

488 SCHULTZE, Maximilian Johann Sigismund. 1825–1874
Observationes nonnulae de ovorum ranarum segmentatione, quae "Furchungsprocess" dicitur. Bonnae, *Formis C. Georgi*, 1863.
Best contemporary description of the segmentation furrowing of the egg.

489 HIS, Wilhelm, *Snr.* 1831–1904
Beobachtungen über den Bau des Säugethier-Eierstockes. *Arch. mikr. Anat.*, 1865, **1**, 151–202.
His was the greatest of the 19th-century embryologists.

490 ——. Die Häute und Höhlen des Körpers. Basel, *Schweighauser*, 1865.
A new classification of tissues based on histogenesis.

491 LANGHANS, Theodor. 1839–1915
Zur Kenntnis der menschlichen Placenta. *Arch. Gynäk.*, 1870, **1,** 317–34.

"Langhans' layer"—the cytotrophoblast, the individual cells of which are termed "Langhans' cells".

492 WALDEYER-HARTZ, Heinrich Wilhelm Gottfried. 1836–1921
Eierstock und Ei. Leipzig, *W. Engelmann,* 1870.

Waldeyer discovered the germinal epithelium.

493 HAECKEL, Ernst Heinrich Philipp August. 1834–1919
Anthropogenie oder Entwicklungsgeschichte des Menschen. Leipzig, *W. Engelmann,* 1874.

Classical work on embryology.

494 HIS, Wilhelm, *Snr.* 1831–1904
Unsere Körperform und das physiologische Problem ihrer Entstehung. Leipzig, *F. C. W. Vogel,* 1874.

In this work His compared the various layers and organs of the embryo to a series of elastic tubes and plates. He thought that the local inequalities of growth and the differences in the consistency of the tissues might account for the various organs and structures. This work led to the idea of "developmental mechanics."

495 HERTWIG, Wilhelm August Oscar. 1849–1922
Beiträge zur Kenntnis der Bildung, Befruchtung und Theilung des thierischen Eies. *Morph. Jb.*, 1876, **1,** 347–434.

Demonstration of the fact that the spermatozoon enters the ovum and that union of the nuclei of the male and female gametes follows. Hertwig was professor of anatomy at Jena and Berlin.

496 BENEDEN, Edouard van. 1846–1910
Le maturation de l'oeuf, la fécondation et les premières phases du développement embryonnaire des mammifères. *Bull. Acad. roy. Sci. Belg.*, 1875, 2 sér., **40,** 686–736.

First detailed description of the segmentation of the mammalian ovum.

497 ——. Contributions à l'histoire de la vésicule germinative et du premier noyau embryonnaire. *Bull. Acad. roy. Sci. Belg.*, 1876, 2 sér., **41,** 38–85.

Independently of Flemming, van Beneden discovered the centrosome.

498 FLEMMING, Walther. 1843–1905
Beobachtungen über die Beschaffenheit des Zellkerns. *Arch. mikr. Anat.*, 1877, **13,** 693–717.

Discovery of the centrosome.

500 BALFOUR, Francis Maitland. 1851–1882
A treatise on comparative embryology. 2 vols. London, *Macmillan & Co.*, 1880–81.

This classical work sums up all the previous knowledge on the subject and includes Balfour's own important contributions. Balfour, a pupil of Michael Foster, became professor of animal morphology in 1882; in the same year he met his death in a mountaineering accident.

501 HIS, Wilhelm, *Snr.* 1831–1904
Anatomie menschlicher Embryonen. 3 pts. and atlas. Leipzig, *F. C. W. Vogel,* 1880–85.

A systematic account of early human embryology that stimulated further investigation in a field in which His stood highest among his contemporaries. He was the first to study the human embryo as a whole.

502 HERTWIG, WILHELM AUGUST OSCAR. 1849–1922, & HERTWIG, KARL WILHELM THEODOR RICHARD. 1850–1937
Die Coelomtheorie; Versuch einer Erklärung des mittleren Keimblatts. Jena, *G. Fischer*, 1881.

503 PFLÜGER, EDUARD FRIEDRICH WILHELM. 1829–1910, & SMITH, WILLIAM J.
Untersuchungen über Bastardirung der anuren Batrachier und die Principien der Zeugung. *Pflüg. Arch. ges. Physiol.*, 1883, **32,** 519–41.
Pflüger was one of the earliest workers in the field of experimental embryology. Above, his first work on the subject, deals with the cross-fertilization of different species of frog.

504 HERTWIG, WILHELM AUGUST OSCAR. 1849–1922
Lehrbuch der Entwicklungsgeschichte des Menschen und der Wirbelthiere. Jena, *G. Fischer*, 1886.

505 MINOT, CHARLES SEDGWICK. 1852–1914
Uterus and embryo. *J. Morph.*, 1889, **2,** 341–462.

507 ——. A theory of the structure of the placenta. *Anat. Anz.*, 1891, **6,** 125–31.

508 ROUX, WILHELM. 1850–1924
Beitrag zur Entwicklungsmechanik des Embryo. *S.B. k. Akad. Wiss. Wien, math.-nat. Cl.*, 1892, **101,** 3 Abt., 27–234.
The name of Roux is especially associated with developmental mechanics ("Entwicklungsmechanik") and he is regarded as the founder of the science of experimental embryology.

511 LOEB, JACQUES. 1959–1924
Ueber die Grenzen der Theilbarkeit der Eisubstanz. *Pflug. Arch. ges. Physiol.*, 1894–95, **59,** 379–94.

512 LILLIE, FRANK RATTRAY. 1870–1947
The embryology of the Unionidae. A study in cell-lineage. *J. Morph.* 1895, **10,** 1–100.

513 KEIBEL, FRANZ KARL JULIUS. 1861–1929
Normentafeln zur Entwicklungsgeschichte der Wirbelthiere. Hrsg. von FRANZ KEIBEL. 16 pts. Jena, *G. Fischer*, 1897–1938.

514 MORGAN, THOMAS HUNT. 1866–1945
The development of the frog's egg; an introduction to experimental embryology. New York, *Macmillan & Co.*, 1897.
First work in English on experimental embryology.

515 SCHAPER, ALFRED. 1863–1905
Die frühesten Differenzirungsvorgänge im Centralnervensystem. *Wilhelm Roux Arch. EntwMech. Org.*, 1897, **5,** 81–132.

516 MALL, FRANKLIN PAINE. 1862–1917
Contributions to the study of the pathology of early human embryos. 3 pts. Baltimore, *etc.*, 1899–1908.

516.1 PETERS, HUBERT. 1859–1934
Ueber die Einbettung des menschlichen Eies und das früheste bisher bekannte menschliche Placentationsstadium. Leipzig, Wien, *F. Deuticke*, 1899.

517 KORSCHELT, EUGEN. 1858–1946, & HEIDER, KARL. 1856–1935
Lehrbuch der vergleichenden Entwicklungsgeschichte der wirbellosen Thiere. Jena, *G. Fischer*, 1902–09.

518 McCLUNG, CLARENCE ERWIN. 1870–1946
The accessory chromosome; sex determination. *Biol. Bull.*, 1902, **3,** 43–84.

The accessory chromosomes were shown by McClung to be the determinants of sex.

519 HARRISON, ROSS GRANVILLE. 1870–1959
Neue Versuche und Beobachtungen über die Entwicklung der peripheren Nerven der Wirbeltiere. *S. B. nied.-rhein. Gesellsch. Nat.- u. Heilk. Bonn*, 1904.

520 WILSON, EDMUND BEECHER. 1856–1939
Experimental studies on germinal localisation. *J. exp. Zool.*, 1904, **1,** 1–73.

521 HERTWIG, WILHELM AUGUST OSCAR. 1849–1922
Handbuch der vergleichenden und experimentellen Entwicklungslehre der Wirbeltheire. Hrsg. von OSCAR HERTWIG. 3 vols. [in 6]. Jena, *G. Fischer*, 1906.

522 LEWIS, WARREN HARMON. 1870–1964
Experiments on the origin and differentiation of the optic vesicle in amphibia. *Amer. J. Anat.*, 1907–08, **7,** 259–77.

523 BRYCE, THOMAS HASTIE. 1862–1946, & TEACHER, JOHN HAMMOND. 1869–1930
Contributions to the study of the early development and imbedding of the human ovum. An early ovum imbedded in the decidua. Glasgow, *J. Maclehose & Sons*, 1908.

The "Bryce-Teacher ovum", age estimated at 13–14 days.

524 LOEB, JACQUES. 1859–1924
Ueber den chemischen Character des Befruchtungvorgangs. Leipzig, *W. Engelmann*, 1908.

525 ——. Die chemische Entwicklungserregung des tierischen Eies; künstliche Parthenogenese. Berlin, *J. Springer*, 1909.

526 KEIBEL, FRANZ KARL JULIUS. 1861–1929, & MALL, FRANKLIN PAINE. 1862–1917
Manual of human embryology. Edited by F. KEIBEL and F. P. MALL. 2 vols. Philadelphia, *J. B. Lippincott*, 1910–12.

The important studies on human embryos, originated by His, were carried on by his pupils, Keibel and Mall.

527 ROUX, WILHELM. 1850–1924
Terminologie der Entwicklungsmechanik. Leipzig, *W. Engelmann*, 1912.

528 PARKER, GEORGE HOWARD. 1864–
The elementary nervous system. Philadelphia, *J. B. Lippincott*, 1919.
Important studies on the survival of primitive types of neuromuscular mechanism in some of the higher vertebrates.

529 GOLDSCHMIDT, RICHARD BENEDICT. 1878–1958
Geschlechtsbestimmung. Berlin, 1921.
English translation, 1923.

530 NEEDHAM, JOSEPH. 1900–
Chemical embryology. 3 vols. Cambridge, *Univ. Press*, 1931.

531 SPEMANN, HANS. 1869–1941
Über den Anteil von Implantat und Wirtskeim an der Orientierung und Beschaffenheit der induzierten Embryonalanlage. *Wilhelm Roux Arch. EntwMech. Org.*, 1931, **123,** 189–517.
Spemann was awarded the Nobel Prize in 1935 for his work on organizers in animal development.

532 ROCK, JOHN. 1890– , & HERTIG, ARTHUR TREMAIN. 1904–
Some aspects of early human development. *Amer. J. Obstet. Gynec.*, 1942, **44,** 973–83; 1943, **45,** 356.
Report of the youngest normal implanted fertilized human ovum, fertilization age about 7½ days. Hertig and Rock published a more detailed study in *Contr. Embryol. Carneg. Instn*, 1945, **31,** 65–84.

History of Embryology

533 NEEDHAM, JOSEPH. 1900–
A history of embryology. Cambridge, *Univ. Press*, 1934.
An exhaustive history of the subject. Deals with embryology from the earliest times to the beginning of the 19th century and includes a valuable bibliography and many illustrations. Second edition, 1959.

534 MEYER, ARTHUR WILLIAM. 1873–
The rise of embryology. Stanford, *California Univ. Press* (1939).
Includes a fine bibliography.

534.1 ADELMANN, HOWARD BERNHARDT. 1898–
Marcello Malpighi and the evolution of embryology. 5 vols. Ithaca, N.Y., *Cornell Univ. Press*, 1966.
Vol. 1 is a biography of Malpighi; the remaining 4 volumes provide an extensive account of the development of embryology.

535–567.2 HISTOLOGY

535 MALPIGHI, MARCELLO. 1628–1694
De viscerum structura exercitatio anatomica. Bononiae, *ex typ. J. Montij*, 1666.
Includes Malpighi's classical essay on the kidney, the "Malpighian bodies" of which have perpetuated his name. The book also includes (pp. 125–26) the first description of Hodgkin's disease. Strangely enough, Malpighi gives no illustration of the kidney in this work. For a reproduction and English translation of this work, see *Ann. med. Hist.*, 1925, **7,** 245–63.

536 ——. Anatome plantarum. 2 pts. Londini, *J. Martyn*, 1675–79.
Malpighi was the founder of microscopic anatomy and a pioneer in the study of plant development. He approached the subject through the study of plant tissues.

537 BICHAT, Marie François Xavier. 1771–1802
Traité des membranes en général et diverses membranes en particulier. Paris, *Richard, Caille & Ravier*, an VIII [1800].

Bichat conceived the idea of a science of anatomy and pathology based upon an accurate classification of the various tissues of the body, their distribution in the various organs and parts, and their particular susceptibilities to disease (Corner). He is regarded as the founder of modern histology and tissue pathology. English translation, Boston, 1813.

538 MÜLLER, Johannes. 1801–1858
De glandularum secernentium structura penitiori. Lipsiae, *sumpt. L. Vossii*, 1830.

Müller's most important histological work. In it he described the microscopic anatomy of a large series of secreting glands. Müller's greatest influence was not so much his own work as the influence he had upon his pupils at Bonn and Berlin. English translation, 1839.

539 HENLE, Friedrich Gustav Jacob. 1809–1885
Symbolae ad anatomiam villorum intestinalium, imprimis eorum epithelii et vasorum lacteorum. Berolini, *A. Hirschwald*, 1837.

Henle first described the epithelia of the skin and intestines, and defined the structure and function of columnar and ciliated epithelium. Modern knowledge of the epithelial tissues starts with Henle.

540 ——. Ueber die Ausbreitung des Epithelium im menschlichen Körper. *Arch. Anat. Physiol. wiss. Med.*, 1838, 103–28.

541 ROSENTHAL, Joseph.
De formatione granulosa in nervis aliisque partibus organismi animalis. Breslau, 1839.

In 1839 Purkinje was the first to use the term "protoplasm", by which he described the embryonic ground substance. This fact is recorded in the inaugural dissertation of one of his students, J. Rosenthal.

542 BOWMAN, *Sir* William. 1816–1892
On the minute structure and movements of voluntary muscle. *Phil. Trans.*, 1840, **130,** 457–501; 1841, **131,** 69–72.

Classical description of striated muscle.

543 HENLE, Friedrich Gustav Jacob. 1809–1885
Allgemeine Anatomie. Leipzig, *L. Voss*, 1841.

Many of the histological discoveries of Henle are described in the above. He classified tissues histologically.

544 HASSALL, Arthur Hill. 1817–1894
The microscopic anatomy of the human body, in health and disease. 2 vols. London, *S. Highley*, [1846]–1849.

First English text-book on microscopical anatomy. His description of the concentric corpuscles of the thymus (p. 9) led to the term "Hassall's corpuscles".

545 SHARPEY, William. 1802–1880
Bone or osseous tissue. In Quain, J.: *Anatomy*. 5th ed., London, 1848, cxxxii–clxiii.

The discovery of the "fibres of Sharpey" is reported on pp. cxlii-cxliii.

546 KÖLLIKER, Rudolph Albert von. 1817–1905
Handbuch der Gewebelehre des Menschen. Leipzig, *W. Engelmann*, 1852.

The first text-book of histology. Kölliker was one of the first to apply Schwann's cell theory to descriptive embryology. He made innumerable contributions to the knowledge of histology and embryology. He founded, and for 50 years edited, the *Zeitschrift für wissenschaftliche Zoologie.*

547 ——. Beiträge zur Kenntniss der glatten Muskeln. *Z. wiss. Zool.*, 1848, **1,** 48–87.

Isolation of smooth muscle.

548 GERLACH, Joseph von. 1820–1896
Mikroskopische Studien aus dem Gebiete der menschlichen Morphologie. Erlangen, *F. Enke*, 1858.

Gerlach introduced several staining methods, the most important of which (a transparent solution of ammonia carmine and gelatin) is called "Gerlach's stain"; it was the first satisfactory histological stain.

549 KLEBS, Theodor Albrecht Edwin. 1834–1913
Die Einschmelzungs-Methode, ein Beitrag zur mikroskopischen Technik. *Arch. mikr. Anat.*, 1869, **5,** 164–6.

Introduction of paraffin embedding.

550 STRICKER, Salomon. 1834–1898
Handbuch der Lehre von den Geweben des Menschen und der Thiere. 2 vols. Leipzig, *W. Engelmann*, 1869–72.

One of the greatest of text-books on histology. English translation, 3 vols., 1870–73.

551 FISCHER, Ernst.
Ueber den Bau der Meissner'schen Tastkörperchen. *Arch. mikr. Anat.*, 1876, **12,** 364–90.

Includes first account of demonstration of nerve endings by means of the gold chloride method.

552 KUPFFER, Karl Wilhelm von. 1829–1902
Ueber Sternzellen der Leber. *Arch. mikr. Anat.*, 1876, **12,** 353–8.

"Kupffer's cells" – stellate cells in the lining of the blood channels in the liver.

553 DUVAL, Mathias Marie. 1844–1907
Technique de l'emploi du collodion humide pour la pratique des coupes microscopiques. *J. Anat. Physiol.* (*Paris*), 1879, **15,** 185–8.

Introduction of collodion for embedding.

554 EHRLICH, Paul. 1854–1915
Ueber die Methylenblaureaction der lebenden Nervensubstanz. *Dtsch. med. Wschr.*, 1886, **12,** 49–52.

Ehrlich's method of intravital staining.

555 HERTWIG, Wilhelm August Oscar. 1849–1922, & HERTWIG, Karl Wilhelm Theodor Richard. 1850–1937
Untersuchungen zur Morphologie und Physiologie der Zelle. 6 pts. Jena, *G. Fischer*, 1884–90.

556 ——. Die Zelle und die Gewebe. 2 pts. Jena, *G. Fischer*, 1893–8.

557 BLUM, F.
Der Formaldehyd als Härtungsmittel. Vorläufige Mittheilung. *Z. wiss. Mikr.*, 1893, **10,** 314–15.
Formalin first used for tissue fixation.

558 HARRISON, Ross Granville. 1870–1959
The outgrowth of the nerve fibre as a mode of protoplasmic movement. *J. exp. Zool.*, 1910, **9,** 787–846.
The inauguration of tissue culture was made possible by Harrison's proof of the outgrowth of nerve-fibres from ganglion cells.

559 CARREL, Alexis. 1873–1944
Rejuvenation of cultures of tissues. *J. Amer. med. Ass.*, 1911, **57,** 1611.
Extra-vital cultivation and rejuvenation of tissue. Carrel was awarded the Nobel Prize in 1912.

560 ——. & BURROWS, Montrose Thomas. 1884–1947
Cultivation of tissues in vitro and its technique. *J. exp. Med.*, 1911, **13,** 387–96; 415–21.
Carrel demonstrated the potential immortality of mammalian tissue. He was able to keep the excised viscera of an animal alive and functioning physiologically *in vitro*. For his later work see the same journal, 1911, **14,** 244–7; 1913, **18,** 155–61.

561 LEWIS, Margaret Reed. 1881– , & LEWIS, Warren Harmon. 1870–1964
Mitochondria and other cytoplasmic structures in tissue cultures. *Amer. J. Anat.*, 1914–15, **17,** 339–401.
Original investigations upon the visible mitochondria.

562 ASCHOFF, Karl Albert Ludwig. 1866–1942
Das reticulo-endotheliale System. *Ergebn. inn. Med.*, 1924, **26,** 1–118.
In an earlier paper on this subject (*Münch. med. Wschr.*, 1922, **69,** 1352–56) Aschoff introduced the term "reticulo-endothelial system"; as early as 1914 he grouped certain phagocytic cells into his system.

563 MÖLLENDORFF, Wilhelm von. 1887–1944
Handbuch der mikroskopischen Anatomie des Menschen. 7 vols. [in 17] Berlin, *J. Springer*, 1927–43.

564 COWDRY, Edmund Vincent. 1888–
General cytology. Chicago, *Univ. Press*, [1924].
This and No. 565 were written by various authorities under the editorship of Cowdry.

565 ——. Special cytology. 2 vols. New York, *P. B. Hoeber*, 1928.

566 RAMÓN Y CAJAL, Santiago. 1852–1934
Degeneration and regeneration of the nervous system. 2 vols. London, *Humphrey Milford*, 1928.
The most complete work on the subject so far written. Ramón y Cajal, great neuroanatomist and histologist, was for many years in charge of the institute bearing his name at Madrid. He gained the Nobel Prize in 1906. Reprinted 1959.

567 BAKER, John Randal. 1900–
The discovery of the uses of colouring agents in biological micro-technique. *J. Quekett micr. Club*, 1943, ser. 4, **1,** 256–75.

567.1 MURRAY, MARGARET RANSOME. 1901– , & KOPECH, GERTRUDE. 1915–
A bibliography of the research in tissue culture 1884–1950. An index to the literature of the living cell cultivated in vitro. 2 vols. New York, *Academic Press*, 1953.

567.2 O'RAHILLY, RONAN. 1918–
Three and one-half centuries of histology. *Irish J. med. Sci.*, 1958, 288–92.

568–664 PHYSIOLOGY: GENERAL

568 ARISTOTLE. 384–322 B.C.
De motu animalium. De incessu animalium. *In his* Works, edited by J. A. SMITH and W. D. ROSS, Oxford, 1912, **5**, 698a–714b.

569 GALEN. 130–200 A.D.
On the natural faculties. With an English translation by A. J. Brock. London, New York, *Putnam*, 1916.

Greek-English bilingual. Before Harvey, Galen was the most important figure in experimental physiology. His system of physiology was accepted until the Middle Ages.

570 ——. De usu partium. *In his* Opera, ed. C. G. KÜHN, Lipsiae, 1822, **3**, 1–939; **4**, 1–366. Translation by M. T. May, 2 vols., Ithaca, N.Y., 1968.

571 NEMESIUS, *Bishop of Emesa. fl.* A.D. 400
De natura hominis liber. Lugduni, *apud Seb. Gryphium*, 1538.

An influential text during the Middle Ages. Nemesius studied man both from the psychological and physiological standpoint. Among the editions of the book may be mentioned that printed by Plantin at Antwerp, 1564, and an English translation by G. Wither, London, 1636.

572 FERNEL, JEAN FRANÇOIS. 1497–1558
De naturali parte medicinae libri septem. Parisiis, *apud Simonem Colinaeum*, 1542.

The earliest work devoted exclusively to physiology and the first to call the subject by that name. It was re-issued in 1554 as part of Fernel's *Medicina* (No. 2271). Fernel suggested that physicians should themselves study the human body and not accept tradition. See Sir Charles Sherrington's *The endeavour of Jean Fernel*, Cambridge, 1946.

573 SANTORIO, SANTORIO [SANCTORIUS]. 1561–1636
De statica medicina. Venetiis, *apud N. Polum*, 1614.

Sanctorius was the founder of the physiology of metabolism. He introduced into physiology exact methods of measurement, pulse counting, temperature determination, and weighing. For description of his experiments, see No. 2668. English translations 1676, 1712, 1842 (J. Quincy).

574 DESCARTES, RENÉ. 1596–1650
De homine figuris et latinitate donatus a Florentio Schuyl. Lugduni Batavorum, *apud F. Moyardum & P. Leffen*, 1662.

Descartes considered the human body a material machine, directed by a rational soul located in the pineal body. This book was the first attempt to cover the whole field of "animal physiology". The work is really a physiological appendix to his *Discourse on method*, 1637, and first appeared in full in 1664, this time in French.

575 CROONE, WILLIAM. 1633–1684
De ratione motus musculorum. Londini, *excud. J. Hayes*, 1664.

Croone accumulated a large fortune from his practice; with it his widow endowed the Croonian Lectures at the Royal College of Physicians, London. He believed muscular contraction to be brought about by the action of a "spirituous liquor" passing from the nerves and interacting with substances in the muscle. Translation of an extract in J. F. Fulton's *Selected readings in the history of physiology*, 2nd ed., 1966, pp. 207–9

576 STENSEN, NIELS [STENO, NICOLAUS]. 1638–1686
De musculis et glandulis observationum specimen. Hafniae, *lit. M. Godiechenii*, 1664.

In this work Steno laid the foundation of our present conception of muscular mechanics. He "at once grasped the significance of the fibrillar structure of skeletal muscle and realised that the tensile forces developed in each individual *fibra motrix* became summated into the response of the muscle as a whole" (Fulton). He proved the muscular nature of the heart.

577 ——. Elementorum myologiae specimen. Florentiae, *ex typ. sub signo Stellae*, 1667.

An expanded edition of No. 576, including some illustrations.

578 MAYOW, JOHN. 1643–1679
Tractatus quinque medico-physici. Oxonii, *e theatro Sheldoniano*, 1674.

Mayow was the first to locate the seat of animal heat in the muscles; he discovered the double articulation of the ribs with the spine and came near to discovering oxygen in his suggestion that the object of breathing was to abstract from the air a definite group of life-giving "particles". He was the first to make the definite suggestion that it is only a special fraction of the air that is of use in respiration. His *Tractatus*, embodying all his brilliant conclusions, is one of the best English medical classics. English translation, Edinburgh, 1907.

579 GLISSON, FRANCIS. 1597–1677
Tractatus de ventriculo et intestinis. Londini, *H. Brome*, 1677.

Glisson introduced the idea of irritability as a specific property of all human tissue, a hypothesis which had no effect upon contemporary physiology, but which was later demonstrated experimentally by Haller (No. 587).

580 KIRCHER, ATHANASIUS. 1602–1680
Physiologia Kircheriana experimentalis. Amstelaedami, *J. Waesberg*, 1680.

Includes the first recorded experiment in hypnotism in animals.

581 BOERHAAVE, HERMAN. 1668–1738
Institutiones medicae in usus annuae exercitationis domesticos digestae. Lugduni Batavorum, *J. van der Linden*, 1708.

One of Boerhaave's best works. The first part deals with physiology, with important observations upon digestion.

582 STAHL, GEORG ERNST. 1660–1734
Theoria medica vera. Halle, *lit. Orphanotrophei*, 1708.

Stahl tried to explain vital phenomena by mystical means. He was the head of the so-called Animistic School which explained disease as caused by misdirected activities on the part of the soul.

583 HOFFMAN, FRIEDRICH. 1660–1742
Fundamenta physiologiae. Halle, 1718.

Hoffman was a writer of extraordinary versatility, and the first to perceive pathology as an aspect of physiology. His *Fundamenta* is an outstanding treatise on physiology.

584 BELCHIER, JOHN. 1706–1785
An account of the bones of animals being changed to a red colour by aliment only. *Phil. Trans.* (1735–6), 1738, **39,** 287–8; 299–300.
Belchier fed animals with madder, noting that new bone formed subsequent to its ingestion was stained red. This was the earliest attempt at vital staining and is also important as making possible the study of osteogenesis.

585 HALLER, ALBRECHT VON. 1708–1777
Primae lineae physiologiae in usum praelectionum academicarum. Gottingae, *A. Vandenhoeck*, 1747.
Haller was one of the most imposing figures in the whole of medicine, besides being a superb bibliographer and the founder of medical bibliography. As a physiologist he was the greatest of his time. Many apparently "new" discoveries of later times had already been accounted for by Haller. The above work includes (p. 259) Haller's resonance theory, similar to that already propounded by Duverney and (more than 100 years later) by Helmholtz (No. 1562). English editions 1754 and later.

586 LA METTRIE, JULIEN OFFRAY DE. 1709–1751
L'homme machine. Leyde, *E. Lusac, fils*, 1748.
La Mettrie attempted among other things to prove the materialism of the soul. The book, published anonymously, was burnt by order of the magistrates of Leyden, owing to its heretical nature. A copy must have escaped, for an English translation appeared in 1749.

587 HALLER, ALBRECHT VON. 1708–1777
De partibus corporis humani sensibilibus et irritabilibus. *Comment. Soc. reg. sci. Gotting.* (1752), 1753, **2,** 114–58.
Glisson in 1677 had introduced the concept of "irritability" as a specific property of all tissues. Haller, in the above work, recorded his experimental proof of this, and distinguished between nerve impulse (sensibility) and muscular contraction (irritability). English translation in *Bull. Hist. Med.*, 1936, **4,** 651–99.

588 ——. Elementa physiologiae corporis humani. 8 vols. Lausanne, Berne, 1757–66.
Haller synthesized the whole physiological knowledge of his time, In the above, probably his greatest work, Haller included some anatomical descriptions which were most valuable. He is said to have written more than 1300 scientific papers.

589 WALSH, JOHN. ?1725–1795
Of the electric property of the torpedo. *Phil. Trans.*, 1773, **63,** 461–77.
The first accurate observations on the torpedo fish were made by Walsh, who was given the Copley Medal of the Royal Society for his work on the subject.

590 BLAGDEN, *Sir* CHARLES. 1748–1820
Experiments and observations in an heated room. *Phil. Trans.*, 1775, **65,** 111–23; 484–94.
First demonstration of the importance of perspiration in the maintenance of constant body temperature.

591 CRAWFORD, ADAIR. 1748–1795
Experiments and observations on animal heat. London, *J. Murray*, 1779.
Earliest experiments upon animal calorimetry.

592 LAVOISIER, ANTOINE LAURENT. 1743–1794, & LA PLACE, PIERRE SIMON DE. 1749–1827
Mémoire sur la chaleur. *Hist. Acad. roy. Sci.* (*Paris*), (1780), 1784, 355–408.
These workers invented an ice calorimeter, with it measured the respiratory quotient of a pig, and demonstrated the analogy between respiration and combustion.

593 GALVANI, Aloysio Luigi. 1737–1798

De viribus electricitatis in motu musculari commentarius. *Bonon. Sci. Art. Inst. Acad. Comment.*, Bologna, 1791, **7**, 363–418.

Galvini's theory of animal electricity (galvanism). English translation by R. M. Green, Cambridge, Mass., 1953

594 SÉGUIN, Armand. 1768–1835, & LAVOISIER, Antoine Laurent. 1743–1794

Premier mémoire sur la respiration des animaux. *Hist. Acad. Sci. (Paris)*, (1789), 1793, 566–84.

Séguin and Lavoisier measured the metabolism of a man (Séguin himself). They made three observations of fundamental importance in this respect: that the intensity of oxidation in man is dependent upon (1) food, (2) environmental temperature, and (3) mechanical work.

595 CRUIKSHANK, William Cumberland. 1745–1800

Experiments on the insensible perspiration of the human body. London, *G. Nicol*, 1795.

Demonstration that carbon dioxide is given off by the skin. This book was first privately printed in 1779; above is the corrected edition.

596 REIL, Johann Christian. 1759–1813

Von der Lebenskraft. *Arch. Physiol. (Halle)*, 1796, **1**, 8–162.

Reil advanced the doctrine of the life-force as the chemical expression of physiological function. Like Glisson and Hunter, he recognised irritability as a specific property of tissue. He founded the *Archiv für die Physiologie*, the first journal of physiology.

597 BICHAT, Marie François Xavier. 1771–1802

Recherches physiologiques sur la vie et la mort. Paris, *Brosson, Gabon et Cie.*, an VIII [1800].

English translation of second edition, Philadelphia, 1809.

598 MAGENDIE, François. 1783–1855

Mémoires sur le mécanisme de l'absorption chez les animaux à sang rouge et chaud. *J. Physiol. exp. path.*, 1821, **1**, 1–17, 18–31.

Magendie, the pioneer of experimental physiology in France, demonstrated the absorption of fluids and semisolids to be a function of the blood-vessels, as well as of the lymphatics. He was the founder, in 1821, of the *Journal de physiologie expérimentale*.

599 BURDACH, Karl Friedrich. 1776–1847

Die Physiologie als Erfahrungswissenschaft. 6 vols. Leipzig, Königsberg, 1826–40.

Burdach's great text-book of physiology was planned to run to 8 vols., but the death of his wife quenched his enthusiasm for the task. Part of the text was written by von Baer, Rathke, Johannes Müller, R. Wagner and others, under the direction of Burdach.

600 SHARPEY, William. 1802–1880

On a peculiar motion excited in fluids by the surfaces of certain animals. *Edinb. med. surg. J.*, 1830, **34**, 113–22.

Sharpey was the first occupant of the chair of anatomy and physiology at University College, London, this chair being the first official recognition of physiology in any English medical school. He wrote a memorable paper on cilia and ciliary motion. Among his pupils were Michael Foster, Burdon-Sanderson and Schäfer.

601 MÜLLER, JOHANNES. 1801–1858
Handbuch der Physiologie des Menschen. 2 vols. Coblenz, *J. Hölscher*, 1834–40.

Müller introduced two new elements into physiology – the psychological and the comparative. For the first time the existing knowledge of comparative chemistry and physics was brought to bear upon physiological problems. Müller was the first to describe the excretory system of the glands as an independent system of tubes, noting that the blood-vessels formed only a capillary network. The *Handbuch* was the first great text-book of physiology in the nineteenth century. English translation 1838–42.

602 PURKINJE, JOHANN EVANGELISTA. 1787–1869, & VALENTIN, GABRIEL GUSTAV. 1810–1883
De phaenomeno generali et fundamentali motus vibratorii continui in membranis. Wratislaviae, *sumpt. A. Schulz et soc.*, 1835.

Classical paper on ciliary epithelial motion. See also *Müller's Arch.*, 1834 391–400.

603 SHARPEY, WILLIAM. 1802–1880
Cilia. In Todd's *Cyclopaedia of anatomy and physiology*. London, 1835–36, **1,** 606–38.

The important discoveries of Purkinje and Valentin, together with additional observations by Sharpey himself were embodied in an article written by him for Todd's *Cyclopaedia.*

604 WEBER, WILHELM EDUARD. 1804–1891, & WEBER, EDUARD FRIEDRICH WILHELM. 1806–1871
Mechanik der menschlichen Gehwerkzeuge. 1 vol. and atlas. Göttingen, *in der Dieterichschen Buchhandlung*, 1836.

The most important contemporary study of the physiology of motion and locomotion.

605 MATTEUCCI, CARLO. 1811–1868
Sur le courant électrique ou propre de la grenouille. *Ann. Chim.*, 1838, **68,** 93–106.

Matteucci established the difference of potential between injured nerve and its muscle.

606 MAYER, JULIUS ROBERT VON. 1814–1878
Bemerkungen über die Kräfte der unbelebten Natur, *Ann. Chem., Pharm.* (*Lemgo*), 1842, **42,** 233–40.

Mayer demonstrated the principle of the conservation of energy as far as physiological processes are concerned.

607 WAGNER, RUDOLPH. 1805–1864
Handwörterbuch der Physiologie . . . hrsg. von R. WAGNER. 4 vols. Braunschweig, *F. Vieweg & Sohn*, 1842–53.

Wagner was professor at Göttingen. His literary output was enormous. In the above work he contributed the sections on sympathetic nerves, nerve-ganglia, and nerve-endings.

608 MATTEUCCI, CARLO. 1811–1868, & HUMBOLDT, FRIEDRICH HEINRICH ALEXANDER VON. 1769–1859
Sur le courant électrique des muscles des animaux vivants ou récemment tués. *C. R. Acad. Sci.* (*Paris*), 1843, **16,** 197–200.

Matteucci's "rheoscopic frog" effect.

609 DU BOIS REYMOND, Emil. 1818–1896
Ueber den sogenannten Froschstrom. *Ann. Physik.* (*Berl.*), 1843, **58,** 1–30.

First description and definition of electrotonus.

610 ——. Untersuchungen über thierische Elektricität. 2 vols. [in 3]. Berlin, *G. Reimer*, 1848–84.

A pupil of J. Müller, Emil du Bois Reymond was the founder of modern electrophysiology. He introduced faradic stimulation and made an exhaustive investigation of physiological tetanus. Above is a collective edition of his writings on the subject.

611 HELMHOLTZ, Hermann Ludwig Ferdinand von. 1821–1894
Ueber die Erhaltung der Kraft, eine physikalische Abhandlung. Berlin, *G. Reimer*, 1847.

An epoch-making work which led the way to the acceptance of the fundamental physical doctrine of the conservation of energy.

612 ——. Ueber die Wärmeentwickelung bei der Muskelaction. *Arch. Anat. Physiol. wiss. Med.*, 1848, 144–64.

Helmholtz showed the muscles to be the principal source of animal heat.

613 MOLESCHOTT, Jacob. 1822–1893
Physiologie des Stoffwechsels in Pflanzen und Thieren. Erlangen, *F. Enke*, 1851.

614 DUCHENNE DE BOULOGNE, Guillaume Benjamin Amand, 1806–1875
De l'électrisation localisée et de son application à la physiologie, à la pathologie et à la thérapeutique. Paris, *J. B. Baillière*, 1855; atlas, 1862.

Duchenne classified the electrophysiology of the entire muscular system and summed up his findings in the above work. The application of his results to pathological conditions marks him as the founder of electrotherapy.

615 BERNARD, Claude. 1813–1878
Leçons de physiologie expérimentale appliquée à la médecine. 2 vols. Paris, *J. B. Baillière*, 1855–56.

Claude Bernard made strenuous efforts to introduce experimental methods into physiology. The above includes his classical work on the function of the liver, pancreas, and gastric glands. (See also No. 634.)

616 ——. Analyse physiologique des propriétés des systèmes musculaire et nerveux au moyen de curare. *C. R. Acad. Sci.* (*Paris*), 1856, **43,** 825–29.

Bernard paralysed motor nerve-endings with curare and demonstrated the independent excitability of muscle; his paper is the classical proof of Haller's doctrine of irritability.

617 FICK, Adolph. 1829–1901
Die medizinische Physik. Braunschweig, *F. Vieweg*, 1856.

618 KÖLLIKER, Rudolph Albert von. 1817–1905, & MÜLLER, Heinrich. 1820–1864
Nachweis der negativen Schwankung des Muskelstroms am natürlich sich contrahirenden Muskel. *Verh. phys.-med. Ges. Würzburg*, 1856, **6,** 528–33.

Kölliker and Müller were the first to measure action currents from cardiac muscle.

619 RAINEY, George. 1801–1884
On the formation of the skeletons of animals, and other hard structures formed in connexion with living tissues. *Brit. for. med.-chir. Rev.*, 1857, **20,** 451–76.
Includes description of "Rainey's tubes" or "corpuscles" in connexion with the process of calcification of tissues.

620 KÜHNE, Willy. 1837–1900
Untersuchungen über Bewegungen und Veränderungen der contraktilen Substanz. *Arch. Anat. Physiol. wiss. Med.,* 1859, 564–642, 748–835.
Proof of the coagulability of muscle proteins.

621 PFLÜGER, Eduard Friedrich Wilhelm. 1829–1910
Untersuchungen über die Physiologie des Electrotonus. Berlin, *A. Hirschwald*, 1859.
One of the most interesting and important works of its time on the physiology of nerve. In it Pflüger first stated the laws governing the make and break stimulation of nerve with the galvanic current. Pflüger was a pupil of Müller and du Bois Reymond.

622 BERNARD, Claude. 1813–1878
Du rôle des actions réflexes paralysantes dans le phénomène des sécrétions. *J. Anat. Physiol.* (*Paris*), 1864, **1,** 507–13.
Studies of the "paralytic secretions" occasioned by section of glandular nerves.

623 FICK, Adolph. 1829–1901
Untersuchungen über elektrische Nervenreizung. Braunschweig, *F. Vieweg*, 1864.
Among the instruments introduced by Fick for the study of muscle and nerve physiology were the myotonograph, the cosine lever and an improved thermopile.

624 DUCHENNE DE BOULOGNE, Guillaume Benjamin Amand. 1806–1875
Physiologie des mouvements demontrée à l'aide de l'expérimentation électrique et de l'observation clinique, et applicable à l'étude des paralysies et des déformations. Paris, *J. B. Baillière*, 1867.
A monumental work, the result of twenty years' study of electro-muscular stimulation "to determine the proper action which the muscles possess in life." English translation by E. B. Kaplan, Philadelphia, 1949.

625 HERMANN, Ludimar. 1838–1914
Untersuchungen über den Stoffwechsel der Muskeln, ausgehend vom Gaswechsel derselben. Berlin, *A. Hirschwald*, 1867.
Hermann's views on nitrogen metabolism in muscular work correctly anticipated the later conclusions of Fletcher, Hopkins and others.

626 FLINT, Austin, *Jnr*. 1836–1915
On the physiological effects of severe and protracted muscular exercise; with especial reference to the influence of exercise upon the excretion of nitrogen. *N.Y. med. J.*, 1871, **13,** 609–97.
Flint made investigations on the nitrogen output of a long-distance walker, before, during, and after the latter's attempt to walk 400 miles in 5 days. The useful data in this paper are often referred to in discussions on the subject.

627 PFLÜGER, Eduard Friedrich Wilhelm. 1829–1910
Ueber die Diffusion des Sauerstoffs, den Ort und die Gesetze der Oxydationsprocesse im thierischen Organismus. *Pflüg. Arch. ges. Physiol.*, 1872, **6,** 43–64, 190.

628 HAUGHTON, Samuel. 1821–1897
Principles of animal mechanics. London, *Longmans, Green & Co.*, 1873.

Haughton stated that the muscular mechanism is so arranged that its work is carried out with the minimum of muscular contraction. This he called the "principle of least action." His opposition to Darwinism is especially noticed in this book.

629 STIRLING, William. 1851–1932
Ueber die Summation elektrischer Hautreize. *Arb. Physiol. Anst. Leipzig*, (1874), 1875, **9,** 223–91.

Stirling, a pupil of Ludwig, became a great teacher of physiology. His paper on the summation of electrical stimuli to the skin was a prize thesis.

630 ECK, Nikolaĭ Vladimirovich. 1849–1908
K voprosu o perevyazkie vorotnoĭ venî. Predvaritelnoye soobshtshenize. [On the ligature of the portal vein.] *Voyenno med. J.*, 1877, **130,** 2, sect., 1.

Eck developed the "Eck fistula" for the experimental study of diseases of the liver and the relation of the liver to metabolism. English translation in *Surg. Gynec. Obstet.*, 1953, **96,** 375.

631 FOSTER, *Sir* Michael. 1836–1907
A text-book of physiology. London, *Macmillan*, 1877.

Foster was one of the greatest of the modern teachers of physiology. He became professor at Cambridge in 1883. Many great scientists are numbered among his pupils.

632 ROMANES, George John. 1848–1894
Observations on the locomotor system of Medusae. *Phil. Trans.*, (1876), 1877, **166,** 269–313; (1877), 1878, **167,** 659–752; (1880), 1881, **171,** 161–202.

633 PFLÜGER, Eduard Friedrich Wilhelm. 1829–1910
Ueber Wärme und Oxydation der lebendigen Materie. *Pflüg. Arch. ges. Physiol.*, 1878, **18,** 247–380.

634 BERNARD, Claude. 1813–1878
Leçons de physiologie opératoire. Paris, *J. B. Baillière*, 1879.

In this, his last work, Bernard showed himself "the unapproachable master in the technique of experimental procedure" (Garrison).

635 VOIT, Carl von. 1831–1908
Handbuch der Physiologie des Gesammt-Stoffwechsels und der Fortpflanzung. Leipzig, *F. C. W. Vogel*, 1881.

Forms vol. 6, pt. 1 of Hermann's *Handbuch der Physiologie.*

636 MOSSO, Angelo. 1846–1910
Les lois de la fatigue étudiées dans les muscles de l'homme. *Arch. ital. Biol.*, 1890, **13,** 123–86.

Mosso invented the ergograph from the study of voluntary contraction. The description of the instrument is on pages 124–41 of the above article.

637 BRAUNE, CHRISTIAN WILHELM. 1831–1892, & FISCHER, OTTO. 1861–1917.
Die Bewegungen des Kniegelenkes. *Abh. math.-phys. Cl. k. sächs. Ges. Wiss. Leipzig*, 1891, **17,** 78–150.
Investigation of the mechanics of motion on mathematical lines. (See also No. 645).

638 CHAUVEAU, JEAN BAPTISTE AUGUSTE. 1827–1917
Le travail musculaire et l'énergie qu'il représente. Paris, *Asselin & Houzeau*, 1891.
Important studies on thermodynamics of muscular work.

639 MOSSO, ANGELO. 1846–1910
La fatica. Milano, *frat. Treves*, 1891.
Moss investigated muscular fatigue with the ergograph of his invention. He showed fatigue to be due to a toxin produced by muscular contraction. English translation, 1906.

640 NOORDEN, CARL HARKO VON. 1858–1944
Beiträge zur Lehre von Stoffwechsel. I. Grundriss einer Methodik der Stoffwechsel-Untersuchungen. Berlin, *A. Hirschwald*, 1892.

641 WOLFF, JULIUS. 1836–1902
Das Gesetz der Transformation der Knochen. Berlin, *A. Hirschwald*, 1892.
"Wolff's law", which stated that every change in form and function of a bone, or in its function alone, is followed by certain definite changes in its internal architecture and equally definite secondary alterations in its mathematical laws.

642 ENGELMANN, THEODOR WILHELM. 1843–1909
Ueber den Ursprung der Muskelkraft. Leipzig, *W. Engelmann*, 1893.

643 MAREY, ÉTIENNE JULES. 1830–1904
Le mouvement. Paris, *G. Masson*, 1894.
Marey, like Muybridge (No. 650–51), was a pioneer in the use of serial pictures as a method of studying the mechanics of locomotion. English translation, 1895.

644 BIEDERMANN, WILHELM. 1852–1929
Elektrophysiologie. Jena, *G. Fischer*, 1895.
First exhaustive treatise on electrophysiology.

645 BRAUNE, CHRISTIAN WILHELM. 1831–1892, & FISCHER, OTTO. 1861–1917
Der Gang des Menschen. *Abh. math.-phys. Cl. k. sächs. Ges. Wiss. Leipzig*, 1895, **21,** 153–322.
Classical study of human locomotion.

646 RICHET, CHARLES ROBERT. 1850–1935
Dictionnaire de physiologie. Vols. 1–10. Paris, *F. Alcan*, 1895–1928.
Covers A–Moelle épinière only.

647 STARLING, ERNEST HENRY. 1866–1927
On the absorption of fluids from the connective tissue spaces. *J. Physiol. (Lond.)*, 1896, **19,** 312–26.
Starling discovered the functional significance of the serum proteins.

648 ATWATER, WILBUR OLIN. 1844–1907, & LANGWORTHY, CHARLES FORD. 1864–

A digest of metabolism experiments in which the balance of income and outgo was determined. Washington, *Govt. Printing Off.*, 1898.

649 SHARPEY-SCHÄFER, *Sir* EDWARD ALBERT. 1850–1935

Text-book of physiology. Edited by E. A. SCHÄFER. 2 vols. Edinburgh, *Y. J. Pentland*, 1898–1900.

A collective work and a classical text-book of physiology. Sharpey-Schäfer is one of the greatest names in British physiology. He was a pupil of Sharpey, and when that great man died without any known descendants Schäfer gave the name to his son, in order to perpetuate it. When his son was killed in the war of 1914–18, Schäfer added it to his own.

649.1 MAGNUS-LEVY, ADOLF. 1865–1955, & FALK, ERNST.

Der Lungengaswechsel des Menschen in den verschiedenen Altersstufen. *Arch. Anat. Physiol., Physiol. Abt.*, 1899, Suppl.-Bd, 314–81.

The first systematic study of the basal metabolism of normal individuals from childhood to old age.

650 MUYBRIDGE, EADWEARD [JAMES EDWARD MUGGERIDGE]. 1830–1904.

Animals in motion. London, *Chapman & Hall*, 1899.

651 ——. The human figure in motion. An electro-photographic investigation of consecutive phases of muscular actions. London, *Chapman & Hall*, 1901.

Muybridge, an Englishman, made exhaustive photographic investigations of consecutive animal movements while he was in America. More than 100,000 photographs were embodied in his *Animal locomotion. An electro-photographic investigation of consecutive phases of animal movements*, 1872–85. Philadelphia, 1887. The great cost of producing this work of 11 folio volumes with 781 photo-engravings restricted its sale to a very few copies and the above two books are abridgements. This pioneer study of serial photography demonstrated the possibilities of motion pictures and foreshadowed the modern cinematograph. Reprinted New York, 1955.

652 LUCIANI, LUIGI. 1840–1919

Fisiologia dell' uomo. 3 vols. Milan, *Società Edit. Libraria*, 1901–11.

5th edition (5 vols.), 1919–21; English translation (5 vols.), London, 1911–21. Luciani was professor of physiology successively at Siena, Florence, and Rome.

653 BERNSTEIN, JULIUS. 1839–1917

Untersuchungen zur Thermodynamik der bioelektrischen Ströme. *Pflüg. Arch. ges. Physiol.*, 1902, **92**, 521–62; 1908, **122**, 129–95; **124**, 462–68.

Bernstein's important studies on the nature of muscular contraction included the observation that changes in surface tension are a controlling factor in the development of the energy of muscular contraction.

654 LOEB, JACQUES. 1859–1924

The dynamics of living matter. New York, *Columbia University Press*, 1906.

655 LAPICQUE, LOUIS. 1866–1952

Définition expérimentale de l'excitabilité. *C. R. Soc. Biol. (Paris)*, 1909, **67**, 280–83.

Lapicque first defined "chronaxia", the duration of excitation of tissue. Partial translation in J. F. Fulton's *Selected readings in the history of physiology*, 2nd ed., 1966, pp. 233–34.

656 WINTERSTEIN, HANS. 1879–1963
Handbuch der vergleichenden Physiologie. Hrsg. von HANS WINTERSTEIN. 4 vols. Jena, *G. Fischer*, 1910–25.

656.1 MACEWEN, *Sir* WILLIAM. 1848–1924
The growth of bone. Glasgow, *J. Maclehose*, 1912
Throughout his life Macewen devoted much time to the study of bone growth. His researches revolutionized ideas concerning osteogenesis.

657 BENEDICT, FRANCIS GANO. 1870– , & CATHCART, EDWARD PROVAN. 1877–1954
Muscular work. A metabolic study. Washington, *Carnegie Inst.*, 1913.
Carnegie Instn Publ. No. 187.

658 BAYLISS, *Sir* WILLIAM MADDOCK. 1860–1924
Principles of general physiology. London, *Longmans, Green*, 1915.
Bayliss's book treats of general physiology from the physical chemical point of view. For some years it remained the most important book of its kind, and to-day is still of great value for its historical information and its accurate bibliography. A fifth edition, edited by L. E. Bayliss, appeared in 1959–60.

659 HILL, ARCHIBALD VIVIAN. 1886– , & HARTREE, WILLIAM. 1870–1943
The four phases of heat-production of muscle. *J. Physiol. (Lond.)*, 1920, **54,** 84–128.
Hill and Hartree made valuable contributions to the knowledge of the thermodynamics of muscle. Hill shared the Nobel Prize with Meyerhof in 1922 for his work on the physiology of muscle. See also *Physiol. Rev.*, 1922, **2,** 310–41.

660 READ, JAY MARION. 1889–
Correlation of basal metabolic rate with pulse rate and pulse pressure. *J. Amer. med. Ass.*, 1922, **78,** 1887–89.
Read's formula for computation of basal metabolic rate.

661 MAGNUS, RUDOLF. 1873–1927
Körperstellung. Berlin, *J. Springer*, 1924.
A classical work on muscle tone and posture, a subject upon which Magnus spent many years of study. He demonstrated among other things that the labyrinth is the one sense organ entirely concerned with posture and equilibrium.

662 BETHE, ALBRECHT. 1872–1954, *et al.*
Handbuch der normalen und pathologischen Physiologie. Hrsg. von A. BETHE, G. BERGMANN, *etc.* 18 vols. Berlin, *J. Springer*, 1925–32.

663 FULTON, JOHN FARQUHAR. 1899–1960
Muscular contraction and the reflex control of movement. Baltimore, *Williams & Wilkins*, 1926.
A detailed study of the physiology of skeletal muscle. A valuable historical introduction will be found on pp. 3–55, and the book includes an extensive bibliography.

663.1 MAGNUS, RUDOLF. 1783–1927
Cameron Prize Lectures on some results of studies in the physiology of posture. *Lancet*, 1926, **2,** 531–36, 585–88.
Magnus demonstrated the function of the otoliths and semicircular canals of the inner ear in regulating the equilibrium of the body.

664 CANNON, Walter Bradford. 1871–1945
The wisdom of the body. New York, *Norton & Co.*, 1932.
A discussion of the regulation of body fluids, hunger, thirst, temperature, oxygen supply, water, sugar, and proteins of the body, and the rôle of the sympathetic-adrenal mechanism.

665–752.7 BIOCHEMISTRY

665 HELMONT, Jean Baptiste van. 1577–1644
Ortus medicinae. Amsterodami, *apud L. Elzevirium*, 1648.
Helmont was one of the founders of biochemistry. He was the first to realize the physiological importance of ferments and gases, and indeed invented the word "gas". He introduced the gravimetric idea in the analysis of urine. The above work is a collection of his writings, issued by his son.

666 BOYLE, Robert. 1627–1691
A defence of the doctrine touching the spring and weight of the air. London, *J. G. for Thomas Robinson*, 1662.
Boyle's law. The above pamphlet was appended to the second edition of Boyle's *The spring and weight of the air*, 1662. The relevant passage is reproduced in J. F. Fulton's *Selected readings in the history of physiology*, 2nd ed., 1966, pp. 8–10. Fulton published a bibliography of Boyle's works in 1956 (2nd ed., 1961).

667 ROUELLE, Hilaire Marie. 1718–1779
Observations sur l'urine humaine. *J. Méd. Chir. Pharm.*, 1773, **40,** 451–68.
Discovery of urea.

668 SCHEELE, Carl Wilhelm. 1742–1786
Undersökning om blåsestenen. *Kongl. Vetenskaps-Acad. Handl.*, 1776, **37,** 327–32.
Discovery of uric acid. English translation in his *Chemical Essays*, London, 1786.

668.1 WOLLASTON, William Hyde. 1766–1828
On cystic oxide, a new species of urinary calculus. *Phil. Trans.*, 1810, **100,** 223–30.
Cystine, the first amino-acid to be isolated, was prepared by Wollaston from a urinary calculus. This was also the first report of cystinuria.

668.2 CHEVREUL, Michel Eugène. 1786–1889
Recherches chimiques sur plusieurs corps gras, et particulièrement sur leurs combinations avec les calculs. Cinquième mémoire. Des corps qu'on a appelés adipocire, c'est-à-dire, de la substance cristallisée des calculs biliaires humains, du spermacéti et de la substance grasse des cadavres. *Ann. Chim. (Paris)*, 1815, **95,** 5–50.
Chevreul characterized cholesterol.

668.3 BRACONNOT, Henri. 1780–1855
Mémoire sur la conversion des matières animales en nouvelles substances par le moyen de l'acide sulfurique. *Ann. Chim. Phys.*, 1820, Sér. 2, **13,** 113–25.
Isolation of glycine and leucine.

669 CHEVREUL, Michel Eugène. 1786–1889
Recherches chimiques sur les corps gras d'origine animale. Paris, *F. G. Levrault*, 1823.
A classical study of animal fats. Chevreul discovered that fats are composed of fatty acids and glycerol.

670 DUTROCHET, RÉNÉ JOACHIM HENRI. 1776–1847
Nouvelles observations sur l'endosmose et l'exosmose. *Ann. Chim. Phys.*, 1827, **35,** 393–400; 1828, **37,** 191–201; 1832, **49,** 411–37; **51,** 159–66; 1835, **60,** 337–68.

The process by which water passes through a membrane from a solution on the one side to another solution on the other side has been known, since the classical work of Dutrochet, as "endosmosis" or "exosmosis"; the pressure due to this passage of water has naturally been called "osmotic".

671 WÖHLER, FRIEDRICH. 1800–1882
Ueber künstliche Bildung des Harnstoffs. *Ann. Phys. Chem.* (*Leipzig*), 1828, **12,** 253–6.

The synthetic preparation of urea was the first occasion that an organic compound has been built up from inorganic materials. Wöhler's discovery led eventually to the brilliant results that have been achieved in attempts to synthesize other organic compounds. A French translation of this article appears in *Ann. Chim.* (*Paris*), 1828, **37,** 330–34.

672 CHEVREUL, MICHEL EUGÈNE. 1786–1889
Neues eigenthümliches stickstoffhaltiges Princip, in Muskelfleisch gefunden. *J. Chem. Physik,* 1832, **65,** 455–56.

Isolation of creatine from muscle.

673 MÜLLER, JOHANNES. 1801–1858
Ueber Knorpel und Knochen. *Ann. Pharm.* (*Heidelberg*), 1837, **21,** 277–82.

Isolation of chondrin and glutin.

674 SCHWANN, THEODOR. 1810–1882
Vorlaüfige Mittheilung betreffend Versuche über die Weingährung und Fäulniss. *Ann. Phys. Chem.* (*Leipzig*), 1837, **41,** 184–93.

Proof that putrefaction is produced by living bodies. Independently of Cagniard-Latour, Schwann discovered the yeast cell. He is regarded as the founder of the germ theory of putrefaction and fermentation.

675 CAGNIARD-LATOUR, CHARLES, *Baron.* 1777–1859
Mémoire sur la fermentation vineuse. *Ann. Chim. Phys.*, 1838, **68,** 206–22.

The earliest demonstration of the true nature of yeast was made by Cagniard-Latour in 1836. All his work on the subject is summed up in this paper.

676 MULDER, GERARD JOHANN. 1802–1880
Action de l'acide hydrochlorique sur la protéine. *Bull. Sci. Phys. nat.* (*Leyde*), 1838, 153.

Mulder gave the name *protéine* to a substance which he believed to be the essential constituent of all organized bodies. Later, with Liebig, he found there was no such definite compound, but the word has remained to designate the nitrogenous products of which it was a mixture.

677 LIEBIG, JUSTUS VON. 1803–1873
Die organische Chemie in ihrer Anwendung auf Physiologie und Pathologie. Braunschweig, *F. Vieweg*, 1842.

First classification of the organic food-stuffs and the processes of nutrition. With this book Liebig introduced the concept of metabolism into physiology.

678 WÖHLER, Friedrich. 1800–1882
Umwandlung der Benzoësäure in Hippursäure im lebenden Organismus. *Ann. Phys. Chem. (Leipzig)*, 1842, **56,** 638–41.
Discovery that benzoic acid taken in with food is excreted in the urine as hippuric acid – a discovery of importance in the chemistry of metabolism. (But see the footnote to p. 474 of Garrison's *History of medicine*, 1929).

679 PETTENKOFER, Max Josef von. 1818–1901
Notiz über eine neue Reaction auf Galle und Zucker. *Ann. Chem. Pharm.*, 1844, **52,** 90–96.
Pettenkofer's test for bile. Previously there had been no means of recognizing the presence of the bile salts.

680 FEHLING, Hermann Christian von. 1812–1885
Quantitative Bestimmung des Zuckers im Harn. *Arch. physiol. Heilk.*, 1848, **7,** 64–73.
Fehling's test for sugar in the urine.

681 STRECKER, Adolph. 1822–1871
Untersuchung der Ochsengalle. *Ann. Chem. Pharm.*, 1848, **65,** 1–37; **67,** 1–60; 1849, **70,** 149–97.

682 LUDWIG, Carl Friedrich Wilhelm. 1816–1895
Ueber die endosmotischen Aequivalente und die endosmotische Theorie. *Z. rat. Med.*, 1849, **8,** 1–52.
In this development of his theory of urinary secretion (see No. 1232) Ludwig made important observations on endosmosis.

683 MILLON, August Nicolas Eugène. 1812–1867
Sur un réactif propre aux composés protéiques. *C. R. Acad. Sci. (Paris)*, 1849, **28,** 40–42.
Millon discovered a special reagent for proteids.

684 FUNKE, Otto. 1828–1879
Atlas der physiologischen Chemie. Leipzig, *W. Engelmann*, 1853.

685 LIEBIG, Justus von. 1803–1873
Ueber einige Harnstoffverbindungen und eine neue Methode zur Bestimmung von Kochsalz und Harnstoff im Harn. *Ann. Pharm. (Heidelberg)*, 1853, **85,** 289–328.
Liebig's method of estimating urea.

685.1 FRERICHS, Friedrich Theodor. 1819–1885, & STAEDELER, Georg. 1821–1871
Ueber das Vorkommen von Leucin und Tyrosin in der menschlichen Leber. *Arch. Anat. Physiol. wiss. Med.*, 1854, 382–92.
Discovery of leucine and tyrosine in the urine.

686 GRAHAM, Thomas. 1805–1869
On osmotic force. *Phil. Trans.*, 1854, **144,** 177–228.
Investigation of osmotic force; provided important information for the physiologists.

687 MARCET, William. 1829–1900
On the immediate principles of human excrements in the healthy state. *Phil. Trans.*, 1857, **147,** 403–13.
First important publication on coprosterol as a product of excretion.

688 GRAHAM, THOMAS. 1805–1869
Liquid diffusion applied to analysis. *Phil. Trans.*, 1861, **151,** 183–224.
Graham's method of separating animal and other fluids by dialysis introduced the distinction between colloidal and crystalloid substances.

690 COHNHEIM, JULIUS FRIEDRICH. 1839–1884
Zur Kenntnis der zuckerbildenden Fermente. *Virchows Arch. path. Anat.*, 1863, **28,** 241–53.
Investigation of the sugar-forming ferments.

691 SCHULTZE, MAXIMILIAN JOHANN SIGISMUND. 1825–1874
Das Protoplasma der Rhizopoden und der Pflanzenzellen. Leipzig, *Engelmann*, 1863.
Schultze showed that protoplasm is practically identical in all living cells.

692 TRAUBE, MORITZ. 1826–1894
Experimente zur Theorie der Zellenbildung und Endosmose. *Arch. Anat. Physiol. wiss. Med.*, 1867, 87–165.
Employing, for the first time, copper ferrocyanide as a semi-permeable membrane Traube investigated osmosis and the permeability of membranes.

693 JAFFÉ, MAX. 1841–1911
Beitrag zur Kenntniss der Gallen- und Harnpigmente. *J. prakt. Chem.*, 1868, **104,** 401–06.
Jaffé discovered urobilin in the urine.

694 ——. Ueber das Vorkommen von Urobilin im Darminhalt. *Zbl. med. Wiss.*, 1871, **9,** 465–66.
Discovery of urobilin in the intestines.

695 MIESCHER, JOHANN FRIEDRICH. 1844–1895
Ueber die chemische Zusammensetzung der Eiterzellen. In: F. HOPPE-SEYLER: *Medicinisch-chemische Untersuchungen*, Berlin, 1871, 441–60.
Miescher discovered nuclein. He demonstrated it in pus cells in 1868. He was also first to suggest the existence of the genetic code (see *Nature, Lond.*, 1967, **215,** 556).

696 VIERORDT, KARL. 1818–1884
Die quantitative Spectralanalyse in ihrer Anwendung auf Physiologie, Physik, Chemie und Technologie. *Tübingen, H. Laupp*, 1876.
Vierordt's spectral analyses of haemoglobin, bile and urine were of great value. He studied the variations in the spectrum of oxyhaemoglobin produced by different dilutions of this substance and was thus able to estimate the haemoglobin content of the blood.

697 JAFFÉ, MAX. 1841–1911
Ueber die Ausscheidung des Indicans unter physiologischen und pathologischen Verhältnissen. *Virchows Arch. path. Anat.*, 1877, **70,** 72–111.
Isolation of indican in the urine.

698 PFEFFER, WILHELM FRIEDRICH PHILIPP. 1845–1920
Osmotische Untersuchungen. Leipzig, *W. Engelmann*, 1877.
The osmotic pressures of solutions were found by Pfeffer to be directly in proportion to the concentration of the solute and to the absolute temperature.

699 WALTER, Friedrich.
Untersuchungen über die Wirkung der Säuren auf den thierischen Organismus. *Arch. exp. Path. Pharmak.*, 1877, **7,** 148–78.

700 BERNARD, Claude. 1813–1878
La fermentation alcoolique. *Rev. sci.* (*Paris*), 1878, **16,** 49–56.
Bernard disbelieved Pasteur's definition of a ferment as "a living form originating from a germ."

701 HOPPE-SEYLER, Ernst Felix Immanuel. 1825–1895
Physiologische Chemie. Berlin, *A. Hirschwald,* 1881.
Hoppe-Seyler, one of the greatest of the physiological chemists, founded the *Zeitschrift für physiologische Chemie* and wrote a classical text-book on the subject.

702 KOSSEL, Albrecht. 1853–1927
Zur Chemie des Zellkerns. *Hoppe-Seyl. Z. physiol. Chem.*, 1882–83, **7,** 7–22; 1886, **10,** 248–64; 1896–97, **22,** 176–87.
Among the many important contributions of Kossel was his study of the chemistry of the cell and cell-nucleus. He was professor of physiology at Marburg and Heidelberg and was awarded the Nobel Prize for Physiology in 1910.

703 KJELDAHL, Johann. 1849–1900
En ny Methode til kvaelstofbestemmelse i organiske Stoffer. *Medd. Carlsberg Lab.* (*Kbh.*), 1883, **2,** 1–27.
Kjeldahl, a Danish chemist, devised a method of determining the amount of nitrogen in an organic compound ("Kjeldahl's method"). A German translation is in *Z. anal. Chem.*, 1883, **22,** 366–82.

704 KÜLZ, Rudolph Eduard. 1845–1895
Ueber eine neue linksdrehende Säure (Pseudooxybuttersäure). *Z. Biol.*, 1884, **20,** 165–78; 1887, **23,** 329–39.
Isolation of β-oxybutyric acid. (Title of second paper: Beiträge zur Kenntniss der activen β-Oxybuttersäure).

705 BRIEGER, Ludwig. 1849–1909
Ueber Ptomaine. 3 vols. Berlin, *A. Hirschwald,* 1885–86.
Brieger isolated and determined the composition of a number of the ptomaines.

706 van't HOFF, Jacobus Hendricus. 1852–1911
Lois d'équilibre chimique dans l'état dilué, gazeux ou dissous. *K. Svenska vetenskAkad. Handl.*, Stockholm, 1885, **21,** No. 17, pp. 1–41.
Van t'Hoff stated that osmotic pressure is proportional to the concentration if the temperature remains invariable, and proportional to the absolute temperature if the concentration remains invariable.

707 HAY, Matthew. 1855–1932
Test for the bile acids. In Landois and Stirling: *Text-book of human physiology*, 2nd ed., London, 1886, **1,** 381.
Hay devised a test for the determination of bile acids in the urine.

708 JAFFÉ, Max. 1841–1911
Ueber den Niederschlag, welchen Pikrinsäure in normalen Harn erzeugt und über eine neue Reaction des Kreatinins. *Hoppe-Seyl. Z. physiol. Chem.*, 1886, **10,** 391–400.
Jaffé's creatinine test.

709 ARRHENIUS, Svante August. 1859–1927
Ueber die Dissociation der in Wasser gelösten Stoffe. *Z. physikal. Chem.*, 1887, **1,** 631–48.
The electrolytic dissociation theory of Arrhenius.

710 BUNGE, Gustav von. 1844–1920
Lehrbuch der physiologischen und pathologischen Chemie. Leipzig, *F. C. W. Vogel*, 1887.

711 van't HOFF, Jacobus Hendricus. 1852–1911
Die Rolle des osmotischen Druckes in der Analogie zwischen Lösungen und Gasen. *Z. physikal. Chem.*, 1887, **1,** 481–508.

712 VAUGHAN, Victor Clarence. 1851–1929, & NOVY, Frederick George. 1864–1957
Ptomaines and leucomaines, or the putrefactive and physiological alkaloids, Philadelphia, *Lea Bros. & Co.*, 1888.

713 ALTMANN, Richard. 1852–1900
Ueber Nucleinsäuren. *Arch. Anat. Physiol., Physiol. Abt.*, 1889, 524–36.

714 BERTHELOT, Pierre Eugène Marcelin. 1827–1907
Fixation de l'azote par la terre végétale nue ou avec le concours des légumineuses. *Rev. sci.* (*Paris*), 1889, **43,** 450–54.
Berthelot showed that bacteria acting in clay soils are able to fix nitrogen.

715 STADELMANN, Ernst. 1853–
Ueber den Einfluss der Alkalien auf den menschlichen Stoffwechsel. Stuttgart, *F. Enke*, 1890.

716 DRECHSEL, Edmund. 1843–1897
Der Abbau der Eiweissstoffe. *Arch. Anat. Physiol., Physiol. Abt.*, 1891, 248–78.
Drechsel discovered that the protein molecule contains both mono- and di-amino acids.

717 HARLEY, Edward Vaughan Berkeley. 1863–1923
The behaviour of saccharine matter in the blood. *J. Physiol.* (*Lond.*), 1891, **12,** 391–408.
Destruction of sugar in the blood.

718 HOPKINS, *Sir* Frederick Gowland. 1861–1947
On the estimation of uric acid in the urine. *J. Path. Bact.*, 1892–93, **1,** 451–59.
Hopkins' method of estimating uric acid in urine.

719 KOSSEL, Albrecht. 1853–1927
Ueber die Nucleinsäure. *Arch. Anat. Physiol., Physiol. Abt.*, 1893, 157–64; 1894, 194–203.
See No. 702.

720 FISCHER, Emil. 1852–1919
Bedeutung der Stereochemie für die Physiologie. *Hoppe-Seyl. Z. physiol. Chem.*, 1898–99, **26,** 60–87.

721 KOSSEL, ALBRECHT. 1853–1927
Ueber die Eiweissstoffe. *Dtsch. med. Wschr.*, 1898, **24,** 581–82.
Kossel forecast the polypeptide nature of the protein molecule.

722 KASTLE, JOSEPH HOEING. 1864–1916, & LOEVENHART, ARTHUR SALOMON. 1878–1929
Concerning lipase, the fat-splitting enzyme, and the reversibility of its action. *Amer. chem. J.*, 1900, **24,** 491–525.
Demonstration of the reversible action of lipase.

723 HOPKINS, *Sir* FREDERICK GOWLAND. 1861–1947, & COLE, SYDNEY WILLIAM. 1877–1952
A contribution to the chemistry of proteids. I. A preliminary study of a hitherto undescribed product of tryptic digestion. *J. Physiol.* (Lond.), 1901, **27,** 418–28.
Isolation of tryptophane.

724 HÖBER, RUDOLF OTTO ANSELM. 1873–1953
Physikalische Chemie der Zelle und Gewebe. Leipzig, *W. Engelmann*, 1902.

725 HAMBURGER, HARTOG JAKOB. 1859–1924
Osmotischer Druck und Ionenlehre in den medicinischen Wissenschaften. 3 vols. Wiesbaden, *J. F. Bergmann*, 1902–04.
Includes an account of all the methods of determining osmotic pressure.

725.1 LEVENE, PHOEBUS AARON THEODORE. 1869–1940
Darstellung und Analyse einiger Nucleinsäuren. *Hoppe-Seyl. Z. physiol. Chem.*, 1903, **39,** 4–8, 133–35, 479–83.
Chemical distinction between DNA and RNA.

726 BOHR, CHRISTIAN. 1855–1911, *et al.*
Ueber einen in biologischer Beziehung wichtigen Einfluss, den die Kohlensäurespannung des Blutes auf dessen Sauerstoffbindung übt. *Skand. Arch. Physiol.*, 1904, **16,** 402–12.
Bohr, Hasselbalch, and Krogh showed, in the experimental animal, that the affinity of blood for oxygen depends upon carbon dioxide pressure.

727 ABDERHALDEN, EMIL. 1877–1950
Abbau und Aufbau der Eiweisskörper im tierischen Organismus. *Hoppe-Seyl. Z. physiol. Chem.*, 1905, **44,** 17–52.

728 KNOOP, FRANZ. 1875–1946
Die Abbau aromatischer Fettsäuren im Tierkörper. *Beitr. chem. Physiol. Path.*, 1905, **6,** 150–62.
β-oxidation theory.

729 ZSIGMONDY, RICHARD ADOLF. 1866–1930
Zur Erkenntnis der Kolloide. Jena, *G. Fischer*, 1905.

730 FISCHER, EMIL. 1852–1919
Untersuchungen über Aminosäuren, Polypeptide und Proteine. Berlin, *J. Springer*, 1906.
In a series of papers, Fischer showed that animal and vegetable proteins are composed of a series of amino-acids united by elimination of water.

730.1 HOWELL, William Henry. 1860–1945
Note upon the presence of amino-acids in the blood and lymph as determined by the β naphthalinsulphochloride reaction. *Amer. J. Physiol.*, 1906, **17**, 273–79.
Demonstration of the presence of amino-acids in the blood.

731 PAVY, Frederick William. 1829–1911
On carbohydrate metabolism. London, *J. & A. Churchill*, 1906.

732 WILLCOCK, Edith Gertrude, & HOPKINS, *Sir* Frederick Gowland. 1861–1947
The importance of individual amino-acids in metabolism. *J. Physiol. (Lond.)*, 1906, **35**, 88–102.
Demonstration of the importance of tryptophane in diet. The pioneer work of Hopkins led eventually to the discovery of vitamins.

733 FLETCHER, *Sir* Walter Morley. 1873–1933, & HOPKINS, *Sir* Frederick Gowland. 1861–1947
Lactic acid in amphibian muscle. *J. Physiol. (Lond.)*, 1907, **35**, 247–309.
Explanation of the production of lactic acid in normal muscular contraction.

734 DAKIN, Henry Drysdale. 1880–1952
The oxidation of butyric acid by means of hydrogen peroxide with formation of acetone, aldehydes, and other products. *J. biol. Chem.*, 1908, **4**, 77–89.
See No. 735.

735 ——. The comparative studies of the mode of oxidation of phenyl derivatives of fatty acids by the animal organism and by hydrogen peroxide. *J. biol. Chem.*, 1908, **4**, 419–35; **5**, 173–85, 303–09; 1909, **6**, 203–43.
Dakin's oxidation theory.

736 GRUBE, Karl Adolph. 1866–
Ueber die kleinsten Moleküle, welche die Leber zur Synthese des Glykogenes verwerten kann. *Pflüg. Arch. ges. Physiol.*, 1908, **121**, 636–40.

737 FREUNDLICH, Herbert. 1880–1941
Kapillarchemie. Leipzig, *Akademische Verlagsgesellschaft*, 1909.

738 OSTWALD, Carl Wilhelm Wolfgang. 1883–1943
Grundriss der Kolloidchemie. Dresden, *Steinkopff*, 1909.

739 KASTLE, Joseph Hoeing. 1864–1916
The oxidases and other oxygen-catalysts concerned in biological oxidations. *Bull. Hyg. Lab. U.S. publ. Hlth Serv.*, No. 59, Washington, 1910.

740 TRAUBE, Isidor. 1860–1943
Die Theorie des Haftdrucks (Oberflächendrucks) und ihre Bedeutung für die Physiologie. *Pflüg. Arch. ges. Physiol.*, 1910, **132**, 511–38; 1911, **140**, 109–34.

741 DAKIN, Henry Drysdale. 1880–1952
Oxidations and reductions in the animal body. London, *Longmans*, 1912.

741.1 FOLIN, Otto Knut Olof. 1876–1934, & FARMER, Chester Jefferson. 1886–
A new method for the determination of total nitrogen in urine. *J. biol. Chem.*, 1912, **11**, 493–501.
Folin introduced several micro-methods for the determination of nitrogen, urea, creatine, etc.

742 HASSELBALCH, Karl Albert. 1874–1962, & LUNDSGAARD, Christen. 1883–
Elektrometrische Reaktionsbestimmung des Blutes bei Körpertemperatur. *Biochem. Z.*, 1912, **38**, 77–91.
Hasselbalch formula for the determination of pH concentration in the blood.

743 WILLSTÄTTER, Richard. 1872–1942, & STOLL, Arthur. 1887–1971
Untersuchungen über Chlorophyll. Berlin, *J. Springer*, 1913.

744 BELL, Richard D., & DOISY, Edward Adelbert. 1893–
Rapid colorimetric methods for the determination of phosphorus in urine and blood. *J. biol. Chem.*, 1920, **44**, 55–67.

745 HOPKINS, *Sir* Frederick Gowland. 1861–1947
On an autoxidisable constituent of the cell. *Biochem. J.*, 1921, **15**, 286–305.
Isolation of glutathione.

746 ROBISON, Robert. 1883–1941
The possible significance of hexosephosphoric esters in ossification. *Biochem. J.*, 1923, **17**, 286–93.
Records an important advance in the knowledge concerning the conversion of blood calcium into the insoluble calcium of bone.

747 JACKSON, Henry. 1892–
Studies in nuclein metabolism. II. The isolation of a nucleotide from human blood. *J. biol. Chem.*, 1924, **59**, 529–34.
Jackson demonstrated the existence of pentose nucleotides in normal blood.

748 MEYERHOF, Otto Fritz. 1884–1951
Chemical dynamics of life phaenomena. Philadelphia, *J. B. Lippincott*, 1924.

749 CLUTTERBUCK, Percival Walter, & RAPER, Henry Stanley. 1882–1951
A study of the oxidation of the ammonium salts of normal saturated fatty acids and its biological significance. *Biochem. J.*, 1925, **19**, 385–96.

750 WARBURG, Otto Heinrich. 1883–1970
Ueber die katalytischen Wirkungen der lebendigen Substanz. Berlin, *J. Springer*, 1928.

751 FISKE, CYRUS HARTWELL. 1890– , & SUBBAROW, YELLAPRAGADA.
Phosphorus compounds of muscle and liver. *Science*, 1929, **70,** 381–382.
Discovery of adenosine-5'-triphosphate (ATP).

751.1 KREBS, *Sir* HANS ADOLF. 1900– , & JOHNSON, WILLIAM ARTHUR.
Citric acid in intermediate metabolism in animal tissues. *Enzymologia*, 1937, **4,** 148–56.
Citric acid cycle of aerobic carbohydrate metabolism. Krebs shared the Nobel Prize with Fritz Lipmann (No. 751.3) in 1953.

751.2 COHN, EDWIN JOSEPH. 1892– , *et al.*
Chemical, clinical, and immunological studies on the products of human plasma fractionation. I. The characterization of the protein fractions of human plasma. *J. clin. Invest.*, 1944, **23,** 417–32.
Fractionation of plasma proteins. With J. L. Oncley, L. E. Strong, W. L. Hughes, and S. H. Armstrong.

751.3 LIPMANN, FRITZ ALBERT. 1899– , & KAPLAN, NATHAN ORAM. 1917–
A common factor in the enzymatic acetylation of sulfanilamide and of choline. *J. biol. Chem.*, 1946, **162,** 743–44.
Coenzyme A.

752 CORI, CARL FERDINAND. 1896–
Enzymatic reactions in carbohydrate metabolism. *Harvey Lect.* (1945–46), 1947, **41,** 253–72.
C. F. Cori and Mrs. G. T. Cori (1896–1957) shared (with Houssay) the Nobel Prize in 1947 for their researches on the course of the catalytic transformation of glycogens.

752.1 WATSON, JAMES DEWEY. 1928– , & CRICK, FRANCIS HARRY COMPTON. 1916–
Molecular structure of nucleic acids. A structure for deoxyribose nucleic acid. *Nature (Lond.)*, 1953, **171,** 737–38.
Watson and Crick shared the Nobel Prize with M. F. H. Wilkins (No. 752.2) for the discovery of the molecular structure of DNA.

752.2 WILKINS, MAURICE HUGH FREDERICK. 1916– , *et al.*
Helical structure of crystalline deoxypentose nucleic acid. *Nature (Lond.)*, 1953, **172,** 759–62.
With W. E. Seeds, A. R. Stokes, and H. R. Wilson. Wilkins discovered the double helix structure of DNA. He shared the Nobel Prize with Crick and Watson in 1962.

752.3 GRUNBERG-MANAGO, MARIANNE, & OCHOA DE ALBORNOZ, SEVERO. 1905–
Enzymatic synthesis and breakdown of polynucleotides; polynucleotide phosphorylase. *J. Amer. chem. Soc.*, 1955, **77,** 3165–66.
Ochoa shared the Nobel Prize with Kornberg in 1959 for their artificial synthesis of nucleic acids by means of enzymes. The above paper describes the discovery of an enzyme able to catalyze the removal of a terminal phosphate group from ribonucleoside diphosphates.

752.4 KORNBERG, ARTHUR. 1918– , *et al.*
Enzymic synthesis of deoxyribonucleic acid. *Biochim. biophys. Acta*, 1956, **21,** 197–98.

With I. R. Lehman, M. J. Bessman, and E. S. Simms. Kornberg shared the Nobel Prize with Ochoa in 1959 for their artificial synthesis of nucleic acids by means of enzymes.

752.5 THEORELL, AXEL HUGO TEODOR. 1903–
The nature and mode of action of oxidation enzymes. Nobel Lecture, December 12, 1955. In *Festschrift Arthur Stoll*, Basel, Birkhäuser, 1957, pp. 35–47.

Theorell was awarded a Nobel Prize in 1955 for his discoveries relating to the nature and mode of action of oxidizing enzymes. The above paper summarizes his work in this field.

752.6 CRICK, FRANCIS HARRY COMPTON. 1916– , *et al.*
General nature of the genetic code for proteins. *Nature* (*Lond.*), 1961, **192,** 1227–32.

With L. Barnett, S. Brenner, and R. J. Watts-Tobin.

752.7 JACOB, FRANÇOIS. 1920– , & MONOD, JACQUES. 1910–
Genetic regulatory mechanisms in the synthesis of proteins. *J. molec. Biol.*, 1961, **3,** 318–56.

Jacob, Monod, and André Lwoff shared the Nobel Prize in 1965 for their discovery of a gene whose function is to regulate the activity of other genes.

For history, see 1584

753–913 CARDIOVASCULAR SYSTEM

753 IBN-AL-NAFIS [ABŪ-L-HASAN ALĀ-ŬD DĪN ALI IBN ABI-L-HAZIN]. 1210–1288
Ibn an Nafis und seine Theorie des Lungenkreislaufs. Von MAX MEYERHOF. *Quell. Stud. Gesch. Med.*, 1933, **4,** 37–88.

Ibn-al-Nafis, a Syrian physician, described the lesser circulation in his commentary on the anatomy of the *Canon* of Avicenna, 1268. This was discovered in three Arabic MSS by Mohyi el Din el Tatawi, who included a German translation in his inaugural dissertation, Freiburg, 1924. Meyerhof includes 28 pages of Arabic text in his paper. A translation of the relevant passage is in *Ann. Surg.*, 1936, **104,** 1–8, and in *Bull med.. Hist.*, 1955, **29,** 430–40.

754 SERVETUS, MICHAEL. 1511–1553
Christianismi restitutio. [Vienne, *Balthasar Arnollet*], 1553.

Contains (p. 170) the first printed description of the lesser circulation. Because of the heretical nature of this book, Servetus was burnt at the stake at Champel, Geneva, by order of Calvin. Most copies of the book were burnt with him; two survive, in Vienna and Paris, and there is an imperfect copy in Edinburgh. It was reprinted page for page in 1790 at Nuremberg. A translation of some of Servetus's writings was published by C. D. O'Malley in 1953; it includes a photographic reproduction of the title page of *Christianismi restitutio*; the passages describing the pulmonary circulation are also translated in J. F. Fulton's *Selected readings in the history of physiology*, 2nd ed., 1966, pp. 44–45.

755 CESALPINO, ANDREA [CAESALPINUS]. 1519–1603
Peripateticarum quaestionum libri quinque. Venetiis, *apud Iuntas*, 1571.

Although some have claimed that Caesalpinus preceded Harvey in the discovery of the circulation, his theories on the subject, unlike Harvey's, were not supported by convincing experimental work, although he came very near to the truth. His ideas are embodied in this and the succeeding work, but they had no influence on his contemporaries or upon Harvey. See the *Bibliotheca Osleriana*, No. 901.

756 ——. Quaestionum peripateticum, libri V. Venetiis, *apud Juntas*, 1593.

The results of tying a vein and the centripetal flow in veins were first recorded in print by Caesalpinus (lib. ii, Qu. xvii, p. 234).

757 FABRIZZI, GIROLAMO [FABRICIUS AB AQUAPENDENTE]. 1537–1619
De venarum ostiolis. Patavii, *ex typ. L. Pasquati*, 1603.

Fabricus, teacher of Harvey at Padua, made important observations on the valves of the veins. He failed to recognize their true function, however, considering this to be merely a delaying of the blood flow. This work must have influenced Harvey in his own attempts at the experimental demonstration of the circulation.

A fascimile edition of the book, with English translation, appeared under the editorship of K. J. Franklin in 1933.

758 HARVEY, WILLIAM. 1578–1657
Praelectiones anatomiae universalis. London, *J. Churchill*, 1886.

Facsimile reprint of Harvey's manuscript notes for a Lumleian Lecture, 1616. These show that at that date Harvey had already completed his demonstration of the circulation of the blood. English translation with annotations, Berkeley, 1961. Edited, with an introduction, translation, and notes by G. Whitteridge, *Edinburgh*, 1964.

759 ——. Exercitatio anatomica de motu cordis et sanguinis in animalibus. Francofurti, *sumpt. Guilielmi Fitzeri*, 1628.

The most important book in the history of medicine. Harvey proved experimentally that in animals the blood is impelled in a circle by the beat of the heart, passing from arteries to veins through pores (i.e., the capillaries, seen by Malphigi with the microscope in 1660). Garrison considers that the importance of Harvey's work lies not so much in the discovery of the circulation as in its quantitative or mathematical demonstration. Probably Harvey chose to have the book printed in Frankfurt because of the famous book fair held there and the consequent greater publicity his book would receive. The book was reprinted in facsimile in 1928 (*Monumenta medica*, Vol. 5, Florence). The Latin text, with an English translation by K. J. Franklin, was published in Oxford, 1957.

760 MALPIGHI, MARCELLO. 1628–1694
De pulmonibus observationes anatomicae. Bononiae, *B. Ferronius*, 1661.

Discovery of the capillary circulation. This book, which is very rare, consists of two letters to Borelli; it is the second letter which contains Malpighi's discovery. It is republished in his *Opera omnia*, Lugduni Batavorum, 1687, ii, 331. It was also published as an appendix to Thomas Bartholin's *De pulmonum substantia et motu diatribe*, 1663. A facsimile was published in Milan in 1958; English translation by J. Young is in *Proc. roy. Soc. Med.*, 1929–30, Sect. Hist. Med., **23,** 1–11.

761 LOWER, RICHARD. 1631–1691
Tractatus de corde. Londini, *J. Allestry*, 1669.

Lower was the first to demonstrate the scroll-like structure of the cardiac muscle. He was one of the first to transfuse blood. Chapter III of the above work records how Lower injected dark venous blood into the insufflated lungs; he concluded that its subsequent bright red colour was due to its absorption of some of the air passing through the lungs. The British Museum copy of this book bears the signature of William Charleton, followed by the date "1668"; it is possible, therefore, that the book actually appeared in that year and not in 1669. Facsimile, with translation, London, 1932.

762 BORELLI, Giovanni Alfonso. 1608–1679
De motu animalium. 2 pts. Romae, *ex typ. A. Bernabo*, 1680–81.

Borelli originated the neurogenic theory of the heart's action and first suggested that the circulation resembled a simple hydraulic system. He was the first to insist that the heart beat was a simple muscular contraction. Borelli was a representative of the Iatro-Mathematical School, which treated all physiological happenings as rigid consequences of the laws of physics and mechanics.

763 THEBESIUS, Adam Christian. 1686–1732
Disputatio medica inauguralis de circulo sanguinis in corde. Lugduni Batavorum, *A. Elzevier*, 1708.

First description of the coronary valves and the venae thebesii.

764 POURFOUR DU PETIT, François. 1664–1741
Mémoire dans lequel il est démontré que les nerfs intercostaux fournissent des rameaux que portent des esprits dans les yeux. *Hist. Acad. roy. Sci. (Paris) (Mém.)*, 1727, 1–19.

Discovery of the vasomotor nerves (see also No. 1313).

765 HALES, Stephen. 1677–1761
Statical essays, containing haemastaticks. Vol. 2. London, *W. Innys & R. Manby*, 1733.

In this work is recorded Hales' invention of the manometer, with which he was the first to measure blood-pressure. His work is the greatest single contribution to our knowledge of the vascular system after Harvey, and led to the development of the blood-pressure measuring instruments now in universal use. For a reprint of part of the work see Willius & Keys, *Cardiac classics*, 1941, pp. 131–55.

765.1 TAUBE, Hartwig Wilhelm Ludwig. 1706–
Dissertationem inauguralem de vera nervi intercostalis origine. Gottingae, *apud Abram Vandenhoeck*, 1743.

Taube described the carotid body and named it "ganglion minutum." See J. Pick, *J. Hist. Med.*, 1959, **14**, 61–73.

766 WEBER, Ernst Heinrich. 1795–1878, & WEBER, Eduard Friedrich Wilhelm. 1806–1871
Wellenlehre. Leipzig, *W. Engelmann*, 1825.

The velocity of the pulse wave was first measured by the Webers.

767 POISEUILLE, Jean Léonard Marie. 1799–1869
Recherches sur la force du coeur aortique. Paris, *Thèse No.* 166, 1828.

Poiseuille was the first after Stephen Hales to make any important addition to the knowledge of the physiology of circulation. In his graduation thesis, above, he described a "haemodynamometer" invented by himself and which he used to repeat some of Hales's blood-pressure experiments. With his haemomanometer, a mercury manometer, which was a great improvement on the long tube used by Hales, Poiseuille showed that the blood-pressure rises and falls on expiration and inspiration, and measured the degree of arterial dilatation produced by each heart beat. English translation in *Edinb. med. surg. J.*, 1829, **32**, 28–38. See also his paper in *J. Physiol. exp. path.*, 1828, **8**, 272–305.

768 ——. Recherches expérimentales sur le mouvement des liquides dans les tubes de très petits diamètres. *C. R. Acad. Sci. (Paris)*, 1840, **11**, 961–67, 1041–48; 1841, **12**, 112–15.

Poiseuille's law of the flow of liquids in tubes – fundamental in blood viscosimetry. Abstract; complete monograph in *Mem. Acad. roy. Sci.* (Paris), 1846, **9**, 433–544.

769 HENLE, Friedrich Gustav Jacob. 1809–1885
Gefässnerven. In his *Allgemeine Anatomie*, Leipzig, 1841, p. 510, 690.
Demonstration of the presence of smooth muscle in the endothelial coat of small arteries.

770 LUDWIG, Carl Friedrich Wilhelm. 1816–1895
Beiträge zur Kenntniss des Einflusses der Respirationsbewegungen auf den Blutlauf im Aortensystem. *Arch. Anat. Physiol. wiss. Med.*, 1847, 242–302.
Ludwig changed Poiseuille's haemodynamometer into the kymograph by the addition of a float and caused this float to write on a recording cylinder.

771 VOLKMANN, Alfred Wilhelm. 1800–1877
Die Hämodynamik nach Versuchen. Leipzig, *Breitkopf & Härtel*, 1850.

772 VIERORDT, Karl. 1818–1884
Die bildliche Darstellung des menschlichen Arterienpulses. *Arch. physiol. Heilk.*, 1854, **13,** 284–87.
Vierordt invented a sphygmograph which acted on the principle that indirect estimation of blood-pressure could be accomplished by measuring the counter-pressure necessary to obliterate the arterial pulsation. This was the first instrument with which a tracing of the human pulse could be made. The paper was expanded into book form in 1855; it is the first record of a study with an instrument of precision of the pulse in health and disease.

773 FAIVRE, J.
Etudes expérimentales sur les lésions organiques du coeur. *Ann. Soc. Méd. Lyon*, 1856, 2 sér., **4,** 180–88.
Faivre made the first accurate estimation of the blood-pressure in man, by connecting the artery with a mercury manometer and making direct readings. These investigations were important, since they established normal values. The paper was republished in book form in 1856.

774 BERNARD, Claude. 1813–1878
De l'influence de deux ordres de nerfs qui déterminent les variations de couleur du sang veineux dans les organes glandulaires. *C. R. Acad. Sci. (Paris)*, 1858, **47,** 245–53; 393–400.
Discovery of the vascoconstrictor and vasodilator nerves and description of their function of regulating the blood supply to the different parts of the body.

775 VIERORDT, Karl. 1818–1884
Die Erscheinungen und Gesetze der Stromgeschwindigkeiten des Blutes. Frankfurt a.M., *Meidinger Sohn & Co.*, 1858.
Vierordt estimated, by means of a "haemotachometer" of his own invention, the rate of the blood flow in various arteries, and also the influence of the blood volume, pulse rate and respiratory rate upon it.

776 MAREY, Etienne Jules. 1830–1904
Recherches sur le pouls au moyen d'un nouvel appareil enregistreur le sphygmographe. Paris, *E. Thunot et Cie.*, 1860.
Invention of the modern sphygmograph.

777 POISEUILLE, Jean Léonard Marie. 1799–1869
Sur la pression du sang dans le système artériel. *C. R. Acad. Sci. (Paris)*, 1860, **51,** 238–42.

778 LUDWIG, CARL FRIEDRICH WILHELM. 1816–1895
Die physiologischen Leistungen des Blutdrucks. Leipzig, *S. Hirzel*, 1865.

Ludwig's inaugural address at Leipzig, in which he introduced the idea of keeping alive excised portions of organs by means of artificial circulation, or perfusion. He suggested that the blood-pressure had a stimulating effect on the vagus.

779 DOGIEL, JAN. 1830–1905
Die Ausmessung der strömenden Blutvolumina. *Arb. physiol. Anst. Lpz.* (1867), 1868, **2,** 196–271.

Invention of the *Stromuhr*, for measurement of the velocity of the blood. Dogiel was a pupil of Ludwig.

780 THANHOFFER, LAJOS VON. 1843–1909
Die beiderseitige mechanische Reizung des Nv. vagus beim Menschen. *Zbl. med. Wiss.*, 1875, **13,** 403–06.

781 KRIES, N. VON.
Ueber den Druck in den Blutcapillaren der menschlichen Haut. *Arb. physiol. Anst. Lpz.* (1875), 1876, **10,** 69–80.

782 STRICKER, SALOMON. 1834–1898
Untersuchungen über die Gefässnerven-Wurzeln des Ischiadicus. *S.B. k. Akad. Wiss. Wien, math.-nat. Cl.*, 1876, 3 Abt., **74,** 173–85.

Stricker was the first to describe vasodilatation on stimulation of the posterior nerve roots.

782.1 ROUGET, CHARLES MARIE BENJAMIN. 1824–1904
Sur le contractilité des capillaires sanguins. *C. R. Acad. Sci.* (*Paris*), 1879, **88,** 916–18.

Rouget made an important investigation of the control of capillary circulation. He described cells ("Rouget's cells") on the outer surfaces of capillary walls, considered to be contractile.

783 MAREY, ETIENNE JULES. 1830–1904
La circulation du sang à l'état physiologique et dans les maladies. Paris, *G. Masson*, 1881.

784 BRAUNE, CHRISTIAN WILHELM. 1831–1892
Das Venensystem des menschlichen Körpers. 2 pts. and atlas. Leipzig, *Veit & Co.*, 1884–89.

Like Braune's other anatomical works, this is notable for its excellent illustrations.

785 MALL, FRANKLIN PAINE. 1862–1917
Der Einfluss der Systems der Vena portae auf die Vertheilung des Blutes. *Arch. Anat. Physiol., Physiol. Abt.*, 1892, 409–53.

786 PORTER, WILLIAM TOWNSEND. 1862–1949
On the results of ligation of the coronary arteries. *J. Physiol.* (*Lond.*), 1893–94, **15,** 121–38; *J. exp. Med.*, 1896, **1,** 46–70.

787 TIGERSTEDT, ROBERT ADOLF ARMAND. 1853–1923
Lehrbuch der Physiologie des Kreislaufes. Leipzig, *Veit & Co.*, 1893.

788 GIBSON, ALEXANDER GEORGE. 1875–1950
The significance of a hitherto undescribed wave in the jugular pulse. *Lancet*, 1907, **2,** 1380–82.
The physiological wave sometimes found in mid-diastole, when the pulse is slow, was first described by Gibson. He termed it the *b*-wave.

789 HARTMANN, HENRI. 1860–1952
Some considerations upon high amputation of the rectum. *Ann. Surg.*, 1909, **50,** 1091–94.
"Hartmann's critical point," the site on the large intestine where the lowest sigmoid artery meets the superior rectal arterial branch.

790 LOMBARD, WARREN PLIMPTON. 1855–1939
The blood-vessels in the arterioles, capillaries and small veins of the human skin. *Amer. J. Physiol.*, 1911–12, **29,** 335–62.
Lombard soaked the skin in cedarwood oil, rendering transparent the superficial epidermal layers, and thus making possible many direct observations on it.

791 SOLLMANN, TORALD HERMANN. 1874–1965, & BROWN, EDGAR DEWIGHT. 1869–
The blood pressure fall produced by traction on the carotid artery. *Amer. J. Physiol.*, 1912, **30,** 88–104.
First description of the carotid sinus depressor reflex.

792 DALE, *Sir* HENRY HALLETT. 1875–1968, & RICHARDS, ALFRED NEWTON. 1876–1966
The vaso-dilator action of histamine and of some other substances. *J. Physiol. (Lond.)*, 1918–19, **52,** 110–65.
Dale and Richards studied the effect of histamine on the control of the circulation and showed its peripheral action to be located in the capillaries and smaller arterioles.

793 KROGH, SCHACK AUGUST STEENBERG. 1874–1949
The anatomy and physiology of the capillaries. New Haven, *Yale Univ. Press*, 1922.
Silliman Lectures. A second edition appeared in 1929. Krogh received the Nobel Prize for Physiology in 1920. His most important work was on the physiology of capillaries.

794 HERING, HEINRICH EWALD. 1866–1948
Der Karotisdruckversuch. *Münch. med. Wschr.*, 1923, **70,** 1287–90.

795 ——. Die Aenderung der Herzschlagzahl durch Aenderung des arteriellen Blutdruckes erfolgt aus reflektorischem Wege; gleichzeitig eine Mitteilung über die Funktion des Sinus caroticus, beziehungsweise der Sinusnerven. *Pflüg. Arch. ges. Physiol.*, 1924, **206,** 721–3.
First description of the structure and function of the sinus nerve and the reflex character of carotid pressure.

795.1 LANDIS, EUGENE MARKLEY. 1901–
The capillary pressure in frog mesentery as determined by micro-injection methods. *Amer. J. Physiol.*, 1926, **75,** 548–70.
Direct measurement of the blood pressure within the capillaries.

796 BLUMGART, HERMAN LUDWIG. 1895– , & WEISS, SOMA. 1898–1942
Studies in the velocity of blood flow. *J. clin. Invest.*, 1927, **4,** 1–13, 15–31, 149–71, 173–97, 199–209, 389–425, 555–74.
First practical method of measuring circulation time.

797 LEWIS, *Sir* THOMAS. 1881–1945
The blood-vessels of the human skin and their responses. London, *Shaw*, 1927.

798 REIN, FRIEDRICH HERMANN. 1898–1953
Die Thermo-Stromuhr. Ein Verfahren zur fortlaufenden Messung der mittleren absoluten Durchflussmengen in uneröffneten Gefässen in situ. *Z. Biol.*, 1928, **87,** 394–418.

Introduction of the *Thermostromuhr*, an instrument for measuring the velocity of the blood flow.

799 WIGGERS, CARL JOHN. 1883–1963
The pressure pulses in the cardiovascular system. London, *Longmans, Green & Co.*, 1928.

Wiggers, professor of physiology at the Western Reserve University, Cleveland, contributed much to the knowledge of the circulation and devised several instruments to promote the study of this subject.

800 STANDARDISATION of methods of measuring the arterial blood pressure. Joint report of the committees appointed by the Cardiac Society of Great Britain and Ireland, and the American Heart Association. *Brit. Heart J.*, 1939, **1,** 261–67.

Anatomy & Physiology of the Heart

801 EUSTACHI, BARTOLOMMEO [EUSTACHIUS]. 1520–1574
Opuscula anatomica. Venetiis, *V. Luchinus*, 1564.

Plate VIII illustrates the "Eustachian valve", the valvula venae cavae in the right auricle.

802 GASSENDI, PIERRE. 1592–1655
Elegans de septo cordis pervio observatio. *In* Pineau, S. [Pinaeus]: De integritatis et corruptionis virginum notis. Lugduni Batavorum, *apud Franciscos Hegerum et Hackium*, 1639.

Gassendi demonstrated the vestigial foramen ovale in the adult heart, settling the question of the perviousness of the septum of the heart. His work was first published in one volume with that of three others, the first being by Pinaeus, as above. Reprint and translation in *Bull. Hist. Med.*, 1939, **7,** 429–57.

802.1 BOTALLO, LEONARDO [BOTALLUS]. 1530–?
Opera omnia medica et chirurgica. Lugduni, *D. & A. à Gaasbeeck*, 1660.

"Botallo's duct", the ductus arteriosus; "Botallo's foramen", the foramen ovale interauriculare; and "Botallo's ligament", the ligamentum arteriosum, are described in this work.

803 VALSALVA, ANTONIO MARIA. 1666–1723
Opera. 2 vols. Venetiis, *apud F. Pitteri*, 1740.

Valsalva described the aortic "sinus of Valsalva".

804 SKODA, JOSEF. 1805–1881
Ueber den Herzstoss und die durch die Herzbewegungen verursachten Töne. *Med. Jb. k. österr. Staates (Wien)*, 1837, N.F., **13,** 227–266.

Skoda's theory of the heart beat.

805 PALICKI, Bogislaus.
De musculari cordis structura. [Breslau,] 1839.
First description of the "Purkinje fibres" of the myocardium, written by one of Purkinje's students.

806 REMAK, Robert. 1815–1865
Neurologische Erläuterungen. *Arch. Anat. Physiol.* (*Lpz.*), 1844, 463–72.
Remak was first to describe the intrinsic ganglia of the heart.

807 WEBER, Eduard Friedrich Wilhelm. 1806–1871, & WEBER, Ernst Heinrich. 1795–1878
Experimenta, quibus probatur nervos vagos rotatione machinae galvano-magneticae irritatos, motum cordis retardare et adeo intercipare. *Ann. univ. Med.* (*Milano*), 1845, 3 ser., **20,** 227–33.
The discovery of the inhibitory power of the vagus. Also published in Wagner's *Handwörterbuch der Physiologie*, 1846, **3,** 45–51. Partial translation in J. F. Fulton's *Selected readings in the history of physiology*, 2nd ed. 1966, p. 296.

808 WILD, F.
Ueber die peristaltische Bewegung des Oesophagus, nebst einigen Bemerkungen über diejenigen des Darms. *Z. rat. Med.*, 1846, **5,** 76–132.
Includes (pp. 76–77) a description of what is probably the first perfusion of the isolated heart.

809 LUDWIG, Carl Friedrich Wilhelm. 1816–1895
Über die Herznerven des Frosches. *Arch. Anat. Physiol. wiss. Med.*, 1848, 139–43.

810 HOFFA, Moritz, & LUDWIG, Carl Friedrich Wilhelm. 1816–1895
Einige neue Versuche über Herzbewegung. *Z. rat. Med.*, 1850, **9,** 107–44.
Experimental ventricular fibrillation.

811 BIDDER, Friedrich Heinrich. 1810–1894
Ueber functionell verschiedene und räumlich getrennte Nervencentra im Froschherzen. *Arch. Anat. Physiol. wiss. Med.*, 1852, 163–177.
Discovery of the ganglion cells at the auriculo-ventricular junction, "Bidder's ganglion".

812 STANNIUS, Friedrich Hermann. 1808–1883
Zwei Reihen physiologischer Versuche. *Arch. Anat. Physiol. wiss. Med.*, 1852, 85–100.
Stannius showed that the apex of the heart ceases to beat rhythmically when separated physiologically by ligature or clamp from the rest of the heart, while the sinus remains unaffected. Partial translation in J. F. Fulton's *Selected readings in the history of physiology*, 2nd ed., 1966, pp. 59–60.

812.1 BERNARD, Claude. 1813–1878
Leçons de physiologie expérimentale appliquée à la médecine. Vol. 1. Paris, *J. B. Baillière*, 1855.
P. 126: Catheterization of the heart of a dog.

813 MAREY, ÉTIENNE JULES. 1830–1904
Loi qui préside à la fréquence des battements du coeur. *C. R. Acad. Sci. (Paris)*, 1861, **53,** 95–8.
Marey's law of the heart. Marey was the first to realize the relationship between the blood pressure and the heart rate.

814 GOLTZ, FRIEDRICH LEOPOLD. 1834–1902
Ueber Reflexionen von und zum Herzen (Klopfversuch). *Königsb. med. Jb.*, 1862, **3,** 271–4.
Rapidly-repeated blows on the belly of a frog caused cessation of the heart-beat, which Goltz concluded was brought about by reflex inhibition through the vagus, an important contribution to the knowledge of the mechanism of shock.

815 BEZOLD, ALBERT VON. 1836–1868
Untersuchungen über die Innervation des Herzens. Leipzig, *W. Engelmann*, 1863.
Discovery of the accelerator or excitatory nerve fibres of the heart (pp. 191–232), "Bezold's ganglia".

816 CHAUVEAU, JEAN BAPTISTE AUGUSTE. 1827–1917, & MAREY, ÉTIENNE JULES. 1830–1904
Appareils et expériences cardiographiques. *Mém. Acad. imp. de Méd. (Paris)*, 1863, **26,** 268–319.
First direct records of the heart impulse by means of a "cardiac sound" and recording tambours, which wrote on a moving drum covered with smoked paper.

817 CZERMAK, JOHANN NEPOMUK. 1828–1873
Ueber mechanische Vagus-Reizung beim Menschen. *Jena. Z. Med. Naturw.*, 1865–66, **2,** 384–6.
"Czermak's vagus pressure." Czermak found that mechanical pressure on a spot in the carotid triangle in the neck produced lowering of the heart rate.

818 TRAUBE, LUDWIG. 1818–1876
Ueber periodische Thätigkeits-Aeusserungen des vasomotorischen und Hemmungs-Nervencentrums. *Zbl. med. Wiss.*, 1865, **3,** 881–5.
First description of the rhythmic variations in tone of the vaso-constrictor centre (Traube–Hering waves).

819 CYON, ELIE DE. 1842–1912, & LUDWIG, CARL FRIEDRICH WILHELM. 1816–1895
Die Reflexe eines der sensiblen Nerven des Herzens auf die motorischen der Blutgefässe. *Arb. physiol. Anst. Leipzig*, (1866), 1867, **1,** 128–49.
Discovery of the vasomotor reflexes.

819.1 BERNSTEIN, JULIUS. 1839–1917
Über den zeitlichen Verlauf der negativen Schwankung des Nervenstroms. *Pflügers Arch. ges. Physiol.*, 1868, **1,** 173–207.
Bernstein introduced the differential rheotome, and the first electrocardiograms were obtained with it by Marchand in 1877 (No. 823.1).

820 FICK, ADOLPH. 1829–1901
Ueber die Messung des Blutquantums in den Herzventrikeln. *S.B. phys.-med. Ges. Würzburg*, 1870, 16.
Fick's principle for the measurement of cardiac output.

821 SCHMIEDEBERG, Johann Ernst Oswald. 1838–1921
Untersuchungen über einige Giftwirkungen am Froschherzen. *Arb. physiol. Anst. Leipzig*, (1870), 1871, **5,** 41–52.
First investigation of the effect of poisons on the frog's heart. In some cases Schmiedeberg found that stimulation of the vagus after administration of poisons produced acceleration of the heart rate.

822 BOWDITCH, Henry Pickering. 1840–1911
Ueber die Eigenthümlichkeiten der Reizbarkeit, welche die Muskelfasern des Herzens zeigen. *Arb. physiol. Anst. Leipzig*, (1871), 1872, **6,** 139–76.
Bowditch established the "all-or-nothing" principle of heart muscle contraction. He founded, at Harvard, the first physiological laboratory in the United States.

823 TALMA, Sape, 1847–1918
Beiträge zur Theorie der Herz- und Arterientöne. *Ditsch. Arch. klin. Med.*, 1874, **15,** 77–98.

823.1 MARCHAND, Richard.
Beiträge zur Kenntniss der Reizwelle und Contractionswelle des Herzmuskels. *Pflügers Arch. ges. Physiol.*, 1877, **15,** 511–36.
Marchand obtained the first electrocardiogram. Using the differential rheotome he measured the time course of the potential variations from the frog's heart.

824 BURDON-SANDERSON, *Sir* John Scott. 1828–1905, & PAGE, Frederick James Montague. 1848–1907
On the time-relations of the excitatory process in the ventricle of the heart of the frog. *J. Physiol.* (*Lond.*), 1879–80, **2,** 384–435.
These workers were among the first to study the action currents of the heart, and made the first records (with the capillary electrometer) of the minute-electrical current produced by the beating of the heart. See also No. 831.

825 TALMA, Sape. 1847–1918
Zur Genese der Herztöne. *Pflüg. Arch. ges. Physiol.*, 1880, **23,** 275–8.

826 RINGER, Sidney. 1834–1910
Regarding the action of hydrate of soda, hydrate of ammonia, and hydrate of potash on the ventricle of the frog's heart. *J. Physiol.* (*Lond.*), 1880–82, **3,** 195–202.
"Ringer's solution."

827 MARTIN, Henry Newell. 1848–1896
On a method of isolating the mammalian heart. *Science*, 1881, **2,** 228.
Martin devised a form of perfusion of the isolated mammalian heart – one of the greatest single contributions ever to come from an American physiological laboratory. This made possible his later work on the heart.

828 ——. Observations on the direct influence of variations of arterial pressure upon the rate of beat of the mammalian heart. *Stud. Biol. Lab. Johns Hopk. Univ.*, 1882, **2,** 213–33.

829 GASKELL, Walter Holbrook. 1847–1914
On the rhythm of the heart of the frog, and on the nature of the action of the vagus nerve. *Phil. Trans.*, 1882, **173,** 993–1033.
Croonian Lectures, 1881. Gaskell's classical memoir on the muscles and nerves of the heart included a description of "Gaskell's nerves", the accelerator nerves of the heart. He showed that the motor impulses from the nerve ganglia in the sinus venosus influence the heart rhythm but do not originate cardiac movements, which are due to the rhythmic contraction of the heart muscle.

830 GASKELL, Walter Holbrook. 1847–1914.
On the innervation of the heart. *J. Physiol. (Lond.)*, 1883–84, **4,** 43–127.
In his important investigation of the innervation of the heart, Gaskell showed that the efferent vasconstrictor fibres originated from the lateral horn of the spinal cord.

831 BURDON-SANDERSON, *Sir* John Scott. 1828–1905, & PAGE, Frederick James Montague. 1848–1907.
On the electrical phenomena of the excitatory process in the heart of the frog and of the tortoise, as investigated photographically. *J. Physiol. (Lond.)*, 1883–84, **4,** 327–38.
See No. 824.

832 MARTIN, Henry Newell. 1848–1896
The direct influence of gradual variations of temperature upon the rate of beat of the dog's heart. *Phil. Trans.*, 1883, **174,** 663–88.
Martin was among the first to study the effect of temperature changes upon the isolated heart.

833 WALLER, Augustus Désiré. 1856–1922
A demonstration in man of electromotive changes accompanying the heart's beat. *J. Physiol. (Lond.)*, 1887, **8,** 229–34.
Waller was first to use electrodes and leads in demonstrating the action currents of the heart, avoiding the necessity of opening the chests of laboratory animals and preparing the way for present-day clinical electrocardiography. He obtained the first electrocardiogram in man.

834 MACKENZIE, *Sir* James. 1853–1925
Pulsation in the veins, with the description of a method for graphically recording them. *J. Path. Bact.*, 1892, **1,** 53–89.
The phlebograph, which developed into the polygraph. With it Mackenzie obtained simultaneous tracings of the pulsations of the jugular vein and radial artery.

835 ROY, Charles Smart. 1854–1897, & ADAMI, John George. 1862–1926
Contributions to the physiology and pathology of the mammalian heart. *Phil. Trans.*, 1892, ser. B., **183,** 199–298.

836 HIS, Wilhelm, *Jnr.* 1863–1934
Die Thätigkeit des embryonalen Herzens und deren Bedeutung für die Lehre von der Herzbewegung beim Erwachsenen. *Arb. med. Klin. Leipzig*, 1893, 14–50.
His described the auriculoventricular bundle which was later named after him. English translation in F. A. Willius and T. E. Keys, *Cardiac classics*, 1941, p. 695.

837 KENT, Albert Frank Stanley. 1863–1958
Researches on the structure and function of the mammalian heart. *J. Physiol. (Lond.)*, 1893, **14,** 233–54.
Kent discovered the auriculoventricular bundle ("bundle of Kent"), a narrow band of muscle between the auricles and ventricles of the heart. Its purpose is to act as a bridge for contractile impulses between the auricles and ventricles.

838 BRAUN, Ludwig. 1867–1936
Ueber Herzbewegung und Herzstoss. Jena, *G. Fischer*, 1898.
First employment of cinematograph to record the cardiac changes during all phases of heart contraction.

839 MacCALLUM, John Bruce. 1876–1906
On the muscular architecture and growth of the ventricles of the heart. In *Contributions to the science of medicine. Dedicated . . . to W. H. Welch.* Baltimore, 1900, pp. 307–35.

A classical account of the development and architecture of the muscular wall of the heart.

840 EINTHOVEN, Willem. 1860–1927
Un nouveau galvanomètre. *Arch. néerl. Sci. exactes nat.*, 1901, 2 sér., **6,** 625–33.

One of the most distinguished of modern physiologists, Einthoven directed much of his research to the development and perfection of recording instruments. His most famous work was in connexion with his string galvanometer, a perfection of the instrument invented by J. S. C. Schweigger, of Halle. Einthoven was awarded the Nobel Prize in 1924.

841 FRIEDENTHAL, Hans Wilhelm Karl. 1870–
Ueber die Entfernung der extracardialen Herznerven bei Säugethieren. *Arch. Anat. Physiol., Physiol. Abt.*, 1902, 135–45.

842 EINTHOVEN, Willem. 1860–1927
The string galvanometer and the human electro-cardiogram. *K. Akad Wet. Amst., Proc. Sect. Sci.*, 1903–04, **6,** 107–15.

Einthoven showed how his string galvanometer could portray the electrical changes occurring in the human heart. Modern electrocardiography became a reality through his work and the string galvanometer finally displaced the capillary electrometer in the measurement of the electric current produced by the contracting heart. Also in *Ann. Physik*, 1903, **12,** 1059.

843 FRANK, Otto. 1865–
Die unmittelbare Registrierung der Herztöne. *Münch. med. Wschr.*, 1904, **51,** 953–4.

The first study.

843.1 CREMER, Max. 1865–1935
Über die direkte Ableitung der Aktionsströme des menschlichen Herzens vom Oesophagus und über das Elektrokardiogramm des Fötus. *Münch. med. Wschr.*, 1906, **53,** 811–13.

Foetal electrocardiogram recorded. Cremer was also the first to record an electrocardiogram with an electrode in the oesophagus.

844 KEITH, *Sir* Arthur. 1866–1955, & FLACK, Martin William. 1882–1931
The form and nature of the muscular connections between the primary divisions of the vertebrate heart. *J. Anat. Physiol. (Lond.)*, 1906–07, **41,** 172–89.

Discovery of the sino-auricular node, the "pacemaker of the heart". Reprinted in Willius & Keys: *Cardiac classics*, 1941, pp. 747–62.

845 TAWARA, Sunao. 1873–
Das Reizleitungssystem des Säugethierherzens. Jena, *G. Fischer*, 1906.

Tawara discovered and described the auriculoventricular node – "node of Tawara".

846 EINTHOVEN, Willem. 1860–1927
Die Registrierung der menschlichen Herztone mittels des Saitengalvanometers. *Pflüg. Arch. ges. Physiol.*, 1907, **117,** 461–72.

Phonocardiography.

847 MACKENZIE, *Sir* JAMES. 1853–1925
The extra-systole. A contribution to the functional pathology of the primitive cardiac tissue. *Quart. J. Med.*, 1907–08, **1,** 131–49, 481–90.

848 EPPINGER, HANS. 1879–1946, & ROTHBERGER, CARL JULIUS. 1871–
Ueber die Folgen der Durchschneidung der Tawaraschen Schenkel der Reizleitungssystems. *Z. klin. Med.*, 1910, **70,** 1–20.
First experimental study of the electrocardiographic changes in bundle-branch block.

849 ABEL, JOHN JACOB. 1857–1938
On the action of drugs and the function of the anterior lymph hearts in cardiectomized frogs. *J. Pharmacol.*, 1913, **3,** 581–608.

850 ——. & TURNER, BENJAMIN BERNARD. 1871–
On the influence of the lymph hearts upon the action of convulsant drugs in cardiectomized frogs. II. *J. Pharmacol.*, 1914, **6,** 91–122.

851 BAINBRIDGE, FRANCIS ARTHUR. 1874–1921
On some cardiac reflexes. *J. Physiol.* (*Lond.*), 1914, **48,** 332–40.
Bainbridge found that cardiac reflex action is produced by inhibition of vagus tone and excitation of the accelerator nerves.

852 SMITH, FRED M. 1888–
The ligation of coronary arteries with electrocardiographic study. *Arch. intern. Med.*, 1918, **22,** 8–27.

853 STARLING, ERNEST HENRY. 1866–1927
The Linacre lecture on the law of the heart. London, *Longmans, Green & Co.*, 1918.
Starling's "law of the heart".

854 LEWIS, *Sir* THOMAS. 1881–1945
The mechanism and graphic registration of the heart beat. London, *Shaw & Sons*, 1920.
Sir Thomas Lewis was a pioneer in the application to clinical medicine of the electrocardiographic method for examination of the heart. His book is both an exhaustive treatise on the subject and a valuable bibliographical source. The above is the second edition of *The mechanism of the heart beat*, 1911; third edition, 1925.

855 GROSS, LOUIS. 1894–
The blood supply to the heart. New York, *P. B. Hoeber*, [1921].

856 SPALTEHOLZ, KARL WERNER. 1861–1940
Die Arterien der Herwand. Leipzig, *S. Hirzel*, 1924.

856.1 DALE, *Sir* HENRY HALLETT. 1875–1968, & SCHUSTER, EDGAR J. H. 1880–1969.
A double perfusion-pump. *J. Physiol.* (*Lond.*), 1928, **64,** 356–64.
Mechanical heart.

857 GROLLMAN, ARTHUR. 1901–
The determination of the cardiac output of man by the use of acetylene. *Amer. J. Physiol.*, 1929, **88,** 432–45.
Grollman introduced the acetylene method of determination of cardiac output.

858 ——. The cardiac output of man in health and disease. Springfield *C. C. Thomas*, 1932.

859 McMICHAEL, *Sir* JOHN. 1904– , & SHARPEY-SCHAFER, EDWARD PETER. 1908–1963
Cardiac output in man by a direct Fick method. *Brit. Heart J.*, 1944, **6,** 33–40.

859.1 DODRILL, FOREST DEWEY. 1902– , *et al.*
Some physiologic aspects of the artificial heart problem. *J. thorac. Surg.*, 1952, **24,** 134–50.
First successful apparatus for the complete bypass of the heart. With E. Hill and R. Gerisch.

Haematology

See also 2011–2028, BLOOD TRANSFUSION; 3048–3161.1, DISORDERS OF THE BLOOD.

860 LEEUWENHOEK, ANTONJ VAN. 1632–1723
Microscopical observations concerning blood, milk, bones, the brain, spittle, and cuticula, etc. *Phil. Trans.*, 1674, **9,** 121–8.
First really accurate description of the red blood corpuscles, which Swammerdam had noted in 1658.

861 BOYLE, ROBERT. 1627–1691
Memoirs for the natural history of humane blood, especially the spirit of that liquor. London, *S. Smith*, 1683.
In this, Boyle's most important medical work, he summarized the contemporary knowledge of blood chemistry.

862 MENGHINI, VINCENZO.
De ferrearum particularum sede in sanguine. *Bonon. Sci. Art. Inst. Acad. Comment.*, 1746, **2,** pt. 2, 244–66.
Discovery of iron in the blood.

863 HEWSON, WILLIAM. 1739–1774
An experimental inquiry into the properties of the blood. Part III. A description of the red particles of the blood. London, *T. Cadell*, 1771.
Hewson established the fact that fibrinogen is responsible for the clotting of blood; he first described the lymphocyte.

863.1 WELLS, WILLIAM CHARLES. 1757–1817
Observations and experiments on the colour of blood. *Phil. Trans.*, 1797, **87,** 416–31.
Wells showed that the colouring matter in the blood was not iron but a complex organic substance subsequently identified as haematin.

864 DONNÉ, ALEXANDRE. 1801–1878
De l'origine des globules du sang, de leur mode de formation et de leur fin. *C.R. Acad. Sci.* (*Paris*), 1842, **14,** 366–68.
Announces the discovery of the blood-platelets.

865 BUCHANAN, ANDREW. 1798–1882
On the coagulation of blood and other fibriniferous liquids. *Lond. med. Gaz.*, 1845, n.s. **1,** 617–21.
Buchanan extracted the fibrin ferment of blood, He showed that it was capable of coagulating blood and other serous fluids not in themselves coagulable.

865.1 REICHERT, KARL BOGISLAUS. 1811–1883
Beobachtungen über eine eiweissartige Substanz in Krystallform. *Müller's Arch. Anat. Physiol. wiss. Med.*, 1849, 197–251.
Reichert obtained haemoglobin crystals in the guinea-pig.

866 FUNKE, OTTO. 1828–1879
Ueber das Milzvenenblut. *Z. rat. Med.*, 1851, n.F. **1,** 172–218; 1852, **2,** 198–217.
Discovery of haemoglobin. (Title of second paper: Neue Beobachtungen über die Krystalle des Milzvenen- und Fisch-Blutes).

867 VIERORDT, KARL. 1818–1884
Neue Methode der quantitativen mikroskopischen Analyse des Blutes. *Arch. physiol. Heilk.*, 1852, **11,** 26–46.
Vierodt was the first to devise an exact method of enumerating the red blood corpuscles. See also his later paper: Zählungen der Blutkörperchen des Menschen, in the same volume, pp. 326–31.

868 WELCKER, HERMANN. 1822–1897
Bestimmungen der Menge des Körperblutes und der Blutfärbekraft, sowie Bestimmungen von Zahl, Maass Oberfläche und Volum des einzelnen Blutkörperchens bei Thieren und bei Menschen. *Z. rat. Med.*, 1858, 3 R., **4,** 145–67; 1863, 3 R., **20,** 257–307.
Welcker was the first to determine the total blood volume and the volume of the normal red blood cells, Earlier paper in *Vjschr. prakt. Heilk.*, 1854, **44,** 63.

869 SCHMIDT, ALEXANDER. 1831–1894
Ueber den Faserstoff und die Ursachen seiner Gerinnung. *Arch. Anat. Physiol. wiss. Med.*, 1861, 545–87, 675–721; 1862, 428–69, 533–564.

870 HOPPE-SEYLER, ERNST FELIX IMMANUEL. 1825–1895
Ueber das Verhalten des Blutfarbstoffe im Spectrum des Sonnenlichtes. *Virchows Arch. path. Anat.*, 1862, **23,** 446–49.
See No. 873.

871 LISTER, JOSEPH, 1*st Baron Lister*. 1827–1912
On the coagulation of the blood. *Proc. roy. Soc.* (*Lond.*), (1862), 1863, **12,** 580–611.
In his Croonian Lecture Lister exploded the theory that blood coagulation is due to ammonia and showed that, in the blood vessels, it depends upon their injury. He further showed that by carrying out the strictest precautions he could keep blood free from putrefaction indefinitely, thus supporting his theory that bacteria were the cause of wound suppuration.

872 STOKES, *Sir* GEORGE GABRIEL. 1819–1903
On the reduction and oxidation of the colouring matter of the blood. *Proc. roy. Soc.* (*Lond.*), 1863–64, **13,** 355–64.
Discovery that oxygen can be removed from haemoglobin by reducing agents.

873 HOPPE-SEYLER, Ernst Felix Immanuel. 1825–1895
Ueber den chemischen und optischen Eigenschaften des Blutfarbstoffs. *Virchows Arch. path. Anat.*, 1864, **29,** 233–35, 597–600.
Hoppe-Seyler obtained haemoglobin in crystalline form and made other importand discoveries in haematology. See also No. 870.

873.1 BIZZOZERO, Giulio. 1846–1901
Sulla funzione ematopoietica del midollo delle ossa. *R. C. R. Ist. Lomb. Sci. Lett.*, 1868, 2 ser., **1,** 815–18.
Bizzozero demonstrated that erythropoiesis and leucopoiesis take place in the bone marrow.

873.2 NEUMANN, Ernst. 1834–1918
Ueber die Bedeutung des Knochenmarkes für die Blutbildung. *Zbl. med. Wiss.*, 1868, **6,** 689; *Arch. Heilk.*, 1869, **10,** 68–102.
Independently of Bizzozero (No. 873.1), Neumann showed that erythropoiesis and leucopoiesis take place in the bone marrow.

874 PREYER, Thierry Wilhelm. 1841–1897
Die Blutkrystalle. Jena, *Mauke*, 1871.

875 OSLER, *Sir* William, *Bart.* 1849–1919
An account of certain organisms occurring in the liquor sanguinis. *Proc. roy. Soc. (Lond.)*, (1873), 1874, **22,** 391–98.
One of the best early descriptions of the blood platelets was given by Osler. He noticed that white thrombi were almost entirely composed of them.

876 MALASSEZ, Louis Charles. 1842–1909
Nouvelle méthode de numération des globules rouges et des globules blancs du sang. *Arch. Physiol. norm. path.*, 1874, 2 sér., **1,** 32–52.
Malassez designed the first haemocytometer, the instrument being given that name by Gowers, who modified it in 1877.

877 HAMMARSTEN, Olof. 1841–1932
Undersökningar af de s.k. fibringeneratorerna fibrinet samt fibrinogenets koagulation. *Upsala LäkFören. Förh.*, 1875–76, **11,** 538–79.
Investigating the mechanism of blood coagulation, Hammarsten showed it to be accomplished by the splitting up of fibrinogen into fibrin and other substances.

878 GOWERS, *Sir* William Richard. 1845–1915
The numeration of blood corpuscles and the effect of iron and phosphorus on the blood. *Practitioner*, 1878, **21,** 1–17.
Gowers invented the modern haemoglobinometer, modified in 1901 by J. S. Haldane (see No. 891). Previously Hoppe-Seyler had used a haematinometer.

879 HAYEM, Georges. 1841–1933
Recherches sur l'évolution des hématies dans le sang de l'homme et des vertébrés. *Arch. Physiol. norm. path.*, 1878, **5,** 692–734.
First accurate counts of the blood platelets.

880 EHRLICH, Paul. 1854–1915
Methodologische Beiträge zur Physiologie und Pathologie der verschiedenen Formen der Leukocyten. *Z. klin. Med.*, 1879–80, **1,** 553–560.
Foundation of the differential blood count technique.

881 BIZZOZERO, Giulio. 1846–1901
Su di un nuovo elemento morfologico del sangue dei mammiferi e della sua importanza nella trombosi e nella coagulazione. *Osservatore*, 1882, **17,** 785–87; **18,** 97–99.

Bizzozero gave the blood-platelets their name and found that they play a part in blood coagulation. A German translation with additions is in *Virchows Arch. path. Anat.*, 1882, **90,** 261–332.

882 GRÉHANT, Nestor. 1838–1910, & QUINQUAUD, Charles Eugène. 1841–1894
Mesure du volume de sang contenu dans l'organisme d'un mammifère vivant. *C. R. Acad. Sci.* (*Paris*), 1882, **94,** 1450–53.

A method of determining blood volume with carbon monoxide.

883 HAYEM, Georges. 1841–1933
Du sang et de ses altérations anatomiques. Paris, *G. Masson*, 1889.

884 ARTHUS, Nicolas Maurice. 1862–1945, & PAGÈS, Calixte.
Nouvelle théorie chimique de la coagulation du sang. *Arch. Physiol. norm. path.*, 1890, 5 *ser.*, **2,** 739–46.

First demonstration of the essential role of calcium in the mechanism of blood coagulation.

885 HEDIN, Sven Gustaf. 1859–1933
Der Hämatokrit, ein neuer Apparat zur Untersuchung des Blutes. *Skand. Arch. Physiol.*, 1890–91, **2,** 134–40.

Hedin's haematocrit. He first briefly described it in *Upsala LäkFören. Förh.*, 1889, **24,** 440.

886 HOWELL, William Henry. 1860–1945
The life history of the formed elements of the blood, especially the red blood corpuscles. *J. Morph.*, 1890–91, **4,** 57–116.

Includes description of "Howell's bodies" seen in mature erythrocytes and called also "Howell-Jolly bodies" after the later description by J. M. J. Jolly.

887 EHRLICH, Paul. 1854–1915
Farbenanalytische Untersuchungen zur Histologie und Klinik des Blutes. Berlin, *A. Hirschwald*, 1891.

Extension of Ehrlich's work on the differential blood count.

888 SCHMIDT, Alexander. 1831–1894
Zur Blutlehre. Leipzig, *F. C. W. Vogel*, 1892.

Schmidt established several new facts regarding blood coagulation.

889 LANDSTEINER, Karl. 1868–1943
Zur Kenntniss der antifermentativen, lytischen und agglutinierenden Wirkungen des Blutserums und der Lymphe. *Zbl. Bakt.*, 1900, **27,** 357–62.

Landsteiner discovered that human blood contains iso-agglutinins capable of agglutinating other human red blood cells. He divided human blood into three groups. He was awarded the Nobel Prize for medicine in 1930

890 TALLQVIST, Theodor Waldemar. 1871–1927
Ein einfaches Verfahren zur directen Schätzung der Färbestärke des Blutes. *Z. klin. Med.*, 1900, **40,** 137–41.

Tallqvist's haemoglobin scale.

891 HALDANE, John Scott. 1860–1936
The colorimetric determination of haemoglobin. *J. Physiol.* (*Lond.*), 1901, 26, 497–504.
Haldane's haemoglobinometer and method for determination of haemoglobin.

892 SAHLI, Hermann. 1856–1933
Über ein einfaches und exactes Verfahren der klinischen Hämometrie. *Verh. dtsch. Congr. inn. Med.*, 1902, **20,** 230–34.
Sahli's method for the determination of haemoglobin.

893 DECASTELLO, Alfred von. 1872– , & STURLI, Adriano.
Ueber die Isoagglutinine im Serum gesunder und kranker Menschen. *Münch. med. Wschr.*, 1902, **49,** 1090–95.
Following Landsteiner's division of human blood into three groups, Decastello and Sturli discovered a fourth (the rarest) group.

894 MORAWITZ, Paul Oskar. 1879–1936
Beiträge zur Kenntniss der Blutgerinnung. *Dtsch. Arch. klin. Med.*, 1903–4, **79,** 1–28, 215–33, 432–42.
Morawitz's theory of blood coagulation.

895 VAUGHAN, Victor Clarence. 1851–1929
On the appearance and significance of certain granules in the erythrocytes of man. *J. med. Res.*, 1903, **10,** 342–66.
Reticulocytes described.

896 JANSKÝ, Jan. 1873–1921
Haematologické studie u psychotiku. *Sborn. Klinický*, 1906–07, **8,** 85–139.
Janský demonstrated that blood could be classified into 4 groups; he named these O, A, B, and AB. His work, published in a little-known journal, was at first overlooked, and in 1910 Moss independently published work on exactly similar lines. A French resumé of the paper is in the above journal, pp. 131–33, and a German summary in *Jb. Neurol. Psychiat.*, 1907, 1028.

897 WRIGHT, James Homer. 1871–1928
The origin and nature of the blood plates. *Boston med. surg. J.*, 1906, **154,** 643–45.
Discovery of the rôle of the megakaryocytes in the formation of the blood platelets.

898 DUNGERN, Emil von. 1876– , & HIRSZFELD, Ludwik. 1884–1954
Ueber Vererbung gruppenspezifischer Strukturen des Blutes. *Z. ImmunForsch.*, 1910, **6,** 284–92.
Proof that blood groups are inherited according to Mendelian laws.

899 HOWELL, William Henry. 1860–1945
The preparation and properties of thrombin, together with observations on antithrombin and prothrombin. *Amer. J. Physiol.*, 1910, **26,** 453–73.

900 MOSS, William Lorenzo. 1876–1957
Studies on isoagglutinins and isohemolysins. *Johns Hopk. Hosp. Bull.*, 1910, **21,** 63–70.
Moss showed that the blood of all individuals could be placed into one of four groups. His classification has been the one most commonly used until recently. The work was similar to that of Janský and completed before the writer learned of the latter's publication.

901 PRICE-JONES, Cecil. 1863–1943
The variation in the sizes of red blood cells. *Brit. med. J.*, 1910, **2,** 1418–19.

Price-Jones described a method for the direct measurement of red blood cells, which has led to the term "Price-Jones curve." See also his book, *Red blood cell diameters*, London, 1933.

902 HOWELL, William Henry. 1860–1945
The role of antithrombin and thromboplastin (thromboplastic substance) in the coagulation of blood. *Amer. J. Physiol.*, 1911–12, **29,** 187–209.

903 KEITH, Norman Macdonnell. 1885– , *et al.*
A method for the determination of plasma and blood volume. *Arch. intern. Med.*, 1915, **16,** 547–76.

N. M. Keith, L. G. Rowntree, and J. T. Geraghty devised a method for determination of plasma and blood volume, which includes the injection of a dye.

904 McLEAN, Jay. 1890–1957
The thromboplastic action of cephalin. *Amer. J. Physiol.*, 1916, **41,** 250–57.

McLean extracted from dog liver a substance which retarded blood coagulation *in vitro* and which, after further work by Howell and Holt (No. 905) was named heparin.

905 HOWELL, William Henry. 1860–1945, & HOLT, Luther Emmett. 1855–1924
Two new factors in blood coagulation – heparin and pro-antithrombin. *Amer. J. Physiol.*, 1918–19, **47,** 328–41.

Isolation of heparin.

906 PAPPENHEIM, Artur. 1870–1916
Morphologische Hämatologie. Hrsg. von H. Hirschfeld. Bd. 1. Leipzig, *W. Klinkhardt*, 1919.

907 HAYEM, Georges. 1841–1933
L'hématoblaste, troisième élement du sang. Paris, *Presse univ. de France*, 1923.

Hayem first named the haematoblasts in 1877 (*Mém. Soc. Biol.* (*Paris*), 1877, **29,** 97). His view, reiterated in 1923, was that they were the early stages of red blood cells and regenerated the blood.

907.1 BERNSTEIN, Felix. 1878–
Ergebnisse einer biostatischen zusammenfassenden Betrachtung über die erblichen Blutstrukturen des Menschen. *Klin. Wschr.*, 1924, **3,** 1495–97.

Bernstein determined the exact method of inheritance of the ABO blood groups.

908 MAXIMOW, Alexander. 1874–1928
Relation of blood cells to connective tissues and endothelium. *Physiol. Rev.*, 1924, **4,** 533–63.

Maximow's blood regeneration theory.

909 DOAN, Charles Austin. 1896– , CUNNINGHAM, Robert Sydney. 1891– , & SABIN, Florence Rena. 1871–1953
Experimental studies on the origin and maturation of avian and mammalian red blood-cells. *Contr. Embryol. Carneg. Instn*, 1925, **16,** 163–226.

910 LANDSTEINER, KARL. 1868–1943, & LEVINE, PHILIP. 1900–
A new agglutinable factor differentiating individual human bloods. *Proc. Soc. exp. Biol.* (*N.Y.*), 1927, **24,** 600–02.

Discovery of M and N agglutinogens. See also the same journal, pp. 941–42.

911 BERGENHEM, BENGT LUDVIG. 1898– , & FÅHRÆUS, ROBERT [ROBIN] SANNO. 1888–
Über spontane Hämolysinbildung im Blut, unter besonderer Berücksichtigung der Physiologie der Milz. *Z. ges. exp. Med.*, 1936, **97,** 555–87.

Lysolecithin found in normal blood.

912 BOYD, WILLIAM CLOUSER. 1903–
Blood groups. *Tab. biol.* (*Amst.*), 1939, **17,** 113–240.

912.1 LEVINE, PHILIP. 1900– , & STETSON, RUFUS E.
An unusual case of intra-group agglutination. *J. Amer. med. Ass.*, 1939, **113,** 126–27.

Discovery of the Rh antigen.

912.2 LANDSTEINER, KARL. 1868–1943, & WIENER, ALEXANDER SOLOMON. 1907–
An agglutinable factor in human blood recognized by immune sera for Rhesus blood. *Proc. Soc. exp. Biol.* (*N.Y.*), 1940, **43,** 223.

Recognition of the Rh antigen.

912.3 MOUREAU, PAUL.
Recherches sur un nouvel hémo-agglutinogène du sang humain. *Acta biol. belg.*, 1941, **1,** 123–28.

Moureau discovered the Rh factor independently of Levine and others whose work was not known to him owing to the military occupation of Belgium. See also his paper in *Amer. J. clin. Path.*, 1946, **16,** 373–79.

912.4 COHN, EDWIN JOSEPH. 1892– , *et al.*
Chemical, clinical, and immunological studies on the products of human plasma fractionation. *J. clin. Invest.*, 1944, **23,** 417–606.

Discovery of the blood derivatives.

912.5 OWREN, PAUL ARNOR. 1905–
The coagulation of blood. Investigations on a new clotting factor. *Acta med. scand.*, 1947, Suppl. 194, 1–327.

Discovery of Factor V. Preliminary account in *Proc. Norwegian Acad. Sci.*, 1941, **17,** 21.

913 WALSH, ROBERT JOHN, & MONTGOMERY, CARMEL M.
A new human *iso*-agglutinin subdividing the *MN* blood groups. *Nature* (*Lond.*), 1947, **160,** 504–5.

S blood-group antigen.

For history, see 1572, 1588.4, 3156

914–971 RESPIRATORY SYSTEM

914 BOYLE, ROBERT. 1627–1691
New experiments physico-mechanicall touching the spring of the air. Oxford, *H. Hall for T. Robinson*, 1660.

Boyle showed the effects of the elasticity, compressibility, and weight of air. He investigated its function in respiration, combustion, and conveyance of sound. The importance of this work in the history of respiration is Boyle's demonstration that air is essential for life.

915 MALPIGHI, Marcello. 1628–1694

De pulmonibus observationes anatomicae. Bononiae, 1661.

Malpighi demonstrated that the pulmonary tissues are vesicular in nature and showed that the trachea ends in bronchial filaments. His *De pulmonibus* includes his demonstration of the capillary anastomosis between arteries and veins (See No. 760).

916 HOOKE, Robert. 1635–1703

An account of an experiment of preserving animals alive by blowing through their lungs with bellows. *Phil. Trans.*, 1667, **2,** 539–40.

By blowing air from a bellows over the exposed lungs of a dog, Hooke proved that respiratory motion is not necessary to maintain life, but that the essential feature of respiration lies in certain blood changes in the lungs. Reprinted in J. F. Fulton's *Selected readings in the history of physiology*, 2nd. ed., 1966, pp. 121–23.

917 HALLER, Albrecht von. 1708–1777

De respiratione experimenta anatomica, quibus aëris inter pulmonem et pleuram absentia demonstratur et musculorum intercostalium internorum officium adseritur. 2 pts. Gottingae, *A. Vandenhoeck*, [1746–1747].

First investigation of the action of the intercostal muscles in respiration.

918 HAMBERGER, Georg Erhard. 1697–1755

De respirationis mechanismo et usu genuino. Jenae, *apud J. C. Croekerum*, 1748.

919 BLACK, Joseph. 1728–1799

Dissertatio medica inauguralis de humore acido a cibis orto, et magnesia alba. Edinburgi, *G. Hamilton & J. Balfour*, 1754.

Isolation of carbon dioxide.

920 PRIESTLEY, Joseph. 1733–1804

Observations on different kinds of air. *Phil. Trans.*, 1772, **62,** 147–264.

The isolation of oxygen was first achieved by Priestley. He also demonstrated that plants immersed in water give off oxygen and that this gas is essential for animal life.

921 RUTHERFORD, Daniel. 1749–1819

De aëre fixo dicto, aut mephitico. Edinburgi, *Balfour & Smellie*, 1772.

Discovery of nitrogen.

922 LAVOISIER, Antoine Laurent. 1743–1794

Mémoire sur la nature du principe qui se combine avec les métaux pendant leur calcination, et qui en augmente le poids. *Hist. Acad. roy. Sci.*, (1775), 1778, 520–26.

Although Priestley isolated oxygen, it was Lavoisier who discovered its real significance. He showed the true nature of the interchange of gases in the lungs and exploded Stahl's phlogiston theory. Lavoisier was guillotined during the French Revolution.

923 ——. Mémoire sur la formation de l'acide, nommé air fixe ou acide crayeux, et que je désignerai désormais sous le nom d'acide du charbon. *Hist. Acad. roy. Sci.*, (1781), 1784, 448–67.

924 ——. Mémoire sur l'affinité du principe oxygine avec les différentes substances auxquelles il est susceptible de s'unir. *Hist. Acad. roy. Sci.*, (1782), 1785, 530–40.

925 CAVENDISH, Henry. 1731–1810
Experiments on air. *Phil. Trans.*, 1784, **74,** 119–53.
Cavendish isolated hydrogen in 1766, and later demonstrated the composition of air.

926 HASSENFRATZ, Jean Henri. 1755–1827
Mémoire sur la combinaison de l'oxigène avec le carbone et l'hydrogène du sang, sur la dissolution de l'oxigène dans le sang, et sur la manière dont le calorique se dégage. *Ann. Chim.*, 1791, **9,** 261–74.
Hassenfratz, a pupil of Lagrange, maintained that the oxidation of carbon and hydrogen took place in the blood, and not in the lungs as taught by others.

927 REISSEISEN, Franz Daniel. 1773–1828, & SOEMMERRING, Samuel Thomas. 1755–1830
Über den Bau der Lungen. Berlin, *in den Vossischen Buchhandlung*, 1808.
In 1804 the Berlin Akademie der Naturwissenschaften offered a prize for the best essay on the structure and function of the lungs. The prize was won by Reisseisen, while Soemmerring received honourable mention. The texts of both works were published in one volume; Soemmerring's essay was entitled "Ueber die Structur, die Verrichtung und den Gebrauch der Lungen".

928 LEGALLOIS, Julien Jean César. 1770–1814
Expériences sur le principe de la vie. Paris, *D'Hautel*, 1812.
Legallois described the action of the vagus nerve on respiration. He showed that bilateral section of the vagus can produce fatal broncho-pneumonia. The above work includes (p. 37) his location of the respiratory centre in the medulla. English translation, Philadelphia, 1813.

929 MAGNUS, Heinrich Gustav. 1802–1870
Ueber die im Blute enthaltenen Gase, Sauerstoffe, Stickstoff, und Kohlensäure. *Ann. Phys. Chem.* (*Leipzig*), 1837, **12,** 583–606.
First quantitative analysis of the blood gases. Magnus proved that the arterial blood contains a higher concentration of oxygen than venous blood and that the latter had a higher carbon dioxide content.

930 HUTCHINSON, John. 1811–1861
On the capacity of the lungs, and on the respiratory functions, with a view of establishing a precise and easy method of detecting disease by the spirometer. *Med.-chir. Trans.*, 1846, **29,** 137–252.
Invention of the spirometer, making possible the determination of the vital capacity of the lungs. Hutchinson's work first appeared in summary form in *Lancet*, 1844, **1,** 390–91, 567–70.

931 SCHIFF, Moritz. 1823–1896
Die Ursache der Lungenveränderung nach Durchschneidung der pneumogastrischen Nerven. *Arch. physiol. Heilk.*, 1847, **6,** 690–721, 769–804.
Study of the effect of section of the vagus on respiration. See also No. 933.

932 REGNAULT, Henri Victor. 1810–1878, & REISET, Jules.
Recherches chimiques sur la respiration des animaux des diverses classes. *Ann. Chim. Phys.*, 1849, 3 sér., **26,** 299–519.
First determination of the respiratory quotient.

933 SCHIFF, Moritz. 1823–1896
Ueber den Einfluss der Vagusdurchschneidung auf das Lungengewebe. *Arch. physiol. Heilk.*, 1850, **9,** 625–62.
See No. 931.

934 MEYER, Lothar. 1830–1895
Die Gase des Blutes. *Z. rat. Med.*, 1857, **8**, 256–316.

Meyer showed that the oxygen in the blood was not held in simple solution but came off in quantity only when the air pressure was reduced to one fiftieth of an atmosphere.

935 ——. De sanguine oxydo carbonico infesto. Wratislaviae, *typ. Grasii, Barthii et soc.*, 1858.

Investigation of the blood gases.

936 SCHULTZE, Maximilian Johann Sigismund. 1825–1874
Untersuchungen über den Bau der Nasenschleimhaut, namentlich die Structur und Endigungsweise der Geruchsnerven bei dem Menschen und den Wirbelthieren. *Abh. naturf. Ges. Halle*, 1862, **7**, 1–100.

Schultze's classical paper on the nerves to the neuro-epithelium in the special sense organs marks an epoch in histology. He describes the cells of the olfactory mucous membrane, "Schultze's cells".

937 PETTENKOFER, Max Josef von. 1818–1901
Ueber die Respiration. *Ann. Chem. Pharm.* (*Heidelberg*), 1862–63, Suppl. 2, 1–52.

938 ——. & VOIT, Carl von. 1831–1908
Untersuchungen über die Respiration. *Ann. Chem. Pharm.* (*Heidelberg*), 1862–63, Suppl. 2, 52–70.

Pettenkofer and Voit devised an apparatus for their important experiments on respiration and metabolism. They were first to estimate the amounts of protein, fat and carbohydrate broken down in the body.

939 PFLÜGER, Eduard Friedrich Wilhelm. 1829–1910
Zur Gasometrie des Blutes. *Zbl. med. Wiss.*, 1866, **4**, 305–8.

Pflüger showed that respiratory changes take place in the tissues.

940 ——. Ueber die Ursache der Athembewegungen, sowie der Dyspnoë und Apnoë. *Pflüg. Arch. ges. Physiol.*, 1868, **1**, 61–106.

941 HERING, Karl Ewald Konstantin. 1834–1918
Die Selbststeuerung der Athmung durch den *Nervus vagus*. *S.B. k. Akad. Wiss., math.-nat. Cl.* (*Wien*), 1868, 2. Abt., **57**, 672–77.

942 BREUER, Joseph. 1842–1925
Die Selbststeuerung der Athmung durch den *Nervus vagus*. *S.B. k. Akad. Wiss., math.-nat. Cl.* (*Wien*), 1868, 2. Abt., **58**, 909–37.

Hering–Breuer reflex"; see also the previous entry.

943 LUSCHKA, Hubert von. 1820–1875
Der Kehlkopf des Menschen. Tübingen, *H. Laupp*, 1871.

944 BERT, Paul. 1833–1886
La pression barométrique. Recherches de physiologie expérimentale. Paris, *G. Masson*, 1878.

Bert proved that high altitude sickness is due to anoxaemia. English translation, 1943.

945 MARTIN, Henry Newell. 1848–1896, & HARTWELL, Edward Mussey. 1850–1922
On the respiratory function of the intercostal muscles. *J. Physiol.* (*Lond.*), 1879–80, **2**, 24–27.

The important work of Martin and Hartwell on the intercostal muscles settled the controversy regarding their function.

946 ZUCKERKANDL, EMIL. 1849–1910
Normale und pathologische Anatomie der Nasenhöhle und ihrer pneumatischen Anhänge. 2 vols. Wien, *W. Braumüller*, 1882–92.

947 HEAD, *Sir* HENRY. 1861–1940.
On the regulation of respiration. *J. Physiol.* (*Lond.*), 1889, **10,** 1–70, 279–90.
Demonstration of the action of the vagus in respiration.

948 HALDANE, JOHN SCOTT. 1860–1936
A new form of apparatus for measuring the respiratory exchange of animals. *J. Physiol.* (*Lond.*), 1892, **13,** 419–30.
The Haldane apparatus for the analysis of the respiratory gases.

949 HÜFNER, CARL GUSTAV VON. 1840–1908
Neue Versuche zur Bestimmung der Sauerstoffcapacität des Blutfarbstoffs. *Arch. Anat. Physiol., Physiol. Abt.*, 1894, 130–76.
Hüfner showed that 1 gm. haemoglobin combines with 1.34 c.c. oxygen.

950 MOSSO, ANGELO. 1846–1910
Fisiologia dell'uomo sulle Alpi. Studii fatti sul Monte Rosa. Milano, *frat. Treves*, 1897.
Mosso made important investigations on respiration at high altitudes. He considered that the respiratory symptoms produced at high altitudes were due to lack of carbon dioxide. English translation, London, 1898.

951 HALDANE, JOHN SCOTT. 1860–1936
A contribution to the chemistry of haemoglobin and its immediate derivatives. *J. Physiol.* (*Lond.*), 1898, **23,** 298–306.
Potassium ferricyanide method for the determination of oxygen in oxyhaemoglobin.

952 MOSSO, ANGELO. 1846–1910
La physiologie de l'apnée étudiée chez l'homme. *Arch. ital. Biol.*, 1903–04, **40,** 1–30.
First studies of the physiology of apnoea in man.

953 TISSOT, JULES.
Nouvelle méthode de mesure et d'inscription du débit et des mouvements respiratoires de l'homme et des animaux. *J. Physiol. Path. gén.*, 1904, **6,** 688–700.
Tissot spirometer.

954 HALDANE, JOHN SCOTT. 1860–1936, & PRIESTLEY, JOHN GILLIES. 1880–1941
The regulation of the lung-ventilation. *J. Physiol.* (*Lond.*), 1905, **32,** 225–66.
Proof of the regulation of respiration by CO_2 concentration of the alveolar air.

955 DOUGLAS, CLAUDE GORDON. 1882–1963
A method for determining the total respiratory exchange in man. *J. Physiol.* (*Lond.*), 1911, **42,** Proc. Physiol. Soc., xvii-xviii.
Douglas bag.

956 PETERS, *Sir* RUDOLPH ALBERT. 1889–
Chemical nature of specific oxygen capacity in haemoglobin. *J. Physiol.* (*Lond.*), 1912, **44,** 131–49.

957 DOUGLAS, CLAUDE GORDON. 1882–1963, *et al.*
Physiological observations made on Pike's Peak, Colorado, with special reference to adaptation to low barometric pressures. *Phil. Trans. B*, 1913, **203,** 185–318.
With J. S. Haldane, Y. Henderson, and E. C. Schneider.

958 CHRISTIANSEN, JOHANNE OSTENFELD. 1882– , *et al.*
The absorption and dissociation of carbon dioxide by human blood. *J. Physiol.* (*Lond.*), 1914, **48,** 244–71.
CO_2 dissociation curves. With C. G. Douglas and J. S. Haldane.

959 MEYERHOF, OTTO FRITZ. 1884–1951
Ueber das Vorkommen des Coferments des alcoholischen Hefegärung im Muskelgewebe und seine muttmassliche Bedeutung im Atmungsmechanismus. *Hoppe-Seyl. Z. physiol. Chem.*, 1918, **101,** 165–75.
Meyerhof shared the Nobel Prize for physiology with A. V. Hill in 1922 for his work on the physiology of muscle.

960 JOFFE, JACK, & POULTON, EDWARD PALMER. 1883–1939
The partition of CO_2 between plasma and corpuscles in oxygenated and reduced blood. *J. Physiol.* (*Lond.*), 1920–21, **54,** 129–51.

961 HALDANE, JOHN SCOTT. 1860–1936
Respiration. New Haven, *Yale Univ. Press*, 1922.
Second edition, 1935, with J. G. Priestley.

962 HARTRIDGE, HAMILTON. 1886– , & ROUGHTON, FRANCIS JOHN WORSLEY. 1899–1972.
The velocity with which carbon monoxide displaces oxygen from combination with haemoglobin. *Proc. roy. Soc. B*, 1923, **94,** 336–67.

963 LUMSDEN, THOMAS WILLIAM.
The regulation of respiration. *J. Physiol.* (*Lond.*), 1923–24, **58,** 81–91, 111–26.
Lumsden introduced the concept of subsidiary respiratory centres in the brain stem.

964 BARCROFT, *Sir* JOSEPH. 1872–1947
The respiratory function of the blood. 2 pts. Cambridge, *Univ. Press*, 1925–28.
Barcroft was professor of physiology at Cambridge 1925–37. His studies of the oxygen-carrying capacity of the blood are recorded in the above monograph.

965 GESELL, ROBERT. 1886–1954
The chemical regulation of respiration. *Physiol. Rev.*, 1925, **5,** 551–95

966 HENRIQUES, OSCAR M.
Die Bindungsweise des Kohlendioxyds im Blute. *Biochem. Z.*, 1928, **200,** 1–24.
Carbamino reaction.

967 HEYMANS, CORNEILLE JEAN FRANÇOIS. 1892–1968
Le sinus carotidien et la zone homologue cardio-aortique. Paris, *Presses univ. de France*, 1929.
His work on the sinus-aorta mechanism in respiration gained Heymans the Nobel Prize in 1938.

968 KEILIN, DAVID. 1887–1963
Cytochrome and respiratory enzymes. *Proc. roy. Soc. B*, 1929, **104,** 206–52.

Keilin discovered cytochrome and laid the foundations of the modern concept of cellular respiration.

969 WARBURG, OTTO HEINRICH. 1883–1970, & NEGELEIN, ERWIN.
Ueber den Absorptionsspektrum des Atmungsferments. *Biochem. Z.* 1929, **214,** 64–100.

Warburg discovered the nature and function of the respiratory ferment. He was awarded the Nobel Prize for physiology in 1931.

970 ——, & CHRISTIAN, WALTER.
Ueber ein neues Oxydationsferment und sein Absorptionsspektrum. *Biochem. Z.*, 1932, **254,** 438–58.

971 MELDRUM, NORMAN URQUHART. 1907–1933, & ROUGHTON, FRANCIS JOHN WORSLEY. 1899–1972.
Carbonic anhydrase. Its preparation and properties. *J. Physiol.* (*Lond.*), 1933, **80,** 113–42.

Isolation of carbonic anhydrase.

972–1092 DIGESTIVE SYSTEM

See also 665–752.7, BIOCHEMISTRY.

972 GLISSON, FRANCIS. 1597–1677
Anatomia hepatis. Londini, *typ. Du-Gardianis*, 1654.

First accurate description of the capsule of the liver (Glisson's capsule) and its blood-supply. He also described the sphincter of the bile duct ("Glisson's sphincter", the sphincter of Oddi).

973 STENSEN, NIELS. [STENO]. 1638–1686
Observationes anatomicae. Lugduni Batavorum, *J. Chouët*, 1662.

Includes the first account of the excretory duct of the parotid gland ("Stensen's duct"), discovered by Stensen. He first reported his discovery in a letter to his teacher, Thomas Bartholin, dated April 22, 1661. Facsimile reproduction, with English translation, Copenhagen. 1951.

974 GRAAF, REGNER DE. 1641–1673
Disputatio medica de natura et usu succi pancreatici. Lugduni Batavorum, *ex off. Hackiana*, 1664.

De Graaf was an early investigator of the pancreatic secretion. He collected the pancreatic juice of dogs by means of artificial pancreatic fistulae, commenting on the small quantity of juice secreted and on its alkaline character. For partial translation see J. F. Fulton, *Selected readings in the history of physiology*, 2nd. ed., 1966, pp. 167–68. Full English translation from 2nd. ed., (1671), London, 1676.

974.1 WEPFER, JOHANN JACOB. 1620–1695
Cicutae aquaticae historia et noxae. Basileae, *J. R König*, 1679.

Discovery of the duodenal (Brunner's) glands (see also No. 975). Wepfer was Brunner's father-in-law.

974.2 BARTHOLIN, CASPAR. 1655–1738
De ductu salivati hactenus non descriptio. Hafniae, *typ. J. P. Bockenhoffer*, 1684.

"Bartholin's duct" and "gland", the sublingual salivary gland and ducts.

975 BRUNNER, Johann Conrad à. 1653–1727
De glandulis in intestino duodeno hominis detectis. Heidelbergae, *C. E. Buchta*, 1687.
"Brunner's glands", earlier described by Wepfer (No. 974.1).

976 VATER, Abraham. 1684–1751
Dissertatio anatomica qua novum bilis diverticulum circa orificium ductus choledochi ut et valvulosam colli vesicae felleae constructionem ad disceptandum proponit. Wittenbergae, *lit. Gerdesianus*, 1720.
Following Vater's classical description of the ampulla of the bile duct, it was named the "ampulla of Vater".

977 POUPART, François. 1661–1709
[Suspenseurs de l'abdomen]. *Hist. Acad. roy. Sci.*, Paris, 1730, 51.
"Poupart's ligament," the inguinal ligament.

978 LIEBERKÜHN, Johann Nathanael. 1711–1756
De fabrica et actione villorum intestinorum tenuium hominis. Lugduni Batavorum, *C. & G. J. Wishof*, 1745.
"Lieberkühn's glands" or "crypts" described. They were discovered by Malpighi in 1688.

979 RÉAUMUR, Réné Antoine Ferchault de. 1683–1757
Sur la digestion des oiseaux. *Hist. Acad. roy. Sci.*, (1752), 1756, 266–307, 461–95.
Using a pet buzzard, de Réaumur succeeded in isolating the gastric juice and demonstrating its solvent effect on foods.

980 STEVENS, Edward.
Dissertatio physiologica inauguralis de alimentorum concoctione. Edinburgi, *Balfour et Smellie*, 1777.
First isolation of human gastric juice. Stevens was also the first successfully to perform an *in vitro* digestion, proving the presence in the gastric juice of the active principle necessary for the assimilation of food. An English translation is included in Spallanzani's *Dissertations relative to the natural history of animals*, 1784, vol. 1, pp. 303–16.

981 SPALLANZANI, Lazaro. 1729–1799
Dissertazioni di fisica animale e vegetabile. Vol. 1. Modena, *Presso la Societá Tipografica*, 1780.
Spallanzani confirmed earlier doctrines of the solvent property of the gastric juice and discovered the action of the saliva in digestion. He stated that gastric juice can act outside the body and can prevent or inhibit putrefaction. He obtained gastric juice by tying a sponge on a piece of string, then allowing it to be swallowed. English translation, 1784.

982 YOUNG, John Richardson. 1782–1804
An experimental inquiry into the principles of nutrition, and the digestive process. Philadelphia, *Eaken & Mecum*, 1803.
Young, one of the first American experimental physiologists, showed the solvent principle in the gastric juice to be an acid, but wrongly inferred that it was phosphoric acid. He also deduced the association and synchrony between gastric juice and saliva. Reprinted, Urbana, Ill., 1959.

983 HESSELBACH, Franz Kaspar. 1759–1816
Anatomisch-chirurgische Abhandlung ueber den Ursprung der Leistenbrüche. Würzburg, *Baumgärtener*, 1806.
Hesselbach's "fascia," "ligament," and "triangle" described.

984 MECKEL, JOHANN FRIEDRICH, *the younger*. 1781–1833
Ueber die Divertikel am Darmkanal. *Arch. Physiol.* (*Halle*), 1809, **9,** 421–53.

"Meckel's diverticulum".

985 MAGENDIE, FRANÇOIS. 1783–1855
Mémoire sur le vomissement. Paris, *Crochard*, 1813.

Physiologists still consult Magendie's classical description of the physiology of deglutition and vomiting. A translation of the above is in *Ann. Phil.*, London, 1813, **1,** 429–38.

986 BRODIE, *Sir* BENJAMIN COLLINS, *Bart.* 1783–1862
Experiments and observations on the influence of the nerves of the eighth pair on the secretions of the stomach. *Phil. Trans.*, 1814, **104,** 102–06.

Before turning to surgery, Brodie did important work in physiology. Above is his study of the influence of the pneumogastric nerve on gastric secretion.

987 PROUT, WILLIAM. 1785–1850
On the nature of the acid and saline matters usually existing in the stomachs of animals. *Phil. Trans.*, 1824, **114,** 45–49.

Proof that the gastric juice contains free hydrochloric acid.

988 TIEDEMANN, FRIEDRICH. 1781–1861, & GMELIN, LEOPOLD. 1788–1853
Die Verdauung nach Versuchen. 2 vols. Heidelberg, *K. Groos*, 1826–27.

Confirmation of the work of Prout.

989 BEAUMONT, WILLIAM. 1785–1853
Experiments and observations on the gastric juice, and the physiology of digestion. Plattsburgh, *F. P. Allen*, 1833.

Alexis St. Martin, a Canadian half-breed who had sustained a gastric fistula, was treated and investigated by Beaumont. With his human medium, Beaumont was the first to study digestion and the movements of the stomach *in vivo*. His work on the subject was the most important before Pavlov. Edinburgh imprint, 1838. Facsimile reprint, Cambridge, *Harvard Univ. Press*, 1929; for preliminary papers see *Med. Recorder*, 1825, **8,** 14–19, 840; 1826, **9,** 94–97.

990 MÜLLER, JOHANNES. 1801–1858, & SCHWANN, THEODOR. 1810–1882
Versuche über die künstliche Verdauung des geronnenen Eiweisses. *Arch. Anat. Physiol. wiss. Med.*, 1836, 66–89.

991 SCHWANN, THEODOR. 1810–1882
Ueber das Wesen des Verdauungsprocesses. *Arch. Anat. Physiol. wiss. Med.*, 1836, 90–138.

Beaumont had considered that the gastric juice contained some other active chemical substance besides hydrochloric acid. Schwann proved this to be pepsin.

992 BOUSSINGAULT, JEAN BAPTISTE. 1802–1887
Analyses comparées des alimens consommés et des produits rendu par une vache laitière. *Ann. Chim.*, 1839, **71,** 113–36.

The first analysis of foodstuffs and fertilizers. Boussingault made a balance of intake and outgo of nutrients in food and excreta.

992.1 BASSOV, Vasili.
Voie artificielle dans l'estomac des animaux. *Bull. Soc. imp. Naturalistes Moscou*, 1843, N.S. **16,** 315–19.
First gastric fistula established specially for the purpose of experimentation.

992.2 BLONDLOT, Nicolas. 1810–1877
Traité analytique de la digestion considérée particulièrement dans l'homme et dans les animaux. Paris, *Fortin, Masson et Cie.*, 1843.
Gastric fistula for experimental purposes.

993 SCHWANN, Theodor. 1810–1882
Versuche um auszumitteln, ob die Galle im Organismus eine für das Leben wesentliche Rolle spielt. *Arch. Anat. Physiol. wiss. Med.*, 1844, 127–59.
Proof of the indispensability of bile to digestion.

994 GERLACH, Joseph. 1820–1896
Beobachtung einer tödlichen Peritonitis, als Folge einer Perforation des Wurmfortsatzes. *Z. rat. Med.*, 1847, **6,** 12–23.
Description of "Gerlach's valve," sometimes seen at the orifice of the appendix.

995 BERNARD, Claude. 1813–1878
De l'origine du sucre dans l'économie animale. *Arch. gén. Méd.*, 1848, 4 sér., **18,** 303–19.
Bernard's first communciation regarding his investigation of the glycogenic function of the liver. Reprinted, with translation, in *Med. Classics*, 1939, **3,** 552–80.

996 ——. Du suc pancréatique et de son rôle dans les phénomènes de la digestion. *C. R. Soc. Biol.* (*Mémoires*), (1849) 1850, **1,** 99–115.
Discovery of the digestive action of the pancreatic juice. Reprinted, with translation, in *Med. Classics*, 1939, **3,** 581–617.

997 MOLESCHOTT, Jacob. 1822–1893
Die Physiologie der Nahrungsmittel. Darmstadt, *C. W. Leske*, 1850.

998 LUDWIG, Carl Friedrich Wilhelm. 1816–1895
Neue Versuche über die Beihilfe der Nerven zur Speichelabsonderung. *Z. rat. Med.*, 1851, n.F. **1,** 254–77.
The innervation of the salivary glands first elucidated.

999 BIDDER, Friedrich Heinrich. 1810–1894, & SCHMIDT, Carl. 1822–1894
Die Verdauungssäfte und der Stoffwechsel. Mitau & Leipzig, *G. A. Reyher*, 1852.
Even after the work of Prout and Beaumont, some physiologists thought that the free acid of the gastric guice was lactic acid; Bidder and Schmidt finally proved that normally the gastric juice always contains HC1 in excess.

999.1 BERNARD, Claude. 1813–1878
Nouvelles recherches expérimentales sur les phénomènes glycogéniques du foie. *C. R. Soc. Biol.* (*Mémoires*), (1857) 1858, 2 sér., **4,** 1–7.
Discovery of glycogen. See also *C. R. Acad. Sci.* (*Paris*), 1857, **44,** 578–86, 1325–31.

1000 ——. Sur le mécanisme de la formation du sucre dans le foie. *C. R. Acad. Sci.* (*Paris*), 1855, **41,** 461–69.

The culmination of Bernard's work on the glycogenic function of the liver. He invented the term "internal secretion" and can be said to have started the scientific investigation of the internal secretions, although for 30 years the significance of his work was not generally realized. By his research on glycogen Bernard showed that the body not only can break down, but can also build up, complex chemical substances.

1001 CORVISART, François Rémy Lucien. 1824–1882
Sur une fonction peu connue du pancréas. La digestion des aliments azotés. 10 pts. Paris, *V. Masson*, 1857–63.

Corvisart showed that pancreatic proteolysis takes place at body temperature, in acid, alkaline, or neutral media.

1002 SAPPEY, Marie Philibert Constant. 1810–1896
Mémoire sur un point d'anatomie pathologique relatif à l'histoire de la cirrhose. *Mém. Acad. imp. Méd.* (*Paris*), 1859, **23,** 269–78.

"Sappey's veins" in the falciform ligament of the liver.

1003 BRÜCKE, Ernst Wilhelm von, *Ritter*. 1819–1892
Beiträge zur Lehre von der Verdauung. *S.B. k. Akad. Wiss. Wien,* 1861, math.-nat. Kl., **43,** Abt. 2, 601–23.

1004 DANILEVSKY, Aleksandr Yakolevič. 1838–?
Ueber specifisch wirkende Körper des natürlichen und künstlichen pancreatischen Saftes. *Virchows Arch. path. Anat.*, 1862, **25,** 279–307.

Discovery of trypsin.

1005 FLINT, Austin, *Jnr*. 1836–1915
Experimental researches into a new excretory function of the liver, consisting in the removal of cholesterine from the blood and its discharge from the body in the form of stercorine. *Amer. J. med. Sci.*, 1862, n.s. **44,** 305–65.

Discovery, in the faeces, of "stercorine" (coprosterol).

1006 AUERBACH, Leopold. 1828–1897
Ueber einen Plexus gangliosus myogastricus. *Jber. schles. Ges. vaterl. Cultur*, (1862), 1863, **40,** 103–04.

Auerbach's plexus and ganglion. See also his book, *Ueber einen Plexus myentericus* Breslau, *Morgenstern*, 1862.

1007 THIRY, Ludwig. 1817–1897
Ueber eine neue Methode den Dünndarm zu isolieren. *S.B. k. Akad. Wiss. Wien*, math.-nat. Kl., 1865, Abt. I, **50,** 77–96.

Thiry – Vella fistula (See also No. 1014).

1008 HEIDENHAIN, Rudolf Peter Heinrich. 1834–1897
Beiträge zur Lehre von der Speichelsecretion. *Stud. physiol. Inst. Breslau*, 1868, **4,** 1–124.

1009 LANGERHANS, Paul. 1847–1888
Beiträge zur mikroskopischen Anatomie der Bauchspeicheldrüse. Inaugural-Dissertation. Berlin, *Gustav Lange*, 1869.

First account of the islands of Langerhans. In 1893 E. Laguesse attached the name of Langerhans to the structures. Langerhans did not suggest any function for them. The book has been reprinted with an English translation by H. Morrison, *Bull. Hist: Med.*, 1937, **5,** 259–97.

1010 PASCHUTIN, VICTOR VASILYEVICH. 1845–1901
Einige Versuche mit Fermenten, welche Stärke und Rohrzucker in Traubenzucker verwandeln. *Arch. Anat. Physiol. wiss. Med.*, 1871, 305–84.

1011 HEIDENHAIN, RUDOLF PETER HEINRICH. 1834–1897
Ueber die Wirkung einiger Gifte auf die Nerven der glandula submaxillaris. *Pflüg. Arch. ges. Physiol.*, 1872, **5,** 309–18.
Study of the effect of poisons on the nerves of the submaxillary gland.

1012 KÜHNE, WILLY. 1837–1900
Ueber das Trypsin. *Verh. naturh.-med. Ver. Heidelberg*, 1874–77, n.F. **1,** 194–98.
Isolation of trypsin.

1012.1 HEIDENHAIN, RUDOLF PETER HEINRICH. 1834–1897
Ueber die Pepsinbildung in den Pylorusdrüsen. *Pflüg. Arch. ges. Physiol.*, 1878, **18,** 169–71.
Heidenhain pouch.

1013 LUCIANI, LUIGI. 1840–1919
Fisiologia del digiuni. Firenze, *Successori Le Monnier*, 1881.
Luciani distinguished three stages of starvation in man – hunger, physiological inanition and pathological inanition.

1014 VELLA, LUIGI. 1825–1886
Nuovo metodo per avere il succo enterico puro, e stabilirne le proprietà fisiologiche. *Mem. r. Accad. Sci. Ist. Bologna*, 1881, **2,** 515–38.
(See No. 1007).

1015 KRONECKER, KARL HUGO. 1839–1914, & MELTZER, SAMUEL JAMES. 1851–1920
Der Schluckmechanismus, seine Erregung und seine Hemmung. *Arch. Anat. Physiol., Physiol. Abt.*, 1883, *Suppl.-Bd.*, 328–62.

1016 KÜHNE, WILLY. 1837–1900, & CHITTENDEN, RUSSELL HENRY. 1856–1943
Ueber die nächsten Spaltungsproducte der Eiweisskörper. *Z. Biol.*, 883, **19,** 159–208.
Kühne and Chittenden isolated and named several new substances during their investigation of the products of digestion. See also the same journal, 1884, **20,** 11–51; 1886, **22,** 409–58; 1889, **25,** 358–67.

1017 ESCHERICH, THEODOR. 1857–1911
Die Darmbakterien des Säuglings und ihre Beziehungen zur Physiologie der Verdauung. Stuttgart, *F. Enke*, 1886.
Includes the first account of *Bact. coli* infection. The organism was later renamed *Escherichia coli.*

1018 ODDI, RUGGERO.
D'une disposition à sphincter spéciale de l'ouverture du canal cholédoque. *Arch. ital. Biol.*, 1887, **8,** 317–22.
"Sphincter of Oddi" of the bile duct, already known to Glisson in 1654. Reprinted as pamphlet, Perugia, 1887.

1018.1 HARTMANN, HENRI. 1860–1952
Quelques points de l'anatomie et de la chirurgie des voies biliaires. *Bull. Soc. anat. Paris*, 1891, 5 sér., **5,** 480–500.
"Hartmann's pouch", a dilatation of the neck of the gall-bladder.

1019 HEIDENHAIN, RUDOLF PETER HEINRICH. 1834–1897
Neue Versuche über die Aufsaugung im Dünndarm. *Pflüg. Arch. ges. Physiol.*, 1894, **56,** 579–631.

1020 NUTTALL, GEORGE HENRY FALKINER. 1862–1937, & THIERFELDER, HANS. 1858–1930
Thierisches Leben ohne Bakterien im Verdauungskanal. *Hoppe-Seyl. Z. physiol. Chem.*, 1895–96, **21,** 109–21; 1896–97, **22,** 62–73; 1897, **23,** 231–35.

Proof that healthy life and perfect digestion are possible without the presence of bacteria in the digestive tract.

1021 KULTSCHITZKY, NIKOLAI. 1856–1925
Zur Frage über den Bau des Darmkanals. *Arch. mikr. Anat.*, 1897, **49,** 7–35.

The "cells of Kultschitzky" in the epithelium of the intestine, between the cells which line the glands of Lieberkühn.

1022 PAVLOV, IVAN PETROVITCH. 1849–1936
Lektsii o rabotïe glavnikh pishtshevarîtelnikh zhelyoz. [Lectures on the work of the principal digestive glands.] St. Petersburg, *I. N. Kushnereff*, 1897.

Pavlov made perhaps the greatest contribution to our knowledge of the physiology of digestion. Especially notable was his method of producing gastric and pancreatic fistulae for the purpose of his experiments. A translation of his description of the stomach pouch devised by him is in J. F. Fulton's *Selected readings in the history of physiology*, 2nd ed., 1966, pp. 192–93. His book was translated into English, a second edition appearing in 1910. He was awarded the Nobel Prize in Physiology in 1904.

1023 ADDISON, CHRISTOPHER, 1*st Viscount Addison of Stallingborough.* 1869–1951
On the topographical anatomy of abdominal viscera in man, especially the gastrointestinal canal. *J. Anat. Physiol.*, 1899, **33,** 565–86.

"Addison's transpyloric plane." Addison was the first British Minister of Health (1919–21).

1024 BAYLISS, *Sir* WILLIAM MADDOCK. 1860–1924, & STARLING, ERNEST HENRY. 1866–1927
The mechanism of pancreatic secretion. *J. Physiol.* (*Lond.*), 1902, **28,** 325–53.

Demonstration of the existence of secretin in the duodenal secretion. Preliminary note in *Lancet,* 1902, **1,** 813.

1025 RUBNER, MAX. 1854–1932
Die Gesetze des Energieverbrauchs bei der Ernährung. Leipzig & Wien, *F. Deuticke*, 1902.

Rubner's classical work on the influence of foodstuffs on metabolism. In it he introduced the term "specific dynamic action of the foodstuffs".

1026 EDKINS, JOHN SYDNEY. 1863–1940
On the chemical mechanism of gastric secretion. *J. Physiol.* (*Lond.*), 1906, **34,** 133–44.

Gastric secretin (gastrin) was first described by Edkins. A preliminary communication is in *Proc. roy. Soc. B,* 1905, **76,** 376.

1027 BENEDICT, FRANCIS GANO. 1870–1957
The influence of inanition on metabolism. Washington, *Carnegie Inst.*, 1907.

1028 LONDON, Efim Semenovič. 1869–1939, & DOBROVOLSKAJA, N.
Studien über die spezifische Anpassung der Verdauungssäfte. *Hoppe-Seyl. Z. physiol. Chem.*, 1910, **68,** 374–77.

1029 CANNON, Walter Bradford. 1871–1945
The mechanical factors of digestion. London, *E. Arnold*, 1911.

1030 CARLSON, Anton Julius. 1875–1956
Contributions to the physiology of the stomach. *Amer. J. Physiol.*, 1912–13, **31,** 151–68, 175–92, 212–22, 318–27; 1913, **32,** 245–63.
Carlson recorded stomach movements by means of a balloon inserted through a gastric fistula. Much of his important work on gastric physiology is summed up in his book (see No. 1033).

1031 GLÉNARD, Roger.
Le mouvement de l'intestin en circulation artificielle. Paris, 1913.
Cinematographic studies of the movements of the intestines in animals. A thesis presented to the Faculty of Science, Paris University.

1032 BABKIN, Boris Petrovich. 1877–1950
Die äussere Sekretion der Verdauungsdrüsen. Berlin, *J. Springer*, 1914.

1033 CARLSON, Anton Julius. 1875–1956
The control of hunger in health and disease. Chicago, *Univ. Press*, (1916).

1034 TRENDELENBURG, Paul. 1884–1931
Physiologische und pharmakologische Versuche über die Dünndarm-peristaltik. *Arch. exp. Path. Pharmak.*, 1917, **81,** 55–129.

1035 ALVAREZ, Walter Clement. 1884–
The mechanics of the digestive tract. New York, *P. H. Hoeber*, 1922.
Includes (p. 111) his smooth diet for duodenal ulcer. Fourth edition entitled *Introduction to gastro-enterology*, 1950.

1036 DuBOIS, Eugene Floyd. 1882–1959
Basal metabolism in health and disease. Philadelphia, *Lea & Febiger*, 1924.

1037 IVY, Andrew Conway. 1893– , & FARRELL, James Irving. 1900–
Contributions to the physiology of gastric secretion. The proof of a humoral mechanism. A new procedure for the study of gastric physiology. *Amer. J. Physiol.*, 1925, **84,** 639–49.

1038 KOSAKA, T., & LIM, Robert Kho-Seng. 1897–
Demonstration of the humoral agent in fat inhibition of gastric secretion. *Proc. Soc. exp. Biol. (N.Y.)*, 1930, **27,** 890–91.
The work of Kosaka and Lim led to the discovery of a hormone inhibiting gastric secretion ("enterogastrone").

1039 ÅGREN, Gunnar. 1907–
Ueber die pharmakodynamischen Wirkungen und chemischen Eigenschaften des Secretins. *Skand. Arch. Physiol.*, 1934, **70,** 10–87.
Preparation of crystalline secretin.

1040 HAHN, Paul Francis. 1908– , *et al.*
Radioactive iron absorption by gastro-intestinal tract. Influence of anemia, anoxia, and antecedent feeding distribution in growing dogs. *J. exp. Med.*, 1943, **78,** 169–88.

An important contribution to the knowledge of iron absorption. With W. F. Bale, J. F. Ross, W. M. Balfour, and G. H. Whipple.

1041 WOLF, Stewart George. 1914– , & WOLFF, Harold George. 1898–1962
Human gastric function. An experimental study of a man and his stomach. New York, *Oxford University Press*, 1943.

Important experiments on gastric function, made on "Tom", a man who had a gastric fistula from the age of 9. Second edition in 1947.

Nutrition; Vitamins

1042 LUNIN, Nikolai Ivanovič. 1853–1937
Ueber die Bedeutung der anorganischen Salze für die Ernährung des Thiers. *Hoppe-Seyl. Z. physiol. Chem.*, 1881, **5,** 31–39.

Working in Bunge's laboratory, Lunin prepared synthetic milk diets and showed that they lacked an unknown factor necessary for animal growth, and that animals cannot live on a chemically pure (i.e. vitamin-free) diet. This was the starting-point of modern research on vitamins.

1043 CHITTENDEN, Russell Henry. 1856–1943
Physiological economy in nutrition. New York, *F. A. Stokes Co.*, 1904.

Chittenden, founder of the first laboratory of physiological chemistry in the U.S.A., made many important experiments in nutrition, especially in connexion with the low protein diet advocated by him.

1044 HOPKINS, *Sir* Frederick Gowland. 1861–1947
The analyst and the medical man. *Analyst*, 1906, **31,** 385–404.

Hopkins predicted the existence of vitamins as early as 1906. He fed animals a diet of zein which failed to maintain growth; however the animals grew at once when casein was substituted. He concluded that "in the organs must appear special, indispensable active substances which the tissues can only make from special precursors in the diet".

1045 LUSK, Graham. 1866–1932
The elements of the science of nutrition. Philadelphia, *W. B. Saunders*, 1906.

Fourth edition, 1928.

1046 STEPP, Wilhelm Otto. 1882–
Versuche über Fütterung mit lipoidfreier Nahrung. *Biochem. Z.*, 1909, **22,** 452–60.

Stepp discovered that removal of fat from the diet greatly reduced its nutritive value but that substitution of pure fats did not make good the deficiency. He thus discovered the existence of fat-soluble vitamins, without fully realizing it. For his later papers, see the same journal, 1911, **57,** 135; 1913, **62,** 405.

1047 FUNK, Casimir. 1884–1967
On the chemical nature of the substance which cures polyneuritis in birds induced by a diet of polished rice. *J. Physiol. (Lond.)*, 1911–12, **43,** 395–400.

One of the earliest attempts to isolate what later became known as vitamin B_1. To Funk we owe the invention of the word "vitamine", later changed to "vitamin".

1048 HOPKINS, *Sir* FREDERICK GOWLAND. 1861–1947
Feeding experiments illustrating the importance of accessory factors in normal dietaries. *J. Physiol. (Lond.)*, 1912, **44**, 425–60.

Hopkins shared the Nobel Prize in Physiology with Eijkman in 1929 for his discovery of the growth-stimulating vitamins.

1048.1 ABEL, JOHN JACOB. 1857–1938, *et al.*
On the removal of diffusible substances from the circulating blood by means of dialysis. *Trans. Ass. Amer. Phycns*, 1913, **28**, 51–54.

Isolation of amino-acids from the blood by vividiffusion. With L. G. Rowntree and B. B. Turner.

1049 McCOLLUM, ELMER VERNER. 1879–1967, & DAVIS, MARGUERITE. 1887–
The necessity of certain lipins in the diet during growth. *J. biol. Chem.*, 1913, **15**, 167–75.

Discovery of "fat-soluble A" (vitamin A). See also *J. biol. Chem.*, 1915, **23**, 181–246, in which the same authors showed the necessity in diet for at least two factors – "fat-soluble A" and "water-soluble B".

1050 OSBORNE, THOMAS BURR. 1859–1929, & MENDEL, LAFAYETTE BENEDICT. 1872–1935
The relation of growth to the chemical constituents of the diet. *J. biol. Chem.*, 1913, **15**, 311–26.

Like McCollum and Davis, Osborne and Mendel showed the necessity in diet of a factor which was later to be known as vitamin A.

1051 FUNK, CASIMIR. 1884–1967
Die Vitamine. Wiesbaden, *J. F. Bergmann*, 1914.

A pioneer work in the study of the vitamins. Much of the previous literature is reviewed. Funk introduced the term "vitamine". In 1912 (*J. State Med.*, **20**, 341) he postulated his theory of the existence of unknown but essential factors in diet.

1052 McCOLLUM, ELMER VERNER. 1879–1967
The newer knowledge of nutrition. New York, *Macmillan Co.*, 1918.

1053 DRUMMOND, *Sir* JACK CECIL. 1891–1952
Note on the role of the antiscorbutic factor in nutrition. *Biochem. J.*, 1919, **13**, 77–80.

In 1920 Drummond suggested the term "vitamin".

1054 STEENBOCK, HARRY. 1886– , *et al.*
Fat-soluble vitamine. VII. The fat-soluble vitamine and yellow pigmentation in animal fats with some observations on its stability to saponification. *J. biol. Chem.*, 1921, **47**, 89–109.

Separation of vitamin A from vitamin D. With M. Sell and M. Van R. Buell.

1054.1 McCOLLUM, ELMER VERNER. 1879–1967, *et al.*
Studies on experimental rickets. XXI. An experimental demonstration of the existence of a vitamin which promotes calcium deposition. *J. biol. Chem.*, 1922, **53**, 293–312.

Discovery of vitamin D. With N. Simmonds, J. E. Becker, and P. G. Shipley.

1055 EVANS, HERBERT MCLEAN. 1882–1971, & BISHOP, KATHARINE SCOTT. 1889–
On the existence of a hitherto unrecognized dietary factor essential for reproduction. *Science*, 1922, **56,** 650–51.
Discovery of vitamin E. See also their later paper in *J. Amer. med. Ass.*, 1923, **81,** 889–92.

1056 STEENBOCK, HARRY. 1886– , *et al.*
Fat-soluble vitamin. XXVI. Antirachitic property of milk and its increase by direct irradiation and by irradiation of the animal. *J. biol. Chem.*, 1925, **66,** 441–49.
Demonstration that the therapeutic properties of ultra-violet light could be effectively stored in foods and later released after consumption. With E. B. Hart, C. A. Hoppert, and A. Black.

1057 GOLDBERGER, JOSEPH. 1874–1929, *et al.*
A further study of butter, fresh beef, and yeast as pellagra preventives, with consideration of the relation of factor P-P of pellagra (and black tongue of dogs) to vitamin B. *U.S. publ. Hlth Rep.*, 1926, **41,** 297–318.
Anti-pellagra vitamin (B_2, riboflavine). With G. A. Wheeler, R. D. Lillie, and L. M. Rogers.

1058 JANSEN, BAREND COENRAAD PETRUS. 1884– , & DONATH, WILLIAM FREDERICK. 1889–
Antineuritisch Vitamine. *Chem. Weekbl.*, 1926, **23**, 201–03.
Isolation of vitamin B_1 (aneurine) in crystalline form.

1059 SZENT-GYÖRGYI, ALBERT. 1893–
Observations on the function of peroxidase systems and the chemistry of the adrenal cortex. Description of a new carbohydrate derivative. *Biochem. J.*, 1928, **22,** 1387–1409.
Isolation of vitamin C, ascorbic acid. Szent-Györgyi was awarded a Nobel Prize in 1937 for his discoveries in connexion with the biological combustion process with special reference to vitamin C and the catalysis of fumaric acid.

1060 WILLIAMS, ROBERT RUNNELS. 1886–1965, & WATERMAN, ROBERT EDWARD. 1899–
The tripartite nature of vitamin B. *J. biol. Chem.*, 1928, **78,** 311–22.
Vitamin B_3.

1061 BOURDILLON, ROBERT BENEDICT. 1889–1971, *et al.*
The absorption spectrum of vitamin D. *Proc. roy. Soc. B*, 1929, **94,** 561–83.
See No. 1065. With C. Fischmann, R. G. C. Jenkins, and T. A. Webster.

1062 DAM, CARL PIETER HENRIK. 1895–
Cholesterinstoffwechsel in Hühnereiern und Hühnchen. *Biochem. Z.*, 1929, **215,** 475–92.
Discovery of the dietary anti-haemorrhagic factor, vitamin K. Dam shared the Nobel Prize with E. A. Doisy in 1943.

1063 BURR, GEORGE OSWALD. 1896– , & BURR, MILDRED M.
On the nature and rôle of the fatty acids essential in nutrition. *J. Biol. Chem.*, 1930, **86,** 587–621.
Demonstration of the need of the body for certain unsaturated fatty acids (vitamin F).

1064 CARTER, CYRIL WILLIAM. 1898– , *et al.*
Maintenance nutrition in the adult pigeon and its relation to torulin (vitamin B_1). *Biochem. J.*, 1930, **24,** 1832–51.
Discovery of vitamin B_5, probably identical with nicotinic acid. With H. W. Kinnersley and R. A. Peters.

1065 BOURDILLON, ROBERT BENEDICT. 1889–1971, *et al.*
The quantitative estimation of vitamin D by radiography. London, *H.M. Stationery Office*, 1931.
Medical Research Council Special Report No. 158. R. B. Bourdillon, H. M. Bruce, C. Fischmann, R. G. C. Jenkins, and T. A. Webster isolated from irradiated ergosterol a crystalline compound, calciferol, which, weight for weight, has 400,000 times the anti-rachitic value of cod liver oil. (See also No. 1061).

1066 BROWNING, ETHEL.
The vitamins. London, *Baillière, Tindall & Cox*, 1931.

1067 ASKEW, FREDERIC ANDERTON, *et al.*
Crystalline vitamin D. *Proc. roy. Soc. B*, 1932, **109,** 488–506.
Written with R. B. Bourdillon, H. M. Bruce, R. K. Callow, J. St. L. Philpot, and T. A. Webster.

1068 REICHSTEIN, TADEUS. 1897– , *et al.*
Synthese der d- und l-Ascorbinsäure (C-Vitamin). *Helv. chim. Acta*, 1933, **16,** 1019–33.
T. Reichstein, A. Grüssner, and R. Oppenauer synthesized vitamin C.

1068.1 WILLIAMS, ROGER JOHN. 1893– , *et al.*
"Pantothenic acid", a growth determinant of universal biological occurrence. *J. Amer. chem. Soc.*, 1933, **55,** 2912–27.
Discovery of pantothenic acid (vitamin B_3). With C. M. Lyman, G. H. Goodyear, J. H. Truesdail, and D. Holaday.

1069 ELLINGER, PHILIPP. 1887–1952, & KOSCHARA, WALTER.
The lyochromes: a new group of animal pigments. *Nature (Lond.)*, 1934, **133,** 553–56.
Chemical formula of riboflavine (vitamin B_2).

1070 EVANS, HERBERT MCLEAN. 1882–1971, *et al.*
Vital needs of the body for certain unsaturated fatty acids. *J. biol. Chem.*, 1934, **106,** 431–50.
Isolation of vitamin F (linolenic acid). With S. Lepkovsky and E. A. Murphy.

1071 ——. The isolation from wheat-germ oil of an alcohol, α-tocopherol, having the properties of vitamin E. *J. biol. Chem.*, 1936, **113,** 319–32.
Isolation of vitamin E. With O. H. Emerson and G. A. Emerson.

1071.1 KÖGL, FRITZ. 1897– , & TÖNNIS, BENNO.
Über das Bios-Problem. Darstellung von krystallisiertem Biotin aus Eigelb. *Hoppe-Seyl. Z. physiol. Chem.*, 1936, **242,** 43–73.
Isolation of biotin.

1072 RUSZNYÁK, STEPHAN, & SZENT-GYÖRGYI, ALBERT. 1893–
Vitamin P: Flavonols as vitamins. *Nature (Lond.)*, 1936, **138,** 27.
Discovery of vitamin P ("citrin").

1073 WILLIAMS, Robert Runnels. 1886–1965, & CLINE, Joseph Kalman. 1908–
Synthesis of vitamin B_1. *J. Amer. chem. Soc.*, 1936, **58,** 1504–05.
Synthesis of aneurine.

1074 HOLMES, Harry Nicholls. 1879–1958, & CORBET, Ruth E.
A crystalline vitamin A concentration. *Science*, 1937, **85,** 103.

1075 TODD, *Sir* Alexander Robertus. 1907– , *et al.*
Studies on vitamin E. The isolation of β-tocopherol from wheat-germ oil. *Biochem. J.*, 1937, **31,** 2257–63.
With F. Bergel and T. S. Work.

1076 KOEHN, Carl James. 1910– , & ELVEHJEM, Conrad Arnold. 1901–1962
Further studies on the concentration of the antipellagra factor. *J. biol. Chem.*, 1937, **118,** 693–99.
Chicken pellagra factor.

1077 ELVEHJEM, Conrad Arnold. 1901–1962, *et al.*
The isolation and identification of the anti-black tongue factor. *J. biol. Chem.*, 1938, **123,** 137–49.
Isolation of nicotinic acid, the pellagra-preventing factor. With R. J. Madden, F. N. Strong, and D. W. Woolley.

1078 HARRIS, Leslie John. 1898–
Vitamins and vitamin deficiencies. Vol. 1. London, *J. & A. Churchill*, 1938.

1079 KARRER, Paul. 1889–1971, *et al.*
α-Tocopherol. *Helv. chim. Acta*, 1938, **21,** 520–25.
P. Karrer, H. Fritzsche, B. H. Ringier, and H. Salomon synthesized vitamin E (α-tocopherol).

1080 DAM, Carl Pieter Henrik. 1895– , *et al.*
Isolierung des Vitamins K in hochgereinigter Form. *Helv. chim. Acta*, 1939, **22,** 310–13.
Isolation of vitamin K_1 from alfalfa. It was isolated independently by R. W. McKee and his co-workers, *J. Amer. chem. Soc.*, 1939, **61,** 1295.

1081 BINKLEY, Stephen Bennett. 1910– , *et al.*
The isolation of vitamin K_1. *J. biol. Chem.*, 1939, **130,** 219–34.
With D. W. MacCorquodale, S. A. Thayer, and E. A. Doisy.

1082 ——. The constitution of vitamin K_2. *J. biol. Chem.*, 1940, **133,** 721–9.
Structural formula of vitamin K_2. With R. W. McKee, S. A. Thayer, and E. A. Doisy. Dam and Doisy shared a Nobel Prize in 1943 for their work on vitamin K.

1083 FIESER, Louis Frederick. 1899–
Synthesis of vitamin K_1. *J. Amer. chem. Soc.*, 1939, **61,** 3467–75.

1084 ANSBACHER, Stefan. 1905–
p-Aminobenzoic acid, a vitamin. *Science*, 1941, **93,** 164–65.
Recognition of β-aminobenzoic acid as a member of the vitamin-B complex.

1085 DU VIGNEAUD, VINCENT. 1901– , *et al.*
On the identity of vitamin H with biotin. *Science*, 1940, **92,** 609–10.
Isolation of β-biotin (formerly known as vitamin H). With D. B. Melville, P. György, and C. S. Rose.

1086 HOGAN, ALBERT GARLAND. 1884– , & PARROTT, ERNEST MILFORD. 1903–
Anaemia in chicks caused by a vitamin deficiency. *J. biol. Chem.*, 1940, **132,** 507–17.
Isolation of vitamin Bc (folic acid, pteroylglutamic acid). Preliminary communication in *J. biol. Chem.*, 1939, **128,** xlvi–xlvii.

1086.1 DRAGSTEDT, LESTER REYNOLD. 1893– , *et al.*
Observations on a substance in pancreas (a fat metabolizing hormone) which permits survival and prevents liver changes in depancreatized dogs. *Amer. J. Physiol.*, 1936, **117,** 175–81.
Lipocaic. With J. Van Prohaska and H. P. Harms.

1087 WAWRA, CECIL Z., & WEBB, JOHN LEYDEN. 1914–1966
The isolation of a new oxidation-reduction enzyme from lemon peel (vitamin P). *Science*, 1942, **96,** 302–03.
Isolation of vitamin P (hesperidin chalcone).

1088 HARRIS, STANTON AVERY. 1902– , *et al.*
Synthetic biotin. *Science*, 1943, **97,** 447–48.
Synthesis of biotin. With D. E. Wolf, R. Mozingo & K. Folkers.

1089 KÖGL, FRITZ. 1897– , & HAM, E.-J. TEN.
Zur Kenntnis des β-Biotins. 34. Mitteilung über pflanzliche Wachstumstoffe. *Hoppe-Seyl. Z. physiol. Chem.*, 1943, **279,** 140–52.
Isolation of α-biotin.

1090 SHORB, MARY SHAW. 1907–
Unidentified growth factors for *Lactobacillus lactis* in refined liver extract. *J. biol. Chem.*, 1947, **169,** 455–56.
Mary Shorb provided a method of biological assay of liver extracts that made possible the isolation of vitamin B_{12}.

1091 RICKES, EDWARD LAWRENCE. 1912– , *et al.*
Crystalline vitamin B_{12}. *Science*, 1948, **107,** 396–97.
With N. G. Brink, F. R. Koniuszy, T. R. Wood, and K. Folkers.

1092 SMITH, ERNEST LESTER. 1904–
Presence of cobalt in the anti-pernicious anaemia factor. *Nature (Lond.)*, 1948, **162,** 144–45.
Independently of Rickes *et al.*, Lester Smith isolated vitamin B_{12} in Britain. See also *Nature (Lond.)*, 1948, **161,** 638.

For history of nutrition, see 1581–2, 1585, 1588.1, 1588.3

1093–1114 LYMPHATIC SYSTEM

1093 EUSTACHI, BARTOLOMMEO [EUSTACHIUS]. 1520–1574
Opuscula anatomica. Venetiis, *V. Luchinus*, 1564.
Eustachius recognized the thoracic duct in the horse and even detected some of its valves. His work on this structure was forgotten until Aselli's description of the lacteals.

1094 ASELLI, CASPARE. 1581–1626
De lactibus sive lacteis venis. Mediolani, *apud Io. B. Bidellium*, 1627.
Records the discovery of the lacteal vessels. Aselli's book has also the distinction of including the first anatomical plates printed in colours (four woodcuts, 16″ × 10″). Reprinted Leipzig, 1969.

1095 PECQUET, JEAN. 1622–1674
Experimenta nova anatomica quibus incognitum chyli receptaculum, et ab eo per thoracem in ramos usque subclavis vasa lactea deteguntur. Paris, 1651.
Pecquet discovered the thoracic duct in dogs and its relation to the lacteals. English translation, London, 1653.

1096 BARTHOLIN, THOMAS. 1616–1680
De lacteis thoracicis in homine brutisque. Hafniae, *M. Martzan*, 1652.
Contains Bartholin's discovery of the thoracic duct. English translation, 1653.

1097 ——. Vasa lymphatica. Hafniae, *Petrus Hakius*, 1653.
Bartholin disputed the claim of Rudbeck as to priority in the discovery of the intestinal lymphatics. Although anticipated in this by Rudbeck, there is no doubt that Bartholinus was the first to appreciate the significance of the lymphatic system as a whole.

1098 RUDBECK, OLOF. 1630–1702
Nova exercitatio anatomica, exhibens ductus hepaticos aquosos, et vasa glandularum serosa. Arosiae, *excud. E. Lauringerus*, 1653.
Rudbeck claimed to have discovered the intestinal lymphatics and their connexion with the thoracic duct in 1651, a claim disputed as to priority by Bartholin (No. 1096–97). This book was reproduced in facsimile in 1930. English translation in *Bull. Hist. Med.*, 1942, **11**, 304–39.

1098.1 GLISSON, FRANCIS. 1597–1677
Anatomia hepatis . . . subjiciuntur nonnulla de lymphae-ductibus nuper repertis. Londini, *typ. Du-Gardianis*, 1654.
Independently of Bartholin and Rudbeck, George Joyliffe (1621–58) observed the lymphatics. He communicated his discovery to Glisson early in 1652 and the latter included an account in the above work (Cap. xxxi).

1099 RUYSCH, FREDERIK. 1638–1731
Dilucidatio valvularum in vasis lymphaticis et lacteis. Hagae-Comitiae, *ex officina H. Gael*, 1665.
First description of the valves of the lymphatics, discovered by Ruysch.

1100 PEYER, JOHANN CONRAD. 1653–1712
Exercitatio anatomico-medica de glandulis intestinorum, earumque usu et affectionibus. Scafhusae, *Onophrius et Waldkirch*, 1677.
Includes a description of "Peyer's patches", the lymphoid follicles in the small intestine which have an important rôle in typhoid. They were first described by J. N. Pechlin (1644–1706) in his *De purgantium medicamentorum facultatibus exercitatio nova*, 1672.

1101 NUCK, ANTONJ. 1650–1692
De ductu salivali novo, saliva, ductibus oculorum aquosis, et humore oculi aqueo. Lugduni Batavorum, *P. vander Aa*, 1685.
Nuck's name has been attached to the glands and duct described by him.

1102 HEWSON, William. 1739–1774
Experimental inquiries: Part the second. Containing a description of the lymphatic system in the human subject and in other animals. Together with observations on the lymph, and the changes which it undergoes in some diseases. London, *J. Johnson*, 1774.

Hewson gave the first complete account of the anatomical peculiarities of the lymphatics. He divided the lymphatics into two groups – superficial and deep. He described the leucocytes as derived from the lymphatic glands and thymus.

1103 CRUIKSHANK, William Cumberland. 1745–1800
The anatomy of the absorbing vessels of the human body. London, *G. Nicol*, 1786.

With Hunter and Hewson, Cruikshank laid the foundation of modern knowledge concerning the lymphatics. He was Dr. Johnson's physician and William Hunter's assistant.

1104 MASCAGNI, Paolo. 1752–1815
Vasorum lymphaticorum corporis humani historia et ichnographia. Senis, *ex typ. P. Carli*, 1787.

Mascagni, professor of anatomy at Siena, made several discoveries regarding the lymphatics. His beautiful atlas contained 41 engravings of the lymphatics and gained him lasting fame. He had previously published a *Prodrome*, in French, 1784; this contained only 4 plates.

1105 WEBER, Ernst Heinrich. 1795–1878
Microscopische Beobachtungen über die sichtbare Fortbewegung der Lymphkörnchen in den Lymphgefässen der Froschlarven. *Arch. Anat. Physiol. wiss. Med.*, 1837, 267–72.

1106 NOLL, Friedrich Wilhelm.
De cursu lymphae in vasis lymphaticis. Marburgi Cattorum, *typ. Elwerti*, 1849.

Noll advanced the theory that lymph is formed by the diffusion of fluids from the blood through the vessel walls into the surrounding tissues.

1107 HIS, Wilhelm, *Snr*. 1831–1904
Untersuchungen über den Bau der Lymphdrüsen. Leipzig, *W. Engelmann*, 1861.

Histology of the lymphatics. His himself drew his illustrations.

1108 RECKLINGHAUSEN, Friedrich Daniel von. 1833–1910
Die Lymphgefässe und ihre Beziehung zum Bindegewebe. Berlin, *A. Hirschwald*, 1862.

"Recklinghausen's canals", the lymph canaliculi.

1109 HIS, Wilhelm, *Snr*. 1831–1904
Ueber das Epithel der Lymphgefässwurzeln und über die von Recklinghausen'schen Saftcanälchen. *Z. wiss. Zool.*, 1863, **13**, 455–73.

1110 SAPPEY, Marie Philibert Constant. 1810–1896
Anatomie, physiologie, pathologie des vaisseaux lymphatiques. Paris, *A. Delahaye & E. Lacrosnier*, 1874–75.

Notable for its illustrations.

1111 WALDEYER-HARTZ, Heinrich Wilhelm Gottfried. 1836–1921
Ueber den lymphatischen Apparat des Pharynx. *Dtsch. med. Wschr.*, 1884, **10**, 313.

1112 STARLING, Ernest Henry. 1866–1927
The influence of mechanical factors on lymph production. *J. Physiol. (Lond.)*, 1894, **16**, 224–67.

1113 SABIN, Florence Rena. 1871–1953
The origin and development of the lymphatic system. Baltimore, *Johns Hopkins Press*, 1913.

1114 YOFFEY, Joseph Mendel. 1902–
The quantitative study of lymphocyte production. *J. Anat.* (*Lond.*), 1933, **67**, 250–62; 1935–36, **70**, 507–14.

1116–1207.1 DUCTLESS GLANDS; INTERNAL SECRETION

See also 3789–3911, Endocrine Disorders

1116 WHARTON, Thomas. 1614–1673
Adenographia: sive, glandularum totius corporis descriptio. Londini, *typ. J. G. impens. Authoris*, 1656.

Wharton described the duct of the submaxillary salivary gland ("Wharton's duct"). He described the thyroid more accurately than his predecessors, naming it. Wharton was one of the few physicians to remain in London during the plague of 1666.

1117 BORDEU, Théophile de. 1722–1776
Recherches sur les maladies chroniques. VI. Analyse médicinale du sang. Paris, 1775.

De Bordeu first conceived the idea of internal secretion by his hypothesis that every organ, tissue and cell discharges into the blood products which influence other parts of the body.

1118 LEGALLOIS, Julien Jean César. 1770–1814
Le sang, est-il identique dans tous les vaisseaux qu'il parcourt? Paris, *Thèse*, [1801].

Like de Bordeu, and more definitely, Legallois anticipated the conception of internal secretions.

1119 COOPER, *Sir* Astley Paston, *Bart.* 1768–1841
The anatomy of the thymus gland. London, *Longman*, 1832.

Cooper, the most popular surgeon in London during the early part of the 19th century, was connected with both Guy's and St. Thomas's Hospital. Among his best works is his description of the thymus; he described the "reservoir" of the thymus as lined by smooth mucous membrane and running spirally, not straight, through the gland.

1120 HEIDENHAIN, Rudolf Peter Heinrich. 1834–1897
Ueber secretorische und trophische Drüsennerven. *Pflüg. Arch. ges. Physiol.*, 1878, **17**, 1–67.

Investigation of the secretory and trophic nerves of glands. Heidenhain considered all secretory phenomena to be intracellular, rather than mechanical, processes.

1121 BAYLISS, *Sir* William Maddock. 1860–1924, & STARLING, Ernest Henry. 1866–1927
The chemical regulation of the secretory process. *Proc. roy. Soc. B*, 1904, **73**, 310–22.

Bayliss and Starling developed the theory of hormonal control of internal secretion.

1122 STARLING, Ernest Henry. 1866–1927
The Croonian Lectures on the chemical correlation of the functions of the body. *Lancet*, 1905, **2**, 339–41, 423–25, 501–03, 579–83.

Starling constructed a general scheme of the "hormones," as he named the internal secretions. This is the first appearance of the word, which was suggested by W. B. Hardy.

1123 BIEDL, Artur. 1869–1933.
Innere Sekretion. Berlin, Wien, *Urban & Schwarzenburg*, 1910.

Biedl showed that the adrenal cortex is essential for life. His book (4th ed., 1922) includes an exhaustive bibliography. An English translation appeared in 1912.

1124 CANNON, Walter Bradford. 1871–1945
Bodily changes in pain, hunger, fear, and rage. New York, *D. Appleton*, 1915.

Cannon showed the close connexion between the endocrine glands and the emotions.

1125 TRENDELENBURG, Paul. 1884–1931
Die Hormone; ihre Physiologie und Pharmakologie. 2 vols. Berlin, *J. Springer*, 1929–34.

Thyroid; Parathyroids

1126 KING, Thomas Wilkinson. 1809–1847
Observations on the thyroid gland, with notes on the same subject by Sir Astley Cooper. *Guy's Hosp. Rep.*, 1836, **1**, 429–56.

King, sometimes referred to as the "father of endocrinology", anticipated the endocrine action of the thyroid.

1126.1 OWEN, *Sir* Richard. 1804–1892
On the anatomy of the Indian rhinoceros (Rh. unicornis *L.*). *Trans. Zool. Soc. Lond.*, 1852, **4**, 31–58.

Owen was among the first to describe the parathyroids.

1127 SANDSTRÖM, Ivar Victor. 1852–1889
Om en ny körtel hos menniskan och åtskilliga däggdjur. *Upsala Läkaref. Förh.*, 1880, **15**, 441–71.

Remak, Owen and Virchow had previously noted the presence of what may have been parathyroids; the first systematic account of them was given by Sandström. An English translation of this paper appeared in *Bull. Inst. Hist. Med.*, Baltimore, 1938, **6**, 192–222; a translation was also published in book form at Baltimore, 1938.

1128 HORSLEY, *Sir* Victor Alexander Haden. 1857–1916
On the function of the thyroid gland. *Proc. roy. Soc.* (*Lond.*), 1884–85, **38**, 5–7; 1886, **40**, 6–9.

From his experimental work Horsley produced evidence to support the view that myxoedema, cretinism and operative cachexia strumipriva are all due to thyroid deficiency.

1129 ——. Functional nervous disorders due to loss of thyroid gland and pituitary body. *Lancet*, 1886, **1**, 5.

First successful experimental hypophysectomy; two dogs survived five and six months respectively after this operation.

1130 GLEY, EUGÈNE. 1857–1930
Sur les fonctions du corps thyroïde. *C.R. Soc. Biol. (Paris)*, 1891, **43,** 841–47.

Gley re-discovered the parathyroids and later come across Sandström's description (see No. 1127). Gley seems to have been the first to understand their real significance; his work showed the necessity of the parathyroids for the maintenance of life.

1131 BAUMANN, EUGEN. 1846–1896
Ueber das normale Vorkommen von Jod im Thierkörper. *Hoppe-Seyl. Z. physiol. Chem.*, 1895–96, **21,** 319–30, 481–93; **22,** 1–17.

Demonstration of the presence of iodine in organic combination in the thyroid. Baumann isolated an iodine-containing compound ("Thyrojodin"). The biochemical research stimulated by this work led eventually to the discovery of thyroxine. Second paper is written with E. Roos.

1132 HUNT, REID. 1870–1948, & SEIDELL, ATHERTON. 1878–
Studies on thyroid. I. The relation of iodine to the physiological activity of thyroid preparations. *Bull. Hyg. Lab. U.S. publ. Hlth. Serv.*, No. 47, 1909.

1133 KENDALL, EDWARD CALVIN. 1886–
The isolation in crystalline form of the compound containing iodin, which occurs in the thyroid; its chemical nature and physiologic activity. *J. Amer. med. Ass.*, 1915, **64,** 2042–43; *Trans. Ass. Amer. Physicians*, 1915, **30,** 420–49.

Kendall isolated in crystalline form the thyroid hormone "thyroxine" on Christmas Day, 1914.

1134 HUNT, REID. 1870–1948
The acetonitril test for thyroid and of some alterations of metabolism. *Amer. J. Physiol.*, 1923, **63,** 257–99.

The acetonitril test was introduced by Hunt in 1905 (*J. biol. Chem.*, **1**, 33) and later modified by him. It shows the activity of thyroid preparations to be proportional to their iodine content.

1135 HANSON, ADOLPH MELANCTHON. 1888–1959
An elementary chemical study of the parathyroid glands of cattle. *Milit. Surg.*, 1923, **52,** 280–84.

Hanson isolated the first really potent parathyroid extract.

1136 COLLIP, JAMES BERTRAM. 1892–1965
The extraction of a parathyroid hormone which will prevent or control parathyroid tetany and which regulates the level of blood calcium. *J. biol. Chem.*, 1925, **63,** 395–438.

Isolation of parathormone, the active principle of the parathyroids.

1137 HARINGTON, *Sir* CHARLES ROBERT. 1897–1972
Chemistry of thyroxine. I. *Biochem. J.*, 1926, **20,** 293–313.

Harington showed that thyroxine is a derivative of tyrosine, and he gave its formula as $C_{15}H_{11}O_4NI_4$.

1138 ——. & BARGER, GEORGE. 1878–1939
Chemistry of thyroxine. III. Constitution and synthesis of thyroxine. *Biochem. J.*, 1927, **21,** 169–81.

Synthesis of thyroxine.

1138.1 GROSS, JACK. 1921– , & PITT-RIVERS, ROSALIND VENETIA. 1907–
3:5:3'-Triiodothyronine. I. Isolation from thyroid gland and synthesis. *Biochem. J.*, 1953, **53,** 645–50.

1138.2 COPP, DOUGLAS HAROLD. 1915– , *et al.*
Evidence for calcitonin – a new hormone from the parathyroid that lowers blood calcium. *Endocrinology*, 1962, **70,** 638–49.
With E. C. Cameron, B. A. Cheney, A. G. F. Davidson, and K. G. Henze.

Adrenals

1139 EUSTACHI, BARTOLOMMEO [EUSTACHIUS]. 1520–1574
Opuscula anatomica. Venetiis, *V. Luchinus*, 1564.
Includes first description of the adrenals.

1140 BROWN-SÉQUARD, CHARLES EDOUARD. 1817–1894
Recherches expérimentales sur la physiologie et la pathologie des capsules surrénales. *C. R. Acad. Sci.* (*Paris*), 1856, **43,** 422–25; 542–46.
Brown-Séquard found that excision of both adrenals in animals invariably proved fatal, thus determining their indispensability. He also believed that they had an antitoxic influence upon the blood. His experimental work was of great importance in the development of our knowledge of the internal secretions.

1141 VULPIAN, EDME FÉLIX ALFRED. 1826–1887
Note sur quelques réactions propres à la substance des capsules surrénales. *C. R. Acad. Sci.* (*Paris*), 1856, **43,** 663–65.
Vulpian discovered adrenaline in the adrenal medulla.

1142 ABELOUS, JACQUES EMILE. 1864–1940, & LANGLOIS, JEAN PAUL. 1862–1923
Des rapports de la fatigue avec les fonctions des capsules surrénales. *Arch. Physiol. norm. path.*, 1893, 5 sér., **5,** 720–28.

1143 OLIVER, GEORGE. 1841–1915, & SHARPEY-SCHÄFER, *Sir* EDWARD ALBERT. 1850–1935
The physiological action of extract of the suprarenal capsules. *J. Physiol.* (*Lond.*), 1895, **18,** 230–76.
These workers demonstrated the existence of a pressor substance (adrenaline) in the adrenal medulla. Preliminary communications regarding the above appeared in the proceedings of the Physiological Society, *J. Physiol.*, 1894, **16**, p. i–v, 1895. **17**, p. ix–xiv.

1144 ABEL, JOHN JACOB. 1857–1983, & CRAWFORD, ALBERT CORNELIUS. 1869–1921
On the blood-pressure-raising constituent of the suprarenal capsule. *Johns Hopk. Hosp. Bull.*, 1897, **8,** 151–57.
Abel and Crawford further investigated the pressor substance of Oliver and Schäfer calling it "epinephrine."

1145 ABEL, JOHN JACOB. 1857–1938
Ueber den blutdruckerregenden Bestandtheil der Nebenniere, das Epinephrin. *Hoppe-Seyl. Z. physiol. Chem.*, 1899, **28,** 318–62.

1146 TAKAMINE, Jôkichi. 1854–1922
The blood-pressure-raising principle of the suprarenal glands. *Therap. Gaz.*, 1901, **17,** 221–24; *Amer. J. Pharm.*, **73,** 523–31.
Isolation of adrenaline.

1147 ALDRICH, Thomas Bell. 1861–
A preliminary report on the active principle of the suprarenal gland. *Amer. J. Physiol.*, 1901, **5,** 457–61.
Independently of Takamine, Aldrich succeeded in isolating adrenaline in a crystalline form. He gave it the formula $C_9H_{13}NO_3$. Adrenaline was the first hormone to be isolated.

1147.1 STOLZ, Friedrich.
Ueber Adrenalin und Alkylaminoacetobrenzcatechin. *Ber. dtsch. chem. Ges.*, 1904, **37,** 4149–54.
Synthesis of adrenaline.

1148 ROGOFF, Julius Moses. 1883–1966, & STEWART, George Neil. 1860–1930
Further studies on adrenal insufficiency in dogs. *Science*, 1927, **66,** 327.
Cortical hormone first obtained.

1149 PFIFFNER, Joseph John. 1903– , & SWINGLE, Wilbur Willis. 1891–
The preparation of an active extract of the suprarenal cortex. *Anat. Rec.*, 1929, **44,** 225.
First practical method of preparing an extract of the active agent of the adrenal cortical hormone. It was named cortin until it was recognized that there are several active agents in the secretion.

1150 KENDALL, Edward Calvin. 1886– , *et al.*
Isolation in crystalline form of the hormone essential to life from the suprarenal cortex; its chemical nature and physiologic properties. *Proc. Mayo Clin.*, 1934, **9,** 245–50.
Together with H. L. Mason, B. F. McKenzie, C. S. Myers, and G. A. Koelsche, Kendall reported the isolation in crystalline form of cortin ($C_{20}H_{30}O_5$).

1151 ——. A physiologic and chemical investigation of the suprarenal cortex. *J. biol. Chem.*, 1936, **114,** lvii–lviii.
Isolation of nine closely related steroid hormones from adrenal cortical extracts; one of these was Compound E ($C_{21}H_{28}O_5$) which in 1939 was renamed cortisone. With H. L. Mason, C. S. Myers, and W. D. Allers. See also the same journal, 1936, **114**, 613,; **116** 267.

1152 WINTERSTEINER, Oskar Paul. 1898– , & PFIFFNER, Joseph John. 1903–
Chemical studies on the adrenal cortex. II. Isolation of several physiologically inactive crystalline compounds from active extracts. III. Isolation of two new physiologically inactive compounds. *J. biol. Chem.*, 1935, **111,** 599–612; 1936, **116,** 291–305.
Isolation of Compound F, identical with Kendall's Compound E (see No. 1151).

1153 REICHSTEIN, Tadeus. 1897–
Über Bestandteile der Nebennieren-Rinde. VI. Trennungsmethoden sowie Isolierung der Substanzen Fa, H, und J. *Helv. chim. Acta*, 1936, **19,** 1107–26.

Isolation of Compound Fa identical with Compounds E and F. Reichstein shared the Nobel Prize with Kendall and Hench in 1950.

1154 FREMERY, P. de, *et al.*
Corticosteron, a crystallized compound with the biological activity of the adrenal-cortical hormone. *Nature* (*Lond.*), 1937, **139,** 26.

Isolation of corticosterone. With E. Laqueur, T. Reichstein, R. W. Spanhoff, and I. E. Uyldert.

1155 STEIGER, Marguerite, & REICHSTEIN, Tadeus. 1897–
Partial synthesis of a crystallized compound with the biological activity of the adrenal-cortical hormone. *Nature* (*Lond.*), 1937, **139,** 925–26.

Isolation of desoxycorticosterone acetate (DOCA).

1155.1 GRUNDY, Hilary M., *et al.*
Isolation of a highly active mineralocorticoid from beef adrenal extract. *Nature* (*Lond.*), 1952, **169,** 795–96.

Isolation of aldosterone. With S. A. Simpson and J. F. Tait.

1155.2 WOODWARD, Robert Burns. 1917– , *et al.*
The total synthesis of steroids. *J. Amer. chem. Soc.*, 1952, **74,** 4223–51.

Synthesis of cortisone. With F. Sondheimer, D. Taub, K. Heusler, and W. M. McLamore.

Pituitary

1156 RATHKE, Martin Heinrich. 1793–1860
Ueber die Entstehung der Glandula pituitaria. *Arch. Anat. Physiol. wiss. Med.*, 1838, 482–85.

Important description of the pituitary.

1157 VASSALE, Giulio. 1862–1912, & SACCHI, Ercole.
Sulla distruzione della ghiandola pituitaria. *Riv. sper. Freniat.*, 1892, **18,** 525–61.

Vassale and Sacchi showed water and mineral metabolism to be affected by hypophysectomy.

1158 PAULESCO, Nicolas. 1869–1931
L'hypophyse du cerveau. I. Physiologie. Paris, *Vigot Frères*, 1908.

Paulesco found that the removal of the anterior pituitary had fatal results, while removal of the posterior lobe had negative results.

1159 DALE, *Sir* Henry Hallett. 1875–1968
The action of extracts of the pituitary body. *Biochem. J.*, 1909, **4**, 427–47.

Oxytocic action of posterior pituitary injection.

1160 CROWE, Samuel James. 1883–1955, *et al.*
Experimental hypophysectomy. *Johns Hopk. Hosp. Bull.*, 1910, **21,** 127–69.

First experimental evidence of the relationship between the pituitary and the reproductive system. With H. W. Cushing and J. Homans.

1161 CUSHING, Harvey Williams. 1869–1939
The functions of the pituitary body. *Amer. J. med. Sci.*, 1910, **139,** 473–84.

1162 ASCHNER, Bernhard. 1883–1960
Über die Funktion der Hypophyse. *Pflüg. Arch. ges. Physiol.*, 1912, **146,** 1–146.
Aschner was able to keep his hypophysectomized dogs alive indefinitely. He found that they developed genital hypoplasia.

1162.1 GAINES, Walter Lee, 1881–
A contribution to the physiology of lactation. *Amer. J. Physiol.*, 1915, **38,** 285–312.
Gaines demonstrated the action of the pituitary in lactation.

1163 EVANS, Herbert McLean. 1882–1971, & LONG, Joseph Abraham. 1879–
The effect of the anterior lobe administered intraperitoneally upon growth, maturity and oestrus cycles of the rat. *Anat. Rec.*, 1921, **21,** 62–63.
Evans and Long showed that continued injections of an anterior pituitary extract produced an acceleration in the growth-rate of laboratory animals.

1164 ABEL, John Jacob. 1857–1938, & ROUILLER, Charles August. 1883–
Evaluation of the hormone of the infundibulum of the pituitary gland in terms of histamine, with experiments on the action of repeated injections of the hormone on the blood pressure. *J. Pharmacol.*, 1922–1923, **20,** 65–84.

1165 ABEL, John Jacob. 1857–1938, *et al.*
Further investigations on the oxytocic-pressor-diuretic principle of the infundibular portion of the pituitary gland. *J. Pharmacol.*, 1923–1924, **22,** 289–316.
With C. A. Rouiller and E. M. K. Geiling.

1166 SMITH, Philip Edward. 1884–
The induction of precocious sexual maturity by pituitary homeo-transplants. *Amer. J. Physiol.*, 1927, **80,** 114–25.
Smith was able to induce precocious sexual maturity in mice and rats by the implantation of pituitary tissue.

1167 ——, & ENGLE, Earl Theron. 1896–1957
Experimental evidence regarding the rôle of the anterior pituitary in the development and regulation of the genital system. *Amer. J. Anat.*, 1927, **40,** 159–217.
Pituitary tissue implanted in the immature mouse was found by these writers to cause precocious sexual maturity. Thus they showed that the activity of the gonads is maintained by the anterior lobe of the pituitary.

1168 ZONDEK, Bernhard. 1891–1966, & ASCHHEIM, Selmar. 1878–
Das Hormon des Hypophysenvorderlappens. *Klin. Wschr.*, 1927 **6,** 348–52; 1928, **7,** 831–35.
Isolation of the gonadotrophic hormone of the anterior pituitary (Prolan A & B).

1168.1 KAMM, Oliver. 1888– , *et al.*
The active principles of the posterior lobe of the pituitary gland. I. The demonstration of the presence of two active principles. II. The separation of the two principles and their concentration in the form of potent solid preparations. *J. Amer. chem. Soc.*, 1928, **50,** 573–601.
Isolation of vasopressin and oxytocin. With T. B. Aldrich, I. W. Grote, L. W. Rowe, and E. P. Bugbee.

1168.2 STRICKER, P., & GRUETER, F.
Action du lobe antérieur de l'hypophyse sur la montée laiteuse. *C. R. Soc. Biol.* (*Paris*), 1929. **99,** 1978–80.
Demonstration of the existence of a pituitary lactogenic hormone (prolactin).

1169 HOUSSAY, Bernardo Alberto. 1887–1971, & BIASOTTI, Alfredo. 1903–
La diabetes pancreática de los perros hipofisoprivos. *Rev. Soc. argent. Biol.*, 1930, **6,** 251–96.
Houssay's depancreatized hypophysectomized dog. This work led to Houssay's demonstration of the importance of the anterior pituitary in sugar metabolism, for which he shared the Nobel Prize in 1947. See also *Endocrinology*, 1931, **15,** 511–23.

1170 COLLIP, James Bertram. 1892–1965, *et al.*
The adrenotropic hormone of the anterior pituitary lobe. *Lancet*, 1933, **2,** 347–48.
Isolation of an impure "adrenotropic hormone" containing adrenocorticotrophic principle. With E. M. Anderson and D. L. Thomson.

1171 RIDDLE, Oscar. 1877– , *et al.*
The preparation, identification and assay of prolactin – a hormone of the anterior pituitary. *Amer. J. Physiol.*, 1933, **105,** 191–216.
With R. W. Bates and S. W. Dykshorn.

1172 VAN DYKE, Harry Benjamin. 1895–
The physiology and pharmacology of the pituitary body. 2 vols. Chicago, *Univ. Press*, 1936–39.
Includes an extensive bibliography.

1173 YOUNG, Frank George. 1908–
Permanent experimental diabetes produced by pituitary (anterior lobe) injections. *Lancet*, 1937, **2,** 372–74.
Anterior pituitary diabetogenic hormone.

1173.1 LI, Choh Hao. 1913– , *et al.*
Interstitial cell stimulating hormone. II. Method of preparation and some physico-chemical studies. *Endocrinology*, 1940, **27,** 803–08.
Isolation of the interstitial cell stimulating (luteinizing) hormone. With M. E. Simpson and H. M. Evans.

1174 ——. Adrenocorticotropic hormone. *J. biol. Chem.*, 1943, **149,** 413–424.
Isolation of pure adrenocorticotrophic hormone (ACTH) from sheep pituitary glands. With H. M. Evans and M. E. Simpson.

1175 SAYERS, George. 1914 , *et al.*
Preparation and properties of pituitary adrenocorticotropic hormone. *J. biol. Chem.*, 1943, **149,** 425–36.
Isolation of ACTH from swine pituitaries. With A. White and C. N. H. Long.

1175.1 LI, CHOH HAO. 1913– , *et al.*
Isolation and properties of the anterior hypophyseal growth hormone. *J. biol. Chem.*, 1945, **159,** 353–66.
Isolation of the anterior pituitary growth hormone. With H. M. Evans and M. E. Simpson.

1175.2 ——. Isolation of pituitary follicle-stimulating hormone (FSH). *Science*, 1949, **109,** 445–46.
With M. E. Simpson and H. M. Evans.

1175.3 DU VIGNEAUD, VINCENT. 1901– , *et al.*
The synthesis of an octapeptide amide with the hormonal activity of oxytocin. *J. Amer. chem. Soc.*, 1953, **75,** 4879–80.
Synthesis of oxytocin. With C. Ressler, J. M. Swan, C. W. Roberts, P. G. Katsoyannis, and S. Gordon. For his work on the synthesis of oxytocin and other posterior pituitary hormones, du Vigneaud was awarded a Nobel Prize (chemistry) in 1955.

1175.4 ——. A synthetic preparation possessing biological properties associated with arginine-vasopressin. *J. Amer. chem. Soc.*, 1954, **76,** 4751–52.
Synthesis of vasopressin. With D. T. Gish and P. G. Katsoyannis.

Gonads; Sex Hormones

1176 BERTHOLD, ARNOLD ADOLPH. 1803–1861
Transplantation der Hoden. *Arch. Anat. Physiol. wiss. Med.*, 1849, 42–46.
Berthold showed that transplantation of a cock's testes to another part of the body prevented atrophy of the comb, the usual sequel to castration. He was thus the first to prove the existence of an internal secretion. English translation in *Bull. Hist. Med.*, 1944, **16** 399–401.

1177 BROWN-SÉQUARD, CHARLES EDOUARD. 1817–1894
Expérience démontrant la puissance dynamogénique chez l'homme d'un liquide extrait de testicules d'animaux. *Arch. Physiol. norm. path.*, 1889, 5 sér., **1,** 651–58.
Brown-Séquard injected into himself a testicular extract in order to bring about rejuvenation. He reported much benefit but his advocacy of this method evoked scepticism and criticism, although it stimulated research on internal secretion, being perhaps the first employment of "male sex hormone". Further papers on this subject were published by Brown-Séquard in the same journal, 1889, 5 sér., **1,** 739–46; 1890, **2,** 201–08, 443–57, 641–48; and 1891, **3,** 747–61.

1178 POEHL, ALEKSANDR VASSILIEVIC [VON PEL]. 1850–1898. [On spermin.]
J. Russk. fis.-chim. Obsh., 1891, **23,** 151–55.
Isolation of spermin from the testis.

1178.1 KNAUER, EMIL. 1867–1935
Einige Versuche über Ovarientransplantation bei Kaninchen. *Zbl. Gynäk.*, 1896, **20,** 524–28.
Knauer implanted ovaries into immature or castrated animals, producing development of sexual characteristics, thus demonstrating the existence of an ovarian hormone.

1179 SOBOTTA, ROBERT HEINRICH JOHANNES. 1869–1945
Ueber die Bildung des Corpus luteum bei der Maus. *Arch. mikr. Anat.*, 1896, **47,** 261–308.

1180 LANE-CLAYPON, JANET ELIZABETH. 1877–1967, & STARLING, ERNEST HENRY. 1866–1927
An experimental enquiry into the factors which determine the growth and activity of the mammary glands. *Proc. roy. Soc. B*, 1905–06, **77,** 505–22.

In their classical paper on the mammary gland, these workers attributed its changes during pregnancy to the foetus.

1181 HITSCHMANN, FRITZ. 1870–1926, & ADLER, LUDWIG. 1876–1958
Der Bau der Uterusschleimhaut des geschlechtsreifen Weibes besonderer Berücksichtigung der Menstruation. *Mschr. Geburt. Gynäk.*, 1908, **27,** 1–82.

First definite description of the cyclical changes in the endometrium, which were shown to be a normal physiological process.

1182 STOCKARD, CHARLES RUPERT. 1879–1939, & PAPANICOLAOU, GEORGE NICHOLAS. 1883–1962
The existence of a typical oestrus cycle in the guinea-pig; with a study of its histological and physiological changes. *Amer. J. Anat.*, 1917, **22,** 225–83.

The vaginal smear test for oestrus; it demonstrates the histological changes occurring in the vagina during the menstrual cycle.

1183 ALLEN, EDGAR. 1892–1943, & DOISY, EDWARD ADELBERT. 1893–
An ovarian hormone. *J. Amer. med. Ass.*, 1923, **81,** 819–21.

Isolation of the active principle of the ovarian hormone (oestrin). More detailed account in *J. biol. Chem.*, 1924, **61**, 711–23.

1184 ——. The induction of a sexually mature condition in immature females by injection of the ovarian follicular hormone. *Amer. J. Physiol.*, 1924, **69,** 577–88.

Test for recognition of the oestrus hormone.

1185 ——. The menstrual cycle of the monkey, *Macacus rhesus*: Observations on normal animals, the effects of removal of the ovaries and the effects of injection of ovarian and placental extracts into the spayed animals. *Contr. Embryol. Carneg. Instn*, 1927, **19,** 1–44.

This paper marks the beginning of modern knowledge of the menstrual cycle. Allen showed that uterine bleeding occurs as a withdrawal effect when oestrogen ceases to act on the endometrium.

1186 LAQUEUR, ERNST. 1880–1947, *et al.*
Über das Vorkommen weiblichen Sexualhormons (Menformon) im Harn von Männern. *Klin. Wschr.*, 1927, **6,** 1859.

Discovery of the oestrogenic activity of male urine. With E. Dingemanse, P. C. Hart, and S. E. de Jongh.

1187 McGEE, LEMUEL CLYDE. 1904–
The effect of the injection of a lipoid fraction of bull testicle in capons. *Proc. Inst. Med. Chicago*, 1927, **6,** 242–54.

McGee prepared the first active male hormone extract from the lipoid fraction of bull testes. His paper includes a preliminary account of the capon-comb test (see No. 1191).

1188 CORNER, George Washington. 1889– , & ALLEN, Willard Myron. 1904–
Physiology of the corpus luteum. *Amer. J. Physiol.*, 1929, **88**, 326–46
Discovery of the corpus luteum hormone, progesterone.

1189 FUNK, Casimir. 1884–1967, & HARROW, Benjamin. 1888–
The male hormone. *Proc. Soc. exp. Biol. (N.Y.)*, 1929, **26**, 325–26.
Funk and Harrow obtained crude active male hormone extracts from male urine.

1190 MARRIAN, Guy Frederic. 1904–
The chemistry of oestrin. I. Preparation from urine and separation from an unidentified solid alcohol. *Biochem. J.*, 1929, **23**, 1090–98.
Isolation of pregnanediol.

1191 MOORE, Carl Richard. 1892–1955, *et al.*
The effects of extracts of testis in correcting the castrated condition in the fowl and in the mammal. *Endocrinology*, 1929, **13**, 367–74.
C. R. Moore, T. F. Gallagher, and F. C. Koch were the first to obtain a potent testicular extract containing the male sex hormone, androsterone, later obtained in crystalline form by Butenandt. They also gave a detailed account of the capon-comb test for the assay of the male hormone.

1192 COLLIP, James Bertram. 1892–1965
The ovary-stimulating hormone of the placenta. *Canad. med. Ass. J.*, 1930, **22**, 215–19, 761–74.
Collip's anterior-pituitary-like (A-L-P) factor.

1193 DOISY, Edward Adelbert. 1893– , *et al.*
The preparation of the crystalline ovarian hormone from the urine of pregnant women. *J. biol. Chem.*, 1930, **86**, 499–509.
Isolation for the first time of a pure crystalline hormone (oestrone). Doisy shared the Nobel Prize with Dam in 1943. Written with C. D. Veler and S. A. Thayer. Preliminary communication in *Amer. J. Physiol.*, 1929, **90**, 329–30.

1194 MARRIAN, Guy Frederic. 1904–
The chemistry of oestrin. III. An improved method of preparation and the isolation of active crystalline material. *Biochem. J.*, 1930, **24**, 435–45.
Crystalline oestriol obtained.

1195 BUTENANDT, Adolf Friedrich Johann. 1903–
Ueber die chemische Untersuchung der Sexualhormone. *Z. angew. Chem.*, 1931, **44**, 905–08.
The male sex hormone, androsterone, was isolated in crystalline form by Butenandt. He shared the Nobel Prize for chemistry with Ruzicka (No. 1201) in 1939.

1196 ZONDEK, Bernhard. 1891–1966
Die Hormone des Ovariums und des Hypophysenvorderlappens. Berlin, *J. Springer*, 1931.
Second edition, 1935.

1197 ALLEN, Edgar. 1892–1943
Sex and internal secretions; a survey of recent research. Baltimore, *Williams & Wilkins*, 1932.
Second edition, 1939, with C. H. Danforth and E. A. Doisy.

1198 BROWNE, John Symonds Lyon. 1904–
Chemical and physiological properties of crystalline oestrogenic hormones. *Canad. J. Res.*, 1933, **8,** 180–97.
Oestriol obtained from placental tissue.

1199 KAUFMANN, Carl.
Die Behandlung der Amenorrhoë mit hohen Dosen der Ovarialhormone. *Klin. Wschr.*, 1933, **12,** 1557–62.
First use of oestrogenic hormone in ovariectomized women, with production of the typical cyclical endometrial changes.

1200 BUTENANDT, Adolf Friedrich Johann. 1903–
Neuere Ergebnisse auf dem Gebiet der Sexualhormone. *Wien. klin. Wschr.*, 1934, **47,** 897–901, 934–36.
Progesterone obtained in crystalline form.

1201 RUZICKA, Leopold. 1887– , *et al.*
Über die Synthese des Testikelhormons (Androsteron) und Stereoisomerer desselben durch Abbau hydrierter Sterine. *Helv. chim. Acta*, 1934, **17,** 1395–1406.
First complete synthesis of a sex hormone (androsterone). With M. W. Goldberg, J. Meyer, H. Brüngger, and E. Eichenberger.

1201.1 DAVID, K., *et al.*
Über krystallinisches männliches Hormon aus Hoden (Testosteron), wirksamer als aus Harn oder aus Cholesterin bereitetes Androsteron. *Hoppe-Seyl. Z. physiol. Chem.*, 1935, **233,** 281–82.
Isolation of testosterone from the testis. With E Dingemanse, J. Freud, and E. Laqueur.

1202 MacCORQUODALE, Donald William. 1898– , *et al.*
Isolation of the principle oestrogenic substance of liquor folliculi. *J. biol. Chem.*, 1936, **115,** 435–48.
Isolation of oestradiol. With S. A. Thayer and E. A. Doisy.

For history, see 1588.2

Pancreas

1203 LANGERHANS, Paul. 1847–1888
Beiträge zur mikroskopischen Anatomie der Bauchspeicheldrüse. Inaugural-Dissertation. Berlin, *Gustav Lange*, 1869.
First account of the "islands of Langerhans". Reprinted with English translation, 1937. See also No. 1009.

1204 MEYER, Jean de. 1878–
Action de la sécrétion interne du pancréas sur différent organes et en particulier sur la sécrétion rénale. *Arch. Fisiol.*, 1909, **7,** 96–99.
De Meyer was apparently the first to suggest the name "insuline" for the substance then believed to be secreted by the pancreas.

1205 BANTING, *Sir* Frederick Grant. 1891–1941, & BEST, Charles Herbert. 1899–
The internal secretion of the pancreas. *J. Lab. clin. Med.*, 1921–22, **7,** 251–66.
Isolation of insulin. The first report on the subject was made by Banting, Best and Macleod at a meeting of the American Physiological Society, Dec. 28, 1921, and published in *Amer. J. Physiol.*, 1922, **59**, 479.

1206 ABEL, JOHN JACOB. 1857–1938
Crystalline insulin. *Proc. nat. Acad. Sci.* (*Wash.*), 1926, **12,** 132–36.
Crystalline insulin first obtained. See also *J. Pharmacol.*, 1927, **31**, 65–85.

1207 RYLE, ANDREW PETER, *et al.*
The disulphide bonds of insulin. *Biochem. J.*, 1955, **60,** 541–56.
Structure of insulin. With F. Sanger, L. F. Smith and R. Kitai.

1207.1 KUNG, YUEH-TING, *et al.*
Total synthesis of crystalline bovine insulin. *Scientia sin.*, 1965, **14,** 1710–16.

1208–1246.1 GENITO-URINARY SYSTEM

1208 FALLOPPIO, GABRIELE [FALLOPIUS]. 1523–1562
Observationes anatomicae. Venetiis, *apud M. A. Ulmum*, 1561.
Fallopius is best remembered for his account of the tubes named after him. He also left excellent descriptions of the ovaries, hymen, clitoris, and round ligaments. He gave to the vagina and the placenta their present scientific names, and definitely proved the existence of the seminal vesicles. Photographic reproduction with annotated Italian version, 2 vols., Modena, 1964.

1209 GRAAF, REGNER DE. 1641–1673
De mulierum organis generationi inservientibus. Lugduni Batavorum, *ex. off. Hackiana*, 1672.
De Graaf demonstrated ovulation anatomically, pathologically and experimentally. In the above work he included the first account of the "Graafian follicle". Translation of Chapter XII, dealing with the ovaries, by G. W. Corner in *Essays in honor of H. M. Evans*, Berkeley, 1943.

1210 ——. De virorum organis generationi inservientibus, de clysteribus et de usu siphonis in anatomia. Lugduni Batavorum, *ex off. Hackiana*, 1668.
Exact and detailed account of the male reproductive system.

1211 SWAMMERDAM, JAN. 1637–1680
Miraculum naturae, sive uteri muliebris fabrica. Lugduni Batavorum, *apud S. Mathaei*, 1672.

1212 MÉRY, JEAN. 1645–1722
Observations anatomiques. *J. Sçavans*, 1684, 129.
Includes a brief description of "Cowper's glands".

1213 NUCK, ANTONJ. 1650–1692
Adenographia curiosa et uteri foeminei anatome nova. Lugduni Batavorum, *apud Jordanum Luchtmans*, 1692.
Description of the "canal of Nuck".

1214 COWPER, WILLIAM. 1666–1709
An account of two new glands and their excretory ducts, lately discovered in human bodies. *Phil. Trans.*, (1699), 1700, **21,** 364–69.
Cowper's description of the glands which bear his name. He was forestalled in their discovery by Jean Méry.

1215 LITTRE, ALEXIS. 1658–1726
Description de l'urèthre de l'homme. *Hist. Acad. roy. Sci.* (*Paris*), (1700), 1719, Mém., 311–16.
"Littre's glands" described.

1216 NABOTH, MARTIN. 1675–1721
De sterilitate mulierum. Leipzig, *A. Zeidler*, 1707.
The Nabothian cysts and glands of the cervix uteri first described.

1217 DOUGLAS, JAMES. 1675–1742
A description of the peritonaeum, and of that part of the membrana cellularis which lies on its outside. With an account of the true situation of all the abdominal viscera, in respect of these two membranes. London, *J. Roberts*, 1730.
Douglas described the peritoneum in detail; his name is perpetuated in the "pouch", "line", and "fold of Douglas". He was a friend of John Hunter and brother of John Douglas the lithotomist.

1218 CRUIKSHANK, WILLIAM CUMBERLAND. 1745–1800
Experiments in which, on the third day after impregnation, the ova of rabbits were found in the Fallopian tubes, and on the fourth day after impregnation in the uterus itself, with the first appearances of the foetus. *Phil. Trans.*, 1797, **87,** 197–214.
Cruikshank showed that the impregnated ovum stayed in the fallopian tube for a period before implantation in the uterus.

1219 KÖLLIKER, RUDOLPH ALBERT VON. 1817–1905
Beiträge zur Kenntniss der Geschlechtsverhältnisse und der Samenflüssigkeit wirbelloser Thiere. Berlin, *W. Logier*, 1841.

1220 ——. Ueber das Wesen der sogenannten Saamenthiere. *N. Notiz. a.d. Geb. d. Natur- und Heilk.*, Weimar, 1841, **19,** 4–8.
Demonstration of the cellular origin of spermatozoa.

1221 RETZIUS, ANDERS ADOLF. 1796–1860
Ueber das Ligamentum pelvoprostaticum oder den Apparat, durch welchen die Harnblase, die Prostata und die Harnröhre an den untern Beckenöffnung befestigt sind. *Müller's Arch. Anat. Physiol. wiss Med.*, 1849, 182–96.
The "cave of Retzius" described.

1222 LEYDIG, FRANZ. 1821–1908
Zur Anatomie der männlichen Geschlechtsorgane und Analdrüsen der Säugethiere. *Z. wiss. Zool.*, 1850, **2,** 1–57.
Leydig was the first to describe the interstitial cells of the testis ("Leydig cells").

1223 ECKHARD, CONRAD. 1822–1915
Untersuchungen über die Erection des Penis beim Hunde. *Beitr. Anat. Physiol.*, 1863, **3,** 123–70.
Important studies of the erector mechanism.

1224 SCHWEIGGER-SEIDEL, FRANZ. 1834–1871
Ueber die Samenkörperchen und ihre Entwicklung. *Arch. mikr. Anat.*, 1865, **1,** 309–35.
Proof that the spermatozöon possesses a nucleus and cytoplasm.

1225 SKENE, ALEXANDER JOHNSTON CHALMERS. 1838–1900
The anatomy and pathology of two important glands of the female urethra. *Amer. J. Obstet.*, 1880, **13,** 265–70.
"Skene's glands" first described.

1226 MACKENRODT, ALWIN KARL. 1859–1925
Ueber die Ursachen der normalen und pathologischen Lagen des Uterus. *Arch. Gynäk.*, 1895, **48,** 393–421.
"Mackenrodt's ligaments," the uterosacral ligaments.

1227 STIEVE, HERMANN. 1886–1952
Die Unfruchtbarkeit als Folge unnatürlicher Lebensweise. München, *J. F. Bergmann*, 1926.
Investigation of the effect of starvation and overfeeding on the gonads and on sexual capacity.

Kidney; Urinary Secretion

1228 EUSTACHI, BARTOLOMMEO [EUSTACHIUS]. 1520–1574
Opuscula anatomica. Venetiis, *V. Luchinus*, 1564.
Several of the plates deal with the structure of the kidney.

1229 BELLINI, LORENZO. 1643–1704
Exercitatio anatomica de structura et usu renum. Florentiae, *ex typ. sub signo Stellae*, 1662.
Classical description of the gross anatomy of the kidney. Bellini discovered the renal excretory ducts ("Bellini's ducts") and advanced a physical theory of the secretion of the urine. A translation of an extract from the 2nd ed. (1663) is in J. F. Fulton's *Selected readings in the history of physiology*, 2nd ed., 1966, pp. 350–52.

1230 MALPIGHI, MARCELLO. 1628–1694
De viscerum structura exercitatio anatomica. Bononiae, *ex typ. J. Montij*, 1666.
Includes (pp. 71–100) his essay, *De renibus*, in which he described the uriniferous tubules, the "Malpighian bodies". The work is reprinted, with translation, in *Ann. med. Hist.*, 1925, **7**, 245–63.

1231 BOWMAN, *Sir* WILLIAM. 1816–1892
On the structure and use of the Malpighian bodies of the kidney. *Phil. Trans.*, 1842, **132,** 57–80.
"Bowman's capsule". He described the structure of the renal corpuscle and its relation to the uriniferous tubule. In the same paper he stated his theory of renal secretion. Reprinted in *Med. Classics*, 1940, **5**, 258–91.

1232 LUDWIG, CARL FRIEDRICH WILHELM. 1816–1895
Beiträge zur Lehre vom Mechanismus der Harnsecretion. Marburg, *N. G. Elwert*, 1843.
Ludwig wrote a classical monograph on renal secretion. He regarded the pressure of the blood as the direct excitant of urinary secretion.

1233 ISAACS, CHARLES EDWARD. 1811–1860
Researches into the structure and physiology of the kidney. *Trans. N. Y. Acad. Med.*, 1857, **1,** 377–435.

1234 ——. On the function of the Malpighian bodies of the kidney. *Trans. N. Y. Acad. Med.*, 1857, **1,** 437–56.
Isaacs confirmed and corrected the findings of Bowman; he introduced dye experiments in the study of the kidney, from which he drew the important conclusion that the Malpighian bodies are the most important agency in the secretion of urine.

1235 HEIDENHAIN, RUDOLF PETER HEINRICH. 1834–1897
Versuche über den Vorgang der Harnabsonderung. *Pflüg. Arch. ges. Physiol.*, 1874, **9,** 1–27.
Heidenhain's "secretion" theory of renal function.

1236 TIGERSTEDT, Robert Adolf Armand. 1853–1923, & BERGMAN, P. G.

Niere und Kreislauf. *Skand. Arch. Physiol.*, 1898, **8,** 223–71.

Discovery that a pressor substance (renin) is produced by the kidneys and enters the circulation by the renal veins.

1237 CUSHNY, Arthur Robertson. 1866–1926

The secretion of the urine. London, *Longmans, Green & Co.*, 1917.

Cushny's theory of urinary secretion was similar to that of Ludwig, with some modifications. Subsequent work of Richards and his co-workers confirmed his theory.

1238 RICHARDS, Alfred Newton. 1876–1966, & SCHMIDT, Carl Frederic. 1893–

A description of the glomerular circulation in the frog's kidney and observations concerning the action of adrenalin and various other substances upon it. *Amer. J. Physiol.*, 1924, **71,** 178–208.

Richards made many experiments concerning the secretion of urine. Among other things he collected and analysed the fluid from a single glomerulus; his work confirmed the theories of Ludwig and Cushny.

1239 WEARN, Joseph Treloar. 1893– , & RICHARDS, Alfred Newton. 1876–1966

Observations on the composition of glomerular urine with particular reference to the problem of reabsorption in the renal tubules. *Amer. J. Physiol.*, 1924, **71,** 209–27.

Experimental proof that certain substances are reabsorbed from the uriniferous tubules.

1240 STARLING, Ernest Henry. 1866–1927, & VERNEY, Ernest Basil. 1894–1967

The secretion of urine as studied on the isolated kidney. *Proc. roy. Soc. B*, 1924–25, **97,** 321–63.

Demonstration that the tubules of the kidney re-absorb water.

1241 REHBERG, Poul Brandt. 1895–

Studies on kidney function. *Biochem. J.*, 1926, **20,** 447–82.

First attempt to determine the glomerular filtration rate in man.

1242 HAYMAN, Joseph Marchant. 1896–

Estimation of afferent arteriole and glomerular capillary pressures in the frog kidney. *Amer. J. Physiol.*, 1927, **79,** 389–409.

1243 MARSHALL, Eli Kennerly. 1889–1966

The aglomerular kidney of the toadfish (Opsanus tau). *Bull. Johns Hopk. Hosp.*, Baltimore, 1929, **45,** 95–101.

1244 RHOADS, Cornelius Packard. 1898–1959

A method for explanation of the kidney. *Amer. J. Physiol.*, 1934, **109,** 324–28.

1245 TRUETA, Joseph. 1897– , *et al.*

Studies of the renal circulation. Oxford, *Blackwell*, 1947.

With A. E. Barclay, P. M. Daniel, K. J. Franklin, and M. M. L. Prichard.

1246 SMITH, HOMER WILLIAM. 1895–1962
The kidney: structure and function in health and disease. New York, *Oxford University Press*, 1951.

1246.1 WIRZ, HEINRICH. 1914– , *et al.*
Lokalisation des Konzentrierungsprozesses in der Niere durch direkte Kryoskopie. *Helv. physiol. pharmacol. Acta*, 1951, **9**, 196–207.
With B. Hargitay and W. Kuhn.

1247–1570.1 NERVOUS SYSTEM

1247 ARIËNS KAPPERS, CORNELIUS UBBO. 1877–1946
Die vergleichende Anatomie des Nervensystems der Wirbeltiere und des Menschen. 2 vols. Haarlem, *Bohn*, 1920–21.
Ariëns Kappers was Professor of Neuroanatomy at Amsterdam. English translation, 1936.

1248 FULTON, JOHN FARQUHAR. 1899–1960
Physiology of the nervous system. London, *Oxford Univ. Press*, 1938.
Includes an excellent bibliography.

Peripheral Nerves (including Nervous Impulses)

1249 MECKEL, JOHANN FRIEDRICH, *the elder*. 1724–1774
Tractatus anatomico-physiologicus de quinto pare nervorum cerebri. Gottingae, *A. Vandenhoeck*, 1748.
Meckel's graduation thesis, a classical description of the sphenopalatine (Meckel's) ganglion and the dural space lodging the Gasserian ganglion ("Meckel's cave").

1250 JOHNSTONE, JAMES. 1730–1802
Essay on the use of the ganglions of the nerves. *Phil. Trans.*, (1764), 1765, **54**, 177–84.
See also his supplementary papers on the subject, in *Phil. Trans.*, (1767), 1768, **57**, 118–31; (1770), 1771, **60**, 30–35.

1251 HIRSCH, ANTON BALTHASAR RAYMUND.
Pars quinti nervorum encephali disquisitio anatomica. Vienna, [n.p.], 1765.
The "Gasserian ganglion", already described by Santorini and others, was named after Johann Ludwig Gasser (*fl.* 1757–65), professor of anatomy at Vienna, by his pupil Hirsch. Also published in Ludwig, C.F., *Scriptores*, 1791, vol. 1, pp. 244–62.

1252 WRISBERG, HEINRICH AUGUST. 1739–1808
Observationes anatomicae de quinto pare nervorum encephali. Gottingae, *J. C. Dieterich*, 1777.
Wrisberg, professor of anatomy at Göttingen, is remembered for his discovery of the nervus intermedius ("nerve of Wrisberg"), described in the above treatise.

1253 SCARPA, ANTONIO. 1747?–1832
Tabulae nevrologicae, ad illustrandum historiam anatomicam cardiacorum nervorum, noni nervorum cerebri, glossopharyngaei et pharyngaei ex octavo cerebri. Ticini, *apud B. Comini*, 1794.
This, Scarpa's greatest work, includes the first proper delineation of the nerves of the heart. Scarpa was a skilful artist and one of the best of those medical men who have illustrated their own books.

1254 BELL, *Sir* CHARLES. 1774–1842
Idea of a new anatomy of the brain. London, *Strahan & Preston*, [1811].

Contains first reference to experimental work on the motor functions of the ventral spinal nerve-roots, without, however, establishing the sensory functions of the dorsal roots. This pamphlet ,which is very rare, is reproduced in *Med. Classics*, 1936, **1**, 105–20. Facsimile reprint, 1966.

1255 ——. On the nerves; giving an account of some experiments on their structure and functions, which lead to a new arrangement of the system. *Phil. Trans.*, 1821, **111**, 398–424.

"Bell's nerve," the long thoracic, described.

1256 MAGENDIE, FRANÇOIS. 1783–1855
Expériences sur les fonctions des racines des nerfs rachidiens. *J. Physiol. exp. path.*, 1822, **2**, 276–79; 366–71.

Magendie definitely established the function of the dorsal spinal nerve roots (Bell's law). This work was confirmed by Müller in 1831. For a translation of the paper, see J. F. Fulton's *Selected readings in the history of physiology*, 2nd ed., 1966, pp. 280–85.

1257 MÜLLER, JOHANNES. 1801–1858
Zur vergleichenden Physiologie des Gesichtssinnes des Menschen und der Thiere. Leipzig, *C. Cnobloch*, 1826.

Includes Müller's law of specific nerve energies. For an English translation, see his *Elements of physiology*, transl. W. Baly, London, 1843, pp. 766–67.

1258 BELL, *Sir* CHARLES. 1774–1842
The nervous system of the human body. [2nd ed.] London, *Longmans*, 1830.

Records Bell's demonstration that the fifth cranial nerve has a sensory-motor function, his discovery of "Bell's nerve" and the motor nerve of the face, lesion of which causes facial paralysis (Bell's palsy). Also includes the first description of myotonia.

1259 MÜLLER, JOHANNES. 1801–1858
Bestätigung des Bell'schen Lehrsatzes. *Notiz. a. d. Geb. d. Natur- u. Heilk.*, Weimar, 1831, **30**, 113–22

Experimental proof of Bell's law (see No. 1254) of the spinal nerve roots.

1260 REMAK, ROBERT. 1815–1865
Vorläufige Mittheilungen microscopischer Beobachtungen über den innern Bau der Cerebrospinalnerven und über die Entwickelung ihrer Formelemente. *Arch. Anat. Physiol. wiss. Med.*, 1836, 145–61.

Discovery of the non-medullated nerve-fibres ("fibres of Remak"). Fuller account in his *Observationes anatomicae* (No. 1262).

1261 BURDACH, ERNST. 1801–1876
Beitrag zur mikroskopischen Anatomie der Nerven. Königsberg, *gebr. Bornträger*, 1837.

1262 REMAK, ROBERT. 1815–1865
Observationes anatomicae et microscopicae de systematis nervosi structura. Berolini, *sumtibus et formis Reimerianis*, 1838.

See No. 1260.

1263 PACINI, Filippo. 1812–1883
Nuovi organi scoperti nel corpo humano. Pistoja, *tipog. Cino*, 1840.
"Pacini's corpuscles", end organs of sensory nerves, earlier described by Vater in 1717.

1264 BERNARD, Claude. 1813–1878
Recherches expérimentales sur les fonctions du nerf spinal, étudié spécialement dans ses rapports avec le pneumogastrique. *Arch. gén. Méd.*, 1844, 4 sér., **4,** 397–426; 1845, **5,** 51–93.

1265 HELMHOLTZ, Hermann Ludwig Ferdinand von. 1821–1894
Vorläufiger Bericht über die Fortpflanzungsgeschwindigkeit der Nervenreizung. *Arch. Anat. Physiol. wiss. Med.*, 1850, 71–73.
Helmholtz succeeded in measuring the velocity of the nervous impulse. This he did by means of a pendulum-myograph of his own invention. A second paper "Messungen über die Fortpflanzungsgeschwindigkeit der Reizung in den Nerven," appeared in the same journal, 1852, 199–216.

1266 WALLER, Augustus Volney. 1816–1870
Experiments on the section of the glossopharyngeal and hypoglossal nerves of the frog, and observations of the alterations produced thereby in the structure of their primitive fibres. *Phil. Trans.*, 1850, **140,** 423–429.
The "law of Wallerian degeneration". The experiments recorded in the above paper were the starting-point of the neuron theory. Waller showed that if glossopharyngeal and hypoglossal nerves are severed, the outer segment, containing the axis-cylinders cut off from the cells, undergoes degeneration, the central stump remaining intact for a long period. From this he inferred that nerve-cells nourish nerve-fibres.

1267 ——. Recherches sur la système nerveux. *C. R. Acad. Sci. (Paris).* 1851, **33,** 370–74; 606–11.

1267.1 TÜRCK, Ludwig. 1810–1868
Ueber den Zustand der Sensibilität nach theilweiser Trennung des Rückenmarkes. *Z. k. k. Ges. Aerzte Wien*, Abt. I, 1851, **7,** 189–201.
Türck showed that degeneration in a nerve track corresponds to the direction in which it conducts nerve impulses – ascending tracts degenerate above the lesion and descending tracks below it.

1268 VIRCHOW, Rudolf Ludwig Karl. 1821–1902
Ueber eine im Gehirn und Rückenmark des Menschen aufgefundene Substanz mit der chemischen Reaction der Cellulose. *Virchows Arch, path. Anat.*, 1854, **6,** 135–38.
Discovery of the neuroglia.

1269 KÜHNE, Willy. 1837–1900
Ueber die peripherischen Endorgane der motorischen Nerven. Leipzig, *W. Engelmann*, 1862.
Kühne described the neuromuscular end organ ("Kühne's spindle") and introduced the term "telolemma" for the outer covering of its sheath.

1270 ——. Die Muskelspindeln. Ein Beitrag zur Lehre von der Entwickelung der Muskeln und Nervenfasern. *Virchows Arch. path. Anat.*, 1863, **28,** 528–38.
The best early description of proprioceptive receptors in muscles.

1271 DEITERS, Otto Friedrich Carl. 1834–1863
Untersuchungen über Gehirn und Rückenmark des Menschen und der Säugethiere. Braunschweig, *F. Vieweg u. Sohn*, 1865.

Deiters discovered glia cells. He showed that each nerve-cell possesses an axis-cylinder or nerve-fibre process. His name is perpetuated in "Deiters' cells" and "nucleus".

1272 DICKINSON, William Howship. 1832–1913
On the changes in the nervous system which follow the amputation of limbs. *J. Anat. Physiol.* (*Lond.*), 1869, **3,** 88–96.

Demonstration that the proximal end of a severed nerve eventually atrophies.

1273 BERNSTEIN, Julius. 1839–1917
Untersuchungen über den Erregungsvorgang im Nerven- und Muskelsysteme. Heidelberg, *C. Winter*, 1871.

1274 ——. Ueber die Ermüdung und Erholung der Nerven. *Pflüg. Arch. ges. Physiol.*, 1877, **15,** 289–327.

After successfully tetanizing a nerve-muscle preparation, Bernstein inferred, from this and additional data, that nerve is exhausted in the process. This conflicted with the findings of Bowditch (No. 1281–82) and Vvedensky (No. 1280).

1275 CATON, Richard. 1842–1926
The electric currents of the brain. *Brit. med. J.*, 1875, **2,** 278.

Caton succeeded in leading off action potentials from the brains of animals, a first step towards the development of the electro-encephalogram. See also *Brit. med. J.*, 1877, **1**, Suppl., 62–75.

1276 RANVIER, Louis Antoine. 1835–1922
Leçons sur l'histologie du système nerveux. 2 vols. Paris, *F. Savy*, 1878.

Includes his description of the "nodes of Ranvier," interruptions of the medullary nerve sheaths.

1277 GOLGI, Camillo. 1844–1926
Sulla struttura delle fibre nervosa midollate periferiche e centrali. *Arch. Sci. med.* (*Torino*), 1880, **4,** 221–46.

"Golgi cells" first described.

1278 TIGERSTEDT, Robert Adolf Armand. 1853–1923
Studien über mechanische Nervenreizung. *Acta Soc. Scient. fenn.*, 1880, **11,** 569–660.

Contains important work on the effects of mechanical stimulation of nerve.

1279 WALLER, Augustus Désiré. 1856–1922, & WATTEVILLE, Armand de. 1846–1925
On the influence of the galvanic current on the excitability of the motor nerves of man. *Phil. Trans.*, (1882), 1883, **173,** 961–91.

1280 VVEDENSKY, Nikolai Igorevich [Wedenskii]. 1844–
Wie rasch ermüdet der Nerv? *Zbl. med. Wiss.*, 1884, **22,** 65–68.

Although Bernstein considered that nerve could be exhausted, Vvedensky was able, in this paper, to show that such is not the case. Further proof was supplied by Bowditch (No. 1281).

1281 BOWDITCH, Henry Pickering. 1840–1911
Note on the nature of nerve-force. *J. Physiol.* (*Lond.*), 1885, **6,** 133–35.

1282 ——. Ueber den Nachweis der Unermüdlichkeit des Säugethiernerven. *Arch. Anat. Physiol., Physiol. Abt.*, 1890, 505–08.

Bowditch demonstrated the indefatigability of nerve ("Bowditch's law").

1283 MARCHI, VITTORIO. 1851–1908, & ALGERI, G.
Sulle degenerazioni discendenti consecutive a lesioni della corteccia cerebrale. *Riv. sper. Freniat.*, 1885, **11,** 492–94.

Marchi's stain, osmic acid, for degenerating myelin sheaths.

1284 BURDON-SANDERSON, *Sir* JOHN SCOTT. 1828–1905
Photographic determination of the time-relations of the changes which take place in muscle during the period of so-called 'latent stimulation'. *Proc. roy. Soc.* (*Lond.*), 1890, **48,** 14–19.

Measurement, by means of photography, of the speed of the nervous impulse.

1285 GOTCH, FRANCIS. 1851–1913, & HORSLEY, *Sir* VICTOR ALEXANDER HADEN. 1857–1916
On the mammalian nervous system, its functions, and their localisation determined by an electrical method. *Phil. Trans. B*, 1891, **182,** 267–526.

Gotch and Horsley showed that electrical currents are produced in the mammalian brain, and they recorded them with the string galvanometer or the capillary electrometer. Their work led eventually to the development of the electroencephalograph.

1286 NISSL, FRANZ. 1860–1919
Ueber die Veränderungen der Ganglienzellen am Fascialiskern des Kaninchens nach Ausreissung der Nerven. *Allg. Z. Psychiat.*, 1892, **48,** 197–98.

1287 RAMÓN Y CAJAL, SANTIAGO. 1852–1934
Nuevo concepto de la histología de los centros nerviosos. *Rev. Cienc. méd.*, 1892, **18,** 457–76.

Ramón y Cajal, son of a struggling Aragonese doctor, lived to become one of the greatest of all histologists. He devised many staining methods for nervous tissue and did work of fundamental importance to neuro-anatomy. He shared the Nobel Prize in Physiology with Golgi in 1906.

1288 SHERRINGTON, *Sir* CHARLES SCOTT. 1857–1952
Notes on the arrangement of some motor fibres in the lumbo-sacral plexus. *J. Physiol.* (*Lond.*), 1892, **13,** 621–772.

Association of the lateral horn cells with the sympathetic outflow.

1289 LENHOSSÉK, MIHÁLY. 1863–1937
Beiträge zur Histologie des Nervensystems und der Sinnesorgane. Wiesbaden, *J. F. Bergmann*, 1894.

1290 LANGLEY, JOHN NEWPORT. 1852–1925, & ANDERSON, *Sir* HUGH KERR. 1865–1928
On reflex action from sympathetic ganglia. *J. Physiol.* (*Lond.*), 1894, **16,** 410–40.

1291 NISSL, FRANZ. 1860–1919
Ueber eine neue Untersuchungsmethode des Centralorgans speciell zur Feststellung der Localisation der Nervenzellen. *Neurol. Zbl.*, 1894, **13,** 507–08.

Nissl's stain.

1292 DOGIEL, Alexander Stanislavovič. 1852–1922
Die sensiblen Nervenendigungen im Herzen und in den Blutgefässen der Säugethiere. *Arch. mkr. Anat.*, 1898, **52,** 44–70.
"Dogiel's end-bulbs" – sensory nerve-endings.

1293 ——. Ueber den Bau der Ganglien in den Geflechten des Darmes und der Gallenblase des Menschen und der Säugethiere. *Arch. Anat. Physiol., Anat. Abt.*, 1899, 130–58.
Classification of the neurones of spinal and other ganglia.

1294 BAYLISS, *Sir* William Maddock. 1860–1924
On the origin from the spinal cord of the vaso-dilator fibres of the hind-limb, and on the nature of these fibres. *J. Physiol.* (*Lond.*), 1901, **26,** 173–209.

1295 HALLIBURTON, William Dobinson. 1860–1931.
The Croonian Lectures on the chemical side of nervous activity. *Lancet*, 1901, **1,** 1659–60, 1741–42.

1296 BIELSCHOWSKY, Max. 1869–1940
Die Silberimprägnation der Axencylinder. *Neurol. Zbl.*, 1902, **21,** 579–84.
Bielschowsky's method of silver staining of nerve fibres. Further paper in the same journal, 1903, 22, 997–1006.

1297 HERRING, Percy Theodore. 1872–1967
The spinal origin of the cervical sympathetic nerve. *J. Physiol.* (*Lond.*), 1903, **29,** 282–85.
Section of the white rami caused retrograde degeneration of the lateral column cells.

1298 HEAD, *Sir* Henry. 1861–1940, *et al.*
The afferent nervous system from a new aspect. *Brain*, 1905, **28,** 99–115.
This paper opened up a new field in the study of the sensory functions of the skin, and the theories put forward in it dominated neurological thought until 1940. With W. H. R. Rivers and J. Sherren.

1299 ——. & SHERREN, James. 1872–1945
The consequences of injury to the peripheral nerves in man. *Brain*, London, 1905, **28,** 116–338.

1300 MACALLUM, Archibald Byron. 1858–1934, & MENTEN, Maud Lenore. 1879–1960
On the distribution of chlorides in nerve cells and fibres. *Proc. roy. Soc. B*, 1906, **77,** 165–93.

1300.1 SHERRINGTON, *Sir* Charles Scott. 1857–1952
On the proprio-ceptive system, especially in its reflex aspect. *Brain*, 1906, **29,** 467–82.
Sherrington investigated and explained the proprioceptive system.

1301 DOGIEL, Alexander Stanislavovič. 1852–1922
Der Bau der Spinalganglien des Menschen und der Säugetiere. Jena, *G. Fischer*, 1908.

1302 RIVERS, William Halse Rivers. 1864–1922, & HEAD, *Sir* Henry. 1861–1940

A human experiment in nerve division. *Brain*, 1908, **31**, 323–450.

Head submitted to the division of his own left radial and external cutaneous nerves. His subsequent study of the loss and restoration of sensation thus brought about led to a re-classification of the sensory pathways. Head was for many years editor of the journal *Brain*.

1302.1 TASHIRO, Shiro. 1882–1963

Carbon dioxide production from nerve fibres when resting and when stimulated; a contribution to the chemical basis of irritability. *Amer. J. Physiol.*, 1913, **32**, 107–36.

Tashiro showed that the production of the nervous impulse depends on the metabolic activity of the nerve fibre.

1303 LUCAS, Keith. 1879–1916

The conduction of the nervous impulse. London, *Longmans, Green & Co.*, 1917.

1304 HEAD, *Sir* Henry. 1861–1940, *et al.*

Studies in neurology. 2 vols. London, *H. Frowde, Hodder & Stoughton*, 1920.

Reprint, with modifications and additions, of seven papers published in the journal *Brain* between 1905 and 1918 by H. Head, W. H. R. Rivers, G. Holmes, J. Sherren, H. T. Thompson, and G. Riddoch.

1305 ERLANGER, Joseph. 1874– , & GASSER, Herbert Spencer. 1888–1963

The compound nature of the action current of nerve as disclosed by the cathode ray oscillograph. *Amer. J. Physiol.*, 1924, **70**, 624–66.

Nobel Prize winners, 1944, for their discoveries regarding the highly differentiated functions of single nerve fibres.

1306 KATO, Genichi. 1890–

The theory of decrementless conduction in narcotised region of nerve. Tokyo, *Nankōdō*, 1924.

A second volume, *Further studies*, appeared in 1926.

1307 ADRIAN, Edgar Douglas, 1*st Baron Adrian*. 1889– , & ZOTTERMAN, Yngve. 1899–

The impulses produced by sensory nerve-endings. Part 2. The response of a single end-organ. *J. Physiol. (Lond.)*, 1926, **61**, 151–71.

The observations of Adrian and Zotterman on the response of single sensory end-organs to a natural stimulus led them to formulate their conception of "adaptation" of receptors to stimuli.

1308 ——. The basis of sensation. The action of the sense organs. London, *Christophers*, 1928.

Adrian shared with Sherrington the Nobel Prize in 1932 for their work on the physiology of the nervous system.

1309 MÜLLER, Ludwig Robert. 1870–

Lebensnerven und Lebenstriebe. 3te. Aufl. Berlin, *J. Springer*, 1931.

1309.1 YOUNG, John Zachary. 1907–
The structure of nerve fibres in Cephalopods and Crustacea. *Proc. roy. Soc. B*, 1936, **121,** 319–37.

Young's discovery of the giant nerve fibres of the squid *Loligo forbesi* made possible the study of the electrical phenomena of the nervous impulse in the interior as well as on the surface of a nerve fibre. It led to the work of Hodgkin and Huxley (No. 1310.1).

1310 KIRKMAN, Hadley. 1901– , & SEVERINGHAUS, Aura Edward. 1894–
A review of the Golgi apparatus. *Anat. Rec.*, 1937–38, **70,** 413–31, 557–73; 1938, **71,** 79–103.

1310.1 HODGKIN, Alan Lloyd. 1914– , & HUXLEY, Andrew Fielding. 1917–
Action potentials recorded from inside a nerve fibre. *Nature* (*Lond.*), 1939, **144,** 710–11.

Hodgkin and Huxley were the first to succeed in inserting electrodes into a living giant nerve fibre and to measure directly the action potential within it. They shared the Nobel Prize with Sir John Eccles in 1963 "for their discoveries concerning the ionic mechanisms involved in the excitation and inhibition in the peripheral and central portions of the nerve cell membrane".

Peripheral Autonomic Nervous System

1311 WILLIS, Thomas. 1621–1675
Practice of physick. London, *T. Dring, C. Harper and J. Leigh*, 1684.

In Treatise III, pp. 128–158 is to be found Willis's description of the intercostal and spinal nerves. Willis described the ganglion chain as the "intercostal nerve" and thought it came from the head.

1312 EUSTACHI, Bartolommeo [Eustachius]. 1520–1574
Tabulae anatomicae. Roma, *F. Gonzaga*, 1714.

Plate XVIII is a drawing of the sympathetic nervous system. Eustachius was the first to describe the ganglion chain but made the mistake of tracing the origin of the cervical portion to the brain-stem.

1313 POURFOUR DU PETIT, François. 1664–1741
Mémoire dans lequel il est démontré que les nerfs intercostaux fournissent des rameaux que portent des esprits dans les yeux. *Hist. Acad. roy. Sci.* (*Paris*), (*Mém.*), 1727, 1–19.

By cutting the intercostal nerves in the neck, du Petit found that disturbances occurred in the eyes and face of the same side; this disproved earlier views of the cerebral origin of the intercostal nerves.

1314 WINSLOW, Jacobus Benignus. 1669–1760
Exposition anatomique de la structure du corps humain. Paris, *G. Desprez*, 1732.

Sect. VI deals with the nerves. Winslow designated the ganglion chain "the grand sympathetic nerve", and the smaller branches "the lesser sympathetic", terms which remain to-day. English translation by G. Douglas, 1733.

1315 BICHAT, Marie François Xavier. 1771–1802
Nerfs de la vie organique. In his *Traité d'anatomie descriptive*, Paris, 1802, **3,** 319–68.

Bichat was the creator of descriptive anatomy. He introduced the terms "animal" and "vegetative" system.

1316 WEBER, Ernst Heinrich. 1795–1878
Anatomia comparata nervi sympathici. Lipsiae, *C. H. Reclam*, 1817.

1317 LOBSTEIN, Jean Georges Chrétien Frédéric Martin. 1777–1835
De nervi sympathetici humani fabrica usu et morbis. Parisiis, *F. G. Levrault*, 1823.

Includes description of "Lobstein's ganglion", an accessory ganglion of the great splanchnic nerve above the diaphragm. English translation, 1831.

1318 BIDDER, Friedrich Heinrich. 1810–1894, & VOLKMANN, Alfred Wilhelm. 1800–1877
Die Selbständigkeit des sympathischen Nervensystems durch anatomische Untersuchungen nachgewiesen. Leipzig, *Breitkopf u. Härtel*, 1842.

These writers showed the sympathetic nervous system to consist largely of small, medullated fibres originating from the sympathetic and spinal ganglia.

1319 BECK, Thomas Snow. 1814–1877
On the nerves of the uterus. *Phil. Trans.*, 1846, **136,** 213–35.

Beck showed that in man the thoracic sympathetic chain receives communications from the last cervical, thoracic and upper 1 or 2 lumbar ganglia.

1320 BERNARD, Claude. 1813–1878
Influence du grand sympathique sur la sensibilité et sur la calorification. *C. R. Soc. Biol.* (*Paris*), (1851), 1852, **3,** 163–64.

Bernard discovered the existence of vasomotor nerves.

1321 ——. Expérience sur les fonctions de la portion céphalique du grand sympathique. *C. R. Soc. Biol.* (*Paris*), (1852), 1853, **4,** 155.

1322 BROWN-SÉQUARD, Charles Edouard. 1817–1894
Experimental researches applied to physiology and pathology. *Med. Exam.* (*Phila.*), 1852, **8,** 481–504.

By applying a galvanic current to the superior part of the divided sympathetic nerve and causing vascular contraction and a fall in temperature, Brown-Séquard inferred that section of the sympathetic paralysed and dilated the blood-vessels (pp. 489–490). (See also Nos. 1325–26).

1323 BUDGE, Julius Ludwig. 1811–1884
Experimenteller Beweis, dass der Nervus sympathicus aus dem Rückenmark entspringt. *Med. Ztg*, 1852, **21,** 161.

1324 BERNARD, Claude. 1813–1878
Recherches expérimentales sur le grand sympathique et spécialement sur l'influence que la section de ce nerf exerce sur la chaleur animal. *C. R. Soc. Biol.* (*Paris*), (*Mémoires*), (1853), 1854, **5,** 77–107.

1325 BROWN-SÉQUARD, Charles Edouard. 1817–1894
Note sur la découverte de quelques-uns des effets de la galvanisation du nerf grand sympathique au cou. *Gaz. méd. Paris*, 1854, 3 sér., **9,** 22–23.

1326 ——. Sur les résultats de la section et de la galvanisation du nerf grand sympathique au cou. *Gaz. méd. Paris*, 1854, 3 sér., **9,** 30–32.

1327 CAMPBELL, HENRY FRASER. 1824–1891
Essays on the secretory and the excito-secretory system of nerves. Philadelphia, *J. B. Lippincott & Co.*, 1857.

Campbell saw in the sympathetic a nervous system related to secretion and nutrition and having intimate connexion with the sensory nerves. He coined the term "excito-secretory" to designate his theory; although this term has fallen into desuetude, the same idea was more recently advanced to explain the action of certain glands of internal secretion.

1328 HORNER, JOHANN FRIEDRICH. 1831–1886
Ueber eine Form von Ptosis. *Klin. Mbl. Augenheilk.*, 1869, **7,** 193–98.

"Horner's syndrome", due to lesion of the cervical sympathetic. The same syndrome was evoked in animals by du Petit in 1727 (see No. 1313). It is a proof that the sympathetic governs the pupillary, vasomotor, sudomotor and pilomotor functions. It was also described by Claude Bernard, *Leçons sur la physiologie et la pathologie du système nerveux*, 1858, **2,** 473–74, and, less impressively, by E. S. Hare, *Lond. med. Gaz.*, 1838–39, **1,** 16–18.

1329 GASKELL, WALTER HOLBROOK. 1847–1914
On the structure, distribution, and function of the nerves which innervate the visceral and vascular system. *J. Physiol. (Lond.)*, 1886, **7,** 1–80.

Gaskell established the origin of the preganglionic neurones (white rami).

1329.1 LANGLEY, JOHN NEWPORT. 1852–1925, & DICKINSON, WILLIAM LEE. 1862–1904
On the local paralysis of peripheral ganglia, and on the connexion of different classes of nerve fibres with them. *Proc. roy. Soc.*, 1889, **46,** 423–31.

Langley and Dickinson studied the effect of nicotine on nerve fibres and were able by this means to make a thorough investigation of the distribution of nerve fibres.

1330 BETHE, ALBRECHT. 1872–1954
Ueber die Primitivfibrillen in den Ganglienzellen von Menschen und andern Wirbelthieren. *Morphol. Arb.*, 1897, **7,** 95–116.

1331 GASKELL, WALTER HOLBROOK. 1847–1914
The involuntary nervous system. Part 1. London, *Longmans, Green & Co.*, 1916.

This book sums up the life work of Gaskell, who laid the histological foundation of the modern study of the autonomic nervous system.

1332 LANGLEY, JOHN NEWPORT. 1852–1925
The autonomic nervous system. Cambridge, *W. Heffer*, 1921.

Langley divided the autonomic nervous system into (1) the orthosympathetic, and (2) the parasympathetic; he defined it as an efferent system.

1333 GAGEL, OTTO. 1899–
Zur Histologie und Topographie der vegetativen Zentren im Rückenmark. *Z. Anat. EntwGesch.*, 1928, **85,** 213–50.

Study of the cells of origin of the white rami.

1334 KUNTZ, ALBERT. 1879–1957
The autonomic nervous system. 2nd ed. Philadelphia, *Lea & Febiger*, 1934.

1335 WHITE, JAMES CLARKE. 1895– , *et al.*
The autonomic nervous system. 3rd ed. New York, *Macmillan Co.*, 1952.

With R. H. Smithwick and F. A. Simeone.

Chemical Mediation of Nervous Impulses

1336 ELLIOTT, THOMAS RENTON. 1877–1961
On the action of adrenalin. *J. Physiol.* (*Lond.*), 1904, **31,** *Proc. Physiol. Soc.*, p. xx–xxi.

The first intimation of the chemical mediation of nerve impulses was given in Elliott's suggestion that when a sympathetic nerve impulse arrives at a smooth-muscle cell it liberates adrenaline, which acts as a chemical stimulator.

1337 HOWELL, WILLIAM HENRY. 1860–1945
Vagus inhibition of the heart in its relation to the inorganic salts of the blood. *Amer. J. Physiol.*, 1905–6, **15,** 280–94.

Howell suggested that nerve impulses act indirectly by increasing the amount of diffusible potassium compounds in the heart tissue.

1338 HUNT, REID. 1870–1948, & TAVEAU, RENÉ DE M.
On the physiological action of certain cholin derivatives and new methods for detecting cholin. *Brit. med. J.*, 1906, **2,** 1788–91.

Discovery of the remarkable hypotensive effect of acetylcholine.

1339 DIXON, WALTER ERNEST. 1871–1931, & HAMILL, PHILIP. 1883–1959
The mode of action of specific substances with special reference to secretin. *J. Physiol.* (*Lond.*), 1908–9, **38,** 314–36.

These workers drew attention to the similarity between the effects of nerve stimulation and certain drugs, especially muscarine, on the heart.

1340 DALE, *Sir* HENRY HALLETT. 1875–1968
The action of certain esters and ethers of choline, and their relation to muscarine. *J. Pharmacol.*, 1914, **6,** 147–90.

Demonstration of the inhibitory action of acetylcholine on the heart. Dale shared the Nobel Prize with Loewi (No. 1343) in 1936 for their work on the chemical mediation of nervous impulses.

1341 EWINS, ARTHUR JAMES. 1882–1958
Acetylcholine, a new active principle of ergot. *Biochem. J.*, 1914, **8,** 44–49.

Isolation of acetylcholine in ergot.

1342 HUNT, REID. 1870–1948
Vasodilator reactions. *Amer. J. Physiol.*, 1918, **45,** 197–267.

Showed that tissues are more sensitive to acetylcholine after treatment with eserine (physostigmine).

1343 LOEWI, OTTO. 1873–1961
Ueber humorale Uebertragbarkeit der Herznervenwirkung. *Pflüg. Arch. ges. Physiol.*, 1921, **189,** 239–42; 1922, **193,** 201–13; 1924, **203,** 408–12; **204,** 361–67, 629–40.

Loewi's important experiments firmly established the theory of chemical intermediaries in nervous reactions. He shared the Nobel Prize for physiology with Dale in 1936.

1344 LOEWI, Otto. 1873–1961, & NAVRATIL, E.
Ueber humorale Uebertragbarkeit der Herznervenwirkung. *Pflüg. Arch. ges. Physiol.*, 1924, **206,** 123–40; 1926, **214,** 678–96.
Established the presence of cholinesterase and that *in vitro* eserine inhibited this esterase.

1345 DALE, *Sir* Henry Hallett. 1875–1968, & DUDLEY, Harold Ward. 1887–1935.
Presence of histamine and acetylcholine in the spleen of ox and horse. *J. Physiol.* (*Lond.*), 1929, **68,** 97–123.
Isolation of acetylcholine from ox and horse spleen.

1346 CANNON, Walter Bradford. 1871–1945, & BACQ, Zénon M.
Studies on conditions of activity in endocrine organs. xxvi. A hormone produced by sympathetic action on smooth muscle. *Amer. J. Physiol.*, 1931, **96,** 392–412.
Cannon and Bacq suggested the name "sympathin" for a substance which they considered to be liberated into the blood stream following nerve stimulation and which acted in the same manner as sympathetic impulses. (See also No. 1350.)

1347 ENGELHART, Erich.
Der humorale Wirkungsmechanismus der Oculomotoriusreizung. *Pflüg. Arch. ges. Physiol.*, 1931, **227,** 220–34.

1348 GIBBS, Owen Stanley. 1898– , & SZELÖCZEY, J.
Die humorale Übertragung der Chorda tympani-Reizung. *Arch. exp. Path. Pharmak.*, 1932, **168,** 64–88.
Production of acetylcholine on stimulation of the chorda tympani nerve.

1349 BAIN, William Alexander. 1905–
Mode of action of vasodilator vasoconstrictor nerves. *Quart. J. exp. Physiol.*, 1933, **23,** 381–89.

1350 CANNON, Walter Bradford. 1871–1945, & ROSENBLUETH, Arturo Stearns. 1900–
Studies on conditions of activity in endocrine organs. xxix. Sympathin E and sympathin I. *Amer. J. Physiol.*, 1933, **104,** 557–74.
Adrenaline and sympathin were suggested to be unidentical substances, and Cannon and Rosenblueth proposed the terms "sympathin E" and "sympathin I."

1351 KIBJAKOW, A. W.
Ueber humorale Uebertragung der Erregung von einem Neuron auf das andere. *Pflüg. Arch. ges. Physiol.*, 1933, **232,** 432–43.
Kibjakow showed that some substance in a muscle perfusate is able to contract muscle during stimulation of nerve.

1352 FELDBERG, Wilhelm Siegmund. 1900– , & GADDUM, *Sir* John Henry. 1900–1965
The chemical transmitter at synapses in a sympathetic ganglion. *J. Physiol.* (*Lond.*), 1933, **80,** 12p–13p.
These workers produced evidence that a chemical agent (acetylcholine) appears in the transfer of nerve impulses from neuron to neuron in sympathetic ganglia.

1353 BROWN, *Sir* George Lindor. 1903–1971, *et al.*
Reactions of the normal mammalian muscle to acetylcholine and to eserine. *J. Physiol.* (*Lond.*), 1936, **87,** 394–424.
With H. H. Dale and W. Feldberg.

1354 CANNON, WALTER BRADFORD. 1871–1945, & ROSENBLUETH, ARTURO STEARNS. 1900–
Autonomic neuro-effector systems. New York, *Macmillan Co.*, 1937.
See No. 1350.

1354.1 EULER, ULF SVANTE VON. 1905–
A specific sympathomimetic ergone in adrenergic nerve fibres (sympathin) and its relations to adrenaline and nor-adrenaline. *Acta physiol. scand.*, 1946, **12,** 73–97.
Noradrenaline shown to be the predominant transmitter of the effects of sympathetic nerve impulses. Shared Nobel Prize, 1970.

For history, see 1583

Spinal cord

1355 BOHN, JOHANN. 1640–1718
Circulus anatomico-physiologicus. Lipsiae, *J. F. Gleditsch*, 1686.
Bohn experimented on the decapitated frog, declaring the reflex phenomena to be entirely material and mechanical, the general view of the time being that "vital spirits" were present in the nerve-fluid. Bohn showed that the nerves do not contain a "nerve juice". (See p. 460 of the book.)

1356 POURFOUR DU PETIT, FRANÇOIS. 1664–1741
Lettres d'un médecin des hôpitaux; un nouveau système du cerveau, *etc.* Namur, 1710.
Theory of contralateral innervation.

1357 UNZER, JOHANN AUGUST. 1727–1799
Erste Gründe einer Physiologie der eigentlichen thierischen Natur thierischer Körper. Leipzig, *bey Weidmanns Erben und Reich*, 1771.
Unzer was probably the first to employ the word "reflex" in connexion with sensory-motor reactions. T. Laycock translated his book into English for the Sydenham Society in 1851.

1358 BURDACH, KARL FRIEDRICH. 1776–1847
Vom Baue und Leben des Gehirns. 3 vols. Leipzig, *in der Dyk'schen Buchhandlung*, 1819–26.
Includes description of "Burdach's column", the posterior column of the spinal cord.

1359 HALL, MARSHALL. 1790–1857
On the reflex function of the medulla oblongata and medulla spinalis. *Phil. Trans.*, 1833, **123,** 635–65.
Marshall Hall established the difference between volitional action and unconscious reflexes. This and subsequent work of Hall gave "reflex action" (a term invented by him) a permanent place in physiology.

1360 CLARKE, JACOB AUGUSTUS LOCKHART. 1817–1880
Researches into the structure of the spinal cord. *Phil. Trans.*, 1851, **141,** 607–21.
Clarke made important researches on the spinal cord. He described the nucleus dorsalis. He introduced the method of mounting sections with Canada balsam.

1361 GOLL, Friedrich. 1829–1903
Beiträge zur feineren Anatomie des menschlichen Rückenmarks. *Denkschr. med.-chir. Ges. Kanton Zürich*, 1860, pp. 130–71.
Includes description of "Goll's column" or "tract", the posterior column of the spinal cord.

1362 SECHENOV, Ivan Mikhailovič. 1829–1905
Physiologische Studien über die Hemmungsmechanischen für die Reflexthätigkeit des Rückenmarks in Gehirne des Frosches. Berlin, *A. Hirschwald*, 1863.
Sechenov discovered the cerebral inhibition of spinal reflexes. He was professor of physiology at St. Petersburg and Moscow, and the "father of Russian physiology".

1363 LOVÉN, Otto Christian. 1835–1904
Ueber die Erweiterung von Arterien in Folge einer Nervenerregung. *Ber. k. sachs. Ges. Wiss. Lpz.*, 1866, **18,** 85–110.
The "Lovén reflex," vasodilatation of an organ when its afferent nerve is stimulated.

1364 GOLTZ, Friedrich Leopold. 1834–1902
Beiträge zur Lehre von den Functionen der Nervencentren des Frosches. Berlin, *A. Hirschwald*, 1869.
Goltz made important observations on the decerebrate frog. He showed it to possess no volitional powers except after stimulation, no memory and no intelligence. His experiments on frogs deprived of their spinal cords showed them to have intelligence but lessened powers of co-ordination and adaptation.

1365 ——. Ueber die Functionen des Lendenmarks des Hundes. *Pflüg. Arch. ges. Physiol.*, 1874, **8,** 460–98.
(See No. 1364.)

1366 LISSAUER, Heinrich. 1861–1891
Beitrag zur pathologischen Anatomie der Tabes dorsalis und zum Faserverlauf in menschlichen Rückenmark. *Neurol. Zbl.*, 1885, **4,** 245–46.
"Lissauer's tract", the marginal tract in the spinal cord.

1367 MITCHELL, Silas Weir. 1829–1914, & LEWIS, Morris James. 1852–
Physiological studies of the knee-jerk. *Med. News (Phila.)*, 1886, **48,** 169–73; 198–203.
Demonstration that the knee-jerk can be reinforced by sensory stimulation.

1368 NANSEN, Fridtjof. 1861–1930
The structure and combination of the histological elements of the central nervous system. *Bergens Mus. Aarsberetning*, 1886, 29–214.
Nansen, better known for his Arctic explorations, was the first to point out that the posterior root fibres divide on entering the spinal cord into ascending and descending branches.

1368.1 HIS, Wilhelm, *Snr.* 1831–1904
Zur Geschichte der menschlichen Rückenmarkes und der Nervenwurzeln. *Abh. math.-phys. Cl. k. sächs. Ges. Wiss. Leipzig*, (1886), 1887, **13,** 477–514.
His clearly stated the neurone theory in 1886.

1369 WALDEYER-HARTZ, Heinrich Wilhelm Gottfried. 1836–1921
Ueber einige neuere Forschungen im Gebiete der Anatomie des Centralnervensystems. *Dtsch. med. Wschr.*, 1891, **17,** 1213–18, 1244–46, 1287–89, 1331–32, 1352–56.

A statement of the neurone theory, to which Waldeyer gave the name.

1370 GOLTZ, Friedrich Leopold. 1834–1902
Der Hund ohne Grosshirn. *Pflüg. Arch. ges. Physiol.*, 1892, **51,** 570–614.

Goltz was able to keep dogs alive for as long as eight months after he had performed sub-total decerebration. He found them incapable of purposive movements but able to walk with adequate co-ordination. Frontal decortication caused restlessness; from his experiments Goltz concluded that the site of integration of pseudo-affective mechanisms is subcortical.

1371 ——, & EWALD, Ernst Julius Richard. 1855–1921
Der Hund mit verkürztem Rückenmark. *Pflüg. Arch. ges. Physiol.*, 1896, **63,** 362–400.

Goltz and Ewald succeeded in impregnating a bitch after its spinal cord had been severed.

1372 FLATAU, Eduard. 1869–1932
Atlas des menschlichen Gehirns und des Faserverlaufes. Berlin, *Karger*, 1894.

Flatau's law – "the greater the length of the fibres in the spinal cord the closer they are situated to the periphery".

1373 BAYLISS, *Sir* William Maddock. 1860–1924
Further researches on antidromic nerve-impulses. *J. Physiol.* (*Lond.*), 1902, **28,** 276–99.

1374 HEAD, *Sir* Henry. 1861–1940, & THOMPSON, Harold Theodore. 1878–1935
The grouping of afferent impulses within the spinal cord. *Brain*, 1906, **29,** 537–741.

1375 MONAKOW, Constantin von. 1853–1930
Der rote Kern, die Haube und die Regio hypothalamica bei einigen Säugetieren und beim Menschen. *Arb. hirnanat. Inst. Zürich*, 1909, **3,** 51–267; 1910, **4,** 103–225.

"Monakow's bundle", the rubrospinal tract.

1376 HEAD, *Sir* Henry. 1861–1940, & RIDDOCH, George. 1888–1947
The automatic bladder, excessive sweating and some other reflex conditions, in gross injuries of the spinal cord. *Brain*, 1917, **40,** 188–263.

Classical studies on "spinal man". Republished in book form, 1918.

1377 RIDDOCH, George. 1888–1947
The reflex functions of the completely divided spinal cord in man, compared with those associated with less severe lesions. *Brain*, 1917, **40,** 264–402.

Riddoch described in detail the results of complete transection of the spinal cord in man. With Head (See No. 1376) he made one of the most painstaking investigations of this subject.

Brain, including Medulla: Cerebrospinal Fluid

1378 WILLIS, THOMAS. 1621–1675
Cerebri anatome: cui accessit nervorum descriptio et usus. Londini, *J. Flesher*, 1664.

The most complete and accurate account of the nervous system which had hitherto appeared. In its preparation Willis was helped by Lower, and its illustrations are by Sir Christopher Wren. Willis's classification of the cerebral nerves held the field until the time of Soemmerring. The book includes (p. 414 and plates 1, 2) the description of the "circle of Willis", and of the eleventh cranial nerve ("nerve of Willis"). Willis recognized the sympathetic system and accepted the brain as the organ of thought. English translation by S. Pordage, 1681, which was reprinted 1965. Wepfer (No. 2703, p. 106) preceded Willis in giving a detailed and complete description of the "circle of Willis".

1379 VIEUSSENS, RAYMOND. 1641–1715
Nevrographia universalis. Lugduni, *J. Certe*, 1684.

Vieussens, professor at Montpellier, was the first correctly to describe the centrum ovale. The publication of the above work threw new light on the subject of the configuration and structure of the brain, spinal cord and nerves. It is considered the best illustrated work on the subject to appear in the 17th century.

1380 PACCHIONI, ANTONIO. 1665–1726
Dissertatio epistolaris ad Lucam Schroeckium de glandulis conglobatis durae meningis humanae. Romae, 1705.

Includes a description of the pacchionian bodies of the arachnoid tissue under the dura, producing by pressure slight depressions ("pacchionian depressions").

1381 WHYTT, ROBERT. 1714–1766
An essay on the vital and other involuntary motions of animals. Edinburgh, *Hamilton, Balfour & Neill*, 1751.

Whytt, famous Edinburgh neurophysiologist, was the first to prove that the response of the pupils to light is a reflex action ("Whytt's reflex"). He described this reflex at length and mentioned that its afferent pathways lie in the optic nerve and the efferent pathways in the third pair.

1382 COTUGNO, DOMENICO [COTUNNIUS]. 1736–1822
De ischiade nervosa commentarius. Neapoli, *apud Frat. Simonios*, 1764.

Valsalva in 1692 briefly mentioned the cerebrospinal fluid, but Cotugno was the first to describe it in any detail, elaborating its pathways. For more information regarding this book and a translation of the section dealing with the cerebrospinal fluid, see the article by H. R. Viets in *Bull. Inst. Hist. Med.*, 1935, **3**, 701–38.

1383 SOEMMERRING, SAMUEL THOMAS. 1755–1830
De basi encephali et originibus nervorum cranio egredientium libri quinque. Gottingae, *apud A. Vandenhoeck vid.*, 1778.

This classification of the cranial nerves superseded that of Willis (No. 1378). Soemmerring is notable for his accuracy in anatomical illustration.

1384 GENNARI, FRANCISCO. 1750–?
De peculiari structura cerebri, nonnulisque ejus morbis. Parmae, *ex reg. typog.*, 1782.

Discovery (in 1776) of the "line of Gennari" ("Gennari's stria") in the cerebral cortex (p. 72).

1385 MONRO, Alexander, *Secundus*. 1733–1817
Observations on the structure and functions of the nervous system. Edinburgh, *W. Creech*, 1783.

Monro discovered the communication between the lateral ventricles of the human brain with each other and with the third ventricle, the "foramen of Monro". Alexander *secundus* was the greatest of the three famous Monros.

1386 PROCHASKA, Georg. 1749–1820
Adnotationum academicarum fasciculi tres. III. De functionibus systematis nervosi, et observationes anatomico-pathologicae. 3 pts. Pragae, *W. Gerle*, 1780–84.

Prochaska introduced the idea of a "sensorium commune" in the central nervous system, the function of which is the reflection to the motor nerves of sensory impressions received by the brain.

1387 REIL, Johann Christian. 1759–1813
Exercitationum anatomicarum fasciculus primus. De structura nervorum. Halle, *Venalis*, 1796.

Description of the "island of Reil". See also *Arch. Physiol.* (*Halle*), 1809, **9**, 136–46; Reil was the editor of this journal, the first periodical devoted to physiology.

1388 ROLANDO, Luigi. 1773–1831
Saggio sopra la vera struttura del cervello dell'uomo e degl'animali e sopra le funzioni del sistema nervoso. Sassari, *Stamp. Privileg.*, 1809.

Includes description of "Rolando's substance", "tubercle", and "funiculus".

1389 GALL, Franz Joseph. 1758–1828, & SPURZHEIM, Johann Caspar. 1776–1832
Anatomie et physiologie du système nerveux en général, et du cerveau en particulier. 4 vols. and atlas. Paris, *F. Schoell*, 1810–19.

Introduced the theory of localization of cerebral function, although in a somewhat fantastic form. This pioneer attempt to map out the cerebral cortex according to function gave rise to the pseudo-science of phrenology. The work also contains some important additions to the knowledge of cerebral anatomy.

1390 MAYO, Herbert. 1796–1852
Anatomical and physiological commentaries. 2 pts. London, *T. & G. Underwood*, 1822–23.

Mayo described the functions of the facial nerves and did much towards the clarification of the idea of reflex action.

1391 FLOURENS, Marie Jean Pierre. 1794–1867
Recherches sur les propriétés et les fonctions du système nerveux dans les animaux vertébrés. *Arch. gén. Méd.*, 1823, **2**, 321–70.

Flourens removed the cerebrum and cerebellum in pigeons, showing maintenance of reflexes with loss of cerebration in the former case and disturbance of equilibrium in the latter case. Thus he demonstrated that the cerebrum is the organ of thought and the cerebellum the organ controlling the co-ordination of body movements and of will-power.

1392 MAGENDIE, François. 1783–1855
Mémoire sur un liquide qui se trouve dans le crâne et le canal vertébral de l'homme et des animaux mammifères. *J. Physiol. exp. path.*, 1825, **5**, 27–37; 1827, **7**, 1–29, 66–82.

First clear description of the cerebrospinal fluid.

1393 ROLANDO, Luigi. 1773–1831
Osservazioni sul cervelletto. *Mem. r. Accad. Sci. Torino*, 1825, **29,** 163–88.

Rolando was the first to investigate the functions of the cerebellum. His name is perpetuated in the "fissure of Rolando", so named by F. Leuret, *Anatomie comparée*, 1839–57, whose attention had been drawn to it previously by Rolando.

1394 ——. Della struttura degli emisferi cerebrali. *Mem. r. Accad. Sci. Torino*, 1829, **35,** 103–47.

1395 BOUILLAUD, Jean Baptiste. 1796–1881
Recherches expérimentales tendant à prouver que le cervelet préside aux actes de la station et de la progression, et non à l'instinct de la propagation. *Arch. gén. Méd.*, 1827, **15**, 64–91; 225–47.

Bouillaud identified the anterior lobes as the speech centre. Refuting Gall, he showed that the brain controls equilibration, station and progression. Title of second paper varies. His earlier *Traité clinique et physiologique de l'encéphalite ou inflammation du cerveau*, Paris, 1825, includes some pathological and clinical studies on loss of articulate speech associated with lesions of the anterior lobes, and gives reasons for the localization of this function in the brain.

1396 PURKINJE, Johann Evangelista [Purkyne]. 1787–1869
Ueber die gangliösen Körperchen in verschiedenen Theilen des Gehirns. *Ber. Versamml. dtsch. Naturf. u. Aerzte*, Prag, (1837), 1838, 179–80.

"Purkinje cells" described.

1397 MAGENDIE, François. 1783–1855
Recherches physiologiques et cliniques sur le liquide céphalo-rachidien ou cérébro-spinal. 1 vol. and atlas. Paris, *Méquignon-Marvis*, 1842.

"Foramen of Magendie" described.

1398 FAIVRE, Ernest.
Des granulations méningiennes. Paris, *Thèse No.* 142, 1853.

See also his paper in *Ann. Sci. nat.*, 1853, **20**, 321–33, (Zool.).

1399 BERNARD, Claude. 1813–1878
Leçons sur la physiologie et la pathologie du système nerveux. 2 vols. Paris, *J. B. Baillière*, 1858.

1400 BROCA, Pierre Paul. 1824–1880
Remarques sur le siège de la faculté du langage articulé, suivie d'une observation d'aphémie (perte de la parole). *Bull. Soc. anat. Paris*, 1861, **36,** 330–57.

Broca claimed the third left frontal convolution of the brain as the centre of articulate speech – a point now disputed. He was first to trephine for a cerebral abscess diagnosed by his theory of localization of function. He introduced the term "aphemia" ("motor aphasia," "Broca's aphasia").

1401 DALTON, John Call. 1825–1889
On the cerebellum, as the centre of co-ordination of the voluntary movements. *Amer. J. med. Sci.*, 1861, n.s. **41,** 83–88.

1401.1 AUBURTIN, Ernest. ?1825–
Considérations sur les localisations cérébrales, et en particulier sur le siège de la faculté du language articulé. *Gaz. hebd. Méd. Chir.*, 1863, **10,** 318–21, 348–51, 397–402, 455–58.

Auburtin did much to establish the principle of cerebral localization. He demonstrated on a patient whose frontal lobe was exposed following a gunshot wound that merely touching the uninjured lobe with a spatula would abolish speech, which would return immediately the spatula was removed.

1402 LUYS, Jules Bernard. 1828–1897
Recherches sur le système nerveux cérébro-spinal; sa structure, ses fonctions, et ses maladies. 1 vol. and atlas. Paris, *J. B. Baillière*, 1865.

Descriptions of the hypothalamus, "nucleus of Luys."

1403 MEYNERT, Theodor Hermann. 1833–1892
Der Bau der Gross-Hirnrinde und seine örtlichen Verschiedenheiten, nebst einem pathologisch-anatomischen Corollarium. *Vjschr. Psychiat.*, 1867, **1,** 77–93, 198–217; 1868, **2,** 88–113.

Meynert described the fountain decussation of the tegmental tract ("Meynert's decussation") and several other structures in the brain. Published in book form, 1868.

1404 MITCHELL, Silas Weir. 1829–1914
Researches on the physiology of the cerebellum. *Amer. J. med. Sci.*, 1869, n.s. **57,** 320–38.

Mitchell, leading American neurologist of his time, performed over 350 experiments upon the cerebellum. He emphasized its co-ordinating function, first postulated by Flourens, and he proposed his "augmentor" theory of cerebellar function.

1405 FRITSCH, Gustav Theodor. 1838–1891, & HITZIG, Eduard. 1838–1907
Ueber die elektrische Erregbarkeit des Grosshirns. *Arch. Anat. Physiol. wiss. Med.*, 1870, 300–32.

These workers showed that electrical stimulation of the frontal cortex in various experimental animals caused movements of the extremities of the opposite side of the body, thus proving the existence of a motor area in the cerebral cortex, predicted earlier in the same year by Hughlings Jackson. Translation in *J. Neurosurg.*, 1963, **20,** 905–16.

1406 GUDDEN, Bernhard Aloys von. 1824–1886
Experimentaluntersuchungen über das peripherische und centrale Nervensystem. *Arch. Psychiat. Nervenkr.*, 1870, **2,** 693–723.

Modern study of the functions of the thalamus began with the important investigations of Gudden. He is remembered eponymically by "Gudden's commissure" and "Gudden's atrophy" – specific thalamic nuclei degenerate when certain areas of the cerebral cortex are destroyed. His collected works were published in 1889. He was drowned in a lake at Starnberg by his patient Ludwig II, the mad king of Bavaria.

1407 BETS, Vladimir Aleksandrovič [Betz, W.]. 1834–1894
Anatomischer Nachweis zweier Gehirncentra. *Zbl. med. Wiss.*, 1874 **12,** 578–80, 595–99.

Discovery of the giant pyramidal cells of the motor cortex.

1408 HITZIG, Eduard. 1838–1907
Untersuchungen über das Gehirn. Berlin, *A. Hirschwald*, 1874.
Hitzig accurately defined the limits of the motor area in the cerebral cortex of the dog and the monkey.

1409 FERRIER, *Sir* David. 1843–1928
The functions of the brain. London, *Smith, Elder & Co.*, 1876.
Ferrier may be said to have laid the foundations of our knowledge concerning the localization of cerebral function. His book includes his earlier work published in the *West Riding Lunatic Asylum Reports*. Facsimile reprint, 1966.

1410 FLECHSIG, Paul Emil. 1847–1929
Die Leitungsbahnen im Gehirn und Rückenmark des Menschen auf Grund entwicklungsgeschichtlicher Untersuchungen. Leipzig, *W. Engelmann*, 1876.
Flechsig mapped out the motor and sensory areas of the cerebral cortex, and named the "pyramidal tract".

1411 FOREL, Auguste Henri. 1848–1931
Untersuchungen über die Haubenregion und ihre oberen Verknüpfungen im Gehirne des Menschen und einiger Säugethiere, mit Beiträgen zu den Methoden der Gehirnuntersuchung. *Arch. Psychiat. Nervenkr.*, 1877, **7**, 393–495.
Forel elucidated the subthalmic region, "campus Foreli".

1412 LEWIS, William Bevan. 1847–1929
On the comparative structure of the cortex cerebri. *Brain*, 1878, **1**, 79–96.
Lewis described the grant cells of the precentral convolution.

1413 EXNER, Siegmund. 1846–1926
Untersuchungen über die Localisation der Funktionen in der Grosshirnrinde des Menschen. Wien, *W. Braumuller*, 1881.
"Exner's plexus".

1414 MUNK, Hermann. 1839–1912
Ueber die Functionen der Grosshirnrinde. Berlin, *A. Hirschwald*, 1881.
Munk made important investigations on the functions of the temporal lobes.

1415 OTT, Isaac. 1847–1916
The relation of the nervous system to the temperature of the body. *J. nerv. ment. Dis.*, 1884, **11**, 141–52.
Ott wrote important papers on the nervous regulation of body temperature. His papers on the heat-centre in the brain and on the thermo-inhibitory apparatus were published in the same journal, 1887, **14**, 150–62, 428–38; 1888, **15**, 85–104.

1415.1 THUDICHUM, Johann Ludwig Wilhelm. 1829–1901
A treatise on the chemical constitution of the brain. London, *Baillière, Tindall & Cox*, 1884.
Thudichum, a German emigré, discovered cephalins and myelins in brain tissue. An enlarged German edition of his book was published at Tübingen, 1901. See biography by D. L. Drabkin, 1958, which includes an annotated bibliography of Thudichum's writings. Reprint of the original work, with historical introduction by Drabkin, 1962.

1416 GOLGI, CAMILLO. 1844–1926
Sulla fina anatomia degli organi centrali del sistema nervoso. Milano, *U. Hoepli*, 1886 [1885].
Golgi was an eminent Italian histologist. The above work contains his valuable discoveries regarding the histology of the nervous system. He demonstrated the existence of multipolar nerve-cells (Golgi cells) by means of his silver nitrate stain, and described the "Golgi apparatus" and "Golgi type II" nerve cells – cells with short axons ramified within the cortex. In 1906 he shared the Nobel prize with Ramón y Cajal. First published as a series of papers in *Riv. sper. Freniat.*, 1882–85.

1416.1 BEEVOR, CHARLES EDWARD. 1854–1907, & HORSLEY, *Sir* VICTOR ALEXANDER HADEN. 1857–1916
A minute analysis (experimental) of the various movements produced by stimulating in the monkey different regions of the cortical centre for the upper limb, as defined by Professor Ferrier. *Phil. Trans. B*, 1887, **178,** 153–68.
Beevor, physician to the National Hospital, Queen Square, London, collaborated with Horsley in an important series of investigations of the localization of cerebral function.

1417 FRANÇOIS-FRANCK, CHARLES EMILE. 1849–1921
Leçons sur les fonctions motrices du cerveau. Paris, *O. Doin*, 1887.
François-Franck's studies on the excitability of the cerebral cortex and the localization of function followed work in collaboration with Pitres; Charcot wrote the preface (see also No. 1423).

1418 WESTPHAL, CARL FRIEDRICH OTTO. 1833–1890
Ueber einen Fall von chronischer progressiver Lähmung der Augenmuskeln (Ophthalmoplegia externa) nebst Beschreibung von Ganglienzellengruppen im Bereiche des Oculomotoriuskerns. *Arch. Psychiat. Nervenkr.*, 1887, **18,** 846–71.
"Westphal's nucleus" – for accommodation – in the third cranial nerve. Called also "Edinger's nucleus" (see the same journal, 1885, **16,** 858–59).

1419 HORSLEY, *Sir* VICTOR ALEXANDER HADEN. 1857–1916, & SHARPEY-SCHÄFER, *Sir* EDWARD ALBERT. 1850–1935
A record of experiments upon the functions of the cerebral cortex. *Phil. Trans. B*, (1888), 1889, **179,** 1–45.
A detailed analysis, by means of faradic stimulation, of the motor responses of the cerebral cortex, internal capsule, and spinal cord of higher primates.

1420 PICK, ARNOLD. 1851–1924
Ueber ein abnormes Faserbündel in der menschlichen Medulla oblongata. *Arch. Psychiat. Nervenkr.*, 1890, **21,** 636–40.
"Pick's bundle" of nerve fibres in the medulla oblongata.

1421 LUCIANI, LUIGI. 1840–1919
Il cervelletto. Nuovi studi di fisiologia normale e patologica. Firenze, *Le Monnier*, 1891.
Luciani succeeded in keeping dogs alive after total extirpation of the cerebellum, and initiated the modern study of cerebellar function.

1422 NISSL, FRANZ. 1860–1919
Ueber den sogenannten Granula der Nervenzellen. *Neurol. Zbl.*, 1894, **13,** 676–85, 781–89, 810–14.
"Nissl's granules".

1423 CHARCOT, JEAN MARTIN. 1825–1893, & PITRES, JEAN ALBERT. 1848–1928
Les centres moteurs corticaux chez l'homme. Paris, *Rueff & Cie.*, 1895.
Three papers by Charcot and Pitres in 1877, 1878, and 1883 left no doubt as to the existence of cortical motor centres n man. These were later published in book form (above).

1424 DEJERINE, JOSEPH JULES. 1849–1917, & DEJERINE-KLUMPKE, AUGUSTA. 1859–1927
Anatomie des centres nerveux. 2 vols. Paris, *Rueff & Cie.*, 1895–1901

1425 DONALDSON, HENRY HERBERT. 1857–1938
The growth of the brain. London, *W. Scott*, 1895.

1426 RETZIUS, MAGNUS GUSTAF. 1842–1919
Das Menschenhirn. Studien in der makroskopischen Morphologie. 2 vols. Stockholm, *P. A. Norstedt*, 1896.
Gross anatomy of the brain.

1427 WERNICKE, CARL. 1848–1905
Atlas des Gehirns. 2 pts. Breslau, *Schletter*, 1897–1900.

1428 LOEB, JACQUES. 1859–1924
Einleitung in die vergleichende Gehirnphysiologie und vergleichende Psychologie. Leipzig, *J. A. Barth*, 1899.

1429 VOGT, OSKAR. 1870–1959
Zur anatomischen Gliederung des Cortex cerebri. *J. Psychol. Neurol. (Lpz.)*, 1903, **2,** 160–80.

1430 CAMPBELL, ALFRED WALTER. 1868–1937
Histological studies on the localisation of cerebral function. Cambridge, *Univ. Press*, 1905.
The precentral area of the cerebral cortex is known as "Campbell's area". Campbell and Brodmann were pioneers in the study of the architectonics of the cerebral cortex.

1431 DEJERINE, JOSEPH JULES. 1849–1917, & ROUSSY, GUSTAVE. 1874–1948
Le syndrome thalamique. *Rev. neurol.*, 1906, **14,** 521–32.
The "thalamic syndrome", investigations of the effect of localized thalamic injury.

1432 SHERRINGTON, *Sir* CHARLES SCOTT. 1857–1952
The integrative action of the nervous system. New Haven, *Yale Univ. Press*, 1906.
Sherrington insisted that the essential function of the nervous system was the co-ordination of activities of the various parts of the organism. His work on the nervous system, especially his experimental studies of reflex action, has had a profound influence upon modern physiology. He shared the Nobel Prize with Adrian in 1932.

1433 SMITH, *Sir* GRAFTON ELLIOT. 1871–1937
A new topographical survey of the human cerebral cortex, being an account of the distribution of the anatomically distinct cortical areas and their relationship to the cerebral sulci. *J. Anat. Physiol. (Lond.)*, 1907, **41,** 237–54.

1434 BRODMANN, Korbinian. 1868–1918
Beiträge zur histologischen Lokalisation der Grosshirnrinde. VI. Die Cortexgliederung des Menschen. *J. Psychol. Neurol.* (*Lpz.*), 1908, **10,** 231–46.
"Brodmann's areas", the occipital and pre-occipital areas of the cerebral cortex.

1435 ——. Vergleichende Lokalisationslehre der Grosshirnrinde in ihren Prinzipien dargestellt auf Grund des Zellenbaues. Leipzig, *J. A. Barth*, 1909.
Brodmann was a pioneer in the study of cytoarchitectonics. His book was republished in 1925. It was the most comprehensive account of the subject. Brodmann's work first appeared as a series of papers in *J. Psychol. Neurol.* (*Lpz.*), 1903–08. His map of the human cortex appeared in the same journal, 1907, **10,** 231–46, 287–334.

1435.1 HORSLEY, *Sir* Victor Alexander Haden. 1857–1916, & CLARKE, Robert Henry. 1850–1926
The structure and functions of the cerebellum examined by a new method. *Brain*, 1908, **31,** 45–124.
Stereotactic apparatus for the accurate location of electrodes in the brain.

1436 KARPLUS, Johann Paul. 1866–1936, & KREIDL, Alois. 1864–1928
Gehirn und Sympathicus. *Pflüg. Arch. ges. Physiol.*, 1909, **129,** 138–144; 1910, **135,** 401–16; 1912, **143,** 109–27.
First experimental studies on the hypothalamus.

1437 SACHS, Ernest. 1879–1958
On the structure and functional relations of the optic thalamus. *Brain*, 1909, **32,** 95–186.

1438 BARBOUR, Henry Gray. 1886–1943, & ABEL, John Jacob. 1857–1938
Tetanic convulsions in frogs produced by acid fuchsin, and their relation to the problem of inhibition in the central nervous system. *J. Pharmacol.*, 1910, **2,** 169–99.

1438.1 MONAKOW, Constantin von. 1853–1930
Die Lokalisation im Grosshirn und der Abbau der Funktion durch kortikale Herde. Wiesbaden, *J. F. Bergmann*, 1914.
A monumental work on cerebral localization.

1439 WEED, Lewis Hill. 1886–1952
Studies on cerebro-spinal fluid. III. The pathways of escape from the subarachnoid spaces with particular reference to the arachnoid villi. *J. med. Res.*, 1914, **31,** 51–117.
Weed mapped out the pathways of the circulation of the cerebrospinal fluid.

1440 ——. The development of the cerebro-spinal spaces in pig and man. *Contr. Embryol. Carneg. Instn*, 1917, **5,** No. 14.

1441 TILNEY, Frederick. 1875–1938, & RILEY, Henry Alsop. 1887–
The form and functions of the central nervous system. New York, *P. B. Hoeber*, 1921.

1442 DUSSER DE BARENNE, JOHANNES GREGORIUS. 1885–1940
Experimental researches on sensory localization in the cerebral córtex of the monkey (Macacus). *Proc. roy. Soc. B*, 1924, **96,** 272–91.

Dusser de Barenne demonstrated the major functional subdivisions of the sensory cortex.

1443 LIDDELL, EDWARD GEORGE TANDY. 1895– , & SHERRINGTON, *Sir* CHARLES SCOTT. 1857–1952
Reflexes in response to stretch (myotatic reflexes). *Proc. roy. Soc. B*, 1924, **96,** 212–42; 1925, **97,** 267–83.

This investigation of the stretch reflex was of value in elucidating muscle tone and posture.

1444 ECONOMO, CONSTANTIN, *Freiherr von San Serff*. 1861–1931, & KOSKINAS, GEORG N.
Die Cytoarchitektonik der Hirnrinde des erwachsenen Menschen. 1 vol. and atlas. Wien & Berlin, *J. Springer*, 1925.

English translation, 1929.

1445 PAVLOV, IVAN PETROVITCH. 1849–1936
Lectures on conditioned reflexes. 2 vols. New York, *International Publishers*, 1928–41.

Besides his important work on digestion, Pavlov is remembered for his investigations upon conditioned reflexes. He is one of the greatest physiologists of all time.

1446 BERGER, JOHANNES ["HANS"]. 1873–1941
Über das Elektrenkephalogramm des Menschen. *Arch. Psychiat. Nervenkr.*, 1929, **87,** 527–70.

First description of the electroencephalogram. Berger showed that the electrical activity of the human brain could be recorded from the intact scalp.

1446.1 LASHLEY, KARL SPENCER. 1890–1958
Brain mechanisms and intelligence: a quantitative study of injuries to the brain. Chicago, *Univ. of Chicago Press*, 1929.

Lashley related nervous function and behaviour with well-defined areas of the brain, particularly in connexion with cerebral lesions.

1446.2 KELLER, ALLEN DUDLEY. 1901– , & HARE, WILLIAM KENDRICK. 1908–
The hypothalamus and heat regulation. *Proc. Soc. exp. Biol. (N.Y.)*, 1932, **29,** 1069–70.

Location of the heat-regulating centre in the hypothalamus.

1447 ADRIAN, EDGAR DOUGLAS, *1st Baron Adrian*. 1889– , & MATTHEWS, *Sir* BRYAN HAROLD CABOT. 1906–
The interpretation of potential waves in the cortex. *J. Physiol. (Lond.)*, 1934, **81,** 440–71.

Confirmation of Berger's findings (No. 1446). See also *Brain*, 1934, **57**, 355–85.

1448 CLARK, *Sir* WILFRID EDWARD LE GROS. 1895–
The structure and connections of the thalamus. *Brain*, 1932, **55,** 406–70.

1449 ——. The topography and homologies of the hypothalamic nuclei in man. *J. Anat. (Lond.)*, 1936, **70,** 203–14.

1450 FOERSTER, Otfrid. 1873–1941
The motor cortex in man in the light of Hughlings Jackson's doctrines. *Brain*, 1936, **59**, 135–59.

In this Hughlings Jackson Lecture, Foerster published his famous cytoarchitectonic map of the human cerebral cortex.

1451 WALKER, Arthur Earl. 1907–
The primate thalamus. Chicago, *Univ. Press*, (1938).

1451.1 HESS, Walter Rudolf. 1881–1973
Die funktionelle Organisation des vegetativen Nervensystems. Basel, *B. Schwabe*, 1948.

Hess shared the Nobel Prize with Egas Moniz in 1949 for his discovery of the functional organization of the interbrain as a co-ordinator of the activities of the internal organs.

For history, see 1574, 1578

1452–1570 ORGANS OF SPECIAL SENSES

1452 SCHNEIDER, Conrad Viktor. 1614–1680
Dissertatio de osse cribriforme, et sensu ac organo odoratus. Wittebergae, *Mevi*, 1655.

"Schneider's membrane", the pituitary membrane of the nasal chamber and sinuses.

1453 SCARPA, Antonio. 1747?–1832
Anatomicae disquisitiones de auditu et olfactu. Ticini, *typog. P. Galeatius*, 1789.

Scarpa made important researches concerning the auditory and olfactory apparatus of fishes, birds, reptiles, and man.

1454 SOEMMERRING, Samuel Thomas. 1755–1830
Abbildungen der menschlichen Organe des Geruches. Frankfurt a.M., *Varrentrapp u. Wenner*, 1809.

1455 ——. Abbildungen der menschlichen Organe des Geschmackes und der Stimme. Frankfurt a.M., *Varrentrapp u. Wenner*, 1806.

1456 MÜLLER, Johannes. 1801–1858
Ueber die phantastischen Gesichtserscheinungen. Coblenz, *J. Hölscher*, 1826.

Müller's early studies on specific nerve energies are included in the above work. Later he stated, in his *Handbuch der Physiologie*, Coblenz, 1840, 2, 258, his law of specific nerve energies – each nerve of special sense, however excited, gives rise to its own peculiar sensation.

1456.1 SCHLEMM, Friedrich. 1795–1858
Arteriarum capitis superficialium icon nova. Berolini, *J. W. Boike*, 1830.

Includes description of the "canal of Schlemm", the circular canal at the junction of the cornea and the sclerotic.

1457 WEBER, Ernst Heinrich. 1795–1878
De pulsu, resorptione, auditu et tactu. Annotationes anatomicae et physiologicae. Lipsiae, *C. F. Koehler*, 1834.

Includes Weber's law on the relationship between stimulus and sensation.

1458 MÜLLER, Johannes. 1801–1858
Ueber die Compensation der physischen Kräfte am menschlichen Stimmorgan, mit Bemerkungen über die Stimme der Säugethiere, Vögel und Amphibien. Berlin, *A. Hirschwald*, 1839.

1459 WEBER, Ernst Heinrich. 1795–1878
Der Tastsinn und das Gemeingefühl. In Wagner's *Handwörterbuch der Physiologie*, Braunschweig, 1846, **3,** Abt. 2, 481–588.

1460 WAGNER, Rudolf. 1805–1864, & MEISSNER, Georg. 1829–1903
Ueber das Vorhandensein bisher unbekannter eigenthümlicher Tastkörperchen (Corpuscula tactus) in den Gefühlswärzchen der menschlichen Haut, und über die End-Ausbreitung sensitiver Nerven. *Nachr. Georg-Augusts Univ. kgl. Ges. Wiss. Göttingen*, 1852, 17–32.
First published account of the tactile nerve endings – "Wagner's corpuscles".

1461 BRÜCKE, Ernst Wilhelm von, *Ritter*. 1819–1892
Grundzüge der Physiologie und Systematik der Sprachlaute für Linguisten und Taubstummenlehrer. Wien, *C. Gerold's Sohn*, 1856.
Classical work on phonetics.

1462 MERKEL, Carl Ludwig. 1812–1876
Anatomie und Physiologie des menschlichen Stimm- und Sprach-Organs (Anthropophonik). Leipzig, *A. Abel*, 1857.

1463 WUNDT, Wilhelm Max. 1832–1920
Beiträge zur Theorie der Sinneswahrnehmung. *Z. rat. Med.*, 1858, **4,** 229–93; 1859, **7,** 279–318, 321–96; 1861, **12,** 145–262; 1862, **14,** 1–77; 1863, **15,** 104–79.
Sensory perception. Wundt was one of the founders of experimental psychology.

1464 FECHNER, Gustav Theodor. 1801–1887
Ueber ein wichtiges psychophysisches Grundgesetz und dessen Beziehung zur Schätzung der Sterngrössen. *Abh. k. sächs. Ges. Wiss.* (*Lpz.*), *math.-phys. Cl.*, (1858), 1859, **4,** 455–532.
Fechner-Weber law on stimulus and sensation (see also No. 1457).

1465 BROWN-SÉQUARD, Charles Edouard. 1817–1894
Recherches sur la transmission des impressions de tact, de chatouillement, de douleur, de température et de contraction (sens musculaire) dans la moëlle épinière. *J. Physiol.* (*Paris*), 1863, **6,** 124–45, 232–48, 581–646.
Among Brown-Séquard's best work was his study of the pathways of conduction in the spinal cord.

1466 TÜRCK, Ludwig. 1810–1868
Ueber die Haut-Sensibilitätsbezirke der einzelnen Rückenmarksnervenpaare. *Denkschr. k. Akad. Wiss.* (*Wien*), *math.-nat. Cl.*, 1868, **29,** 299–326.
Investigation of the cutaneous distribution of the separate pairs of spinal nerves.

1467 DONDERS, Frans Cornelis. 1818–1889
De physiologie der spraakklanken. Utrecht, *C. van der Post, jr.*, 1870.
Donders' most important work was performed in the field of ophthalmology, but he wrote a classical treatise on the physiology of speech.

1468 BLIX, MAGNUS GUSTAV. 1849–1904
Experimentelle Beiträge zur Lösung der Frage über die specifische Energie der Hautnerven. *Z. Biol.*, 1884, **20,** 141–56; 1885, **21,** 145–60.

Besides his investigation of the specific energies of cutaneous nerves, Blix is remembered for his work on the thermodynamics of muscular contraction; he designed a muscle indicator diagram; he was also the first to suggest centrifugal force in the separation of red and white blood cells.

1469 GOLDSCHEIDER, JOHANNES KARL AUGUST EUGEN ALFRED. 1858–1935
Die spezifische Energie der Temperaturnerven. *Mh. prakt. Derm.*, 1884, **3,** 198–208, 225–41.

1470 ——. Neue Thatsachen über die Hautsinnesnerven. *Arch. Anat. Physiol., Physiol. Abt.*, 1885, Suppl.-Bd., 1–110.

Goldscheider recorded important investigations on the nerves conveying the sensation of temperature and on the nerves of cutaneous sensation.

1471 TARCHANOFF, IVAN ROMANOVICH [TARKHANOFF]. 1848–1909
Ueber die galvanischen Erscheinungen in der Haut des Menschen bei Reizungen der Sinnesorgane und bei verschiedenen Formen der psychischen Thätigkeit. *Pflüg. Arch. ges. Physiol.*, 1890, **46,** 46–55.

Psycho-galvanic reflex described.

1472 EWALD, ERNST JULIUS RICHARD. 1855–1921
Physiologische Untersuchungen über das Endorgan des Nervus octavus. Wiesbaden, *J. F. Bergmann*, 1892.

1473 FERRY, ERVIN SIDNEY. 1868–
Persistence of vision. *Amer. J. Sci.*, 1892, 3 ser. **44,** 192–207.

Ferry modified Weber's law on the relationship between stimulus and sensation. Following the work of Porter, *Proc. roy. Soc.* (*Lond.*), 1898, **63**, 347; 1902, **70,** 313 the term "Ferry–Porter Law" came into being.

1474 ZWAARDEMAKER, HENDRIK. 1857–1930
Die Physiologie des Geruchs. Leipzig, *W. Engelmann*, 1895.

1475 FREY, MAX VON. 1852–1932
Untersuchungen über die Sinnesfunctionen der menschlichen Haut. I. Druckempfindung und Schmerz. *Abh. k. sächs. Ges. Wiss.* (*Lpz.*), *math.-phys. Cl.*, (1896), 1897, **23,** 169–226.

In his investigations on cutaneous sensibility Frey introduced his method of testing the sensitiveness of pressure points by means of bristles mounted in a handle.

1476 WINKLER, CORNELIS. 1855–1941
The central course of the nervus octavus and its influence on motility. *Verh. kon. Akad. Wet.* (*Amst.*), 1907, **14,** 1–202.

Winkler was professor of neurology and psychiatry at Amsterdam and Utrecht. He published more than 200 papers, among the most important being that on the central pathways of the eighth nerve.

1477 HOFFMANN, ERICH. 1868–1959
Ueber eine nach innen gerichtete Schützfunktion der Haut (Esophylaxie) nebst Bemerkungen über die Entstehung der Paralyse. *Dtsch. med. Wschr.*, 1919, **45**, 1233–36.

Hoffman stressed the rôle of the skin as a secretory organ, producing hormone-like substances; he suggested the term "esophylaxis" for this function.

Eye; Vision

1478 VAROLIO, Constanzo. 1543–1575
De nervis opticis. Patavii, *apud P. et A. Meiettos fratres*, 1573.

In his day Varolio was an eminent anatomist, and his book on the optic nerve is his best work. His name is perpetuated in medical terminology by the "pons varolii".

1479 CARCANO LEONE, Giovanni Battista. 1536–1606
Anatomici libri II . . . In altero de musculis, palpebrarum atque oculorum motibus deservientibus, accurate disseritur. Ticini, *apud H. Bartholum*, 1574.

First exact description of the lacrimal duct. Carcano gave the true position of the lacrimal gland and showed the route taken by the tears.

1480 SCHEINER, Christoph. 1575–1650
Oculus, hoc est: fundamentum opticum. Oeniponti, *apud D. Agricolam*, 1619.

Scheiner, a Jesuit astronomer, was a pioneer in physiological optics. He demonstrated how images fall on the human retina, noting the changes in curvature of the lens during accommodation, and devised the pin-hole test ("Scheiner's test") to illustrate accommodation and refraction.

1481 MEIBOM, Heinrich. 1638–1700
De vasis palpebrarum novis epistola. Helmstadi, *typ. H. Mulleri*, 1666.

Meibom described the conjunctival (Meibomian) glands; they were, however, already known to Galen and were figured by Casserius in 1609.

1482 DUDDELL, Benedict.
A treatise of the diseases of the horny coat of the eye, and the various kinds of cataracts. London, *J. Clark*, 1729.

"Descemet's membrane" was first described by Duddell. Descemet described it in 1758; see No. 1484.1.

1483 ZINN, Johann Gottfried. 1727–1759
De ligementis ciliaribus. Gottingae, *typ. J. C. L. Schulzii*, 1753.

1484 ——. Descriptio anatomica oculi humani. Gottingae, *apud vid. A. Vandenhoeck*, 1755.

Zinn published a fine atlas of the human eye; he was the first adequately to describe the "zonule of Zinn" and the "annulus of Zinn".

1484.1 DESCEMET, Jean. 1732–1810
An sola lens crystallina cataracte sedes? [Paris], *Veuve de Quillau*, 1758.

"Descemet's membrane"; see No. 1482.

1484.2 PORTERFIELD, William. 1695–1771
A treatise on the eye. The manner and phenomena of vision. 2 vols. Edinburgh, *G. Hamilton & J. Balfour*, 1759.

Porterfield was professor of the institutes and practice of medicine at Edinburgh from 1724–26. His book included many original observations. It was the first important British work on the anatomy and physiology of the eye.

1485 FONTANA, Felice. 1730–1805
Ricerche de motu del iride. Lucca, *Giusta*, 1765.

"Fontana's canal" or "space" described.

1486 YOUNG, Thomas. 1773–1829
Observations on vision. *Phil. Trans.*, 1793, **83,** 169–81.

The versatile Young is regarded as one of the greatest of all scientists. In the above work he showed that the act of accommodation is due to a change of curvature of the crystalline lens, whereby light rays of various lengths can be brought to a focus on the retina.

1487 ——. On the mechanism of the eye. *Phil. Trans.*, 1801, **91,** 23–88.

Includes the first description of astigmatism, with measurements and optical constants.

1488 ——. On the theory of light and colours. *Phil. Trans.*, 1802, **92,** 12–48.

Young, the "Father of physiological optics", established the wave theory of light, explaining the phenomena of interference and dispersion.

1489 SOEMMERRING, Samuel Thomas. 1755–1830
Abbildungen des menschlichen Auges. Frankfurt a.M., *Varrentrapp u. Wenner*, 1801.

Soemmerring is best remembered for his fine anatomical illustrations, of which those devoted to the human eye are a good example. In 1791 he made important observations on the macula lutea: De foramine centrali limbo luteo cincto retinae humanae, *Comment. Soc. reg. Sci. Gotting.*, 1795–98 (1799), **13**, 3–13; on p. 4 he states that he made these observations on January 27, 1791.

1490 TENON, Jacques René. 1724–1816
Observations anatomiques sur quelques parties de l'oeil et des paupières. In his *Mémoires et observations sur l'anatomie, la pathologie, et la chirurgerie*, Paris, *Nyon*, 1806, pp. 193–207.

Although Tenon did not discover the fibrous capsule and the interfascial space of the orbit, they are named after him.

1491 JACOB, Arthur. 1790–1874
An account of a membrane in the eye, now first described. *Phil. Trans.*, 1819, **109,** 300–07.

"Jacob's membrane", the layer of the retina containing the rods and cones.

1492 PURKINJE, Johann Evangelista [Purkyně]. 1787–1869
Beiträge zur Kenntniss des Sehens in subjectiver Hinsicht. Prag, *Fr. Vetterl von Wildenkron*, 1819.

Purkinje's graduation dissertation on the subjective visual phenomena earned for him the friendship of Goethe and the chair of physiology at Breslau.

1493 FLOURENS, Marie Jean Pierre. 1794–1867
Recherches expérimentales sur les propriétés et les fonctions du système nerveux, dans les animaux vertébrés. Paris, *Crevot*, 1824.

Experimental proof that vision depends on the integrity of the cerebral cortex.

1494 HORNER, William Edmonds. 1793–1853
Description of a small muscle of the internal commissure of the eyelids. *Philad. J. med. phys. Sci.*, 1824, **8,** 70–80.

Horner described the tensor tarsi (Horner's) muscle, supplying the lacrimal apparatus. It was first described by Duvernay in 1749.

1495 MÜLLER, Johannes. 1801–1858
Zur vergleichenden Physiologie des Gesichtssinnes des Menschen und der Thiere. Leipzig, *C. Cnobloch*, 1826.

Includes (p. 73) his explanation of the colour sensations produced by pressure upon the retina.

1496 FIELDING, George Hunsley. 1801–1871
On a new membrane in the eye. Hull, *I. Wilson*, 1832.
"Fielding's membrane," the tapetum of the retina.

1497 DALRYMPLE, John. 1804–1852
The anatomy of the human eye. London, *Longmans*, 1834.
First English work on ocular anatomy.

1498 WHEATSTONE, *Sir* Charles. 1802–1875 ,
Contributions to the physiology of vision. *Phil. Trans.*, 1838, **128,** 371–94; 1852, **142,** 1–17.

1499 BREWSTER, *Sir* David. 1781–1868
On the conversion of relief by inverted vision. *Trans. roy. Soc. Edinb.*, 1840–44, **15,** 657–62.

1500 ——. On the knowledge of distance given by binocular vision. *Trans. roy. Soc. Edinb.*, 1840–44, **15,** 663–75.

1501 BRUCH, Karl Wilhelm Ludwig. 1819–1884
Untersuchungen zur Kentniss des körnigen Pigments der Wirbelthiere in physiologischer und pathologischer Hinsicht. *Zürich, Meyer u. Zeller*, 1844.
Includes a description of "Bruch's membrane" of the choroid.

1502 KUSSMAUL, Adolf. 1822–1902
Die Farbenerscheinungen im Grunde des menschlichen Auges. Heidelberg, *K. Groos*, 1845.
An important description of colour phenomena in the fundus oculi. This paper won for Kussmaul the Karl Friedrich Medal of the University of Heidelberg.

1503 LISTING, Johann Benedict. 1808–1882
Beitrag zur physiologischen Optik. Göttingen, *Vandenhoeck & Rupprecht*, 1845.

1504 MACKENZIE, William. 1791–1868
On the vision of objects on and in the eye. *Edinb. med. surg. J.*, 1845, **64,** 38–97.
An introduction to the then little-known subject of catoptrics.

1505 BOWMAN, *Sir* William. 1816–1892
Lectures on the parts concerned in the operations on the eye, and on the structure of the retina. London, *Longman*, 1849.
Bowman did more than any other man to advance ophthalmic surgery in England. The above work is the first to include a sound description of the microscopical anatomy of the eye and the ciliary ("Bowman's") muscle. The book consists of several lectures given at the London Ophthalmic Hospital and published in the *Lond. med. Gaz.* in 1847. Part of it is reprinted in *Med. Classics*, 1940, **5**, 292–336.

1506 MÜLLER, Heinrich. 1820–1864
Zur Histologie der Netzhaut. *Z. wiss. Zool.*, 1851, **3,** 234–37.
Discovery of visual purple.

1507 BUDGE, Julius Ludwig. 1811–1884
Ueber den Einfluss des Nervensystems auf die Bewegung der Iris. *Arch. physiol. Heilk.*, 1852, **11,** 773–826.

1508 HELMHOLTZ, HERMANN LUDWIG FERDINAND VON. 1821–1894
Ueber die Theorie der zusammengesetzten Farben. *Arch. Anat. Physiol. wiss. Med.*, 1852, 461–82; *Ann. Phys. Chem.*, 1852, **87,** 45–66.
Helmholtz's theory of colour vision.

1509 ——. Ueber die Accommodation des Auges. *v. Graefes Arch. Ophthal.*, 1854–55, **1,** 2 Abt., 1–74.
Helmholtz determined the optical constants and explained the mechanism of accommodation, with the help of the ophthalmometer which he had invented in 1852.

1510 BUDGE, JULIUS LUDWIG. 1811–1884
Ueber die Bewegung der Iris. Braunschweig, *F. Vieweg u. Sohn*, 1855.

1511 PANIZZA, BARTOLOMEO. 1785–1867
Osservazioni sul nervo ottico. *G. r. Ist. Lomb. Sci.*, 1855, **7,** 237–52.
Panizza localized visual function in the posterior part of the cerebellum.

1512 SCHULTZE, MAXIMILIAN JOHANN SIGISMUND. 1825–1874
Zur Anatomie und Physiologie der Retina. Bonn, *M. Cohen u. Sohn*, 1866.
One of the greatest of all histologists, Max Schultze is remembered by ophthalmologists for his monograph on the nerve-endings in the retina.

1513 HELMHOLTZ, HERMANN LUDWIG FERDINAND VON. 1821–1894
Handbuch der physiologischen Optik. 1 vol. and atlas. Leipzig, *L. Voss*, 1867.
One of the greatest books on physiological optics. It includes Helmholtz's revival of the Young theory of colour vision.

1514 HOLMGREN, ALARIK FRITHIOF. 1831–1897
Om retinaströmmen. *Upsala LäkFören. Förh.*, 1870–71, **6,** 419–55.
First demonstration of retinal action currents.

1515 HERING, KARL EWALD KONSTANTIN. 1834–1918
Zur Lehre vom Lichtsinne. *S.B. k. Akad. Wiss.* (*Wien*), *math.-nat. Cl.*, 3 Abt., 1872, **66,** 5–24; 1873, **68,** 186–201, 229–44; 1874, **69,** 85–104, 179–217; 1875, **70,** 169–204.
Hering's theory of colour sense.

1515.1 LEBER, THEODOR. 1840–1917
Studien über den Flüssigkeitswechsel im Auge. *v. Graefes Arch. Ophthal.*, 1873, **19,** Abt. II, 87–185.
Leber discovered how the ciliary body excretes intraocular fluid.

1516 GUDDEN, BERNHARD ALOYS VON. 1824–1886
Ueber die Kreuzung der Fasern im Chiasma nervorum opticorum. *v. Graefes Arch. Ophthal.*, 1874, **20,** 2 Abt., 249–68; 1879, **25,** 1 Abt., 1–56.
Important studies on the partial decussation of optic paths.

1517 BOLL, FRANZ CHRISTIAN. 1849–1879
Zur Physiologie des Sehens und der Farbenempfindung. *Mber. k. preuss. Akad. Wiss. Berlin*, 1877, 2–7, 72–74.
Boll noted that visual purple is bleached on exposure to light.

1518 SATTLER, Hubert. 1844–1928
Ueber den feineren Bau der Chorioidea des Menschen nebst Beiträgen zur pathologischen und vergleichenden Anatomie der Aderhaut. *v. Graefes Arch. Ophthal.*, 1876, **22,** Abt. 2, 1–100.
"Sattler's layer" of the choroid.

1519 KÜHNE, Willy. 1837–1900
Ueber den Sehpurpur. *Untersuch. physiol. Inst. Univ. Heidelberg,* 1878, **1,** 15–103.
Kühne was professor of physiology at Amsterdam and Heidelberg. Among his best work is his investigation of visual purple (rhodopsin) which he was first to extract from the retina. Several other papers by him on the same subject appear in the above volume.

1520 LOCKWOOD, Charles Barrett. 1856–1914
The anatomy of the muscles, ligaments and fasciae of the orbit, including an account of the capsule of Tenon, the check ligaments of the recti, and the suspensory ligaments of the eye. *J. Anat. Physiol.* (*Lond.*), 1885, **20,** 1–25.
"Lockwood's suspensory ligament" of the globe of the eye.

1521 HENSCHEN, Salomon Eberhard. 1847–1930
Kort öfversigt af läran om lokalisationen i hjernbarken. *Upsala LäkFören. Förh.*, 1888, **27,** 507–25, 601–12.
Discovery of the cortical visual centre.

1522 LADD-FRANKLIN, Christine. 1847–1930
Eine neue Theorie der Licht-Empfindung. *Z. Psychol. Physiol. Sinnesorg.*, 1893, **4,** 211–21.
Ladd-Franklin theory of vision.

1523 RAMÓN Y CAJAL, Santiago. 1852–1934
Die Retina der Wirbelthiere. Wiesbaden, *J. F. Bergmann,* 1894.
Classical account of the vertebrate retina.

1524 KRIES, Johannes Adolf von. 1853–1928
Ueber die Funktion der Netzhautstäbchen. *Z. Psychol. Physiol. Sinnesorg.*, 1896, **9,** 81–123.
Important paper on the function of the retinal rods.

1525 EDRIDGE-GREEN, Frederick William. 1863–1953
Some observations on the visual purple of the retina. *Trans. ophthal. Soc. U.K.*, 1902, **22,** 300–02.
Edridge-Green first put forward his theories on the function of the retinal rods and of the visual purple about 1889. See also his *Physiology of vision,* 1920.

1525.1 GULLSTRAND, Alvar. 1862–1930
Demonstration eines Instrumentes zur Erzeugung von Strahlengebilden um leuchtende Punkte. *Ber. ophthal. Ges.* (1902), 1903, 290–92.
Gullstrand invented the slit-lamp, making possible the microscopic study of the living eye.

1526 ——. Einführung in die Methoden der Dioptrik des Auges des Menschen. Leipzig, *S. Hirzel,* 1911.
Discovery of the intracapsular mechanism of accommodation. Gullstrand received the Nobel Prize in 1911 for his work on the dioptrics of the eye.

1527 VOGT, ALFRED. 1879–1943
Atlas der Spaltlampenmikroskopie des lebenden Auges. Berlin, *J. Springer*, 1921.

An important work on the biomicroscopy of the eye. English translation, Berlin, 1921. Second edition, vol. 1–2 (in German), 1930–31; vol. 3 (in English), Zürich, 1941.

1528 ADRIAN, EDGAR DOUGLAS, 1*st Baron Adrian*. 1889– , & MATTHEWS, RACHEL.
The action of light on the eye. *J. Physiol.* (*Lond.*), 1927, **63,** 378–414; **64,** 279–301; 1928, **65,** 273–308.

Adrian and Matthews made important researches on the electrical discharges from the vertebrate optic nerve.

1529 PARSONS, *Sir* JOHN HERBERT. 1868–1957
An introduction to the theory of perception. Cambridge, *University Press*, 1927.

1530 DUKE-ELDER, *Sir* WILLIAM STEWART. 1898–
The nature of the intra-ocular fluids. London, *G. Pulman*, 1927.

1531 ——. Text-book of ophthalmology. Vol. 1. The development, form, and function of the visual apparatus. London, *H. Kimpton*, 1932.

1532 HARTLINE, HALDAN KEFFER. 1903–
The responses of single optic nerve fibers of the vertebrate eye to illumination of the retina. *Amer. J. Physiol.*, 1938, **121,** 400–15.

Hartline continued and extended the work initiated by Adrian and Matthews on electrical discharges from the optic nerve. See also his later papers in the same journal, 1940, **130**, 690–711.

1533 POLYAK, STEPHEN. 1889–1955
The anatomy and the histology of the retina in man, ape, and monkey. Chicago, *Univ. Press*, (1941).

1534 GRANIT, RAGNAR ARTHUR. 1900–
Sensory mechanisms of the retina: with an appendix on electroretinography. London, *Geoffrey Cumberlege*, 1947.

An account of twenty years' work on the electrical responses of the retina, a discussion of visual purple and visual violet, and an exposition of Granit's hypothesis of colour vision. His researches have done much to elucidate the mechanism of visual processes.

1535 MANN, IDA CAROLINE. 1893–
The development of the human eye. 2nd ed. London, *British Medical Association*, 1949.

Ear; Hearing

1536 MASSA, NICCOLÒ. 1499–1569
Anatomiae liber introductorius. Venetiis, *F. Bindoni ac M. Pasini*, 1536.

Massa described the action of the ossicles.

1537 FALLOPPIO, GABRIELE [FALLOPIUS]. 1523–1562
Observationes anatomicae. Venetiis, *apud M. A. Ulmum*, 1561.

Includes first clear description of the membrana tympani. Fallopius discovered the aqueduct of Fallopius.

1538 EUSTACHI, BARTOLOMMEO [EUSTACHIUS]. 1520–1574
De auditus organis. In his *Opuscula anatomica*, Venetiis, 1564, pp. 148–64.

Eustachius is credited with several anatomical discoveries, among them the tensor tympani muscle and the Eustachian tube. In the last respect, however, he was anticipated by Alcmaeon, about 500 B.C. Eustachius was the first to describe the chorda tympani as a nerve.

1539 COITER, VOLCHER. 1534–1600
De auditus instrumento. In his *Externarum et internarum principalium humani corporis partium tabulae*, Noribergae, *in off. T. Gerlatzeni*, 1573, 88–105.

The first monograph on the ear. A compendium of contemporary knowledge of the anatomy and physiology of the ear.

1540 CASSERIO, GIULIO [JULIUS CASSERIUS *Placentinus*]. 1552–1616
De vocis auditusque organis historia anatomica. 2 pts. Ferrariae, *exc. V. Baldinus, typ. Cameralis*, 1600–01.

Important early monograph on the comparative anatomy of the ear.

1541 INGRASSIA, GIOVANNI FILIPPO. 1510–1580
In Galeni librum de ossibus. Panormi, *ex typog. J. B. Maringhi*, 1603.

Ingrassia is by some accredited with the discovery of the stapes; he also observed the sound-conducting capacity of the teeth.

1542 FOLLI, CECILIO [FOLIUS]. 1615–1660
Nova auris internae delineatio. Venetiis, 1645.

Announces the discovery of the long process of the malleus. Folius "accurately discussed the general configuration of the middle ear, described the round and oval windows, delineated the three ossicles with the so-called fourth ossicle, the semicircular canals and cochlea" (Mettler). Also in A. Haller, *Disputationes ad morborum historiam*, etc., 1749, **4**, 365–68.

1543 STENSEN, NIELS [STENO]. 1638–1686
Observationes anatomicae, quibus varia oris, oculorum, et narium vasa describuntur. Lugduni Batavorum, *J. Chouët*, 1662.

Ceruminous glands first mentioned.

1544 WILLIS, THOMAS. 1621–1675
De anima brutorum. London, *R. Davis*, 1672.

Chap. XIV is devoted to the sense of hearing; in it Willis described the "paracusis of Willis". English translation, 1684.

1545 DUVERNEY, JOSEPH GUICHARD. 1648–1730
Traité de l'organe de l'ouïe, contenant la structure, les usages et les maladies de toutes les parties de l'oreille. Paris, *E. Michallet*, 1683.

First scientific account of the structure, function and diseases of the ear. Duverney showed that the bony external meatus develops from the tympanic ring and that the mastoid air cells communicate with the tympanic cavity. It was Duverney who first suggested the theory of hearing later developed by, and accredited to, Helmholtz. English translation, 1737.

1546 VALSALVA, ANTONIO MARIA. 1666–1723
De aure humana tractatus. Bononiae, *typ. C. Pisarii*, 1704.

Valsalva, a pupil of Malpighi and teacher of Morgagni, is best remembered for his work upon the ear, in which he described and depicted its most minute muscles and nerves. He divided the ear into "external", "middle", and "internal"; his method of inflating the middle ear (Valsalva's manoeuvre) is still practised. The book includes a description of "Valsalva's dysphagia".

1547 CASSEBOHM, Johann Friedrich. 1699?–1743
Tractatus quatuor anatomici de aure humana. Halae Magdeburgi, *sumtibus Orphanotrophei*, 1734.

Important tracts on the anatomy and physiology of the ear. Cassebohm wrote two further tracts in 1735.

1548 PYL, Theodor.
Dissertatio medica de auditu in genere et de illo que fit per os in specie. Gryphiswald, 1742.

Pyl was the first (page 20) to record the labryinthine fluid and to discuss its rôle in the transmission of sound.

1549 COTUGNO, Domenico [Cotunnius]. 1736–1822
De aquaeductibus auris humanae internae. Neapoli, *ex typ. Simoniana*, 1761.

Cotugno is sometimes accredited with the discovery of the *liquor Cotunnii*, the labyrinthine fluid, first noted by Pyl in 1742. He did, however, make important contributions to the knowledge on the structure and function of the ear, including the discovery of the aural aqueducts. The naso-palatine nerve and the columns in the osseous spiral lamina are named after him.

1550 SCARPA, Antonio. 1747?–1832
De structura fenestrae rotundae auris, et de tympano secundario anatomicae observationes. Mutinae, *apud Soc. typog.*, 1772.

Scarpa, who was a master of anatomic illustration, discovered the membranous labyrinth. (See also No. 1553.)

1551 GEOFFROY, Étienne Louis, *le comte*. 1725–1810
Dissertations sur l'organe de l'ouie. 1. De l'homme. 2. Des reptiles. 3. Des poissons. Amsterdam & Paris, *Cavelier*, 1778.

1552 COMPARETTI, Andrea. 1746–1801
Observationes anatomicae de aure interna comparata. Patavii, *S. Bartholomaeus*, 1789.

1553 SCARPA, Antonio. 1747?–1832
De penitiori ossium structura commentarius. Lipsiae, *J. F. Hartknoch*, 1799.

1554 SOEMMERRING, Samuel Thomas. 1755–1830
Abbildungen des menschlichen Hoerorganes. Frankfort a.M., *Varrentrapp u. Wenner*, 1806.

1555 JACOBSON, Ludwig Levin. 1783–1843
Supplementa ad otojatriam. Supplementum primum de anastomosi nervorum nova in aure detecta. *Acta. reg. Soc. Med. Havnien.*, 1818, **5**, 293–303.

Jacobson described the tympanic canal, nerve, and plexus, all of which are named after him. In 1809 he discovered "Jacobson's organ", as reported two years later by G. Cuvier.

1556 WEBER, Ernst Heinrich. 1795–1878
De aure et auditu hominis et animalium. Lipsiae, *apud G. Fleischerum*, 1820.

1557 FLOURENS, MARIE JEAN PIERRE. 1794–1867
Expériences sur les canaux semi-circulaires de l'oreille. *Mém. Acad. roy. d. Sci.* (*Paris*), 1830, **9**, 455–77.

Flourens showed that lesion of the semicircular canals produces motor incoordination and loss of equilibrium.

1558 SHRAPNELL, HENRY JONES. *d.* 1834
On the form and structure of the membrana tympani. *Lond. med. Gaz.*, 1832, **10**, 120–24.

Description of the pars flaccida ("Shrapnell's membrane") of the tympanic membrane.

1559 CORTI, ALFONSO, *Marchese*. 1822–1888
Recherches sur l'organe de l'ouïe des mammifères. *Z. wiss. Zool.*, 1851, **3**, 109–69.

Corti made important investigations on the finer anatomy of the mammalian cochlea. The "organ of Corti" in the cochlea is named after him.

1560 REISSNER, ERNST. 1824–1878
De auris internae formatione. Dorpati Livonorum, *H. Laakmann*, 1851.

Description of the vestibular membrane ("Reissner's membrane").

1561 SCHULTZE, MAXIMILIAN JOHANN SIGISMUND. 1825–1874
Ueber die Endigungsweise des Hörnerven im Labyrinth. *Arch. Anat. Physiol. wiss. Med.*, 1858, 343–81.

Schultze's great monographs on the nerve-endings of the sense organs were of prime importance in the development of the science of histology. Besides that dealing with the internal ear, he wrote others dealing with the nose and the retina (See Nos. 936, 1512).

1562 HELMHOLTZ, HERMANN LUDWIG FERDINAND VON. 1821–1894
Die Lehre von der Tonempfindungen als physiologische Grundlage für die Theorie der Musik. Braunschweig, *F. Vieweg u. Sohn*, 1863.

Helmholtz's theory of hearing, upon which all modern theories of resonance are based. This exhaustive study of acoustics ranks as one of the greatest books on the subject and shows that Helmholtz was, besides being a great physicist and physician, an accomplished musician. English translation of 3rd edition, London, 1875.

1563 ——. Die Mechanik der Gehörknöchelchen und des Trommelfells. Bonn, *M. Cohen & Sohn*, 1869.

Helmholtz's study of the mechanism of the tympanum and ossicles of the middle ear did much to elucidate the phenomenon of audition. It includes a description of "Helmholtz's ligament" of the malleus. English translation, 1874.

1564 GOLTZ, FRIEDRICH LEOPOLD. 1834–1902
Ueber die physiologische Bedeutung der Bogengänge des Ohrlabyrinths. *Pflüg. Arch. ges. Physiol.*, 1870, **3**, 172–92.

Goltz demonstrated the relation of vertigo and vestibular disturbance, showing that the former is a result of disease or irritation of the semicircular canals.

1565 HARTMANN, ARTHUR. 1849–1931
Eine neue Methode der Hörprüfung mit Hülfe elektrischer Ströme. *Arch. Anat. Physiol., Physiol. Abt.*, 1878, 155–57.

First audiometer.

1566 RETZIUS, MAGNUS GUSTAF. 1842–1919
Das Gehörorgan der Wirbelthiere. 2 vols. Stockholm, *Samson & Wallin*, 1881–84.

1567 STEIN, STANISLAV ALEKSANDR FYODOROVICH. 1855–
Die Lehren von den Funktionen der einzelnen Theile des Ohrlabyrinths. Jena, *G. Fischer*, 1894.

1568 EWALD, ERNST JULIUS RICHARD. 1855–1921
Zur Physiologie des Labyrinths. 3. Mittheilung. Das Hören der labyrinthlosen Tauben. *Pflüg. Arch. ges. Physiol.*, 1894, **59,** 258–75.

1569 ——. Zur Physiologie des Labyrinths. 4. Mittheilung. Die Beziehungen des Grosshirns zum Tonuslabyrinth. *Pflüg. Arch. ges. Physiol.*, 1895, **60,** 492–508.

1570 WILKINSON, GEORGE. 1867–1956, & GRAY, ALBERT ALEXANDER. 1869–1936
The mechanism of the cochlea. A restatement of the resonance theory of hearing. London, *Macmillan & Co.*, 1924.

1570.1 BÉKÉSY, GEORG VON. 1899–1972
Uber den Knall und die Theorie des Hörens. *Phys. Z.*, 1933, **34,** 577–82.
In 1961 Békésy was awarded a Nobel Prize for his discoveries concerning the physical mechanisms of stimulation within the cochlea.

History of Physiology

1571 DALTON JOHN CALL. 1825–1889
The experimental method in medical science. New York, *G. P. Putnam's Sons*, 1882.
Dalton, professor of physiology at the universities of Buffalo and Vermont, and the College of Physicians and Surgeons, New York, was the first American to devote his time exclusively to that subject. He was present at the first demonstration of ether as an anaesthetic, Oct. 16, 1846, and was quick to see its possibilities as a means of illustrating his lectures with experiments on living animals. As a result of the opposition to this method of teaching he published the above book.

1572 ——. Doctrines of the circulation. Philadelphia, *H. C. Lea's Son & Co.*, 1884.

1573 MARCET, WILLIAM. 1829–1900
A contribution to the history of the respiration of man. London, *J. & A. Churchill*, 1897.

1574 NEUBURGER, MAX. 1868–1955
Die historische Entwicklung der experimentellen Gehirn- und Rückenmarksphysiologie vor Flourens. Stuttgart, *F. Enke*, 1897.

1575 FOSTER, *Sir* MICHAEL. 1836–1907
Lectures on the history of physiology. Cambridge, *Univ. Press*, 1901.
Reprinted 1924.

1576 STIRLING, WILLIAM. 1851–1932
Some apostles of physiology. London, *Waterlow & Sons*, 1902.
This handsome volume contains biographical sketches of the important figures in the history of physiology, together with a fine collection of portraits.

1577 BORUTTAU, HEINRICH JOHANNES. 1869–1923
Geschichte der Physiologie. In Puschmann's *Handbuch der Geschichte der Medizin*, Jena, 1903, **2,** 327–456.

1578 FEARING, FRANKLIN. 1892–
Reflex action. A study in the history of physiological psychology. Baltimore, *Williams & Wilkins*, 1930.

1580 FULTON, JOHN FARQUHAR. 1899–1960
Physiology. New York, *P. B. Hoeber*, 1931.
A short history of the subject, published in the "Clio Medica" series.

1581 SALMONSEN, ELLA MAUD. 1885–1971
Bibliographical survey of vitamins 1650–1930, with a section on patents by M. H. Wodlinger. Chicago, *M. H. Wodlinger*, 1932.

1582 LUSK, GRAHAM. 1866–1932
Nutrition. New York, *P. B. Hoeber*, 1933.
Clio Medica series. A brief history of the subject. Lusk was a great figure in the study of nutrition; he died before the book was ready for publication, and it was completed by E. F. DuBois.

1583 CANNON, WALTER BRADFORD. 1871–1945
The story of the development of our ideas of chemical mediation of nerve impulses. *Amer. J. med. Sci.*, 1934, **188,** 145–59.

1584 LIEBEN, FRITZ. 1890–
Geschichte der physiologischen Chemie. Leipzig, *Deuticke*, 1935.

1585 DRUMMOND, *Sir* JACK CECIL. 1891–1952, & WILBRAHAM, ANNE, *Lady Drummond*. ?–1952
The Englishman's food. A history of five centuries of English diet. London, *Jonathan Cape*, (1939).
Revised edition, 1958.

1586 FRANKLIN, KENNETH JAMES. 1897–1966
A short history of physiology. 2nd ed. London, *Staples Press*, 1949.

1587 BASTHOLM, EGVIND BØRGE MARTIN MARIUS. 1904–
The history of muscle physiology from the natural philosophers to Albrecht von Haller. Copenhagen, *Munksgaard*, 1950.
Acta Historica Scientiarum Naturalium et Medicinalium, Vol. 7.

1588 ROTHSCHUH, KARL EDUARD. 1908–
Geschichte der Physiologie. Berlin, *J. Springer*, 1953.
Revised and enlarged English translation, Huntington, N.Y., 1972.

1588.1 McCOLLUM, ELMER VERNER. 1879–
A history of nutrition. Boston, *Houghton Mifflin Co.*, 1957.

1588.2 BÖTTCHER, HELMUTH MAXIMILIAN. 1895–
Hormone: Die Geschichte der Hormonforschung. Köln, *Kiepenheuer & Witsch*, 1963.

1588.3 ——. Das Vitaminbuch. Die Geschichte der Vitaminforschung. Köln, *Kiepenheuer & Witsch*, [1965].

1588.4 FISHMAN, ALFRED PAUL. 1918– , & RICHARDS, DICKINSON WOODRUFF. 1895–
Circulation of the blood: men and ideas. New York, *Oxford University Press*, 1964.

1588.5 FULTON, JOHN FARQUHAR. 1899–1960
Selected readings in the history of physiology. Compiled by JOHN F. FULTON, completed by LEONARD G. WILSON. Springfield, *C. C. Thomas*, 2nd ed., 1966.

These readings extend from Aristotle to contemporary writers; they give access to many classical works that might otherwise be unobtainable to students of the history of physiology. Foreign material is translated into English. First edition 1930.

STATE MEDICINE: PUBLIC HEALTH: HYGIENE

1589–1671.5

1589 FRONTINUS, SEXTUS JULIUS. A.D. 35–104
The two books on the water supply of the city of Rome of Sextus Julius Frontinus, water commissioner of the city of Rome, A.D. 97. A photographic reproduction of the sole original Latin manuscript and its reprint in Latin; also, a translation into English, and explanatory chapters by Clemens Herschel. Boston, *Dana, Estes & Co.*, 1899.

The *De aquis urbis Romae* of Frontinus gives a history and description of the water supply of ancient Rome, and the laws governing its use and maintenance.

1590 PHAER, THOMAS [PHAYER; PHAYR]. 1510–1560
A new booke entyteled the regiment of lyfe. London, *E. Whytchurch*, 1544.

Translation of a book by Jehan Goeurot published in 1530. Garrison states that it is a version of the *Regimen Sanitatis*.

1591 BOORDE, ANDREW [BORDE]. ?1490–1549
The breviary of helthe, for all manner of syckenesses and diseases the whiche may be in man, or woman doth folowe. London, *W. Middleton*, 1547.

This, probably the earliest "modern" work on hygiene, throws some light on the condition of that subject in the sixteenth century.

1592 CORNARO, LUIGI. 1467–1566
Trattato de la vita sobria. Padova, *G. Perchacino*, 1558.

Garrison considers this "the best treatise on personal hygiene and the simple life in existence". A good English edition was published in 1903.

1594 HARINGTON, *Sir* JOHN. 1560–1612
A new discourse of a stale subject, called the Metamorphosis of Aiax. Written by Misacmos to his friend Philostilpnos. London, *R. Field*, 1596.

Harington invented a water-closet in which the disposal of excreta was for the first time controlled by mechanical means. He published several tracts on the device, the first appearing in 1596. These were reprinted at Chiswick, 1814. "Ajax" is a pun on "a jakes", an Elizabethan name for a privy. Annotated edition by Elizabeth S. Donno, London, 1962.

1595 FLOYER, *Sir* John. 1649–1734
Medicina gerocomica; or, the Galenic art of preserving old men's healths. London, *F. Isted*, 1724.
First book devoted to geriatrics.

1596 HALES, Stephen. 1677–1761
A description of ventilators. London, *W. Innys*, 1743.
Hales devised a ventilator, by means of which fresh air could be introduced into gaols, mines, hospitals, the holds of ships, etc. The invention met with immediate approval and contributed much towards the health of those for whom it was employed. Hales was the inventor of artificial ventilation.

1597 TISSOT, Simon André. 1728–1797
Avis au peuple sur la santé. Lausanne, *J. Zimmerli pour F. Grasset*, 1761.
A tract on medicine written for the lay public; it ran through several editions and was translated into all European languages. English translation in 1765.

1598 HOWARD, John. 1726–1790
The state of the prisons in England and Wales. Warrington, *W. Eyres*, 1777.
Howard devoted much of his life to the improvement of the conditions then prevailing in prisons. The publication of his book led to legislation abolishing abuses in prisons and providing for their proper cleaning. The Howard League for Penal Reform is one result of his charitable work.

1599 FRANK, Johann Peter. 1745–1821
System einer vollständigen medicinischen Polizey. 9 vols. Mannheim, Tübingen, Wien, 1779–1827.
First systematic treatise on public hygiene. In his classical work, Frank, the "Father of Public Hygiene," considered the ruler of a state to stand in the relation of a father to his children, among his duties being the safeguarding of the people's health and the preservation of a healthy race by appropriate laws. The last two volumes were edited by G. C. G. Voigt.

1600 TENON, Jacques René. 1724–1816
Mémoires sur les hôpitaux de Paris. Paris, *P. D. Pierres*, 1788.
Reforms quickly followed Tenon's disclosures of the dreadful conditions prevailing in the hospitals of Paris in the 18th century. He was also instrumental in the foundation of a special hospital for children.

1601 HOWARD, John. 1726–1790
An account of the principle lazarettos in Europe. Warrington, *T. Cadell*, 1789.
Following on his work for the improvement of the conditions in prisons, Howard travelled extensively in Europe, carrying out an elaborate investigation into the conditions of hospitals.

1602 HUFELAND, Christoph Wilhelm. 1762–1836
Die Kunst das menschliche Leben zu verlängern, Jena, *Akad. Buchhandlung*, 1797.
Hufeland's "Makrobiotik," one of the most popular books of its time on personal hygiene. It was translated into all European languages. Hufeland was court physician at Weimar.

1603 ROBERTON, John.
A treatise on medical police. 2 vols. Edinburgh, *J. Moir*, 1809.
First notable work on the subject in English.

1604 WELLS, William Charles. 1757–1817
An essay on dew. London, *Taylor & Hessay*, 1814.

For this important work, Wells was awarded the Rumford Medal of the Royal Society. His researches on the subject were of major importance in the development of the science of ventilation, particularly in its relation to relative humidity and the influence of the latter on the comfort of the occupants of factories, ships, theatres, etc. Wells was physician to St. Thomas's Hospital, London, from 1800 until his death.

1605 FODÉRÉ, François Emmanuel. 1764–1835
Leçons sur les épidémies et l'hygiène publique. 4 vols. Paris, *F. G. Levrault*, 1822–24.

1606 PARENT-DUCHÂTELET, Alexandre Jean Baptiste. 1790–1836
Hygiène publique. 2 vols. Paris, *J. B. Baillière*, 1836.

1607 ——. De la prostitution dans la ville de Paris. 2 vols. Paris, *J. B. Baillière*, 1836.

1608 CHADWICK, *Sir* Edwin. 1800–1890
Report on the sanitary condition of the labouring population of Great Britain. London, *W. Clowes & Sons*, 1843.

Chadwick was secretary to the Poor Law Commission when he made this report to Parliament. It was reprinted in Edinburgh, 1965. See also No. 1625.

1609 MASSACHUSETTS.
Report of a general plan for the promotion of public and personal health, devised, prepared, and recommended by the commissioners appointed under a resolve of the legislature of Massachusetts relating to a sanitary survey of the State. Boston, *Dutton & Wentworth*, 1850.

L. Shattuck, N. P. Banks, and J. Abbott produced a report with proposals regarding public health organization in Massachusetts. A Board of Health was not set up until 1869, however. Shattuck has been called "the Chadwick of America". An abridged version of this famous Report appears in G. C. Whipple's *State sanitation*, Cambridge, [Mass.,] 1917; a facsimile reproduction was published in 1948.

1610 CHEVALLIER, Jean Baptiste Alphonse. 1793–1879
Dictionnaire des altérations et falsifications des substances alimentaires, médicamenteuses et commerciales. 2 vols. Paris, *Béchet jeune*, 1850.

Chevallier, a famous chemist, was a prolific writer. Above is probably his most important publication.

1610.1 INTERNATIONAL SANITARY CONFERENCE.
Procès-verbaux de la conférence sanitaire internationale ouverte à Paris le 27 juillet 1851. Paris, *Imprimerie Nationale*, 1852.

First international sanitary conference; it prepared an international sanitary code dealing with cholera, plague, and yellow fever.

1611 NIGHTINGALE, Florence. 1820–1910
Notes on hospitals. London, *John W. Parker & Son*, 1859.

Includes four plans of hospitals. A third edition, completely revised, was published by Longmans, Green & Co., London, 1863.

1612 NIGHTINGALE, FLORENCE. 1820–1910. Notes on nursing: what it is, and what it is not. London, *Harrison & Sons*, [1859].

After receiving training in Germany and France, Florence Nightingale had some nursing experience in England. The Crimean war gave her an opportunity to demonstrate the value of trained nurses. Within a few months of her arrival at Scutari, the mortality rate among soldiers there fell from 42% to 2%. Florence Nightingale lived to become the greatest figure in the history of nursing. Facsimile reproduction (? of first edition), Philadelphia, 1946. Biographies by Sir E. T. Cook, 1913, and Cecil Woodham-Smith, 1950. See also ***Bio-bibliography of** Florence Nightingale*, by W. J. Bishop, 1962.

1613 PETTENKOFER, MAX JOSEF VON. 1818–1901

Ueber eine Methode die Kohlensäure in der atmosphärischen Luft zu bestimmen. *J. prakt. Chem.*, 1862, **85,** 165–84.

Pettenkofer was the founder of experimental hygiene; he was the first to institute a laboratory for hygienic investigation.

1614 PARKES, EDMUND ALEXANDER. 1819–1876

A manual of practical hygiene. London, *John Churchill & Sons*, 1864.

First important English treatise on hygiene.

1615 BAZALGETTE, *Sir* JOSEPH WILLIAM. 1819–1891

Metropolitan Board of Works. Report on experiments with respect to the ventilation of sewers. 3 parts. London, *Brickhill & Bateman*, [1866–69].

Bazalgette planned the sewers of London.

1616 VIRCHOW, RUDOLF LUDWIG KARL. 1821–1902

Ueber die Canalisation von Berlin. *Vjschr. gerichtl. öff. Med.*, 1868, n.F. **9,** 1–43.

Virchow advocated a canal sewer system for Berlin. Such a system was constructed by Hobrecht (see No. 1624).

1617 ——. Ueber gewisse, die Gesundheit benachtheiligende Einflüsse der Schulen. *Virchows Arch. path. Anat.*, 1869, **46,** 447–70.

Improvements in school hygiene and the regular inspection of school children were brought about by the efforts of Virchow.

1618 PETTENKOFER, MAX JOSEF VON. 1818–1901

Das Kanal- oder Siel-System in München. München, *H. Manz*, 1869.

Pettenkofer was responsible for the installation of the modern system of sewage disposal in Munich, and thus succeeded in almost completely ridding that city of typhoid.

1619 LISTER, JOSEPH, 1*st Baron Lister*. 1827–1912

On the effects of the antiseptic system of treatment upon the salubrity of a surgical hospital. *Lancet*, 1870, **1,** 4–6, 40–42.

Reprinted in *Med. Classics*, 1937, **2,** 84–101.

1620 BELGRAND, MARIE FRANÇOIS EUGÈNE. 1810–1878

La Seine. Etudes hydrologiques. Régime de la pluie, des sources, des eaux courantes. (Les travaux souterrains de Paris.) 4 vols. and atlas. Paris, *Vve. C. Dunod*, 1872–87.

Belgrand designed the Paris sewers.

1621 GALTON, *Sir* DOUGLAS STRUTT. 1822–1899

Observations on the construction of healthy dwellings. Oxford, *Clarendon Press*, 1880.

Galton spent some years in the army; he had a variety of interests, chief among them being railways, education, and sanitary science. He designed the Herbert Hospital at Woolwich and he invented a ventilating fire grate.

1622 COHN, HERMANN LUDWIG. 1838–1906
Die Hygiene des Auges in den Schulen. Wien, Leipzig, *Urban & Schwarzenberg*, 1883.

Cohn did much to promote school hygiene. He advocated regular examination of the eyes of school-children, an idea which was put into practice in 1885. An English translation of the book appeared in 1886.

1623 BOLTON, *Sir* FRANCIS JOHN. 1831–1887
London water supply, including a history and description of the London waterworks. London, *W. Clowes*, 1884.

1624 HOBRECHT, JAMES. 1825–1902
Die Canalisation von Berlin. Berlin, *Ernst u. Korn*, 1884.

Hobrecht was responsible for the construction of the Berlin sewers.

1625 RICHARDSON, *Sir* BENJAMIN WARD. 1828–1896
The health of nations. A review of the works of Edwin Chadwick. 2 vols. London, *Longmans, Green & Co.*, 1887.

Chadwick may be said to have initiated the public health era. Largely through his efforts the Public Health Act 1848 came into existence in England. He was the greatest sanitarian of the 19th century; among other things he was responsible for the introduction of glazed earthenware pipes for drains. See also R. A. Lewis's *Edwin Chadwick and the public health movement, 1832–54*, London, 1952. Facsimile reprint, 1965.

1626 SIMON, *Sir* JOHN. 1816–1904
Public health reports. 2 vols. London, *J. & A. Churchill*, 1887.

Simon was the first medical officer for the City of London. Together with his *English sanitary institutions*, the above work played a great part in paving the way for modern reforms in the sphere of hygiene and public health. Next to Chadwick, Simon was the greatest sanitary reformer of the 19th century. (See also No. 1650.) Biography by R. Lambert, 1963.

1627 BILLINGS, JOHN SHAW. 1838–1913
Description of the Johns Hopkins Hospital. Baltimore, *I. Friedenwald*, 1890.

Billings was responsible for the designing of the Johns Hopkins Hospital, Baltimore.

1628 BURDETT, *Sir* HENRY CHARLES. 1847–1920
Hospitals and asylums of the world. 4 vols. and atlas. London, *J. & A. Churchill*, 1891–93.

This great work deals with the history, administration, and planning of hospitals, and includes a bibliography.

1629 STEVENSON, *Sir* THOMAS. 1838–1908, & MURPHY, SHIRLEY FOSTER. 1849–1923
A treatise on hygiene and public health. Edited by T. STEVENSON and S. F. MURPHY. 3 vols. London, *J. & A. Churchill*, 1892–94.

A co-operative work.

1630 GALTON, *Sir* DOUGLAS STRUTT. 1822–1899
Healthy hospitals. Oxford, *Clarendon Press*, 1893.

1631 DIBDIN, WILLIAM JOSEPH. 1850–1925
The purification of sewage and water. London, *Sanitary Publ. Co.*, 1897.

Dibdin introduced the bacterial system of sewage purification. Previously he had devised the contact system.

1632 STODDART, FREDERICK WALLIS. 1860–1917
Some points in the construction of the continuous sewage filter. *Proc. incorp. Ass. munic. County Engrs*, 1901, **28**, 278–90.

1633 GREAT BRITAIN. *Parliament.*
Royal Commission on sewage disposal. Reports 1–8. London, *Eyre & Spottiswoode*, 1902–12.

1634 CALMETTE, LÉON CHARLES ALBERT. 1863–1933
Recherches sur l'épuration biologique et chimique des eaux d'égout. 8 vols. Paris, *Masson & Cie.*, 1905–08.

1635 FOREL, AUGUSTE HENRI. 1848–1931
Die sexuelle Frage. München, *E. Reinhardt*, 1905.
Forel's best work; translated into 16 languages; 16th edition in 1931.

1636 WASSERMANN, AUGUST VON. 1866–1925
Die Bedeutung der Bakterien für die Gesundheitspflege. München, *R. Oldenbourg*, 1905.

1637 WINSLOW, CHARLES-EDWARD AMORY. 1877–1957, & PHELPS, EARLE BERNARD. 1876–
Investigation on the purification of Boston sewage, with a history of the sewage-disposal problem. Washington, *Govt. Printing Office*, 1906.

1638 HENRI, VICTOR, *et al.*
Stérilisation de grandes quantités d'eau par les rayons ultraviolets. *C. R. Acad. Sci.* (*Paris*), 1910, **150,** 932–34; **151,** 677–80.
With A. Helbronner and M. de Recklinghausen.

1639 RUBNER, MAX. 1854–1932, *et al.*
Handbuch der Hygiene. 6 vols. Leipzig, *S. Hirtzel*, 1911–13.
With Max Gruber and P. M. Ficker.

1640 FOWLER, GILBERT JOHN. 1868–1953
Sewage disposal by oxidation methods. *Trans. XV. Int. Congr. Hyg. Demog.*, 1912, Washington, 1913, **4,** 375–83.

1641 ROSENAU, MILTON JOSEPH. 1869–1946
Preventive medicine and hygiene. New York, *D. Appleton & Co.*, 1913.
6th edition, 1935.

1642 IMHOFF, KARL. 1876–
Fortschritte der Abwasserreinigung. Berlin, 1925.
In 1909 Imhoff devised the system of sewage purification which bears his name.

1643 MACEACHERN, MALCOLM THOMAS. 1882–1956
Hospital organization and management. 2nd ed. Chicago, *Physicians' Record Co.*, 1946.

1644 STONE, JOSEPH EDMUND. 1888–
Hospital organization and management. 4th ed. London, *Faber & Faber*, 1952.

History of State Medicine, Public Health, and Hygiene

1645 SANGER, WILLIAM W.
The history of prostitution. New York, *American Med. Press*, 1858.
Reprinted in 1919.

1646 VIOLLET LE DUC, EUGÈNE EMMANUEL. 1814–1879
Histoire de l'habitation humaine. Paris, 1875.

1647 UFFELMANN, JULIUS AUGUST CHRISTIAN. 1837–1894
Die öffentliche Hygiene im alten Rom. Berlin, 1881.

1648 FORT, GEORGE FRANKLIN.
Medical economy during the Middle Ages; a contribution to the history of European morals, from the time of the Roman Empire to the close of the fourteenth century. New York, *J. W. Bouton*, 1883.

1649 KOTELMANN, LUDWIG WILHELM JOHANNES. 1839–1908
Gesundheitspflege im Mittelalter. Hamburg, Leipzig, *L. Voss*, 1890.

1650 SIMON, *Sir* JOHN. 1816–1904
English sanitary institutions, reviewed in their course of development, and in some of their political and social relations. London, *Cassell & Co.*, 1890.
One of the best accounts of the development of public health in Great Britain in the 19th century. It is a mine of information and greatly influenced modern developments and legislation on public health.

1651 RUBNER, MAX. 1854–1932
Zur Vorgeschichte der modernen Hygiene. Berlin, *O. Francke*, 1905.

1652 DELAUNAY, HENRI. 1865–
L'hygiène publique à travers les âges. Paris, *Vigot frères*, 1906.

1653 MORRIS, *Sir* MALCOLM ALEXANDER. 1849–1924
The story of English public health. London, *Cassell & Co.*, 1919.

1654 RÁVENEL, MAZYCK PORCHER. 1861–1946
A half-century of public health. Jubilee historical volume of the American Public Health Association. New York, *Amer. Publ. Health Assoc.*, 1921.

1654.1 LA CROIX, PAUL. 1806–1884
History of prostitution among all the peoples of the world, from the most remote antiquity to the present day. Translated from the original French by SAMUEL PUTNAM. 3 vols. Chicago, *Pascal Covici*, 1926.

1655 GARRISON, FIELDING HUDSON. 1870–1935
The history of heating, ventilation, and lighting. *Bull. N. Y. Acad. Med.*, 1927, 2 ser., **3**, 57–67.

1656 NEWSHOLME, *Sir* ARTHUR. 1857–1943
Evolution of preventive medicine. London, *Baillière, Tindall & Cox*, 1927.

1657 McCURRICH, HUGH JAMES. 1890–
The treatment of the sick poor of this country and the preservation of the health of the poor in this country. London, *Humphrey Milford*, 1929.

1658 WILLIAMS, JOHN HARGREAVES HARLEY. 1901–
A century of public health in Britain, 1832–1929. London, *A. & C. Black*, 1932.

1659 FILBY, FREDERICK A.
A history of food adulteration and analysis. London, *Allen & Unwin*, 1934.

1660 NEWSHOLME, *Sir* ARTHUR. 1857–1943
Fifty years in public health: a personal narrative with comments. London, *George Allen & Unwin*, (1935).

1661 ——. The last thirty years in public health. London, *Allen & Unwin*, (1936).

1662 HIMES, NORMAN EDWIN. 1899–
Medical history of contraception. Baltimore, *Williams & Wilkins*, 1936.
Reprinted with updating preface, 1963.

1663 NEWMAN, *Sir* GEORGE. 1870–1948
The building of a nation's health. London, *Macmillan & Co.*, 1939.

1664 CANADIAN PUBLIC HEALTH ASSOCIATION.
The development of public health in Canada: a review of the history and organization of public health in the provinces of Canada, with an outline of the present organization of the National Health Section of the Department of Pensions and National Health, Canada. Edited by R. D. DEFRIES. Toronto, *Canad. Pub. Hlth. Assoc.*, (1940).

1665 REYNOLDS, REGINALD. 1905–
Cleanliness and godliness. London, *Allen & Unwin*, 1943.
Includes a history of the privy.

1666 WINSLOW, CHARLES-EDWARD AMORY. 1877–1957
The conquest of epidemic diseases. A chapter in the history of ideas. Princeton, *University Press*, 1943.

1667 ROBINS, FREDERICK WILLIAM.
The story of water supply. London, *Oxford University Press*, 1946.

1668 LEONARD, FRED EUGENE. 1866–1922
A guide to the history of physical education. 3rd edition, revised and enlarged by GEORGE AFFLECK. Philadelphia, *Lea & Febiger*, 1947.

1669 FERGUSON, THOMAS. 1900–
The dawn of Scottish social welfare. A survey from medieval times to 1863. London, *Nelson*, 1948.

1670 SAND, RENÉ. 1877–1953
Vers la médecine sociale. Paris, *J. B. Baillière*, 1948.
English translation, 1952.

1671 FRAZER, William Mowll. 1888–1958
A history of English public health, 1834–1939. London, *Baillière, Tindall & Cox*, 1950.

1671.1 WILLIAMS, Ralph Chester. 1888–
The United States public health service, 1798–1950. Washington, *Commissioned Officers Association of the United States Public Health Service*, 1951.

1671.2 BROCKINGTON, Colin Fraser. 1903–
A short history of public health. London, *Churchill*, 1956.
2nd edition, 1966.

1671.3 ROSEN, George. 1920–
A history of public health. New York, *MD Publications*, 1958.

1671.4 HENRIQUES, Louis Fernando. 1916–
Prostitution and society. A survey. 3 vols. London, *MacGibbon & Kee*, 1962–68.
Vol. 1: Primitive, classical and oriental. Vol. 2: Prostitution in Europe and the New World. Vol. 3: Modern sexuality.

1671.5 FINCH, Bernard Ephraim, & GREEN, Hugh.
Contraception through the ages. London, *Peter Owen*, 1963.

1672–1685 EPIDEMIOLOGY

See also 1767–1782.1, CLIMATIC & GEOGRAPHICAL FACTORS IN MEDICINE.

1672 HIPPOCRATES, 460–375 B.C.
Epidemics. *In*: *Hippocrates, with an English translation.* By W. H. S. Jones and E. T. Withington. London, *W. Heinemann*, 1923, **1,** 139–287.
Hippocrates introduced the inductive method of studying epidemics. Above is a Greek-English bilingual text; an English text will also be found in *Med. Classics*, 1938, **3**, 100–44.

1673 BAILLOU, Guillaume de [Ballonius]. 1538–1616
Epidemiorum et ephemeridum libri duo. Paris, *J. Quesnel*, 1640.
De Baillou was a follower of Hippocrates in his advancement of the doctrine of "epidemic constitutions". Crookshank regards him as the first modern epidemiologist.

1674 CLEGHORN, George. 1716–1789
Observations on the epidemical diseases in Minorca. From the year 1744 to 1749. London, *D. Wilson*, 1751.
Cleghorn left a good account of several diseases and conditions not previously observed, among them epidemic jaundice. He included in his book accounts of many post-mortems.

1675 HUXHAM, John. 1692–1768
Observationes de aëre et morbis epidemicis. 3 vols. Londini, *J. Hinton*, 1752–70.
Huxham made daily records of the weather and prevailing diseases; his aim was to establish a relationship between atmospheric conditions and disease. The work was first published in 1728; vol. 1 and 2 of the edition given above are second edition, which was rounded off by a third volume published posthumously. English translation of vol. 1–2, 1758–67.

1676 VILLALBA, JOAQUIN DE.
Epidemiologia española. 2 vols. Madrid, *M. Repullés*, 1802.
A chronological history of epidemics occurring in Spain to the end of the 17th century.

1677 HAESER, HEINRICH. 1811–1884
Bibliotheca epidemiographica. Jenae, *F. Mauke*, 1843.
A second edition was published in 1862.

1678 HECKER, JUSTUS FRIEDRICH KARL. 1795–1850
Die grossen Volkskrankheiten des Mittelalters. Historisch-pathologische Untersuchungen. Gesammelt und in erweiteter Bearbeitung hrsg. von A. HIRSCH. Berlin, *T. C. F. Enslin*, 1865.
A collection of essays on the black death, the dancing mania, and the English sweat, published 1832–34 and later in a collective English edition, *The epidemics of the Middle Ages*, 1837, with new editions in 1844 and 1854.

1679 HAESER, HEINRICH. 1811–1884
Geschichte der epidemischen Krankheiten. Jena, *H. Dufft*, 1882.
Forms vol. 3 of his *Lehrbuch der Geschichte der Medizin*, 3te. Aufl.

1680 CREIGHTON, CHARLES. 1847–1927
A history of epidemics in Britain. 2 vols. Cambridge, *University Press*, 1891–94.
The most important work on the subject and a classical contribution to modern epidemiology, of which Creighton may be said to have been the founder. Reprinted 1965.

1681 STICKER, GEORG. 1860–1960
Abhandlungen aus der Seuchengeschichte und Seuchenlehre. 2 vols. [in 3]. Giessen, *A. Töpelmann*, 1908–12.

1682 PRINZING, FRIEDRICH. 1859–
Epidemics resulting from wars. Edited by HARALD WESTERGAARD. Oxford, *Clarendon Press*, 1916.

1683 GREENWOOD, MAJOR. 1880–1949
Epidemiology, historical and experimental. Baltimore, *Johns Hopkins Press*, 1932.

1683.1 ——. Epidemics and crowd diseases; an introduction to the history of epidemiology. London, *Williams & Norgate*, 1935.

1684 MAJOR, RALPH HERMON. 1884–
War and disease. London, *Hutchinson*, (1943).

1685 WINSLOW, CHARLES-EDWARD AMORY. 1877–1957, *et al.*
The history of American epidemiology. St. Louis, *C. V. Mosby*, 1952.
With W. G. Smillie, J. A. Doull, J. E. Gordon, and F. H. Top.

1686–1716 STATISTICS

1686 GRAUNT, JOHN. 1620–1674
Natural and political observations mentioned in a following index, and made upon the Bills of Mortality. London, *T. Roycroft for J. Martin, J. Allestry and T. Dicas*, 1662.
The first book on vital statistics. Graunt, a draper, studied the Bills of Mortality, which began as weekly lists of deaths and their causes, and were compiled by parish clerks. They gained much in importance after Graunt's work, and in 1838 merged into the Registrar-General's returns. Graunt was a friend of Sir William Petty, and some authorities attribute the authorship of the above work to the latter.

1687 HALLEY, EDMUND. 1656–1742

An estimate of the degrees of mortality of mankind, drawn from curious tables of the births and funerals at the city of Breslaw, with an attempt to ascertain the price of annuities upon lives. *Phil. Trans.*, 1693, **17**, 596–610.

Halley, the astronomer, compiled the "Breslau tables" to show "the proportion of men able to bear arms . . . to estimate mortality rates, to ascertain the price of annuities upon lives, and was thus the virtual founder of vital statistics" (Garrison). The data on which Halley based his conclusions were supplied to him by Caspar Neumann, a pastor of Breslau.

1688 PETTY, *Sir* WILLIAM. 1623–1687

Several essays in political arithmetic. London, *Robert Clavel and Henry Mortlock*, 1699.

A pioneer statistician, Petty took the first census of Ireland. He was professor of anatomy at Oxford and later Graham professor of music.

1689 JURIN, JAMES. 1684–1750

A letter . . . containing, a comparison between the mortality of the natural small pox, and that given by inoculation. London, *W. & J. Innys*, 1723.

Jurin was an enthusiastic supporter of inoculation against smallpox and statistically proved its efficacy. During the last few months of his life he was President of the Royal College of Physicians of London.

1690 MOIVRE, ABRAHAM DE. 1667–1754

Annuities upon lives; or, the valuation of annuities upon any number of lives; as also, of reversions. To which is added, an appendix concerning the expectations of life and probabilities of survivorship. London, *F. Fayram, B. Motte, and W. Pearson*, 1725.

De Moivre, French Huguenot mathematician and demographer, formulated the hypothesis that among a body of persons over a certain age the successive annual decreases by death are nearly equal.

1691 SÜSSMILCH, JOHANN PETER. 1707–1767

Die göttliche Ordnung in denen Veränderungen des menschlichen Geschlechts. Berlin, *D. A. Gohl*, 1742.

Süssmilch, a German army chaplain, produced an important book on vital statistics. Among other things, he showed the necessity of a healthy and industrious population for the survival of a nation. His work was the most important until the time of Malthus.

1691.1 DEPARCIEUX, ANTOINE. 1703–1768

Essai sur les probabilités de la durée de la vie humaine: d'où l'on déduit la manière de déterminer les rentes viagères, tant simples qu'en tontines. Paris, *Guérin Frères*, 1746.

Deparcieux was the first to construct correct life tables. Appendix in 1760.

1692 SHORT, THOMAS. 1690?–1772

New observations, natural, moral, civil, political, and medical, on city, town, and country Bills of Mortality. London, *T. Longman & A. Millar*, 1750.

Original and suggestive work on vital statistics, showing vividly the changing conditions of life as he saw it (Greenwood).

1693 MALTHUS, Thomas Robert. 1766–1834
An essay on the principle of population, as it affects the future improvement of society. London, *J. Johnson*, 1798.

Malthus laid down the principle that populations increase in geometrical ratio, but that subsistence increases only in arithmetical ratio. He argued that a stage is reached where increase of populations must be limited by sheer want, and he advocated checks on population increase in order to reduce misery and want. His work suggested to Darwin and Wallace the idea of the "survival of the fittest" and had a profound influence on the decrease in size of families down to the present time. The book was at first published anonymously, but Malthus attached his name to the greatly altered edition of 1803.

1694 KING, Gregory. 1648–1712
Natural and political observations and conclusions upon the state and condition of England. *In*: Chalmers, G.: *An estimate of the comparative strength of Great Britain.* 2nd ed., London, *J. Stockdale*, 1802.

King attempted to estimate the population by statistical methods. The above paper was written in 1696 but not published until 1802, when it appeared as an appendix to Chalmers's books. As a statistician King surpassed Petty.

1695 DUVILLARD, E. E.
Analyse et tableaux de l'influence de la petite vérole sur la mortalité à chaque âge, et de celle qu'un préservatif tel que la vaccine peut avoir sur la population et la longevité. Paris, *Imprimerie Impériale*, 1806.

Duvillard showed statistically the effect of smallpox vaccination on the mortality rate.

1696 CASPER, Johann Ludwig. 1796–1864
Beiträge zur medizinischen Statistik und Staatsarzneikunde. 2 vols. Berlin, *F. Dümmler*, 1825–35.

1697 HAWKINS, Francis Bisset. 1796–1894
Elements of medical statistics. London, *Longman*, 1829.

First English book devoted specifically to medical statistics. Hawkins was instrumental in obtaining the insertion of a column for the names of diseases or other causes of deaths, in connexion with the first Act for the registration of births and deaths.

1698 LOUIS, Pierre Charles Alexandre. 1787–1872
Recherches sur les effets de la saignée dans quelques maladies inflammatoires, et sur l'action de l'émétique et des vésicatoires dans la pneumonie. Paris, *J. B. Baillière*, 1835.

Broussais's system of medicine, his "médecine physiologique", was refuted by Louis, who, by his introduction of statistical methods into medicine, exposed its fallacies. Besides his important work on tuberculosis, Louis was instrumental in establishing medicine as an exact science by the introduction of the numerical or statistical method. English translation, Boston, 1836.

1699 FARR, William. 1807–1883
Vital statistics. *In* McCulloch, J. R., *A statistical account of the British Empire*, 2nd ed. London, 1839, **2,** 521–90.

Ranks with Graunt's *Observations* as an original contribution to medical statistics. First edition, 1837.

1700 GAVARRET, Louis Denis Jules. 1809–1890
Principes généraux de statistique médicale. Paris, *Bechet jeune & Labé*, 1840.

In his work on medical statistics Gavarret improved and systematized the method of Louis and gave special consideration to therapeutic problems.

1701 KÖRÖSI, JOSEF VON. 1844–1906
Plan einer Mortalitäts-Statistik für Grossstädte. Wien, *C. Gerold*, 1873.

The modern methods of interpreting vital statistics of large cities were devised by von Körösi.

1702 RUMSEY, HENRY WYLDBORE. 1809–1876
Essays and papers on some fallacies of statistics concerning life and death, health and disease. London, *Smith, Elder & Co.*, 1875.

1703 FARR, WILLIAM. 1807–1883
Supplement to the thirty-fifth annual report of the Registrar-General of Births and Marriages in England. London, *Eyre & Spottiswoode*, 1875.

Includes statistical calculations of the effect on life expectation if certain preventible diseases were eliminated.

1704 ——. Vital statistics. London, *E. Stanford*, 1885.

Farr applied statistical methods to epidemiology and was the first mathematically to express the rise and fall of epidemic diseases, thus making possible the more accurate prediction of the occurrence of epidemics.

1705 BILLINGS, JOHN SHAW. 1838–1913
On vital and medical statistics. New York, *Trow*, 1889.

1706 PEARSON, KARL. 1857–1936
The chances of death and other studies in evolution. 2 vols. London, *E. Arnold*, 1897.

1707 DAVENPORT, CHARLES BENEDICT. 1866–1944
Statistical methods, with special reference to biological variation. New York, *J. Wiley & Sons*, 1899.

1709 GALTON, *Sir* FRANCIS. 1822–1911
Probability the foundation of eugenics. Oxford, *H. Frowde*, 1907.

1710 BERTILLON, JACQUES. 1851–1914
La dépopulation de la France. Paris, *F. Alcan*, 1911.

1711 PEARSON, KARL. 1857–1936
On the handicapping of the first-born. London, *Dulau & Co.*, 1914.

1712 PEARL, RAYMOND. 1879–1940, & REED, LOWELL JACOB. 1886–1966
On the rate of growth of the population of the United States since 1790 and its mathematical representation. *Proc. nat. Acad. Sci.* (*Wash.*), 1920, **6,** 275–88.

1713 CARR-SAUNDERS, *Sir* ALEXANDER MORRIS. 1886–
The population problem; a study in human evolution. Oxford, *Clarendon Press*, 1922.

1714 PEARL, RAYMOND. 1879–1940
The natural history of population. Oxford, *University Press*, 1939.

1715 WESTERGAARD, HARALD.
Contributions to the history of statistics. London, *P. S. King*, 1932.

1716 GREENWOOD, MAJOR. 1880–1949
Medical statistics from Graunt to Farr. Cambridge, *University Press*, 1948.
FitzPatrick Lectures, 1941 and 1943.

1717–1757 MEDICAL JURISPRUDENCE

See also 2069–2117, TOXICOLOGY.

1717 CONSTITUTIO CRIMINALIS CAROLINA. 1533
Kaiser Karl's des Fünften Peinliche Gerichtsordnung . . . Hrsg. von R. SCHMID. Jena, *A. Schmid*, 1835.
The Constitutio Criminalis of Charles V is probably the oldest European document of any importance dealing with medical jurisprudence. It authorized judges to call expert witnesses in medico-legal cases.

1718 CODRONCHI, GIOVANNI BATTISTA. 1547–1628
Methodus testificandi, inquibusvis casibus medicis oblatis. In his: *De vitiis vocis, libri duo*, Francofurti, *A. Wechel*, 1597, pp. 148–232.
First important work on forensic medicine.

1719 FIDELI, FORTUNATO. 1550–1630
De relationibus medicorum. Panormi, *apud I. A. de Franciscis*, 1602.

1720 ZACCHIAS, PAOLO. 1584–1659
Quaestiones medico-legales. 9 vols. Romae, Amstelaedami, 1621–61.
Zacchias, a Papal physician, was one of the founders of medical jurisprudence. His treatise includes information concerning injuries of the eye, etc., and contains section on the medico-legal aspects of insanity. The last two volumes were published in Amsterdam.

1721 SEBITZ, MELCHIOR [SEBIZIUS]. 1578–1674
De notis virginitatis. Lipsiae, 1630.
Details the methods of previous and contemporary writers concerning the determination of virginity.

1722 WELSCH, GOTTFRIED. 1618–1690
Rationale vulnerum lethalium judicium. Lipsiae, *sumpt. Ritzschianis*, 1660.

1723 GARMANN, CHRISTIAN FRIEDERICH. 1640–1708
De gemellis et partu numerosiore. Lipsiae, *typ. vid. H. Coleri*, 1667.
Medico-legal aspects of multiple births.

1724 SWAMMERDAM, JAN. 1637–1680
Tractatus physico-anatomico-medicus de respiratione usuque pulmonum. Lugduni Batavorum, *apud Danielem, Abraham. et Adrian. à Gaasbeeck*, 1667.
Swammerdam's earliest published work. In it he recorded his discovery that the lungs of newborn infants will float on water if respiration has taken place, an important medico-legal point.

1725 BLÉGNY, NICOLAS DE. 1652–1722
La doctrine des rapports de chirurgie, fondée sur les maximes d'usage et sur la disposition des nouvelles ordonnances. Lyon, *T. Amaubry*, 1684.
Medico-legal aspects of surgery. De Blégny was the first Frenchman to contribute anything of importance to forensic medicine.

1726 BOHN, Johann. 1640–1718
De renunciatione vulnerum, seu vulnerum lethalium examen. Lipsiae, *J. F. Gleditsch*, 1689.

1727 SCHREYER, Johann.
Erörterung und Erläuterung der Frage: Ob es ein gewiss Zeichen, wenn eines todten Kindes Lunge im Wasser untersincket, dass solches in Mutter-Leibe gestorben sey? Zu Rettung seiner Ehre in Druck befördert. Zeitz, *J. H. Ammersbachen*, 1690.

Swammerdam's discovery that the foetal lungs will float on water if respiration has taken place was first put to practical use by Schreyer, who thereby secured the acquittal of a girl accused of infanticide.

1728 VALENTINI, Michael Bernhard. 1657–1729
Corpus juris medico-legale. Francofurti ad M., *sumpt. J. A. Jungii*, 1722.

First systematic work on forensic medicine.

1729 ALBERTI, Michael. 1682–1757
Systema jurisprudentiae medicae. 6 vols. Halae, *imp. Orphanotrophei*, 1736–47.

A work covering the whole field of medical jurisprudence as then understood, and ranking in importance with the work of Valentini.

1730 LOUIS, Antoine. 1723–1792
Mémoire sur une question anatomique relative à la jurisprudence; dans lequel on établit les principes pour distinguer, à l'inspection d'un corps trouvé pendu, les signes du suicide d'avec ceux de l'assassinat. Paris, *P. G. Cavelier*, 1763.

Louis was a pioneer of French medical jurisprudence. Above is a classical discussion on the differential signs of murder and suicide in cases of hanging.

1731 ——. Mémoire contre la légitimité des naissances prétendues tardives. Paris, *P. G. Cavelier*, 1764.

An attempt to set the minimum and maximum time limits of duration of human pregnancy. Supplement published in 1764.

1732 HUNTER, William. 1718–1783
On the uncertainty of the signs of murder, in the case of bastard children. *Med. Obs. & Inqu.*, London, 1784, **6**, 266–90.

This essay on the signs of murder in illegitimate children is, in Garrison's view, the most important early contribution to forensic medicine by a British writer.

1733 FARR, Samuel. 1741–1795
Elements of medical jurisprudence. London, *T. Becket*, 1788.

First textbook in English on medical jurisprudence.

1734 FODÉRÉ, François Emmanuel. 1764–1835
Les lois éclairées par les sciences physiques, ou traité de médecine légale et hygiène publique. 3 vols. Paris, *chez Croullebois et chez Deterville*, an VII [1799].

This important publication was for many years the authoritative textbook on the subject in France.

1735 BECK, Theodoric Romeyn. 1791–1855
Elements of medical jurisprudence. 2 vols. Albany, *Websters & Skinners*, 1823.

First notable American text on forensic medicine.

1736 HEINROTH, JOHANN CHRISTIAN AUGUST. 1773–1843
System der psychisch-gerichtlichen Medizin. Leipzig, *C. H. F. Hartmann*, 1825.

Medico-legal aspects of insanity.

1737 GROSS, SAMUEL DAVID. 1805–1884
Observations on manual strangulation, illustrated by cases and experiments. *West. J. med. phys. Sci.*, 1836, **9**, 25–38.

1738 TAYLOR, ALFRED SWAINE. 1806–1880
Elements of medical jurisprudence. London, *Deacon*, 1836.

One of the best-known English texts on the subject; twelfth edition, *Principles and practice of medical jurisprudence*, appeared in 1965.

1739 RAY, ISAAC. 1807–1881
A treatise on the medical jurisprudence of insanity. London, *G. Henderson*, 1839.

First modern treatise on the medico-legal aspects of insanity.

1740 GUY, WILLIAM AUGUSTUS. 1810–1885
Principles of forensic medicine. London, *H. Renshaw*, 1844.

1741 CASPER, JOHANN LUDWIG. 1796–1864
Gerichtliche Leichenöffnungen. Berlin, *A. Hirschwald*, 1850.

Casper was a great authority on forensic medicine. He also wrote on medical statistics. Above is an important compilation on judicial post-mortems.

1742 HAMILTON, FRANK HASTINGS. 1813–1886
Deformities after fractures. *Trans. Amer. med. Ass.*, 1855, **8**, 347–443.

Hamilton was a medical inspector of the U. S. Army and later became Professor of Surgery at Bellevue Hospital.

1743 CASPER, JOHANN LUDWIG. 1796–1864
Practisches Handbuch der gerichtlichen Medicin. 2 vols. Berlin, *A. Hirschwald*, 1857–58.

Casper was the greatest name in forensic medicine in his time. His book was published in English by the New Sydenham Society in 1861–65; it was unsurpassed for many years.

1744 ——. Klinische Novellen zur gerichtlichen Medizin. Berlin, *A. Hirschwald*, 1863.

1745 TARDIEU, AUGUSTE AMBROISE. 1818–1879
Etude médico-légale et clinique sur l'empoisonnement. Paris, *J. B. Baillière*, 1867.

1746 DRAGENDORFF, GEORG JOHANN NOËL. 1836–1898
Die gerichtlich-chemische Ermittelung von Giften in Nahrungsmitteln, Luftgemischen, Speiseresten, Körpertheilen, *etc.* St. Petersburg, *H. Schmitzdorff*, 1868.

Dragendorff, professor of pharmacy at Dorpat, Marburg, and Vienna, contributed an important book on forensic chemistry. He was responsible for the introduction of several methods for the detection of poisons in the human body.

1747 ——. Beiträge zur gerichtlichen Chemie einzelner organischer Gifte. St. Petersburg, *H. Schmitzdorff*, 1872.

1748 KRAFFT-EBING, RICHARD VON. 1840–1902
Lehrbuch der gerichtlichen Psychopathologie. Stuttgart, *F. Enke*, 1875.

1749 HOFMANN, EDUARD VON, *Ritter*. 1837–1897
Lehrbuch der gerichtlichen Medicin. Wien, *Urban & Schwarzenberg*, 1877–78.

An important German work on the subject, Hofmann's book went through many editions and was translated into several European languages.

1750 MANN, JOHN DIXON. 1840–1912
Forensic medicine and toxicology. London, *C. Griffin & Co.*, 1893.

1751 BROUARDEL, PAUL CAMILLE HIPPOLYTE. 1837–1906
La mort et la mort subite. Paris, *J. B. Baillière*, 1895.

Brouardel was Professor of Forensic Medicine, Paris. He was to a great extent responsible for the development of that subject in France; he instituted courses of practical instruction at the Paris morgue, and wrote several monographs on forensic medicine.

1752 ——. L'infanticide. Paris, *J. B. Baillière*, 1897.

1753 ——. La pendaison, la strangulation, la suffocation, la submersion. Paris, *J. B. Baillière*, 1897.

1754 UHLENHUTH, PAUL THEODOR. 1870–1957
Eine Methode zur Unterscheidung der verschiedenen Blutarten, im besonderen zum differentialdiagnostischen Nachweise des Menschenblutes. *Dtsch. med. Wschr.*, 1901, **27**, 82–83, 260–61.

Uhlenhuth was the first to use precipitins in medico-legal tests for human blood.

1755 MERCIER, CHARLES ARTHUR. 1852–1919
Criminal responsibility. Oxford, *Clarendon Press*, 1905.

1756 OTTENBERG, REUBEN. 1882–
Medicolegal application of human blood grouping. *J. Amer. med. Ass.*, 1921, **77,** 682–83; 1922, **78,** 873–77; **79,** 2137–43.

An important series of papers on blood-grouping and the jurisprudence of paternity. Ottenberg performed the first matched-blood transfusion.

1757 McINDOE, *Sir* ARCHIBALD HECTOR. 1900–1960, & FRANCESCHETTI, ADOLPHE. 1896–
Reciprocal skin homografts in a medico-legal case of familial identification of exchanged identical twins. *Brit. J. plast. Surg.*, 1950, **2,** 283–89.

Skin grafting used to decide the relationship of identical twins who had been accidentally separated at birth.

1758–1766 MEDICAL ETHICS

1758 JONES, WILLIAM HENRY SAMUEL. 1876–1963
The doctor's oath, an essay in the history of medicine. Cambridge, *Univ. Press*, 1924.

The Hippocratic Oath forms the basis of medical ethics. It was probably an ancient temple oath of the Asclepiadae, and not a genuine Hippocratic document. In the above work the various manuscripts of the Oath are enumerated and critically discussed. A translation of the Oath of Hippocrates is also to be found in *Med. Classics*, 1938, **3**, facing p. 1.

1759 CASTRO, Rodericus a. 1546–1627
Medicus-politicus: sive de officiis medico-politicis tractatus. Hamburgi, *ex bibl. Frobeniano*, 1614.
One of the first "modern" works on medical ethics.

1760 HOERNIGK, Ludwig von. 1600–1667
Politia medica. Franckfurt a.M., *bey C. Schleichen u. Mitverwandten*, 1638.

1761 HARVEY, Gideon. 1640–?1700
The conclave of physicians, detecting their intrigues, frauds, and plots, against their patients. London, *J. Partridge*, 1683.

1762 FRITSCH, Ahasuerus. 1629–1701
Medicus peccans, sive tractatus de peccatis medicorum. Norimbergae, *apud W. M. Endterum*, 1684.

1763 BARD, Samuel. 1742–1821
A discourse upon the duties of a physician. New York, *A. & J. Robertson*, 1769.
Samuel Bard was one of the founders of King's College, New York.

1764 PERCIVAL, Thomas. 1740–1804
Medical ethics; or, a code of institutes and precepts, adapted to the professional conduct of physicians and surgeons. Manchester, *printed by S. Russell for J. Johnson and R. Bickerstaff, London*, 1803.
First published for private circulation, 1794. The British and American medical professions have adopted much of "Percival" in their ethical codes. An edition of the book published in 1927 was edited by C. D. Leake.

1765 BELL, John. 1763–1820
Letters on professional character and manners. Edinburgh, *J. Moir*, 1810.

1766 PAGEL, Julius Leopold. 1851–1897
Medicinische Deontologie. Berlin, *O. Coblentz*, 1897.

CLIMATIC & GEOGRAPHICAL FACTORS IN MEDICINE
1767–1782.1

1767 HIPPOCRATES, 460–275 b.c.
On airs, waters and places. *In his* Works, edited by W. H. S. Jones and E. T. Withington. London, 1923, **1**, 65–137.
English and Latin text. English text also in *Med. Classics*, 1938, **3**, 19–42. "The first book ever written on medical geography, climatology, and anthropology" (Garrison).

1768 ABDOLLATIF [Abu Muhammad Abdu'l-Latif]. 1162–1231
Historiae Aegypti compendium. Oxonii, *typ. Academicis*, 1800.
Arabic-Latin bilingual text. Abdollatif gave a good description of the fauna and flora of Egypt, its inhabitants and some of its diseases. He was the first writer, according to Hirsch, to dispute the accuracy of Galen. The first printed version of his work appeared in 1789 (Tübingen, Arabic text).

1769 CLERMONT, Charles [Claromontius].
De aere, locis, et aquis terrae Angliae; deque morbis Anglorum vernaculis. Londini, *T. Roycroft et J. Martyn*, 1672.
An outline of the medical topography of England.

1770 HILLARY, William. 1697–1763
Observations on the changes of the air and the concomitant epidemical diseases, in the Island of Barbados. London, *C. Hitch & L. Hawes*, 1759.
Hillary included good accounts of lead colic and infective hepatitis, and probably the first description of sprue.

1771 CASAL Y JULIAN, Caspar. 1679–1759
Historia natural, y medica de el Principado de Asturias. Madrid, *M. Martin*, 1762.
Includes the first clear description of pellagra. Casal wrote the book in 1735, but it was not published until 1762; a reprint was published in Oviedo in 1900.

1772 RUTTY, John. 1698–1775
A chronological history of the weather and seasons, and of the prevailing diseases in Dublin. London, *Robinson & Roberts*, 1770.
Rutty's book includes a description of relapsing fever.

1773 CHALMERS, Lionel. 1715–1777
An account of the weather and diseases of South-Carolina. 2 vols. London, *E. & C. Dilly*, 1776.
Originally published in the *Gentleman's Magazine*, 1751–54.

1774 FOTHERGILL, John. 1712–1780
Observations on the weather and diseases of London. In his *Works*. London, 1783, **1,** 145–240.

1775 CURRIE, William. 1754–1828
An historical account of the climates and diseases of the United States of America. Philadelphia, *T. Dobson*, 1792.

1776 FINKE, Leonhard Ludwig. 1747–1837
Versuch einer allgemeinen medicinisch-praktischen Geographie. 3. vols. Leipzig, *Weidmann*, 1792–95.

1777 DRAKE, Daniel. 1785–1852
A systematic treatise, historical, etiological, and practical, on the principal diseases of the interior valley of North America. 2 vols. Cincinnati, *W. B. Smith & Co.*, 1850–55.
This classical contribution to the social history of North America includes the most important work on the natural history of malaria published up to that time

1778 HIRSCH, August. 1817–1894
Handbuch der historisch-geographischen Pathologie. 2 vols. Erlangen, *F. Enke*, 1860–64.
This is perhaps the greatest work on the subject. An English translation by Charles Creighton in 3 vols. was published by the New Sydenham Society in 1883–86.

1779 LOMBARD, Henri Clermond. 1803–1895
Traité de climatologie médicale. 4 vols. and atlas. Paris, *J. B. Baillière*, 1877–80.

1780 McKINLEY, Earl Baldwin. 1894–1938
A geography of disease. Washington, *George Washington Univ. Press*, 1935.

Published as supplement to *Amer. J. trop. Med.*, 1935, **15,** No. 5.

1781 PETERSEN, William Ferdinand. 1887–
The patient and the weather. With the assistance of Margaret E. Milliken. 4 vols. [in 7]. Ann Arbor, *Edwards Bros.*, 1934–38.

1782 KÖPPEN, Wladimir Peter, & GEIGER, Rudolf.
Handbuch der Klimatologie. Vol. 1–5. Berlin, *Gebr. Bornträger*, 1930–38.

1782.1 BARKHUS, Arne.
Medical geographies. *Ciba Symp.*, 1945, **6,** 1997–2016.

A historical survey of the classical works.

1783–1958 MATERIA MEDICA: PHARMACY PHARMACOLOGY

For drugs with specific action, see under the diseases concerned

1783 THEOPHRASTUS *of Eresos.* 380–286 B.C.
De historia plantarum. [Treviso], (*imp. B. Confalonerium de Salodio*, 1483).

Theophrastus was a pupil of Aristotle and inherited the latter's library. His work is important as probably representing the teaching of Aristotle, who left no botanical works. Part of the book is devoted to plant-lore and the gathering of drugs for medicinal purposes. Theophrastus collated and systematized the existing botanical knowledge and described about 500 plants. Aldus printed a Greek edition of the book in 1497, and a Greek-English bilingual edition appeared in the *Loeb Classics* series in 1916, in 2 vols., edited by Sir A. Hort.

1784 KRATEUAS [Cratevas]. *fl.* 100 B.C.
[Singer, C.: Drawings illustrating the Rhizotomikon from the Julia Aniciana Codex, A.D. 512]. *J. Hellen. Stud.*, 1927, **47,** 8–17.

Only fragments of the works of Krateuas have come down to us, second-hand, through the writings of others, particularly Dioscorides. The MS of Dioscorides known as the *Codex Aniciae Julianae* contained some of the drawings of Krateuas, and these have been reproduced in Singer's paper.

1785 SCRIBONIUS LARGUS. *fl.* A.D. 40
De compositionibus medicamentorum liber unus. Parisiis, *ap. C. Wechel*, 1528.

First written in A.D. 47. This is an important compilation of drugs and prescriptions. Among other things, it records the drinking of one's own blood as a therapeutic rite. Scribonius was the first to describe accurately the preparation of true opium. G. Helmreich edited a Latin edition of the book, published in 1887, while a German version by W. Schonack appeared in 1913.

1786 DIOSCORIDES, Pedanius, *Anazarbeus. fl.* A.D. 54–68
De materia medica. Edidit Max Wellmann. 3 vols. Berolini, *Weidmann*, 1906–14.

Dioscorides was the originator of the materia medica; his work is the authoritative source on the materia medica of antiquity. He described over 600 plants and plant principles. His work was first printed in Greek by Aldus Manutius in 1499; the first Latin translation was published in 1478. John Goodyer made an English translation between 1652–55, which remained in manuscript form until 1934, when R. T. Gunther edited and published it—the first English edition of the Great Herbal. The above also contains the *Fragmenta* of Krateuas.

1787 THOMPSON, Reginald Campbell. 1876–1941
The Assyrian herbal. London, *Luzac & Co.*, 1924.

A study of ancient Assyrian medical drugs.

1788 ABU MANSUR MUWAFFAK BIN ALI HARAWI. *fl.* 970
Liber fundamentorum pharmacologiae . . . Primus Latio donavit R. Seligmann. 2 pts. Vindobonae, *Antonius Nob. de Schmid*, 1830–1833.

The most important Persian pharmacological work. It was written about A.D. 970. The above epitome is taken from a MS of 1055; a German version appeared in 1893 under the direction of R. Kobert.

1789 NICOLAUS *Salernitanus.* *fl.* 1140
Antidotarium. Venetiis, *N. Jensen*, 1471.

This work, which first appeared in 1140, was the first formulary to be printed. It consists of 139 prescriptions and includes the original formula for the "anaesthetic sponge" (spongia somnifera), the earliest sources of which are MSS of the 8th century, and a table of weights and measures which formed the basis of the modern grain, scruple, drachm, etc. The book must have been of great contemporary value, as it was one of the first medical works to be printed.

1790 PLATEARIUS, Matthaeus. *fl.* 1130–1150
De simplici medicina seu Circa instans. *In* Nicolaus Praepositus, *Dispensarium*, Lugduni, 1537, ff. 70–96.

The original of the first French herbal, this derived from Dioscorides and first appeared about 1140. A French translation was published by P. Dorveaux in 1913.

1791 MACER, Aemilius. *circa* 70–16 B.C.
De naturis qualitatibus et virtutibus octuaginta octo herbarum Neapoli, *imp. per Arnoldum de Bruxella*, 1477.

Macer Floridus, a poem describing the virtues of 88 simples. It was written in the 12th century and is ascribed variously to Aemilius Macer, Hugo of Tours, and to Odo of Meudon. It was the original of the earliest known Scandinavian medical writing, the *Laegebog* of Henrik Harpestreng. Many editions and translations are available.

1792 ALBERTUS MAGNUS [Albert von Bollstädt]. 1193–1280
De vegetabilibus libri vii. Berolini, *G. Reimeri*, 1867.

One of Albertus' most important publications and the best work on natural history produced during the Middle Ages. It was written about 1250, and is based on his own accurate botanical observations, containing also some therapeutic material. C. Jessen edited the above edition.

1793 NICOLAUS *Myrepsus.* *circa* 1280
Medicamentorum opus. Basileae, *apud I. Oporinum*, 1549.

The "Antidotarium magnum" of Nicolaus Myrepsus. It was the largest strictly pharmaceutical work that had appeared (it was written about 1270–1280) and contained more than 2,500 formulae. The above is a Latin translation by Leonhart Fuchs.

1794 ORTOLFF VON BAYRLANT. *circa* 1400
Artzneibuch. [Augsburg, ?*G. Zainer*], 1477.

First German pharmacopoeia. Ortolff was a physician in Würzburg. The book was an important German text of popular medicine in its day. See also Hain 12111

1795 HERBARIUS MOGUNTINUS
Herbarius Moguntie impressus. Mainz, *P. Schoeffer*, 1484.

First printed herbal with illustrations.

1796 HERBAL.

Herbarius zu Teutsch. [Mainz, *P. Schoeffer*, 1485].

One of the fundamental botanical works. It was probably compiled by Johann von Caub and contains some good illustrations, together with some very fanciful pictures of animals. (See also No. 95). Reproduced in facsimile, Munich, 1924.

1797 HORTUS SANITATIS.

Ortus sanitatis. Moguntiae, *J. Meydenbach*, 1491.

In part based on the German *Ortus sanitatis*, but dealing at greater length with many herbs. It is one of the most important of the early herbals. See also No. 96). Available in facsimile in W. L. Schreiber's *Die Kräuterbücher des XV. and XVI. Jahrhunderts*, Munich, 1924. An English translation of *c.* 1521 (S.T.C. 22367) was reprinted London, *Quaritsch*, 1954, edited by N. Hudson.

1798 LEONICENO, Niccolo. 1428–1524

De Plinii et plurium aliorum in medicina erroribus. (Ferrara, *L. de Valentia et A. de Castronovo*, 1492.)

A correction of the botanical errors of Pliny. Remembering the times in which Leoniceno lived, Garrison considers this work "a feat of the rarest intellectual courage." It was accepted by later botanists and thus made possible scientific description of the materia medica.

1799 BANCKES' HERBAL.

Here begynnyth a new mater, the whiche sheweth and treateth of ye vertues & proprytes of herbes, the whiche is called an Herball. London, *Rycharde Banckes*, 1525.

Earliest English printed herbal. Published anonymously, it is usually referred to as "Banckes' Herbal". Only two copies are known. Reproduced with modern transcription, New York, 1941.

1800 OVIEDO Y VALDÉS, *Don* Gonçalo Fernández de. 1478–1557

Sumaria de la historia natural de las Indias. Toledo, *R. de Petras*, 1525.

First known description of the medicinal plants of Central America. Oviedo first described *chigoe* ("jiggers"?) in this book. A 3-volume edition was published at Madrid in 1851–53.

1801 GRAND HERBIER.

Le grand herbier en Francoys: contenant les qualitez, vertus et proprietez des herbes, arbres, gommes, *etc.* Paris, *Pierre Sergent*, [before 1526].

The "Grand Herbier" or "Arbolayre" was probably derived from Platearius (No. 1790). It is not dated, but the "Grete Herbal" (No. 1802) is a translation of it.

1802 GREAT HERBAL.

The grete herball whiche geveth parfyt knowlege and understandyng of all maner of herbes and there gracyous vertues. Southwarke, *P. Treveris*, 1526.

First illustrated English herbal. It is mainly a translation of the French "Grand Herbier".

1803 BRUNFELS, Otto. 1488–1534

Herbarum vivae eicones. 3 vols. Argentorati, *apud I. Schottum*, 1530–40.

Brunfels was first in time and importance among the German botanists of the 16th century. For the illustrations in this work he went direct to nature instead of to the earlier writers. The result was a new standard in botanical illustration and a book on the subject which relied wholly on personal observation. The drawings were by Hans Weiditz.

1804 BRASAVOLA, Antonio Musa. 1500–1555
Examen omnium simplicium medicamentorum, quorum in officinis usus est. (Romae, *A. B. de Asula*), 1536.

Brasavola introduced some new drugs into the pharmacopoeia. The book is written in the form of a dialogue.

1805 TURNER, William. 1510–1568
Libellus de re herbaria novus. Londini, *apud Ioannem Byddellum*, 1538.

Turner, the "Father of English Botany", treated plants as simples, and did not attempt to show their relationships. He was a much travelled man and a friend of Conrad Gesner. He introduced lucerne into England. Reproduced in facsimile, London, 1877.

1806 TRAGUS, Hieronymus [Bock (Jerome)]. 1498–1554
New Kreütter Bůch. Strassburg, *W. Rihel*, 1539.

Although his figures are not as good as those of Brunfels, Bock escaped some of his errors. His work gave a fresh impetus to plant description, which had languished since the time of Theophrastus.

1807 GESNER, Conrad. 1516–1565
Historiae plantarum et vires ex Dioscoride, Paulo Aegineta, *etc.* Parisiis, *apud Ioannem Lodoicum Tiletanum*, 1541.

A pocket dictionary of plants. Gesner, the "German Pliny", is remarkable for his encyclopaedic bibliographies. He attempted a *Historia plantarum*, which was unfinished at his death.

1808 FUCHS, Leonhart. 1501–1566
De historia stirpium commentarii. Basileae, *in off. Isingriniana*, 1542.

The most famous herbal of the 16th century. Besides its accurate and detailed account of medical plants, it contains over 500 fine woodcuts, some of which are of interest as being the first European figures of certain American plants. A Flemish edition of the book, 1543, contains woodcuts of such excellence that many prefer it to the earlier edition. The name of Fuchs is preserved in the American "fuchsias".

1809 GESNER, Conrad. 1516–1565
Enumeratio medicamentorum purgantium. Basileae, *per H. Frobenium*, 1543.

An index of purgatives.

1810 CORDUS, Valerius. 1515–1544
Pharmacorum omnium, quae quidem in usu sunt, conficiendorum ratio, vulgo vocant dispensatorium pharmacopolarum. Norimbergae, *apud J. Petreium*, 1546.

The first real pharmacopoeia to be published. It was recognized as the official pharmacopoeia of Nuremberg. A facsimile was published under the direction of L. Winkler in 1934.

1811 TURNER, William. 1510–1568
A new herball. 3 pts. London, *S. Mierdman*; Collen, *A. Birckman*, 1551–68.

Turner's great herbal was the only original English herbal written in the sixteenth century, and was the most profusely illustrated. Parts 2 and 3 were produced in 1562 and 1568, while Turner was an exile in Germany.

1812 DODOENS, Rembert [Dodonaeus]. 1517–1585
Crŭÿdeboeck. Tantwerpen, *Jan van der Loe*, 1554.

Dodoens was the first Belgian botanist of international repute. Many of the blocks used to illustrate the above work were borrowed from Fuchs.

1813 ANGUILLARA, Luigi. *circa* 1512–1570
Semplici dell'eccellente . . . liquali in piu pareri à diversi nobili huomini scritti appaiono, et nuovamente da G. Marinello mandati in luce. Vinegia, *V. Valgrisi*, 1561.

Anguillara was one of the best of many commentators of Dioscorides.

1814 CORDUS, Valerius. 1551–1544
Annotationes in Pedacii Dioscoridis Anazarbei de medica materia. Argentorati, *excud. I. Rihelius*, 1561.

This work not only modernises the species listed by Dioscorides, but in addition lists about 500 new species of plants. Published posthumously, the work was carefully edited by Conrad Gesner. Cordus was the inventor of phytography and the discoverer of ethyl (sulphuric) ether.

1815 GARCIA D'ORTA. 1501–1568
Coloquios dos simples, e drogas he cousas mediçinais da India. Goa, *Joannes*, 1563.

The first account of Indian materia medica and the first text-book on tropical medicine written by a European. It includes a classical account of cholera. It is the third book printed in India and is almost priceless. For an account of its author, see L. H. Roddis, *Ann. med. Hist.*, 1929, **1**, 198–207. English translation by Sir Clements R. Markham, London, 1913.

1816 OCCO, Adolph. 1524–1606
Enchiridion, sive ut vulgo vocant dispensatorium, compositorum medicamentorum, pro Reipub. Augstburgensis pharmacopoeis. [Augsburg, 1564].

One of the earliest pharmacopoeias, and one which exerted a great influence on later pharmacopoeias. Several new editions followed the first, and that of 1613 was adopted as the official pharmacopoeia of Augsburg, the famous *Pharmacopoeia Augustana*. Occo, the third of a famous medical family, was town physician of Augsburg. The book has been reprinted in facsimile, with notes, by the State Historical Society of Wisconsin, 1927, and is edited by T. Husemann.

1817 MONARDES, Nicolas. 1493–1588
Dos libros. El uno trata de todas las cosas que traen nuestras Indias Occidentales, *etc.* Sevilla, *S. Trugillo*, 1565.

First treatise on Central American drugs, and for many years the most important work on the medicinal plants of the New World. A second part to the book appeared in 1571, and a third, together with the first two, in 1574. English translation by John Frampton: *Joyfull newes out of the newe found world*, 1577 (reprinted 1925).

1818 BOMBASTUS AB HOHENHEIM, Aurelius Philippus Theophrastus [Paracelsus]. 1493–1541
Septem libri de gradibus, de compositionibus, de dosibus receptorum ac naturalium. Basileae, *P. Perna*, 1568.

Paracelsus has been called by some "the pioneer of modern chemists" and by others "uncouth, boorish, vain, ignorant and pretentious". His *De gradibus* contains most of his innovations in chemical therapeutics. A definitive edition of the works of Paracelsus was published by K. Sudhoff.

1819 ACOSTA, Cristóvão. ?1515–1580 or 1594
Tractado delas drogas, y medicinas de las Indias Orientales, con sus plantas. Burgos, *M. de Victoria*, 1578.

In the main this is a translation of Garcia d'Orta's *Coloquios*, with the addition of some illustrations. Acosta travelled to India, where he met Garcia d'Orta.

1820 GERARDE, JOHN. 1545–1612
The herball or generall historie of plantes. London (*E. Bollifant for B.* and *J. Norton*), 1597.

Gerarde is perhaps the best remembered of all the English herbalists. The most important edition of his book is the second, published by T. Johnson in 1633. Johnson greatly enlarged the book, correcting many mistakes and bringing the number of plants included to a total of 2850. Osler (*Bibliotheca*, No. 2722) states that Gerarde used for this work a translation of Dodoens (see No. 1812) without acknowledgement. See also the statement to this effect in A. Arber, *Herbals*, 2nd ed., 1938, p. 129.

1821 PHARMACOPOEIA.
Pharmacopoeia Londinensis. London, *E. Griffin for J. Marriott*, 1618.

The first London pharmacopoeia, issued by the (Royal) College of Physicians. The first edition was published on May 7, but contained many typographical errors; a corrected edition appeared on December 7, 1618. In the first issue the name of the publisher is printed "Marriot". Facsimile reprint of both versions, with introduction by G. Urdang, Madison, 1944.

1822 PARKINSON, JOHN. 1567–1650
Paradisi in sole paradisus terrestris or a garden of flowers with a kitchen garden and an orchard. London, *H. Lownes and R. Young*, 1629.

The title is a pun on the author's name (park-in-sun).

1823 ——. Theatrum botanicum: The theater of plants. Or, an herball of a large extent. London, *T. Cotes*, 1640.

Parkinson, the last of the old English herbalists, was Apothecary to James I. His massive herbal of 1,755 pages describes nearly 3,800 plants and is one of the pillars of English botany.

1824 PHARMACOPOEIA.
Codex medicamentarius seu pharmacopoeia Parisiensis. Lutetiae Parisiorum, *sumpt. Olivarii de Varennes*, 1639.

First Paris pharmacopoeia.

1825 PISO, WILLEM [LE POIS, (GUILLAUME)]. 1611–1678
De Indiae utriusque re naturali et medica libri quatuordecim. Amstelaedami, *apud L. et D. Elzevirios*, 1658.

Piso introduced ipecacuanha into Europe. Reproduced in part, with translation, in *Opuscula Selecta Neerlandicorum de Arte Medica*, 1937, No. 14.

1826 BADO, SEBASTIANO [BALDI]. *fl.* 1640–1676
Anastasis corticis Peruviae, seu chinae defensio. Genuae, *typ. P. I. Calenzani*, 1663.

A defence of the virtues of Peruvian bark. Bado includes evidence to show that "fever bark" was introduced into Spain in 1632.

1827 WELSCH, GOTTFRIED. 1618–1690
De medicis et medicamentis Germanorum. Lipsiae, 1688.

1828 RIVINUS, AUGUSTUS QUIRINUS. 1652–1723
Censura medicamentorum officinalium. Lipsiae, *J. Fritsch*, 1701.

A list of officially recognized drugs, with a classification of useless and undesirable ones. Rivinus also noted incompatibles.

1829 LINNÉ, CARL VON [LINNAEUS]. 1707–1778
Genera plantarum. Lugduni Batavorum, *apud Conradum Wishoff*, 1737.

Linnaeus's botanical classification, the starting-point of modern systematic botany. The book is dedicated to Boerhaave. English translation, 1771.

1830 GAUB, HIERONYMUS DAVID. 1705–1780
Libellus de methodo concinnandi formulas medicamentorum. Lugduni Batavorum, *C. Wishoff*, 1739.
A treatise on prescriptions. Gaub was professor of chemistry at Leyden.

1831 HEBERDEN, WILLIAM, *Snr.* 1710–1801
Αντìθηρìακά; an essay on mithridatium and theriaka. [London], 1745.
Heberden's first printed work. His criticism of current superstitions concerning these two concoctions resulted ultimately in their removal from the pharmacopoeia.

1832 BARTRAM, JOHN. 1699–1777
Descriptions, virtues, and uses of sundry plants of these northern parts of America. [Philadelphia], 1751.
Bartram founded the first botanical garden in America (at Kingsessing). Linnaeus refers to him as the "greatest natural botanist in the world".

1833 HALLER, ALBRECHT VON. 1708–1777
Bibliotheca botanica. 2 vols. Tiguri, *apud Orell, Gessner, Fuessli, et socc.*, 1771–72.
This was the first of the several bibliographies compiled by Haller, one of the greatest figures in the history of medicine. The work contains the most exhaustive and thorough information of the writings in the field of botany then extant. Choulant considered that the bibliographies on botany and anatomy were the best of Haller's works.

1834 BROWN, WILLIAM. 1752–1792
Pharmacopoeia simpliciorum et efficaciorum. Philadelphiae, *ex off. Styner & Cist*, 1778.
First pharmacopoeia published in the U.S.A. Reproduced in facsimile, with translation, in *The Badger Pharmacist*, 1938. No. 22–25.

1835 PERCIVAL, THOMAS. 1740–1804
Observations on the medical uses of the oleum jecoris aselli, or cod liver oil, in the chronic rheumatism, and other painful disorders. *Lond. med. J.*, 1782, **3**, 392–401.
First record of the clinical use of cod-liver oil in England.

1836 WITHERING, WILLIAM. 1741–1799
An account of the foxglove, and some of its medical uses. Birmingham, *G. G. J. & J. Robinson*, 1785.
Withering practised near Birmingham. He learned that digitalis was good for dropsy and began trying it on heart disease. By 1783 it was introduced into the Edinburgh pharmacopoeia. Withering was one of the greatest medical botanists and his book is a pharmacological classic. Before his time digitalis was occasionally mentioned in the literature. but it was due to him that its action in dropsy and on the heart became generally recognized. He did not know of the distinction between renal and cardiac dropsy. Facsimile reprint, London, 1949.

1837 SCHOEPFF, JOHANN DAVID. 1752–1800
Materia medica Americana, potissimum regni vegetabilis. Erlangae, *J. J. Palmii*, 1787.
Schoepff went as an army surgeon to America with the British Forces in 1777. He returned to Germany in 1784 and compiled his comprehensive work on the American materia medica.

1838 CULLEN, WILLIAM. 1710–1790
A treatise of the materia medica. 2 vols. Edinburgh, *C. Elliot*, 1789.
An expansion of Cullen's "Lectures on materia medica".

1838.1 DEROSNE, Charles Louis. 1780–1846
Sur l'opium. *Ann. Chim.*, 1802, **45,** 257–85.
Isolation of alkaloids from opium.

1839 SERTÜRNER, Friedrich Wilhelm Adam. 1783–1841
Darstellung der reinen Mohnsäure (Opiumsäure); nebst einer chemischen Untersuchung des Opiums, mit vorzüglicher Hinsicht auf einen darin neu entdeckten Stoff. *J. Pharm.* (*Lpz.*), 1806, **14,** 47–93.
Isolation of morphine.

1840 GOMES, Bernardino Antonio. 1769–1823
Ensaio sobre o cinchonino, e sobre sua influencia em a virtude da quina, e de outras cascas. *Mem. Acad. reale Sci. Lisboa*, 1810, **3,** 202–217.
Gomes obtained a substance, which he named *cinchonino*, from cinchona bark. That it contained the active principle of cinchona was later proved by Pelletier and Caventou. For an English translation of the paper, see *Edinb. med. surg. J.*, 1811, 7, 420–31.

1841 BARTON, William Paul Crillon. 1786–1856
Vegetable materia medica of the United States. 2 vols. Philadelphia, *M. Carey & Son*, 1817–18.
Barton served as a naval surgeon and, in 1815, became professor of botany at Philadelphia.

1842 BIGELOW, Jacob. 1786–1879
American medical botany. 3 vols. Boston, *Cummings & Hilliard*, 1817–20.
Bigelow, one of America's greatest botanists, was professor of materia medica at Harvard.

1843 PELLETIER, Pierre Joseph. 1788–1842, & MAGENDIE, François. 1783–1855
Recherches chimiques et physiologiques sur l'ipécacuanha. *Ann. Chim. Phys.*, (*Paris*), 1817, **4,** 172–85.
Isolation of emetine.

1844 ——& CAVENTOU, Joseph Bienaimé. 1795–1877
Mémoire sur un nouvel alcali végétal (la strychnine) trouvé dans la fève de Saint-Ignace, la noix vomique, *etc.* *J. Pharm.* (*Paris*), 1819, **5,** 145–174.
Isolation of strychnine.

1845 PHARMACOPOEIA.
Pharmacopoeia of the United States of America. Boston, *C. Ewer*, 1820.
First official U.S. pharmacopoeia.

1846 MAGENDIE, François. 1783–1855
Formulaire pour la préparation et l'emploi de plusieurs nouveaux médicamens, tels que la noix vomique, la morphine, *etc.* Paris, *Méquignon-Marvis*, 1822.
Magendie was the pioneer of experimental physiology in France. His *Formulaire* introduced into medical practice several of the newly discovered alkaloids, notably morphine, veratrine, brucine, piperine, emetine, as well as quinine and strychnine. An English translation of this book appeared in 1824.

1847 SCHENK, JOHANN HEINRICH.
Erfahrungen über die grossen Heilkräfte des Leberthrans gegen chronische Rheumatismen und besonders gegen das Hüft- und Lendenweh. *J. pract. Heilk.*, 1822, **55,** 6 St., 31–58; 1826, **62,** 3 St., 3–40.
Schenk's account of his experience with cod-liver oil led to its general use on the continent of Europe. Author's name incorrectly given as Scherer in original.

1848 SÉRULLAS, GEORGES SIMON. 1774–1832
Mémoire sur l'iodure de potassium, l'acide hydriodique et sur un composé nouveau de carbone, d'iode et d'hydrogène. *Ann. Chim. Phys.*, 1822, 2 sér., **20,** 163–68.
Iodoform discovered.

1849 RAFINESQUE, CONSTANTIN SAMUEL. 1783–1840
Medical flora. 2 vols. Philadelphia, *Atkinson, etc.*, 1828–30.
Rafinesque was a great botanist, conchologist, archaeologist and economist. He died in extreme poverty in Philadelphia and, but for the intervention of a few friends, his body would have been sold for dissection purposes.

1849.1 LUGOL, JEAN GUILLAUME AUGUST. 1786–1851
Mémoire sur l'emploi de l'iode dans les maladies scrofuleuses. Paris, *Baillière*, 1829.
Lugol's solution.

1850 GUTHRIE, SAMUEL. 1782–1848
New mode of preparing a spirituous solution of chloric ether. *Amer. J. Sci. Arts*, 1832, **21,** 64–65; **22,** 105–06.
Guthrie, Liebig and Soubeiran discovered chloroform independently of one another. Guthrie discovered the modern method of making chloroform by distilling alcohol with chlorinated lime. Second paper has title: On pure chloric ether.

1851 SOUBEIRAN, EUGÈNE. 1793–1858
Recherches sur quelques combinaisons du chlore. *Ann. Chim. (Paris)*, 1831, 2 sér., **48,** 113–57.
Soubeiran, like Liebig and Guthrie, discovered chloroform; it is difficult to determine who was first, as each may have allowed an interval of time to elapse between discovery and publication.

1852 LIEBIG, JUSTUS VON. 1803–1873
Ueber die Verbindungen, welche durch die Einwirkung des Chlors auf Alkohol, Aether, ölbildenes Gas und Essiggeist entstehen. *Ann. Pharm. (Heidelberg)*, 1832, **1,** 182–230.
Discovery, in 1831, of chloroform and chloral. Independently chloroform was discovered by Soubeiran and by Guthrie.

1853 ROBIQUET, PIERRE JEAN. 1780–1840
Nouvelles observations sur les principaux produits de l'opium. *Ann. Chim. (Paris)*, 1832, 2 sér., **51,** 225–67.
Isolation of codeine.

1854 GEIGER, PHILIPP LORENZ. 1785–1836, & HESSE, HERMANN.
Darstellung des Atropins. *Ann. Pharm. (Heidelberg)*, 1833, **5,** 43–81; **6,** 44–65.
Isolation of atropine.

1855 RUNGE, FRIEDLIEB FERDINAND. 1795–1867
Ueber einige Producte der Steinkohlendestillation. *Ann. Phys. Chem. (Lpz.)*, 1834, **31,** 65–77, 513–24; **32,** 308–32.
Carbolic acid first prepared from coal-tar.

1856 PEREIRA, JONATHAN. 1804–1853
The elements of materia medica. 2 vols. London, *Longman*, 1839–40.
The first great English work on the subject. Pereira was Professor of Materia Medica at the School of Pharmacy set up by the Pharmaceutical Society of Great Britain.

1857 PIRIA, RAFFAELE. 1815–1865
Recherches sur la salicine et les produits qui en dérivent. *C. R. Acad. Sci. (Paris)*, 1839, **8,** 479–85.
Isolation of salicin.

1858 BENNETT, JOHN HUGHES. 1812–1875
Treatise on the oleum jecoris aselli, or cod liver oil. Edinburgh, *Maclachlan, Stewart & Co.*, 1841.
Bennett visited Paris and Germany, and learned there of the beneficial effects of cod-liver oil. His book drew the attention of English medical men to the value of the oil. He also discovered bromine.

1859 BALARD, ANTOINE JÉROME. 1802–1876
Mémoire sur l'alcool amylique. *C. R. Acad. Sci. (Paris)*, 1844, **19,** 634–41.
Discovery of amyl nitrite.

1860 HOMOLLE, AUGUSTIN EUGENE. 1808–1875
Mémoire sur la digitale pourprée. *J. Pharm. Chim.*, 1845, 3me. sér., **7,** 57–83.
Isolation of an active principle in digitalis, amorphous digitalin, more potent than the plant itself.

1861 MERCK, GEORG FRANZ. 1825–1873
Vorläufige Notiz über eine neue organische Base im Opium. *Ann. Phys. Chem. (Lpz.)*, 1848, **66,** 125–28.
Isolation of papaverine.

1861.1 GERLAND, H.
New formation of salicylic acid. *J. chem. Soc.*, 1852, **5,** 133–35.
Synthesis of salicylic acid.

1862 PORCHER, FRANCIS PEYRE. 1825–1895
The medicinal, poisonous and dietetic properties of the cryptogamic plants of the United States. New York, *Baker, Godwin & Co.*, 1854.

1862.1 BUCHHEIM, RUDOLF. 1820–1879
Lehrbuch der Arzneimittellehre. Leipzig, *L. Voss*, 1856.
Buchheim was the most important of the early teachers of pharmacology.

1863 BERNARD, CLAUDE. 1813–1878
Leçons sur les effets des substances toxiques et médicamenteuses. Paris, *J. B. Baillière*, 1857.

1864 LEMAIRE, FRANÇOIS JULES. 1814–?
Du coaltar saponiné, désinfectant énergique. Paris, *Germer-Baillière*, 1860.
Lemaire was first to point out the antiseptic properties of carbolic acid.

1865 NIEMANN, ALBERT. 1834–1861
Ueber eine neue organische Base in den Cocablättern. Göttingen, *E. A. Huth*, 1860.
Isolation of cocaine, 1859, from the coca leaf, brought from Peru by Scherzer.

1866 PHARMACOPOEIA.
British Pharmacopoeia, published pursuant to the Medical Act, 1858 London, *General Medical Council*, 1864.
First official British pharmacopoeia.

1866.1 FRASER, *Sir* THOMAS RICHARD. 1841–1919
On the physiological action of the Calabar bean (Physostigma venenosum, *Balf.*). *Trans. roy. Soc. Edinb.* (1866), 1867, **24,** 715–88.
Isolation of eserine (physostigmine).

1867 BROWN, ALEXANDER CRUM. 1838–1922, & FRASER, *Sir* THOMAS RICHARD. 1841–1919
On the connection between chemical constitution and physiological action. *Trans. roy. Soc. Edinb.*, 1868–69, **25,** 151–203, 693–739.
Brown and Fraser were the first to investigate the relationship between the chemical constitution of substances and their action upon the body.

1868 MORÉNO Y MAÏZ, THOMAS.
Recherches chimiques et physiologiques sur l'Erythroxylum coca du Pérou et la cocaïne. Paris, *L. Leclerc*, 1868.
This, the first study of the pharmacological action of cocaine, contains the earliest suggestion of its use as a local anaesthetic.

1869 LIEBREICH, OSCAR. 1839–1908
Das Chloral, ein neues Hypnoticum. *Arch. dtsch. Ges. Psychiat.*, 1869, **16,** 237.
Demonstration of the value of chloral hydrate as a hypnotic. See also his monograph *Das Chloralhydrat*, Berlin, 1869.

1869.1 SCHMIEDEBERG, JOHANN ERNST OSWALD. 1838–1921
Untersuchungen über die pharmakologisch wirksamen Bestandtheile der Digitalis purpurea *L.* *Arch. exp. Path. Pharmak.*, 1875, **3,** 16–43.
Schmiedeberg isolated digitoxin from digitalis.

1870 BENTLEY, ROBERT. 1825–1893, & TRIMEN, HENRY. 1843–1896
Medicinal plants, being descriptions with original figures of the principal plants employed in medicine. 4 vols. London, *J. & A. Churchill*, 1880.

1871 ANREP, VASILI KONSTANTINOVICH. 1852–1918
Ueber die physiologische Wirkung des Cocaïn. *Pflüg. Arch. ges. Physiol.*, 1880, **21,** 38–77.
Anrep studied the action of cocaine and, like Moréno y Maiz, suggested that it might be used as a local anaesthetic.

1872 KOCH, ROBERT. 1843–1910
Ueber Desinfection. *Mitt. k. GesundhAmte*, 1881, **1,** 234–82.
Important report on disinfection.

1873 LADENBURG, ALBERT.
Die natürlich vorkommenden mydriatisch wirkenden Alkaloïde. *Ann. Chem. Pharm.*, 1881, **206,** 274–307.
Isolation of hyoscine (scopolamine).

1874 MARTINDALE, WILLIAM. 1840–1902
The extra pharmacopoeia of unofficial drugs . . . With references to their use abstracted from the medical journals by W. WYNN WESTCOTT. London, *H. K. Lewis*, 1883.
25th edition, 1967.

1875 SCHMIEDEBERG, JOHANN ERNST OSWALD. 1838–1921
Grundriss der Arzneimittellehre. Leipzig, *F. C. W. Vogel*, 1883.

Schmiedeberg, leading German pharmacologist, was professor at Dorpat and Strassburg. Among his many valuable investigations may be mentioned his study of the effect of drugs on the circulation.

1877 CERVELLO, VINCENZO. 1854–1919
Recherches cliniques et physiologiques sur la paraldéhyde. *Arch. ital. Biol.*, 1884, **6,** 113–34.

Introduction of paraldehyde into therapeutics as a narcotic.

1878 FILEHNE, WILHELM. 1844–1927
Ueber das Antipyrin, ein neues Antipyreticum. *Z. klin. Med.*, 1884, **7,** 641–42.

Introduction of antipyrin.

1879 UNNA, PAUL GERSON. 1850–1929
Eine neue Form medicamentöser Einverleibung. *Fortschr. Med.*, 1884, **2,** 507–09.

Unna introduced specially coated pills for local absorption in the intestine.

1880 BINZ, CARL. 1832–1913
Vorlesungen über Pharmakologie. Berlin, *A. Hirschwald*, 188[4]–86.

Includes his test for quinine in urine. English translation of second edition, 1895–97. Binz was professor of pharmacology at Bonn. His most important work was perhaps the demonstration that quinine in low concentrations kills numerous micro-organisms.

1881 BRUNTON, *Sir* THOMAS LAUDER, *Bart.* 1844–1916
A text-book of pharmacology, therapeutics and materia medica. London, *Macmillan & Co.*, 1885.

Brunton was physician to St. Bartholomew's Hospital and an eminent pharmacologist. He is notable for his introduction of amyl nitrite in the treatment of angina pectoris and for a vast amount of other work concerning the action of drugs on the cardiovascular system.

1882 BAUMANN, EUGEN. 1846–1896
Ueber Disulfone. *Ber. dtsch. chem. Ges.*, 1886, **19,** 2806–14.

Preparation of sulphonal.

1883 UNNA, PAUL GERSON. 1850–1929
Ichthyol und Resorcin als Repräsentanten der Gruppe reduzierender Heilmittel. Hamburg, Leipzig, *L. Voss*, 1886.

Unna introduced ichthyol and resorcinol into medicine. Supplement to *Mh. prakt. Derm.*, No. 1.

1883.1 NAGAI, NAGAJOSI. 1844–1929
Ephedrin. *Pharm. Ztg*, 1887, **32,** 700.

Isolation of ephedrine.

1884 KAST, ALFRED. 1856–1903
Sulfonal, ein neues Schlafmittel. *Berl. klin. Wschr.*, 1888, **25,** 309–14.

Introduction of sulphonal, previously discovered by Baumann.

1885 FRASER, *Sir* THOMAS RICHARD. 1841–1919
Strophanthus hispidus; its natural history, chemistry, and pharmacology. *Trans. roy. Soc. Edinb.*, 1890, **35,** 955–1027; 1892, **36,** 343–457.

Introduction of strophanthus hispidus.

1886 CASH, John Theodore. 1854–1936, & DUNSTAN, *Sir* Wyndham Rowland. 1861–1949

The physiological action of the nitrites of the paraffin series, considered in connection with their chemical constitution. *Phil. Trans. B*, (1893), 1894, **184,** 505–639.

1887 PAUL, Benjamin Horatio. 1828–1902, & COWNLEY, Alfred John.

The chemistry of ipecacuanha. *Pharm. J.*, 1894–95, **54,** 111–15, 373–374, 690–92.

Emetine first obtained in pure form.

1888 FISCHER, Emil. 1852–1919, & ACH, Lorenz.

Neue Synthese der Harnsäure und ihrer Methylderivate. *Ber. dtsch. chem. Ges.*, 1895, **28,** 2473–80.

1889 FILEHNE, Wilhelm. 1844–1927

Ueber das Pyramidon, ein Antipyrinderivat. *Berl. klin. Wschr.*, 1896, **33,** 1061–63.

Filehne was responsible for the introduction of amidopyrine (pyramidon).

1890 KRÖNIG, Claus Ludwig Theodor Bernhard. 1863–1918, & PAUL, Theodor. 1862–1928

Die chemischen Grundlagen der Lehre von der Giftwirkung und Desinfection. *Z. Hyg. InfektKr.*, 1897, **25,** 1–112.

Krönig and Paul described a new method for the quantitative study of disinfection and laid the foundation of modern knowledge of disinfectants.

1890.1 HEFFTER, Karl Wilhelm Arthur. 1859–1925

Ueber Pellote. Beiträge zur chemischen und pharmakologischen Kenntniss der Cacteen. Zweite Mitteilung. *Arch. exp. Path. Pharmak.*, 1898, **40,** 385–429.

Isolation of mescaline.

1891 FRÄNKEL, Sigmund. 1868–

Die Arzneimittel-Synthese auf Grundlage der Beziehungen zwischen chemischem Aufbau und Wirkung. Berlin, *J. Springer*, 1901.

1892 FISCHER, Emil. 1852–1919, & MERING, Joseph von. 1849–1908

Ueber eine neue Klasse von Schlafmitteln. *Therap. Gegenw.*, 1903, **44,** 97–101.

Synthesis of barbitone.

1893 RIDEAL, Samuel. 1863–1929, & WALKER, J. T. Ainslie. 1868–1930

Standardisation of disinfectants. *J. sanit. Inst.*, 1903, **24,** 424–41.

Rideal–Walker method for testing disinfectants.

1893.1 CLOETTA, Max. 1868–1940

Ueber Digalen (Digitoxinum solubile). *Münch. med. Wschr.*, 1904, **51,** 1466–68.

Introduction of digalen.

1894 MELTZER, SAMUEL JAMES. 1851–1920, & AUER, JOHN. 1875–1948
Physiological and pharmacological studies of magnesium salts. *Amer. J. Physiol.*, 1905, **14,** 366–88; 1906, **15,** 387–405; **16,** 233–51.
A study of the anaesthetic and other effects of magnesium salts.

1895 BARGER, GEORGE. 1878–1939, *et al.*
An active alkaloid from ergot. *Brit. med. J.*, 1906, **2,** 1792.
Isolation of ergotoxine. With F. H. Carr and H. H. Dale.

1895.1 WINDAUS, ADOLF. 1876–1959, & VOGT, KARL. 1880–
Synthese des Imidazolyläthylamins. *Ber. dtsch. chem. Ges.*, 1907, **40,** 3691–95.
Synthesis of histamine.

1896 ABEL, JOHN JACOB. 1857–1938, & ROWNTREE, LEONARD GEORGE. 1883–
On the pharmacological action of some phthaleins and their derivatives. *J. Pharmacol.*, 1909, **1,** 231–64.
This work led to the universal clinical use of phenolsulphonephthalein in renal function tests and of phenoltetrachlorphthalein in hepatic function tests.

1897 HUNT, REID. 1870–1948, & TAVEAU, RENÉ DE M.
On the relation between the toxicity and chemical constitution of a number of derivatives of choline and analogous compounds. *J. Pharmacol.*, 1909, **1,** 303–39.

1898 BARGER, GEORGE. 1878–1939, & DALE, *Sir* HENRY HALLETT. 1875–1968
Chemical structure and sympathomimetic action of amines. *J. Physiol.* (*Lond.*), 1910, **41,** 19–59.
Discovery of histamine in an ergot extract.

1899 DALE, *Sir* HENRY HALLETT. 1875–1968, & LAIDLAW, *Sir* PATRICK PLAYFAIR. 1881–1940
The physiological action of β-iminoazolylethylamine. *J. Physiol.* (*Lond.*), 1910, **41,** 318–44.
Study of the effect of histamine.

1900 MEYER, HANS HORST. 1853–1939, & GOTTLIEB, RUDOLPH. 1864–1924
Die experimentelle Pharmakologie als Grundlage der Arzneibehandlung. Berlin, *Urban & Schwarzenberg*, 1910.

1901 ABEL, JOHN JACOB. 1857–1938, & MACHT, DAVID ISRAEL. 1882–1961
Two crystalline pharmacological agents obtained from the tropical toad, *Bufo agua*. *J. Pharmacol.*, 1911–12, **3,** 319–77.
Isolation of bufagin. Preliminary communication in *J. Amer. med. Ass.*, 1911, **56,** 1531–35.

1901.1 BARGER, GEORGE. 1878–1939, & DALE, *Sir* HENRY HALLETT. 1875–1968
β-iminazolylethylamine a depressor constituent of intestinal mucosa. *J. Physiol.* (*Lond.*), 1911, **41,** 499–503.
Isolation of histamine from animal tissues.

1902 MORGENROTH, Julius. 1871–1924, & LEVY, Richard. 1882–
Chemotherapie der Pneumokokkeninfektion. *Berl. klin. Wschr.*, 1911, **48,** 1560–61, 1979–83.

First clinical use of optochin, a quinine derivative, specific in pneumococcal infections.

1903 BOURQUELOT, Émile. 1851–1921
La synthèse des glucosides par les ferments. *J. Pharm. Chim.*, 1913, 7 sér., **8,** 337–59.

Bourquelot did important work on the synthesis of glucosides; several more papers followed the one given above.

1903.1 HENRY, Thomas Anderson. 1873–1958
The plant alkaloids. London, *J. & A. Churchill*, 1913.

1903.2 DAKIN, Henry Drysdale. 1880–1952
On the use of certain antiseptic substances in the treatment of infected wounds. *Brit. med. J.*, 1915, **2,** 318–20.

Eusol and chloramine-T.

1904 STRAUB, Walter. 1874–1944
Digitaliswirkung am isolierten Vorhof des Frosches. *Arch. exp. Path. Pharmak.*, 1916, **79,** 19–29.

An important analysis of the action of digitalis on the isolated heart.

1905 BROWNING, Carl Hamilton. 1881–1972, *et al.*
Flavine and brilliant green, powerful antiseptics with low toxicity to the tissues: their use in the treatment of infected wounds. *Brit. med. J.*, 1917, **1,** 73–79.

Introduction of acriflavine. With R. Gulbransen, E. L. Kennaway, and L. H. D. Thornton.

1906 TSCHIRCH, Alexander. 1856–1939
Handbuch der Pharmakognosie. 3 vols. and Register. Leipzig, *C. H. Tauchnitz*, 1917–27.

Includes detailed accounts of the history of each drug.

1907 JACOBS, Walter Abraham. 1883– , & HEIDELBERGER, Michael. 1888–
Chemotherapy of trypanosome and spirochete infections. Chemical series. I. N-phenylglycineamide-*p*-arsonic acid. *J. exp. Med.*, 1919, **30,** 411–15.

Introduction of tryparsamide.

1908 YOUNG, Hugh Hampton. 1870–1945, *et al.*
A new germicide for use in the genito-urinary tract; "mercurochrome–220." *J. Amer. med. Assoc.*, 1919, **73,** 1483–91.

Introduction of mercurochrome. With E. C. White and E. O. Swartz.

1909 HEFFTER, Karl Wilhelm Arthur. 1859–1925
Handbuch der experimentellen Pharmakologie . . . Hrsg. von A. Heffter. Vol. 1– . Berlin, *J. Springer*, 1920– .

1910 SPIRO, Karl. 1867–1932, & STOLL, August.
Ueber die wirksamen Substanzen des Mutterkorns. *Schweiz. med. Wschr.*, 1921, **2,** 525–29.

Isolation of ergotamine.

1911 CHURCHMAN, John Woolman. 1877–1937
Intravenous use of dyes. *J. Amer. med. Ass.*, 1925, **85,** 1849–53.
Churchman demonstrated the selective bactericidal action of gentian violet against staphylococci. See also *J. exp. Med.*, 1912, **16**, 221–47; *J. Urol.*, 1924, **11**, 1–18.

1913 GOTTLIEB, Rudolf. 1864–1924
Vergleichende Messungen über die Gewöhnung des Atemzentrums an Morphin, Dicodid und Dilaudid. *Münch. med. Wschr.*, 1926, **73,** 595–96.
Introduction of dilaudid.

1914 HANZLIK, Paul John. 1885–
Actions and uses of the salicylates and cinchophen in medicine. *Medicine*, 1926, **5,** 197–373.

1915 LOEVENHART, Arthur Salomon. 1878–1929, & STRATMAN-THOMAS, Warren Kidwell. 1894–
On the chemotherapy of neurosyphilis and trypanosomiasis. *J. Pharmacol.*, 1926, **29,** 69–82.
Study of the effect of 12 different substances in neurosyphilis and trypanosomiasis.

1915.1 BEST, Charles Herbert. 1899– , *et al.*
The nature of the vaso-dilator constituents of certain tissue extracts. *J. Physiol.* (*Camb.*), 1927, **62,** 397–417.
Proof that histamine occurs in certain organs in amounts sufficient to account for the depressant action of extracts of these organs. With H. H. Dale, H. W. Dudley, and W. V. Thorpe.

1916 CUSHNY, Arthur Robertson. 1866–1926
The action and uses in medicine of digitalis and its allies. London, *Longmans, Green & Co.*, 1925.

1917 SOLIS-COHEN, Solomon. 1857–1948, & GITHENS, Thomas Stotesbury. 1878–
Pharmacotherapeutics. New York, *D. Appleton & Co.*, 1928.

1918 CHEN, Ko Kuei. 1898– , & SCHMIDT, Carl Frederic. 1893–
Ephedrine and related substances. Baltimore, *Williams & Wilkins Co.*, 1930.
A digest of the literature, together with an excellent bibliography. By their earlier work (*J. Pharmacol.*, 1924, **24**, 339–57) Chen and Schmidt aroused world-wide interest in ephedrine.

1919 FELDBERG, Wilhelm Siegmund. 1900– , & SCHILF, Erich.
Histamin: seine Pharmakologie und Bedeutung für die Humoralphysiologie. Berlin, *J. Springer*, 1930.

1920 SMITH, Sydney.
Digoxin, a new digitalis glucoside. *J. chem. Soc.*, 1930, 508–10.
Isolation of digoxin from *Digitalis lanata*.

1921 FISCHL, Viktor, & SCHLOSSBERGER, Hans. 1887–
Handbuch der Chemotherapie. 2 vols. Leipzig, *Fischer*, 1932–34.

1922 FLEMING, *Sir* Alexander. 1881–1955
Lysozyme. *Proc. roy. Soc. Med.*, 1932, **26,** 71–84.

Fleming found a bacteriolytic substance in tears, nasal secretions, and many tissues; he called it "lysozyme". For his earlier papers on the subject, see *Proc. roy. Soc. B*, 1922, **93**, 306–17; *Lancet*, 1929, **1**, 217–20.

1923 CHOPRA, Ram Nath. 1882– , *et al.*
The pharmacological action of an alkaloid obtained from *Rauwolfia serpentina* Benth. A preliminary note. *Indian J. med. Res.*, 1933, **21,** 261–71.

R. N. Chopra, J. C. Gupta, and B. Mukherjee demonstrated the sedative and hypotensive effect of an alkaloid isolated from *Rauwolfia serpentina.*

1924 CLARK, Alfred Joseph. 1885–1941
The mode of action of drugs on cells. London, *E. Arnold & Co.*, 1933.

1925 UNGAR, Georges. 1906– , *et al.*
Inhibition des effets de l'histamine sur l'intestin isolé du cobaye par quelques substances sympathicomimétiques et sympathicolytiques. *C. R. Soc. Biol.* (*Paris*), 1937, **124,** 445–46.

First antihistamine ("933 F"). With J. L. Parrot and D. Bovet.

In 1957 Bovet (see also Nos. 1950, 4727, 5725, 5728) received the Nobel Prize for his work on the synthesis of antihistamines and certain muscle relaxants.

1926 BUTTLE, Gladwin Albert Hurst. 1899– , *et al.*
The action of substances allied to 4:4'-diaminodiphenylsulphone in streptococcal and other infections in mice. *Biochem. J.*, 1938, **32,** 1101–10.

G. A. H. Buttle, T. Dewing, G. E. Foster, W. H. Gray, S. Smith, and D. Stephenson discovered the potency of dapsone.

1927 EISLER, O, & SCHAUMANN, O.
Dolantin, ein neuartiges Spasmolytikum und Analgetikum. (Chemisches und pharmakologisches.) *Dtsch. med. Wschr.*, 1939, **65,** 967–69.

Synthesis of pethidine (dolantin).

1928 GUNN, James Andrew. 1882–1958
The pharmacological actions and therapeutic uses of some compounds related to adrenaline. *Brit. med. J.*, 1939, **2,** 155–60, 214–19.

1928.1 STOLL, August, & HOFMANN, Albert. 1906–
Partialsynthese von Alkaloiden vom Typus des Ergobasins. *Helv. chim. Acta*, 1943, **26,** 944–65.

Synthesis of lysergic acid diethylamide (LSD).

1928.2 DODD, Matthew Charles. 1910– , & STILLMAN, William Barlow. 1904–
The in vitro bacteriostatic action of some simple furan derivatives. *J. Pharmacol.*, 1944, **82,** 11–18.

Nitrofuran (nitrofurazone).

1928.3 LÄUGER, P., *et al.*
Über Konstitution und toxische Wirkung von natürlichen und neuen synthetischen insektentötenden Stoffen. *Helv. chim. Acta*, 1944, **27**, 892–928.
With H. Martin and P. Müller. Dichlordiphenyltrichlorethane (DDT) was introduced as an insecticide by Paul Müller (1889–1965). He received the Nobel Prize in 1948 for his discovery of the high efficacy of DDT against several varieties of arthropod.

1929 PETERS, *Sir* RUDOLPH ALBERT. 1889– , *et al.*
British anti-lewisite (*BAL*). *Nature* (*Lond.*), 1945, **156**, 616–19.
With L. A. Stocken and R. H. S. Thompson. BAL (dimercaprol) was discovered during the 1939–45 war.

1929.1 SNYDER, MARSHALL LOVEJOY. 1907– , *et al.*
Effectiveness of a nitrofuran in the treatment of infected wounds. *Milit. Surg.*, 1945, **97**, 380–84.
First clinical use of "furacin" (nitrofuran). With C. L. Kiehn and J. W. Christopherson.

1929.2 ROCHA E SILVA, MAURICIO. 1910– , *et al.*
Bradykinin, a hypotensive and smooth muscle stimulating factor released from plasma globulin by snake venoms and by trypsin. *Amer. J. Physiol.*, 1949, **156**, 261–73.
Discovery of bradykinin. With W. T. Beraldo and G. Rosenfeld.

1930 PHARMACOPOEIA.
Pharmacopoea internationalis. Editio prima. 2 vols. and supplement. Geneva, *World Health Organization*, 1951–59.
2nd ed., 1967, with title *Specifications for the quality control of pharmaceutical preparations;* English, French, Russian, and Spanish editions.

1931 MÜLLER, J. M., *et al.*
Reserpin, der sedative Wirkstoff aus *Rauwolfia serpentina* Benth. *Experientia* (*Basel*), 1952, **8**, 338.
Isolation of reserpine. With E. Schlittler and H. J. Bein.

1931.1 ERSPAMER, VITTORIO. 1909– , & ASERO, B.
Identification of enteramine, the specific hormone of the enterochromaffin cell system, as 5-hydroxytryptamine. *Nature* (*Lond.*), 1952, **169**, 800–1.

1931.2 COURVOISIER, S., *et al.*
Propriétés pharmacodynamiques du chlorhydrate de chloro-3(diméthylamino-3'propyl)-10 phénothiazine (4.560 R.P.). *Arch. int. Pharmacodyn.*, 1953, **92**, 305–61.
Chlorpromazine. With J. Fournel, R. Ducrot, M. Kolsky, and P. Koetschet.

Antibiotics

1932 TYNDALL, JOHN. 1820–1893
The optical deportment of the atmosphere in relation to the phenomena of putrefaction and infection. *Phil. Trans.*, 1876, **166**, 27–74.
Tyndall observed the selective bacteria-inhibiting effect of *Penicillium* and the resistance of *Ps. pyocanea* to it.

1932.1 PASTEUR, LOUIS. 1822–1895, & JOUBERT, JULES FRANÇOIS.
Charbon et septicémie. *C. R. Acad. Sci.* (*Paris*), 1877, **85,** 101–15.

Pasteur and Joubert were probably the first to realize the practical implications of antibiosis. They noted the antagonism between *Bacillus anthracis* and other bacteria in cultures.

1932.2 EMMERICH, RUDOLF. 1852–1914, & LÖW, OSCAR. 1844–
Bakteriolytische Enzyme als Ursache der erworbenen Immunität und die Heilung von Infectionskrankheiten durch dieselben. *Z. Hyg. Infekt.-Kr.*, 1889, **31,** 1–65.

Emmerich and Löw prepared a water-soluble antibiotic substance, pyocyanase, from *Psuedomonas aeruginosa.* It inhibited pathogenic cocci and the organisms responsible for diphtheria, plague, cholera, and typhoid.

1933 FLEMING, *Sir* ALEXANDER. 1881–1955
On the antibacterial action of cultures of a penicillium, with special reference to their use in the isolation of *B. influenzae. Brit. J. exp. Path.*, 1929, **10,** 226–36.

Discovery of the growth-inhibiting action of *Penicillium* on certain bacteria. Nobel Prize (with Florey and Chain) 1945.

1933.1 DUBOS, RENÉ JULES. 1901–
Bactericidal effect of an extract of a soil bacillus on gram-positive cocci. *Proc. Soc. exp. Biol.* (*N. Y.*), 1939, **40,** 311–12.

Isolation of gramicidin.

1933.2 OXFORD, ALBERT EDWARD, *et al.*
Studies in the biochemistry of micro-organisms. LX. Griseofulvin, $C_{17}H_{17}O_6Cl$, a metabolic product of *Penicillium griseo-fulvum* Dierckx. *Biochem. J.*, 1939, **33,** 240–48.

Isolation of griseofulvin. With H. Raistrick and P. Simonart.

1934 CHAIN, ERNST BORIS. 1906– , *et al.*
Penicillin as a chemotherapeutic agent. *Lancet*, 1940, **2,** 226–28.

Clinical application of penicillin. With H. W. Florey, A. D. Gardner, N. G. Heatley, M. A. Jennings, J. Orr-Ewing, and A. G. Sanders. Chain and Florey shared the Nobel Prize with Fleming (No. 1933) in 1945.

1935 SCHATZ, ALBERT. 1920– , *et al.*
Streptomycin, a substance exhibiting antiobiotic activity against Gram-positive and Gram-negative bacteria. *Proc. Soc. exp. Biol.* (*N. Y.*), 1944, **55,** 66–69.

Introduction of streptomycin. With E. Bugie and S. A. Waksman.

1936 JOHNSON, BALBINA A., *et al.*
Bacitracin: a new antibiotic produced by a member of the *B. subtilis* group. *Science*, 1945, **102,** 376–77.

With H. Anker and F. L. Meleney.

1937 AINSWORTH, GEOFFREY CLOUGH. 1905– , *et al.*
"Aerosporin," an antibiotic produced by *Bacillus aerosporus* Greer. *Nature* (*Lond.*), 1947, **160,** 263.

Discovery of aerosporin (polymyxin). With A. M. Brown and G. Brownlee.

1938 EHRLICH, JOHN. 1907– , *et al.*
Chloromycetin, a new antibiotic from a soil actinomycete. *Science*, 1947, **106,** 417.
Production of chloramphenicol from *Streptomyces venezuelae*. With Q. R. Bartz, R. M. Smith, D. A. Joslyn, and P. R. Burkholder.

1939 HERRELL, WALLACE EDGAR. 1909– , *et al.*
Procaine penicillin G (duracillin); a new salt of penicillin which prolongs the action of penicillin. *Proc. Mayo Clin.*, 1947, **22,** 567–70.
With D. R. Nichols and F. R. Heilman.

1940 SMADEL, JOSEPH EDWIN. 1907–1963, & JACKSON, ELIZABETH B.
Chloromycetin, an antibiotic with chemotherapeutic activity in experimental rickettsial and viral infections. *Science*, 1947, **106,** 418–19.
Introduction of chloramphenicol.

1941 STANSLY, PHILIP GERALD. 1912– , *et al.*
Polymyxin: a new chemotherapeutic agent. *Bull. Johns Hopk. Hosp.*, 1947, **81,** 43–54.
With R. G. Shepherd and H. J. White.

1942 DUGGAR, BENJAMIN MINGE. 1872–1956, *et al.*
Aureomycin: a product of the continuing search for new antibiotics. *Ann. N.Y. Acad. Sci.*, 1948, **51,** 177–342.
Discovery and clinical application of chlortetracycline (aureomycin).

1943 CLARKE, HANS THACHER. 1887– , *et al.*
The chemistry of penicillin. Report of a collaborative investigation by American and British chemists. Princeton, *University Press*, 1949.

1944 FLOREY, HOWARD WALTER, *Baron Florey*. 1898–1968, *et al.*
Antibiotics. 2 vols. London, Oxford, *University Press*, 1949.
Written in collaboration with a number of colleagues at the Oxford School of Pathology.

1944.1 WAKSMAN, SELMAN ABRAHAM. 1888–1973, & LECHEVALIER, HUBERT ARTHUR. 1926–
Neomycin, a new antibiotic active against streptomycin-resistant bacteria, including tuberculosis organisms. *Science*, 1949, **109, 305–07.**
Isolation of neomycin.

1945 FINLAY, ALEXANDER CARPENTER. 1906– , *et al.*
Terramycin, a new antibiotic. *Science*, 1950, **111,** 85.
Oxytetracycline (terramycin).

1945.1 EBLE, THOMAS EUGENE. 1923– , & HANSON, FREDERICK REUBEN. 1921–
Fumagillin, an antibiotic from *Aspergillus fumigatus* H-3. *Antibiot. & Chemother.*, 1951, **1,** 54–58.
Isolation of fumagillin, an antibiotic with amoebicidal properties.

1945.2 FINLAY, ALEXANDER CARPENTER. 1906– , *et al.*
Viomycin, a new antibiotic active against mycobacteria. *Amer. Rev. Tuberc.*, 1951, **63,** 1–3.
Isolation of viomycin.

1945.3 HAZEN, ELIZABETH LEE. 1888– , & BROWN, RACHEL FULLER. 1898–
Fungicidin, an antibiotic produced by a soil actinomycete. *Proc. Soc. exp. Biol. (N.Y.)*, 1951, **76,** 93–97.
Isolation of nystatin (fungicidin).

1946 McGUIRE, JAMES MYRLIN. 1909– , *et al.*
"Ilotycin," a new antibiotic. *Antibiot. and Chemother.*, 1952, **2,** 281–83.
Discovery of erythromycin. With R. L. Bunch, R. C. Anderson, H. E. Boaz, E. H. Flynn, H. M. Powell, and J. W. Smith.

1947 WAKSMAN, SELMAN ABRAHAM. 1888–1973
The literature on streptomycin 1944–1952. New Brunswick, *Rutgers Univ. Press*, 1952.
Waksman (see also No. 1935) was awarded the Nobel Prize in 1952 for his work on streptomycin.

Sulphonamides

1948 GELMO, PAUL. 1879–
Ueber Sulfamide der *p*-Amidobenzolsulfonsäure. *J. prakt. Chem.*, 1908, **77,** 369–82.
Para-aminobenzenesulphonamide (sulphanilamide) first prepared.

1949 DOMAGK, GERHARD. 1895–1964
Ein Beitrag zur Chemotherapie der bakteriellen Infektionen. *Dtsch. med. Wschr.*, 1935, **61,** 250–53.
Prontosil, the first drug containing sulphanilamide, was introduced into medicine by Domagk. He was awarded the Nobel Prize in 1939.

1950 TRÉFOUËL, J., *et al.*
Activité du *p*-aminophénylsulfamide sur les infection streptococciques expérimentales de la souris et du lapin. *C. R. Soc. Biol. (Paris)*, 1935, **120,** 756–58.
J. Tréfouël, Mme Tréfouël, F. Nitti, and D. Bovet assumed that the sulphonamide group was responsible for the results obtained with Domagk's prontosil. Their work led them to introduce sulphanilamide.

1951 WHITBY, *Sir* LIONEL ERNEST HOWARD. 1895–1956
Chemotherapy of pneumococcal and other infections with 2-(*p*-aminobenzenesulphonamido) pyridine. *Lancet*, 1938, **1,** 1210–12.
Experimental proof of the efficacy of sulphapyridine (M & B 693) in pneumococcal pneumonia.

1952 EVANS, GLADYS MARY, *Mrs. Jenks*, & GAISFORD, WILFRID FLETCHER. 1902–
Treatment of pneumonia with 2-(*p*-aminobenzenesulphonamido) pyridine. *Lancet*, 1938, **2,** 14–19.
Clinical proof of the value of sulphapyridine.

1953 GSELL, OTTO.
Chemotherapie akuter Infektionskrankheiten durch Ciba 3714 (Sulfanilamidothiazol). *Schweiz. med. Wschr.*, 1940, **70,** 342–50.
First important clinical trial of sulphathiazole.

1954 MARSHALL, ELI KENNERLY. 1889–1966, *et al.*
Sulfanilylguanidine: a chemotherapeutic agent for intestinal infections. *Bull. Johns Hopk. Hosp.* 1940, **67,** 163–88.
Sulphaguanidine was introduced by E. K. Marshall, A. C. Bratton, H. J. White, and J. T. Litchfield.

1955 ROBLIN, RICHARD OWEN. 1907– , *et al.*
Chemotherapy, II. Some sulfanilamido heterocycles. *J. Amer. chem. Soc.*, 1940, **62,** 2002–05.
Synthesis of sulphamerazine, by R. O. Roblin, J. H. Williams, P. S. Winnek & J. P. English.

1955.1 WOODS, DONALD DEVEREUX. 1912–1964
The relation of *p*-aminobenzoic acid to the mechanism of the action of sulphanilamide. *Brit. J. exp. Path.*, 1940, **21,** 74–90.
Isolation of *p*-aminobenzoic acid, a structural analogue of sulphanilamide.

1956 FINLAND, MAXWELL. 1902– , *et al.*
Sulfadiazine. Therapeutic evaluation and toxic effects on four hundred and forty-six patients. *J. Amer. med. Ass.*, 1941, **116,** 2641–47.
Introduction of sulphadiazine. With E. Strauss and O. L. Peterson.

1957 POTH, EDGAR JACOB. 1899– , & KNOTTS, FRANK LOUIS. 1912–
Succinyl sulfathiazole, a new bacteriostatic agent locally active in the gastrointestinal tract. *Proc. Soc. exp. Biol. (N.Y.)*, 1941, **48,** 129–30.
Introduction of sulphasuxidine.

1958 MACARTNEY, DONALD WILLIAM, *et al.*
Sulphamethazine: clinical trial of a new sulphonamide. *Lancet*, 1942, **1,** 639–41.
Sulphadimidine; with G. S. Smith, R. W. Luxton, W. A. Ramsay, and J. Goldman.

For history of pharmacy and pharmacology, see 2029–2068.9

1959–2068.9 THERAPEUTICS

1959 GALEN. A.D. 130–200
De methodo medendi. *In his*: Opera, ed. C. G. KÜHN, Lipsiae, 1825, **10,** 1–1021.

1960 PETRUS HISPANUS, *Pope John XXI.* ?1226–1277
Thesaurus pauperum. [Florence, *F. Bonaccorsi, circa* 1485.]
One of the most popular medical books of the Middle Ages; first written about 1260. After its first printing about 1485 it was many times reprinted in the next 100 years. Petrus Hispanus was the only medical man to become Pope.

1961 ISAAC *Judaeus* [ISHÂQ IBN SULAIMÂN AL ISRÂ'ILI]. ?880–932
De particularibus diaetis. Padua, *Cerdonis*, 1487.
First separately printed work on diet.

1962 ELSHOLTZ, JOHANN SIGMUND. 1623–1688
Clysmatica nova; oder newe Clystier-Kunst. Berlin, *D. Reichel*, 1665.
Elsholtz's book on the venous infusion of medicaments was one of the first works to deal with blood transfusion. Latin edition in 1667; English translation in 1677.

1963 MAJOR, Johann Daniel. 1634–1693
Chirurgia infusoria. Kiloni, *J. Reumannus*, 1667.

Major, the first professor of medicine at Kiel, was the first to make successful intravenous injections of drugs into the human body, in 1662. Sir Christopher Wren in 1656 had injected wine and ale into the veins of a dog.

1964 STOLL, Maximilian. 1742–1788
Rationis medendi in Nosocomio practico Vindobonensi. 7 pts. Viennae Austriae, 1777–90.

1965 FRANK, Johann Peter. 1745–1821
De curandis hominum morbis epitome. 7 vols. (in 10). Mannhemii Tubingae, Viennae, Taurini), 1792–1825.

1966 HAHNEMANN, Christian Friedrich Samuel. 1755–1843
Organon der rationellen Heilkunde. Dresden, *Arnold*, 1810.

Hahnemann, the founder of homoeopathy, embodied his theories in the *Organon*. The minute doses set down by him did much to correct the evils of the polypharmacy of his time. He professed to base medicine on a knowledge of symptoms, regarding investigation of the causes of symptoms as useless; he thus rejected all the lessons of pathology and morbid anatomy. There are several English translations, the first of which appeared in 1833.

1967 TROUSSEAU, Armand. 1801–1867, & PIDOUX, Hermann. 1808–1882
Traité de thérapeutique et de matière médicale. 2 vols. Paris, *Béchet jeune*, 1836–39.

"A valuable work of reference, containing a large amount of information on the various articles of the materia medica, collected from the best authorities, interspersed with much original matter" (Waring).

1968 RYND, Francis. 1801–1861
Neuralgia – introduction of fluid to the nerve. *Dublin med. Press*, 1845, **13,** 167–68.

The first hypodermic infusions were made possible by an invention of Rynd. The description of his instrument is given in *Dublin Quart. J. med. Sci.*, 1861, **32,** 13.

1969 WOOD, Alexander. 1817–1884
New method of treating neuralgia by the direct application of opiates to the painful joints. *Edinb. med. surg. J.*, 1855, **82,** 265–81.

Wood of Edinburgh was the first (1853) to employ hypodermic injection as a therapeutic procedure. See also *Brit. med. J.*, 1858, 721–23, for a later paper by him. A full account of his work is given by Howard-Jones (No. 2063).

1970 HALL, Marshall. 1790–1857
On a new mode of effecting artificial respiration. *Lancet*, 1856, **1,** 229.

Marshall Hall's method of artificial respiration.

1971 SILVESTER, Henry Robert. 1828–1908
A new method of resuscitating still-born children, and of restoring persons apparently drowned or dead. *Brit. med. J.*, 1858, 576–79.

Silvester's method of artificial respiration.

1972 WOOD, Horatio Charles. 1841–1920
A treatise on therapeutics. Philadelphia, *J. B. Lippincott*, 1874.

Wood was professor of botany (1866–76), therapeutics (1876–1907) and nervous diseases (1875–1901) in the University of Pennsylvania. In his book the effects of various drugs in small doses was first discussed; it also contains a standard classification of drugs.

1973 BRUNTON, *Sir* THOMAS LAUDER, *Bart.* 1844–1916
An introduction to modern therapeutics, being the Croonian Lectures on the relationship between chemical structure and physiological action. London, *Macmillan & Co.*, 1892.
One of the best known of Lauder Brunton's works.

1974 SHARPEY-SCHÄFER, *Sir* EDWARD ALBERT. 1850–1935
Description of a simple and efficient method of performing artificial respiration in the human subject especially in cases of drowning. To which is appended instructions for the treatment of the apparently drowned. *Med.-chir. Trans.*, 1904, **87,** 609–23.
Schafer's method of artificial respiration.

1975 HUCHARD, HENRI. 1844–1910, & FIESSINGER, CHARLES ALBERT. 1857–1942
La thérapeutique en vingt medicaments. Paris, *A. Maloine*, 1910.
Huchard and Fiessinger suggested that actual drug therapy should be limited to 20 medicaments.

1976 ABEL, JOHN JACOB. 1857–1938, *et al.*
Plasma removal with return of corpuscles (plasmaphaeresis), *J. Pharmacol.*, 1914, **5,** 625–41.
Report of a method of removal of plasma from the living animal, with return of the corpuscles after washing and separation by centrifugalization. With L. G. Rowntree and B. B. Turner. See also their earlier papers in the same journal, 1914, **5**, 275–316, 611–23.

1977 HALDANE, JOHN SCOTT. 1860–1936
The therapeutic administration of oxygen. *Brit. med. J.*, 1917, **1,** 181–83.
Haldane initiated modern oxygen therapy.

1978 PETERSEN, WILLIAM FERDINAND. 1887–
Protein therapy and nonspecific resistance. New York, *Macmillan Co.*, 1922.

1979 EVE, FRANK CECIL. 1871–1952
Actuation of the inert diaphragm by a gravity method. *Lancet*, 1932, **2,** 995–97.
Eve's method of artificial respiration.

1980 NIELSEN, HOLGER. 1866–1955
En oplivningsmethode. *Ugeskr. Læg.*, 1932, **94,** 1201–03.
Holger Nielsen ("arm-lift") method of artificial respiration.

1981 LOVELACE, WILLIAM RANDOLPH. 1907–1965
Oxygen for therapy and aviation: an apparatus for the administration of oxygen or oxygen and helium by inhalation. *Proc. Mayo Clin.*, 1938, **13,** 646–54.

1982 BULBULIAN, ARTHUR H. 1900–
Design and construction of the masks for the oxygen inhalation apparatus. *Proc. Mayo Clin.*, 1938, **13,** 654–56.
The B. L. B. (Boothby-Lovelace-Bulbulian) mask. See also the previous entry.

1983 TOCANTINS, LEANDRO MAUES. 1901–
Rapid absorption of substances injected into the bone marrow. *Proc. Soc. exp. Biol.* (*N.Y.*), 1940, **45**, 292–96.

Tocantins demonstrated the possibility of transfusion of fluids via the bone marrow. See also later paper with J. F. O'Neill, *Surg. Gynec. Obstet.*, 1941, **73** 281–87.

1984–2010.2 PHYSICAL THERAPY: HYDROTHERAPY

1984 ASCLEPIADES *of Bithynia*. 124–56 B.C.
Ὑγιεινὰ παραγγέλματα. Gesundheitsvorschriften . . . bearbeitet . . . von Robert Ritter von Welz. Würzburg, *Vogt u. Mocker*, 1842.

The Greek physician Asclepiades acquired a great reputation in Rome. His remedies included change of diet, friction, bathing, and exercise. The above edition includes Greek, Latin, and German texts.

1985 GALEN. A.D. 130–200
De sanitate tuenda. In his *Opera* . . . ed. C. G. KÜHN, Lipsiae, 1823, **6**, 1–748.

Translation by R. M. Green, Springfield, Ill., 1951.

1986 DE BALNEIS.
De balneis omnia quae extant apud Graecos, Latinos, et Arabas. Venetiis, *apud Iuntas*, 1553.

This is a collective work, incorporating the writings of more than 70 authorities, among whom may be mentioned Avicenna, Averroes, Avenzohar, Guainerio, Gesner, Savonarola, Petrus de Abano, and Maimonides. It gives an extensive history of balneology and an exact description of all the then known watering-places (about two hundred).

1986.1 MERCURIALI, GERONIMO. 1530–1606
Artis gymnasticae apud antiquos celeberrimae, nostris temporibus ignoratae. Venetiis, *apud Iuntas*, 1569.

First illustrated book on gymnastics. It is the foundation-stone of later work on the subject and is important for the study of gymnastics among the ancients. It includes some excellent woodcuts.

1987 HAHN, JOHANN SIGMUND. 1696–1773
Unterricht von der wunderbare Heilkraft des frischen Wassers bei dessen innerlichem und äusserlichem Gebrauche durch die Erfahrung bestätigt. Breslau, Leipzig, *D. Pietsch*, 1737.

The treatment of fevers by means of the cold pack was revived by S. Hahn and by his son J. S. Hahn; in his treatise, the latter advised the use of water in all diseases. A seventh edition of the book appeared as recently as 1938.

1987.1 TISSOT, CLÉMENT JOSEPH. 1750–1826
Gymnastique médicinale et chirurgicale, ou essai sur l'utilité du mouvement, ou des différens exercices du corps, et du repos dans la cure des maladies. Paris, *Bastien*, 1780.

The first book on therapeutic exercise as the term is understood to-day.

1988 CURRIE, JAMES. 1756–1805
Medical reports, on the effects of water, cold and warm, as a remedy in fever and febrile diseases. Liverpool, *Cadell & Davies*, 1797.

Currie was the first in Great Britain to use cold water packs in the treatment of fever. He made some original observations on the clinical use of the thermometer. It was Currie who first edited Robert Burns's Collected Works.

1988.1 GRAPENGIESSER, Carl Johann Christian. 1773–1813
Versuche des Galvanismus zur Heilung einiger Krankheiten. Berlin, *Myliussi*, 1801.

Grapengiesser was one of the first to employ galvanic currents in treatment.

1989 CARPUE, Joseph Constantine. 1764–1846
An introduction to electricity and galvanism. London, *A. Phillips*, 1803.

A pioneer work in electrotherapy.

1990 DÖBEREINER, Johann Wolfgang. 1780–1849
Anleitung zur Darstellung und Anwendung aller Arten der kräftigsten Bäder und Heilwässer welche von Gesunden und Kranken gebraucht werden. Jena, 1816.

Döbereiner was the first to treat the subject of light therapy on a scientific basis.

1991 EDWARDS, William Frédéric. 1777–1849
De l'influence des agens physiques sur la vie. Paris, *Crochard*, 1824.

Includes account of Edwards' important experimental work regarding the effect of light on the body. English translation in 1832.

1992 PRIESSNITZ, Vincenz. 1799–1851
The coldwater cure, its principles, theory, and practice. London, *W. Strange*, [183–?].

Priessnitz, a layman, became famous for his successful use of cold water as a therapeutic.

1993 LING, Per Henrik. 1776–1839
Gymnastikens allmänna grunder. Upsala, *Palmblad & Co.*, 1840.

Gymnastics and therapeutic massage were first developed in Sweden by Ling. In 1813 a central institute for training teachers in gymnastics was established in Stockholm, largely through his efforts.

1994 CRUSELL, Gustaf Samuel. 1810–1858
Ueber den Galvanismus als chemisches Heilmittel gegen örtliche Krankheiten. St. Petersburg, *K. Kray*, 1841–43.

The first successful use of galvanism as a therapeutic measure is recorded by Crusell.

1995 DUCHENNE DE BOULOGNE, Guillaume Benjamin Amand. 1806–1875
De l'électrisation localisée et de son application à la physiologie, à la pathologie, et à la thérapeutique. Paris, *J. B. Baillière*, 1855; atlas, 1862.

Duchenne, most famous of the electrotherapists, employed faradic current in treating patients as early as 1830. An English translation of his book appeared in 1871. (See also No. 614.)

1996 ZIEMSSEN, Hugo Wilhelm von. 1829–1902
Die Electricität in der Medicin. Berlin, *A. Hirschwald*, 1857.

1996.1 BUSQUÉ y TORRO, Sebastian
Gimnástica, hygiénica, medica, y ortopédica. Madrid, *M. Galiano*, 1865.

Busqué developed the modern concept of rehabilitation.

1996.2 ALTHAUS, Julius. 1833–1900
On the electrolytic treatment of tumors, and other surgical diseases. London, *J. Churchill*, 1867.
Althaus was the first to employ electrolysis for medical purposes.

1997 DOWNES, *Sir* Arthur Henry. 1851–1938, & BLUNT, Thomas Porter.
Researches on the effect of light upon bacteria and other organisms. *Proc. roy. Soc.* (*Lond.*), 1877, **26,** 488–500.
Downes and Blunt were the first to demonstrate the bactericidal action of sunlight; they regarded the germicidal property of light as depending on oxidation.

1998 WINTERNITZ, Wilhelm. 1835–1917
Die Hydrotherapie. 2 vols. Wien, *Urban & Schwarzenberg*, 1877.

1999 D'ARSONVAL, Jacques Arsène. 1851–1940
Récherches d'électrothérapie: la voltaisation sinusoïdale. *Arch. Physiol. norm. path.*, 1892, 5 sér., **4,** 69–80.
Introduction of high-frequency currents in electrotherapy.

2000 FINSEN, Niels Ryberg. 1860–1904
Om anvendelse medicinen af koncentrerede kemiske lysstraaler. Kjøbenhavn, *Gyldendal*, 1896.
Finsen was the founder of modern phototherapy. He demonstrated the value of invisible light, the actinic or chemical ray, the ultra-violet ray, as therapeutic measures. He received the Nobel Prize for Medicine in 1903.

2001 BECQUEREL, Antoine Henri. 1852–1908
Sur les radiations émises par phosphorescence. *C. R. Acad. Sci.* (*Paris*), 1896, **122,** 420–21.
The discovery of radioactivity. Becquerel shared the Nobel Prize for Physics in 1903 with Pierre and Marie Curie.

2002 FREUND, Leopold. 1868–1944
Demonstration eines mit Röntgenstrahlen behandelten Falles von Naevus pigmentosus pilosus. *Wien. klin. Wschr.*, 1897, **10,** 73–74.
First use of *x* rays for deep irradiation therapy.

2003 CURIE, Pierre. 1859–1906, & CURIE, Marie Sklodowska. 1867–1934
Sur une substance nouvelle radio-active, contenue dans la pechblende. *C. R. Acad. Sci.* (*Paris*), 1898, **127,** 175–78, 1215–17.
The Curies, studying the radioactivity of minerals containing uranium and thorium, isolated from pitchblende a substance which they called radium and which they showed to possess an astonishing degree of radioactivity. Since then radium has proved to be a valuable agent in the treatment of cancer. They shared the Nobel Prize for Physics with Becquerel in 1903 and Marie Curie received the Nobel Prize for Chemistry in 1911.

2003.1 LEDUC, Stephane Armand Nicolas. 1853–1939
Introduction électrolytique des ions dans l'organisme vivant. *C. R. Ass. franç. Avance. Sci.* (1900), 1901, **29,** pt. 2, 1111–25.
Introduction of ionic medication.

2003.2 ——. L'électrisation cérébrale. *Rev. int. Électrothér.*, 1903–04, **13,** 143–49.
Leduc reported the effects of a galvanic current on the brain. His work led the way to electric convulsion therapy, introduced by Cerletti and Bini (No. 4962).

2004 PERTHES, GEORG CLEMENS. 1869–1927
Ueber den Einfluss der Röntgenstrahlen auf epitheliale Gewebe, insbesondere auf das Carcinom. *Arch. klin. Chir.*, 1903, **71,** 955–1000.
Perthes was one of the first to study the inhibitory effect of *x* rays on carcinoma; he was a pioneer in radiotherapy.

2005 BERGONIÉ, JEAN. 1857–1925, & TRIBONDEAU, L.
Interprétation de quelques résultats de la radiothérapie et essai de fixation d'une technique rationelle. *C. R. Acad. Sci.* (*Paris*), 1906, **143,** 983–85.
Bergonié–Tribondeau law, "the sensitivity of cells to radiation varies directly with the reproductive capacity of the cells and inversely with their degree of differentiation" (Dorland).

2006 WEBER, *Sir* HERMANN DAVID. 1823–1918, & WEBER, FREDERICK PARKES. 1863–1962
Climatotherapy and balneotherapy. London, *Smith, Elder & Co.*, 1907.

2007 NAGELSCHMIDT, KARL FRANZ. 1875–1952
Ueber Diathermie. (Transthermie, Thermopenetration.) *Münch. med. Wschr.*, 1909, **56,** 2575–76.
Nagelschmidt employed high frequency currents in treatment after the suggestions of Tesla and the work of Nernst, claiming priority over the latter in the use of this method. Nagelschmidt named this form of treatment "diathermy".

2008 ——. Lehrbuch der Diathermie. Berlin, *J. Springer*, 1913.

2009 SCHLIEPHAKE, ERWIN. 1894–
Therapeutische Versuche im elektrischen Kurzwellenfeld. *Klin. Wschr.*, 1930, **9,** 2333–36.
Introduction of short-wave diathermy.

2010 PIÉRY, ANTOINE MARIUS. 1873–
Traité de climatologie biologique et médicale. Publié sous la direction de M. Piéry. 3 vols. Paris, *Masson*, 1934.

2010.1 POHLMANN, R., *et al.*
Ueber die Ausbreitung und Absorption des Ultraschalls im menschlichen Gewebe und seine therapeutische Wirkung an Ischias und Plexusneuralgie. *Dtsch. med. Wschr.*, 1939, **65,** 251–54.
First therapeutic use of ultrasonics. With R. Richter and E. Parow.

2010.2 WAKIM, KHALIL GEORGES. 1907– , *et al.*
Therapeutic possibilities of microwaves. *J. Amer. med. Ass.*, 1949, **139,** 989–93.
Introduction of microwave radiation therapy. With J. F. Herrick, G. M. Martin, and F. H. Krusen.

For history of physical therapy, see 2029, 2043, 2046–7, 2057.1

2011–2028 BLOOD TRANSFUSION

See also 860–913, HAEMATOLOGY.

2011 COLLE, GIOVANNI. 1558–1631
Methodus facile parandi iucunda tuta et nova medicamenta. Venetiis, 1628.
Page 170 includes the first definite description of a blood transfusion.

2012 LOWER, Richard. 1631–1691
The method observed in transfusing the blood out of one live animal into another. *Phil. Trans.*, 1665–66, **1,** 353–58.
In February 1665 Lower successfully transfused dogs with blood.

2013 DENIS, Jean Baptiste [Denys]. *c.* 1625–1704
Lettre . . . touchant deux expériences de la transfusion faites sur des hommes. Paris, *J. Cusson*, 1667.
The first transfusion of blood into a human being was performed by Denis, when, on June 15, 1667, he transfused lamb's blood into a youth. A later subject of Denis proved a failure – probably the first recorded case of incompatible blood transfusion. The work is summarized in *J. Sçavans*, 1667, 93–96.

2014 LOWER, Richard. 1631–1691, & KING, *Sir* Edmund. 1629–1707
An account of the experiment of transfusion, practised upon a man in London. *Phil. Trans.*, 1667, **2,** 557–64.
First transfusion of blood performed on a human in England, Nov. 23, 1667.

2015 BLUNDELL, James. 1790–1877
Experiments on the transfusion of blood by the syringe. *Med.-chir. Trans.*, 1818, **9,** 56–92.
(See No. 2017.)

2016 PRÉVOST, Jean Louis. 1790–1850, & DUMAS, Jean Baptiste André. 1800–1884
Examen du sang et de son action dans les divers phénomènes de la vie. *Ann. Chim.* (*Paris*), 1821, **18,** 280–97.
First successful use of defibrinated blood for animal transfusions. This was the first attempt to prevent coagulation during transfusion.

2017 BLUNDELL, James. 1790–1877
Observations on transfusion of blood. *Lancet*, 1828–29, **2,** 321–24.
Blundell revived interest in blood transfusion through his attempts to alleviate post-partum haemorrhage by this means. His investigations showed that transfusion between animals of different species was impracticable, pointed out the difficulties of direct transfusion, and led him to the invention of a funnel and syringe for performing indirect transfusion.

2018 LANDOIS, Leonard. 1837–1902
Auflösung der rothen Blutzellen. *Zbl. med. Wiss.*, 1874, **12,** 419–22.
Landois discovered the haemolyzing effect of blood serum of one species when transfused into another.

2019 HUSTIN, Albert. 1882–
Note sur une nouvelle méthode de transfusion. *Bull. Soc. roy. Sci. méd. Brux.*, 1914, **72,** 104–11.
Hustin demonstrated the anticoagulant powers of sodium citrate and glucose in blood transfusion.

2020 AGOTE, Luis. 1868–1954
Nuevo procédimiento para la transfusion del sangre. *An. Inst. mod. Clin. méd.* (*B. Aires*), 1914–15, **1,** 24–31.
Agote was the first to transfuse citrated blood. Text in Spanish and French.

2021 LEWISOHN, Richard. 1875–1962
A new and greatly simplified method of blood transfusion. A preliminary report. *Med. Rec.* (*N.Y.*), 1915, **87,** 141–42.
About the same time as Agote, Lewisohn introduced the citrate method of blood transfusion. See also his later paper in *Surg. Gynec. Obstet.*, 1915, **21,** 37–47.

2021.1 ROBERTSON, OSWALD HOPE. 1886–
Transfusion with preserved red blood cells. *Med. Bull.* (*Paris*), 1917–1918, **1,** 436–40.
Robertson stored blood and used it with good results to treat casualties on the battlefield.

2022 FLOSDORF, EARL WILLIAM. 1904–1958, & MUDD, STUART. 1893–
Procedure and apparatus for preservation in "lyophile" form of serum and other biological substances. *J. Immunol.*, 1935, **29,** 389–425.

2023 MARRIOTT, HUGH LESLIE. 1900– , & KEKWICK, ALAN. 1909–1974
Continuous drip blood transfusion. *Lancet*, 1935, **1,** 977–81.
Introduction of the slow-drip method of blood transfusion.

2024 HEDENIUS, PER JOHANNES. 1906–
A new method of blood transfusion. *Acta med. scand.*, 1936, **89,** 263–267.
Heparin used in blood transfusion. See also the same journal, **88**, 443–49.

2025 YUDIN, SERGEI SERGEIEVICH. 1891–1954
Transfusion of cadaver blood. *J. Amer. med. Ass.*, 1936, **106,** 997–99.
Cadaver blood used in human transfusions. Prof. Samov of Kharkov carried out the first experimental work on transfusion of cadaver blood in 1927.

2026 FANTUS, BERNARD. 1874–1940
The therapy of the Cook County Hospital. Blood preservation. *J. Amer. med. Ass.*, 1937, **109,** 128–31.
Describes the establishment of the first blood bank (at the Cook County Hospital).

2027 GOODALL, JAMES ROBERT. 1878–1947, *et al.*
An inexhaustible source of blood for transfusion, and its preservation. Preliminary report. *Surg. Gynec. Obstet.*, 1938, **66,** 176–78.
J. R. Goodall, F. O. Anderson, G. T. Altimas, and F. L. MacPhail pointed out the possibility of using placental blood for transfusion purposes.

2028 GRÖNWALL, ANDERS JOHAN TROED. 1912– , & INGLEMAN, BJÖRN.
Untersuchungen über Dextran und sein Verhalten bei parenteraler Zufuhr. *Acta physiol. scand.*, 1944, **7,** 97–107.
Introduction of dextran as plasma substitute.

For history of blood transfusion, see 2029.1, 2068.1

History of Pharmacology & Therapeutics

2029 FLOYER, *Sir* JOHN. 1649–1734
The ancient ψυχρολουσία revived; or, an essay to prove cold bathing both safe and useful. London, *S. Smith & B. Walford*, 1702.
A history of cold bathing.

2029.1 SCHEEL, PAUL. 1773–1811
Die Transfusion des Blutes und Einsprützung der Arzeneyen in die Adern. Historisch und in Rücksicht auf die practische Heilkunde bearbeitet. 2 vols. Copenhagen, *F. Brummer*, 1802–03.
An excellent early history of the subject. A third volume was published by J. F. Dieffenbach, Berlin, 1828.

2030 GUIBOURT, Nicholas Jean Baptiste Gaston. 1790–1867
Histoire abrégée des drogues simples. 2 vols. Paris, *L. Colas*, 1820.

2031 HOEVEN, Cornelis Pruys van der. 1792–1871
De historia medicamentorum. Lugduni Batavorum, *S. & J. Luchtmans*, 1846.

2032 FLÜCKIGER, Friedrich August. 1828–1894, & HANBURY, Daniel. 1825–1875
Pharmacographia. A history of the principal drugs of vegetable origin, met with in Great Britain and British India. London, *Macmillan & Co.*, 1874.

2033 PETERSEN, Jacob Julius. 1840–1912
Hauptmomente in der geschichtlichen Entwickelung der medicinischen Therapie. Kopenhagen, *A. F. Höst*, 1877.

2034 WARING, Edward John. 1819–1891
Bibliotheca therapeutica, or bibliography of therapeutics, chiefly in reference to articles of the materia medica, with numerous critical, historical, and therapeutical annotations, and an appendix containing the bibliography of British mineral waters. 2 vols. London, *New Sydenham Soc.*, 1878–79.

2035 BELL, Jacob. 1810–1859, & REDWOOD, Theophilus. 1806–1892
Historical sketch of the progress of pharmacy in Great Britain. London, *Butler & Tanner*, 1880.

2036 PETERS, Hermann. 1847–1920
Aus pharmazeutischer Vorzeit in Bild und Wort. 2 vols. Berlin, *J. Springer*, 1889–91.
English translation, Chicago, 1899.

2037 FIESSINGER, Charles Albert. 1857–1942
La thérapeutique des vieux maîtres. Paris, *Soc. d'Editions Sci.*, 1897.

2038 BERENDES, Julius. 1837–1914
Geschichte der Pharmazie. Leipzig, *E. Gunther*, 1898.

2039 DRAGENDORFF, Georg Johann Noël. 1836–1898
Die Heilpflanzen der verschiedenen Völker und Zeiten. Stuttgart, *F. Enke*, 1898.

2040 ANDRÉ-PONTIER, L.
Histoire de la pharmacie. Paris, *O. Doin*, 1900.

2041 SCHELENZ, Hermann. 1846–1922
Geschichte der Pharmazie. Berlin, *J. Springer*, 1904.

2043 MARTIN, Ferdinand Heinrich Alfred. 1874–
Deutsches Badewesen in vergangenen Tagen. Jena, *E. Diederichs*, 1906.

2044 HOEFLER, Max. 1848–1914
Die volkmedizinische Organotherapie und ihr Verhältnis zum Kultopfer. Stuttgart, [1908?].

2045 WOOTTON, A. C. 1843–1910
Chronicles of pharmacy. 2 vols. London, *Macmillan & Co.*, 1910.

2046 GRASSET, HECTOR.
La médecine naturiste à travers les siècles. Histoire de la physiothérapie. Paris, *J. Rousset*, 1911.

2047 COLWELL, HECTOR ALFRED. 1875–1946
An essay on the history of electrotherapy and diagnosis. London, *W. Heinemann*, 1922.

2048 ROHDE, ELEANOR SINCLAIR. *d.* 1950
The old English herbals. London, *Longmans, Green & Co.*, 1922.

2049 BENEDICENTI, ALBERICO.
Malati medici e farmacisti. Storia dei rimedi traverso i secoli e delle teorie che ne spiegano l'azione sull'organismo. 2 vols. Milano, *V. Hoepli*, 1924–25.
Second edition 1947–51.

2050 KLEBS, ARNOLD CARL. 1870–1943
Catalogue of early herbals. Lugano, *l'Art Ancien*, 1925.

2051 URDANG, GEORGE. 1882–1960
Der Apotheker als Subjekt und Objekt der Literatur. Berlin, *J. Springer*, 1926.

2052 LA WALL, CHARLES HERBERT. 1871–1937
Four thousand years of pharmacy; an outline history of pharmacy. Philadelphia, *J. B. Lippincott*, 1927.
First history of pharmacy by an American. Reprinted as *The curious lore of drugs and medicines*, New York, Garden City Publ. Co., 1936.

2053 SINGER, CHARLES JOSEPH. 1876–1960
The herbal in antiquity and its transmission to later ages. *J. Hellen. Stud.*, 1927, **47**, 1–52.
In this paper Singer showed the methods by which ancient herbals are studied and the results achieved by such study.

2054 THOMPSON, CHARLES JOHN SAMUEL. 1862–1943
The mystery and art of the apothecary. London, *John Lane*, [1929].

2055 REUTTER DE ROSEMONT, LOUIS. 1876–
Histoire de la pharmacie à travers les âges. 2 vols. Paris, *Peyronnet*, 1931.

2056 COULTER, JOHN STANLEY. 1885–1949
Physical therapy. New York, *P. B. Hoeber*, 1932.
Clio Medica series.

2056.1 TISCHNER, RUDOLF, 1879–
Geschichte der Homöopathie. 1 vol. [in 4]. Leipzig, *B. Schwabe*, 1932–39.

2057 ADLUNG, ALFRED. 1875– , & URDANG, GEORGE. 1882–1960
Grundiss der Geschichte der deutschen Pharmazie. Berlin, *J. Springer*, 1935.

2057.1 BRAUCHLE, Alfred
Naturheilkunde in Lebensbildern. Leipzig, *Reclam*, 1937.
Mainly 19th–20th century: includes hydrotherapy, massage, and dietetics. Second edition, 1951.

2058 GRIER, James.
A history of pharmacy. London, *Pharmaceutical Press*, 1937.

2059 ARBER, Agnes Robertson. 1879–1960
Herbals: their origin and evolution. A chapter in the history of botany, 1470–1670. 2nd edition. Cambridge, *University Press*, 1938.
Includes an invaluable bibliography. Reprinted 1953.

2061 TAYLOR, Norman. 1883–
Cinchona in Java: the story of quinine. New York, *Greenberg*, [1945].

2062 BUESS, Heinrich. 1911–
Die Injektion. *Ciba Z.*, 1946, **9**, 3594–3642.
Deals exhaustively with the history of intravenous and intramuscular injection.

2063 HOWARD-JONES, Norman. 1909–
A critical study of the origins and early development of hypodermic medication. *J. Hist. Med.*, 1947, **2**, 201–49.

2064 BOUSSEL, Patrice.
Histoire illustrée de la pharmacie. Paris, *Guy Le Prat*, [1949].

2065 JARAMILLO-ARANGO, Jaime. 1897–1962
A critical review of the basic facts in the history of cinchona. *J. Linn. Soc.* (*Botany*), 1949, **53**, 272–309.

2067 URDANG, George. 1882–1960
The development of pharmacopoeias. *Bull. Wld Hlth Org.*, 1951, **4**, 577–603.

2068 MOLDENKE, Harold Norman. 1909– , & MOLDENKE, Alma Lance. 1908–
Plants of the Bible. Waltham, Mass., *Chronica Botanica Co.*, 1952.
The most comprehensive treatise available on plants and plant products mentioned in the Bible.

2068.1 MALUF, Noble Suydam R. 1913–
History of blood transfusion. *J. Hist. Med.*, 1954, **9**, 59–107.

2068.2 MATTHEWS, Leslie Gerald.
History of pharmacy in Britain. Edinburgh, *E. & S. Livingstone*, 1962.

2068.3 BÖTTCHER, Helmuth Maximilian. 1895–
Miracle drugs. A history of antibiotics. London, *Heinemann*, 1963.
First published in German, 1959.

2068.4 HOLMSTEDT, Bo, & LILJESTRAND, Goran.
Readings in pharmacology. Selected and edited by B. Holmstedt and G. Liljestrand. Oxford, *Pergamon Press*, 1963.
An anthology of outstanding achievements in the growth of pharmacology.

2068.5 KREMERS, Edward. 1865–1941, & URDANG, George. 1882–1960
History of pharmacy. 3rd ed. Philadelphia, *Lippincott*, 1963.

2068.6 THOMAS, KENNETH BRYN.
Curare, its history and usage. London, *Pitman*, [1964].

2068.7 TREASE, GEORGE EDWARD. 1902–
Pharmacy in history. London, *Baillière, Tindall and Cox*, 1964.
Traces the origins of pharmacy in ancient civilizations and its development in England from mediaeval to modern times.

2068.8 VELLARD, J.
Histoire du curare. Les poisons de chasse en Amérique du Sud. Paris, *Gallimard*, [1965].

2068.9 HEILMANN, KARL EUGEN.
Kräuterbücher in Bild und Geschichte. München-Allach, *K. Kölbl*, 1966.

2069–2117 TOXICOLOGY

See also 1717–1757, MEDICAL JURISPRUDENCE.

2069 NICANDER [NIKANDER]. 185–135 B.C.
Theriaca et alexipharmaca. Venetiis, *apud Aldum Manutium*, 1499.
Nicander was a Greek poet and physician. His *Theriaca* deal in 958 hexameters with the symptoms and treatment of poisoning by the bites of poisonous animals; the *Alexipharmaca* consider intoxications through animal, vegetable and mineral poisoning and their suitable antidotes. He is the first writer to mention the medicinal use of the leech. The above work has a Greek text; a Latin translation appeared at Cologne in 1531.

2070 PETRUS *de Abano*. 1250–1315
Tractatus de venenis. Mantua, [*Thomas of Hermannstadt*], 1472.
One of the earliest of the important treatises on toxicology, and one of the finest, typographically, of medical incunabula. For an English translation, see *Ann. med. Hist.*, 1924, **6**, 26–53.

2071 LETTSOM, JOHN COAKLEY. 1744–1815
Some remarks on the effects of lignum quassiae amarae. *Mem. med. Soc. Lond.*, 1779–87, **1**, 128–65.
Includes (p. 151) "original account of alcoholism, which is incidentally the first paper on the drug habit" (Garrison).

2072 ORFILA, MATHIEU JOSEPH BONAVENTURE. 1787–1853
Traité des poisons. 2 vols. Paris, *Crochard*, 1814–15.
Orfila, pioneer toxicologist, was the leading medico-legal expert of his time. He was born in Minorca, studied at Valencia, Barcelona and Paris, and was one of the founders of the Académie de Médicine. He was a popular teacher, and is particularly remembered for his writings on toxicology. English translation, 1815–17.

2073 PARIS, JOHN AYRTON. 1875–1856
Pharmacologia; or the history of medicinal substances, with a view to establish the art of prescribing. 3rd ed. London, *W. Phillips*, 1820.
First description of arsenic cancer (p. 133).

2074 WATERTON, CHARLES. 1782–1865
Wanderings in South America. London, *J. Mawman*, 1825.
Includes a detailed description of the paralysing effects of curare.

2075 ADDISON, Thomas. 1793–1860, & MORGAN, John. 1797–1847
An essay on the operation of poisonous agents upon the living body. London, *Longman, Rees*, 1829.

First book in English on the action of poisons on the living body.

2076 CHRISTISON, *Sir* Robert. 1797–1882
A treatise on poisons. Edinburgh, *A. Black*, 1829.

Christison, famous toxicologist, was professor of medical jurisprudence at Edinburgh. During the trial of Burke and Hare he performed an autopsy on the body of one of the victims and gave evidence as to the cause of death.

2077 MARSH, James. 1794–1846
Account of a method of separating small quantities of arsenic from substances with which it may be mixed. *Edinb. new phil. J.*, 1836, **21,** 229–36.

Marsh method for the detection of arsenic.

2077.1 SLEEMAN, *Sir* William Henry. 1788–1856
Rambles and recollections of an Indian official. Vol. 1. London, *Hatchard & Sons*, 1844.

Lathyrism was known to Hippocrates. Sleeman, who had no special knowledge of medicine, gave the first detailed account.

2078 KÖLLIKER, Rudolph Albert von. 1817–1905
Physiologische Untersuchungen über die Wirkung einiger Gifte. *Virchows Arch. path. Anat.*, 1856, **10,** 3–77, 235–96.

First investigation of the effects of poisons on muscular contraction.

2079 BERNARD, Claude. 1813–1878
Analyse physiologique des propriétés des systèmes musculaires et nerveux au moyen du curare. *C. R. Acad. Sci. (Paris)*, 1856, **43,** 825–829.

Bernard showed that curare acted by stopping the transmission of impulses from motor nerves to voluntary muscles.

2080 WORMLEY, Theodor George. 1826–1897
Micro-chemistry of poisons. New York, *Bailliere Bros.*, 1867.

2081 LEWIN, Louis. 1850–1929
Die Nebenwirkungen der Arzneimittel. Berlin, *A. Hirschwald*, 1881.

This is the only book of its kind. It deals with the borderline between the pharmacological and the toxicological action of drugs with the untoward or side-side-effects of all kinds of medicaments. For details regarding this book and its author, see D. I. Macht, *Ann. med. Hist.*, 1931, **3,** 179–94, which includes a bibliography of Lewin's writings.

2082 KUNKEL, Adam Josef. 1848–1905
Handbuch der Toxikologie. Jena, *G. Fischer*, 1899–1901.

2083 KOBERT, Eduard Rudolf. 1854–1918
Lehrbuch der Intoxikationen. 2te. Aufl. 2 vols. Stuttgart, *F. Enke*, 1902–06.

2084 ABEL, John Jacob. 1857–1938, & FORD, William Webber. 1871–1941
On the poisons of Amanita phalloides. *J. biol. Chem.*, 1906–07, **2,** 273–88.

Abel and Ford showed that there were two poisons in the fungus *Amanita phalloides* and that immunity against them could be attained. A further study on the subject by them is in *Arch. exp. Path. Pharmak.*, 1908, Suppl., 8–15.

2085 SCOTT, *Sir* HENRY HAROLD. 1874–1956
On the 'vomiting sickness' of Jamaica. *Ann. trop. Med. Parasit.*, 1916, **10,** 1–78.
Discovery of the cause of the "vomiting sickness of Jamaica", ackee poisoning.

2086 LEWIN, LOUIS. 1850–1929
Phantastica. Berlin, *G. Stilke*, 1924.
A monograph on narcotic drugs. English translation, 1931.

2089 LESCHKE, ERICH FRIEDRICH WILHELM. 1877–1933
Die wichtigsten Vergiftungen. Fortschritte in deren Erkennung und Behandlung. München, *J. F. Lehmann*, 1933.

2090 McINTYRE, ARCHIBALD ROSS. 1902–
Curare, its history, nature, and clinical use. Chicago, *University Press*, 1947.

2091 HALD, JENS, *et al.*
The sensitizing effect of tetraethylthiuramdisulphide (Antabuse) to ethylalcohol. *Acta pharmacol.* (*Kbh.*), 1948, **4,** 285–96.
Introduction of "antabuse" in the treatment of alcoholism. With E. Jacobsen and V. Larsen. See also *Lancet*, 1948, **2**, 1004.

2092–2101 LEAD POISONING

See also 2118–2138, INDUSTRIAL HYGIENE AND MEDICINE; 2069–2091, TOXICOLOGY.

2092 CITOIS, FRANÇOIS [CITESIUS]. 1572–1652
De novo et populari apud Pictones dolore colico bilioso diatriba. Augustoriti Pictonum, *apud Antonium Mesnier*, 1616.
Citois described Poitou colic, "colica Pictonum", in great detail, and it was this description which was responsible for the condition being recognized as a definite syndrome.

2093 HUXHAM, JOHN. 1692–1768
De morbo colico Damnoniensi. Londini, *S. Austen*, 1739.
Huxham left a vivid account of the "Devonshire colic". He was at fault, however, in ascribing it to the tartar extracted from apples in the process of making cider.

2094 CADWALADER, THOMAS. 1708–1779
An essay on the West-India dry-gripes . . . to which is added, an extraordinary case in physick. Philadelphia, *B. Franklin*, 1745.
Cadwalader, a pupil of Cheselden, left a classical account of lead colic and lead palsy. This was later shown by Benjamin Franklin to be due to the consumption of Jamaica rum which had been distilled through lead pipes. The "extraordinary case" mentioned in the title, refers to a case of osteomalacia.

2095 TRONCHIN, THÉODORE. 1709–1781
De colica pictonum. Genevae, *apud fratres Cramer*, 1757.
Tronchin, sometime physician to Voltaire, showed that the so-called "Poitou colic" was caused by drinking water which had passed through lead gutters. Tronchin introduced inoculation into Holland, France, and Switzerland; he was Boerhaave's favourite pupil and became a very wealthy practitioner.

2096 BAKER, *Sir* GEORGE. 1722–1809
An essay concerning the cause of the endemial colic of Devonshire. London, *J. Hughs*, 1767.

Baker demonstrated that the cider of Devonshire contained lead, while that made in other parts of England did not. He further showed that it was common practice in Devon to line cider presses with lead. He proved that lead poisoning was the cause of Devonshire colic. He was responsible for the abandonment of lead in the making of cider presses, and thus for the disappearance of the colic. See also his paper in *Med. Trans. Coll. Phys. Lond.*, 1768, 1, 175–256.

2097 MÉRAT DE VAUMARTOISE, FRANÇOIS VICTOR. 1780–1851
Sur la colique, vulgairement appelée colique des peintres, des plombiers, du plomb, etc. Paris, *P. F. Rigot*, an XI [1803].

2098 TANQUEREL DES PLANCHES, LOUIS JEAN CHARLES MARIE. 1810–1862
Traité des maladies de plomb ou saturnines. 2 vols. Paris, *Ferra*, 1839.

Classical description of the diseases found among lead workers. English translation, 1848.

2099 BURTON, HENRY. 1799–1849
On a remarkable effect upon the human gums produced by the absorption of lead. *Med.-chir. Trans.*, 1840, **23,** 63–79.

Burton was the first to note the blue line on the gums in lead poisoning – "Burton's blue line" – an important diagnostic sign. He was physician to St. Thomas's Hospital, London.

2100 DEJERINE-KLUMPKE, AUGUSTA. 1859–1927
Des polynévrites en général et des paralysies et atrophies saturnines en particulier. Paris, *F. Alcan*, 1889.

Madame Dejerine-Klumpke, famous neurologist, contributed an important work on lead palsies.

2101 LEGGE, *Sir* THOMAS MORISON. 1863–1932, & GOADBY, *Sir* KENNETH WELDON. 1873–1958
Lead poisoning and lead absorption. London, *E. Arnold*, 1912.

2102–2115 VENOMS

2102 REDI, FRANCESCO. 1626–1697
Osservazioni intorno alle vipere. Firenze, *Stella*, 1664.

The first methodical work on snake-poison. Redi demonstrated for the first time that, for the poison to produce its effects, it must be injected under the skin.

2103 FONTANA, FELICE. 1730–1805
Richerche fisiche sopra il veleno della vipera. Lucca, *J. Giusti*, 1767.

The starting point of modern investigations of serpent venoms. English translation, 1787.

2104 MITCHELL, SILAS WEIR. 1829–1914, & REICHERT, EDWARD TYSON. 1855–
Researches upon the venom of the rattlesnake. Washington, *Smithsonian Inst.*, 1860.

See 2106.

2105 FAYRER, *Sir* JOSEPH. 1824–1907
The thanatophidia of India. London, *J. & A. Churchill*, 1872.
Describes all the venomous snakes of India. One of the finest books on the subject.

2106 MITCHELL, SILAS WEIR. 1829–1914, & REICHERT, EDWARD TYSON. 1855–
Researches upon the venoms of poisonous serpents. Washington, *Smithsonian Inst.*, 1886.
Mitchell (see also No. 2104) and Reichert showed snake venom to be protein in nature, and demonstrated the presence of toxic albumins. Mitchell was one of the first to investigate the snake venoms.

2107 CALMETTE, LÉON CHARLES ALBERT. 1863–1933
Contribution à l'étude du vénin des serpents. *Ann. Inst. Pasteur*, 1894, **8,** 275–91; 1895, **9,** 225–51; 1898, **12,** 343–47.
Calmette carried out extensive investigations on the immunization of animals to venoms. He obtained antivenom sera with therapeutic properties.

2108 FRASER, *Sir* THOMAS RICHARD. 1841–1919
On the rendering of animals immune against the venom of the cobra and other serpents; and on the antidotal properties of the blood serum of the immunised animals. *Brit. med. J.*, 1895, **1,** 1309–12.
Fraser investigated the possibilities of immunization against cobra venom and obtained "antivenene", an antivenom serum.

2109 CALMETTE, LÉON CHARLES ALBERT. 1863–1933
Le vénin des serpents. Paris, *Soc. d'éd. Scient.*, 1896.

2110 FLEXNER, SIMON. 1863–1946, & NOGUCHI, HIDEYO. 1876–1928
Snake venom in relation to haemolysis, bacteriolysis, and toxicity. *J. exp. Med.*, 1902, **6,** 277–301.

2111 KYES, PRESTON. 1875–
Ueber die Wirkungsweise des Cobragiftes. *Berl. klin. Wschr.*, 1902, **39,** 886–90; 918–22.
While in Germany Kyes published an important series of papers on venoms. He showed lecithin to be a complement of cobra-haemolysin.

2112 ——. & SACHS, HANS. 1877–1945
Zur Kenntniss der Cobragift activirenden Substanzen. *Berl. klin. Wschr.*, 1903, **40,** 21–23, 57–60, 82–85.

2113 ——. Ueber die Isolirung von Schlangengift-Lecithiden. *Berl. klin. Wschr.*, 1903, **40,** 956–59, 982–84.

2114 NOGUCHI, HIDEYO. 1876–1928
Snake venoms. Washington, *Carnegie Inst.*, 1909.

2115 BRAZIL, VITAL. 1865–1950
A defensa contra o ophidismo. Sao Paulo, 1911.
Brazil founded the Instituto Butantan, São Paulo, one of the first institutes to produce antivenin sera on a large scale. French translation, 1911.

History of Toxicology

2116 LEWIN, Louis. 1850–1929
Die Gifte in der Weltgeschichte. Berlin, *J. Springer*, 1920.

Lewin was a prolific writer, producing more than 200 books and papers. The above is perhaps his best work, and contains a history of poisonings from the most ancient times to the present century.

2117 ——. Die Pfeilgifte, nach eigenen toxikologischen und ethnologischen Untersuchungen. Leipzig, *J. A. Barth*, 1923.

2118–2138 INDUSTRIAL HYGIENE AND MEDICINE

See also 2069–2117, Toxicology.

2118 ELLENBOG, Ulrich. 1440–1499
Von den gifftigen besen Tempffen und Reuchen. Augsburg, *M. Ramminger*, 1524.

Written in 1473 but not published until 1524, this is the first known work on industrial hygiene and toxicology. A reprint of the text appears in *Münch. Beitr. Lit. Naturwiss. Med.*, 1927, **2**, Sonderheft; and an English translation in *Lancet*, 1932, **1**, 270–71.

2119 PANSA. Martin.
Consilium peripneumoniacum. Leipzig, *T. Schürer*, 1614.

Martin Pansa, a pupil of Georg Agricola, wrote the most important work on occupational disease before Ramazzini. He described the symptoms of the lung diseases of miners and smelters.

2120 STOCKHUSEN, Samuel.
Libellus de lythargyrii fumo morbifico. Goslar, 1656.

Stockhusen had considerable experience in treating the diseases of miners. His book on industrial diseases did much to clarify contemporary knowledge regarding the relative toxicity of lead, mercury, arsenic, cobalt and other metals, although he claimed that lead colic was caused only by lead fumes. French translation of the book, 1776.

2121 RAMAZZINI, Bernardino. 1633–1714
De morbis artificum diatriba. Mutinae, *A. Capponi*, 1700.

Ramazzini was the first to deal adequately with occupational diseases; his book was the first systematic treatise on the subject. It deals with pneumoconiosis and other diseases of miners, with lead poisoning in potters, with silicosis in stonemasons, diseases among metal workers, and even a chapter devoted to the "diseases of learned men". It was translated into English in 1705; a new English translation by Wilmer Cave Wright appeared in 1940.

2122 POTT, Percivall. 1714–1788
Chirurgical observations relative to the cataract, the polypus of the nose, the cancer of the scrotum, *etc*. London, *for L. Hawes, W. Clarke and R. Collins*, 1775.

First description of an occupational cancer (chimney-sweeps' cancer of the scrotum).

2123 THACKRAH, CHARLES TURNER. 1795–1833
The effects of the principal arts, trades and professions, and of civic states and habits of living on health and longevity. London, *Longman*, 1831.

The first systematic publication in Great Britain on industrial disease and its prevention. Thackrah took an active part in the foundation of the Leeds School of Medicine. Although he must have followed to some extent Ramazzini's work, Thackrah dealt with several diseases incident to trades peculiar to England. A reprint of the 2nd (1832) edition, with a life of the author by A. Meiklejohn, was published in 1957.

2124 POL, B., & WATELLE, T. J. J.
Mémoire sur les effets de la compression de l'air. *Ann. Hyg. publ.*, 1854, 2 sér., **1**, 241–79.

An early paper on "caisson sickness".

2125 THIERSCH, CARL. 1822–1895
De maxillarum necrosi phosphorica. Lipsiae, *apud A. Edelmannum*, 1867.

A classical description of phosphoric necrosis of the jaw.

2126 VOLKMANN, RICHARD VON. 1830–1889
Beiträge zur Chirurgie, anschliessend an einen Bericht über die Thätigkeit der chirurgischen Universitäts-Klinik zu Halle im Jahre 1873. Leipzig, *Breitkopf u. Härtel*, 1875.

Contains (pp. 370–81) first description of industrial tar and paraffin cancer.

2127 HIRT, LUDWIG. 1844–1907
Die Krankheiten der Arbeiter. 4 vols. Breslau, Leipzig, *F. Hirt u. Sohn*, 1871–78.

2128 HÄRTING, FRIEDRICH HUGO, & HESSE, WALTHER.
Der Lungenkrebs, die Bergkrankheit in den Schneeberger Gruben. *Vjschr. gerichtl. Med.*, 1879, n.F. **30,** 296–309; **31,** 102–32, 313–37.

First description of miners' cancer.

2129 OLIVER, *Sir* THOMAS. 1853–1942
Dangerous trades; the historical, social, and legal aspects of industrial occupations as affecting health, by a number of experts. Edited by T. OLIVER. London, *John Murray*, 1902.

2130 ——. Diseases of occupation, from the legislative, social, and medical points of view. London, *Methuen & Co.*, 1908.

2131 HILL, *Sir* LEONARD ERSKINE. 1866–1952
Caisson sickness, and the physiology of work in compressed air. London, *E. Arnold*, 1912.

2132 MOCK, HARRY EDGAR. 1880–1959
Industrial medicine and surgery. Philadelphia, *W. B. Saunders*, 1919.

2133 VERNON, HORACE MIDDLETON. 1870–1951
Industrial fatigue and efficiency. London, *G. Routledge*, 1921.

2134 HAMILTON, ALICE. 1869–
Industrial poisons in the United States. New York, *Macmillan Co.*, 1925.

2135 BREZINA, Ernst.
Die gewerblichen Vergiftungen und ihre Bekämpfung. Stuttgart, *F. Enke*, 1932.

History of Industrial Hygiene and Medicine

2136 ROSEN, George, 1910–
The history of miners' diseases. A medical and social interpretation. New York, *Schuman's*, 1943.

2137 TELEKY, Ludwig. 1872–1957
History of factory and mine hygiene. New York, *Columbia University Press*, 1948.

2138 FULTON, John Farquhar. 1899–1960
Aviation medicine in its preventive aspects: an historical survey. London, *Oxford University Press*, 1948.
Heath Clark Lectures, 1947.

MILITARY AND NAVAL HYGIENE AND MEDICINE

2139–2188

See also 5547–5813.7, Surgery.

2139 PARÉ, Ambroise. 1510–1590
La méthode de traicter les playes faictes par hacquebutes et aultres bastons à feu: et de celles qui sont faictes par flèches, dardz et semblables. Paris, *Chés viuant Gaulterot*, 1545.
Among Paré's most important works is his treatise on gunshot wounds. He is one of the greatest of the military surgeons, and is particularly remembered for his abandonment of the practice of cauterization of gunshot wounds with boiling oil, until his time a universal procedure.

2139.1 MAGGI, Bartolomeo. 1477–1552
De vulnerum sclopetorum et bombardarum curatione tractatus Bononiae, *per B. Bonardum*, 1552.
Maggi, professor of surgery at Bologna, wrote an important work on military surgery. He showed that not all gunshot wounds suppurated and he discarded cauterization, treating such wounds with white of egg and salt water.

2140 GALE, Thomas. 1507–1587
An excellent treatise of wounds made with gonneshot. London, *R. Hall*, (1563).
Gale, a contemporary of Paré, was surgeon in Henry VIII's army at Montreuil. His book supported the views of Paré regarding the treatment of gunshot wounds, denying the poisonous effect of bullets; Gale, however, applied messy and complicated unguents to wounds, doing more harm than good. Forms part 3 of his *Certaine workes of chirurgerie* (No. 2371).

2141 CLOWES, William. 1544–1604
A prooved practise for all young chirurgians, concerning burnings with gunpowder, and woundes made with gunshot. London, *T. Orwyn for T. Cadman*, 1588.
An interesting picture of Elizabethan surgery is given by William Clowes in this book on gunshot wounds. Clowes, the best surgical writer in Elizabethan times, was surgeon to St. Bartholomew's Hospital. In amputation he covered the stump with integument – an earlier form of the flap method. The *Selected Writings of William Clowes* were edited by F. N. L. Poynter, London, 1949.

2142 FABRY, Wilhelm [Fabricius *Hildanus*]. 1560–1634
New Feldt Arztny Buch von Kranckheiten und Schäden, so in Kriegen den Wundartzten gemeinlich fürfallen. Basel, *L. König*, 1615.

Fabry's book includes an early description of a field drug chest for army use. He was one of the most eminent surgeons of his time, although not prepared to adopt all the teachings of Paré. He had considerable mechanical ingenuity and devised many pieces of apparatus.

2143 MAGATI, Cesare. 1579–1647
De rara medicatione vulnerum. Venetiis, *apud A. & B. Dei, fratres*, 1616.

Like Paré, Magati believed that gunshot wounds were not in themselves poisonous. He suggested a bandage moistened with plain water in place of the various salves then in vogue.

2144 WOODALL, John. 1556–1643
The surgions mate. London, *E. Griffin*, 1617.

One of the earliest books on naval medicine, this contained much sound advice for the ship's surgeon. Woodall was an early advocate of limes and lemons as a preventive measure against scurvy. He was surgeon to St. Bartholomew's Hospital.

2145 MINDERER, Raymund. *c.* 1570–1621
Medicina militaris, seu libellus castrensis. Augspurg, *A. Aperger*, 1620.

Minderer's book gives a good idea of the position of military surgery during the Thirty Years' War. He published a pharmacopoeia in 1621; he also discovered ammonium acetate. An English edition of the above book appeared in 1674.

2146 PURMANN, Matthäus Gottfried. 1649–1711
Der rechte und warhafftige Feldscher. Franckfurt & Leipzig, *M. Rohrlach*, 1690.

Purmann was a skilful army surgeon – one of the most famous of the period. Despite this he believed in the efficacy of the weapon-salve and the sympathetic powder.

2147 COCKBURN, William. 1669–1739
An account of the nature, causes, symptoms and cure of the distempers that are incident in seafaring people. With observations on the diet of the sea-men in his Majesty's navy. London, *Hugh Newman*, 1696.

Cockburn studied medicine at Leyden; he became famous on account of his secret remedy for dysentery. The book is a record of two years spent as a ship's doctor.

2148 ATKINS, John. 1685–1757
The navy-surgeon, or a practical system of surgery. London, *C. Ward*, 1734.

Atkins was an English naval surgeon. His book includes some useful case reports and contains the first English description of African trypanosomiasis.

2149 LE DRAN, Henri François. 1685–1770
Traité ou reflexions tirées de la pratique sur les playes d'armes à feu. Paris, *C. Osmont*, 1737.

English translation, 1743.

2150 PRINGLE, *Sir* John. 1707–1782
Observations on the diseases of the army. London, *A. Millar & D. Wilson*, 1752.

Pringle, founder of modern military medicine, was Physician-General of the British Army from 1744 to 1752. His books lay down the principles of military sanitation and the ventilation of barracks, gaols, hospital ships, etc. He did much to improve the lot of soldiers, and it was due to remarks in his book that foot-soldiers were given blankets when on service. The preface of the book includes an account of the origin of the Red Cross idea (the neutrality of military hospitals on the battlefield); for a further note on this, see *Lancet*, 1943, 2, 234.

2151 LIND, James. 1716–1794
An essay on the most effectual means, of preserving the health of seamen, in the Royal Navy. London, *A. Millar*, 1757.

Lind is regarded as the founder of naval hygiene in England. Besides his work on scurvy (See 3713), he is notable for the above book, which deals not only with the men but also with the appalling conditions in which they lived afloat. He advocated measures to improve ships' ventilation and to prevent the spread of disease aboard ship. He also caused great improvements to be made in the food on board ships of the British Navy. L. H. Roddis published a biography of Lind in 1951.

2152 SWIETEN, Gerard L. B. van. 1700–1772
Kurze Beschreibung und Heilungsart der Krankheiten, welche am öftesten in dem Feldlager beobachtet werden. Wien, Prag, Triest, *J. T. Trattnern*, 1758.

An essay on diseases of military camps. English translation, 1762.

2153 BROCKLESBY, Richard. 1722–1797
Oeconomical and medical observations . . . tending to the improvement of military hospitals, and to the cure of camp diseases, incident to soldiers. London, *T. Becket & P. A. De Hondt*, 1764.

The best book of the century regarding military sanitation.

2154 RAVATON, Hugues.
Chirurgie d'armée. Paris, *P. F. Didot le jeune*, 1768.

One of the most important works on military surgery during the 18th century. Ravaton, a skilful army surgeon, was the first to employ a tin boot, suspended on four rings, for the "hanging" position of broken bones. He was also first to adopt the double-flap method in amputations.

2155 JONES, John. 1729–1791
Plain, concise, practical remarks, on the treatment of wounds and fractures; to which is added an appendix, on camp and military hospitals. Philadelphia, *R. Bell*, 1776.

The appendix is the first American work on military medicine.

2156 PRINGLE, *Sir* John. 1707–1782
A discourse upon some late improvements of the means for preserving the health of mariners. London, *Royal Society*, 1776.

Besides his pioneer work in military medicine, Pringle did much to improve the conditions of sailors afloat. (See also No. 2150.)

2157 RUSH, Benjamin. 1745–1813
Directions for preserving the health of soldiers: recommended to the consideration of the officers of the Army of the United States. Published by order of the Board of War. Lancaster, *John Dunlap*, 1778.

A reprint from the *Philadelphia Packet*, No. 284. The pamphlet was reprinted by the Massachesetts Temperance Alliance in Boston, 1865, for distribution to the Union soldiers.

2158 BLANE, *Sir* GILBERT. 1749–1834
Observations on the diseases incident to seamen. London, *J. Cooper*, 1785.

William Hunter recommended Blane as private physician to Admiral Rodney; Blane sailed with him to the W. Indies and became physician to the British Fleet. He was held in great esteem in the Navy and was instrumental in effecting improvements in living conditions among seamen. He strongly supported Lind's views on scurvy. In 1799 he made recommendations which formed the basis of the Quarantine Act of that year. Later he became physician to St. Thomas's Hospital. With Lind he stands predominant in the history of naval medicine.

2159 TROTTER, THOMAS. 1761–1832
Medicina nautica; an essay on the diseases of seamen. 3 vols. London, *T. Cadell, jun. and W. Davies* (*T. N. Longman and O. Rees*), 1797–1803.

Trotter has left an excellent account of the conditions of seamen at the beginning of the 19th century. His book includes an interesting theory of the causation of fevers. He worked hard to improve the conditions of the ship's medical officer and the seaman.

2160 LARREY, DOMINIQUE JEAN, *le baron.* 1766–1842
Mémoires de chirurgie militaire, et campagnes. 4 vols. Paris, *J. Smith*, 1812–17.

Larrey was the greatest military surgeon in history. Of him Napoleon said: "C'est l'homme le plus vertueux que j'ai connu." He was present at all Napoleon's great battles and one of the few who stood by him on his abdication, and was waiting for him on his return in 1815. Larrey was one of the first to amputate at the hip-joint (No. 4442), the first to describe the therapeutic effect of maggots on wounds, gave the first description of "trench foot", invented the "ambulante volonte", used advanced first-aid posts on the battlefield, and devised several new operations. He was familiar with the stomach tube, with *débridement*, and with the infectious nature of granular conjunctivitis (See No. 5837). He was a kindly man, who devoted much of his life to the well-being of the soldiers, among whom not even Napoleon commanded more love and respect.

2161 GUTHRIE, GEORGE JAMES. 1785–1856
On gun-shot wounds of the extremities, requiring the different operations of amputation, with their after treatment. London, *Longman*, 1815.

Guthrie was the leading British military surgeon during the first half of the 19th century. He served in the Napoleonic Wars; his book is one of the most important in the history of the subject.

2162 HENNEN, JOHN. 1779–1828
Observations on some important points in the practice of military surgery. Edinburgh, *A. Constable & Co.*, 1818.

"A valuable surgical record of the Napoleonic period" (Garrison).

2163 DUPUYTREN, GUILLAUME, *le baron.* 1777–1835
Traité théorique et pratique des blessures par armes de guerre. 2 vols. Paris, *J. B. Baillière*, 1834.

2164 STROMEYER, GEORG FRIEDRICH LUDWIG. 1804–1876
Maximen der Kriegsheilkunst. Hannover, *Hahn*, 1855.

A landmark in military surgery, written by the founder of modern military surgery in Germany. Stromeyer, surgeon-general to the army of Hanover, is also notable for his important contributions to orthopaedics.

2165 GREAT BRITAIN. War Office. *Medical Services.*
Medical and surgical history of the British Army which served in Turkey and the Crimea during the war against Russia, in the years 1854–6. 2 vols. London, *Harrison & Sons*, 1858.

First official medical and surgical history of a war.

2166 DUNANT, JEAN HENRI. 1828–1910
Un souvenir de Solferino. Genève, *J. G. Fick*, 1862.

Dunant's account of the great sufferings endured by the wounded at Solferino resulted in the Geneva Convention of 1864. In 1901 he was awarded the first Nobel Peace Prize. English translation, London, 1947.

2167 MITCHELL, SILAS WEIR. 1829–1914, *et al.*
Gunshot wounds and other injuries of nerves. Philadelphia, *J. B. Lippincott & Co.*, 1864.

Mitchell, G. R. Morehouse, and W. W. Keen were army surgeons during the American civil war; their book was the first exhaustive study of the traumatic neuroses.

2168 ESMARCH, JOHANN FRIEDRICH AUGUST VON. 1823–1908
Der erste Verband auf dem Schlachtfelde. Kiel, *Schwers*, 1869.

Esmarch introduced the first-aid bandage on the battlefield.

2169 MAAS, HERMANN. 1842–1886
Kriegschirurgische Beiträge aus dem Jahre 1866. Breslau, *Maruschke & Berendt*, 1870.

A surgical history of the Seven Weeks War between Germany and Austria.

2170 LISTER, JOSEPH, 1*st Baron Lister*. 1827–1912
A method of antiseptic treatment applicable to wounded soldiers in the present war. *Brit. med. J.*, 1870, **2**, 243–44.

In 1870, for the first time on the battlefield, French and German army surgeons applied antiseptic methods in the management of wounds. Lister published the above short paper describing the simplest method he could devise to use carbolic as an antiseptic.

2171 UNITED STATES. War Dept. *Surgeon-General's Office.*
The medical and surgical history of the War of the Rebellion, 1861–65. 6 vols. Washington, *Govt. Printing Office*, 1870–88.

Written by J. J. Woodward, C. Smart, G. A. Otis, and D. L. Huntington.

2172 VIRCHOW, RUDOLF LUDWIG KARL. 1821–1902
Ueber Lazarette und Barracken. *Berl. klin. Wschr.*, 1871, **8**, 109–11, 121–24, 133–35, 157–59.

2173 KLEBS, THEODOR ALBRECHT EDWIN. 1834–1913
Beiträge zur pathologischen Anatomie der Schusswunden. Leipzig, *F. C. W. Vogel*, 1872.

Klebs filtered the discharges from gunshot wounds, found the filtrate to be non-infectious, and from that reasoned that traumatic septicaemia is of bacterial origin. He was the first to filter bacteria and to experiment with the filtrate.

2174 LANGENBECK, BERNHARD RUDOLPH CONRAD VON. 1810–1887
Chirurgische Beobachtungen aus dem Kriege. Berlin, *A. Hirschwald*, 1874.

2175 LAVERAN, CHARLES LOUIS ALPHONSE. 1845–1922
Traité des maladies et épidémies des armées. Paris, *G. Masson*, 1875.

2176 FRÖLICH, FRANZ HERMANN. 1839–1900
Militärmedicin. Braunschweig, *F. Wreden*, 1887.

2177 GRAY, HENRY MCILREE WILLIAMSON. 1870–1938
Treatment of gunshot wounds by excision and primary suture. *Brit. med. J.*, 1915, **2**, 317.

Gray revived *débridement* of wounds, with primary suture, a procedure with which Desault and Larrey were familiar.

2178 GREAT BRITAIN. War Office. *Medical Services.*
History of the Great War. Medical Services. 12 vols. London, *H.M. Stationery Office*, 1921–31.

General history. 4 vols. 1921–24; Diseases of the war. 2 vols. 1922–23; Hygiene. 2 vols. 1923; Pathology. 1923; Surgery. 2 vols. 1922; Casualties and medical statistics. 1931.

2179 UNITED STATES. War Dept. *Surgeon-General's Office.*
The medical department of the U.S. army in the World War. Prepared under the direction of M. W. Ireland. 15 vols. [in 17]. Washington, *Govt. Printing Office*, 1921–29.

2180 GREAT BRITAIN.
History of the second world war. Medical series. 13 vols. London, *H.M. Stationery Office*, 1952–62.

History of Military & Naval Hygiene & Medicine

2181 BILLROTH, CHRISTIAN ALBERT THEODOR. 1829–1894
Historische Studien über die Beurtheilung und Behandlung der Schusswunden vom funfzehnten Jahrhundert bis auf die neueste Zeit. Berlin, *G. Reimer*, 1859.

English translation in *Yale J. Biol. Med.*, 1931, **4**, 16–36, 119–48, 225–57; reprinted in book form, New Haven, 1933.

2182 KÖHLER, ALBERT. 1850–1936
Grundriss einer Geschichte der Kriegschirurgie. Berlin, *A. Hirschwald*, 1901.

2183 BRUNNER, CONRAD. 1859–1927
Die Verwundeten in den Kriegen der alten Eidgenossenschaft. I. *Beitr. klin. Chir.*, 1903, **37**, 1–174.

History of the care of the wounded during the Wars of the Swiss Confederation. Brunner shows that the Swiss were the first nation in Europe to organize state care of the wounded. Part 2 of the above work was published in book form, Tübingen, 1903.

2184 CABANÈS, AUGUSTIN. 1862–1928
Chirurgiens et blessés à travers l'histoire. Paris, *A. Michel*, [1918].

In this well-illustrated book Cabanès deals exhaustively with the transportation and surgical treatment of the wounded.

2185 GARRISON, FIELDING HUDSON. 1870–1935
Notes on the history of military medicine. Washington, *Assoc. Mil. Surg.*, 1922.

2186 ASHBURN, PERCY MOREAU. 1872–1940
A history of the Medical Department of the United States Army. Boston, *Houghton Mifflin*, 1929.

2187 RODDIS, LOUIS HARRY. 1886–
A short history of nautical medicine. New York, *P. B. Hoeber*, (1941).

2188 KEEVIL, JOHN JOYCE. 1901–1957
Medicine and the navy, 1200–1900. 4 vols. Edinburgh, *E. & S. Livingstone Ltd.*, 1957–63.
Vol. 3–4 by C. Lloyd and J. L. S. Coulter.

2189–2243.3 MEDICINE: GENERAL WORKS

See also 1–86.4, COLLECTED WORKS; OPERA OMNIA.

2189 GALEN. A.D. 130–200
Galen on medical experience. First edition of the Arabic version with English translation and notes, by R. WALZER. London, *Oxford University Press*, 1934.

2190 RABANUS MAURUS, *Archbishop of Mayence*. 776?–856
De sermonum proprietate, seu de universo. [Strassburg, *Adolf Rusch*, 1467?]
This is the earliest known printed book to include a section dealing with medicine. It is a general encyclopaedia – the first of all printed encyclopaedias – and devotes Book 18, Chap. V to medicine and diseases. It is known to have been printed by Rusch, the "R" printer, before July 20, 1467, from the first roman type ever cast. For an interesting paper on the book, including a translation of the chapter dealing with medicine, see E. C. Jessup, *Ann. med. Hist.* 1934, n.s., **6**, 35–41.

2191 JOHN *of Gaddesden* [JOHANNES ANGLICUS]. 1280?–1361
Rosa anglica practica medicina a capite ad pedes. (Papie, *J. A. Birreta*, 1492.)
First printed medical book of an Englishman. John of Gaddesden was a prebendary of St. Paul's and physician to Edward II. The work, to quote Garrison, "consists mainly of Arabist quackeries and countryside superstitions"; it was compiled in 1314. For information regarding the various printed editions, see the article by Dock in *Janus (Amsterdam)*, 1907, **51**, 425.

2192 FERRARI DA GRADI (GIOVANNI MATTEO). 1392?–1472
Practica, sive commentarium textuale in Nonum Almansoris cum ampliationibus et additionibus materierum. 2 vols. [Pavia, 1472.]
For bibliographical and other details regarding this, the first large medical book to be printed, see the essay by Arnold C. Klebs in: *Essays on the history of medicine presented to Karl Sudhoff, on his seventieth birthday*, 1923, London, 1924.

2193 DE FEBRIBUS.
De febribus opus sane aureum non magis utile, quam rei medicae profitentibus necessarium. Venetiis, *apud Gratiosum Perchacinum*, 1576.
Includes writings on fever by Hippocrates, Galen, Paul of Aegina, Alexander of Tralles, Aetius, Oribasius, Nonus, Actuarius, Avicenna, Rhazes, Avenzoar, Averroes, Isaac Judaeus, Serapion, Haly Abbas, Celsus, Serenus, Pliny, Gariopontus, Constantinus Africanus, Gordon, Peter of Abano, Arnold of Villanova, Nicolaus Nicolus, and the medical writings attributed to Philonius.

2194 ALPINO, PROSPERO [ALPINUS]. 1553–1617
De praesagienda vita et morte aegrotantium. Venetiis, *M. Sessa*, 1601.
A classical work on prognosis. English translation, London, 1746.

2195 PLATTER, Felix [Plater]. 1536–1614

Praxeos seu de cognoscendis, praedicendis, praecavendis, curandisque affectibus homini incommodantibus. 2 vols. Basileae, *typ. C. Waldkirchius*, 1602–03.

The first attempt at a classification of diseases according to symptoms. Over a period of 50 years Platter dissected more than 300 bodies and made many observations of value to pathological anatomy.

2196 SENNERT, Daniel. 1572–1637

De febribus libri iv. Accessit ad calcem; ejusdem de dysenteria tractatus. Lugduni, *J. Lautret*, 1627.

An important monograph on fevers.

2197 LE BOË, Franciscus de [Sylvius]. 1614–1672

Praxeos medicae idea nova. 4 vols. Lugduni Batavorum, *apud viduam J. Le Carpentier* (Hagae Comitum, *apud Henricum Scheuleer*), 1671–74.

Sylvius was a supporter of the Iatrochemical School. He established at Leyden the first chemical laboratory in Europe.

2198 SYDENHAM, Thomas. 1624–1689

Observationes medicae circa morborum acutorum historiam et curationem. Londini, *G. Kettilby*, 1676.

Sydenham recorded important observations on dysentery, scarlet fever, scarlatina, measles and other conditions. He stressed the clinical study of medicine and kept careful case records. The above book is really a third edition of his *Methodus curandi febres*, 1666.

2199 BOERHAAVE, Herman. 1668–1738

Aphorismi de cognoscendis et curandis morbis. Lugduni Batavorum, *J. vander Linden*, 1709.

The *Aphorisms* represent one of Boerhaave's best works. English translation, 1715.

2200 SWIETEN, Gerard L. B. van. 1700–1772

Commentaria in Hermanni Boerhaave aphorismos, de cognoscendis et curandis morbis. 6 vols. Lugduni Batavorum, *J. & H. Verbeek*, 1742–76.

A pupil of Boerhaave, van Swieten transplanted the latter's method of teaching to Vienna and founded the Vienna School of Medicine. He spent many years on the preparation of his great *Commentaria*. English translation, 18 vols., 1771–76.

2201 HUXHAM, John. 1692–1768

An essay on fevers. London, *S. Austen*, 1750.

Huxham's best work. He was well known in the west of England and wrote important monographs on diphtheria and on Devonshire colic. Huxham seemed to appreciate that a difference existed between typhus and typhoid, at that time usually regarded as one condition. The second edition of this book included the first use of the word "influenza" by an English physician.

2202 LINNÉ, Carl von [Linnaeus]. 1707–1778

Genera morborum in auditorum usum. Upsaliae, *C. E. Steinert*, 1763.

Linnaeus's classification of disease.

2203 SAUVAGES DE LA CROIX, François Boissier de. 1706–1767

Nosologia methodica, sistens morborum classes, genera et species. 5 vols. Amstelodami, *frat. de Tournes*, 1768.

Sauvages adopted the botanical system of Linnaeus for a classification of diseases; his book exerted a wide influence on his contemporaries. He enumerated 2,400 different diseases.

2204 CULLEN, WILLIAM. 1710–1790

Synopsis nosologiae methodicae. Edinburgi, 1769.

This work made Cullen's reputation. In it he divided diseases into fevers, neurosis, cachexias and local disorders. Cullen was the foremost British clinical teacher of his time, and one of the first to give clinical lectures in Great Britain. (See also No. 76.) Several English translations are available.

2205 CLARK, JOHN. 1744–1805

Observations on fevers. London, *T. Cadell*, 1780.

2207 HEBERDEN, WILLIAM, *Snr.* 1710–1801

Commentarii de morborum historia et curatione. Londini, *T. Payne*, 1802.

Samuel Johnson called Heberden "the last of our learned physicians". The above work included all his important papers which had earned him his great reputation and which are dealt with elsewhere in the present book (see Nos. 2887, 4491, 5438, 5831).

The book was published by Heberden's son and at once acquired a European reputation; "it had the distinction of being the last important medical treatise written in Latin" (Rolleston). An English translation which appeared in the same year as the original work was reprinted in 1962.

2208 PINEL, PHILIPPE. 1745–1826

Adynamie. *Dict. Sci. méd.*, Paris, 1812, **1**, 161–63.

2209 BLACKALL, JOHN. 1771–1860

Observations on the nature and cure of dropsies. London, *Longman*, 1813.

Blackall was before Bright in detecting albuminuria in association with dropsy. His book, of which the second edition is more important than the first, includes reports on cases of angina pectoris.

2210 PARRY, CALEB HILLIER. 1755–1822

Collections from the unpublished writings. 2 vols. London, *Underwoods*, 1825.

Includes Parry's interesting description of 8 cases of exophthalmic goitre, the first of which was observed in 1786 (see No. 3813), and his notes on 4 cases of angina pectoris. Parry was a copious note-taker, and many of these notes are here published for the first time. His careful records of many years' observation in practice were intended to form a large work, *Elements of pathology and therapeutics*, of which only the first volume appeared, in 1815; this was republished, together with the unfinished vol. 2, in 1825.

2211 SMITH, THOMAS SOUTHWOOD. 1788–1861

A treatise on fever. London, *Longman, etc.*, 1830.

2212 BIGELOW, JACOB. 1786–1879

A discourse on self-limited diseases. Boston, *N. Hale*, 1835.

Bigelow was attached to the Massachusetts General Hospital. The above "did more than any other work or essay in our own language to rescue the practice of medicine from the slavery of the drugging system which was a part of the inheritance of the profession" (Oliver Wendell Holmes).

2213 STOKES, WILLIAM. 1804–1878

A treatise on the diagnosis and treatment of diseases of the chest. Dublin, *Hodges & Smith*, 1837.

Stokes, most prominent of the Irish school of medicine, established his reputation by his book on diseases of the chest. Important among its contents are his discovery of a stage of pneumonia prior to that described by Laennec as the first, his observations that contraction of the side has sometimes followed the cure of pneumonia and that paralysis of the intercostal muscles and diaphragm may result from pleurisy, and his employment of the stethoscope as an aid to the detection of foreign bodies in the air passages.

2215 BRIGHT, RICHARD. 1789–1858, & ADDISON, THOMAS. 1793–1860
Elements of the practice of medicine. Vol. 1, pts. 1–3. London, *Longmans*, [1836]–39.

No more published.

2216 CANSTATT, CARL FRIEDRICH. 1807–1850
Die Krankheiten des höheren Alters und ihre Heilung. 2 vols. Erlangen, *Enke*, 1839.

Canstatt's book is one of the most important in the history of geriatrics, summarizing all previous work on the subject.

2217 MAGENDIE, FRANÇOIS. 1783–1855
Leçons sur les phénomènes physiques de la vie. 4 vols. Paris, *J. B. Baillière*, 1836–38.

Magendie, pioneer experimental physiologist, regarded pathology as only a modification of physiology, "medicine the physiology of the sick man". By him clinical medicine was reconstructed on physiological lines.

2218 GRAVES, ROBERT JAMES. 1796–1853
A system of clinical medicine. Dublin, *Fannin & Co.*, 1843.

Graves was one of the founders of the Irish school of medicine and one of the most important figures in Irish medicine at the middle of the 19th century. Second edition of the book (as *Clinical lectures on the practice of medicine*) in 1848.

2219 WATSON, *Sir* THOMAS, *Bart.* 1792–1882
Lectures on the principles and practice of physic. 2 vols. London, *J. W. Parker*, 1843.

First published in the *Medical Times & Gazette*, 1840–42, Watson's famous lectures appeared in book form and formed the most important treatise of medicine for a quarter-century. Watson wrote in a fine style and his book was recognized as a sound guide to clinical medicine. Watson suggested (vol. 2, p. 349) rubber gloves for antisepsis; he also instructed his students to wash their hands in a solution of chloride of lime before assisting at deliveries.

2220 MURCHISON, CHARLES. 1830–1879
A treatise on the continued fevers of Great Britain. London, *Parker, Son, & Bourn*, 1862.

Murchison was one of the greatest clinical teachers London has ever known; of his many writings his book on the continued fevers is probably the most important.

2221 TROUSSEAU, ARMAND. 1801–1867
Clinique médicale de l'Hôtel-Dieu de Paris. 2 vols. Paris, *J. B. Baillière*, 1861.

Trousseau, great clinician of the Hôtel-Dieu, made important advances in the treatment of diphtheria, typhoid, scarlet fever and other conditions. In his book he emphasized the value of bedside observation. He supported the doctrine of the specific nature of disease and realized the significance of Pasteur's work on fermentation. English translation, 1868–72.

2222 CHARCOT, JEAN MARTIN. 1825–1893
Leçons sur les maladies des vieillards et les maladies chroniques. Paris, *A. Delahaye*, 1867.

Charcot inaugurated a course of study of geriatrics, at the Salpêtrière, in 1866; his lectures are embodied in the above work. English translation, 1881.

2223 ADDISON, THOMAS. 1793–1860
A collection of the published writings. London, *New Sydenham Soc.*, 1868.

Addison was a contemporary of Bright at Guy's Hospital and a fine lecturer.

2224 TRAUBE, Ludwig. 1818–1876
Zur Fieberlehre. In his *Gesammelte Beiträge*, Berlin, 1871, **2**, pt. 1, 624–56, 679–83; 1878, **3**, 503–05, 582–87.

2225 SENATOR, Hermann. 1834–1911
Untersuchungen über den fieberhaften Process und seine Behandlung. Berlin, *A. Hirschwald*, 1873.

Senator was a director of the Charité Hospital in Berlin and later at the university polyclinic. His study of fever represents his best work.

2226 LIEBERMEISTER, Carl von. 1833–1901
Handbuch der Pathologie und Therapie des Fiebers. Leipzig, *F. C. W. Vogel*, 1875.

2227 LATHAM, Peter Mere. 1789–1875
The collected works. 2 vols. London, *New Sydenham Soc.*, 1876–78.

Latham, successively physician to the Middlesex and St. Bartholomew's hospitals, was an authority on cardiac disease and among the earliest in England to advocate auscultation. He held progressive views on medical education and championed clinical study in the wards. His clinical lectures are among the very best.

2228 CHARCOT, Jean Martin. 1825–1893
Leçons sur les maladies du foie, des voies biliaires et des reins. Paris, *Progrès Médical*, 1877.

2229 STRÜMPELL, Ernst Adolf Gustav Gottfried. 1853–1925
Lehrbuch der speciellen Pathologie und Therapie der inneren Krankheiten. 2 vols. Leipzig, *F. C. W. Vogel*, 1883–84.

More than 30 editions of this book appeared, many translated into other languages. English translation in 1887.

2230 FAGGE, Charles Hilton. 1838–1883
The principles and practice of medicine. 2 vols. London, *J. & A. Churchill*, 1886.

Fagge was physician to Guy's Hospital and editor of *Guy's Hospital Reports*. His important text-book was published posthumously.

2231 OSLER, *Sir* William, *Bart.* 1849–1919
The principles and practice of medicine. New York, *D. Appleton*, 1892.

Osler's text-book was the best English work on medicine of its time. He became Regius professor of medicine at Oxford in 1904. Besides being one of the greatest of all clinicians, he was possessed of a fine literary style and an extensive knowledge of medical bibliography. Garrison has written of him: "When he came to die, Osler was, in a very real sense, the greatest physician of our time . . . Good looks, distinction, blithe, benignant manners, a sunbright personality, radiant with kind feeling and good will toward his fellow men, an Apollonian poise, swiftness and surety of thought and speech, every gift of the gods was his; and to these were added careful training, unsurpassed clinical ability, the widest knowledge of his subject, the deepest interest in everything human, and a serene hold upon his fellows that was as a seal set upon them." For Osler's own account of the preparation of his text-book, see the *Bibliotheca Osleriana* (No. 6772), item 3544.

2232 GULL, *Sir* William Withey. 1816–1890
A collection of the published writings. 2 vols. London, *New Sydenham Soc.*, 1894–96.

Gull, one of the best clinicians of his time, spent most of his working life at Guy's Hospital. He described the spinal lesion of tabes and left an important account of aneurysm. His best works are his description of myxoedema and his original description of arteriolosclerotic atrophy of the kidney.

2233 STILLER, Berthold. 1837–1922
Die asthenische Konstitutionskrankheit. Stuttgart, *F. Enke*, 1907.
"Stiller's disease" – habitus asthenicus.

2234 EPPINGER, Hans. 1879–1946, & HESS, Leo. 1879–1963
Vagotonie: klinische Studie. Berlin, *A. Hirschwald*, 1910.
English translation, 1915.

2235 HURRY, Jamieson Boyd. 1857–1930
Vicious circles in disease. London, *J. Churchill*, 1911.

2236 OTT, Isaac. 1847–1916
Fever: its thermotaxis and metabolism. New York, *P. B. Hoeber*, 1914.

2237 KLEMPERER, Paul. 1887–1964, *et al.*
Diffuse collagen disease; acute disseminated lupus erythematosus and diffuse scleroderma. *J. Amer. med. Ass.*, 1942, **119**, 331–32.
P. Klemperer, A. D. Pollack, and G. Baehr combined a number of diseases, hitherto regarded as unrelated, into an entity which they termed diffuse collagen disease.

2238 SELYE, Hans. 1907–
The physiology and pathology of exposure to stress. Montreal, *Acta Inc.*, 1950.
In his study of the aetiology of the collagen diseases Selye developed the idea that animals react to stress or injury by a certain sequence of physiological reactions – the "general adaptation syndrome".

History of Internal Medicine

See also 6376–6703.1, History of Medicine, *and under individual subjects.*

2239 FABER, Knud Helge. 1862–1956
Nosography in modern internal medicine. New York, *P. B. Hoeber*, 1923.
A well-illustrated and reliable account of the evolution of internal medicine.

2240 ROLLESTON, *Sir* Humphry Davy, *Bart.* 1862–1944
Internal medicine. New York, *P. B. Hoeber*, 1930.
A short history of the subject; one of the *Clio Medica* series.

2241 MAJOR, Ralph Hermon. 1884–
Classic descriptions of disease. Springfield, *C. C. Thomas*, 1932.
A collection of classical descriptions of disease by 179 different writers, from ancient times to the present. Foreign papers are translated into English. A second edition of this most interesting and useful book appeared in 1939, the principal additions being on the subjects of malaria and yellow fever, and a third edition in 1945.

2242 SHOCK, Nathan Wetherill. 1906–
A classified bibliography of gerontology and geriatrics. Stanford, *University Press*, (1951).
Supplements in 1957 and 1963.

2243 BETT, Walter Reginald. 1903–1968
The history and conquest of common diseases. Edited by Walter R. Bett. Norman, *Univ. of Oklahoma Press*, 1954.

2243.1 BLOOMFIELD, Arthur Leonard. 1888–
A bibliography of internal medicine. Selected diseases. Chicago, *University of Chicago Press*, 1960.
Attempts to list and annotate every reference of fundamental importance in the development of 21 selected diseases.

2243.2 KEELE, Kenneth David. 1909–
The evolution of clinical methods in medicine. London, *Pitman*, [1963].
FitzPatrick Lectures 1960–61. This book traces the changing clinical methods throughout the centuries to show how they arose and how they have grown into their present forms.

2243.3 LÜTH, Paul.
Geschichte der Geriatrie. Dreitausend Jahre Physiologie, Pathologie und Therapie des alten Menschen. Stuttgart, *Ferdinand Enke*, 1965.

2244–2261 CONDITIONS DUE TO PHYSICAL FACTORS

2244 ACOSTA, Jose de. 1539–1600
Historia natural y moral de las Indias. Sevilla, *Juan de León*, 1590.
Lib. 3, chap. 9 contains his description of mountain sickness, "Acosta's disease", which he experienced during his crossing of the Peruvian Andes. English translation, London, 1604.

2245 FABRY, Wilhelm [Fabricius *Hildanus*]. 1560–1634
De combustionibus. Basileae, *sumpt. Ludovici Regis*, 1607.
Fabricius was the first to classify burns. English translation, London, 1643.

2246 HORST, Georg. ?–1688
De siriasi. Basileae, *typ. J. J. Deckeri*, 1665.
A treatise on sunstroke.

2247 DUPUYTREN, Guillaume, *le baron*. 1777–1835
Leçons orales de clinique chirurgicale. Tom. 1. Paris, *Germer-Baillière*, 1832.
Dupuytren's classification of burns (p. 424).

2248 LONGMORE, *Sir* Thomas. 1816–1895
Remarks upon a tabular return (No. 1), or synopsis of sixteen cases of heat-apoplexy. *Indian Ann. med. Sci.*, 1859, **6**, 396–406.
Longmore was an army surgeon in India; he gave an excellent account of heat-stroke.

2249 BARCLAY, Alexander. 1822–1874
Contributions to the natural history of insolatio. *Madras quart. J. med. Sci.*, 1860, **1**, 347–95.
Barclay, an army surgeon, wrote an important paper on heat-stroke.

2250 WOOD, Horatio Charles. 1841–1920
Thermic fever, or sunstroke. Philadelphia, *J. B. Lippincott*, 1872.
A study of the pathology of sunstroke. Wood held the chairs of botany, therapeutics, and neurology at the University of Pennsylvania.

2251 BARTHE DE SANDFORT, Edmond.
La kérithérapie (nouvelle balnéation thermocireuse). *J. Méd. intern.*, 1913, **17,** 211–14.
Treatment of burns with ambrine (paraffin-resin solution); keritherapy.

2252 UNDERHILL, Frank Pell. 1877–1932, *et al.*
Blood concentration changes in extensive superficial burns, and their significance for systemic treatment. *Arch. intern. Med.*, 1923, **32,** 31–49.
F. P. Underhill, G. L. Carrington, R. Kapsinow, and G. T. Pack made important studies on the blood concentration following burns.

2253 DAVIDSON, Edward Clark. 1894–1933
Tannic acid in the treatment of burns. *Surg. Gynec. Obstet.*, 1925, **41,** 202–21.
Introduction of tannic acid in the treatment of burns.

2254 RIEHL, Gustav. 1855–1943
Zur Therapie schwerer Verbrennungen. *Wien. klin. Wschr.*, 1925, **38,** 833–34.
Riehl was an early advocate of blood transfusion in the treatment of shock after burns.

2255 GOLDBLATT, David. 1894–
Contribution to the study of burns, their classification and treatment. *Ann. Surg.*, 1927, **85,** 490–501.
Goldblatt's classification of burns.

2256 PACK, George Thomas. 1898– , & DAVIS, Andrew Hobson, 1899–
Burns. Types, pathology and management. Philadelphia, *Lippincott, Co.*, 1930.

2257 JELLINEK, Stefan. 1871–
Elektrische Verletzungen: Klinik und Histopathologie. Leipzig, *J. A. Barth*, 1932.

2258 ALDRICH, Robert Henry. 1902–
The role of infection in burns; the theory and treatment with special reference to gentian violet. *New Engl. J. Med.*, 1933, **208,** 299–309.
Introduction of gentian violet in the treatment of burns.

2259 BETTMAN, Adalbert Goodman. 1883–
The tannic acid-silver nitrate treatment of burns: a method of minimizing shock and toxemia and shortening convalescence. *Northw. Med.*, 1935, **34,** 46–51.
Bettman introduced the tannic acid-silver nitrate method of treating burns.

2260 BUNYAN, John.
Envelope method of treating burns. *Proc. roy. Soc. Med.*, 1940, **34,** 65–70.
Bunyan bag.

2261 HARKINS, Henry Nelson. 1905–
The treatment of burns. Springfield, Baltimore, *C. C. Thomas*, 1942.
Contains some history of the subject and includes a valuable bibliography of 1,320 entries.

2262–2268 TROPICAL MEDICINE

See also under the names of individual tropical diseases

2262 WATESON, GEORGE, 1544–?
The cures of the diseased, in remote regions. Preventing mortalitie, incident in forraine attempts, of the English nation. London, *F. K(ingston) for H. L(ownes)*, 1598.

Attributed to Wateson, Elizabethan poet, soldier, and traveller, this book is the earliest work in English devoted to tropical medicine. It is available in a facsimile reproduction, with introduction and notes by Charles Singer, Oxford, 1915.

2262.1 ABREU, ALEXO DE, 1568–1630
Tratado de las siete enfermedades, de la inflammacion universal del higado, zirbo, pyloron, y riñones, y de la obstrucion, de la satiriasi, de la terciana y febre maligna, y passion hipocondriaca. Lleva otros tres tratados, del mal de Loanda, del guzano, y de las fuentes y sedales. Lisboa, *P. Craesbeeck*, 1623.

The first important work on tropical diseases. Only six copies of this book are known. It includes full accounts of malaria, typhoid, and scurvy, and the first accurate descriptions of yellow fever, amoebic hepatitis, dracontiasis, trichuriasis, and tungiasis. For a study of the book see F. Guerra, *Clio Medica,* 1968,**1**, 59–60.

2263 BONTIUS, JACOBUS. 1592–1631
De medicina Indorum. Lugduni Batavorum, *F. Hackium*, 1642.

Bontius was probably the first to regard tropical medicine as an independent branch of medical science. He spent the last four years of his life in the Dutch East Indies, and his book incorporates the experience he gained there. It is the first Dutch work on tropical medicine and includes the first modern descriptions of beri-beri and cholera. English translation, 1769.

2264 LIND, JAMES. 1716–1794
An essay on diseases incidental in Europeans in hot climates. London, *T. Becket & P. A. De Hondt*, 1768.

Lind came near to discovering the connexion between malaria and mosquitoes. He is best remembered for his work on scurvy, but the above book is one of the more important early works on tropical medicine.

2265 PRUNER-BEY, FRANZ. 1808–1882
Die Krankheiten des Orient's. Erlangen, *Palm u. Enke*, 1847.

2266 MANSON, *Sir* PATRICK. 1844–1922
Tropical diseases. London, *Cassell & Co.*, 1898.

Manson has been called the "Father of modern tropical medicine". He had a vast experience of disease in the Tropics and himself made many valuable contributions to the knowledge of this subject. He described tinea nigra and tinea imbricata, found filaria in elephantiasis and discovered *Filaria hominis*. In 1898 he founded the London School of Tropical Medicine. The 16th edition of his book, edited by P. H. Manson-Bahr, appeared in 1966.

2267 CASTELLANI, ALDO. 1877–1971, & CHALMERS, ALBERT JOHN. 1870–1920.
Manual of tropical medicine. London, *Baillière, Tindall & Cox*, 1910.

Castellani has made several discoveries of great importance in tropical medicine. The above work is a standard text on tropical medicine in English. Third edition, 1919.

History of Tropical Medicine

2268 SCOTT, *Sir* HENRY HAROLD. 1874–1956

A history of tropical medicine. 1 vol. [in 2]. London, *Arnold*, 1939.

Based on the FitzPatrick Lectures, 1937–38; this is an exhaustive history of the subject, and one of the best histories of special subjects yet produced. The book is furnished with a most useful bibliography.

2269–2319.2 PATHOLOGY

See also 2606–2662, TUMOURS.

2269 GALEN, A.D. 130–200

De locis affectis. In his *Opera*, ed. C. G. KÜHN, Lipsiae, 1824, **8,** 1–452.

Galen devoted six books of his works to pathology. His ideas on inflammation and on tumours led him to make many valuable deductions. He was familiar with cholera, hydrophobia, and malaria, the relations of urinary calculi to the kidney, ureter, and bladder. He recognized bronchitis, empyema, consumption, and pyuria.

2270 BENIVIENI, ANTONIO. 1443–1502

De abditis nonnulis ac mirandis morborum et sanationum causis. Florentiae, *P. Giuntae*, 1507.

Benivieni was a pioneer in the field of pathology, living at a time hardly ready for his work. His book records many of his autopsy findings. He attempted to explain the hidden or internal causes of disease; as a pathologist he ranks almost as high as Morgagni, and he has been called "the father of pathological anatomy". Facsimile reproduction and translation, 1954.

2271 FERNEL, JEAN FRANÇOIS. 1497–1558

Medicina. 3 pts. [in 1]. Lutetiae Parisiorum, *apud A. Wechelum*, 1554.

Part 2 of this work introduced the term "pathology" in its modern sense. It is the first explicit treatise on the subject. Fernel was the first to describe appendicitis, endocarditis, etc. He believed aneurysms to be produced by syphilis, and differentiated true from false aneurysms. He was physician to Henri II of France.

2272 SCHENCK, JOHANN, *von Grafenberg*. 1530–1598

Observationum medicarum, rararum, novarum, *etc.* 2 vols. Francofurti, *sumpt. J. Rhodii*, 1600.

Schenck was the greatest compiler of his day. His *Observationes* form the easiest source-book for the pathological observations of Sylvius, Vesalius, and Columbus, and represent a life-time of medical reading and experience. They were first published at Basle, 1584–97.

2273 SEVERINO, MARCO AURELIO. 1580–1656

De recondita abscessuum natura. Neapoli, 1632.

The first text-book of surgical pathology. It treats of all kinds of swellings under the term "abscess" and describes neoplasms of the genital organs and sarcomata of bones. Tumours of the breast are classified into four groups, the section devoted to them being one of the most important in the book. This was also the first book to include illustrations of lesions with the text.

2274 BONET, THÉOPHILE. 1620–1689

Sepulchretum, sive anatomia practica ex cadaveribus morbo denatis. Genevae, *L. Chouët*, 1679.

This is the first collection of systematized pathological anatomy. It contains clinical and pathological descriptions of nearly 3,000 cases selected from the literature from the time of Hippocrates, but mainly from the 16th and 17th centuries. It is a most useful reference book to early descriptions of pathological conditions.

2275 HOFFMANN, FRIEDRICH. 1660–1742
De metastasi sive sede morbo mutata. Halae, **1731.**

In Allbutt's opinion Hoffmann was the first to perceive that pathology is an aspect of physiology.

2276 MORGAGNI, GIOVANNI BATTISTA. 1682–1771
De sedibus, et causis morborum per anatomen indagatis libri quinque. 2 vols. Venetiis, *typog. Remondiniana*, 1761.

By this great work, one of the most important in the history of medicine, Morgagni was the true founder of modern pathological anatomy. The work was completed in Morgagni's 79th year and consists of a series of 70 letters reporting about 700 cases and necropsies. As best he could, he correlated the clinical record with the post-mortem finding. Morgagni gave the first descriptions of several pathological conditions. He was Professor of Anatomy at Padua. Selections from the above work are reproduced in *Med. Classics*, 1940, **4**, 640–839. English translation by B. Alexander, 3 vols., London, 1769. Selections published, Stuttgart, 1967.

2277 HUNTER, JOHN. 1728–1793
On the digestion of the stomach after death. *Phil. Trans.*, 1772, **62,** 447–54.

2278 SANDIFORT, EDUARD. 1742–1814
Observationes anatomicae-pathologicae. 4 vols. Lugduni Batavorum, *P. v. d. Eyk & D. Vygh*, 1777–81.

Sandilfort's beautifully illustrated work on pathological anatomy included records of ulcerative aortic endocarditis, renal calculi, herniae, bony ankyloses, and congenital abnormalities. His work is comparable with that of Morgagni.

2279 WALTER, JOHANN GOTTLIEB. 1734–1818
Von den Krankheiten des Bauchfells und dem Schlagfluss. Berlin, *G. J. Decker*, 1785.

Text in Latin and German. Includes an accurate description of peritonitis.

2280 BAILLIE, MATTHEW. 1761–1823
An account of a remarkable transposition of the viscera. *Phil. Trans.*, 1788, **78,** 350–63.

Baillie recorded a case of congenital dextrocardia with complete situs inversus viscerum. Reprinted in F. A. Willius & T. E. Keys, *Cardiac classics*, 1941, pp. 257–62.

2281 ——. The morbid anatomy of some of the most important parts of the human body. London, *J. Johnson & G. Nicol*, 1793.

Baillie was a nephew and pupil of W. Hunter. The above is the first systematic text-book of morbid anatomy, treating the subject for the first time as an independent science. The work is well written and notable for its fine illustrations on copper-plates, the work of William Clift (who did so much to preserve John Hunter's museum). Baillie was the last and most eminent owner of the famous gold-headed cane.

2282 ——. A series of engravings, accompanied with explanations, which are intended to illustrate the morbid anatomy of some of the most important parts of the human body. London, *W. Bulmer & Co.*, 1799–1802.

Atlas for No. 2281.

2283 HUNTER, John. 1728–1793

A treatise on the blood, inflammation, and gun-shot wounds. London, *G. Nicol*, 1794.

It was while serving with the army at Belle Isle during the Seven Years' War that Hunter collected the material for his epoch-making book on inflammation and gun-shot wounds. His studies on inflammation in particular are fundamental for pathology.

2284 MECKEL, Johann Friedrich, *the younger*. 1781–1833

Tabulae anatomico-pathologicae. 4 pts. Lipsiae, *I. F. Gleditsch*, 1817–26.

First systematic work on human abnormalities. Meckel's work on embryology brought a better understanding of congenital malformations, which had previously been attributed by many to supernatural influence. He was the greatest comparative anatomist in Germany before Johannes Müller.

2285 BRIGHT, Richard. 1789–1858

Reports of medical cases, selected with a view of illustrating the symptoms and cure of diseases by a reference to morbid anatomy. 2 vols. [in 3]. London, *Longmans*, 1827–31.

Although the name of Bright is perpetuated by his classical description of chronic non-suppurative nephritis, he made many other valuable contributions to medical knowledge in the above work. He differentiated renal from cardiac dropsy and was first to correlate this and the previously observed albuminuria with the nephritic changes observed at autopsy. The work contains some fine illustrations.

2286 CRUVEILHIER, Jean. 1791–1874

Anatomie pathologique du corps humain. 2 vols. Paris, *J. B. Baillière*, 1829–42.

The fine illustrations of gross pathology make this one of the greatest works of its kind. Cruveilhier, first professor of pathological anatomy in Paris, gave the first description of disseminated sclerosis (in vol. 2 above), and an early description of "Cruveilhier's palsy" (see No. 4734). Hypertrophic pyloric stenosis and ulceration of the stomach due to hyperacidity were also for the first time described in the above work; to each the name "Cruveilhier's disease" has been attached.

2287 HORNER, William Edmonds. 1793–1853

A treatise on pathological anatomy. Philadelphia, *Carey*, 1829.

First American work on the subject. Horner was professor of anatomy at Pennsylvania, and made several anatomical discoveries.

2288 LOBSTEIN, Jean George Chrétien Frédéric Martin. 1777–1835

Traité d'anatomie pathologique. 2 vols. and atlas. Paris, *F. G. Levrault*, 1829–33.

Includes a historical review of the subject from the time of the Ancient Egyptians to Corvisart, and shows the advances in pathology during the preceding 50 years. Lobstein was the first to use the word "arteriosclerosis". He was professor at Strasbourg.

2289 HOPE, James. 1801–1841

Principles and illustrations of morbid anatomy. London, *Whittaker & Co.*, 1834.

Hope left a fine pathological atlas with brilliantly coloured lithographs from his own drawings. While the book does not equal the atlases of Cruveilhier and Carswell, it is important as being a great stimulus to the study of pathology in England.

2290 HODGKIN, THOMAS. 1798–1866
Lectures on the morbid anatomy of the serous and mucous membranes. 2 vols. London, *Simpkin, Marshall & Co.*, 1836–40.

Important work which stimulated the study of tissue pathology in England.

2291 CARSWELL, *Sir* ROBERT. 1793–1857
Illustrations of the elementary forms of disease. London, *Longman, etc.*, 1838.

Carswell was professor of morbid anatomy at University College, London, and one of the leading English pathologists of his day. His great pathological atlas contains plates selected from 2,000 water-colours painted and lithographed by himself.

2292 GROSS, SAMUEL DAVID. 1805–1884
Elements of pathological anatomy. 2 vols. Boston, *Marsh*, 1839.

In his day Gross was the most famous surgeon in the U.S.A. He was for a time professor of pathological anatomy at Cincinnati Medical College and while there published his *Elements*, the first exhaustive study in English of the subject; Horner's book (No. 2287) was the only important work on pathology to precede it in America.

2293 ROKITANSKY, CARL, *Freiherr von.* 1804–1878
Handbuch der pathologischen Anatomie. 3 vols. Wien, *Braumüller u. Seidel*, 1842–46.

Rokitansky ranks with Morgagni as among the greatest of all writers on gross pathology. He is said to have performed over 30,000 autopsies himself. His *Handbuch* was for many years pre-eminent among its contemporaries. Although Rokitansky embraced more than one false doctrine, he was quick to admit and correct his mistakes. Virchow's criticism of the first edition of the *Handbuch* led Rokitansky to re-write it. He foresaw the eventual importance of chemical pathology, at that time non-existent. English translation, 4 vols., London, 1849–54.

2294 ADDISON, WILLIAM. 1802–1881
Experimental and practical researches on the structure and function of blood corpuscles; on inflammation; and on the origin and nature of tubercles in the lungs. *Trans. prov. med. surg. Ass.*, 1843, **11**, 233-306.

Addison gave an important account of the process of inflammation. See also his book (No. 3059).

2295 ROYAL COLLEGE OF SURGEONS OF ENGLAND.
Descriptive catalogue of the pathological specimens. 7 vols. London, *W. Clowes, Taylor & Francis*, 1846–64.

2296 VIRCHOW, RUDOLF LUDWIG KARL. 1821–1902
Die pathologischen Pigmente. *Virchows Arch. path. Anat.*, 1847, **1,** 379–404, 407–86.

2297 MOREL, BENEDICT AUGUSTIN. 1809–1873
Traité des dégénérescences physiques, intellectuelles et morales de l'espèce humaine. 1 vol. and atlas. Paris, *Baillière*, 1857.

2298 LISTER, JOSEPH, 1*st Baron Lister.* 1827–1912
On the early stages of inflammation. *Phil. Trans.*, 1858, **148,** 645–702

This paper reports the results of one of Lister's most valuable researches; his conclusions still hold to-day.

2299 VIRCHOW, Rudolph Ludwig Karl. 1821–1902
Die Cellularpathologie in ihrer Begründung auf physiologische und pathologische Gewebelehre. Berlin, *A. Hirschwald*, 1858.

Virchow was the greatest figure in the history of pathology. His best work *Die Cellularpathologie*, is one of the most important books in the history of medicine, and the foundation stone of cellular pathology. Reprinted Hildesheim, 1966. English translation, 1860. Virchow, professor of pathology at Würzburg and Berlin, founded the *Archiv für pathologische Anatomie und Physiologie* (*"Virchow's Archiv"*). Biography by E. H. Ackerknecht, 1953.

2300 CORNIL, André Victor. 1837–1908, & RANVIER, Louis Antoine. 1835–1922
Manuel d'histologie pathologique. 3 pts. Paris, *Germer-Baillière*, 1869–76.

2301 BERNARD, Claude. 1813–1878
Leçons de pathologie expérimentale. Paris, *J. B. Baillière*, 1872.

An elaboration of his lectures on the subject at the Collège de France.

2302 COHNHEIM, Julius Friedrich. 1839–1884
Neue Untersuchungen über die Entzündung. Berlin, *A. Hirschwald*, 1873.

Cohnheim was the master experimental pathologist of the 19th century. He was a pupil of Virchow and Kölliker; in contradiction of the former, he showed the essential feature of inflammation to be the passage of leucocytes through the capillary walls and their accumulation at the site of injury—"ohne Gefässe keine Entzündung". His first article on the subject will be found in *Virchows Arch. path. Anat.*, 1867, **40**, 1–79.

2303 ——. Vorlesungen über allgemeine Pathologie. 2 vols. Berlin, *A. Hirschwald*, 1877–80.

Apart from Virchow's *Cellularpathologie*, this was the most influential text-book of pathology during the 19th century. An English translation was published by the New Sydenham Society in 1889–90.

2304 VIRCHOW, Rudolf Ludwig Karl. 1821–1902
Die Sections-Technik im Leichenhause des Charité-Krankenhauses. Berlin, *A. Hirschwald*, 1876.

2305 ZIEGLER, Ernst. 1849–1905
Lehrbuch der allgemeinen und speciellen pathologischen Anatomie und Pathogenese. Jena, *G. Fischer*, 1881–82.

An outstanding text-book which to-day remains of value to pathologists. Ziegler was professor of pathology at Freiburg, and founded the *Beiträge zur pathologischen Anatomie* (*"Ziegler's Beiträge"*).

2306 WILD, Carl.
Beitrag zur Kenntnis der amyloiden und der hyalinen Degeneration des Bindegewebes. *Beitr. path. Anat. Physiol.*, 1886, **1**, 175–200.

First reported case of primary amyloidosis.

2307 METCHNIKOFF, Elie [Mechnikov, Ilya Ilyich]. 1845–1916
Lektsii o sravnitelnoi patologii vospaleniy. St. Petersburg, *K. L. Rikker*, 1892.

Metchnikoff's classical lectures on the pathology of inflammation. The book was translated into French in the same year, and in 1893 an English version appeared.

2308 WELCH, WILLIAM HENRY. 1850–1934
Adaptation in pathological processes. *Trans. Congr. Amer. Phys. Surg.* 1897, **4,** 284–310; also in *Amer. J. med. Sci.*, 1897, **113,** 631–55.
Reproduced in *Bibliotheca Medica Americana*, Baltimore, 1937, Vol. 3.

2309 ADAMI, JOHN GEORGE. 1862–1926
The principles of pathology. 2 vols. London, *H. Frowde,* 1909–10.
Vol. 2 written with A. G. Nicholls.

2310 MARCHAND, FELIX JACOB. 1846–1928
Ueber die Entzündung. *Med. Klin.*, 1911, **7,** 1921–27.
A notable paper on inflammation. Marchand succeeded Ziegler as editor of the latter's *Beiträge.*

2311 HENKE, FRIEDRICH. 1868– , & LUBARSCH, OTTO. 1860–1933
Handbuch der speziellen pathologischen Anatomie und Histologie. 12 vols. Berlin, *J. Springer*, 1924–52.

2312 CAMERON, *Sir* GORDON ROY. 1899–1966
Pathology of the cell. Edinburgh, *Oliver & Boyd*, 1952.

History of Pathology

2313 CHIARI, HANS. 1851–1916
Geschichte der pathologischen Anatomie des Menschen. *In:* Puschmann, T.: *Handbuch der Geschichte der Medizin*, 1903, **2,** 473–559.
Considered by Garrison the best modern history of pathology.

2314 RUFFER, *Sir* MARC ARMAND. 1859–1917
Studies in the palaeopathology of Egypt. Edited by R. L. MOODIE. Chicago, *Univ. Press*, 1921.
A collection of papers previously published in various journals. Ruffer spent many years in Egypt in the study of palaeopathology and this work, together with the later writings of the editor, form the most important contributions to the subject.

2315 MOODIE, ROY LEE. 1880–1934
Palaeopathology; an introduction to the study of ancient evidences of disease. Urbana, *Univ. of Illinois Press*, 1923.

2316 GOLDSCHMID, EDGAR. 1881–1957
Entwicklung und Bibliographie der pathologisch-anatomischen Abbildung. Leipzig, *K. W. Hiersemann*, 1925.
Traces the development of pathological anatomical illustration and includes a chronological bibliography of all important publications containing illustrations of pathological conditions, and an index of artists, printers, and publishers.

2317 LONG, ESMOND RAY. 1890–
A history of pathology. Baltimore, *Williams & Wilkins*, 1928.
The first systematic history of the subject in the English language. Revised edition, New York, *Dover Publications*, 1965.

2318 ——. Selected readings in pathology. Springfield, *C. C. Thomas*, 1929.
This work makes it possible to read many of the classical writings on the subject which previously, through language difficulties, were beyond the reach of many. The book forms a valuable companion to Dr. Long's history of the subject.

2319 KRUMBHAAR, EDWARD BELL. 1882–1966
Pathology. New York, *P. B. Hoeber*, 1937.

Krumbhaar edited the *Clio Medica* series of volumes on the history of medicine, and contributed a history of pathology to it.

2319.1 FOSTER, WILLIAM DEREK.
A short history of clinical pathology. Edinburgh, *E. & S. Livingstone Ltd.*, 1961.

2319.2 BROTHWELL, DON REGINALD, & SANDISON, ANDREW TAWSE.
Diseases in antiquity; a survey of the diseases, injuries and surgery of early populations. Springfield, *C. C. Thomas*, [1967].

2320–2361.1 TUBERCULOSIS

See also 3216–3243, PULMONARY TUBERCULOSIS, *and under the names of the various organs.*

2320 SMITH, *Sir* GRAFTON ELLIOT. 1871–1937, & RUFFER, *Sir* MARC ARMAND. 1859–1917
Pott'sche Krankheit an einer ägyptischen Mumie. Giessen, *A. Töpelmann*, 1910.

The fact that tuberculosis was present among the ancient Egyptians was proved when Elliot Smith and Ruffer described a genuine case of Pott's disease in a mummy of 1000 B.C.

2321 LE BOË, FRANCISCUS DE [SYLVIUS]. 1614–1672
Opera medica. Amstelodami, *apud D. Elsevirium et A. Wolfgang*, 1679.

Tuberculosis was known to the ancients only in its advanced form, and little progress was made in the knowledge of the condition until the time of Sylvius. He asserted that tubercles are often to be found in the lung and that they softened and suppurated to form cavities.

2322 BAYLE, GASPARD LAURENT. 1774–1816
Recherches sur la phthisie pulmonaire. Paris, *Gabon*, 1810.

Bayle gave the best description to date of the varieties of tuberculosis. He was first to use the term "miliary" to describe small tubercles and first to speak of a tuberculosis diathesis. He left an original description of the course character of tubercle and its identity with the pulmonary, granular, and other varieties of tuberculosis. He recognized six types of pulmonary lesion. English translation, Liverpool, 1815.

2323 KLENCKE, PHILIPP FRIEDRICH HERMANN. 1813–1881
Ueber die Ansteckung und Verbreitung der Scrophelkrankheit bei Menschen durch den Genuss der Kuhmilch. Leipzig, *C. E. Kollmann*, 1846.

Klencke showed the possibility of the transmission of tuberculosis to man by cow's milk. In 1843 he succeeded in inoculating rabbits with tuberculosis.

2324 VILLEMIN, JEAN ANTOINE. 1827–1892
Etudes sur la tuberculose; preuves rationnelles et expérimentales de sa spécificité et de son inoculabilité. Paris, *J. B. Baillière*, 1868.

Villemin inoculated guinea-pigs and rabbits with sputum, caseous material, and miliary tubercles, with resulting development of tuberculosis. His brilliant experimental work proved tuberculosis to be a specific infection transmissible by an inoculable agent.

2325 BUHL, LUDWIG VON. 1816–1880
Lungenentzündung, Tuberkulose und Schwindsucht. München, *R. Oldenbourg*, 1872.

Buhl stated that disseminated miliary tuberculosis is always associated with the presence of a caseous focus in some part of the body, which is the centre from which infection starts (Buhl–Dittrich law). English translation, 1874.

2326 GRANCHER, JACQUES JOSEPH. 1843–1907
De l'unité de la phthisie. Paris, *Thèse No.* 50, 1873.

Confirmation of Villemin. Grancher in 1903 instituted the "Grancher system" – the boarding out of children from tuberculous households in France.

2327 KLEBS, THEODOR ALBRECHT EDWIN. 1834–1913
Die künstliche Erzeugung der Tuberkulose. *Arch. exp. Path. Pharmak.*, 1873, **1**, 163–80.

Klebs was the first to produce experimental bovine tuberculosis (by feeding cattle with infected milk). His work confirmed the earlier researches of Villemin.

2328 THAON, LOUIS ALBERT. 1846–1886
Recherches sur l'anatomie pathologique de la tuberculose. Paris, *Thèse No.* 45, 1873.

2329 COHNHEIM, JULIUS FRIEDRICH. 1839–1884
Die Tuberkulose vom Standpunkte der Infectionslehre. Leipzig, *A. Edelmann*, 1880.

Cohnheim, a pioneer pathologist, was Virchow's most distinguished pupil. Among his many valuable experiments the greatest was perhaps his successful inoculation of tuberculosis in the anterior chamber of the rabbit's eye, 1877, an account of which is included in the above work. This proved that tuberculous material derived from different sources owed its infectiveness to the same contagious factor. The book first appeared in quarto, 29 pp., 1879, with a Latin imprint: Lipsiae, *typis A. Edelmanni*. This scarce version was followed by the more common octavo (44 pp.) recorded above. An English translation is included in D. U. Cullimore's *Consumption as a contagious disease*, London, [1880].

2330 CONCATO, LUIGI MARIA. 1825–1882
Sulla poliorromennite scrofolosa, o tisi delle sierose. *G. int. Sci. med.*, 1881, n.s. **3**, 1037–53.

Concato's excellent description of tuberculous inflammation of the serous membranes resulted in the eponym "Concato's disease".

2330.1 ZIEHL, FRANZ. 1859–1926
Zur Färbung des Tuberkelbacillus. *Dtsch. med. Wschr.*, 1882, **8**, 451.

Ziehl–Neelsen stain.

2331 KOCH, ROBERT. 1843–1910
Die Aetiologie der Tuberkulose. *Berl. klin. Wschr.*, 1882, **19**, 221–30.

Discovery of the tubercle bacillus, announced March 24, 1882. This paper also contains the first statement of "Koch's postulates". Koch published a fuller account in *Mitt. k. GesundhAmte*, 1884, 2, 1–88, in which he reported how he had succeeded in producing experimental tuberculosis in animals after cultivating the bacillus. Reprinted with translation in *Med. Classics*, 1938, 2, 821–80. Koch received the Nobel Prize in 1905.

2332 ——. Weitere Mittheilungen über ein Heilmittel gegen Tuberkulose. *Dtsch. med. Wschr.*, 1890, **16**, 1029–32; 1891, **17**, 101–02, 1189–92.

Introduction of tuberculin in the treatment of tuberculosis. The second paper describes "Koch's phenomenon".

2333 ——. Ueber neue Tuberkulinpräparate. *Dtsch. med. Wschr.*, 1897, **23,** 209–13.
Koch's new tuberculin (Tuberculin R).

2334 ARLOING, SATURNIN. 1846–1911
Sur l'obtention de cultures et d'émulsions homogènes du bacille de la tuberculose humaine en milieu liquide et "sur une variété mobile de ce bacille". *C. R. Acad. Sci.* (*Paris*), 1898, **126,** 1319–21.
Sero-agglutination for the diagnosis of presence of tubercle bacillus.

2335 SMITH, THEOBALD. 1859–1934
A comparative study of bovine tubercle bacilli and of human bacilli from sputum. *J. exp. Med.*, 1898, **3,** 451–511.
First clear differentiation between the bovine and human types of tubercle bacillus.

2336 CALOT, JEAN FRANÇOIS. 1861–1944
Les maladies qu'on soigne à Berck. Paris, *Masson*, 1900.
An account of the work of the Rothschild Hospital at Berck-sur-Mer, where Calot specialized in the treatment of surgical tuberculosis in children.

2337 CALMETTE, LÉON CHARLES ALBERT. 1863–1933
Sur un nouveau procédé de diagnostic de la tuberculose chez l'homme par l'ophtalmo-réaction à la tuberculine. *C. R. Acad. Sci.* (*Paris*), 1907, **144,** 1324–26.
Calmette's conjunctival reaction test for tuberculosis.

2338 PIRQUET VON CESENATICO, CLEMENS PETER. 1874–1929
Der diagnostische Wert der kutanen Tuberkulinreaktion bei der Tuberkulose des Kindesalters auf Grund von 100 Sektionen. *Wien. klin. Wschr.*, 1907, **20,** 1123–28.
Introduction of von Pirquet's test – a cutaneous reaction employed in the diagnosis of tuberculosis.

2339 MORO, ERNST. 1874–1951
Ueber eine diagnostisch verwertbare Reaktion der Haut auf Einreibung mit Tuberkulinsalbe. *Münch. med. Wschr.*, 1908, **55,** 216–18; 2025–28.
Moro's percutaneous tuberculin reaction, employed as a diagnostic measure.

2340 WOLFF-EISNER, ALFRED. 1877–1948
Die kutane und konjunktivale Tuberkulinreaktion, ihre Bedeutung für Diagnostik und Prognose der Tuberkulose. *Z. Tuberk.*, 1908, **12,** 21–25.
Wolff-Eisner's conjunctival tuberculin reaction.

2341 MANTOUX, CHARLES. 1877–1947
Intradermo-réaction de la tuberculine. *C. R. Acad. Sci. (Paris)*, 1908, **147,** 355–57.
Mantoux's intradermal tuberculin skin test.

2342 ROLLIER, AUGUSTE. 1874–1954
Die Heliotherapie der Tuberkulose. Berlin, *J. Springer*, 1913.
In 1903 Rollier introduced ultra-violet light and Alpine sunlight in the treatment of surgical tuberculosis. Heliotherapy for chronic affections was advocated as early as the 5th century A.D. by Caelius Aurelianus.

2343 CALMETTE, Léon Charles Albert. 1863–1933, *et al.*
Essai d'immunisation contre l'infection tuberculeuse. *Bull. Acad. Méd.* (*Paris*), 1924, 3 sér., **91,** 787–96.

With C. Guérin and B. Weill-Hallé. B.C.G. (Bacille Calmette-Guérin) vaccine was first produced in 1906 and subcultured for 13 years. It was used as a prophylactic against tuberculosis in children in 1921. See also No. 2346.

2344 MØLLGAARD, Holger. 1885–
Ueber die experimentellen Grundlagen für die Sanocrysin-Behandlung der Tuberkulose. *Tuberk.-Bibl.*, 1925, Heft 20, 1–72.

Møllgaard was responsible for the introduction of sanocrysin.

2345 SAUERBRUCH, Ernst Ferdinand. 1875–1951, *et al.*
Ueber Versuche, schwere Formen der Tuberkulose durch diätetische Behandlung zu beeinflussen. *Münch. med. Wschr.*, 1926, **73,** 47–51.

Gerson introduced a salt-restricted diet in the treatment of tuberculosis; this was subsequently modified by Sauerbruch and Herrmannsdorfer, becoming known as the "Gerson–Sauerbruch–Herrmannsdorfer diet". With A. Herrmannsdorfer and M. Gerson.

2346 CALMETTE, Léon Charles Albert. 1863–1933, *et al.*
Sur la vaccination préventive des enfants nouveau-nés contre la tuberculose par le B.C.G. *Ann. Inst. Pasteur*, 1927, **41,** 201–32.

With C. Guérin, L. Négre, and A. Boquet.

2347 WELLS, Henry Gideon. 1875–1943, & LONG, Esmond Ray. 1890–
The chemistry of tuberculosis. Second edition. Baltimore, *Williams & Wilkins*, 1932.

2348 VOLLMER, Hermann. 1896–1959, & GOLDBERGER, Esther White. 1905–
A new tuberculin patch test. *Amer. J. Dis. Child.*, 1937, **54,** 1019–24.

2349 FELDMAN, William Hugh. 1892– , *et al.*
The effect of promin (sodium salt of P.P'-diamino-diphenyl-sulfone-N, N'-dextrose sulfonate) on experimental tuberculosis: a preliminary report. *Proc. Mayo Clin.*, 1940, **15,** 695–99.

Experimental evidence of the value of promin (sodium glucosulphone) in tuberculosis. With H. C. Hinshaw and H. E. Moses. See also *Amer. Rev. Tuberc.*, 1942, **45**, 303–33.

2350 HINSHAW, Horton Corwin. 1902– , & FELDMAN, William Hugh. 1892–
Streptomycin in treatment of clinical tuberculosis: a preliminary report. *Proc. Mayo Clin.*, 1945, **20,** 313–18.

2351 DOMAGK, Gerhard. 1895–1964, *et al.*
Ueber eine neue, gegen Tuberkelbazillen in vitro wirksame Verbindungsklasse. *Naturwissenschaften*, 1946, **33,** 315.

Introduction of thiosemicarbazone in treatment of tuberculosis. With R. Behnisch, F. Mietzsch, and H. Schmidt.

2352 FRAPPIER, Armand. 1904– , & GUY, Roland. 1913–
A new and practical B.C.G. skin test (the B.C.G. scarification test) for the detection of the total tuberculous allergy. *Canad. J. publ. Hlth*, 1950, **41,** 72–83.

2352.1 HEAF, FREDERICK ROLAND GEORGE. 1894–1973
The multiple-puncture tuberculin test. *Lancet*, 1951, **2**, 151–53.
The Heaf multiple-puncture tuberculin test.

2353 ROBITZEK, EDWARD HEINRICH. 1912– , *et al.*
Chemotherapy of human tuberculosis with hydrazine derivatives of isonicotinic acid. (Preliminary report of representative cases.) *Quart. Bull. Sea View Hosp.*, 1952, **13**, 27–51.
Introduction of isoniazid. With I. J. Selikoff and G. G. Ornstein. See also *Amer. Rev. Tuberc.*, 1952, **65**, 257–442.

History of Tuberculosis

2354 FLICK, LAWRENCE FRANCIS. 1856–1938
Development of our knowledge of tuberculosis. Philadelphia, 1925.

2355 PIÉRY, ANTOINE MARIUS. 1873– , & ROSHEM, JULIEN.
Histoire de la tuberculose. Paris, *G. Doin*, 1931.

2356 MEACHEN, GEORGE NORMAN. 1876–
A short history of tuberculosis. London, *Bale*, 1936.

2357 WEBB, GERALD BERTRAM. 1871–1948
Tuberculosis. New York, *P. B. Hoeber*, 1936.
Clio Medica series.

2358 KAYNE, GEORGE GREGORY. 1901–1945
The control of tuberculosis in England, past and present. London, *Oxford University Press*, 1937.

2359 CUMMINS, STEVENSON LYLE. 1873–1949
Tuberculosis in history from the 17th century to our own times. London, *Baillière, Tindall & Cox* 1949.

2360 MOORMAN, LEWIS JEFFERSON. 1875–1954
Tuberculosis and genius. Chicago, *University Press*, 1940.

2361 HART, PHILIP MONTAGU D'ARCY. 1900–
Chemotherapy of tuberculosis. Researches during the past 100 years. *Brit. med. J.*, 1946, **2**, 805–10, 849–55.

2361.1 BURKE, RICHARD MICHAEL. 1903–
Historical chronology of tuberculosis. 2nd ed. Springfield, *C. C. Thomas*, 1955.

2362–2432.1 SYPHILIS

See also 4772–4806, NEUROSYPHILIS; 5195–5227, VENEREAL DISEASES.

2362 GRÜNPECK, JOSEPH. 1473–1532
Tractatus de pestilentia scorra. [? Leipzig, *Boettiger*, 1496].
Grünpeck was first to record mixed primary lesions, multiple primary lesions, and to note the second incubation period of syphilis. A translation of the above is in *Arch. Derm. Syph. (Chicago)*, 1930, **22**, 430.

2363 LEONICENO, NICCOLÒ. 1428–1524
Libellus de epidemia, quam vulgo morbum Gallicum vocant. Venetiis *in domo Aldi Manutii*, 1497.

One of the earliest treatises on the subject. Leoniceno includes a good description of syphilitic hemiplegia. He believed that syphilis was known to classical writers. English translation in R. H. Major, *Classic descriptions of disease*, 3rd ed., 1945, p. 15.

2363.1 VILLALOBOS, FRANCISCO LOPEZ DE. 1473–1560
El sumario de la medicina, con un tratado sobre las pestiferas buuas. Salamanca, *Antonio de Barreda*, 1498.

H. Goodman considers this among the best of all works on the subject in the 15th and 16th centuries. For English translation see *Bull. Inst. Hist. Med.*, 1939, **7**, 1129–37. An English translation was also published in London, 1870.

2364 FRACASTORO, GIROLAMO [FRACASTORIUS]. 1478–1553
Syphilis sive morbus gallicus. Veronae, [*S. Nicolini da Sabbio*], 1530.

The most famous of all medical poems. It epitomized contemporary knowledge of syphilis, gave to it its present name, and recognized a venereal cause. Fracastorius refers to mercury as a remedy. First complete English translation by Nahum Tate (later Poet Laureate) was published in 1686; recent translation by W. van Wyck (1934). L. Baumgartner and J. F. Fulton published a handlist of editions of the poem in 1933 and a bibliography of the poem in 1935.

2365 MASSA, NICCOLÒ. 1499–1569
Liber de morbo gallico. [n.p. ?Venice,] 1532.

Includes a description of the neurological manifestations of syphilis. Massa was professor of anatomy in Venice.

2366 MATTIOLI, PIETRO ANDREA. 1500–1577
Morbi gallici novum ac utilissimum opusculum quo vera et omnimoda ejus cura percipi potest. [Bononiae, *imp. haered. Hieronymi de Benedictis*, 1533].

Mattioli considered mercury a specific in the treatment of syphilis. He was probably the first to work extensively on syphilis of the newborn. He is better known for his commentary on Dioscorides.

2367 DIAZ DE ISLA, RODRIGO RUIZ. 1462–1542
Tractado cótra el mal serpentino. (Sevilla, *D. de Robertis*, 1539.)

Diaz de Isla, a Barcelonese surgeon, wrote of a disease "previously unknown, unseen and undescribed", which appeared in Barcelona in 1493 and which was obviously syphilis. This is probably the earliest reference to the West Indian origin of syphilis (the writer believed that the disease originated in Haiti) and the book is the chief source of the opinions of those who believe in the American origin of syphilis. Text reproduced with German translation in *Janus*, 1901, **6**, 653–55; 1902, **7**, 31–40.

2368 HÉRY, THIERRY DE. ?1500–1599
La methode curatoire de la maladie venerienne. Paris, *M. David*, 1552.

De Héry made a fortune from treating syphilitic patients. He recommended mercurial inunctions and guaiac internally.

2369 PARACELSUS, [BOMBASTUS AB HOHENHEIM (AUREOLUS PHILIPPUS THEOPHRASTUS)]. 1493–1541
Von der frantzösischen kranckheit drey Bücher. Franckfurt a.M., *H. Gülfferichen*, 1553.

Paracelsus suggested the hereditary transmission of syphilis and advocated mercury internally, as an antisyphilitic. He called the disease "French gonorrhoea" and thus started the confusion which lasted until the 19th century.

2370 FALLOPPIO, GABRIELE [FALLOPIUS]. 1523–1562
De morbo gallico. Patavii, *apud C. Gryphium*, 1563.
Fallopius was one of the first prominent opponents of the use of mercury in syphilis. He distinguished between syphilitic and non-syphilitic condylomata.

2371 GALE, THOMAS. 1507–1587
Certaine works of chirurgerie. London, *R. Hall*, (1563).
Includes the first mention of syphilis in the English literature.

2372 LUVIGNI, ALOISIO [LUISINUS].
De morbo gallico omnia quae extant. 2 vols. Venetiis, *apud J. Zilettum*, 1566–67.
A collection of important writings on syphilis to 1500. Luvigni was born about the beginning of the 16th century. Boerhaave published a revision of this work in 1728, covering the period 1495–1566.

2373 CLOWES, WILLIAM. 1540–1604
A short and profitable treatise touching the cure of the morbus gallicus by unctions. London, *J. Daye*, 1579.
William Clowes, the greatest of the Elizabethan surgeons, published the first original English treatise on syphilis. It was his first work; it demonstrates the prevalence of the disease at that time (Clowes says that of every 20 persons admitted to St. Bartholomew's Hospital, 15 were found to be suffering from syphilis).

2374 FERNEL, JEAN FRANÇOIS. 1497–1558
De luis venereae curatione perfectissima liber. Antverpiae, *ex. off. C. Plantini*, 1579.
French translation, Paris, 1879.

2375 ABERCROMBY, DAVID. 1621–1695
Tuta, ac efficax luis venereae. Londini, *S. Smith*, 1684.
Abercromby advanced the idea that syphilis was caused by a parasite.

2376 GRUNER, CHRISTIAN GOTTFRIED. 1744–1815
Morborum antiquitates. Vratislaviae, *J. F. Korn*, 1774.
Pp. 85–100: "Lists 191 semeiological varieties of syphilis described in the period" (Garrison).

2377 HUNTER, JOHN. 1728–1793
A treatise on the venereal disease. London, 1786.
In Hunter's day the venereal diseases were thought to be due to a single poison. To test this theory, Hunter inoculated himself with matter taken from a gonorrhoeal patient who, unknown to Hunter, also had syphilis. Hunter contracted the latter disease and maintained that gonorrhoea and syphilis were caused by a single pathogen. Backed by the weight of Hunter's authority, this experiment retarded the development of knowledge regarding the two diseases. The hard ("Hunterian") chancre eponymizes Hunter.

2378 BELL, BENJAMIN. 1749–1806
A treatise on gonorrhoea virulenta, and lues venerea. 2 vols. Edinburgh, *J. Wartson & G. Mudie*, 1793.
Bell was the first to differentiate between gonorrhoea and syphilis.

2378.1 BERTIN, RENÉ JOSEPH HYACINTHE. 1757–1828
Traité de la maladie vénérienne chez les enfans nouveau-nés, les femmes enceintes et les nourrices. Paris, *Chez Gabon*, 1810.
First systematic work on congenital syphilis.

2379 WALLACE, William. 1791–1837
Treatment of the venereal disease by the hydriodate of potash, or iodide of potassium. *Lancet*, 1835–36, **2**, 5–11.

Wallace introduced potassium iodide in the treatment of syphilis, reporting good results in 139 patients.

2380 COLLES, Abraham. 1773–1843
Practical observations on the venereal disease, and on the use of mercury. London, *Sherwood, Gilbert & Piper*, 1837.

In this work (p. 304) is stated "Colles' law". Colles introduced small doses of mercury in the treatment of syphilis. He was professor of surgery at Dublin.

2381 RICORD, Phillippe. 1800–1889
Traité pratique des maladies vénériennes. Paris, *De Just Rouvier & E. Le Bouvier*, 1838.

Includes the description of "Ricord's chancre", the initial lesion in syphilis. Ricord re-demonstrated the specific character of syphilis and divided it into the three stages, primary, secondary, and tertiary. See also No. 5202.

2383 DIDAY, Charles Joseph Paul Edouard. 1812–1894
Traité de la syphilis des nouveau-nés et des enfants à la mamelle. Paris, *V. Masson*, 1854.

An important work on congenital syphilis. English translation, 1859.

2384 BETTINGER, Julius. 1802–1887
Aerztliches Intelligenz-Blatt, 1856, **3**, 425–28.

First demonstration of the experimental inoculability of syphilis. The information is given in a discussion on the subject by the Society of Physicians of the Palatinate; it appeared anonymously, without title, and identity of the writer was not disclosed until fifty years later. See the footnote on page 585 of Garrison's *Introduction* for further details; a biographical note appears in *Derm. Z.*, 1913, **20**, 220–23.

2385 VIRCHOW, Rudolf Ludwig Karl. 1821–1902
Ueber die Natur der constitutionell-syphilitischen Affectionen. *Virchows Arch. path. Anat.*, 1858, **15**, 217–336.

Virchow's great work on the pathology of syphilis confirmed the fact that it was a disease which involved all organs and tissues of the body, and showed that the causal organism was transferred through the blood to the various organs and tissues. Republished in book form, Berlin, 1859.

2386 HUTCHINSON, *Sir* Jonathan. 1828–1913
Report on the effects of infantile syphilis in marring the development of the teeth. *Trans. path. Soc. Lond.*, 1858, **9**, 449–55.

Hutchinson, of St. Bartholomew's Hospital, is memorable for his original description of the notched incisors ("Hutchinson's teeth") in congenital syphilis. His name is also associated with "Hutchinson's triad" (interstitial keratitis, notched incisors and labyrinthine disease) in congenital syphilis.

2387 KUSSMAUL, Adolf. 1822–1902
Untersuchungen über den constitutionellen Mercurialismus und sein Verhältniss zur constitutionellen Syphilis. Würzburg, *Stahel*, 1861.

2388 PELLIZZARI, Pietro. 1823–1892
Della trasmissione delle sifilide mediante l'inoculazione del sangre. [Florence, 1862].

Proof of the possibility of transmission of syphilis by blood transfusion.

2389 WILKS, *Sir* SAMUEL, *Bart.* 1824–1911
On the syphilitic affections of internal organs. *Guy's Hosp. Rep.* 1863, **24,** 1–63.

Wilks' outstanding work was on visceral syphilis, a subject which he was one of the first to study.

2390 PROFETA, GIUSEPPE. 1840–1911
Sulla sifilide per allattamento. *Sperimentale,* 1865, 4 ser., **15,** 328–38, 339–418.

Profeta's law – a non-syphilitic child born of syphilitic parents is immune.

2390.1 LANCEREAUX, ÉTIENNE. 1829–1910
Traité historique et pratique de la syphilis. Paris, *J. B. Baillière,* 1866.

A complete review of contemporary knowledge. English translation, 2 vols., 1868–69.

2391 MOON, HENRY. 1845–1892
On irregular and defective tooth development. *Trans. odont. Soc. G. B.,* 1876–77, n.s. **9,** 223–43.

"Moon's molars", the first molars in congenital syphilitics.

2392 KLEBS, THEODOR ALBRECHT EDWIN. 1834–1913
Das Contagium der Syphilis. Eine experimentelle Studie. *Arch. exp. Path. Pharmak.,* 1878–79, **10,** 161–221.

Klebs inoculated syphilis into apes, and probably saw the spirochaete before Schaudinn and Hoffmann.

2393 FOURNIER, JEAN ALFRED. 1832–1915
La syphilis héréditaire tardive. Paris, *G. Masson,* 1886.

Fournier, one of the greatest syphilologists, did more than any other person to develop the knowledge regarding congenital syphilis. Through his writings, the importance of syphilis as a cause of degenerative diseases was recognized.

2394 BALZER, FÉLIX. 1849–1929
Expériences sur la toxicité du bismuth. *C. R. Soc. Biol.* (*Paris*), 1889, 9 sér., **1,** 537–44.

Balzer was the first to suggest bismuth in the treatment of syphilis.

2395 FOURNIER, JEAN ALFRED. 1832–1915
Les chancres extra-génitaux. Paris, *Rueff & Cie.,* 1897.

2396 JARISCH, ADOLF. 1850–1902
Therapeutische Versuche bei Syphilis. *Wien. med. Wschr.,* 1895, **45,** 720–21.

Jarisch–Herxheimer reaction; see also No. 2397.

2397 HERXHEIMER, KARL. 1861–1944
Ueber eine bei Syphilitischen vorkommende Quecksilberreaktion. *Dtsch. med. Wschr.,* 1902, **28,** 895–97.

See No. 2396.

2398 METCHNIKOFF, ELIE. 1845–1916, & ROUX, PIERRE PAUL EMILE. 1853–1933
Etudes expérimentales sur la syphilis. *Ann. Inst. Pasteur,* 1903, **17,** 809–21; 1904, **18,** 1–6.

Metchnikoff and Roux successfully transmitted syphilis from man to the higher apes. Although not the first to do this, they recorded much new information concerning the disease.

2399 SCHAUDINN, Fritz Richard. 1871–1906, & HOFFMANN, Erich. 1868–1959
Vorläufiger Bericht über das Vorkommen von Spirochaeten in syphilitischen Krankheitsprodukten und bei Papillomen. *Arb. k. GesundhAmte*, 1905, **22,** 527–34.

On March 3, 1905, Schaudinn discovered the causal organism of syphilis, *Spirochaeta pallida*, in serum obtained from a genital lesion by Hoffmann. Schaudinn later re-named the spirochaete *Treponema pallidum*.

2399.1 BERTARELLI, Ernesto. 1873–
Ueber die Transmission der Syphilis auf das Kaninchen. Vorläufiger Bericht. *Zbl. Bakt.*, 1906, I Abt. Orig., **41,** 320–26.

Transmission of syphilis to rabbits.

2400 LANDSTEINER, Karl. 1868–1943, & MUCHA, Viktor. 1877–
Zur Technik der Spirochaetenuntersuchung. *Wien. klin. Wschr.*, 1906, **19,** 1349–50.

Dark field method of diagnosis for presence of *T. pallidum*.

2401 LEVADITI, Constantin. 1874–1953
A propos de l'imprégnation au nitrate d'argent des spirochètes sur coupes. *C. R. Soc. Biol.* (*Paris*), 1906, **60,** 67–68.

Levaditi's method of staining *T. pallidum*.

2402 WASSERMANN, August von. 1866–1925, *et al.*
Eine serodiagnostische Reaktion bei Syphilis. *Dtsch. med. Wschr.*, Berlin, 1906, **32,** 745–46.

The "Wassermann reaction," a specific diagnostic blood test for syphilis, and a modification of the complement-fixation reaction of Bordet and Gengou. With A. Neisser and C. Bruck.

2403 EHRLICH, Paul. 1854–1915, & HATA, Sahachiro. 1873–1938
Die experimentelle Chemotherapie der Spirillosen (Syphilis, Rückfallfieber, Hühnerspirillose, Frambösie). Berlin, *J. Springer*, 1910.

After many experiments on the action of synthetic drugs upon spirochaetal diseases, Ehrlich and Hata in 1909 discovered salvarsan ("606"), specific in the treatment of syphilis and yaws.

2404 NOGUCHI, Hideyo. 1876–1928
A method for the pure cultivation of pathogenic Treponema pallidum (Spirochaeta pallida). *J. exp. Med.*, 1911, **14,** 99–108.

Pure cultures of *T. pallidum* first obtained.

2405 EHRLICH, Paul. 1854–1915
Ueber Laboratoriumsversuche und klinische Erprobung von Heilstoffen. *Chem. Ztg*, 1912, **36,** 637–38.

Introduction of neoarsphenamine (neosalvarsan).

2406 LANGE, Karl Friedrich August. 1883–
Die Ausflockung kolloidalen Goldes durch Zerebrospinalflüssigkeit bei luetischen Affektion des Zentralnervensystems. *Z. Chemother.*, 1913, **1,** 44–78.

Lange's colloidal gold test for the diagnosis of cerebrospinal syphilis. See also *Berl. klin. Wschr.*, 1912, **49,** 897–901.

2407 MEINICKE, Ernst. 1878–1945
Ueber ein neue Methode der serologischen Luesdiagnose. *Berl. klin. Wschr.*, 1917, **54,** 613–14.
Meinicke diagnostic reaction.

2408 SACHS, Hans. 1877–1945, & GEORGI, Walter. 1889–1920
Zur Kritik des serologischen Luesnachweises mittels Ausflockung. *Münch. med. Wschr.*, 1919, **66,** 440–42.
Sachs–Georgi diagnostic reaction.

2409 WEICHARDT, Julius Wolfgang. 1875– , & SCHRADER, Erich.
Über die Serodiagnostik der Syphilis mittels Ausflockung durch cholesterinierte Extrakte. *Med. Klin.*, 1919, **15,** 139–40.
Weichardt's reagent.

2410 WARTHIN, Aldred Scott. 1866–1931, & STARRY, Allen Chronister. 1890–
A more rapid and improved method of demonstrating spirochetes in tissues (Warthin and Starry's cover-glass method). *Amer. J. Syph.*, 1920, **4,** 97–103.
Warthin and Starry's method.

2411 SAZERAC, Robert, 1875– , & LEVADITI, Constantin. 1874–1953
Traitement de la syphilis par le bismuth. *C. R. Acad. Sci. (Paris)*, 1921, **173,** 338–40.
Introduction of sodium-potassium bismuth tartrate in the treatment of syphilis.

2412 KAHN, Reuben Leon. 1887–
A simple quantitative precipitation reaction for syphilis. *Arch. Derm. Syph. (Chicago)*, 1922, **5,** 570–78.
Kahn test.

2413 KOLMER, John Albert. 1886–1962
Studies in the standardization of the Wassermann reaction. XXX. A new complement-fixation test for syphilis based upon the results of studies in the standardization of technic. *Amer. J. Syph.*, 1922, **6,** 82–110.
Kolmer test.

2414 STOKES, John Hinchman. 1885– , & CHAMBERS, Stanley Owen. 1897–
Bismuth arsphenamine sulphate. *J. Amer. med. Ass.*, 1927, **89,** 1500–1505.
Clinical introduction of bismarsen, synthesized by G. W. Raiziss in 1924.

2414.1 EAGLE, Harry. 1905–
Studies in the serology of syphilis. VIII. A new flocculation test for the serum diagnosis of syphilis. *J. Lab. clin. Med.*, 1932, **17,** 787–91.
Eagle flocculation test.

2415 TATUM, Arthur Lawrie. 1884–1955, & COOPER, Garrett Arthur. 1904–
An experimental study of mapharsen (meta-amino para-hydroxy phenyl arsine oxide) as an antisyphilitic agent. *J. Pharmacol.*, 1934, **50,** 198–215.
Introduction of mapharsen.

2416 FOERSTER, Otto Hottinger. 1876–1965, *et al.*
Mapharsen in the treatment of syphilis. A preliminary report. *Arch. Derm. Syph.* (*Chicago*), 1935, **32,** 868–92.
Clinical use of mapharsen. With R. L. McIntosh, L. M. Wieder, H. R. Foerster, and G. A. Cooper.

2417 PANGBORN, Mary Candace. 1907–
Isolation and purification of a serologically active phospholipid from beef heart. *J. Biol. Chem.*, 1942, **143,** 247–56.
Introduction of cardiolipin antigens for the serological diagnosis of syphilis.

2418 MAHONEY, John Friend. 1889–1957, *et al.*
Penicillin treatment of early syphilis. A preliminary report. *Vener. Dis. Inform.*, 1943, **24,** 355–57; also in *Amer. J. publ. Hlth*, 1943, **33,** 1387–91.
Introduction of penicillin in treatment of syphilis. With R. C. Arnold and A. Harris.

2419 NELSON, Robert Armstrong. 1922– , & MAYER, Manfred Martin. 1916–
Immobilization of *Treponema pallidum in vitro* by antibody produced in syphilitic infection. *J. exp. Med.*, 1949, **89,** 369–93.
Nelson's treponemal immobilization test.

History of Syphilis

See also 5226–5227, History of Venereal Diseases.

2420 FUCHS, Conrad Heinrich. 1803–1855
Die ältesten Schriftsteller über die Lustseuche in Deutschland, von 1495 bis 1510. Göttingen, *Dieterich*, 1843.
Gives texts of German tracts on syphilis published between 1495 and 1510.

2421 ROSENBAUM, Julius. 1807–1874
Geschichte der Lustseuche in Alterthume. Halle, *Lippert u. Schmidt*, 1845.
Second impression; first published 1839. French translation, 1847; English version, 1901. 4th edition (1904) reprinted 1971.

2422 BURET, Frédéric.
Syphilis today and among the ancients. 2 vols. Philadelphia, *F. A. Davis*, 1891–95.

2423 BLOCH, Iwan. 1872–1922
Der Ursprung der Syphilis. 2 pts. Jena, *G. Fischer*, 1901–11.
Bloch is the chief modern supporter of the theory of the Columbian origin of syphilis.

2424 SUDHOFF, Karl Friedrich Jakob. 1853–1938
Aus der Frühgeschichte der Syphilis. Leipzig, *Barth*, 1912.
Sudhoff, one of the greatest of medical historians, believed in the pre-Columbian existence of syphilis.

2425 ——. Mal Franzoso in Italien in der ersten Hälfte des 15. Jahrhunderts. Giessen, *A. Töpelmann*, 1912.
Forms Heft 5 of K. Sudhoff & G. Sticker: *Zur historischen Biologie der Krankheitserreger.*

2426 DOHI, Keizo. 1866–1931
Beiträge zur Geschichte der Syphilis; insbesondere über ihren Ursprung und ihre Pathologie in Ostasien. Tokio, *Nankodo*, 1923.
Gives, in an appendix, a list of writers on syphilis from 1495 to 1829.

2427 SUDHOFF, Karl Friedrich Jakob. 1853–1938
The earliest printed literature on syphilis. Being ten tractates from the years 1495–98 . . . Adapted by Charles Singer. Florence, *R. Lier & Co.*, 1925.

2428 JEANSELME, Antoine Edouard. 1858–1935
Histoire de la syphilis. Paris, *G. Doin*, 1931.
Forms tome I of *Traité de la syphilis*, ed. by E. Jeanselme and E. Schulmann.

2429 PUSEY, William Allen. 1865–1940
The history and epidemiology of syphilis. Springfield, Baltimore, *C. C. Thomas*, 1933.

2430 HOLCOMBE, Richmond Cranston. 1874–
Who gave the world syphilis? The Haitian myth. New York, *Froben Press*, 1937.

2431 WHITWELL, James Richard. 1863–1945
Syphilis in earlier days. London, *H. K. Lewis*, 1940.

2432 GOODMAN, Herman. 1894–
Notable contributors to the knowledge of syphilis. New York, *Froben Press*, 1944.

2432.1 DENNIE, Charles Clayton. 1883–
A history of syphilis. Springfield, *C. C. Thomas*, 1962.

2433–2447 LEPROSY

2433 ARETAEUS *the Cappadocian*. A.D. 81–138?
On elephas, or elephantiasis. In his *Extant Works*, edited by Francis Adams, London, 1856, 366–73, 494–98.
Classical description of "elephantiasis Aretaei," nodous leprosy.

2434 DANIELSSEN, Daniel Cornelis. 1815–1894, & BOECK Carl, Wilhelm. 1808–1875
Om spedalskhed. Udgivet efter Foranstaltning af den Kongelige Norske Regjerings Departement for det Indre. 1 vol. and atlas. Christiania (Bergen), *trykt. hos C. Gröndahl*, 1847.
First modern description of leprosy ("Danielssen-Boeck disease"). Danielssen, physician to the leprosy hospital at Bergen, was the founder of scientific leprology. The extremely rare *Atlas* was published in Bergen; it consists of 24 plates and two pages of text. French translation, Paris, *J. B. Baillière*, 1848; the atlas was also reproduced in French in 1946.

2435 MOUAT, Frederic John. 1816–1897
Notes on native remedies. No. 1. The chaulmoogra. *Indian Ann. med. Sci.*, 1854, **1**, 646–52.
Chaulmoogra oil was first introduced into Western medicine by Mouat, having been used for many centuries previously by the Chinese.

2436 HANSEN, GERHARD HENRIK ARMAUER. 1841–1912
Indberetning til det Norske mediciniske Selskab i Christiania om en med understøttelse af selskabet foretagen reise for at anstille undersøgelser angående spedalskhedens årsager, tildels udførte sammen med forstander Hartwig. *Norsk Mag. f. Laegevidensk.*, 1874, 3 R., **4,** 9 Heft, 1–88.

Hansen discovered the leprosy bacillus in 1871, publishing his findings three years later. He had been stimulated by the previous work of Danielssen and Boeck, and his own demonstration of the leprosy bacillus is one of the earliest observations of pathogenic bacteria. For an English translation of the paper, see *Brit. for. med.-chir. Rev.*, 1875, **55**, 459–89.

2436.1 NEISSER, ALBERT LUDWIG SIEGMUND. 1855–1916
Über die Ätiologie des Aussatzes. *Jber. akad. nat. Vereins Breslau*, 1879, **57,** 65–72.

Neisser obtained leprosy tissue from Hansen and was able to demonstrate the leprosy bacillus more convincingly than Hansen.

2437 POWER, FREDERICK BELDING. 1853–1927, & GORNALL, FRANK HOWORTH.
The constituents of chaulmoogra seeds. *J. chem. Soc.*, 1904, **85,** 838–51.

2438 ROST, ERNEST REINHOLD. 1872–
The cultivation of the Bacillus leprae. *Indian med. Gaz.*, 1904, **39,** 167–69.

Rost cultivated the leprosy bacillus and he prepared leprolin.

2439 UNNA, PAUL GERSON. 1850–1929
Histotechnik der leprösen Haut. Hamburg, Leipzig, 1910.

2440 ROGERS, *Sir* LEONARD. 1868–1962, & MUIR, ERNEST. 1880–
Leprosy. Bristol, *J. Wright & Co.*, 1925.

Third edition 1946.

2441 FAGET, GUY HENRY. 1891–1947, *et al.*
The promin treatment of leprosy. A progress report. *Publ. Hlth Rep.* (*Wash.*), 1943, **58,** 1729–41.

Promin (sodium glucosulphone) introduced in the treatment of leprosy. With R. C. Pogge, F. A. Johansen, J. F. Dinan, B. M. Prejean, and C. G. Eccles.

2442 MUIR, ERNEST. 1880–
Preliminary report on diasone in the treatment of leprosy. *Int. J. Leprosy*, 1944, **12,** 1–6.

Muir found diasone (a sulphone) valuable in the treatment of leprosy.

2442.1 HARKNESS, ARTHUR HERBERT, & BROWNLEE, G.
Leprosy treated with sulphetrone in 1943. *Proc. roy. Soc. Med.*, 1948, **41,** 309–10.

Clinical use of solapsone (sulphetrone).

2442.2 SHEPARD, CHARLES CARTER. 1914–
Acid-fast bacilli in nasal excretions in leprosy, and results of inoculation of mice. *Amer. J. Hyg.*, 1960, **71,** 147–57.

Transmission of leprosy to animals. See also *J. exp. Med.*, 1960, **112,** 445.

History of Leprosy

2443 ZAMBACO, DÉMÉTRIUS ALEXANDRE, *Pasha*. 1830–1913
La lèpre à travers les siècles et les contrées. Paris, *Masson & Cie.*, 1914.

2444 MERCIER, CHARLES ARTHUR. 1852–1919
Leper houses and mediaeval hospitals. London, *H. K. Lewis*, 1915.
FitzPatrick Lectures, 1914.

2445 ROGERS, *Sir* LEONARD. 1868–1962
Recent advances in the treatment and prophylaxis of leprosy. *Edinb. med. J.*, 1930, **37**, 1–27.
Cameron Prize Essay.

2446 WEYMOUTH, ANTHONY [*Pseudonym*].
Through the leper-squint. A study of leprosy from pre-Christian times to the present day. London, *Selwyn & Blount*, (1938).

2447 KEFFER, LUIZA.
Indice bibliográfico de lepra, 1560–1943. 3 vols. São Paulo, 1944–48.
Supplements 1–5, 1952–62.

2448–2463.1 PARASITOLOGY

2448 REDI, FRANCESCO. 1626–1697
Osservazioni . . . intorno agli animali viventi che si trovano negli animali viventi. Firenze, *per P. Matini*, 1684.
Redi was among the first of the parasitologists. He demonstrated the reproductive organs of *Ascaris lumbricoides* and also ascaris eggs. The results of his experiments appear in the above work, which also records his study and description of 108 different species of parasites.

2449 RUDOLPH, KARL ASMUND. 1771–1832
Entozoorum, sive verminum intestinalium, historia naturalis. 2 vols. Amstelodami, 1808–10.
A system of helminthology. Rudolphi gave the name "echinococcus" to the common vesicular hydatid, describing three species.

2450 KÜCHENMEISTER, GOTTLOB FRIEDRICH HEINRICH. 1821–1890
Ueber Cestoden im allgemeinen und die des Menschen insbesondere. Zittau, *W. Pahl*, 1853.

2451 DAVAINE, CASIMIR JOSEPH. 1812–1882
Traité des entozoaires et des maladies vermineuses. Paris, *J. B. Baillière*, 1860.

2452 COBBOLD, THOMAS SPENCER. 1828–1886
Entozoa. 2 pts. London, *Groombridge & Sons*, 1864–69.
Cobbold was the most distinguished helminthologist of his time. He named *Filaria bancrofti*, *Bilharzia haematobia*, and several other parasites. He was a friend of Manson, several of whose papers he communicated to the Linnean Society and the Quekett Microscopical Club.

2453 LEUCKART, Karl Georg Friedrich Rudolf. 1823–1898
Die menschlichen Parasiten und die von ihnen herrührenden Krankheiten. 2 vols. Leipzig, *F. C. Winter*, 1863–76.
English translation, Edinburgh, 1886.

2454 BRAUN, Maximilian Gustav Christian Carl. 1850–1930
Die thierischen Parasiten des Menschen. Würzburg, *A. Stuber*, 1883.

2455 MANSON, *Sir* Patrick. 1844–1922
The Filaria sanguinis hominis and certain new form of parasitic disease in India, China and warm countries. London, *H. K. Lewis*, 1883.
A collection of several papers written by Manson.

2456 BLANCHARD, Raphaël Anatole Emile. 1857–1919
Traité de zoologie médicale. 2 vols. Paris, *J. B. Baillière*, 1886–90.

2457 KOCH, Robert. 1843–1910
Reise-Bericht über Rinderpest, Bubonenpest in Indien und Afrika, Tsetse- oder Surrakrankheit, Texasfieber, tropische Malaria, Schwarzwasserfieber. Berlin, *J. Springer*, 1898.

2458 CLARKE, James Jackson. 1860–1940
Protozoa and disease. 4 vols. London, *Baillière, Tindall & Cox*, 1903–15.

2459 LEIDY, Joseph. 1823–1891
Researches in helminthology and parasitology. With a bibliography of his contributions to science. Washington, *Smithsonian Inst.*, 1904.
In vol. 46 of *Smithsonian Miscellaneous Collections.* Leidy was the greatest descriptive naturalist in America.

2460 PROWAZEK, Stanislaus Joseph Matthias von. 1875–1915
Handbuch der pathogenen Protozoen. 3 vols. Leipzig, *J. A. Barth*, 1912–31.

2461 STILES, Charles Wardell. 1867–1941, & HASSALL, Albert. 1862–1942
Key-catalogue of the protozoa reported for man. Washington, *Govt. Printing Office*, 1925.

2462 WENYON, Charles Morley. 1878–1948
Protozoology. 2 vols. London, *Baillière, Tindall & Cox*, 1926.

2463 LEIPER, Robert Thomson. 1881–1969
Landmarks in medical helminthology. *J. Helminth.*, 1929, **7**, 101–18.

2463.1 FOSTER, William Derek.
A history of parasitology. Edinburgh, *E. & S. Livingstone Ltd.*, 1965.

2464–2527 MICROBIOLOGY

2464 WILLIS, Thomas. 1621–1675
Diatribae duae medico-philosophicae quarum prior agit de fermentatione sive de motu intestino particularum in quovis corpore. Londini, *T. Roycroft*, 1659.
Contains the earliest suggestion that fermentation is an intestinal or internal motion of particles; the analogy between putrefaction and fermentation is also noted.

2465 GLEICHEN, Wilhelm Friedrich von [*Called* Russworm]. 1717–1783
Abhandlung über die Saamen- und Infusionsthierchen, und über die Erzeugung: nebst mikroskopischen Beobachtungen des Saamens der Thiere, und verschiedener Infusionen. Nürnberg, *A. W. Winterschmidt*, 1778.
Gleichen was probably the first to attempt to stain bacteria; he used carmine and indigo.

2466 MÜLLER, Otto Friedrich. 1730–1784
Animalcula infusoria fluviatilia et marina, quae detexit, systematice descripsit et ad vivum delineari. Hauniae, *N. Mölleri*, 1786.
Müller was the first to attempt a systematic classification of bacteria. He published several papers on the subject, the best being the above posthumous work.

2467 FABBRONI, Giovanni Valentino Mattia. 1752–1822
Dell' arte de fare il vino. Firenze, 1787.
Fabbroni is considered the first to promote modern ideas on the nature of fermentation. He showed that air was not necessary for fermentation to take place; he was first to regard the ferment as an albumenoid substance. Several of the names used by him are in use to-day.

2468 KERNER, Christian Andreas Justinus. 1786–1862
Neue Beobachtungen über die in Würtemberg so häufig vorfallenden tödtlichen Vergiftung durch den Genuss geräuchter Würste. Tübingen, *C. F. Osiander*, 1820.
Botulism first described.

2469 EHRENBERG, Christian Gottfried. 1795–1876
Die Infusionsthierchen als vollkommene Organismen. 1 vol. and atlas. Leipzig, *L. Voss*, 1838.
Includes (p. 80) first description of *B. subtilis*.

2470 DUJARDIN, Félix. 1801–1860
Histoire naturelle des zoophytes. Paris, *Lib. encyclopéd. de Roret*, 1841.
Further modification of and improvements in the classification of bacteria.

2471 GOODSIR, John. 1814–1867
History of a case in which a fluid periodically ejected from the stomach contained vegetable organisms of an undescribed form. *Edinb. med. surg. J.*, 1842, **57**, 430–43.
First description of *Sarcina ventriculi*, discovered by Goodsir.

2472 PASTEUR, Louis. 1822–1895
Mémoire sur la fermentation appelée lactique. *C. R. Acad. Sci. (Paris)*, 1857, **45**, 913–16.

2473 PASTEUR, Louis. 1822–1895.
Nouveaux faits pour servir à l'histoire de la levure lactique. *C. R. Acad. Sci.* (*Paris*), 1859, **48,** 337–38.

This and the preceding entry mark Pasteur's commencement of the study of fermentation. He found that the conversion of sugar to lactic acid in fermentation is due to small corpuscles, isolated or grouped.

2474 ——. Expériences relatives aux générations dites spontanées. *C. R. Acad. Sci.* (*Paris*), 1860, **50,** 303–07, 849–54; **51,** 348–52, 675–78.

2475 ——. Mémoire sur les corpuscles organisés qui existent dans l'atmosphere. Examen de la doctrine des générations spontanées. *Ann. Sci. nat.* (*Zool.*), 1861, **16,** 5–98.

The success of experiments recorded in the above paper marks the downfall of the theory of spontaneous generation. Pasteur's researches on fermentation led him to the discovery of the bacteria and yeasts and hence to the germ theory of disease; from this all modern bacteriology and immunology have developed.

2476 ——. Nouvel exemple de fermentation determinée par des animalcules infusoires pouvant vivre sans gaz oxygène libre, et en dehors de tout contact avec l'air de l'atmosphere. *C. R. Acad. Sci.* (*Paris*), 1863, **56,** 416–21.

Pasteur confirmed the fact, established by Schwann (No. 674) that putrefaction was a biological process.

2477 ——. Examen du rôle attribué au gaz oxygène atmosphérique dans la destruction des matières animales et végétales après la mort. *C. R. Acad. Sci.* (*Paris*), 1863, **56,** 734–40.

2478 ——. Recherches sur la putréfaction. *C. R. Acad. Sci.* (*Paris*), 1863, **56,** 1189–94.

Pasteur was the first to differentiate between aerobic and anaerobic organisms. (See also Nos. 2476–77.)

2479 ——. Études sur le vin. Paris, *Imp. impériale,* 1866.

2480 ——. Études sur le vinaigre. Paris, *Gauthier-Villars,* 1868.

Pasteur discovered that spoiling of wine by micro-organisms could be prevented by partial heat sterilization (pasteurization) at a temperature of 55–60° C.

2481 ——. Études sur la maladie des vers à soie. 2 vols. Paris, *Gauthier-Villars,* 1870.

Pasteur spent five years investigating silkworm disease before he discovered its cause.

2482 WEIGERT, Carl. 1845–1904
Ueber Bakterien in der Pockenhaut. *Zbl. med. Wiss.,* 1871, **9,** 609–11.

Weigert, famous as pathologist and histologist, was the first to stain bacteria. He introduced many of the best staining methods in use to-day. Weigert discovered bacteria in haemorrhagic smallpox. In the same paper is described how carmine will colour cocci.

2483 COHN, Ferdinand Julius. 1828–1898
Untersuchungen über Bacterien. *Beitr. Biol. Pflanzen,* 1872, **1,** Heft 2, 127–224; Heft 3, 141–207; 1876, **2,** Heft 2, 249–76.

Cohn's morphological classification of bacteria. He founded the *Beiträge.*

2484 LISTER, JOSEPH, *1st Baron Lister.* 1827–1912
A further contribution to the natural history of bacteria and the germ theory of fermentative changes. *Quart. J. micr. Sci.*, 1873, n.s. **13,** 380–408.
Isolation of *Bact. lactis.*

2485 PASTEUR, LOUIS. 1822–1895
Études sur la bière, ... avec une théorie nouvelle de la fermentation. Paris, *Gauthier-Villars,* 1876.
Pasteur resumed his studies on fermentation in 1876, and in this book takes into account the developments in this field since his previous publications on the subject. Facsimile reproduction in 1920; English translation, 1879.

2486 WEIGERT, CARL. 1845–1904
Ueber eine Mykose bei einem neugeborenen Kinde (Bakterienfärbung mit Anilinfarben). *Jber. schles. Ges. vaterl. Cultur,* (1875), 1876, **53,** 229.
In this paper Weigert showed that methyl violet will reveal cocci in tissues.

2487 EHRLICH, PAUL. 1854–1915
Beitrag zur Kenntnis der Anilinfärbungen und ihrer Verwendung in der mikroskopischen Technik. *Arch. mikr. Anat.*, 1877, **13,** 263–77.
Ehrlich's first paper on the staining of specific granulations in white blood corpuscles by means of aniline dyes. His work immensely affected subsequent technical methods of staining.

2488 KOCH, ROBERT. 1843–1910
Verfahrungen zur Untersuchung, zum Conserviren und Photographiren der Bacterien. *Beitr. Biol. Pflanzen,* 1877, **2,** 399–434.
Koch greatly improved staining methods; he laid the foundations of the technical procedures employed to-day. In the above paper he described his method of making films of bacteria on cover slips and fixing them by gentle heat; he also gave details of his method of photographing bacteria. In some of his plates the cilia are clearly perceptible.

2489 LISTER, JOSEPH, *1st Baron Lister.* 1827–1912
On the lactic fermentation and its bearings on pathology. *Trans. path. Soc. Lond.*, 1877–78, **29,** 425–67.
Lister was the first to obtain a pure culture of a bacterium (*Bact. lactis*).

2490 PASTEUR, LOUIS. 1822–1895, & JOUBERT, JULES FRANÇOIS.
Charbon et septicémie. *C. R. Acad. Sci.* (*Paris*), 1877, **85,** 101–15.
Discovery of *Vibrion septique* (*Cl. septicum*), the first pathogenic anaerobe to be found.

2491 TYNDALL, JOHN. 1820–1893
Fermentation and its bearings on the phenomena of disease. Glasgow, *W. Collins,* 1877.
See No. 2495.

2492 MAGNIN, ANTOINE.
Les bactéries. Paris, *F. Savy,* 1878.
English translation by G. M. Sternberg, 1880.

2493 EHRLICH, PAUL. 1854–1915
Ueber das Methylenblau und seine klinisch-bakterioskopische Verwerthung. *Z. klin. Med.*, 1881, **2,** 710–13.
Introduction of methylene blue in bacteriological staining.

2494 OGSTON, *Sir* ALEXANDER. 1844–1929
Report upon micro-organisms in surgical diseases. *Brit. med. J.*, 1881, **1,** 369–75.

Ogston showed micrococci to be constantly present in acute and chronic abscesses. He discovered *Staph. aureus.*

2495 TYNDALL, JOHN. 1820–1893
Essays on the floating-matter of the air in relation to putrefaction and infection. London, *Longmans, Green & Co.*, 1881.

Tyndall interested himself in atmospheric germs and dust. His experiments on sterilization by heat led him to the discovery in 1877 of fractional sterilization (Tyndallization). His work on the subject is included in the above book, in which he also described the bactericidal effects of moulds. The researches of Tyndall, even more than those of Pasteur, dealt the final blow to the doctrine of spontaneous generation; they were fundamental for the progress of bacteriology.

2496 FEHLEISEN, FRIEDRICH. 1854–1924
Ueber Erysipel. *Dtsch. Z. Chir.*, 1882, **16,** 391–97.

Discovery of *Strep. pyogenes.* English translation, 1886.

2497 GESSARD, CARLE. 1850–1925
Sur les colorations bleue et verte des linges à pansements. *C. R. Acad. Sci. (Paris)*, 1882, **94,** 536–38.

Isolation of *Pseudomonas aeruginosa* (*Ps. pyocyanea*).

2498 FLÜGGE, CARL GEORG FRIEDRICH WILHELM. 1847–1923
Fermente und Mikroparasiten. Leipzig, *F. C. W. Vogel*, 1883.

English translation of second edition, 1890.

2498.1 MALASSEZ, LOUIS CHARLES. 1842–1909, & VIGNAL, W.
Sur une forme de tuberculose sans bacilles. *C. R. Soc. Biol.*, 1883, 7 sér., **5,** 338–41.

Isolation of *Pasteurella pseudotuberculosis.*

2499 GRAM, HANS CHRISTIAN JOACHIM. 1853–1938
Ueber die isolirte Färbung der Schizomyceten in Schnitt- und Trockenpräparaten. *Fortschr. Med.*, 1884, **2,** 185–89.

Gram's method of staining bacteria – one of the most widely used to-day.

2500 BARY, HEINRICH ANTON DE. 1831–1888
Vorlesungen über Bacterien. Leipzig, *W. Engelmann*, 1885.

2501 CORNIL, ANDRÉ VICTOR. 1837–1908, & BABÈS, VICTOR. 1854–1926
Les bactéries et leur rôle dans l'anatomie et l'histologie pathologiques des maladies infectieuses. 1 vol. and atlas. Paris, *F. Alcan*, 1885.

2502 HAUSER, GUSTAV. 1856–1935
Ueber Fäulnissbacterien. Leipzig, *F. C. W. Vogel*, 1885.

Isolation of *Proteus vulgaris.*

2503 HUEPPE, FERDINAND ADOLF THEOPHIL. 1852–1938
Die Methoden der Bakterienforschung. Wiesbaden, *Kriedel*, 1885.

Hueppe, a colleague of Koch, wrote an admirable manual on bacteriological methods, a subject to which he gave several original contributions.

2503.1 MAYER, Adolf Eduard Maydolf. 1843–
Ueber die Mosaikkrankheit des Tabaks. *Landw. VersSta.*, 1886, **32,** 450–67.

Mayer was first to describe and name the mosaic disease of tobacco and to demonstrate its infectious nature. Translation in *Phytopathological Classics*, No. 7, pp. 9–24, Ithaca, 1942.

2504 CROOKSHANK, Edgar March. 1858–1928
An introduction to practical bacteriology based upon the methods of Koch. London, *H. K. Lewis*, 1886.

Crookshank studies under Koch, and later became professor of bacteriology at King's College, London.

2505 SALMON, Daniel Elmer. 1850–1914, & SMITH, Theobald. 1859–1934.
The bacterium of swine-plague. *Amer. monthly micr. J.*, 1886, **7,** 204–05.

Discovery of *Salmonella cholerae-suis*. The Salmonelleae tribe was named after Salmon.

2506 GAERTNER, August Anton Hieronymus. 1848–1934
Ueber die Fleischvergiftung in Frankenhausen a.K. und den Erreger derselben. *Korrespbl. ärztl. Ver. Thüringen*, 1888, **17,** 573–600.

Discovery of *Salmonella enteritidis*, a cause of food poisoning.

2506.1 IVANOVSKI, Dmitri Alexievich. 1864–1920
Ueber die Mosaikkrankheit der Tabakspflanze. *Bull. Acad. imp. Sci. St. Petersburg*, 1892, **3,** 67–70.

The Russian botanist Ivanovski demonstrated that the agent responsible for tobacco mosaic disease could pass through the finest filter then available. This was the starting point of research into the aetiology of virus diseases. An English version is in *Phytopathological classics* (American Phytopathological Society), No. 7, pp. 25–30. Ithaca, N.Y., 1942.

2507 LOEFFLER, Friedrich August Johann. 1852–1915
Ueber Epidemieen unter den im hygienischen Institute zu Greifswald gehaltenen Mäusen und über die Bekämpfung der Feldmausplage. *Zbl. Bakt.*, 1892, **11,** 129–41.

Isolation of *Salm. typhi-murium*.

2508 WELCH, William Henry. 1850–1934, & NUTTALL, George Henry Falkiner. 1862–1937
A gas-producing bacillus (Bacillus aërogenes capsulatus nov. spec.) capable of rapid development in the blood-vessels after death. *Johns Hopk. Hosp. Bull.*, 1892, **3,** 81–91.

Discovery of the gas gangrene bacillus (Welch bacillus) *Cl. perfringens*. Reprinted in *Med. Classics*, 1941, **5,** 852–85.

2509 STERNBERG, George Miller. 1838–1915
A manual of bacteriology. New York, *W. Wood & Co.*, 1893.

Sternberg, U.S. Surgeon General 1893–1902, was a pioneer bacteriologist. Independently of Pasteur he discovered the pneumoccus and was first in America to photograph the tubercle baccillus. He it was who sent Reed off to make his great discoveries regarding yellow fever.

2510 ERMENGEM, EMILE PIERRE MARIE VAN. 1851–1932
Contribution à l'étude des intoxications alimentaires. Recherches sur des accidents à caractères botuliniques provoqués par du jambon. *Arch. Pharmacodyn.*, 1897, **3,** 213–350, 499–601.

Cl. botulinum was discovered in cases of food poisoning by van Ermengem.

2511 LOEFFLER, FRIEDRICH AUGUST JOHANN. 1852–1915, & FROSCH, PAUL. 1860–1928
Summarischer Bericht über die Ergebnisse der Untersuchungen der Commission zur Erforschung der Maul- und Klauenseuche. *Dtsch. med. Wschr.*, 1897, **23,** 617; 1898, **24,** 80–83, 97–100.

Loeffler and Frosch proved that foot-and-mouth disease is caused by a filter-passing virus; this is the first recognition of a filtrable virus as the cause of animal disease.

2512 BEIJERINCK, MARTINUS WILLEM. 1851–1931
Ueber ein Contagium vivum fluidum als Ursache der Fleckenkrankheit der Tabaksblätter. *Verh. k. Akad. Wet. Amst.*, 1898, Sect. 2, Deel 6, No. 5.

Beijerinck confirmed the findings of Ivanovski. He showed that the tobacco mosaic virus would diffuse through agar.

2513 DURHAM, HERBERT EDWARD. 1866–1945
On an epidemic of gastro-enteritis associated with the presence of a variety of the Bacillus enteritidis (Gaertner), and with positive sero-diagnostic evidence (in vivo and in vitro). *Brit. med. J.*, 1898, **2,** 600–01.

Discovery of *Salm. aertycke* in patients suffering from food poisoning.

2514 NOBELE, JULES DE. 1865–
Du séro-diagnostic dans les affections gastro-intestinales d'origine alimentaire. *Ann. Soc. Méd. Gand*, 1898, **77,** 281–306.

Discovery of *Salmonella aertrycke*, independently of Durham.

2515 MORO, ERNST. 1874–1951
Ueber die nach Gram färbbaren Bacillen des Säuglingsstuhles. *Wien. klin. Wschr.*, 1900, **13,** 114–15.

Isolation of *Lactobacillus acidophilus*.

2516 WELCH, WILLIAM HENRY. 1850–1934
Morbid conditions caused by Bacillus aërogenes capsulatus. *Johns Hopk. Hosp. Bull.*, 1900, **11,** 185–204.

Welch grouped together the diseases caused by *Cl. perfringens*, earlier discovered by him in association with Nuttall (see No. 2508).

2517 KOLLE, WILHELM. 1868–1935, & WASSERMANN, AUGUST VON. 1866–1925
Handbuch der pathogenen Mikroorganismen. 6 vols. Jena, *G. Fischer*, 1903–09.

Third edition, 10 vols. [in 19], 1929–31.

2518 SMITH, ERWIN FRINK. 1854–1927
Bacteria in relation to plant diseases. 3 vols. Washington, *Carnegie Inst.*, 1905–14.

One of the most careful investigations of the bacterial diseases in plants was made by Smith, who conclusively demonstrated the existence of such diseases and proposed a scheme of classification for the bacteria concerned.

2518.1 MORGAN, Harry de Riemer. 1863–1931
Upon the bacteriology of the summer diarrhoea of infants. *Brit. med. J.*, 1906, **1,** 908–12.
Morgan's bacillus, *Proteus morgani.*

2519 NOGUCHI, Hideyo. 1876–1928
Pure cultivation of Spirochaeta refringens. *J. exp. Med.*, 1912, **15,** 466–69.
Noguchi obtained pure cultures of spirochaetae. See also his later papers in the same journal, 1912, **16**, 199–210, 620–28.

2520 WEINBERG, Michel. 1868–1940, & SÉGUIN, P.
Notes bactériologiques sur les infections gazeuses. *C. R. Soc. Biol. (Paris)*, 1915, **78,** 274–79.
Isolation of *Cl. oedematiens.*

2521 ——. Contribution à l'étiologie de la gangrène gazeuse. *C. R. Acad. Sci. (Paris)*, 1916, **163,** 449–51.
Isolation of *Cl. histolyticum.*

2522 BERGEY, David Hendricks. 1860–1937
Manual of determinative bacteriology. Baltimore, *Williams & Wilkins Co.*, 1923.
The Society of American Bacteriologists appointed in 1920 a Committee on Characterization and Classification of Bacterial Types. Their reports were incorporated in the above *Manual* issued under the names of Bergey and his associated. A 7th edition appeared in 1957.

2522.1 MURRAY, Everitt George Dunne. 1890–1964, *et al.*
A disease of rabbits characterised by a large mononuclear leucocytosis, caused by a hitherto undescribed bacillus *Bacterium monocytogenes* (n.sp.). *J. Path. Bact.*, 1926, **29,** 407–39.
Isolation of *Listeria monocytogenes.* With R. A. Webb and M. B. R. Swann.

2523 TOPLEY, William Whiteman Carlton. 1886–1944, & WILSON, *Sir* Graham Selby. 1895–
The principles of bacteriology and immunity. 2 vols. London, *E. Arnold*, (1929).
Fifth edition, 1964.

2524 GREAT BRITAIN. *Medical Research Council.*
A system of bacteriology. 9 vols. London, *H.M. Stationery Office*, 1929–31.

2524.1 WOODRUFF, Alice Miles, & GOODPASTURE, Ernest William. 1886–1960
The susceptibility of the chorio-allantoic membrane of chick embryos to infection with the fowl-pox virus. *Amer. J. Path.*, 1931, **7,** 209–22.
By their demonstration of the infection of the chorio-allantoic membrane with the virus of fowl pox, Woodruff and Goodpasture initiated widespread adaption of this host for the study of viruses.

2524.2 LANCEFIELD, Rebecca Craighill. 1895–
A serological differentiation of human and other groups of hemolytic streptococci. *J. exp. Med.*, 1933, **57,** 571–95.
Lancefield determined the principal pathogenic strains of haemolytic streptococci and subdivided them into types. All important strains pathogenic to humans fall into Lancefield's Group A.

2524.3 GRIFFITH, FREDERICK. 1879?–1941
The serological classification of *Streptococcus pyogenes*. *J. Hyg. (Camb.)*, 1934, **34,** 542–84.

Griffith's classification of streptococci.

2524.4 KLIENEBERGER, EMMY. 1892–
The natural occurrence of pleuropneumonia-like organisms in apparent symbiosis with *Streptobacillus moniliformis* and other bacteria. *J. Path. Bact.*, 1935, **40,** 93–105.

Klieneberger isolated typical strains of pleuropneumonia-like organisms from *Strep. moniliformis.*

2524.5 STANLEY, WENDELL MEREDITH. 1904–
Isolation of a crystalline protein possessing the properties of tobacco-mosaic virus. *Science*, 1935, **81,** 644–45.

Isolation of a virus in the form of a crystalline material, subsequently shown to be a nucleoprotein.

2524.6 SCHLESINGER, MAX. 1906–1937
The Feulgen reaction of the bacteriophage substance. *Nature (Lond.)*, 1936, **138,** 508–09.

Schlesinger showed the fundamental constituents of bacteriophages to consist mainly of nucleic acid and protein.

2525 McCOY, ELIZABETH FLORENCE. 1903– , & McCLUNG, LELAND SWINT. 1910–
The anaerobic bacteria and their activities in nature and disease. A subject bibliography. 2 vols. Berkeley, *Univ. of California Press*, 1939.

2526 MacCALLUM, *Sir* PETER. 1885– , *et al.*
A new mycobacterial infection in man. *J. Path. Bact.*, 1948, **60,** 93–122.

Myco. ulcerans first described. With J. C. Tolhurst, G. Buckle, and H. A. Sissons.

2527 FRAENKEL-CONRAT, HEINZ LUDWIG. 1910– , & WILLIAMS, ROBLEY COOK. 1908–
Reconstitution of active tobacco mosaic virus from its inactive protein and nucleic acid components. *Proc. nat. Acad. Sci. (Wash.)*, 1955, **41,** 690–98.

First reconstitution of a virus.

For history of microbiology, see 2579–2581.6

2528–2578.12 INFECTION; IMMUNOLOGY; SEROLOGY

2528 FRACASTORO, GIROLAMO [FRACASTORIUS]. 1478–1553
De sympathia et antipathia rerum liber unus. De contagione et contagiosis morbis et curatione. Venetiis, *apud heredes L. Iuntae*, 1546.

This book represents a landmark in the development of our knowledge of infectious disease. Fracastorius was the first to state the germ theory of infection. He recognized typhus and suggested the contagiousness of tuberculosis. Haeser describes him as the "founder of scientific epidemiology". An English translation by W. C. Wright appeared in 1930.

2529 NEEDHAM, Marchmont. 1620–1678

Medela medicinae. London, *R. Lownds*, 1665.

Needham was one of the earliest – if not the first – Englishman to write on the germ theory. In his book he included an account of Kircher's experiments with the microscope.

2530 GASPARD, Marie Humbert Bernard. 1788–1871

Mémoire physiologique sur les maladies purulentes et putrides, sur la vaccine, *etc. J. Physiol. exp. path.*, 1822, **2,** 1–45; 1824, **4,** 1–69.

Gaspard was one of the first to make experimental studies on pyaemia following the injection of putrid fluids. He experimented on dogs, sheep, foxes, and pigs, injecting putrid infusions pus, vaccine, lymph, blood, bile, urine, saliva, carbonic acid, hydrogen or sulphuretted hydrogen.

2531 MARX, Karl Friedrich Heinrich. 1796–1877

Origines contagii. Caroliruhae et Badae, *D. R. Marx*, 1824.

A supplementary "Additamenta" was published in 1826.

2532 BASSI, Agostino. 1773–1856

Del mal del segno calcinaccio o moscardino, malattia che affligge i bachi da seta e sul modo di liberarne le bigattaje anche le più infestate. 2 vols. Lodi, *Orcesi*, 1835–36.

By his demonstration of the parasitic nature of the muscardine disease of silkworms, Bassi is regarded as the founder of the doctrine of pathogenic micro-organisms. He is rather neglected by medical historians. Facsimile reprint, Pavia, 1956. His *Opere* were published in 1925.

2533 HENLE, Friedrich Gustav Jacob. 1809–1885

Von den Miasmen und Contagien. In his *Pathologische Untersuchungen*, Berlin, 1840, pp. 1–82.

Bassi's work on the muscardine disease of silkworms (No. 2532), with its prophecy of the discovery of microbes as the causal agents of other diseases, inspired Henle to write his famous essay on miasms and contagions. He laid down postulates on the aetiological relation of microbes to disease which became fundamentals of bacteriology and which did much to check the reckless speculation which had arisen regarding microbes. English translation in *Bull. Hist. Med.*, 1938, **6**, 911–983.

2534 PANUM, Peter Ludvig. 1820–1885

Bidrag til Laeren om den saakaldte putride eller septiske Infection. *Bibl. Læger*, 1856, 4 R., **8,** 253–85.

Panum was the first to investigate the chemical products of putrefaction. His work had great significance for the doctrine of putrid intoxication. An abstract of the above paper is in *Jb. in- u. ausländ. ges. Med.*, 1859, **101, 213–17.**

2535 KLEBS, Theodor Albrecht Edwin. 1834–1913

Die Ursache der infectiösen Wundkrankheiten. *Cor.-Bl. d. schweiz. Aerzte*, 1871, **1,** 241–46.

Klebs, professor of pathology at Berne, Würzburg, Prague, Zurich, and Chicago, preceded Koch in investigations of the pathology of traumatic infection. He found bacteria in gunshot wounds, granulation tissue, etc., and developed his theory of a single organism, *Microsporon septicum*, as the cause of all pathological changes.

2536 KOCH, Robert. 1843–1910

Untersuchungen über die Aetiologie der Wundinfectionskrankheiten. Leipzig, *F. C. W. Vogel*, 1878.

Koch's epochal work on the aetiology of traumatic infectious disease established his reputation. He inoculated animals with material from various sources and produced six types of infection, each due to micro-organisms. He carried these infections through several generations of animals. His great work determined the rôle of bacteria in the aetiology of wound infections and demonstrated for the first time the specificity of infection. English translation (New Sydenham Society), 1880.

2537 PASTEUR, Louis. 1822–1895
Sur les maladies virulentes, et en particulier sur la maladie appelée vulgairement choléra des poules. *C. R. Acad. Sci.* (*Paris*), 1880, **90,** 239–48.

This paper marked the beginning of Pasteur's work on the attenuation of the infective organism. Noting that fowls inoculated with an attenuated form of the chicken cholera bacterium acquired immunity, he developed the idea of a protective inoculation by attenuated living cultures, and subsequently adopted this principle with anthrax, rabies, and swine erysipelas. His work laid the foundations of the science of immunology. See also his later paper in the same journal, 1880, **91,** 673–80.

2538 METCHNIKOFF, Elie. 1845–1916
Über eine Sprosspilzkrankheit der Daphnien. Beitrag zur Lehre über den Kampf der Phagocyten gegen Krankheitserreger. *Virchows Arch. path. Anat.*, 1884, **96,** 177–95.

Metchnikoff originated the theory of phagocytosis. He described phagocytes in leucocytes and showed their function as scavengers.

2539 SALMON, Daniel Elmer. 1850–1914, & SMITH, Theobald. 1859–1934
On a new method of producing immunity from contagious diseases. *Proc. biol. Soc. Wash.*, 1884–86, **3,** 29–33.

An important discovery regarding the process of immunity was made when Salmon and Smith found that dead virus can induce immunity against the living virulent virus.

2540 EHRLICH, Paul. 1854–1915
Das Sauerstoff-Bedürfniss des Organismus. Eine farbenanalytische Studie. Berlin, *A. Hirschwald,* 1885.

2541 PASTEUR, Louis. 1822–1895
Méthode pour prévenir la rage après morsure. *C. R. Acad. Sci.* (*Paris*), 1885, **101,** 765–74; 1886, **102,** 459–69; 835–8; **103,** 777–85.

Pasteur's papers describing his rabies vaccine and the results he attained with it gave further proof of the value of attenuated virus as a protective inoculum against infective diseases in man and animals. This is considered Pasteur's greatest triumph. A grateful public subscribed two and a half million francs and made possible the erection of the Institut Pasteur, Paris.

2542 NUTTALL, George Henry Falkiner. 1862–1937
Experimente über die bacterienfeindlichen Einflüsse des thierischen Körpers. *Z. Hyg. InfektKr.* 1888, **4,** 353–94.

Demonstration of the bactericidal power of the defibrinated blood of certain animals.

2543 BUCHNER, Hans. 1850–1902
Ueber die bakterientödtende Wirkung des zellenfreien Blutserums. *Zbl. Bakt.*, 1889, **5,** 817–23; **6,** 1–11.

Following Nuttall's work, Buchner demonstrated that the bactericidal power of defibrinated blood was possessed by the cell-free serum, and was lost on heating the serum to 55° C. for 1 hour.

2544 BEHRING, EMIL ADOLF VON. 1854–1917, & KITASATO, SHIBASABURO. 1856–1931
Ueber das Zustandekommen der Diphtherie-Immunität und der Tetanus-Immunität bei Thieren. *Dtsch. med. Wschr.*, 1890, **16,** 1113–1114.

Discovery of diphtheria and tetanus antitoxins, the basis of serotherapy. Behring was the first recipient (1900) of the Nobel Prize for Medicine.

2545 ——. Gesammelte Abhandlungen zur ätiologischen Therapie von ansteckenden Krankheiten. Leipzig, *G. Thieme*, 1893.

2545.1 STERNBERG, GEORGE MILLER. 1838–1915
Practical results of bacteriological researches. *Trans. Ass. Amer. Phycns*, 1892, **7,** 68–86.

Sternberg demonstrated that the serum of an animal recovered from vaccinia possesses the property of neutralizing the activity of the causative virus. His test was readily adaptable for use in various virus-host systems.

2546 PFEIFFER, RICHARD FRIEDRICH JOHANNES. 1858–1945, & ISAYEV, VASILIY ISAYEVICH. 1854–1911
Ueber die specifische Bedeutung der Choleraimmunität (Bakteriolyse). *Z. Hyg. InfektKr.*, 1894, **17,** 355–400; **18,** 1–16.

Pfeiffer and Isayev recorded the occurrence of bacteriolysis in cholera vibrios under certain conditions ("Pfeiffer's phenomenon").

2547 BORDET, JULES JEAN BAPTISTE VINCENT. 1870–1961
Contribution à l'étude du sérum chez les animaux vaccinés. *Ann. Soc. roy. Sci. méd. nat. Brux.*, 1895, **4,** 455–530.

Bordet's classical paper on the properties of the sera of immunized animals. He showed two different substances (now known as sensitizing antibody and complement) to be involved in the phenomenon of bacteriolysis. He was awarded the Nobel Prize in 1919.

2548 METCHNIKOFF, ELIE. 1845–1916
Sur la destruction extracellulaire des bactéries dans l'organisme. *Ann. Inst. Pasteur*, 1895, **9,** 433–61.

See No. 2538.

2549 GRUBER, MAX. 1853–1927, & DURHAM, HERBERT EDWARD. 1866–1945
Eine neue Methode zur raschen Erkennung des Choleravibrio und des Typhusbacillus. *Münch. med. Wschr.*, 1896, **43,** 285–86.

The discovery of bacterial agglutination. Gruber and Durham discovered the agglutinating action of the serum of typhoid patients upon the typhoid bacillus.

2550 WIDAL, GEORGES FERNAND ISIDOR. 1862–1929, & SICARD, ARTHUR.
Recherches de la réaction agglutinante dans le sang et le sérum desséchés des typhiques et dans la sérosité des vésicatoires. *Bull. Mém. Soc. méd. Hôp. Paris*, 1896, 3 sér., **13,** 681–82.

Developing the work of Gruber and Durham, Widal noted that a patient's serum could be tested with bacteria of known type and his disease identified by this means. The "Gruber–Widal test" was the outcome of this work.

2551 BORDET, JULES JEAN BAPTISTE VINCENT. 1870–1961
Sur l'agglutination et la dissolution des globules rouges par le sérum d'animaux injectés de sang défibriné. *Ann. Inst. Pasteur*, 1898, **12,** 688–95; 1899, **13,** 225–50.

Bordet's important work on bacterial haemolysis turned the attention of many investigators towards the subject.

2552 ——. Les sérums hémolytiques, leurs antitoxines et les théories des sérums cytolytiques. *Ann. Inst. Pasteur*, 1900, **14,** 257–96; 1901, **15,** 303–18.

2553 ——, & GENGOU, OCTAVE. 1875–1959
Sur l'existence de substances sensibilisatrices dans la plupart des sérums antimicrobiens. *Ann. Inst. Pasteur*, 1901, **15,** 289–302.

The Bordet–Gengou complement-fixation reaction is the basis of many tests for infection, notably the Wassermann test for syphilis, and reactions for gonococcus infection, glanders, hydatid disease.

2554 NUTTALL, GEORGE HENRY FALKINER. 1862–1937
On the rôle of insects, arachnids and myriapods, as carriers in the spread of bacterial and parasitic diseases of man and animals. A critical and historical study. *Johns Hopk. Hosp. Rep.*, 1900, **8,** 1–154.

2555 METCHNIKOFF, ELIE. 1845–1916
L'immunité dans les maladies infectieuses. Paris, *Masson*, 1901.

A classical study of the mechanisms concerned in specific antibacterial immunity, and one of Metchnikoff's best works. He was awarded the Nobel Prize in 1908.

2556 WASSERMANN, AUGUST VON. 1866–1925
Hämolysine, Cytotoxine und Präcipitine. *Samml. klin. Vortr.*, 1902, n.F. 331 (Chir. Nr. 94), 339–84.

2558 WRIGHT, *Sir* ALMROTH EDWARD. 1861–1947, & DOUGLAS, STEWART RANKEN. 1871–1936
An experimental investigation of the rôle of the blood fluids in connection with phagocytosis. *Proc. roy. Soc.* (*Lond.*), 1903–04, **72,** 357–370; 1904, **73,** 128–42.

Wright and Douglas showed the existence of thermolabile substances (opsonins) in normal and immune serum.

2559 EHRLICH, PAUL. 1854–1915
Gesammelte Arbeiten über Immunitätsforschung. Berlin, *A. Hirschwald*, 1904.

2560 NEUFELD, FRED. 1861–1945, & RIMPAU, WILLI. 1877–
Ueber die Antikörper des Streptokokken- und Pneumokokken-Immunserums. *Dtschr. med. Wschr.*, 1904, **30,** 1458–60.

Bacteriotropins named and described.

2561 NUTTALL, GEORGE HENRY FALKINER. 1862–1937
Blood immunity and blood relationship, a demonstration of certain blood relationships amongst animals by means of the precipitin test for blood. Cambridge, *Univ. Press*, 1904.

2562 KOLLE, WILHELM. 1868–1935, & HETSCH, HEINRICH. 1873–
Die experimentelle Bakteriologie und die Infektionskrankheiten. Berlin, Wein, *Urban & Schwarzenberg*, 1906.

2563 METCHNIKOFF, ELIE. 1845–1916
Quelques remarques sur le lait aigri. Paris, *A. Maloine*, 1906.
Metchnikoff's theory regarding the effect of lactic acid on bacteria.

2564 RICKETTS, HOWARD TAYLOR. 1871–1910
Infection, immunity and serum therapy. Chicago, *A. M. A. Press*, 1906.

2565 EHRLICH, PAUL. 1854–1915
Beiträge zur experimentellen Pathologie und Chemotherapie. Leipzig, *Akad. Verlag.*, 1909.

2566 WOLFF-EISNER, ALFRED. 1877–1948
Handbuch der experimentellen Serumtherapie. München, *J. F. Lehmann*, 1910.

2567 MUCH, HANS. 1880–1932
Die Immunitätswissenschaft. Würzburg, *C. Kabitzsch*, 1911.

2568 ZINSSER, HANS. 1878–1940
Infection and resistance. New York, *Macmillan Co.*, 1914.

2569 HEKTOEN, LUDVIG. 1863–1951
The influence of the x-ray on the production of antibodies. *J. infect. Dis.*, 1915, **17,** 415–22.
Proof that *x* rays suppress antibody response.

2570 BILLINGS, FRANK. 1854–1932
Focal infection. New York, *D. Appleton*, 1916.
Billings developed the doctrine of focal infection. See also his earlier paper in *Arch. intern. Med.*, 1912, **9**, 484–98.

2571 TWORT, FREDERICK WILLIAM. 1877–1950
An investigation on the nature of ultra-microscopic viruses. *Lancet*, 1915, **2,** 1241–43.
The transmissible lysis of bacteria by viruses (Twort–d'Herelle phenomenon) was first pointed out by Twort. The lytic agent has been named *bacteriophage*. See also No. 2572.

2571.1 SANARELLI, GIUSEPPE. 1864–1940
Pathogénie du choléra. Reproduction expérimentale de la maladie. *C. R. Acad. Sci. (Paris)*, 1916, **163,** 538–40.
Sanarelli claimed priority in observing the Shwartzman phenomenon (No. 2576). See *Ann. Inst. Pasteur*, 1939, **63**, 105.

2572 D'HERELLE, FELIX HUBERT. 1873–1949
Le bactériophage. Paris, *Masson*, 1921.
The bacteriophage discovered by d'Herelle was considered by him to be a filtrable substance capable of bacteriolysis and is similar to, if not identical with, Twort's pre-cellular ultra-microscopic virus. D'Herelle wrote several papers on the subject, the first of which appeared in *C. R. Acad. Sci.* (Paris), 1917, **165**, 373–75; all are embodied in the above book. A bibliography covering the years 1917–1956 was published by H. Raettig in Stuttgart, 1958.

2573 ROSENOW, Edward Carl. 1875–
Results of experimental studies on focal infection and elective localization. *Med. Clin. N. Amer.*, 1921, **5,** 573–92.

Rosenow and Billings (No. 2570) showed that focal infection could be caused by bacteria in teeth, etc.

2573.1 LITTLE, Clarence Cook. 1888–
The genetics of tissue transplantation in mammals. *J. Cancer Res.*, 1924, **8,** 75–95.

Little established that the homograft reaction was due to genetic differences between donor and recipient.

2574 BESREDKA, Alexandre. 1870–1940
Immunisation locale; pansements spécifiques. Paris, *Masson & Cie.*, 1925.

Besredka's vaccine, sensitized vaccine.

2575 WELLS, Harry Gideon. 1875–1943
The chemical aspects of immunity. New York, *Chem. Catalog Co.*, 1925.

2576 SHWARTZMAN, Gregory. 1896–
Studies on Bacillus typhosus toxic substances. I. Phenomenon of local skin reactivity to B. typhosus culture filtrate. *J. exp. Med.*, 1928, **48,** 247–68.

"Shwartzman phenomenon."

2576.1 ELFORD, William Joseph. 1900–1952, & ANDREWES, *Sir* Christopher Howard. 1896–
The sizes of different bacteriophages. *Brit. J. exp. Path.*, 1932, **13,** 446–56.

Method of estimating the sizes of a number of bacteriophages by means of a series of graded collodion membranes.

2576.2 LANDSTEINER, Karl. 1868–1943
Die Spezifizität der serologischen Reaktionen. Berlin, *Springer*, 1933.

English translation 1936 (revised 1945).

2576.3 HOSKINS, Meredith.
A protective action of neurotropic against viscerotropic yellow fever virus in *Macacus rhesus*. *Amer. J. trop. Med.*, 1935, **15,** 675–80.

One of the first examples of an animal virus interference phenomenon was demonstrated by Hoskins.

2576.4 MARRACK, John Richardson. 1886–
The chemistry of antigens and antibodies. *Spec. Rep. Ser. med. Res. Coun. (Lond.)*, 1938, **230,** 1–194.

2576.5 TISELIUS, Arne Wilhelm Kauren. 1902–1971, & KABAT, Elvin Abraham. 1914–
An electrophoretic study of immune sera and purified antibody preparations. *J. exp. Med.*, 1939, **69,** 119–31.

Antibodies shown to be gamma globulins.

2577 HIRST, George Keble. 1909–
The agglutination of red cells by allantoic fluid of chick embryos infected with influenza virus. *Science*, 1941, **94,** 22–23.

Discovery of virus haemagglutination.

2578 McCLELLAND, Laurella. 1912– , & HARE, Ronald. 1899–
The absorption of influenza virus by red cells and a new in vitro method of measuring antibodies for influenza virus. *Canad. publ. Hlth J.*, 1941, **32,** 530–38.

Independently of Hirst, McClelland and Hare discovered virus haemagglutination.

2578.1 FREUND, Jules Thomas. 1891– , & McDERMOTT, Katherine.
Sensitization to horse serum by means of adjuvants. *Proc. Soc. exp. Biol. (N.Y.)*, 1942, **49,** 548–53.

Freund's adjuvant.

2578.2 MEDAWAR, *Sir* Peter Brian. 1915–
The behaviour and fate of skin autografts and skin homografts in rabbits. *J. Anat. (Lond.)*, 1944, **78,** 176–99.

Demonstration that the mechanism of rejection of transplanted tissue is immunological in character.

2578.3 BURNET, *Sir* Frank Macfarlane. 1899– , & FENNER, Frank John. 1914–
The production of antibodies. 2nd ed. Melbourne, *Macmillan*, 1949.

Burnet and Fenner introduced the "self-marker" concept. For his work on immunological tolerance Burnet shared the Nobel Prize for physiology and medicine with Medawar in 1960.

2578.4 COONS, Albert Hewett. 1912– , & KAPLAN, Melvin H 1920–
Localization of antigen in tissue cells. II. Improvements in a method for the detection of antigen by means of fluorescent antibody. *J. exp. Med.*, 1950, **91,** 1–13.

Fluorescent antibody technique.

2578.5 BRUTON, Ogden Carr. 1908–
Agammaglobulinemia. *Pediatrics*, 1952, **9,** 722–27.

First report.

2578.6 BILLINGHAM, Rupert Everett. 1921– , *et al.*
'Actively acquired tolerance' of foreign cells. *Nature (Lond.)*, 1953, **172,** 603–06.

Proof of Burnet and Fenner's theory of immunity. With L. Brent and P. B. Medawar. See also *Proc. roy. Soc. B*, 1954, **143**, 58–80. For their discovery of acquired immunological tolerance Medawar and Burnet (No. 2578.3) shared the Nobel Prize in 1960.

2578.7 ——. Quantitative studies on tissue transplantation immunity. I. The survival times of skin homografts exchanged between members of different inbred strains of mice. *Proc. roy. Soc. B*, 1954, **143,** 43–58.

Experimental production of immunological tolerance. With L. Brent, P. B. Medawar, and E. M. Sparrow.

2578.8 MAYER, Manfred Martin. 1916– , & LEVINE, Lawrence. 1924–
Kinetic studies on immune hemolysis. III–IV. *J. Immunol.*, **1954, 72,** 511–30.

Complement fixation.

2578.9 PORTER, RODNEY ROBERT. 1917–
The fractionation of rabbit γ-globulin by partition chromatography. *Biochem. J.*, 1955, **59,** 405–10.
Preliminary note in *Biochem. J.*, 1954, **58,** xxxix–xl.

2578.10 GIERER, ALFRED, & SCHRAMM, GERHARD.
Infectivity of ribonucleic acid from tobacco mosaic virus. *Nature (Lond.)*, 1956, **177,** 702–03.
Proof that nucleic acid produces infectivity. See also *Z. Naturf.*, 1956, **11B,** 138–42.

2578.11 ROITT, IVAN MAURICE, *et al.*
Autoantibodies in Hashimoto's disease (lymphadenoid goitre). *Lancet*, 1956, **2,** 820–21.
Demonstration of autoantibodies. With D. Doniach, P. N. Campbell and R. V. Hudson.

2578.12 ISAACS, ALICK. 1921–1967, & LINDENMANN, JEAN. 1924–
Virus interference. I. The interferon. *Proc. roy. Soc. B*, 1957, **147,** 258–67.
Discovery of interferon, a protein produced from the interaction of virus and cells and having the property of interfering with the multiplication of viruses.

History of Microbiology

2579 LOEFFLER, FRIEDRICH AUGUST JOHANN. 1852–1915
Vorlesungen über die geschichtliche Entwickelung der Lehre von den Bacterien. Teil 1. Leipzig, *F. C. W. Vogel*, 1887.
Loeffler, professor of hygiene at Greifswald, made many discoveries in bacteriology. His history of the subject was unfortunately left unfinished.

2580 BULLOCH, WILLIAM. 1868–1941
The history of bacteriology. London, *Oxford Univ. Press*, 1938.
An expansion of the Heath Clark Lectures, delivered by Bulloch in 1936. The writer brought into the light many forgotten and almost forgotten pioneers in bacteriology. The book includes brief biographical notes of the more important workers (arranged in a separate section), and an extensive bibliography.

2581 FORD, WILLIAM WEBBER. 1871–1941
Bacteriology. New York, *Hoeber*, 1939.
In this volume of the *Clio Medica* series Ford acknowledges his indebtedness to the work of Bulloch, but has himself done a great service in producing in a small compass a great array of facts supported with a bibliography as exhaustive and accurate as Bulloch's.

2581.1 GRAINGER, THOMAS HUTCHINSON. 1913–
A guide to the history of bacteriology. New York, *Ronald Press*, 1958.
A selective annotated bibliography.

2581.2 DOETSCH, RAYMOND NICHOLAS. 1920–
Microbiology. Historical contribution from 1776–1908. New Brunswick, *Rutgers University Press*, [1960].

2581.3 BROCK, Thomas Dale. 1926–
Milestones in microbiology. Englewood Cliffs, N.J., *Prentice-Hall*, 1961.

2581.4 HAHON, Nicholas. 1924–
Selected papers on virology. Englewood Cliffs, N.J., *Prentice-Hall*, 1964.
A source of not-readily available early material.

2581.5 LECHEVALIER, Hubert Arthur. 1926– , & SOLOTOROVSKY, Morris.
Three centuries of microbiology. New York, *McGraw Hill*, 1965.

2581.6 PARISH, Henry James.
A history of immunization. Edinburgh and London, *E. & S. Livingstone*, 1965.

2581.7–2605 ALLERGY AND ANAPHYLAXIS

2581.7 BOTALLO, Leonardo. 1500–?
De catarrho commentarius. Parisiis, *apud B. Turrisanum*, 1564.
Summer catarrh (hay fever) first described.

2582 BOSTOCK, John. 1773–1846
Case of periodical affection of the eyes and chest. *Med.-chir. Trans.*, 1819, **10,** 161–65.
Bostock's classical description of the "catarrhus aestivus", hay fever. The condition is sometimes referred to as "Bostock's catarrh". He was physician to Guy's Hospital, London.

2583 ——. Of the catarrhus aestivus, or summer catarrh. *Med.-chir. Trans.*, 1828, **14,** 437–46.

2584 ELLIOTSON, John. 1791–1868
Hay fever. *Lond. med. Gaz.*, 1831, **8,** 411–16; 1832–33, **12,** 164–71.
Elliotson was the first to ascertain that pollen was the cause of hay fever.

2585 MAGENDIE, François. 1783–1855
Lectures on the blood. Philadelphia, *Harrington, Barrington & Haswell*, 1839.
Pp. 244–49: Magendie showed that secondary or subsequent injections of egg-albumin caused death in rabbits who had tolerated an initial injection. This was the first experiment in anaphylaxis, though Jenner in 1798 had observed the phenomenon in variolous inoculations.

2586 SALTER, Henry Hyde. 1823–1871
On asthma: its pathology and treatment. London, *J. Churchill*, 1860.
The best work on asthma to appear during the 19th century. Salter called special attention to asthma from animal emanations (cats, rabbits, horses, dogs, cattle, etc.).

2587 LIVEING, Edward. 1832–1919
On megrim, sick-headache, and some allied disorders. London, *J. & A. Churchill*, 1873.
See No. 4549.

2588 BLACKLEY, Charles Harrison. 1820–1900
Experimental researches on the causes and nature of catarrhus aestivus. London, *Baillière, Tindall & Cox*, 1873.

Blackley showed that pollen can produce hay fever in both the asthmatic and catarrhal forms; he also showed that skin reactions were evoked in sensitive persons. Facsimile reproduction, 1959.

2589 ——. Hay fever. London, *Baillière, Tindall & Cox*, 1880.

2590 PORTIER, Paul. 1866–1962, & RICHET, Charles Robert. 1850–1935.
De l'action anaphylactique de certains venins. *C. R. Soc. Biol. (Paris)*, 1902, **54**, 170–72.

First full description of the phenomenon of "anaphylaxis", the name itself being coined by Richet.

2591 ARTHUS, Nicolas Maurice. 1862–1945
Injections répétées de sérum de cheval chez le lapin. *C. R. Soc. Biol. (Paris)*, 1903, **55**, 817–20.

The "Arthus phenomenon" – a symptom of anaphylaxis.

2592 DUNBAR, William Philipps. 1863–1922
Ursache und Behandlung des Heufiebers. Leipzig, *J. J. Weber*, 1905.

Dunbar studied the relationship of pollen to hay fever, separated the active substances responsible for producing the condition, and introduced a specific therapy.

2593 PIRQUET VON CESENATICO, Clemens Peter. 1874–1929, & SCHICK, Bela. 1877–1967
Die Serumkrankheit. Wien, *F. Deuticke*, 1905.

An excellent description of serum sickness and its significance.

2594 OTTO, Richard. 1872–1952
Das Theobald Smithsche Phänomen der Serum-Ueberfindlichkeit. In *Gedenkschr. f. d. verstorb. Generalstabsarzt . . . von Leuthold*, Berlin, 1906, **1**, 153–72.

The "Theobald Smith phenomenon" was not reported by Smith, but communicated by him to Ehrlich. Later Otto published details of the results obtained in his study of the phenomenon.

2595 ROSENAU, Milton Joseph. 1869–1946, & ANDERSON, John F. 1873–1958
A study of the cause of sudden death following the injection of horse serum. Washington, *Govt. Printing Office*, 1906.

Forms No. 29 of the Bulletin of the Hygienic Laboratory, U.S. Marine Hospital Service. Rosenau and Anderson drew attention to the fact that animals receiving an injection of a foreign protein became sensitive to a second dose of the same protein. This reaction is similar to the anaphylaxis of Richet and the "Theobald Smith phenomenon".

2596 BESREDKA, Alexandre. 1870–1940, & STEINHARDT, Edna.
De l'anaphylaxie et de l'anti-anaphylaxie vis-à-vis du sérum de cheval. *Ann. Inst. Pasteur*, 1907, **21**, 117–27, 384–91.

"Anti-anaphylaxis" was the term given by Besredka and Steinhardt to the specific desensitization of sensitized animals.

2597 NICOLLE, Maurice. 1862–1932
Contribution à l'étude du "phénomène d'Arthus". *Ann. Inst. Pasteur*, 1907, **21**, 128–37.
"Passive" anaphylaxis first demonstrated.

2598 PIRQUET VON CESENATICO, Clemens Peter. 1874–1929
Klinische Studien über Vakzination und vakzinale Allergie. Leipzig, Wien, *F. Deuticke*, 1907.
Pirquet suggested the word "Allergie"; see also his paper with this title in *Münch. med. Wschr.*, 1906, **53**, 1457–58.

2599 RICHET, Charles Robert. 1850–1935
De l'anaphylaxie en général et de l'anaphylaxie par la mytilocongestine en particulier. *Ann. Inst. Pasteur*, 1907, **21**, 497–524; 1908, **22**, 465–495.
Nobel Prizewinner, 1913, in recognition of his work on anaphylaxis.

2600 AUER, John. 1875–1948, & LEWIS, Paul A. 1879–1929
The physiology of the immediate reaction of anaphylaxis in the guinea-pig. *J. exp. Med.*, 1910, **12**, 151–75.
First adequate account of the physiological reactions leading to fatal anaphylactic shock.

2600.1 MELTZER, Samuel James. 1851–1920
Bronchial asthma as a phenomenon of anaphylaxis. *J. Amer. med. Ass.*, 1910, **55**, 1021–24.
The work of Auer and Lewis (No. 2600) led Meltzer to the conclusion that bronchial asthma was due to anaphylaxis, although he did not appreciate that not all cases of asthma were so caused.

2600.2 SCHULTZ, William Henry. 1873–1947
Physiological studies in anaphylaxis. I. The reaction of smooth muscle of the guinea-pig sensitized with horse serum. *J. Pharmacol.*, 1910, **1**, 549–67.
Schultz-Dale test for anaphylaxis. See also No. 2600.5

2600.3 NOON, Leonard. 1878–1913
Prophylactic inoculation against hay fever. *Lancet*, 1911, **1**, 1572–73.
Noon and Freeman introduced the treatment of hay fever by means of injections of pollen extract.

2600.4 FREEMAN, John. 1877–1962
Further observations on the treatment of hay fever by hypodermic inoculations of pollen vaccine. *Lancet*, 1911, **2**, 814–17.
See No. 2600.3.

2600.5 DALE, *Sir* Henry Hallett. 1875–1968
The anaphylactic reaction of plain muscle in the guinea-pig. *J. Pharmacol.*, 1913, **4**, 167–223.
See No. 2600.2.

2601 BESREDKA, Alexandre. 1870–1940
Anaphylaxie et antianaphylaxie. Paris, *Masson & Cie.*, 1917.
English translation, 1919.

2601.1 PRAUSNITZ, Otto Carl Willy. 1876–1963, & KÜSTNER, Heinz. 1897–

Studien über die Ueberempfindlichkeit. *Zbl. Bakt., I Abt. Orig.*, 1921, **86,** 160–69.

Prausnitz-Küstner reaction. These workers demonstrated antibodies in the blood of persons suffering from atopic allergic diseases. They produced local passive sensitization by intracutaneous injection of serum from a hypersensitive subject. Prausnitz spent his later years in England, where he adopted the surname Prausnitz Giles.

2602 LEWIS, *Sir* Thomas. 1881–1945, & GRANT, Ronald Thomson. 1892–

Vascular reactions of the skin to injury. II. The liberation of a histamine-like substance in injured skin; the underlying cause of factitious urticaria and of wheals produced by burning; and observations upon the nervous control of certain skin reactions. *Heart*, 1924, **11,** 209–65.

Lewis postulated that a histamine-like substance ("H-substance") was responsible for the anaphylaxis symptom-complex. See also *The blood-vessels of the human skin and their responses*, 1927.

2603 STORM VAN LEEUWEN, Willem. 1882–1933

Allergic diseases; diagnosis and treatment of bronchial asthma, hay-fever, and other allergic diseases. Philadelphia, *J. B. Lippincott*, 1925.

In his important studies of asthma, Storm van Leeuwen demonstrated that in the great majority of patients allergens are the cause of the condition and also that patients are sensitive to mould spores. He experimented with an allergen-proof chamber and showed the benefit of high altitude to asthmatics.

2604 FRANKLIN, Philip. 1880–1951

Treatment of hay fever by intranasal zinc ionization. *Brit. med. J.*, 1931, **1,** 1115–16.

Introduction of the method.

2605 DRAGSTEDT, Carl Albert. 1895– , & GEBAUER-FUELNEGG, Erich.

Studies in anaphylaxis. *Amer. J. Physiol.*, 1932, **102,** 512–26.

Detection of the release of histamine into the circulation during anaphylactic reaction. Thereafter histamine was identified as Lewis's "H-substance".

2606–2662 TUMOURS IN GENERAL

2606 GALEN. A.D. 130–200

De tumoribus praeter naturam. In his *Opera*, Ed. C. G. Kühn, Leipzig, 1824, **7,** 705–32.

Galen's classification of tumours persisted for more than 1,000 years. He considered neoplasms to be due to an excess of black bile, which solidified in certain sites. He advocated purges to dissolve the black bile, and if these were unsuccessful the knife. He was not familiar with internal tumours. He employed the term "sarcoma" for any fleshy-like superficial swelling. On p. 729 occurs the description of "Galen's sarcocele". German translation by P. Richter, Leipzig, 1913.

2607 LE DRAN, Henri François. 1685–1770

Mémoire avec un précis de plusieurs observations sur le cancer. *Mém. Acad. roy. Chir. (Paris)*, 1757, **7,** 224–310.

Le Dran's important discussion on cancer for the first time discarded the humoral theory of the disease.

2608 PEYRILHE, Bernard. 1735–1804
Dissertatio academica de cancro. Parisiis, *De Hansy Jeune*, 1774.
Peyrilhe was the first to attempt an experimental study to determine the nature of cancer. He injected fluid from human mammary cancer into a dog. French edition, 1776.

2609 POTT, Percivall. 1714–1788
Chirurgical observations relative to the cataract, the polypus of the nose, the cancer of the scrotum, *etc.* London, *T. J. Carnegy*, 1775.
First description of an occupational cancer (chimney-sweeps' cancer of the scrotum).

2610 RÉCAMIER, Joseph Claude Anthelm. 1774–1852
Recherches sur le traitement du cancer par la compression méthodique. 2 vols. Paris, *Gabon*, 1829.
Récamier was the first to recognize the process of metastasis. He also described for the first time invasion of veins by cancer.

2611 HOME, *Sir* Everard. 1756–1832
A short tract on the formation of tumours. London, *Longman*, 1830.
Contains the first illustrations of microscopic sections of cancer. Home drew no worthwhile conclusion from his microscopic studies.

2611.1 WARREN, John Collins. 1778–1856
Surgical observations on tumours, with cases and operations. Boston, *Crocker & Brewster*, 1837.
First North American book on tumours.

2612 MÜLLER, Johannes. 1801–1858
Ueber den feinern Bau und die Formen der krankhaften Geschwülste. Lief. 1. Berlin, *G. Reimer*, 1838.
This classical work showed that Müller realized the necessity of the cell theory for the comprehension of the nature of cancer. He recognized cells, their nuclei and nucleoli, and could distinguish various types of tumours microscopically. Only Lieferung 1 of the book was published; C. West translated it into English in 1840.

2613 VIRCHOW, Rudolf Ludwig Carl. 1821–1902
Zur Entwickelungsgeschichte des Krebses. *Virchows Arch. path. Anat.*, 1847, **1**, 94–201.
While still a young man Virchow founded the above journal. He wrote a fine paper on cancer and suggested that the exciting cause is local irritation.

2614 LEIDY, Joseph. 1823–1891
Transplantation of malignant tumors. *Proc. Acad. nat. Sci. Philad.*, 1851, **5**, 212.
First experimental transplantation of tumours.

2615 HANNOVER, Adolph. 1814–1894
Das Epithelioma. Leipzig, *L. Voss*, 1852.
Hannover coined the word "epithelioma". He did not recognize its malignant character but maintained that metastases were produced by cancer cells arriving by way of the blood stream.

2616 BRIGHT, Richard. 1789–1858
Clinical memoirs on abdominal tumours and intumescence. London, *New Sydenham Soc.*, 1860.

2617 VIRCHOW, RUDOLF LUDWIG KARL. 1821–1902
Die krankhaften Geschwülste. Vol. 1–3, Heft 1. Berlin, *A. Hirschwald*, 1863–67.

This work was not completed, Virchow stopping when he reached the subject of carcinoma. It is one of the most important source books on cancer but it also records one of Virchow's mistakes – his theory of the connective-tissue origin of carcinoma.

2618 THIERSCH, CARL. 1822–1895
Der Epithelialkrebs namentlich der Haut. 1 vol. and atlas. Leipzig, *W. Engelmann*, 1865.

Thiersch, professor of surgery at Erlangen and inventor of the method of skin grafting which bears his name, also made an important contribution to the knowledge of the histogenesis of cancer. He disproved Virchow's theory of the connective-tissue origin of cancer, and advanced evidence of its epithelial cell origin.

2619 MOORE, CHARLES HEWITT. 1821–1870
On the influence of inadequate operations on the theory of cancer. *Med.-chir. Trans.*, 1867, **50**, 245–80.

Modern surgical treatment of cancer is based upon principles laid down by Moore.

2620 WALDEYER-HARTZ, HEINRICH WILHELM GOTTFRIED. 1836–1921
Die Entwicklung der Carcinome. *Virchows Arch. path. Anat.*, 1867, **41**, 470–523; 1872, **55**, 67–159.

Waldeyer confirmed the work of Thiersch (No. 2618) on the epithelial origin of cancer, disproving Virchow's theory. So great was the authority of the latter that it was not until the appearance of the second of the above papers that Virchow's error was finally recognized.

2620.1 NOVINSKY, MSTISLAV ALEXANDROVICH. 1841–1914
O privivanii rakovikh novoobrazovanii. [On the inoculation of cancerous neoplasms.] *Med. Vestn.*, 1876, **16**, 289–90.

Novinsky successfully transplanted two tumours in dogs. German translation in *Zbl. med. Wiss.*, 1876, **14**, 790–91.

2621 HANAU, ARTHUR NATHAN. 1858–1900
Erfolgreiche experimentelle Uebertragung von Carcinom. *Fortschr. Med.*, 1889, **7**, 321–39.

Hanau successfully transplanted cancer in mammals.

2622 RUSSELL, WILLIAM. 1852–1940
An address on a characteristic organism of cancer. *Brit. med. J.*, 1890, **2**, 1356–60.

"Russell's bodies."

2622.1 MORAU, HENRI. 1860–
Inoculation en série d'une tumeur épithéliale de la souris blanche. *C. R. Soc. Biol.*, 1891, **43**, 289–90.

In 1889 Morau transferred epitheliomata in mice and by 1893 had carried his experiments through 17 generations, the first systematic survey of tumour-host relationships from a purely biological viewpoint.

2623 KUNDRAT, HANS. 1845–1893
Ueber Lympho-Sarkomatosis. *Wien. klin. Wschr.*, 1893, **6**, 211–13, 234–39.

"Kundrat's lymphosarcoma."

2623.1 REHN, Ludwig. 1849–1930
Blasengeschwülste bei Fuchsin-Arbeitern. *Arch. klin. Chir.*, 1895, **50,** 588–600.
Rehn noted the frequent appearance of papilloma and carcinoma of the bladder among men employed in the aniline dye industry.

2624 SJÖGREN, Tage Anton Ultimus. 1859–1939
Fall af epiteliom behandladt med Roentgenstråler. *Förh. Svenska Läkare-Sallskapets Sammankomster*, Stockholm, 1899, p. 208.
In June 1899 Sjögren was the first successfully to use Roentgen rays in the treatment of cancer.

2624.1 LOEB, Leo. 1865–1959
On transplantation of tumors. *J. med. Res.*, 1901, **6,** 28–38.
Loeb successfully transplanted cystic sarcoma of the thyroid in rats. He established the fact that growth of the transplant occurred through proliferation of its peripheral cells.

2625 BORST, Maximilian. 1869–1946
Die Lehre von den Geschwülsten. 2 vols. Wiesbaden, *J. F. Bergmann*, 1902.

2625.1 FRIEBEN, Ernst August Franz Albert. 1875–
Cancroid des rechten Handrückens. *Dtsch. med. Wschr.*, 1902, **28,** Vereins-Beilage, 335.
Frieben reported the carcinogenic effect of *x* rays in man.

2626 HANSEMANN, David Paul von. 1858–1920
Die mikroskopische Diagnose der bösartigen Geschwülste. 2te. Aufl. Berlin, *A. Hirschwald*, 1902.
Hansemann originated the theory of anaplasia.

2627 GOLDBERG, S. W., & LONDON, Efim Semenovic. 1869–1939
Zur Frage der Beziehungen zwischen Becquerelstrahlen und Hautaffectionen. *Derm. Z.*, 1903, **10,** 457–62.
Records the first successful employment of radium in the treatment of cancer.

2628 JENSEN, Carl Oluf. 1864–1934
Experimentelle Untersuchungen über Krebs bei Mäusen. *Zbl. Bakt.*, 1903, Abt. I, Orig., **34,** 28–34, 122–43.
Jensen carried rat sarcoma through as many as 40 generations of rodents without change in microscopic structure. His classical study discredited the theory of the infectivity of cancer, and established its inoculability. See also *Z. Krebsforsch.*, 1909, **7**, 45–54.

2629 SCHMIDT, Martin Benno. 1863–1949
Die Verbreitungswege der Karzinome und die Beziehung generalisierter Sarkome zu den leukämischen Neubildungen. Jena, *G. Fischer*, 1903.
Schmidt supported the theory of the haematogenous origin of carcinoma metastases.

2630 SJÖGREN, Tage Anton Ultimus. 1859–1939
Om Röntgenbehandling af sarkom. *Hygiea*, 1904, 2 F., **4,** 1142–49.
See No. 2624.

2631 SJÖGREN, TAGE ANTON ULTIMUS. 1859–1939.
Om Röntgenbehandling af maligna svulster. *Nord. T. Terapi*, 1904–05, **3**, 8–23.
See No. 2624.

2632 RIBBERT, MORITZ WILHELM HUGO. 1855–1920
Die Entstehung des Carcinoms. Bonn, *F. Cohen*, 1905.
Ribbert was the modern protagonist of the theory of the embryonal origin of cancer.

2633 TYZZER, ERNEST EDWARD. 1875–1965
A study of heredity in relation to the development of tumors in mice. *J. med. Res.*, 1907–08, **17**, 199–211.
First experimental study of the heredity of mouse cancer.

2634 SCHLOFFER, HERMANN. 1868–1937
Chronisch entzündliche Bauchdeckengeschwülste nach Bruchoperationen. *Zbl. Chir.*, 1908, **35**, Beilage, 113–15.
"Schloffer's tumour" – an inflammatory tumour of the abdomen following herniotomy.

2635 LAZARUS-BARLOW, WALTER SYDNEY. 1865–1950
The Croonian Lectures on radioactivity and carcinoma. *Brit. med. J.*, 1909, **1**, 1465–70, 1536–44.

2636 CARREL, ALEXIS. 1873–1944, & BURROWS, MONTROSE THOMAS. 1884–1947
Cultures de sarcome en dehors de l'organisme. *C. R. Soc. Biol. (Paris)*, 1910, **69**, 332–34.
Using the Rous chicken sarcoma, Carrel and Burrows were the first to grow tumour tissue *in vitro*.

2637 ROUS, FRANCIS PEYTON. 1879–
A transmissible avian neoplasm (sarcoma of the common fowl). *J. exp. Med.*, 1910, **12**, 696–705; 1911, **13**, 397–411.
Original description of the chicken sarcoma (Rous sarcoma), transmissible by cell-free filtrates or desiccates. More than 50 years later (1966) Rous shared the Nobel Prize with Charles Huggins for work on cancer.

2637.1 CLUNET, JEAN. 1878–1917
Le cancer expérimental. *J. méd. franç.*, 1911, **5**, 299–305.
Experimental production of malignant tumours by means of *x* rays.

2638 FREUND, ERNST. 1863–1946, & KAMINER, GISA. 1883–1941
Zur Diagnose des Karzinoms. *Wien. klin. Wschr.*, 1911, **24**, 1759–64.
A serum reaction, employed by Freund and Kaminer in 1910 for the diagnosis of cancer.

2639 BAYON, HENRY PETER GEORGE. 1876–1952
Epithelial proliferation induced by the injection of gasworks tar. *Lancet*, 1912, **2**, 1579.
Experimental production of cancer by the injection of tar.

2640 FIBIGER, JOHANNES. 1867–1928
Untersuchungen über eine Nematode (Spiroptera sp. n.) und deren Fähigkeit papillomatöse und carcinomatöse Geschwulstbildungen im Magen der Ratte hervorzurufen. *Z. Krebsforsch.*, 1913, **13,** 217–80; 1914, **14,** 295–326.

Fibiger demonstrated in rodents the effect of nematodes in the development of carcinoma. He was awarded the Nobel Prize in 1926. His results have subsequently not been confirmed and are no longer accepted.

2641 HOFFMAN, FREDERICK LUDWIG. 1865–1946
The mortality from cancer throughout the world. Newark, N.J., *Prudential Press*, 1915.

2642 LATHROP, A. E. C., & LOEB, LEO. 1869–1959
Further investigations on the origin of tumors in mice. III. On the part played by internal secretion in the spontaneous development of tumors. *J. Cancer Res.*, 1916, **1,** 1–19.

Demonstration of the influence of an internal secretion on the development of spontaneous cancer. Castration of female mice of a strain in which mammary cancer was frequent reduced its incidence and delayed its growth.

2643 YAMAGIWA, KATSUSABURO. 1863–1930, & ICHIKAWA, KOKICHI. 1887–
Ueber die künstliche Erzeugung von Karzinom. *Verh. jap. path. Ges.*, 1916, **6,** 169–78; 1917, **7,** 191–96.

First experimental production of tar cancer in rabbits by painting with tar products.

2644 EWING, JAMES. 1866–1943
Neoplastic diseases. Philadelphia, *W. B. Saunders*, 1919.

Fourth edition, 1940.

2645 BRODERS, ALBERT COMPTON. 1885–1964
Squamous-cell epithelioma of the lip. A study of five hundred and thirty-seven cases. *J. Amer. med. Ass.*, 1920, **74,** 656–64.

Broders' classification of tumours, an index of malignancy.

2645.1 BULLOCK, FREDERICK DABNEY. 1878– , *et al.*
A preliminary report on the experimental production of sarcoma of the liver of rats. *Proc. Soc. exp. Biol.* (*N.Y.*), 1920, **18,** 29–30.

Proof that cancer can be caused by a parasite, *Cysticercus fasciolaris*, the larval stage of *Taenia crassicolis*. With M. R. Curtis and G. L. Rohdenberg. See also *Proc. N. Y. path. Soc.*, 1920, **20**, 149–75.

2646 KENNAWAY, *Sir* ERNEST LAURENCE. 1881–1958
The formation of a cancer-producing substance from isoprene (2-methyl-butadiene). *J. Path. Bact.*, 1924, **27,** 233–38.

Kennaway produced carcinogenic tars by submitting acetylene or isoprene to high temperatures in an atmosphere of hydrogen, thus proving that some carcinogens are pure hydrocarbons.

2647 GYE, WILLIAM EWART. 1884–1952
The aetiology of malignant new growths. *Lancet*, 1925, **2,** 109–17.

Gye advanced the theory that an ultramicroscopic virus combined with an intrinsic chemical factor were concerned in the production of the Rous sarcoma.

2648 BARNARD, JOSEPH EDWIN. 1870–1949
The microscopical examination of filterable viruses associated with malignant new growths. *Lancet*, 1925, **2,** 117–23.

Barnard supported, with photomicrographs, Gye's theory concerning the origin of cancer.

2649 DAWSON, JAMES WALKER. 1870–1927
The melanomata. *Edinb. med. J.*, 1925, **32,** 501–732.

A classical account.

2650 BENDIEN, S. G. T.
Haemagglutinegehalte van het bloedserum bij carcinoompatiënten. *Ned. T. Geneesk.*, 1926, **70,** i, 2856–58.

Bendien test for the diagnosis of cancer. He published books in German and English on this subject in 1931.

2651 WARBURG, OTTO HEINRICH. 1883–
Ueber den Stoffwechsel der Tumoren. Berlin, *J. Springer*, 1926.

In his important studies of the metabolism of tumours, Warburg was first to observe that malignant tissue utilizes glucose by glycolysis, whether or not oxygen is available (aerobic glycolysis). English translation, 1930.

2652 SLYE, MAUD. 1879–
Cancer and heredity. *Ann. intern. Med.*, 1928, **1,** 951–76.

By selective breeding over a period of 15 years, Maud Slye produced generations of mice absolutely resistant to, or particularly susceptible to, cancer. She demonstrated that resistance is a Mendelian dominant and susceptibility a recessive, either of which can be bred into or out of susceptible or resistant generations, according to the laws of genetics. Her earlier papers are in *J. med. Res.*, 1914, **25,** 281; 1915, **27,** 159; *J. Cancer Res.*, 1916, **1,** 479, 503; 1921, **6,** 139; 1922, **7,** 107.

2653 PIRQUET VON CESENATICO, CLEMENS PETER. 1874–1929
Allergie des Lebensalters, die bösartigen Geschwülste. Leipzig, *G. Thieme*, 1930.

Important study of the age and sex incidence of cancer.

2654 COOK, *Sir* JAMES WILFRED. 1900– , *et al.*
The production of cancer by pure hydrocarbons. *Proc. roy. Soc. B*, 1932, **111,** 455–96.

Discovery of the carcinogenic properties of dibenzanthracene compounds. With I. Hieger, E. L. Kennaway, and W. V. Mayneord.

2655 PANCOAST, HENRY KHUNRATH. 1875–1939
Superior pulmonary sulcus tumor. Tumor characterized by pain. Horner's syndrome, destruction of bone and atrophy of hand muscles. *J. Amer. med. Ass.*, 1932, **99,** 1391–96.

"Pancoast's tumour."

2656 SHOPE, RICHARD EDWIN. 1901–1966
A transmissible tumor-like condition in rabbits. *J. exp. Med.*, 1932, **56,** 793–802.

Shope papilloma, a benign infectious tumour due to a virus.

2657 LACASSAGNE, ANTOINE MARCELLIN. 1884–1971
Apparition de cancers de la mamelle chez la souris mâle, soumise à des injections de folliculine. *C. R. Acad. Sci. (Paris)*, 1932, **195,** 630–632.

2658 BITTNER, JOHN JOSEPH. 1904–
Some possible effects of nursing on the mammary gland tumor incidence in mice. *Science*, 1936, **84,** 162.

Bittner's milk factor in the transmission of mammary cancer in mice. See also *Amer. J. clin. Path.*, 1937, 7, 430–35.

2659 BONSER, GEORGIANA MAY, *et al.*
The carcinogenic action of oestrone: induction of mammary carcinoma in female mice of a strain refractory to the spontaneous development of mammary tumours. *J. Path. Bact.*, 1937, **45,** 709–14.

With L. H. Stickland and K. I. Connal.

2659.1 LEUCHTENBERGER, CECILIE. 1906– , *et al.*
"Folic acid" a tumor growth inhibitor. *Proc. Soc. exp. Biol.* (*N.Y.*), 1944, **55,** 204–05.

Inhibition of tumour growth by a folic acid concentrate. With R. Lewisohn, D. Laszlo, and R. Leuchtenberger. These workers later (*Proc. Soc. exp. Biol. N.Y.*, 1944, **56,** 144–45) obtained similar results with xanthopterin.

2659.2 HADDOW, *Sir* ALEXANDER. 1907– , *et al.*
Influence of synthetic oestrogens upon advanced malignant disease. *Brit. med. J.*, 1944, **2,** 393–98.

Administration of synthetic oestrogens in advanced mammary cancer caused regression of tumours. With J. M. Watkinson, E. Paterson, and P. C. Koller.

2659.3 GOODMAN, LOUIS SANFORD. 1906– , *et al.*
Nitrogen mustard therapy. Use of methyl-bis (beta-chloroethyl(amine) hydrochloride and tris (beta-chloroethyl)amine hydrochloride for Hodgkin's disease, lymphosarcoma, leukemia and certain allied and miscellaneous disorders. *J. Amer. med. Ass.*, 1946, **132,** 126–32.

With M. M. Wintrobe, W. Dameshek, M. J. Goodman, A. Gilman, and M. T. McLennan.

2660 BEARD, HOWARD HORACE. 1894– , *et al.*
Effect of intraperitoneal injection of malignant urine extracts in normal and hypophysectomized rats. *Science*, 1947, **105,** 475–76.

Test for diagnosis of cancer. With B. Halperin and S. H. Libert.

2660.1 STEWART, SARAH ELIZABETH. 1906– , *et al.*
The induction of neoplasms with a substance released from mouse tumors by tissue culture. *Virology*, 1957, **3,** 380–400.

Isolation of polyoma, a tumour-inducing virus. With B. E. Eddy, A. M. Gochenour, N. G. Borgese, and G. E. Grubbs.

2660.2 BURKITT, DENNIS.
A sarcoma involving the jaws in African children. *Brit. J. Surg.*, 1958–59, **46,** 218–23.

"Burkitt's tumour" (African lymphoma), first described in detail by Dr. Alfred Cook, but not published by him.

History of Tumours

2661 WOLFF, JACOB. 1861–1938
Die Lehre von der Krebskrankheit von den ältesten Zeiten bis zur Gegenwart. 4 vols. Jena, *Fischer*, 1907–28.

Exhaustive and accurate review of all the available information on cancer.

2662 HAAGENSEN, Cushman Davis. 1900–
An exhibit of important books, papers, and memorabilia illustrating the evolution of the knowledge of cancer. *Amer. J. Cancer*, 1933, **18,** 42–126.

2663–2702.2 PHYSICAL DIAGNOSIS IN GENERAL

See also under the names of individual organs and regions

2663 GALEN. A.D. 130–200
De pulsuum usu. In his *Opera*, ed, C. G. Kühn, Lipsiae, 1823, **5,** 149–210.

Galen established a system of medicine on the minutiae of pulse variations, which persisted into the 18th century. Herophilus of Chalcedon is said to have counted the pulse with a water-clock.

2664 ——. De morborum differentiis. In his *Opera*, ed. C. G. Kühn, Lipsiae, 1823, **6,** 836–80.

2665 ——. De symptomatum differentiis. In his *Opera*, ed. C. G. Kühn, Lipsiae, 1823, **7,** 42–84.

2666 ACTUARIUS, Johannes. ?–1283
De urinis libri vii. Basileae, *apud A. Cratandrum*, [1529].

An elaborate treatise on urinoscopy. Actuarius was first to use a graduated glass for its examination. He described paroxysmal haemoglobinuria.

2667 SILVATICO, Giambattista. 1550–1621
De iis, qui morborum simulant deprehendendis liber. Mediolani, *ex off quondam P. Pontii*, 1595.

The first treatise on feigned diseases.

2668 SANTORIO, Santorio [Sanctorius]. 1561–1636
Commentaria in primam fen primi libri canonis Avicennae. Venetiis, *apud M. A. Brogiollum*, 1625.

Records the first application of the thermometer in the study of disease and the first description of a pulsilogium, or pulse-clock, devised by Sanctorius. Illustrations of both are included.

2670 FLOYER, *Sir* John. 1649–1734
The physician's pulse-watch. 2 vols. London, *S. Smith & B. Walford*, 1707–10.

Before watches had hands to record the seconds, Floyer invented a pulse-watch which divided the minute. He was the first to count the pulse with the aid of a watch and to make regular observations on the pulse-rate.

2671 MARTINE, George. 1702–1741
Essays medical and philosophical. London, *A. Millar*, 1740.

First important work on clinical thermometry.

2672 AUENBRUGGER, Leopold, *Edler von Auenbrugg*. 1722–1809
Inventum novum ex percussione thoracis humani ut signo abstrusos interni pectoris morbos detegendi. Vindobonae, *J. T. Trattner*, 1761.

The greatness of Auenbrugger's discovery of the value of immediate percussion of the chest as a diagnostic measure was not at first recognized. His little book met with a cold reception, while a French translation by Rozière de la Chassagne in 1770 attracted little notice. But Auenbrugger lived to see the appearance in 1808 of J. N. Corvisart's classical translation of the book, after which the value of percussion was universally recognized. English translation by J. Forbes, 1824 (reprinted in F. A. Willius and T. E. Keys: *Cardiac classics*, 1941, pp. 193–213); also with introduction by H. E. Sigerist, in *Bull. Hist. Med.*, 1936, **4**, 373–403. For bibliography of the *Inventum novum* see P. J. Bishop, *Tubercle*, 1961, **42**, 78.

2673 LAENNEC, René Théophile Hyacinthe. 1781–1826
De l'auscultation médiate. 2 vols. Paris, *J. A. Brosson & J. S. Chaudé*, 1819.

Auscultation in the instrumental sense dates from Laennec's invention of the stethoscope (at first merely a roll of stiff paper) with a view to amplifying the sound of the heart's action. The publication of this book revolutionized the study of diseases of the thoracic organs. The second edition, 1826, is even more important, since it gives not only the various physical signs elicited in the chest, but adds the pathological anatomy, diagnosis, and treatment of each disease encountered. Laennec, perhaps the greatest clinician of his time, died of tuberculosis. Reprinted, 1962. English translation by J. Forbes, 1821.

2674 STOKES, William. 1804–1878
An introduction to the use of the stethoscope. Edinburgh, *Maclachlan & Stewart*, 1825.

Stokes, famous member of the Irish school of medicine, published the first systematic treatise on the use of the stethoscope – and this before his qualification at Edinburgh. His name is perpetuated in medical literature in connexion with "Cheyne–Stokes respiration" and the "Stokes–Adams syndrome".

2675 PIORRY, Pierre Adolphe. 1794–1879
De la percussion médiate. Paris, *J. S. Chaudé*, 1828.

Piorry, pioneer of mediate percussion, introduced the percussor and the pleximeter in 1826.

2676 SKODA, Josef. 1805–1881
Abhandlung über Perkussion und Auskultation. Wien, 1839.

Skoda classified the various sounds obtained on percussion according to their musical pitch and tone. "Skoda's resonance" is an important diagnostic sign in pneumonia and pericardial effusion. Following Skoda's work percussion at last gained general acceptance as a diagnostic procedure. English translation, 1853.

2676.1 NEUMANN, Ernst. 1834–1918
Ueber das verschiedene Verhalten gelähmter Muskeln gegen den constanten und inducirten Strom und die Erklärung desselben. *Dtsch. Klinik*, 1864, **16**, 65–69.

First publication on electrodiagnosis.

2677 WUNDERLICH, Carl Reinhold August. 1815–1877
Das Verhalten der Eigenwärme in Krankheiten. Leipzig, *O. Wigand*, 1868.

This classical work on temperature in disease laid the foundation of modern knowledge regarding clinical thermometry. Garrison has said of Wunderlich that he "found fever a disease and left it a symptom". The book was translated into English and published by the New Sydenham Society in 1871.

2678 WILKS, *Sir* SAMUEL, *Bart.* 1824–1911
On markings or furrows on the nails as the result of illness. *Lancet*, 1869, **1,** 5–6.

2679 ALLBUTT, *Sir* THOMAS CLIFFORD. 1836–1925
Medical thermometry. *Brit. for. med.-chir. Rev.*, 1870, **45,** 429–41.
Allbutt introduced the modern clinical thermometer.

2680 BROADBENT, *Sir* WILLIAM HENRY, *Bart.* 1835–1907
The pulse. London, *Cassell & Co.*, 1890.

2681 KRIES, JOHANNES ADOLF VON. 1853–1928
Studien zur Pulslehre. Freiburg i. B., *J. C. B. Mohr*, 1892.

2682 BARKER, LEWELLYS FRANKLIN. 1867–1943
The clinical diagnosis of internal diseases. 3 vols. New York, *Appleton & Co.*, 1916.

Diagnostic Roentgenology

2683 RÖNTGEN, WILHELM CONRAD. 1845–1923
Ueber eine neue Art von Strahlen. *S. B. phys.-med. Ges. Würzburg*, 1895, 132–41.
The discovery of *x* rays, which Kölliker later re-named "Roentgen rays"; the foundation stone of the science of roentgenology. For his work Röntgen was awarded the Nobel Prize for Physics in 1901. Reproduced in facsimile in *Isis*, 1936, **26**, 249–69. English translation in *Nature*, 1896, **53**, 274 and 377.

2684 JONES, *Sir* ROBERT. 1858–1933, & LODGE, *Sir* OLIVER JOSEPH. 1851–1940
The discovery of a bullet lost in the wrist by means of the Roentgen rays. *Lancet*, 1896, **1,** 476–77.
This was probably the first published report of the clinical use of *x* rays (February 22).

2685 PUPIN, MICHAEL IDVORSKY. 1858–1935
A few remarks on experiments with Roentgen rays. *Electricity*, New York, 1896, **10,** 68–69.
Introduction of the intensifying screen.

2686 THOMSON, ELIHU. 1853–1937
Stereoscopic Roentgen pictures. *Electrical World*, New York, 1896, **27,** 280.
Invention of the Roentgen stereoscope.

2687 MACINTYRE, JOHN. 1857–1928
X-ray records for the cinematograph. *Arch. Skiagraphy*, 1897, **1,** 37.
Macintyre was the first to demonstrate *x*-ray cinematography.

2688 HOLZKNECHT, GUIDO. 1872–1931
Eine neue, einfache Dosirungsmethode in der Radiotherapie (das Chromoradiometer). *Wien. klin. Rdsch.*, 1902, **16,** 685–87.
Holzknecht did important work on Roentgen-ray dosimetry.

2689 ALBERS-SCHÖNBERG, HEINRICH ERNST. 1865–1921
Die Röntgen-Technik. Hamburg, *L. Gräfe & Sillem*, 1903.
Albers-Schönberg invented the compression diaphragm, the function of which is to intensify the object by cutting out secondary rays.

2690 GROEDEL, FRANZ MAXIMILIAN. 1881–1951
Die Technik der Roentgenkinematographie. *Dtsch. med. Wschr.*, 1909, **35,** 434–35.
First of an important series of papers by Groedel on Roentgen-cinematography.

2691 BUCKY, GUSTAV. 1880–1963
A grating-diaphragm to cut off secondary rays from the object. *Arch. Roentgen Ray*, 1913–14, **18,** 6–9.
Bucky devised a diaphragm for roentgenography which, by preventing the secondary rays from reaching the plate, secured better contrast and definition.

2692 COOLIDGE, WILLIAM DAVID. 1873–1975
A powerful Roentgen ray tube with a pure electron discharge. *Amer. J. Roentgenol.*, 1913–14, n.s. **1,** 115–24.
Coolidge invented a vacuum tube for the generation of Roentgen rays.

2693 SICARD, JEAN ATHANASE. 1872–1929, & FORESTIER, JACQUES. 1890–
Méthode radiographique d'exploration de la cavité épidurale par le lipiodol. *Rev. neurol.*, 1921, **28,** 1264–66.
Lipiodol first used in radiology.

2694 HOLZKNECHT, GUIDO. 1872–1931
Einstellung der Röntgenologie. Wien, *J. Springer*, 1927.

2695 OKA, MITSUTOMO.
Eine neue Methode zur röntgenologischen Darstellung der Milz. *Fortschr. Röntgenstr.*, 1929, **40,** 497–501.
Thorium dioxide ("thorotrast") first used in radiological diagnosis.

2696 STUMPF, PLEIKART. 1888–
Archiv und Atlas der normalen und pathologischen Anatomie in typischen Röntgenbildern. Das röntgenographische Bewegungsbild und seine Anwendung (Flachenkymographie und Kymoskopie). *Fortschr. Röntgenstr.*, 1931, Ergänzungsband 41.
Introduction of roentgenkymography.

2697 GIANTURCO, CESARE. 1905– , & ALVAREZ, WALTER CLEMENT. 1884–
Roentgen ray motion pictures of the stomach. *Proc. Mayo Clin.*, 1932, **7,** 669–71.
Camera used for direct Roentgen-cinematography.

2698 BARTELINK, D. L.
Röntgenschnitte. *Fortsch. Röntgenstr.*, 1933, **47,** 399–407.
Tomography first described.

2699 GROSSMANN, G.
Tomographie. *Fortschr. Röntgenstr.*, 1935, **51,** 61–80, 191–208.
Grossmann improved the tomograph.

2700 SHANKS, Seymour Cochrane. 1893– , & KERLEY, Peter James. 1900–
A text-book of x-ray diagnosis by British authors. Edited by S. C. Shanks and P. J. Kerley. 2nd ed. 4 vols. London, *H. K. Lewis*, 1950–51.

History of Radiology

2701 GOCHT, Hermann. 1869–1938
Die Röntgen-Literatur. 2 vols. Stuttgart, *F. Enke*, 1911–12.

2702 GLASSER, Otto. 1895–1964
The science of radiology. Edited by Otto Glasser. Springfield, *C. C. Thomas*, 1933.
Gives details of the development of all branches of the subject, together with a useful bibliography.

2702.1 BRUWER, André Johannes. 1918–
Classic descriptions in diagnostic roentgenology. 2 vols. Springfield, *C. C. Thomas*, 1964.
A compilation of pioneer contributions to the technology and methodology of diagnostic roentgenology.

2702.2 GRIGG, Emanuel Radu Newman. 1916–
The trail of the invisible light. From X-Strahlen to radio(bio)logy. Springfield, *C. C. Thomas*, 1965.

2703–3161.1 DISEASES OF THE CARDIOVASCULAR SYSTEM

2703 WEPFER, Johann Jacob. 1620–1695
Observationes anatomicae, ex cadaveribus eorum, quos sustulit apoplexia. Schaffhusii, *J. C. Suteri*, 1658.
Wepfer showed apoplexy to be a result of haemorrhage into the brain. He described four cases, with clinical and post-mortem findings.

2704 RAYNAUD, Maurice. 1834–1881
De l'asphyxie locale et de la gangrene symétrique des extrémités. Paris, *Rignoux*, 1862.
First description of "Raynaud's disease". For a translation by T. Barlow see *Selected Monographs*, London, 1888, pp. 1–199 (New Sydenham Society Publication), which also contains a translation of Raynaud's second paper on the subject.

2705 NOTHNAGEL, Carl Wilhelm Hermann. 1841–1905
Zur Lehre von den vasomotorischen Neurosen. *Dtsch. Arch. klin. Med.*, 1867, **2**, 173–91.
Nothnagel described the vasomotor type of acroparaesthesia, sometimes called after him.

2706 MITCHELL, Silas Weir. 1829–1914
Clinical lecture on certain painful affections of the feet. *Philad. med. Times*, 1872, **3**, 81, 113.
First complete description of erythromelalgia, "Weir Mitchell's disease". See also his paper in *Amer. J. med. Sci.*, 1878, **76**, 17–36.

2707 LEGG, JOHN WICKHAM. 1843–1921
A case of haemophilia complicated with multiple naevi. *Lancet*, 1876, **2**, 856.
First description of multiple hereditary telangiectasis ("Rendu–Osler–Weber disease").

2708 OERTEL, MAX JOSEPH. 1835–1897
Therapie der Kreislauf-Störungen. Leipzig, *F. C. W. Vogel*, 1884.

2709 SCHULTZE, FRIEDRICH. 1848–1934
Ueber Akroparästhesie. *Dtsch. Z. Nervenheilk.*, 1893, **3**, 300–18.
"Schultze's acroparaesthesia." Schultze described the simple form of acroparaesthesia.

2710 RENDU, HENRI JULES LOUIS. 1844–1902
Épistaxis répétes chez un sujet porteur de petits angiomes cutanés et muqueux. *Gaz. Hop. (Paris)*, 1896, **69**, 1322–23.
Rendu's account of multiple hereditary telangiectasis ("Rendu–Osler–Weber disease").

2711 TREUPEL, GUSTAV. 1867–1926, & EDINGER, A.
Untersuchungen über Rhodan-Verbindungen. *Münch. med. Wschr.*, 1900, **47**, 717–20.
Introduction of thiocyanates in treatment of hypertension.

2712 OSLER, *Sir* WILLIAM, *Bart.* 1849–1919
On a family form of recurring epistaxis, associated with multiple telangiectases of the skin and mucous membranes. *Johns Hopk. Hosp. Bull.*, 1901, **12**, 333–37.
"Rendu–Osler–Weber disease". Multiple hereditary telangiectasis was first described by Legg (No. 2707) in 1876, and later by Rendu (No. 2710) and Weber (No. 2714). Reprinted in *Med. Classics*, 1939, **4**, 243–53.

2713 PAL, JAKOB. 1863–1936
Gefässkrisen. Leipzig, *S. Hirzel*, 1905.

2714 WEBER, FREDERICK PARKES. 1863–1962
Multiple hereditary developmental angiomata (telangiectases) of the skin and mucous membranes associated with recurring haemorrhages. *Lancet*, 1907, **2**, 160–62.
"Rendu–Osler–Weber disease."

2715 MOSCHCOWITZ, ELI. 1879–1964
Hypertension of the pulmonary circulation. *Amer. J. med. Sci.*, 1927, **174**, 388–406.

2716 KEITH, NORMAN MACDONNELL. 1885– , *et al.*
Some different types of essential hypertension: their course and prognosis. *Amer. J. med. Sci.*, 1929, **197**, 332–43.
The Keith–Wagener–Barker classification of hypertension. With H. P. Wagener and N. W. Barker.

2717 HINES, EDGAR ALPHONSO. 1906– , & BROWN, GEORGE ELGIE. 1885–1935
A standard stimulus for measuring vasomotor reactions: its application in the study of hypertension. *Proc. Mayo Clin.*, 1932, **7**, 332–35.
Cold-pressor test.

2718 TARR, LEONARD. 1901– , *et al.*
The circulation time in various clinical conditions determined by the use of sodium dehydrocholate. *Amer. Heart J.*, 1933, **8,** 766–86.
Use of decholin sodium for estimation of circulation time. With B. S. Oppenheimer and R. V. Sagar.

2719 GOLDBLATT, HARRY. 1891– , *et al.*
Studies on experimental hypertension. 1. The production of persistent elevation of systolic blood pressure by means of renal ischemia. *J. exp. Med.*, 1934, **59,** 347–79.
The first of Goldblatt's important papers on experimental hypertension. Written with J. Lynch, R. F. Hanzal, and W. W. Summerville.

2720 BARKER, MARION HERBERT. 1899–1947
Blood cyanates in the treatment of hypertension. *J. Amer. med. Ass.*, 1936, **106,** 762–67.
Barker made thiocyanate treatment a practical proposition in hypertension.

2721 HOUSSAY, BERNARDO ALBERTO. 1887–1971, & FASCIOLO, JUAN CARLOS. 1911–
Secreción hipertensora del rinón isquemiado. *Rev. Soc. argent. Biol.*, 1937, **13,** 284–94.
Houssay and Fasciolo transplanted an ischaemic kidney into an animal from which both kidneys had been removed. Hypertension resulted after establishment of circulation, supporting the view that hypertension is due to a chemical substance with pressor action produced in the ischaemic kidney. They later showed that the ischaemic kidneys of hypertensive dogs contained an excess of renin. See also *Bol. Acad. nac. Med. B. Aires*, 1937, **34**, 342; *J. Physiol.* (*Lond.*), 1938, **94**, 281.

2722 HOMANS, JOHN. 1877–
Circulatory diseases of the extremities. New York, *Macmillan Co.*, 1939.

2723 WAGENER, HENRY PATRICK. 1890– , & KEITH, NORMAN MACDONNELL. 1885–
Diffuse arteriolar disease with hypertension and the associated retinal lesions. *Medicine*, 1939, **18,** 317–430.
Wagener and Keith classified essential hypertension into four grades.

2724 WILSON, CLIFFORD. 1906– , & BYROM, FRANK BURNET.
Renal changes in malignant hypertension; experimental evidence. *Lancet*, 1939, **1,** 136–39.
Production of hypertension in rats by constriction of one renal artery, and important studies of the renal changes produced, which included degeneration of the renal arterioles.

2725 KEMPNER, WALTER. 1903–
Treatment of kidney disease and hypertensive vascular disease with rice diet. *N. Carol. med. J.*, 1944, **5,** 125–33.
Kempner rice diet for the treatment of hypertension.

2725.1 ABEATICI, S., & CAMPI, L.
La visualizzazione radiologica della porta per via splenica. *Minerva med.* (*Torino*), 1951, **42,** i, 593–94.
Introduction of portal venography for investigation of portal hypertension.

2726–2883.1 HEART AND AORTA

2726 MAYOW, John. 1643–1679
Tractatus . . . de motu musculari et spiritibus animalibus. Oxonii, *e theatro Sheldoniano*, 1674.
In the second edition of the "Tractatus quinque" Mayow recorded a case of mitral stenosis, probably the first description. Reprinted in his "Medico-physical works," Edinburgh, 1907, pp. 295–97.

2727 RIVIÈRE, Lazare [Riverius]. 1589–1655
Opera medica universa. Francofurti, *J. P. Zubrodt*, 1674.
Riverius was the first to note aortic stenosis (page 638 of the above).

2728 GERBEZIUS, Marcus. ?–1718
Pulsus mira inconstantia. *Misc. cur. Ephem. nat. cur.*, 1691, Norimbergae, 1692, **10**, 115–18.
First reported case of temporary cardiac arrest with syncopal attacks, the syndrome to which the names of Stokes (No. 2756) and Adams (No. 2745) were later attached.

2729 VIEUSSENS, Raymond. 1641–1715
Novum vasorum corporis humani systema. Amstelodami, *P. Marret*, 1705.
Vieussens was among the first to describe the morbid changes in mitral stenosis, the throbbing pulse in aortic insufficiency, and the first correctly to describe the structure of the left ventricle, the course of the coronary vessels and the valve in the large coronary vein. He was the first to diagnose thoracic aneurysm during the life of the patient. Vieussens included a classical description of the symptoms of aortic regurgitation in his book.

2730 COWPER, William. 1666–1709
Of ossifications or petrifactions in the coats of arteries, particularly in the valves of the great artery. *Phil. Trans.*, 1706, **24**, 1970–77.
First description of aortic insufficiency. Reproduced in F. A. Willius & T. E. Keys: *Cardiac classics*, 1941, pp. 109–14.

2731 LANCISI, Giovanni Maria. 1654–1720
De subitaneis mortibus libri duo. Romae, *J. F. Buagni*, 1707.
In the above work Lancisi noted cardiac hypertrophy and dilatation as causes of sudden death. He was the first to describe valvular vegetation, and his book gives a classification of the cardiac diseases then recognized. Lancisi's work laid the foundation for a true understanding of cardiac pathology.

2732 HALLER, Albrecht von. 1708–1777
De aortae venaeque cavae gravioribus quibusdam morbis. Gottingae, *A. Vandenhoeck*, [1749].

2733 SENAC, Jean Baptiste. 1693–1770
Traité de la structure du coeur, de son action, et de ses maladies. 2 vols. Paris, *chez Briasson*, 1749.
Senac's valuable treatise on the heart added much to the knowledge of the anatomy and diseases of that organ; he mentioned the leucocytes, which he considered to belong to the chyle, and he described pericarditis. Senac was the first to use quinine for palpitation.

2734 MORGAGNI, Giovanni Battista. 1682–1771
De sedibus, et causis morborum per anatomen indagatis. 2 vols. Venetiis, *typ. Remondiniana*, 1761.

Classical descriptions of mitral stenosis (Letter III) and heart block, Stokes-Adams syndrome (vol. 1, p. 70) are reprinted in English translation in F. A. Willius and T. E. Key's *Cardiac classics*, 1941, pp. 177–82.

2734.1 NICHOLLS, Frank. 1699–1778
Observations concerning the body of his late Majesty, October 26, 1760. *Phil. Trans.* (1761), 1762, **52**, 265–75.

Nicholls was first to describe dissecting aneurysm of the aorta, the patient being King George II, to whom he was physician from 1753–60. Nicholls was also the first to give a correct description of the mode of production of aneurysm.

2734.2 SANDIFORT, Eduard. 1742–1814
Observationes anatomico-pathologicae. Vol. 1. Lugduni Batavorum *P. v. d. Eyk & D. Vygh*, 1771.

A good account of the "tetralogy of Fallot" (No. 2792) is given on pp. 1–38. For English translation see *Amer. Heart J.*, 1956, **51**, 9–25.

2734.3 UNDERWOOD, Michael. 1737–1820
A treatise on the diseases of children. A new edition. 2 vols. London, *J. Mathews*, 1789.

In this edition of Underwood's book appeared for the first time mention, in a treatise on children's diseases, of congenital heart disease, (vol. 2, pp. 122–27).

2735 SPENS, Thomas. 1764–1842
History of a case in which there took place a remarkable slowness of the pulse. *Med. Commentaries*, (1792), Edinburgh, 1793, **7**, 458–65.

Morgagni described a case of "epilepsy with slow pulse" (see No. 2734), but Adams has been given the credit for reporting the first clear case of heart block (No. 2745). There is no doubt that Spens reported such a case in 1792.

2736 BAILLIE, Matthew. 1761–1823
The morbid anatomy of some of the most important parts of the human body. 2nd ed. London, *J. Johnson & G. Nicol*, 1797.

P. 46: Baillie suggested a relationship between rheumatic fever and valvular heart disease.

2737 CORVISART DES MAREST, Jean Nicolas, *Baron*. 1755–1821
Essai sur les maladies et les lésions organiques du coeur et des gros vaisseaux. Paris, *Méquignon-Marvis*, 1806.

Corvisart really created cardiac symptomatology and made possible the differentiation between cardiac and pulmonary disorders. He was first to explain heart failure mechanically and to describe the dyspnoea of effort. His translation of Auenbrugger's book on percussion resulted in the universal adoption of that procedure. Corvisart was Napoleon's favourite physician. English translation, 1812, reproduced 1962.

2738 BURNS, Allan. 1781–1813
Observations on some of the most frequent and important diseases of the heart. Edinburgh, *Bryce & Co.*, 1809.

Burns described endocarditis and reported three cases of mitral stenosis. He recognized the thrill present in the latter condition and seems to have understood the mechanism of a cardiac murmur. He also described unilateral paralysis of the diaphragm resulting from pressure on the phrenic nerve by a thoracic aneurysm. Biography by J. B. Herrick, 1935.

2739 DUNDAS, David.
An account of a peculiar disease of the heart. *Med.-chir. Trans.*, 1809, **1**, 37–46.
Account of nine cases of rheumatic endocarditis.

2740 WELLS, William Charles. 1757–1817
On rheumatism of the heart. *Trans. Soc. Improve. med. chir. Knowl.*, 1812, **3**, 373–424.
David Pitcairn is accredited with the first reference to rheumatism as a cause of cardiac disease, in a lecture given in 1788. Jenner read a paper on the same subject in 1789, but the first clinical report on the subject to be published was that by Wells. The paper is reprinted in F. A. Willius & T. E. Keys: *Cardiac classics*, 1941, pp. 294–312.

2741 HODGSON, Joseph. 1788–1869
A treatise on the diseases of arteries and veins. London, *T. Underwood* 1815.
Includes the best illustrations of aneurysms and of aortic valvular endocarditis so far published and, the first description of non-sacculated dilatation of the aortic arch ("Hodgson's disease").

2742 PARRY, Caleb Hillier. 1755–1822
An experimental inquiry into the nature, cause and varieties of the arterial pulse. London, *Underwood*, 1816.

2743 CHEYNE, John. 1777–1836
A case of apoplexy in which the fleshy part of the heart was converted into fat. *Dublin Hosp. Rep.*, 1818, **2**, 216–23.
First accurate description of the condition which later became known as "Cheyne–Stokes respiration". Reprinted in F. A. Willius & T. E. Keys: *Cardiac classics*, 1941, pp. 317–20.

2744 ROSTAN, Léon. 1790–1866
Mémoire sur cette question, l'asthme des vieillards est-il une affection nerveuse? *Nouv. J. Méd. Chir. Pharm.*, 1817, **3**, 3–30.
Rostan gave an early description of cardiac ("Rostan's") asthma.

2745 ADAMS, Robert. 1791–1875
Cases of diseases of the heart, accompanied with pathological observations. *Dublin Hosp. Rep.*, 1827, **4**, 353–453.
On p. 396 commences a classical account of heart block with syncopal attacks, the first complete description of this condition. Following the paper by Stokes (No. 2756) the eponym "Stokes–Adams syndrome" was employed to describe this state. Adams recognized a thrill in mitral regurgitation (p. 423). Adams also understood tricuspid incompetence (p. 436). The paper is reproduced in full in *Med. Classics*, 1939, 3, 633–96.

2746 HODGKIN, Thomas. 1798–1866
On the retroversion of the valves of the aorta. *Lond. med. Gaz.*, 1828–29, **3**, 433–43.
Aortic insufficiency is usually associated with the name of Corrigan but Hodgkin's account antedates Corrigan by three years. This is one of Hodgkin's best publications.

2747 HOPE, JAMES. 1801–1841

A treatise on the diseases of the heart and great vessels. London, *W. Kidd*, 1831.

Hope did much to advance the knowledge of heart murmurs, valvular disease, and aneurysm; he described the second sound of the heart on the left side of the sternum in mitral stenosis as "altered" – losing its short, flat clear sound and becoming a prolonged bellows murmur. From his description this became known as "Hope's early diastolic murmur". His classical descriptions of cardiac asthma, valvular disease (pp. 307–45 above), and cardiac neurosis are reprinted in F. A. Willius & T. E. Keys: *Cardiac classics*, 1941, pp. 405–15.

2748 CORRIGAN, *Sir* DOMINIC JOHN. 1802–1880

On permanent patency of the mouth of the aorta, or inadequacy of the aortic valves. *Edinb. med. surg. J.*, 1832, **37**, 225–45.

In his wonderfully clear account of aortic insufficiency, Corrigan described the "water-hammer pulse" now commonly known as "Corrigan's pulse". He recognized that the hypertrophy of the heart present in this condition is compensatory and not a disease. Corrigan was the last of the famous band forming the "Irish School of Medicine" in the 19th century. Reprinted in *Med. Classics*, 1937, **1**, 703–27.

2748.1 HÉRISSON, JULES.

Le sphygmomètre; instrument qui traduit à l'oeil toute l'action des artères. Paris, *Crochard*, 1834.

Hérisson invented an instrument for recording blood pressure.

2749 BOUILLAUD, JEAN BAPTISTE. 1796–1881

Traité cliniques des maladies du coeur. 2 vols. Paris, *J. B. Baillière*, 1835.

Vol. 2, page 238: "Bouillaud's disease" – rheumatic endocarditis. Although not first to note the cardiac manifestations of acute rheumatism, Bouillaud was the first to demonstrate the frequency and importance of heart disease co-incident with acute articular rheumatism. The above work includes the first description of a case of mitral disease with articular rheumatism. In 1836 Bouillaud published his *Nouvelles recherches* which contain his "law of coincidence" between rheumatism and cardiac disease. Translation of the section on the pathology of endocarditis in *Cardiac classics*, by F. A. Willius and T. E. Keys, 1941, pp. 446–55.

2750 SOBERNHEIM, JOSEPH FRIEDRICH. 1803–1846

Akute idiopathische Herzentzündung. In his: *Praktische Diagnostik*, Berlin, 1837, pp. 118–20.

Sobernheim first used the term "myocarditis".

2750.1 MERCIER, LOUIS AUGUSTE. 1811–1882

Rétrécissement avec oblitération presque complète de la portion thoracique de l'aorte. *Bull. Soc. anat. Paris*, 1839, **14**, 158–60.

Diagnosis of coarctation of aorta during life. Translation in *Amer. J. Cardiol.*, 1965, **16**, 253–55.

2751 PIGEAUX, ANTOINE LOUIS JULES. 1807–?

Traité pratique des maladies du coeur. Paris, *J. Rouvier*, 1839.

2752 CHEVERS, NORMAN. 1818–1886

Observations on the diseases of the orifice and valves of the aorta. *Guy's Hosp. Rep.*, 1842, **7**, 387–442.

First clear account of chronic constrictive pericarditis.

2753 BARLOW, George Hilaro. 1806–1866, & REES, George Owen. 1813–1889
Account of observations . . . on patients whose urine was albuminous. *Guy's Hosp. Rep.*, 1843, n.s. **1,** 189–316.

An early description of a case of subacute bacterial endocarditis is reported on pp. 227–32 (Case 8).

2754 FAUVEL, Sulpice Antoine. 1813–1884
Mémoire sur les signes stethoscopiques du rétricissement de l'orifice auriculo-ventriculaire gauches du coeur. *Arch. gén. Méd.*, 1843, 4 sér., **1,** 1–16.

First description of the presystolic murmur in mitral stenosis.

2755 BRICHETEAU, Isidore. 1789–1861
Observation d'hydropneumopéricarde, accompagnée d'un bruit de fluctuation perceptible à l'oreille. *Arch. gén. Méd.*, 1844, 4 sér., **4,** 334–39.

First adequate description of pneumopericardium.

2756 STOKES, William. 1804–1878
Observations on some cases of permanently slow pulse. *Dublin quart. J. med. Sci.*, 1846, **2,** 73–85.

Stokes' celebrated account of heart block with syncopal attacks – the Stokes–Adams syndrome (see also No. 2745). Stokes was most interested in the diagnostic value of this condition. The paper is reprinted in *Med. Classics*, 1939, **3**, 727–38.

2757 WALSHE, Walter Hayle. 1812–1892
A practical treatise on the diseases of the heart and the great vessels. London, *Taylor, Walton & Maberly*, 1851.

Walshe, physician to University College Hospital, London, was one of the first to recognize the presystolic character of the direct mitral murmur in mitral stenosis.

2758 KIRKES, William Senhouse. 1823–1864
On some of the principal effects resulting from the detachment of fibrinous deposits from the interior of the heart, and their mixture with the circulating blood. *Med.-chir. Trans.*, 1852, **35,** 281–324.

A classical description of embolism resulting from intracardiac coagula. Reprinted in Willius & Keys: *Cardiac classics*, 1941, pp. 474–82.

2759 VIERORDT, Karl. 1818–1884
Die bildliche Darstellung des menschlichen Arterienpulses. *Arch. physiol. Heilk.*, 1854, **13,** 284–87.

Vierordt invented a sphygmograph which acted on the principle that the indirect estimation of the blood-pressure could be accompanied by measuring the counter-pressure necessary to obliterate the arterial pulsation. This was the first instrument with which a tracing of the human pulse could be made. The paper was expanded into book form in 1855 and is the first record of a study with an instrument of precision of the pulse in health and disease.

2760 STOKES, William. 1804–1878
The diseases of the heart and aorta. Dublin, *Hodges & Smith*, 1854.

On pp. 320–27 is to be found Stokes' account of fatty degeneration of the heart, in which he so well described the periodic form of respiration now known as "Cheyne–Stokes breathing". Stokes also gave the first description of paroxysmal tachycardia (p. 161).

2761 PEACOCK, THOMAS BEVILL. 1812–1882
On malformations, etc., of the human heart. London, *J. Churchill*, 1858.
Includes an account of the "tetralogy of Fallot" (see No. 2792).

2762 DUROZIEZ, PAUL LOUIS. 1826–1897
Du double souffle intermittent crural, comme signe de l'insuffisance aortique. *Arch. gén. Méd.*, 1861, 5 sér., **17,** 417–43, 588–605.
The double intermittent murmur over the femoral arteries, diagnostic of aortic insufficiency, has become known as "Duroziez's sign."

2763 GAIRDNER, *Sir* WILLIAM TENNANT. 1824–1907
Short account of cardiac murmurs. *Edinb. med. J.*, 1861, **7,** 438–53.
The murmur which Fauvel (No. 2754) had called "presystolic" was described by Gairdner, who called it "auricular-systolic." This paper is important as being largely responsible for the recognition in Great Britain of the presystolic murmur, previously discounted by most authorities.

2764 FLINT, AUSTIN. 1812–1886
On cardiac murmurs. *Amer. J. med. Sci.*, 1862, n.s., **44,** 29–54.
First description of the "Austin Flint murmur", present at the apex beat in aortic regurgitation. Reprinted in *Med. Classics*, 1940, **4**, 864–900.

2765 FRIEDREICH, NIKOLAUS. 1825–1882
Krankheiten des Herzens. 2te. Aufl. Erlangen, *F. Enke*, 1867.
First appeared in Virchow's *Handbuch der speciellen Pathologie und Therapie*, Erlangen, 1854, **5**, 1 Abt., 385–530.

2766 POTAIN, PIERRE CARL ÉDOUARD. 1825–1901
Des mouvements et des bruits qui se passent dans les veines jugulaires. *Bull. Soc. méd. Hôp. Paris* (*Mémoires*), 1867, 2 sér., **4,** 3–27.
Classical account of the movements and murmurs in the jugular veins, important in the diagnosis of heart diseases. Potain's writings were models of clarity and style. A translation of this paper is to be found in Willius & Keys: *Cardiac classics*, 1941, pp. 533–56.

2767 WINGE, EMANUEL FREDRIK HAGBARTH. 1827–1894
[Mycosis endocardii.] *Norsk Mag. Laegevid.* (*Förh. Norske med. Selskab*), 1869, **23,** 78–82.
Winge first suggested that endocarditis was due to microbial infection. A translation of part of his paper is in R. H. Major, *Classic descriptions of disease*, 3rd ed., 1945, p. 472.

2768 MYERS, ARTHUR BOWEN RICHARDS. 1838–1921
On the etiology and prevalence of diseases of the heart among soldiers. London, *J. Churchill*, 1870.
First description of "Da Costa's syndrome" – the "effort syndrome" of Sir Thomas Lewis.

2769 WILKS, *Sir* SAMUEL, *Bart.* 1824–1911
Capillary embolism or arterial pyaemia. *Guy's Hosp. Rep.*, 1870, 3 sér., **15,** 29–35.
One of the first accounts of bacterial endocarditis was given by Wilks, who, in his classical paper on the subject, called the condition "arterial pyaemia". Reprinted in Willius & Keys: *Cardiac classics*, 1941, pp. 579–84.

2770 DA COSTA, JACOB MENDES. 1833–1900
On irritable heart; a clinical study of a form of functional cardiac disorder and its consequences. *Amer. J. med. Sci.*, 1871, n.s. **61,** 17–52.

"Da Costa's syndrome." This was first described by Myers (No. 2768) and is now known as "effort syndrome", "soldier's heart", "disordered action of the heart".

2771 FAGGE, CHARLES HILTON. 1838–1883
On the murmurs attendant on mitral contraction. *Guy's Hosp. Rep.*, 1871, 3 ser., **16,** 247–342.

Important and exhaustive account of the knowledge of presystolic murmurs. Fagge's paper also includes many clinical observations relating to the rhythm of heart murmurs and the state of the sounds of the heart in 67 cases at Guy's Hospital.

2772 BÄUMLER, CHRISTIAN. 1836–1933
Cases of partial and general idiopathic pericarditis. *Trans. clin. Soc. Lond.*, 1872, **5,** 8–22.

Pericarditis epistenorcardiaca described.

2773 BAMBERGER, HEINRICH. 1822–1888
Ueber zwei seltene Herzaffektionen, mit Bezugnahme auf die Theorie des ersten Herztons. *Wien. med. Wschr.*, 1872, **22,** 1–4, 25–28.

"Bamberger's disease" (Pick's disease, No. 2803).

2774 HEIBERG, HJALMAR. 1837–1897
Ein Fall von Endocarditis ulcerosa puerperalis mit Pilzbildungen im Herzen (Mycosis endocardii). *Virchows Arch. path. Anat.*, 1872, **56,** 407–14.

Heiberg suggested the microbic nature of endocarditis. He described what appeared to him to be the mycelia of *Leptothrix* in the vegetations of a case of ulcerative endocarditis.

2775 TRAUBE, LUDWIG. 1818–1876
Ein Fall von Pulsus bigeminus nebst Bemerkungen über die Leberschwellungen bei Klappenfehlern und über acute Leberatrophie. *Berl. klin. Wschr.*, 1872, **9,** 185–88, 221–24.

First clear description of pulsus bigeminus. Translated in Willius & Keys: *Cardiac classics*, 1941, pp. 590–99.

2776 KUSSMAUL, ADOLF. 1822–1902
Ueber schwielige Mediastino-Pericarditis und den paradoxen Puls. *Berl. klin. Wschr.*, 1873, **10,** 433–35, 445–49, 461–64.

Kussmaul introduced the concept of the "paradoxical pulse".

2777 POTAIN, PIERRE CARL ÉDOUARD. 1825–1901
Du rhythme cardiaque appelé bruit de galop, de son mécanisme et de sa valeur séméiologique. *Bull. Soc. méd. Hôp. Paris*, (1875), 1876, **12,** (Mém.), 137–66.

Analysis of "gallop rhythm".

2778 ROKITANSKY, CARL, *Freiherr von*. 1804–1878
Die Defecte der Scheidewände der Herzens. Wien, *W. Braumüller*, 1875.

Rokitansky's memoir on defects of the septum of the heart was his last work, and probably his greatest. It represented 14 years' study of the subject.

2779 BALFOUR, George William. 1823–1903
Clinical lectures on diseases of the heart and aorta. London, *J. & A. Churchill*, 1876.
Includes "Balfour's test" to ascertain whether the heart is still active, in cases of apparent death.

2780 DUROZIEZ, Paul Louis. 1826–1897
Du retrécissement mitral pur. *Arch. gén. méd.*, 1877, 6 sér., **30,** 32–54, 184–97.
First description of congenital mitral stenosis, "Duroziez's disease".

2781 HAMMER, Adam. 1818–1878
Ein Fall von thrombotischem Verschlusse einer der Kranzarterien des Herzens. *Wien. med. Wschr.*, 1878, **28,** 97–102.
First description of coronary thrombosis with diagnosis before death.

2782 ROGER, Henri. 1809–1891
Recherches cliniques sur la communication congénitale des deux coeurs par inocclusion du septum interventriculare. *Bull. Acad. Méd. (Paris)*, 1879, 2 sér., **8,** 1074–94, 1189–91.
Roger drew attention to an important anomaly of the septum, interventricular patency ("maladie de Roger"), demonstrating the presence of a murmur in this condition. This is sometimes called "Roger's murmur", although it had been noted by earlier writers. Translated in Willius & Keys: *Cardiac classics*, 1941, pp. 624–38.

2783 WEIGERT, Carl. 1845–1904
Ueber die pathologische Gerinnungs-Vorgänge. *Virchows Arch. path. Anat.*, 1880, **79,** 87–123.
First description (p. 106) of cardiac infarction.

2784 BASCH, Samuel Siegfried von. 1837–1905
Ueber die Messung des Blutdrucks am Menschen. *Z. klin. Med.*, 1881, **2,** 79–96.
Basch's important modifications of the methods of blood-pressure recording mark the beginning of clinical sphygmomanometry.

2785 CONCATO, Luigi Maria. 1825–1882
Sulla poliorromennite scrofolosa, o tisi delle sierose. *G. int. Sci. med.*, 1881, n.s. **3,** 1037–53.
"Concato's disease" – inflammation of the serous membranes. Involvement of the pericardium was later described by Pick (No. 2803).

2786 LEYDEN, Ernst von. 1832–1910
Ueber Fettherz. *Z. klin. Med.*, 1882, **5,** 1–25.
Fatty infiltration of the heart first described.

2787 BASCH, Samuel Siegfried von. 1837–1905
Ein Metall-Sphygmomanometer. *Wien. med. Wschr.*, 1883, **33,** 673–675.
First clinical use of the sphygmomanometer.

2788 PETER, Charles Félix Michel. 1824–1893
Traité clinique et pratique des maladies du coeur et de la crosse de l'aorte. Paris, *J. B. Baillière*, 1883.

2789 PAUL, Constantin Charles Théodore. 1833–1896
Diagnostic et traitement des maladies du coeur. Paris, *Asselin & Cie.*, 1883.
English translation, 1884.

2790 OSLER, *Sir* WILLIAM, *Bart.* 1849–1919
The Gulstonian Lectures, on malignant endocarditis. *Brit. med. J.*, 1885, **1,** 467–70, 522–26, 577–79.
Subacute bacterial endocarditis.

2791 MACWILLIAM, JOHN ALEXANDER. 1857–1937
Fibrillar contraction of the heart. *J. Physiol.* (*Lond.*), 1887, **8,** 296–310.
MacWilliam discovered that fibrillar contraction of the heart is due to "a rapid succession of incoordinated peristaltic contractions". He clearly described auricular and ventricular fibrillation, and showed that ventricular fibrillation could be caused by the injection of certain poisons into the blood stream. His paper is included, with an account of his life, in Willius and Keys: *Cardiac classics*, 1941, pp. 666–678.

2792 FALLOT, ETIENNE LOUIS ARTHUR. 1850–1911
Contribution à l'anatomie pathologique de la maladie bleu (cyanose cardiaque). *Marseille méd.*, 1888, **25,** 77–93, 138–58, 207–23, 270–86, 341–54, 403–20.
The "tetralogy of Fallot". He gave an important, but not the first, account of this condition (see No. 2734.2). Abstract translation in F. A. Willius and T. E. Keys: *Cardiac classics*, 1941, pp. 689–90.

2793 ROY, CHARLES SMART. 1854–1897, & ADAMI, JOHN GEORGE. 1862–1926
Remarks on failure of the heart from overstrain. *Brit. med. J.*, 1888, **2,** 1321–26.
Important experimental work on cardiac overstrain was carried out by Roy and Adami who considered that mechanical overstrain caused chronic thickening of the cardiac valves.

2794 STEELL, GRAHAM. 1851–1942
The murmur of high-pressure in the pulmonary artery. *Med. Chron.* (*Manch.*), 1888–89, **9,** 182–88.
First description of the pulmonary diastolic murmur – the "Graham Steell murmur". Reproduced in Willius & Keys: *Cardiac classics*, 1941, pp. 680–85.

2795 BOUVERET, LÉON. 1851–1929
De la tachycardie essentielle paroxystique. *Rev. Médecine*, 1889, **9,** 753–93, 837–55.
Bouvert introduced the term "paroxysmal tachycardia".

2796 HUCHARD, HENRI. 1844–1910
Maladies du coeur et des vaisseaux. Paris, *O. Doin*, 1889.
In his important monograph on disorders of the cardiovasculat system, Huchard was apparently the first to use the designation "Stokes-Adams disease".

2797 MACWILLIAM, JOHN ALEXANDER. 1857–1937
Cardiac failure and sudden death. *Brit. med. J.*, 1889, **1,** 6–8.
First description of a case of death from ventricular fibrillation.

2798 POTAIN, PIERRE CARL ÉDOUARD. 1825–1901
Du sphygmomanomètre et de la mesure de la pression artérielle chez l'homme à l'état normale et pathologique. *Arch. Physiol. norm. path.*, 1889, 5 sér., **1,** 556–69.
Potain devised a simple portable air sphygmomanometer for blood-pressure estimation.

2799 ROSENBACH, OTTOMAR. 1851–1907
Die Krankheiten des Herzens und ihre Behandlung. Wien, Leipzig, *Urban & Schwarzenberg*, 1893–97.

2800 BROADBENT, WALTER. 1868–1951
An unpublished physical sign. *Lancet*, 1895, **2**, 200–01.
"Broadbent's sign" – recession of the intercostal spaces as a sign of adherent pericardium.

2801 MOSSO, ANGELO. 1846–1910
Sphygmomanomètre pour mesurer la pression du sang chez l'homme. *Arch. ital. Biol.*, 1895, **23**, 177–97.
A sphygmomanometer for registering the blood-pressure in the finger was invented by Mosso.

2802 EWART, WILLIAM. 1848–1929
Practical aids in the diagnosis of pericardial effusion, in connection with the question as to surgical treatment. *Brit. med. J.*, 1896, **1**, 717–21.
Pulmonary collapse at the left base in pericardial effusion – "Ewart's sign."

2803 PICK, FRIEDEL. 1867–1926
Ueber chronische unter dem Bilde der Leberzirrhose verlaufende Perikarditis (perikarditische Pseudoleberzirrhose) nebst Bemerkungen über die Zuckergussleber. *Z. klin. Med.*, 1896, **29**, 385–410.
"Pick's disease" – pericardial pseudocirrhosis of the liver.

2804 RIVA-ROCCI, SCIPIONE. 1863–1937
Un nuovo sfigmomanometro. *Gaz. med. Torino*, 1896, **47**, 981–96, 1001–17.
Riva-Rocci's sphygmomanometer marked the end of the search for a simple clinical method of estimating the blood-pressure.

2805 BROADBENT, *Sir* WILLIAM HENRY, *Bart.* 1835–1907, & BROADBENT, *Sir* JOHN FRANCIS HARPIN, *Bart.* 1865–1946
Heart disease. London, *Baillière, Tindall & Cox*, 1897.
Chapter 17 includes J. Broadbent's classical description of adherent pericardium. See F. A. Willius and T. E. Keys: *Cardiac classics*, 1941, pp. 712–5, for reproduction of part of this chapter.

2806 EISENMENGER, VICTOR.
Die angeborenen Defecte der Kammerscheidewand des Herzens. *Z. klin. Med.*, 1897, **32**, Suppl.-Heft, 1–28.
"Riding aorta," patent interventricular septum and right ventricular enlargement – the "Eisenmenger syndrome".

2807 HILL, *Sir* LEONARD ERSKINE. 1866–1952, & BARNARD, HAROLD LESLIE. 1868–1908
A simple and accurate form of sphygmomanometer or arterial pressure gauge contrived for clinical use. *Brit. med. J.*, 1897, **2**, 904.
Hill and Barnard made an important modification to the Riva-Rocci sphygmomanometer when they substituted a pressure gauge in place of the mercury manometer used for pressure readings.

2808 GIBSON, GEORGE ALEXANDER. 1854–1913
Diseases of the heart and the aorta. Edinburgh, *Y. J. Pentland*, 1898.

2809 RUMMO, GAETANO. 1853–1917
Sulla cardioptosi; primo abbozzo anatomo-clinico. *Arch. Med. int. (Palermo)*, 1898, **1**, 161–83.
Rummo drew attention to a downward displacement of the heart – "Rummo's disease".

2809.1 WENCKEBACH, Karel Frederik. 1864–1940
Zur Analyse des unregelmässigen Pulses. *Z. klin. Med.*, 1899, **36**, 181–99.
"Wenckebach phenomenon", a form of arrhythmia.

2809.2 FIEDLER, Carl Ludwig Alfred. 1835–1921
Ueber akute interstitielle Myokarditis. Dresden, *W. Baensch*, 1899.
"Fiedler's myocarditis."

2810 GAERTNER, Gustav. 1855–1937
Ueber einen neuen Blutdruckmesser (Tonometer). *Wien. med. Wschr.*, 1899, **49**, 1412–18.
Gaertner, an Austrian physician, invented an instrument for measuring blood pressure by means of a compressing ring applied to the finger.

2811 HUCHARD, Henri. 1844–1910
Traité clinique des maladies du coeur et de l'aorte. 3 vols. Paris, *O. Doin*, 1899–1903.

2812 MACKENZIE, *Sir* James. 1853–1925
The study of the pulse. Edinburgh, *Y. J. Pentland*, 1902.
In his classical monograph Mackenzie included (p. 10) a description and illustration of his polygraph, with which he made simultaneous tracings of the pulse, apex beat, etc.

2813 MORITZ, Friedrich. 1861–1938
Ueber orthodiagraphische Untersuchungen am Herzen. *Münch. med. Wschr.*, 1902, **49**, 1–8.
Orthodiagraphy of the heart.

2814 BONNET, L. M.
Sur la lésion dite sténose congénitale de l'aorte dans la région de l'isthme. *Rev. Médecine*, 1903, **23**, 108–26.
Distinction of infantile and adult types of coarctation of the aorta.

2815 CHIARI, Hans. 1851–1916
Ueber die syphilitischen Aortenerkrankungen. *Verh. dtsch. path. Ges.*, (1903), 1904, **6**, 137–63.

2816 ASCHOFF, Karl Albert Ludwig. 1866–1942
Zur Myocarditisfrage. *Verh. dtsch. path. Ges.*, 1904, **8**, 46–53.
In his classical work on rheumatic myocarditis, Aschoff described the characteristic lesion (Aschoff body or nodule) and presented a histopathological picture of myocarditis that was to exert a great influence on the classification of the disease. The paper is translated in Willius & Keys: *Cardiac classics*, 1941, pp. 733–39.

2817 KÖHLER, Alban. 1874–1947
Technik der Herstellung fast orthodiagraphischer Herzphotogramme vermittelst Röntgeninstrumentarien mit kleiner Elektrizitätsquelle. *Wien. klin. Rdsch.*, 1905, **19**, 279–82.
Introduction of teleradiography of the heart.

2818 KOROTKOV, Nikolai Sergeievich. 1874–1920
[On methods of studying blood pressure.] *Izvest. imp. voyenno-med. Akad. St. Petersburg*, 1905, **11**, 365.
Korotkov introduced the modern method of applying the stethoscope to the brachial artery during blood-pressure examination with Riva-Rocci's sphygmomanometer, for the purpose of investigating the sounds made by the blood after release of the air-pressure cuff. For an English translation of the paper see *Bull. N.Y. Acad. Med.*, 1941, **17**, 877–79.

2819 MACKENZIE, *Sir* JAMES. 1853–1925
New methods of studying affections of the heart. *Brit. med. J.*, 1905, **1,** 519–21, 587–89, 702–05, 759–62, 812–15.
Mackenzie established the remarkable action of digitalis in auricular fibrillation.

2820 MARTIN, *Sir* CHARLES JAMES. 1866–1955
The determination of arterial blood-pressure in a clinical practice. *Brit. med. J.*, 1905, **1,** 865–70.

2821 RITCHIE, WILLIAM THOMAS. 1873–1945
Complete heart-block, with dissociation of the action of the auricles and ventricles. *Proc. roy. Soc. Edinb.*, 1905–06, **25,** 1085–91.
Auricular flutter in man first recognized.

2822 CUSHNY, ARTHUR ROBERTSON. 1866–1926, & EDMUNDS, CHARLES WALLIS. 1873–1941
Paroxysmal irregularity of the heart and auricular fibrillation. In: *Studies in pathology written . . . to celebrate the quatercentenary of Aberdeen University.* Edited by W. BULLOCH, Aberdeen, 1906, pp. 95–110.
First recognition of auricular fibrillation in man. Cushny and Edmunds had a case under their care in 1901. Hering described the condition in man in *Prag. med. Wschr.*, 1903, **28**, 377.

2823 KRILOFF, DMITRI DMITRIYEVICH. 1879–
[Estimation of blood-pressure by Korotkov's auditory method.] *Izvest. Imp. voyenno-med. Akad. St. Petersburg*, 1906, **13,** 113, 221, 319.
Kriloff made extensive observations on the sounds which Korotkov had shown to be emitted by the blood after removal of the Riva-Rocci air-pressure cuff during blood-pressure measurement.

2824 REUTER, KARL.
Ueber Spirochaete pallida in der Aortenwand bei Hellerscher Aortitis. *Münch med. Wschr.*, 1906, **53,** 778.
Treponema pallidum first discovered in the diseased aorta.

2825 FELLNER, BRUNO, *jnr.*
Neuerung zur Messung des systolischen und diastolischen Druckes. *Verh. Kongr. inn. Med.*, 1907, **24,** 404–07.
Fellner suggested the use of the stethoscope in the measurement of systolic and diastolic pressure.

2826 MACKENZIE, *Sir* JAMES. 1853–1925
Diseases of the heart. London, *H. Frowde*, 1908.
Chapter 30 includes Mackenzie's classical description of the clinical picture of "nodal rhythm" (auricular fibrillation). Reprinted in F. A. Willius & T. E. Keys: *Cardiac classics*, 1941, pp. 769–93.

2827 OSLER, *Sir* WILLIAM, *Bart.* 1849–1919
Chronic infectious endocarditis. *Quart. J. Med.*, 1908–09, **2,** 219–30.
The tender subcutaneous nodes in subacute bacterial endocarditis ("Osler's nodes") were first observed by Osler in 1888, and reported in 1909. This paper is the first definite clinical description of subacute bacterial endocarditis.

2828 BRACHT, ERICH. 1882– , & WÄCHTER.
Beitrag zur Aetiologie und pathologischen Anatomie der Myokarditis rheumatica. *Dtsch. Arch. klin. Med.*, 1909, **96,** 493–514.
"Bracht–Wächter bodies" in the myocardium in bacterial endocarditis.

2829 HORDER, THOMAS JEEVES, *1st Baron Horder*. 1871–1955
Infective endocarditis, with an analysis of 150 cases. *Quart. J. Med.*, 1909, **2,** 289–324.

Classical description of subacute bacterial endocarditis.

2830 LEWIS, *Sir* THOMAS. 1881–1945
Auricular fibrillation; a common clinical condition. *Brit. med. J.*, 1909, **2,** 1528.

First description of auricular fibrillation as a cause of clinical perpetual arrhythmia. See also the paper in *Heart*, London, 1909–10, **1**, 306–72.

2831 ROTHBERGER, CARL JULIUS. 1871– , & WINTERBERG, HEINRICH. 1867–1929
Vorhofflimmern und Arhythmia perpetua. *Wien. klin. Wschr.*, 1909, **22,** 839–44.

Independently of Lewis (No. 2830) these workers claimed auricular fibrillation to be the cause of perpetual arrhythmia.

2832 EPPINGER, HANS. 1879–1946, & STOERK, OSCAR. 1870–1926
Zur Klinik des Elektrokardiogramms. *Z. klin. Med.*, 1910, **71,** 157–164.

First clinical and pathological description of bundle-branch block.

2833 JOLLY, WILLIAM ADAM. 1878–1939, & RITCHIE, WILLIAM THOMAS. 1873–1945
Auricular flutter and fibrillation. *Heart*, 1910, **2,** 177–221.

Auricular flutter first described.

2834 LIBMAN, EMANUEL. 1872–1946, & CELLER, HERBERT LOUIS. 1878–1928
The etiology of subacute infective endocarditis. *Amer. J. med. Sci.*, 1910, **140,** 516–27.

Libman and Celler found *Strep. endocarditidis* to be the most common cause of subacute bacterial endocarditis.

2835 OBRASTZOW, W. P., & STRAZHESKO, NIKOLAI DIMITRIEVICH. 1876–
Zur Kenntniss der Thrombose der Koronararterien des Herzens. *Z. klin. Med.*, 1910, **71,** 116–32.

First complete description of coronary thrombosis, diagnosed *ante mortem* and proved at necropsy.

2836 SCHOTTMÜLLER, HUGO. 1867–1936
Endocarditis lenta. Zugleich ein Beitrag zur Artunterscheidung der pathogenen Streptokokken. *Münch. med. Wschr.*, 1910, **57,** 617–20, 697–99.

First to isolate *Strep. viridans* in cases of bacterial endocarditis, Schottmüller named the condition Endocarditis lenta.

2837 VAQUEZ, LOUIS HENRI. 1860–1936
Les arythmies. Paris, *J. B. Baillière*, 1911.

2838 BAEHR, GEORGE. 1887–
Glomerular lesions of subacute bacterial endocarditis. *J. exp. Med.*, 1912, **15,** 330–47.

Baehr drew attention to the renal lesions in subacute bacterial endocarditis.

2839 HERRICK, JAMES BRYAN. 1861–1954
Clinical features of sudden obstruction of the coronary arteries. *J. Amer. med. Ass.*, 1912, **59**, 2015–20.

Best extant description of coronary thrombosis. Herrick showed that sudden coronary occlusion is not necessarily fatal. Reprinted in Willius & Keys: *Cardiac classics*, 1941, pp. 817–29.

2840 LEWIS, *Sir* THOMAS. 1881–1945
Electro-cardiography and its importance in the clinical examination of heart affections. *Brit. med. J.*, 1912, **1**, 1421–23, 1479–82; **2**, 65–67.

2841 LIBMAN, EMANUEL. 1872–1946
A study of the endocardial lesions of subacute bacterial endocarditis. *Amer. J. med. Sci.*, 1912, **144**, 313–27.

2842 HUISMANS, L.
Der Ersatz des Orthiodiagraphen durch der Teleröntgen. *Verh. dtsch. Kongr. inn. Med.*, 1913, **30**, 266–69.

Instantaneous radiography of the heart.

2843 RITCHIE, WILLIAM THOMAS. 1873–1945
Auricular flutter. Edinburgh, London, *W. Green & Son*, 1914.

2844 WENCKEBACH, KAREL FREDERIK. 1864–1940
Die unregelmässige Herztätigkeit und ihre klinische Bedeutung. Leipzig, Berlin, *W. Engelmann*, 1914.

Wenckebach was the first to demonstrate (pp. 173–75) the value of quinine ("Wenckebach's pills") in the treatment of paroxysmal fibrillation. The same work contains a number of excellent descriptions of various forms of cardiac arrhythmia. A second edition, written in co-operation with H. Winterberg, appeared in 1927.

2845 CRANE, AUGUSTUS WARREN. 1868–1937
Roentgenology of the heart. *Amer. J. Roentgenol.*, 1916, **3**, 513–24.

Introduction of kymography in clinical cardiology.

2846 LUTEMBACHER, RENÉ. 1884–
De la sténose mitrale avec communication interauriculaire. *Arch. Mal. Coeur*, 1916, **9**, 237–60.

"Lutembacher syndrome."

2847 LEWIS, *Sir* THOMAS. 1881–1945
Report upon soldiers returned as cases of "disordered action of the heart" (D.A.H.) or "valvular disease of the heart" (V.D.H.). London *H.M. Stationery Off.*, 1917.

Medical Research Committee Special Rept. No. 8. Sir Thomas Lewis described as "effort syndrome" the condition of disordered action of the heart known as "Da Costa's syndrome".

2848 FREY, WALTER. 1884–
Ueber Vorhofflimmern beim Menschen und seine Beseitigung durch Chinidin. *Berl. klin. Wschr.*, 1918, **55**, 450–52.

Following Wenckebach's discovery of the efficacy of quinine in the restoration of normal rhythm in auricular fibrillation, Frey showed that quinidine was the most effective of the cinchona alkaloids in this respect.

2849 ZONDEK, HERMANN. 1887–
Das Myxödemherz. *Münch. med. Wschr.*, 1918, **65**, 1180–82.

"Myxoedema heart" first recorded.

2850 VELDEN, Reinhard von den. 1880–1941
Die intrakardiale Injektion. *Münch. med. Wschr.*, 1919, **66,** 274–75.
First attempt to restore the heart's action by intracardiac injection.

2851 LEWIS, *Sir* Thomas. 1881–1945
The mechanism and graphic registration of the heart beat. London, *Shaw & Sons*, 1920.
See No. 854. Third edition, 1925.

2852 PARDEE, Harold Ensign Bennett. 1886–
An electrocardiographic sign of coronary artery obstruction. *Arch. intern. Med.*, 1920, **26,** 244–57.
First description of the typical changes in the electrocardiogram in coronary thrombosis.

2853 SAXL, Paul. 1880–1932
Verhandlungen ärtzlicher Gesellschaften und Kongressberichte. *Wien. klin. Wschr.*, 1920, **33,** 179–80.
Saxl injected a mercurial compound (Novasurol), a powerful diuretic, for the treatment of cardiac failure.

2854 COOMBS, Carey Franklin. 1879–1932
Rheumatic heart disease. Bristol, *John Wright*, 1924.

2855 LIBMAN, Emanuel. 1872–1946, & SACKS, Benjamin. 1896–
A hitherto undescribed form of valvular and mural endocarditis. *Arch. intern. Med.*, 1924, **33,** 701–37.
"Libman–Sacks disease."

2856 ABBOTT, Maude Elizabeth Seymour. 1869–1940
Congenital cardiac disease. In: Osler & McCrea: *Modern medicine*, 3rd ed., Philadelphia, 1927, **4,** 612–812.

2857 ERDHEIM, Jakob. 1874–1937
Medionecrosis aortae idiopathica (cystica). *Virchows Arch. path. Anat.*, 1929, **273,** 454–79; 1930, **276,** 187–229.
Classical description of aortic medionecrosis.

2858 FORSSMANN, Werner Theodor Otto. 1904–
Die Sondierung des rechten Herzens. *Klin. Wschr.*, 1929, **8,** 2085–87, 2287.
Cardiac catheterization. Forssmann catheterized his own heart. In 1956 he shared the Nobel Prize with Cournand (No. 2871) and Richards (No. 2883.1) for his work on cardiac catheterization. See also historical note in *Lancet*, 1949, **1,** 746.

2859 SANTOS, Reynaldo dos. 1880– , *et al.*
L'artériographie des membres de l'aorte et de ses branches abdominales. *Med. contemp.* (*Lisboa*), 1929, **47,** 93–96.
Aortography. With A. C. Lamas and J. Pereira Caldas. Also published in *Bull. Soc. med.-chir. Paris*, 1929, **55,** 587–601.

2860 WOLFF, Louis. 1898– , PARKINSON, *Sir* John. 1885– , & WHITE, Paul Dudley. 1886–
Bundle-branch block with short P–R interval in healthy young people prone to paroxysmal tachycardia. *Amer. Heart J.*, 1930, **5,** 685–704.
Wolff–Parkinson–White syndrome.

2861 GROLLMAN, ARTHUR. 1901–
The cardiac output of man in health and disease. Springfield, *C. C. Thomas*, 1932.

2862 LEWIS, *Sir* THOMAS. 1881–1945
A lecture on vaso-vagal syncope and the carotid sinus mechanism. *Brit. med. J.*, 1932, **1,** 873–76.
Vaso-vagal syncope.

2863 WOLFERTH, CHARLES CHRISTIAN. 1887–1965, & WOOD, FRANCIS CLARK. 1901–
The electrocardiographic diagnosis of coronary occlusion by the use of chest leads. *Amer. J. med. Sci.*, 1932, **183,** 30–35.
Introduction of chest leads.

2864 WILSON, FRANK NORMAN. 1890–1952, *et al.*
Electrocardiograms that represent the potential variations of a single electrode. *Amer. Heart J.*, 1934, **9,** 447–58.
Unipolar leads. With F. D. Johnson, A. G. MacLeod, and P. S. Barker.

2865 ABBOTT, MAUDE ELIZABETH SEYMOUR. 1869–1940
Atlas of congenital cardiac disease. New York, *Amer. Heart Assoc.*, 1936.
Reprinted 1954.

2865.1 SCHELLONG, FRITZ.
Elektrographische Diagnostik der Herzmuskelerkrankungen. *Verh. Dtsch. Ges. inn. Med.*, 1936, **48,** 288–310.
Introduction of the vectorcardiogram.

2866 ROESLER, HUGO. 1899–
Clinical roentgenology of the cardiovascular system. Springfield, *C. C. Thomas*, 1937.
Radiological measurements of the heart size.

2867 LEVY, ROBERT LOUIS. 1888– , *et al.*
Effects of induced oxygen want in patients with cardiac pain. *Amer. Heart J.*, 1938, **15,** 187–200.
Diagnosis of cardiac pain. With A. L. Barach and H. G. Bruenn.

2868 PRAECORDIAL LEADS.
Praecordial leads in electrocardiography. A joint memorandum of a committee of the Cardiac Society of Gt. Britain and Ireland, and the Committee of the American Heart Association. *Brit. med. J.*, 1938, **1,** 187 (only).
Also in *Amer. Heart J.*, 1938, **15**, 107–08, 235–39.

2869 ROBB, GEORGE PORTER. 1898– , & STEINBERG, ISRAEL. 1902–
A practical method of visualization of the chambers of the heart, the pulmonary circulation, and the great vessels in man. *J. clin. Invest.*, 1938, **17,** 507.
Introduction of angiocardiography. A fuller account by the same authors is in *Amer. J. Roentgenol.*, 1939, **41**, 1–17.

2870 STARR, Isaac. 1895– , *et al.*
Studies on the estimation of cardiac output in man, and of abnormalities in cardiac function, from the heart's recoil and the blood's impacts; the ballistocardiogram. *Amer. J. Physiol.*, 1939, **127,** 1–28.
Introduction of the ballistocardiogram. With A. J. Rawson, H. A. Schroeder, and N. R. Joseph.

2871 COURNAND, André Frédéric. 1895– , & RANGES, Hilmert Albert. 1906–
Catheterization of the right auricle in man. *Proc. Soc. exp. Biol. (N.Y.)*, 1941, **46,** 462–66.
First investigations with the cardiac catheter as a clinical method of investigation. For his work in this field Cournand in 1956 shared the Nobel Prize with Forssmann (No. 2858) and Richards (No. 2883.1).

2873 SCHROEDER, Henry Alfred. 1906–
Studies on congestive heart failure. I. The importance of restriction of salt as compared to water. *Amer. Heart J.*, 1941, **22,** 141–53.
Low-sodium diet in heart failure.

2874 STEWART, William Holmes. 1868– , *et al.*
Cineroentgenographic diagnosis of congenital and acquired heart disease. *Amer. J. Roentgenol.*, 1941, **46,** 636–40.
Angiocardiography. With C. W. Breimer and H. C. Maier.

2875 GOLDBERGER, Emanuel. 1913–
A simple indifferent electrocardiographic electrode of zero potential and a technique of obtaining augmented, unipolar, extremity leads. *Amer. Heart J.*, 1942, **23,** 483–92.
Augmented unipolar leads.

2876 HENNY, George Christian. 1899– , *et al.*
Electrokymograph for recording heart motion, improved type. *Amer. J. Roentgenol.*, 1947, **57,** 409–16.
With B. R. Boone and W. E. Chamberlain.

2877 McMICHAEL, *Sir* John. 1904–
Circulatory failure studied by means of venous catheterization. *Advanc. intern. Med.*, 1947, **2,** 64–101.

2878 TAUSSIG, Helen Brooke. 1898–
Congenital malformations of the heart. New York, *Commonwealth Fund*, 1947.

2879 BRODÉN, Bror Leonhard Johan. 1910– , *et al.*
Thoracic aortography. Preliminary report. *Acta radiol. (Stockh.)* 1948, **29,** 181–88.
With H. E. Hanson and J. Karnell.

2880 CHRISTIE, Ronald Victor. 1902–
Penicillin in subacute bacterial endocarditis. Report to the Medical Research Council on 269 patients treated in 14 centres appointed by the Penicillin Clinical Trials Committee. *Brit. med. J.*, 1948, **1,** 1–4.

2881 PRINZMETAL, Myron. 1908– , *et al.*
Mechanism of the auricular arrhythmias. *Circulation*, 1950, **1**, 241–45.
With E. Corday, I. C. Brill, A. L. Seller, R. W. Oblath, W. A. Flieg, and H. E. Kruger.

2882 WOOD, Paul Hamilton. 1907–1962
Congenital heart disease. *Brit. med. J.*, 1950, **2**, 639–45, 693–98.
A new classification proposed.

2883 ZOLL, Paul Maurice. 1911–
Resuscitation of the heart in ventricular standstill by external electric stimulation. *New Engl. J. Med.*, 1952, **247**, 768–71.
External cardiac pacemaker.

2883.1 RICHARDS, Dickinson Woodruff. 1895–
The contributions of right heart catheterization to physiology and medicine, with some observations on the physiopathology of pulmonary heart disease. *Amer. Heart J.*, 1957, **54**, 161–71.
See No. 2858.

Angina Pectoris

See also 3021–3047.3, Cardiovascular Surgery.

2884 HYDE, Edward, 1*st Earl of Clarendon.* 1609–1674
Life of Edward, 1st Earl of Clarendon, by himself. Oxford, 1759, **1**, 9.
From the description given by the Earl of Clarendon in his autobiography, his father, Henry Hyde, almost certainly suffered from, and died of, angina pectoris. If this is really so, it is the first recorded case. The description is reproduced in *Ann. med. Hist.*, 1922, **4**, 210.

2885 MORGAGNI, Giovanni Battista. 1682–1771
De sedibus, et causis morborum. Venetiis, *typ. Remondiniana*, 1761, **1**, 282.
An authentic case of angina pectoris is recorded by Morgagni; he observed it in 1707.

2886 ROUGNON DE MAGNY, Nicolas François. 1727–1799
Lettre de M. Rougnon à M. Lorry, touchant les causes de la mort de feu Monsieur Charles, ancien capitaine de cavalerie, arrivée à Besançon le 23 février 1768. Besançon, *J. F. Charmet*, 1768.
Osler, Allbutt and several other authorities believe this to be the description of an authentic case of angina, thus preceding Heberden's classical account. Other eminent authorities consider the patient to have suffered from pulmonary emphysema. This little book of 55 pages is extremely rare; the whereabouts of only 2 copies is known.

2887 HEBERDEN, William, *Snr.* 1710–1801
Some account of a disorder of the breast. *Med. Trans. Coll. Phys. Lond.*, 1772, **2**, 59–67.
This classical description of angina pectoris is the substance of a paper read on July 21, 1768. Although descriptions of angina are to be found in the works of earlier writers, these mention only dyspnoea in their cases. The merit of Herberden's account (in which, incidentally, he used the name "angina pectoris") lies in the fact that he was the first to include a description of the paroxysmal oppression in the thorax. His account is so perfect that it might well have been written to-day.

2888 PARRY, Caleb Hillier. 1755–1822
An inquiry into the symptoms and causes of the syncope anginosa, commonly called angina pectoris. Bath, *R. Cruttwell*; London, *Cadell & Davis*, 1799.

This was a paper read before the Gloucester Medical Society in 1788, but not published until 1799. Largely confirming the earlier work of Heberden on the condition, Parry stated his conclusion that disease of the coronary arteries is the responsible factor in angina pectoris (which he called "syncope anginosa"). He was the first to observe the slowing of the heart rate following pressure on the carotid artery.

2889 BURNS, Allan. 1781–1813
Observations on some of the most frequent and important diseases of the heart. Edinburgh, *Bryce & Co.*, 1809.

Burns was among the first to suggest (see p. 136) that angina pectoris is an expression of coronary obstruction.

2890 BRUNTON, *Sir* Thomas Lauder. 1844–1916
On the use of nitrite of amyl in angina pectoris. *Lancet*, 1867, **2**, 97–98.

Lauder Brunton was responsible for the introduction of amyl nitrite for the alleviation of angina. Reprinted in F. A. Willius & T. E. Keys: *Cardiac classics*, 1941, pp. 561–64.

2891 NOTHNAGEL, Carl Wilhelm Hermann. 1841–1905
Angina pectoris vasomotoria. *Dtsch. Arch. klin. Med.*, 1867, **3**, 309–322.

Nothnagel, himself a victim of angina, described the vasomotor form of the disease.

2892 MURRELL, William. 1853–1912
Nitro-glycerine as a remedy for angina pectoris. *Lancet*, 1879, **1**, 80–81, 113–15, 151–52, 225–27.

Murrell introduced trinitrin (nitroglycerin, glyceryl trinitrate) in the treatment of angina.

2893 ASKANAZY. S.
Klinisches über Diuretin. *Dtsch. Arch. klin. Med.*, 1895, **56**, 209–30.

In 1895 Askanazy proposed diuretin as a remedy for anginal pain.

2894 ALLBUTT, *Sir* Thomas Clifford. 1836–1925
Diseases of the arteries, including angina pectoris. 2 vols. London, *Macmillan & Co.*, 1915.

Includes his suggestion of the aortic genesis of angina pectoris, and (vol. 2, p. 368) his mechanical theory of cardiac pain in coronary occlusion.

2894.1 BOUSFIELD, Guy William John. 1893–
Angina pectoris: changes in electrocardiogram during paroxysm. *Lancet*, 1918, **2**, 457–58.

First electrocardiogram recorded (1917) from a patient with angina pectoris.

2895 JONNESCO, Thomas. 1860–1926
Angine de poitrine guérie par la résection du sympathique cervico-thoracique. *Bull. Acad. Méd.* (*Paris*), 1920, 3 sér., **84**, 93–102.

Cervical sympathectomy for the treatment of angina pectoris was first carried out by Jonnesco in 1916.

2896 LAEWEN, ARTHUR. 1876–1958
Paravertebrale Novokaininjektionen zur Differentialdiagnose intra-abdomineller Erkrankungen. *Zbl. Chir.*, 1922, **49,** 1510–12.
First paravertebral injection for treatment of angina pectoris.

2897 MACKENZIE, *Sir* JAMES. 1853–1925
Angina pectoris. London, *H. Frowde*, 1923.
A classical description of angina by "the beloved physician", one of the greatest of all cardiologists. Mackenzie considered the disease to be due to cardiac failure.

2898 BRUNN, FRITZ, & MANDL, FELIX. 1892–1957
Die paravertebrale Injektion zur Bekämpfung visceraler Schmerzen. *Wien. klin. Wschr.*, 1924, **37,** 511–14.
Paravertebral injection of alcohol first used as a method of treating angina pectoris.

2899 BLUMGART, HERRMAN LUDWIG. 1895– , *et al.*
Congestive heart failure and angina pectoris: the therapeutic effect of thyroidectomy on patients without clinical or pathologic evidence of thyroid toxicity. *Arch. intern. Med.*, 1933, **51,** 866–77.
Angina pectoris treated by thyroidectomy. With S. A. Levine and D. D. Berlin.

2900 RAAB, WILHELM. 1895–
Thiouracil treatment of angina pectoris; rationale and results. *J. Amer. med. Ass.*, 1945, **128,** 249–56.

2901–2993.1 ARTERIES

2901 LOBSTEIN, JEAN GEORGES CHRÉTIEN FRÉDÉRIC MARTIN. 1777–1835
Traité d'anatomie pathologique. Paris, *F. G. Levrault*, 1833.
Vol. 2, pp. 553–600 deals with diseases of the arteries. Lobstein wrote an important section on ossification of arteries, and was first to use the word "artério-sclérose" (on p. 550).

2902 BRODIE, *Sir* BENJAMIN COLLINS, *Bart.* 1783–1862
Lectures illustrative of various subjects in pathology and surgery. London, *Longman*, 1846.
Page 361 contains the first description of intermittent claudication in man. This was first reported (in the horse) by "Boullay" [? J. Bouley] in *Arch. gén. Méd.*, 1831, **27**, 425.

2903 VIRCHOW, RUDOLF LUDWIG KARL. 1821–1902
Ueber die acute Entzündung der Arterien. *Virchows Arch. path. Anat.*, 1847, **1,** 272–378.

2904 ROKITANSKY, CARL, *Freiherr von.* 1804–1878
Ueber einige der wichtigsten Krankheiten der Arterien. *Denkschr. k. Akad. Wiss. Wien*, 1852, **4,** 1–72.
One of Rokitansky's best works.

2905 CHARCOT, JEAN MARTIN. 1825–1893
Sur la claudication intermittente. *C. R. Soc. Biol.* (*Paris*), (1858), *Mémoires*, 1859, 2 sér., **5,** 225–38.
Charcot was among the first to report intermittent claudication in man.

2906 KUSSMAUL, Adolf. 1822–1902, & MAIER, Rudolf. 1824–1888
Ueber eine bisher noch nicht beschriebene eigenthümliche Arterienerkrankung (Periarteritis nodosa), die mit Morbus Brightii und rapid fortschreitender allgemeiner Muskellähmung einhergeht. *Dtsch. Arch. klin. Med.*, 1866, **1,** 484–518.

First description of periarteritis nodosa.

2907 FRIEDLÄNDER, Carl. 1847–1887
Ueber Arteriitis obliterans. *Zbl. med. Wiss.*, 1876, **14,** 65–70.

First description of thrombo-angiitis obliterans, which Friedländer called "arteriitis obliterans".

2908 HUCHARD, Henri. 1844–1910
L'artério-sclérose subaiguë dans ses rapports avec les spasmes vasculaires et son traitement par la trinitrine (nitroglycérine). *Gaz. Hôp (Paris)*, 1887, **60,** 1034–35.

"Huchard's disease" – continued hypertension causing arteriosclerosis. Huchard did much to develop the knowledge concerning arteriosclerosis and summarized his work in a classical monograph published in 1909.

2909 CARREL, Alexis. 1873–1944
La technique opératoire des anastomoses vasculaires et la transplantation des viscères. *Lyon méd.*, 1902, **98,** 859–64.

Carrel perfected the operation of arterial suture, end-to-end anastomosis of severed vessels with triple-threaded sutures. See also No. 3026.

2910 JOSUÉ, Otto. 1869–1923
Athérôme aortique expérimental par injections répétées d'adrénaline dans les veines. *C. R. Soc. Biol. (Paris)*, 1903, **55,** 1374–76.

Experimental production of arteriosclerosis.

2911 MÖNCKEBERG, Johann Georg. 1877–1925
Ueber die reine Mediaverkalkung der Extremitätenarterien und ihr Verhalten zur Arteriosklerose. *Virchows Arch. path. Anat.*, 1903, **171,** 141–67.

"Mönckeberg's sclerosis." He described a form of medial sclerosis of the blood-vessels of the extremities. See also his later papers in *Klin. Wschr.*, 1924, **52,** 1473–78, 1521–26.

2912 BUERGER, Leo. 1879–1943
Thrombo-angiitis obliterans; a study of the vascular lesions leading to presenile spontaneous gangrene. *Amer. J. med. Sci.*, 1908, **136,** 567–580.

Buerger's important paper on thrombo-angiitis obliterans gives the first comprehensive report of the clinical and pathological aspects of the disease. Buerger gave the condition its present name; it is also known as "Buerger's disease".

2913 KLOTZ, Oskar. 1878–1936
Arteriosclerosis; diseases of the media and their relation to aneurysm. Lancaster, Pa., 1911.

2914 ARRILAGA, Francisco C.
Cardiacos negros. Buenos Aires, *Thesis No.* 2536, 1912.

A classical description of "Ayerza's disease" (cor pulmonale), to which Arrilaga gave the name. Corvisart mentioned the condition in 1806. See No. 2917.

2915 ANITSCHKOW, Nikolaus. 1885– , & CHALATOW, S. S. 1884–
Ueber experimentelle Cholesterinsteatose und ihre Bedeutung für die Entstehung einiger pathologischer Prozesse. *Zbl. allg. Path. path. Anat.*, 1913, **24,** 1–9.

Experimental production of arteriosclerosis with cholesterol-rich diet.

2916 LJUNGDAHL, Malte Johan Julius. 1882–
Untersuchungen über die Arteriosklerose des kleinen Kreislaufs. Wiesbaden, *J. F. Bergmann,* 1915.

2917 AYERZA, Luis.
Consideraciones sobre la denominación de "Enfermedad de Ayerza." *Semana méd.*, 1925, **32,** pt. 2, 386–88.

In 1901 Abel Ayerza lectured on the syndrome of chronic cyanosis, dyspnoea, erythraemia, and sclerosis of the pulmonary artery, "Ayerza's disease" (cor pulmonale). He did not publish this work, but an important discussion on the nomenclature has been given by Luis Ayerza in the above paper and in a previous paper in the same journal, 1925, **32**, pt. 1, 43.

2918 KLOTZ, Oskar. 1878–1936
Concerning the pathology of some arterial diseases. *Ann. clin. Med.*, 1925–26, **4,** 814–28.

Klotz, eminent Canadian pathologist, is particularly remembered for his contributions to the subject of arteriosclerosis. (See also No. 2913.)

2919 SCHMIDT, Max. 1898–
Intracranial aneurysms. *Brain*, 1930, **53,** 498–540.

Temporal arteritis is first described in Case 24 (p. 532). Schmidt's paper also appeared in *Bibl. Laeger*, 1930, **122**, 269 (Case 24, p. 320). Temporal arteritis was also described as a new condition by B. T. Horton, T. B. Magath, and G. E. Brown, *Proc. Mayo Clin.*, 1932, **7**, 700–01.

2920 SANTOS, Reynaldo dos. 1880– , & CALDAS, J.
Les dérivés du thorium dans l'artériographie des membres. *Medicina contemp.* (*Lisboa*), 1931, **49,** 234–36.

Thorotrast first used in arteriography.

2921 WEISS, Soma. 1898–1942, & BAKER, James Porter. 1913–
The carotid sinus in health and disease: its rôle in the causation of fainting and convulsions. *Medicine*, 1933, **12,** 297–354.

The carotid sinus syndrome.

2922 WAGENER, Henry Patrick. 1890– , & KEITH, Norman Macdonnell. 1885–
Diffuse arteriolar disease with hypertension and the associated retinal lesions. *Medicine*, 1939, **18,** 317–430.

The Keith–Wagener classification of fundal lesions.

2923 LAUBRY, Charles. 1872–1941, *et al.*
Grosse pulmonaire. Petite aorte. Affection congénitale. *Bull. Soc. méd. Hôp. Paris*, 1940, **56,** 847–50.

Idiopathic dilatation of the pulmonary artery reported. With D. Routier and R. Heim de Balsac.

2924 RICH, Arnold Rice. 1893–
The rôle of hypersensitivity in periarteritis nodosa; as indicated by seven cases developing during serum sickness and sulfonamide therapy. *Bull. Johns Hopk. Hosp.*, 1942, **71**, 123–35.
Rich considered hypersensitivity to be an important factor in the aetiology of periarteritis nodosa.

Ligations of Arteries

2925 HOME, *Sir* Everard. 1756–1832
An account of Mr. Hunter's method of performing the operation for the popliteal aneurism. *Lond. med. J.*, 1786, **7**, 391–406.
First description of John Hunter's method of treating popliteal aneurysm. This consisted in a single ligature of the artery at a distance high in the healthy tissues. Recorded by his brother-in-law. See also *Trans. Soc. Improve. med. Knowl.*, 1793, **1**, 138. Reprinted in *Med Classics*, 1940, **4**, 449–57.

2926 BELL, John. 1763–1820
The principles of surgery. Edinburgh, 1801, **1**, 421–26.
First ligation of the gluteal artery.

2927 DESAULT, Pierre Joseph. 1744–1795
Remarques et observations sur l'opération de l'anévrisme. In his *Oeuvres chirurgicales*, Paris, 1801, **2**, 553–80.
Desault developed the technique of tying blood-vessels for the treatment of aneurysm.

2928 ABERNETHY, John. 1764–1831
Surgical observations. London, *Longmans*, 1809, pp. 234–92.
First ligation of the external iliac artery for aneurysm. Abernethy performed the operation in 1796.

2929 COOPER, *Sir* Astley Paston, *Bart.* 1768–1841
A case of aneurism of the carotid artery. *Med.-chir. Trans.*, 1809, **1**, 1–12, 222–33.
Cooper ligated the common carotid artery on Nov. 1, 1805; the patient died, but a second case (June 22, 1808) proved successful. (See also No. 2955.)

2930 DORSEY, John Syng. 1783–1818
Inguinal aneurism cured by tying the external iliac artery in the pelvis. *Eclectic Repert.*, 1811, **2**, 111–15.
First successful ligation of the external iliac artery in America (Aug. 19, 1811).

2931 TRAVERS, Benjamin. 1783–1858
A case of aneurism by anastomosis in the orbit, cured by the ligature of the common carotid artery. *Med.-chir. Trans.*, 1811, **2**, 1–16.

2932 GOODLAD, William.
Case of inguinal aneurism cured by tying the external iliac artery. *Edinb. med. surg. J.*, 1812, **8**, 32–39.
Goodlad successfully ligated the external iliac on July 29, 1811.

2933 ONDERDONK, Henry U.
A case in surgery. *Amer. med. phil. Reg.*, 1814, **4**, 176–81.
Successful ligation of the femoral artery, Jan. 17, 1813.

2934 POST, WRIGHT. 1766–1828

Successful ligation of the femoral artery; 1796. *Amer. med. phil. Reg.*, 1814, **4**, 452.

Wright Post, professor of surgery and anatomy at Columbia College, New York, was the first in America to ligate the femoral artery successfully (for popliteal aneurysm), according to John Hunter's method.

2935 STEVENS, WILLIAM. 1786–1868

A case of aneurism of the glutaeal artery, cured by tying the internal iliac. *Med.-chir. Trans.*, 1814, **5**, 422–34.

First successful ligation of the internal iliac, Dec. 27, 1812. The patient died in 1822 and an account of the autopsy is given by Richard Owen in *Med.-chir. Trans.*, 1830, **16**, 219–35.

2936 COLLES, ABRAHAM. 1773–1843

On the operation of tying the subclavian artery. *Edinb. med. surg. J.*, 1815, **11**, 1–25.

Colles tied the subclavian artery in 1811 and again in 1813. Garrison reminds us that Colles is accredited with the first successful ligation of the innominate artery in Europe, but is unable to verify this. The paper is reprinted in *Med. Classics*, 1940, **4**, 1043–72.

2937 GUTHRIE, GEORGE JAMES. 1785–1856

Case of a wound of the peroneal artery successfully treated by a ligature. *Med.-chir. Trans.*, 1816, **7**, 330–37.

On July 2, 1815, Guthrie successfully ligated the peroneal artery of a German soldier wounded at the Battle of Waterloo.

2938 SODEN, JOHN SMITH. 1780–1863

Case of inguinal aneurism cured by tying the external iliac artery. *Med.-chir. Trans.*, 1816, **7**, 536–40.

2939 POST, WRIGHT. 1766–1828

Case of brachial aneurism, cured by tying the subclavian artery above the clavicle. *Tr. phys.-med. soc. N.Y.*, 1817, **1**, 387–94.

Post was the first successfully to ligate the subclavian artery outside the scaleni (Sept. 8, 1817).

2940 SCARPA, ANTONIO. 1747–1832

Memoria sulla legature delle principali arterie degli arti. Pavia, *P. Bizzoni*, 1817.

2941 COOPER, *Sir* ASTLEY PASTON, *Bart.* 1768–1841, & TRAVERS, BENJAMIN. 1783–1858

Surgical essays. London, *Cox & Son*, 1818, **1**, 101–30.

In 1817 Cooper ligated the abdominal aorta. The patient died next day, but examination showed that his aorta was so diseased that he could never have recovered, while the ligation was so well performed that with a less degree of aortic disease the man would probably have survived.

2942 MOTT, VALENTINE. 1785–1865

Reflections on securing in a ligature the arteria innominata, to which is added a case in which the artery was tied by a surgical operation. *Med. surg. Register*, 1818, **1**, 9–54.

First ligation of the innominate artery, May 11, 1818. The artery was tied off half an inch below its bifurcation and the patient suffered no respiratory or circulatory embarrassment. The ligature separated from the artery on the 14th day, but on the 20th day the patient was able to walk downstairs. A fatal haemorrhage occurred from the wound, however, and the patient died on the 26th day.

2943 DUPUYTREN, GUILLAUME, *le baron.* 1777–1835
Account of the tying of the subclavian artery. *Edinb. med. surg. J.*, 1819, **15,** 476.
Dupuytren successfully ligated the subclavian artery on March 7, 1819.

2944 GIBSON, WILLIAM. 1788–1868
Case of a wound of the common iliac artery. *Amer. med. Recorder*, 1820, **3,** 185–93.
Gibson was the first to ligate the common iliac, July 27, 1812.

2945 COGSWELL, MASON FITCH. 1761–1830
Account of an operation for the extirpation of a tumor in which a ligature was applied to the carotid artery. *New Engl. J. Med. Surg.*, 1824, **13,** 357–60.
Cogswell ligated the primitive carotid on Nov. 4, 1803.

2946 MACGILL, WILLIAM D. 1802–1833
Account of a case in which both carotids were successfully tied. *N.Y. med. phys. J.*, 1825, **4,** 576.
In 1823 Macgill successfully ligated in continuity both primitive carotid arteries in the same subject within a month. He was the first American to do so.

2947 DUPUYTREN, GUILLAUME, *le baron.* 1777–1835
Observation sur un cas de ligature de l'artère iliaque externe. *Repert. gén. Anat. Physiol. path.*, 1826, **2,** 230–50.
Successful ligation of the external iliac, Oct. 16, 1815.

2948 KEY, CHARLES ASTON. 1793–1849
Case of axillary aneurism successfully treated by tying the subclavian artery. *Med.-chir. Trans.*, 1827, **13,** 1–11.
In 1823 Key successfully ligated the subclavian artery for aneurysm at the axilla.

2949 WARDROP, JAMES. 1782–1869
Case of carotid aneurism, successfully treated by tying the artery above the aneurismal tumor. *Med.-chir. Trans.*, 1827, **13,** 217–26.
Wardrop successfully treated aneurysm of the carotid artery by distal ligation, a procedure suggested by Pierre Brasdor.

2950 MOTT, VALENTINE. 1785–1865
Ligature of the arteria iliaca communis, at its origin. *Philad. J. med. phys. Sci.*, 1827, **14,** 176.
Successful ligation of the common iliac.

2951 ——. Aneurism of the arteria innominata involving the subclavian and the root of the carotid; successfully treated by tying the carotid artery. *Amer. J. med. Sci.*, 1829, **5,** 297–300.
Second report, 1830, **6,** 532.

2952 ——. Case of diffused femoral aneurism, for which the external iliac artery was tied. *Amer. J. med. Sci.*, 1831, **8,** 393–97.

2953 ——. Case of aneurism of the right subclavian artery, in which that vessel was tied within the scaleni muscles. *Amer. J. med. Sci.*, 1833, **12** 354–59.
In his day Mott was the ablest exponent of vascular surgery in the U.S.A.

2954 COOPER, *Sir* ASTLEY PASTON, *Bart.* 1768–1841
Case of a femoral aneurism, for which the external iliac artery was tied, with an account of the preparation of the limb, dissected at the expiration of eighteen years. *Guy's Hosp. Rep.*, 1836, **1,** 43–52.
The artery was tied in 1808, and the patient died in 1826.

2955 ——. Account of the first successful operation, performed on the carotid artery, for aneurism, in the year 1808; with the post-mortem examination, in 1821. *Guy's Hosp. Rep.*, 1836, **1,** 53–58.
See No. 2929.

2956 ——. Some experiments and observations on tying the carotid and vertebral arteries, and the pneumo-gastric, phrenic, and sympathetic nerves. *Guy's Hosp. Rep.*, 1836, **1,** 457–75, 654.

2957 KEY, CHARLES ASTON. 1793–1849
Femoral aneurism successfully treated by a ligature of the external iliac artery. *Guy's Hosp. Rep.*, 1836, **1,** 68–70.
Successful ligation of external iliac artery for femoral aneurysm, 1822.

2958 MOTT, VALENTINE. 1785–1865
A case of aneurism of either the ischiatic or gluteal artery, in which the right internal iliac artery was successfully tied. *Amer. J. med. Sci.*, 1837, **20,** 13–15.

2959 TWITCHELL, AMOS. 1781–1850
Gun-shot wound of the face and neck; ligature of the carotid artery. *New Engl. quart. J. med. Surg.*, 1842–43, **1,** 188–93.
First successful ligature of the carotid artery (for secondary haemorrhage) Oct. 18, 1807, eight months before Sir Astley Cooper (No. 2929).

2960 BUCK, GURDON. 1807–1877
Case of aneurism of the femoral artery for which ligatures were successively applied to the femoral, profunda, external and common iliac. *N.Y. J. Med.*, 1858, 3 ser., **5,** 305–11.

2961 SYME, JAMES. 1799–1870
Case of iliac aneurism. *Med.-chir. Trans.*, 1862, **45,** 381–87.
Syme treated a case of iliac aneurysm by opening the sac and ligating the common iliac and the internal and external iliac arteries.

2962 PARKER, WILLARD. 1800–1884
Ligature of the left subclavian inside the scalenus muscle, together with common carotid and vertebral arteries for subclavian aneurism; hemorrhage from the distal end of the subclavian; death on 42nd day. *Amer. Med. Times*, 1864, **8,** 114–16.

2963 SMYTH, ANDREW WOODS. 1832–1916
Successful operation for subclavian aneurism. *Amer. J. med. Sci.*, 1866, **52,** 280–82.
First successful ligation of the innominate artery, 1864. A report on the condition of the patient in 1869 is given in *New Orleans J. Med.*, 1869, 22, 464–69.

2964 LISTER, JOSEPH, *1st Baron Lister*. 1827–1912
Observations on ligature of arteries on the antiseptic system. *Lancet*, 1869, **1,** 451–55.

Lister evolved a carbolized catgut ligature, better than any previously produced. He was able to cut short the ends of his ligature, closing the wound tightly and eliminating the necessity for bringing the ends of ligatures out through the wound.

2965 BALLANCE, *Sir* CHARLES ALFRED. 1865–1936, & EDMUNDS, WALTER. 1850–1930
A treatise on the ligation of the great arteries in continuity. London, *Macmillan & Co.*, 1891.

Includes Ballance's scale of measurement of calibre of arteries.

2966 HALSTED, WILLIAM STEWART. 1852–1922
Ligation of the first portion of the left subclavian artery and excision of a subclavio-axillary aneurism. *Johns Hopk. Hosp. Bull.*, 1892, **3,** 932–94.

First successful ligation of the left subclavian artery.

2967 MURPHY, JOHN BENJAMIN. 1857–1916
Resection of arteries and veins injured in continuity—end to end suture—experimental and clinical research. *Med. Rec.* (*N.Y.*), 1897, **51,** 73–88.

Successful suture of femoral artery, 1896.

2968 KEHR, HANS.
Der erste Fall von erfolgreicher Unterbindung der Art. hepatica propria gegen Aneurysma. *Münch. med. Wschr.*, 1903, **50,** 1861–67.

Successful ligation of the hepatic artery.

2969 HALSTED, WILLIAM STEWART. 1852–1922
Partial, progressive and complete occlusion of the aorta and other large arteries in the dog by means of the metal band. *J. exp. Med.*, 1909, **11,** 373–91.

Halsted introduced a metal band in place of a ligature for the occlusion of arteries.

2970 VAUGHAN, GEORGE TULLY. 1859–1948
Ligation (partial occlusion) of the abdominal aorta for aneurism. *Ann. Surg.*, 1921, **74,** 308–12.

First successful ligation of the abdominal aorta.

Aneurysms

See also 2726–2883.1, HEART AND AORTA; 2925–2970, LIGATIONS OF ARTERIES.

2971 SAPORTA, ANTOINE. ?–1573
De tumoribus praeter naturam libri V. Lugduni, *P. Ravaud*, 1624.

Saporta, in 1554, gave the earliest description of an aortic aneurysm. The manuscript of his book was discovered many years after his death, and was published by a Lyons doctor, named Gras.

2972 VESALIUS, ANDREAS. 1514–1564
In: WELSCH, G. H. *Sylloge curationum et observationum medicinalium centurias iv complectens*. Augustae Vindelicorum, *G. Goebelii*, 1667, pt. 4, p. 46.

In 1555 Vesalius was the first to diagnose aneurysm of the thoracic and abdominal aorta in a living person. This was confirmed at autopsy two years later.

2973 LANCISI, Giovanni Maria. 1654–1720
De motu cordis et aneurysmatibus. Romae, *J. M. Salvioni*, 1728.

Lancisi noted the frequency of cardiac aneurysm and showed the importance of syphilis, asthma, palpitation, violent emotions and excess as causes of aneurysm. He was the first to describe cardiac syphilis. Revision of 1745 edition of *De aneurysmatibus*, with translation and notes, by W. C. Wright, 1952.

2974 HUNTER, William. 1718–1783
The history of an aneurysm of the aorta, with some remarks on aneurysms in general. *Med. Obs. Inqu.*, 1757, **1**, 323–57.

First recorded case of arteriovenous aneurysm.

2975 SCARPA, Antonio. 1747–1832
Sull' aneurisma. Pavia, *tipog. Bolzani*, 1804.

Scarpa distinguished true from false aneurysms. English translation, Edinburgh, 1808.

2976 DUPUYTREN, Guillaume, *le baron*. 1777–1835
[Anévrisme à l'artère poplitée guéri par la compression.] *Bull. Fac. Méd. Paris*, 1818, **6**, 242.

Dupuytren was the first successfully to treat aneurysm by compression.

2977 VELPEAU, Alfred Armand Louis Marie. 1795–1867
Mémoire sur la piqûre ou l'acupuncture des artères dans le traitement des anévrismes. *Gaz. méd. Paris*, 1831, **2**, 1–4.

First attempt at operative treatment of aneurysm.

2978 BELLINGHAM, O'Bryen. 1805–1857
Observations on aneurism, and its treatment by compression. London, *J. Churchill*, 1847.

Bellingham introduced the "Dublin method" of treating aneurysm by slow compression.

2979 DONDERS, Frans Cornelis. 1818–1889, & JANSEN, Jan Hissink. 1816–1885
Untersuchungen über die Natur der krankhaften Veränderungen der Arterienwände, die als Ursachen der spontanen Aneurysmen zu betrachten sind. *Arch. physiol. Heilk.*, 1848, **7**, 359–402, 530–60.

2980 MOORE, Charles Hewitt. 1821–1870, & MURCHISON, Charles. 1830–1879
On a new method of procuring the consolidation of fibrin in certain incurable aneurisms. *Med.-chir. Trans.*, 1864, **47**, 129–49.

Moore and Murchison introduced the method of treating aneurysm by passing wire into the aneurysmal sac.

2981 RASMUSSEN, Fritz Valdemar. 1833–1877
Om Haemoptyse navnlig den lethale, i anatomisk og klinisk Henseende. *Hospitalstidende*, 1868, **11**, 33–36, 37–40, 41–43, 45–46, 49–52; 1869, **12**, 41–42, 45–48.

Tuberculous aneurysm of the lung ("Rasmussen's aneurysm"). English translation in *Edinb. med. J.*, 1868, **14**, 385–401, 486–503; 1869, **15**, 97–104, 228–36.

2982 QUINCKE, Heinrich Irenaeus. 1842–1922
Ein Fall von Aneurysma der Leberarterie. *Berl. klin. Wschr.*, 1871, **8**, 349–52, 386.

Quincke observed aneurysm of the hepatic artery in 1870.

2983 WELCH, Francis Henry. 1839–1910
On aortic aneurism in the army, and the conditions associated with it. *Med.-chir. Trans.*, 1876, **59,** 59–77.
Welch, an Army surgeon, supported the theory of a causal connexion between syphilis and aneurysm.

2984 EPPINGER, Hans. 1846–1916
Pathogenese (Histogenese und Aetiologie) der Aneurysmen einschliesslich des Aneurysma equi verminosum. *Arch. klin. Chir.*, 1887, **35,** Suppl.-Heft, 1–563.

2985 MATAS, Rudolph. 1860–1957
Traumatic aneurism of the left brachial artery. Failure of direct and indirect pressure; ligation of the artery immediately above tumor; return of pulsation on the tenth day; ligation immediately below tumor; failure to arrest pulsation; incision and partial excision of sac; recovery. *Med. News* (*Phila*), 1888, **53,** 462–66.
First aneurysmorrhaphy, April 6, 1888. See also *Trans. Amer. surg. Ass.*, 1902, **20**, 396–434.

2985.1 DÖHLE, Karl Gottfried Paul. 1855–1928
Ueber Aortenerkrankung bei Syphilitischen und deren Beziehung zur Aneurysmenbildung. *Dtsch. Arch. klin. Med.*, 1895, **55,** 190–210.
Döhle clearly defined a specific syphilitic lesion of the aorta as a prerequisite of aortic aneurysm.

2986 CHURTON, Thomas. 1839–1926
Multiple aneurysms of the pulmonary artery. *Brit. med. J.*, 1897, **1,** 1223.
Churton was the first to recognize this condition at necropsy.

2987 HELLER, Arnold. 1840–1913
Die Aortensyphilis als Ursache von Aneurysmen. *Münch. med. Wschr.*, 1899, **46,** 1669–71.
Heller established the fact that syphilis is a cause of aortic aneurysm.

2988 BABCOCK, William Wayne. 1872–1963
A new treatment for thoracic aneurysm. *Ann. clin. Med.*, 1926, **4,** 933–42.
Babcock's operation for thoracic aneurysm. See also *Amer. J. Surg.*, 1932, **16,** 401–07.

2989 ——. Operative decompression of aortic aneurysm by carotid-jugular anastomosis. *Surg. Clin. N. Amer.*, 1929, **9,** 1031–41.
Babcock's operation for aortic aneurysm.

2990 SAUERBRUCH, Ernst Ferdinand. 1875–1951
Erfolgreiche operative Beseitigung eines Aneurysma der rechten Herzkammer. *Arch. klin. Chir.*, 1931, **167,** 586–88.
First successful surgical intervention in cardiac aneurysm.

2991 SMITH, Harry LeRoy. 1887– , & HORTON, Bayard Taylor. 1895–
Arteriovenous fistula of the lung associated with polycythemia vera: report of a case in which the diagnosis was made clinically. *Amer. Heart J.*, 1939, **18,** 589–92.
Pulmonary arteriovenous aneurysm; first description of the clinical syndrome.

2992 HEPBURN, JOHN. 1888– , & DAUPHINEE, JAMES ARNOLD. 1903–
Successful removal of hemangioma of the lung followed by the disappearance of polycythemia. *Amer. J. med. Sci.*, 1942, **204,** 681–85.
First successful excision of arteriovenous aneurysm of lung.

2993 POPPE, JOHN KARL. 1911–
Cellophane treatment of syphilitic aneurysms with report of results in six cases. *Amer. Heart J.*, 1948, **36,** 252–56.

2993.1 DUBOST, CHARLES. 1914– , *et al.*
A propos du traitement des anévrysmes de l'aorte. Ablation de l'anévrysme. Rétablissement de la continuité par greffe d'aorte humaine conservée. *Mem. Acad. Chir.* (*Paris*), 1951, **77,** 381–83.
Resection of abdominal aortic aneurysm and closure with homologous graft. With M. Allary and N. Oeconomos.

2994–3005 VEINS

2994 BRODIE, *Sir* BENJAMIN COLLINS, *Bart.* 1783–1862
Observations on the treatment of varicose veins of the legs. *Med.-chir. Trans.*, 1816, **7,** 195–210.
Brodie first operated for varicose veins in 1814.

2995 ——. Lectures illustrative of various subjects in pathology and surgery. London, *Longman*, 1846.
P. 186: Brodie's test for insufficiency of the valves in varicose veins, later associated with the name of Trendelenburg.

2996 PAGET, *Sir* JAMES, *Bart.* 1814–1899
On gouty and some other forms of phlebitis. *St. Barth. Hosp. Rep.*, 1866, **2,** 82–92.
Paget-Schroetter syndrome, venous obstruction in the upper extremity.

2997 TRENDELENBURG, FRIEDRICH. 1844–1924
Ueber die Unterbindung der Vena saphena magna bei Unterschenkelvaricen. *Beitr. klin. Chir.*, 1890, **7,** 195–210.
"Trendelenburg's operation" – ligation of the great saphenous vein for the treatment of varicose veins in the leg. Reprinted, with translation, in *Med. Classics*, 1940, **4,** 989–1023. The paper also describes his test for insufficiency of the valves, a procedure previously described by Brodie (No. 2995).

2998 MOORE, W.
The operative treatment of varicose veins, with especial reference to a modification of Trendelenburg's operation. *Intercolon. med. J. Aust.*, 1896, **1,** 393–407.
Moore's operation of high resection of the saphenous vein for treatment of varicosities.

2999 SCHIASSI, BENEDETTO.
La cure des varices du membre inférieur par l'injection intraveineuse d'une solution d'iode. *Sem. méd.* (*Paris*), 1908, **28,** 601–02.
Schiassi combined operative and sclerosant methods in the treatment of varicose veins. Translation in *Med. Press*, 1909, **87,** 377.

3000 LINSER, Paul. 1871–
Ueber die konservative Behandlung der Varicen. *Med. Klin.*, 1916, **12,** 897–98.
Injection treatment of varicose veins was introduced by Linser.

3001 GÉNÉVRIER, J.
Du traitement des varices par les injections coagulantes, concentrées de sels de quinine. *Soc. méd. mil. franç., Bull.*, 1921, **15,** 169–71.
Injection of quinine urethane for the treatment of varicose veins.

3002 SICARD, Jean Athanase. 1872–1929, *et al.*
Traitement des varices par les injections phlébo-sclérosantes du salicylate de soude. *Gaz. Hôp. Paris*, 1922, **95,** 1573–75.
Introduction of sodium salicylate injections for the treatment of varicose veins. With J. Paraf and J. Lermoyez.

3003 LINSER, Karl.
Die Behandlung der Krampfadern mit intravarikösen Kochsalz-injektionen. *Derm. Wschr.*, 1925, **81,** 1345–51.
Sodium chloride first used in the injection treatment of varicose veins.

3004 NOBL, Gabor. 1864–1938
Die Calorose als Verödungsmittel varikös entarteter Venen. *Wien. klin. Wschr.*, 1926, **39,** 1217–19.
Nobl used dextrose in the injection treatment of varicose veins.

3004.1 BIRLEY, James Leatham. 1884–1934
Traumatic aneurysm of the intracranial portion of the internal carotid artery. With a note by Wilfred Trotter. *Brain*, 1928, **51,** 184–208.
In 1924 Wilfred Trotter (1872–1939) performed the first planned operation for intracranial aneurysm diagnosed pre-operatively.

3005 COOPER, William Morris. 1894–
Treatment of varicose veins. *Ann. Surg.*, 1934, **99,** 799–805.
Cooper combined ligation with subsequent injection of 5 per cent. sodium morrhuate in the treatment of varicose veins.

For history, see No. 3161

3006–3020 THROMBOSIS; EMBOLISM

3006 VIRCHOW, Rudolf Ludwig Karl. 1821–1902
Thrombose und Embolie. Gefässentzündung und septische Infektion. In his *Gesammelte Abhandlungen zur wissenschaftlichen Medicin*, Frankfurt a.M., *Meidinger, Sohn u. Co.*, 1856, pp. 219–732.
Reprints of papers published between 1846 and 1853. Virchow gave the first clear description of thrombosis and embolism (see especially *Beitr. exp. Path.*, 1846, 2, 227–380).

3007 ZENKER, Friedrich Albert. 1825–1898
Beiträge zur normalen und pathologischen Anatomie der Lungen. Dresden, *G. Schönfeld's Buchhandlung*, 1862.
First description of pulmonary fat embolism in man.

3008 PANUM, Peter Ludvig. 1820–1885
Experimentelle Untersuchungen zur Physiologie und Pathologie der Embolie; Transfusion und Blutmenge. Berlin, *G. Reimer*, 1864.

3009 FELTZ, Victor Timothée. 1835–1893
Traité clinique et expérimental des embolies capillaires. Paris, *J. B. Baillière*, 1870.

3010 COHNHEIM, Julius Friedrich. 1839–1884
Untersuchungen über die embolischen Processe. Berlin, *A. Hirschwald*, 1872.

Cohnheim developed the doctrine of infarction as a result of occlusion of terminal arteries. He explained the haemorrhagic nature of certain infarcts on the basis of a reflux flow and diapedesis through the altered capillaries of the infarcted area.

3011 WELCH, William Henry. 1850–1934
Thrombosis and embolism. In Allbutt, C.: *System of medicine*, London, 1899, **4**, 284–310; and in 2nd ed., 1909, **6**, 691–821.

3012 TRENDELENBURG, Friedrich. 1844–1924
Ueber die operative Behandlung der Embolie der Lungenarterie. *Arch. klin. Chir.*, 1908, **86**, 686–700.

Pulmonary embolectomy first attempted, "Trendelenburg's operation" – first successfully performed by Kirschner (see No. 3016).

3013 MOSNY, Ernest. 1861–1918, & DUMONT, J.
Embolie fémorale au cours d'un rétrécissement mitral pur. Arteriotomie. Guérison. *Bull. Acad. Méd.* (*Paris*), 1911, 3 sér., **66**, 358–61.

First successful embolectomy; operation carried out by G. Labey, November 16, 1911.

3014 KEY, Einer Samuel Henrik. 1872–1954
Ein Fall operierter Embolie der Arteria femoralis. *Wien. klin. Wschr.*, 1913, **26**, 936–39.

Key performed his first successful embolectomy on December 4, 1912, and reported it to a meeting of the Svenska Läkaresällskapet on January 28, 1913. See also his review in *Ergebn. Chir. Orthop.*, 1929, **22**, 1–94.

3014.1 BAUER, Fritz.
Fall von Embolus aortae abdominalis, Operation, Heilung. *Zbl. Chir.*, 1913, **40**, 1945–46.

First successful aortic embolectomy.

3015 WARTHIN, Aldred Scott. 1866–1931
Traumatic lipaemia and fatty embolism. *Int. Clin.*, 1913, 23 ser., **4**, 171–227.

Classical clinical description of pulmonary fat embolism.

3016 KIRSCHNER, Martin. 1879–1942
Ein durch die Trendelenburgsche Operation geheilter Fall von Embolie der Art. pulmonalis. *Arch. klin. Chir.*, 1924, **133**, 312–59.

First successful surgical treatment of pulmonary embolism, a procedure suggested by Trendelenburg in 1908 (see No. 3012).

3017 JEFFERSON, *Sir* Geoffrey. 1886–
Report of a successful case of embolectomy. *Brit. med. J.*, 1925, **2**, 985–87.

First successful embolectomy in Britain.

3018 DUCUING, Jean. 1889–
Phlébites, thromboses et embolies post-opératoires. Paris, *Masson*, 1929.

3019 MURRAY, Donald Walter Gordon. 1896– , *et al.*
Heparin and the thrombosis of veins following injury. *Surgery*, 1937, **2,** 163–87.

Clinical use of heparin as anticoagulant. With L. B. Jaques, T. S. Perrett, and C. H. Best.

3020 WRIGHT, Irving Sherwood. 1901– , *et al.*
Report of the Committee for the Evaluation of Anticoagulants in the Treatment of Coronary Thrombosis with Myocardial Infarction. *Amer. Heart J.*, 1948, **36,** 801–15.

With C. D. Marple and D. F. Beck.

3021–3047.3 CARDIOVASCULAR SURGERY

See also 2925–2970, Ligations of Arteries; 2971–2993.1, Aneurysms; 3006–3020, Thrombosis and Embolism.

3021 ROMERO, Francisco.
Sur l'hydrothorax et l'hydropéricarde. *Bull. Fac. Méd. Paris*, 1814–1815, **4,** 373–76.

First successful pericardiocentesis. The above reference is not to his first writing on the subject, which cannot be traced. See also *Dict. Sci. med.*, 1819, **40,** 370.

3022 HILSMANN, Friedrich Alexander. 1849–
Ueber die Paracentese des Perikardiums. *Schriften Univ. Kiel*, (1875), 1876, Diss. Nr. 2, pp. 20.

Account of first pericardiocentesis for suppurative pericarditis.

3023 REHN, Ludwig. 1849–1930
Fall von penetrirender Stichverletzung des rechten Ventrikel's. Herznaht. *Zbl. Chir.*, 1896, **23,** 1048–49.

Rehn was the first successfully to suture a wound of the human heart.

3024 JABOULAY, Mathieu. 1860–1913
Chirurgie du grand sympathique et du corps thyroïde. Paris, *O. Doin*, 1900.

Jaboulay was the first to perform the operation of sympathectomy for the relief of vascular disease.

3025 BRAUER, Ludolph. 1865–1951
Ueber chronisch adhäsive Mediastino-Perikarditis und deren Behandlung. *Münch. med. Wschr.*, 1902, **49,** 1072, 1732.

Brauer was first to suggest the operation of cardiolysis, a procedure carried out by Petersen.

3025.1 MUNRO, John Cummings. 1858–1910
Ligation of the ductus arteriosus. *Ann. Surg.*, 1907, **46,** 335–38.

Munro was first to suggest the feasibility of ligation of a patent ductus arteriosus.

3026 CARREL, Alexis. 1873–1944
The surgery of blood vessels, etc. *Johns Hopk. Hosp. Bull.*, 1907, **18,** 18–28.

Carrel's remarkable technique of end-to-end anastomosis of blood vessels; *see also* No. 2909.

3027 CARREL. ALEXIS. 1873–1944.
Results of the transplantation of blood vessels, organs and limbs. *J. Amer. med. Ass.*, 1908, **51,** 1662–67.

Carrel showed that arteries kept for days or weeks outside the body can be transplanted successfully.

3028 ——. Latent life of arteries. *J. exp. Med.*, 1910, **12,** 460–86.

Carrel's experiments showed that it was possible to preserve portions of blood-vessels in cold storage for long periods before using them in transplantation. For an appreciation of Carrel, see Garrison's *History,* p. 733.

3028.1 DOYEN, EUGÉNE LOUIS. 1859–1916
Chirurgie des malformations congénitales ou acquises du coeur. *Congr. franç. Chir., Proc.-verb.*, 1913, **26,** 1062–65; *Presse méd.*, 1913, **21,** 860.

First attempt at surgical relief of valvular disease of the heart (congenital pulmonary stenosis).

3029 TUFFIER, THÉODORE. 1857–1929
Etude expérimentelle sur la chirurgie des valvules du coeur. *Bull. Acad Méd.* (*Paris*), 1914, 3 sér., **71,** 293–95.

Tuffier carried out the first successful experimental operation for the relief of chronic valvular disease.

3030 HALLOPEAU, PAUL. 1876–1924
Un cas de cardiolyse. *Bull. Mém. Soc. Chir. Paris*, 1921, **47,** 1120–21.

First pericardiectomy, for constrictive pericarditis.

3030.1 CUTLER, ELLIOTT CARR. 1888–1947, & LEVINE, SAMUEL ALBERT. 1891–
Cardiotomy and valvulotomy for mitral stenosis. Experimental observations and clinical notes concerning an operated case with recovery. *Boston med. surg. J.*, 1923, **188,** 1023–27.

Successful section of mitral valve for relief of mitral stenosis.

3031 VOLHARD, FRANZ. 1872–1950, & SCHMIEDEN, VIKTOR. 1874–1945
Ueber Erkennung und Behandlung der Umklammerung des Herzens durch schwielige Perikarditis. *Klin. Wschr.*, 1923, **2,** 5–9.

First complete pericardiectomy for constrictive pericarditis.

3032 SOUTTAR, *Sir* HENRY SESSIONS. 1875–1964
The surgical treatment of mitral stenosis. *Brit. med. J.*, 1925, **2,** 603–06.

Report of successful case.

3033 BLUMGART, HERRMAN LUDWIG. 1895– , *et al.*
Congestive heart failure and angina pectoris: the therapeutic effect of thyroidectomy on patients without clinical or pathologic evidence of thyroid toxicity. *Arch. intern. Med.*, 1933, **51,** 866–77.

Thyroidectomy for the treatment of congestive heart failure and angina pectoris. With S. A. Levine and D. D. Berlin.

3034 BECK, CLAUDE SCHAEFFER. 1894–1971
The development of a new blood supply to the heart by operation. *Ann. Surg.*, 1935, **102,** 801–13.

By implantation of the pectoral muscle into the pericardium Beck provided a collateral circulation to the heart.

3035 ——, & TICHY, Vladimir Leslie. 1899–
The production of a collateral circulation to the heart. I. An experimental study. *Amer. Heart J.*, 1935, **10,** 849–73.
First cardio-omentopexy.

3036 PEET, Max Minor. 1885–1949
The surgical treatment of hypertension. *Proc. Calif. Acad. Med.*, 1935–36, **5,** 58–90.
Peet operation for hypertension. Preliminary communication in *Univ. Hosp. Bull.* (*Ann Arbor*), 1935, **1**, 17–18.

3037 O'SHAUGHNESSY, Laurence. 1900–1940
An experimental method of providing a collateral circulation to the heart. *Brit. J. Surg.*, 1936, **23,** 665–70.
By attaching a pedicled omental graft to the surface of the heart (cardio-omentopexy), thus providing a collateral circulation to that organ, O'Shaughnessy made an important advance in the treatment of angina and cardiac ischaemia generally.

3038 LERICHE, René. 1879–1955, *et al.*
Arteriectomy. *Surg. Gynec. Obstet.*, 1937, **64,** 149–55.
Arteriectomy in arterial thrombosis. With R. Fontaine and S. M. Dupertuis.

3038.1 GIBBON, John Heysham. 1903–
An oxygenator with a large surface-volume ratio. *J. Lab. clin. Med.*, 1939, **24,** 1192–98.
First heart-lung machine used successfully on an animal.

3039 GROSS, Robert Edward. 1905– , & HUBBARD, John Perry. 1903–
Surgical ligation of a patent ductus arteriosus: report of first successful case. *J. Amer. Med. Ass.*, 1939, **112,** 729–31.
See also later paper in *Ann. Surg.*, 1939, **110**, 321–56.

3040 LERICHE, René. 1879–1955
De la résection du carrefour aortico-iliaque avec double sympathectomie lombaire pour thrombose artéritique de l'aorte; le syndrome de l'oblitération termino-aortique par artérite. *Presse méd.*, 1940, **48,** 601–04.
Obliteration of the abdominal aorta.

3041 SMITHWICK, Reginald Hammerick. 1899–
A technique for splanchnic resection for hypertension; preliminary report. *Surgery*, 1940, **7,** 1–8.
Smithwick operation for hypertension.

3042 KING, Edgar Samuel John.
Surgery of the heart. London, *E. Arnold & Co.*, (1941).
Includes valuable information regarding the history of the subject.

3043 BLALOCK, Alfred. 1899–1964, & TAUSSIG, Helen Brooke. 1898–
The surgical treatment of malformations of the heart in which there is pulmonary stenosis or pulmonary atresia. *J. Amer. med. Ass.*, 1945, **128,** 189–202.
The "Blalock–Taussig operation" for the relief of congenital defects of the pulmonary artery.

3044 CRAFOORD, Clarence. 1899– , & NYLIN, Karl Gustav Vilhelm. 1892–
Congenital coarctation of the aorta and its surgical treatment. *J. thorac. Surg.*, 1945, **14,** 347–61.

3045 POTTS, Willis John. 1895– , *et al.*
Anastomosis of the aorta to a pulmonary artery. Certain types in congenital heart disease. *J. Amer. med. Ass.*, 1946, **132,** 627–31.
With S. Smith and S. Gibson.

3046 BROCK, Russell Claude, *Baron Brock of Wimbledon.* 1903–
Pulmonary valvulotomy for the relief of congenital pulmonary stenosis. Report of three cases. *Brit. med. J.*, 1948, **1,** 1121–26.

3046.1 HARKEN, Dwight Emary. 1910– , *et al.*
The surgical treatment of mitral stenosis. 1. Valvuloplasty. *New Engl. J. Med.*, 1948, **239,** 801–09.
Valvuloplasty for mitral stenosis. With L. B. Ellis, P. F. Ware, and L. R. Norman.

3047 BLAND, Edward Franklin. 1901– , & SWEET, Richard Harwood. 1901–
A venous shunt for marked mitral stenosis. *Amer. Practit.*, 1948, **2,** 756–61.
First pulmonary-azygos shunt operation for relief of mitral stenosis. Two further patients were operated upon later the same year; all three are reported in *J. Amer. med. Ass.*, 1949, **140**, 1259. A similar procedure was successfully employed independently by F. d'Allaines and his colleagues in 1949 (*Mém. Acad. Chir., Paris*, 1949, **75**, 318–19).

3047.1 GROSS, Robert Edward. 1905–
Surgical treatment for coarctation of the aorta. Experiences from 60 cases. *J. Amer. med. Ass.*, 1949, **139,** 285–92.
Resection of coarctation of aorta and closure of defect with homologous graft.

3047.2 GIBBON, John Heysham. 1903–
Application of a mechanical heart and lung apparatus to cardiac surgery. *Minn. Med.*, 1954, **37,** 171–80, 185.
First pump oxygenator used on humans.

3047.3 LILLEHEI, Clarence Walton. 1918–
Controlled cross circulation for direct-vision intracardiac surgery; correction of ventricular septal defects, atrioventricularis communis, and tetralogy of Fallot. *Postgrad. Med.*, 1955, **17,** 388–96.
Controlled cross circulation for intracardiac surgery.

3048–3155 DISORDERS OF THE BLOOD

3048 ALBUCASIS [Abul-Qasim]. 936–1013
Liber theoricae. Augustae Vindelicorum, *imp. S. Grimm & M. Vuirsung*, 1519.
The *Altasrif* of Albucasis was a great treatise on medicine and surgery. The medical part, above, contains what is probably the earliest description of haemophilia (fol. 145).

3049 AMATUS *Lusitanus* [Rodriguez de Castello Branco (João)]. 1511–1568
Curationum medicinalium centuriae quatuor. Basileae, [*H. Frobenius*], 1556.
Contains (Cent. iii, curat. 70, p. 286) first recorded case of purpura as a separate entity, not associated with fever. An English translation of this section is included in R.H. Major, *Classic descriptions of disease,* 3rd ed., 1945, p. 514.

3050 PANAROLI, Domenico. ?–1657
Iatrologismorum seu medicinalium observationum pentecostae quinque utilibus praeceptis. Romae, *F. Moneta,* 1652.
Panaroli described haemolytic jaundice of the newborn.

3051 BEHRENS, Rudolph August. ?–1747
Epistolica dissertatio altera pro spicilegio observationum de morbo maculoso haemorrhagico et noxiis nonnulis mytulis perscripta. Brunsvigae, 1735.
Behrens gave the name "morbus maculosus haemorrhagicus" to the disease purpura haemorrhagica. His paper is reprinted in Werlhof's *Opera medica,* Hannover, 1775, **2**, 615–36.

3052 WERLHOF, Paul Gottlieb. 1699–1767
Disquisitio medica et philologica de variolis et anthracibus. Hannoverae, *sumt. haered. Nicolai Foersteri,* 1735.
Werlhof gave a classical description of purpura haemorrhagica ("Werlhof's disease").

3053 WILLAN, Robert. 1757–1812
On cutaneous diseases. Vol. 1, p. 457. London, *J. Johnson,* [1796]–1808.
Abdominal purpura (Henoch) first described.

3054 OTTO, John Conrad. 1774–1844
An account of an haemorrhagic disposition existing in certain families. *Med. Reposit.,* 1803, **6,** 1–4.
Otto recognized and adequately described haemophilia, noting that females are not affected but may transmit the disease. His paper is one of the first great contributions to medicine in North America. Reproduced in R. H. Major, *Classic descriptions of disease,* 3rd ed., 1945, p. 522.

3055 BURNS, Allan. 1781–1813
Observations on the surgical anatomy of the head and neck. Edinburgh, *Bryce,* 1811.
First recorded case of chloroma is to be found on p. 369 of this book.

3056 NASSE, Christian Friedrich. 1778–1851
Von einer erblichen Neigung zu tödtlichen Blutungen. *Arch. med. Erfahr.,* 1820, **1,** 385–434.
In his description of haemophilia Nasse stressed the immunity of females, despite their ability to transmit the disease. This fact has become known as "Nasse's law".

3057 BOUILLAUD, Jean Baptiste. 1796–1881
Observations sur l'état des veines dans les infiltrations des membres. *J. Physiol. exp. path.,* 1823, **3,** 89–93.
Description of venous obstruction and dropsy.

3058 SCHÖNLEIN, JOHANN LUCAS. 1793–1864
Peliosis rheumatica. In his *Allgemeine und specielle Pathologie und Therapie*, 1837, **2,** 48–49.
"Schönlein's disease" (purpura) first described.

3059 ADDISON, WILLIAM. 1802–1881
Experimental and practical researches on inflammation and on the origin and nature of tubercles of the lungs. London, *J. Churchill*, 1843.
Addison made important observations on the blood corpuscles. He is by some considered "the world's first haematologist". He gave the first description of leucocytosis, so named by Virchow in 1858, and he anticipated Cohnheim's conception of inflammation. He was first to observe diapedesis. *See Lancet*, 1907, **1**, 182–83.

3060 ANDRAL, GABRIEL. 1797–1876
Essai d'hématologie pathologique. Paris, *Fortin, Masson & Cie.*, 1843.
Andral invented the terms "anaemia" and "hyperaemia". He analysed the blood fibrin and albumin. He recognized several forms of anaemia, including that due to lead poisoning. English translation, 1844.

3061 BENNETT, JOHN HUGHES. 1812–1875
Case of hypertrophy of the spleen and liver, in which death took place from suppuration of the blood. *Edinb. med. surg. J.*, 1845, **64,** 413–23.
First definite description of leukaemia; a case under the care of Sir R. Christison but reported by Bennett. On p. 400 of the same journal is a report of a case by D. Craigie, referring to a patient seen in 1841 but not recognized as leukaemia until Craigie heard of Bennett's case in the same hospital. Bennett published a monograph on leucocythaemia in 1852, in which he included the first illustrations of the microscopic appearance of the blood in leukaemia.

3062 VIRCHOW, RUDOLF LUDWIG KARL. 1821–1902
Weisses Blut. *N. Notiz. Geb. Natur- u. Heilk.*, 1845, **36,** 151–56.
Only six weeks after Bennett, Virchow independently published a report on the necropsy of a case of leukaemia. He gave the condition its present name. For translation, see R. H. Major, *Classic descriptions of disease*, 3rd ed., 1945, p. 510.

3062.1 FULLER, HENRY WILLIAM. 1820–1873
Particulars of a case in which enormous enlargement of the spleen and liver, together with dilatation of all the blood vessels of the body, were found coincident with a peculiarly altered condition of the blood. *Lancet*, 1846, **2,** 43–44.
Leukaemia diagnosed during life as the result of a blood examination.

3063 GRANDIDIER, JOHANN LUDWIG. 1810–?
Die Haemophilie oder die Bluterkrankheit. Leipzig, *O. Wigand*, 1855.
First full clinical description of haemophilia.

3064 VIRCHOW, RUDOLF LUDWIG KARL. 1821–1902
Ueber farblose Blutkörperchen und Leukämie. In his *Gesammelte Abhandlungen zur wissenschaftlichen Medicin*, Frankfort a.M., *Meidinger*, 1856, pp. 147–218.
Includes his paper on "weisses Blut" (see No. 3062) and three later papers on leukaemia.

3064.1 FRIEDREICH, NIKOLAUS. 1825–1882
Ein neuer Fall von Leukämie. *Virchows Arch. path. Anat.*, 1857, **12,** 37–58.
Acute leukaemia first described.

3064.2 BABINGTON, Benjamin Guy. 1794–1866
Hereditary epistaxis. *Lancet*, 1865, **2**, 362–63.

3065 HENOCH, Eduard Heinrich. 1820–1910
Über den Zusammenhang von Purpura und Intestinalstörungen. *Berl. klin. Wschr.*, 1868, **5**, 517–19.

"Henoch's purpura." Henoch described a form of purpura with abdominal symptoms first mentioned by Willan. *See also* the same journal, 1874, **11**, 622, 641–43.

3066 NEUMANN, Ernst. 1834–1918
Ein Fall von Leukämie mit Erkrankung des Knochenmarkes. *Arch. Heilk.* (*Lpz.*), 1870, **11**, 1–14.

Neumann was the first to note changes in the bone marrow in leukaemia, and he proposed the term "myelogenous leukaemia".

3067 ORTH, Johannes. 1847–1923
Ueber das Vorkommen von Bilirubinkrystallen bei neugebornen Kindern. *Virchows Arch. path. Anat.*, 1875, **63**, 447–62.

Kernicterus first described.

3068 HENOCH, Eduard Heinrich. 1820–1910
Ueber Purpura fulminans. *Berl. klin. Wschr.*, 1887, **24**, 8–10.

First description.

3069 WILSON, Claude. 1860–1937
Some cases showing hereditary enlargement of the spleen. *Trans. clin. Soc. Lond.*, 1890, **23**, 162–72.

A classical clinical account of congenital haemolytic jaundice in six relatives in four generations.

3069.1 EHRLICH, Paul. 1854–1915
Farbenanalytische Untersuchungen zur Histologie und Klinik. Berlin, *A. Hirschwald*, 1891.

By means of his methods of staining blood cells Ehrlich differentiated two types of leukaemia, lymphatic and myelogenous.

3070 VAQUEZ, Louis Henri. 1860–1936
Sur une forme spéciale de cyanose s'accompagnant d'hyperglobulie excessive et persistante. *C. R. Soc. Biol.* (*Paris*), 1892, **44**, 384–88.

Vaquez first described polycythaemia vera (erythraemia). Osler's paper on the subject (No. 3073) made it generally known in the English-speaking world, and the condition has since been named "Vaquez–Osler disease". For translation, see R. H. Major, *Classic descriptions of disease*, 3rd ed., 1945, p. 497.

3071 HAYEM, Georges. 1841–1933
Leçons sur les maladies du sang. Paris, *Masson & Cie.*, 1900.

3072 BROWN, Philip King. 1869–1940, & OPHÜLS, William. 1871–1933
A fatal case of acute primary infectious pharyngitis. *Trans. Med. Soc. Calif.*, 1901, 93–101.

First recorded case of extreme leucopenia.

3073 OSLER, *Sir* William, *Bart.* 1849–1919
Chronic cyanosis, with polycythaemia and enlarged spleen: a new clinical entity. *Amer. J. med. Sci.*, 1903, **126**, 187–201.

When describing polycythaemia with cyanosis, Osler thought it a new entity, but later acknowledged the priority of Vaquez's description (No. 3070). Reprinted in *Med. Classics*, 1939, **4**, 254–75.

3074 WOLFF, ALFRED.
Ueber eine Methode zur Untersuchung des lebenden Knochenmarks von Thieren und über das Bewegungsvermögen der Myelocyten. *Dtsch. med. Wschr.*, 1903, **29,** 165–67.

Wolff trephined the tibia and femur of experimental animals and suggested biopsy of bone marrow as a clinical procedure.

3075 ARNETH, JOSEPH. 1873–1955
Die neutrophilen weissen Blutkörperchen bei Infektions-Krankheiten. Jena, *G. Fischer*, 1904.

"Arneth count." Arneth distinguished 5 groups of polymorphonuclear leucocytes and advocated the estimation of these groups as a valuable aid in the determination of bone-marrow reaction to infective and other agents (plate 8, p. 37).

3076 GEISBÖCK [GAISBOCK], FELIX
Die Bedeutung der Blutdruckmessung für die Praxis. *Dtsch. Arch. klin. Med.*, 1905, **83,** 363–409.

Includes (p. 396) description of "Geisböck's disease" – polycythemia hypertonica.

3077 STERNBERG, CARL. 1872–1935
Pathologie der Primärerkrankungen des lymphatischen und hämatopoetischen Apparates. Wiesbaden, *J. F. Bergmann*, 1905.

Includes (p. 151) Sternberg's description of lymphogranulomatosis, which has been given the eponym "Sternberg's disease".

3078 NÄGELI, OTTO. 1871–1938
Blutkrankheiten und Blutdiagnostik. Leipzig, *Veit & Co.*, 1907–08.

3079 TÜRK, WILHELM. 1871–1916
Septische Erkrankungen bei Verkümmerung des Granulozytensystems *Wien. klin. Wschr.*, 1907, **20,** 157–62.

First reported case of complete agranulocytosis.

3079.1 ELLERMANN, VILHELM. 1871–1924, & BANG, O.
Experimentelle Leukämie bei Hühnern. *Zbl. Bakt.*, 1908, Abt. I, Orig., **46,** 595–609.

Cell-free transmission of fowl leukaemia.

3080 GHEDINI, GIOVANNI. 1877–
Per la patogenesi e per la diagnosi delle malattie del sangue e degli organi emopoietici. Puntura esplorativa del midollo osseo. *Clin. med. ital.*, 1908, **47,** 724–36.

Introduction of bone marrow biopsy by puncturing the shaft of the tibia.

3081 BULLOCH, WILLIAM. 1868–1941, & FILDES, *Sir* PAUL. 1882–1971
Haemophilia. London, *Dulau & Co.*, 1911.

Bulloch and Fildes, in their detailed account of haemophilia, claimed to have established the fact of immunity in females, and denied the authenticity of published cases of female haemophilia. They confirmed the law of Nasse. This work, one of the most important on the subject, was issued as Memoir XII of the Eugenics Laboratory, University of London, and forms parts V–VI of the *Treasury of Human Inheritance* series.

3082 PAPPENHEIM, ARTUR. 1870–1916
Grundriss der hämatologischen Diagnostik. Leipzig, *W. Klinkhardt*, 1911.

One of the leaders in modern haematology, Papperheim improved the methods of staining blood cells.

3082.1 RESCHAD, Hassan, & SCHILLING-TORGAU, V.
Ueber eine neue Leukämie durch echte Uebergangsformen (Splenozytenleukämie) und ihre Bedeutung für die Selbständigkeit dieser Zellen. *Münch. med. Wschr.*, 1913, **60,** 1981–84.
Monocytic leukaemia reported.

3083 FRANK, Alfred Erich. 1884–1957
Die essentielle Thrombopenie (konstitutionelle Purpura – Pseudo-Hämophilie). *Berl. klin. Wschr.*, 1915, **52,** 454–58, 490–94.
Frank's essential thrombopenia.

3084 EPPINGER, Hans. 1880–1946, & KLOSS, Karl.
Zur Therapie der Polyzythämie. *Therap. Mh.*, 1918, **32,** 322–26.
Phenylhydrazine hydrochloride first used in the treatment of polycythaemia.

3085 WESTERGREN, Alf Vilhelm. 1891–
Studies of the suspension stability of the blood in pulmonary tuberculosis. *Acta med. scand.*, 1921, **54,** 247–82.
Westergren's method of measuring the erythrocyte sedimentation rate.

3086 SCHULTZ, Werner. 1878–1947
Gangräneszierende Prozesse und Defekt des Granulocytensystems. *Dtsch. med. Wschr.*, 1922, **48,** 1495–96.
"Schultz's syndrome" – first description of agranulocytic angina. Schultz reported 4 cases of necrotic ulcerative infection of the throat with complete or almost complete disappearance of polymorphonuclears. To describe the blood change he introduced the term "agranulocytosis".

3087 SEYFARTH, Carly Paul. 1890–
Die Sternumtrepanation, ein einfache Methode zur diagnostischen Entnahme von Knochenmark bei Lebenden. *Dtsch. med. Wschr.*, 1923, **49,** 180–81.
Bone marrow biopsy by sternal puncture.

3088 ARINKIN, Mikhail. 1876–1948
[Methodology of examining bone marrow in live patients, with haemopoietic disease.] *Vestn. Khir.*, 1927, No. 30, 57–60.
Needle puncture for bone marrow biopsy. German account in *Folia haemat. (Lpz.)*, 1929, **38,** 233–40.

3089 PELGER, Karel. 1885–1931
Demonstratie van een paar zeldzaam voorkomende typen van bloedlichaampjes en bespreking der patiënten. *Ned. T. Geneesk.*, 1928, **72,** 1178.
See No. 3092.

3090 WEISS, Soma. 1898–1942, *et al.*
The velocity of blood flow in health and disease as measured by the effect of histamine on the minute vessels. *Amer. Heart J.*, 1929, **4,** 664–91.
Measurement of circulation time. With G. P. Robb and H. L. Blumgart.

3091 WINTERNITZ, M., *et al.*
Eine klinisch brauchbare Bestimmungsmethode der Blutumlaufszeit mittels Decholininjektion. *Med. Klin.*, 1931, **27,** 986–88.
The decholin method for estimation of circulation time. With J. Deutsch and Z. Brull.

3092 HUËT, G. J.
Over een familiaire anomalie der leucocyten. *Ned. T. Geneesk.*, 1931, **75,** 5956–59.
Pelger-Huët anomaly of the nuclei of the leucocytes; see also No. 3089. German translation in *Klin. Wschr.*, 1932, **11**, 1264–66.

3093 MACFARLANE, ROBERT GWYN. 1907– , & BARNETT, BURGESS.
The haemostatic possibilities of snake-venom. *Lancet*, 1934, **2,** 985–987.
Snake venom used in the treatment of haemophilia.

3094 SALAH, M.
Sternal puncture; preliminary note. *J. Egypt. med. Ass.*, 1934, **17,** 846–50.
Needle for sternal puncture.

3095 QUICK, ARMAND JAMES. 1894–
The prothrombin in hemophilia and in obstructive jaundice. *J. biol. Chem.*, 1935, **109,** lxxiii–lxxix.
Quick's method for determination of prothrombin clotting time. See also *Amer. J. med. Sci.*, 1935, **190**, 501–11.

3096 WINTROBE, MAXWELL MYER. 1901– , & LANDSBERG, J. WALTER. 1907–
A standardized technique for the blood sedimentation test. *Amer. J. med. Sci.*, 1935, **189,** 102–15.
Wintrobe's method for the determination of the erythrocyte sedimentation rate.

3096.1 PATEK, ARTHUR JACKSON. 1904– , & TAYLOR, FRANCIS HENRY LASKEY. 1900–1959
Hemophilia. II. Some properties of a substance obtained from normal human plasma effective in accelerating the coagulation of hemophilic blood. *J. clin. Invest.*, 1937, **16,** 113–24.
Antihaemophilic globulin (factor VIII).

3097 BUTT, HUGH ROLAND. 1910– , & SNELL, ALBERT MARKLEY. 1896–1960
The use of vitamin K and bile in treatment of the hemorrhagic diathesis in cases of jaundice. *Proc. Mayo Clin.*, 1938, **13,** 74–80.
Vitamin K used in the treatment of haemorrhagic disease.

3098 LAWRENCE, JOHN HUNDALE. 1904– , *et al.*
Studies on leukemia with the aid of radioactive phosphorus. *New int. Clin.*, 1939, n.s., **2,** vol. 3, 33–58.
Therapeutic use of radioactive isotopes. With K. G. Scott and L. W. Tuttle.

3099 ——. Nuclear physics and therapy: preliminary report on a new method for the treatment of leukemia and polycythemia. *Radiology*, 1940, **35,** 51–60.
Radio-phosphorus in treatment of leukaemia.

3100 LEVINE, PHILIP. 1900– , *et al.*
The rôle of iso-immunization in the pathogenesis of erythroblastosis fetalis. *Amer. J. Obstet. Gynec.*, 1941, **42,** 925–37.
Erythroblastosis foetalis due to rhesus incompatibility between mother and child. With L. Burnham, E. M. Katzin, and P. Vogel.

3102 STAHMANN, MARK ARNOLD. 1914– , *et al.*
Studies on the hemorrhagic sweet clover disease. V. Identification and synthesis of the hemorrhagic agent. *J. biol. Chem.*, 1941, **138,** 513–27.

Isolation of dicoumarol (3:3-methylene-bis-4-hydroxycoumarin). With C. F. Huebner and K. P. Link.

3103 COMLY, HUNTER HALL. 1919–
Cyanosis in infants caused by nitrates in well water. *J. Amer. med. Ass.*, 1945, **129,** 112–16.

Methaemoglobinaemia. Comly first suggested the above hypothesis, since proved valid.

3104 COOMBS, ROBIN ROYSTON AMOS, *et al.*
Detection of weak and "incomplete" Rh agglutinins: a new test. *Lancet*, 1945, **2,** 15–16.

Coombs's test. With A. E. Mourant and R. R. Race. A fuller description appears in *Brit. J. exp. Path.*, 1945, **26**, 255–66.

3105 WIENER, ALEXANDER SOLOMON. 1907–
Conglutination test for Rh sensitization. *J. Lab. clin. Med.*, 1945, **30,** 662–67.

Conglutination test.

3106 PATERSON, EDITH, *et al.*
Leukaemia treated with urethane compared with deep *x*-ray therapy. *Lancet*, 1946, **1,** 677.

Urethane in treatment of leukaemia. With A. Haddow, I. Ap Thomas, and J. M. Watkinson.

3107 SOULIER, JEAN PIERRE. 1913– , & GUEGUEN, JEAN.
Action hypoprothrombinémiante (anti-K) de la phényl-indanedione étudiée expérimentalement chez le lapin. Son application chez l'homme. *C. R. Soc. Biol. (Paris)*, 1947, **141,** 1007–11.

Introduction of phenylindanedione.

3108 REINIŠ, Z., & KUBÍK, MIRKO.
Klinische Erfahrungen mit einem neuen Präparat der Cumarinreihe. *Schweiz. med. Wschr.*, 1948, **78,** 785–90.

Introduction of ethyl biscoumacetate ("tromexan").

Anaemia and Chlorosis

3109 LANGE, JOHANN. 1485–1565
Medicinalium epistolarum miscellanea. Basileae, *J. Oporinus*, 1554.

Epistle xxi, pp. 74–77, contains the first definite description of chlorosis, "De morbo virgineo".

3110 HOFFMANN, FRIEDRICH. 1660–1742
De genuina chlorosis indole, origine et curatione. Halis, 1731.

Classical description of chlorosis. Lange accurately diagnosed this condition, but it was left to Hoffmann to separate it as a definite clinical entity.

3111 LETTSOM, JOHN COAKLEY. 1744–1815
Hints respecting the chlorosis of boarding schools. London, *C. Dilly*, 1795.

3112 COMBE, James Scarth. 1796–1883
History of a case of anaemia. *Trans. med.-chir. Soc. Edinb.*, 1824, **1**, 194–204.

First description of pernicious anaemia. Paper read May 1, 1822.

3113 BLAUD, Pierre. 1774–1858
Sur les maladies chlorotiques et sur un mode de traitement spécifique dans ces affections. *Rev. méd. franç. étrang.*, 1832, **45**, 337–67.

For the treatment of chlorosis Blaud prescribed a pill (Blaud's pill), composed of sulphate of iron and carbonate of potassium. Preliminary report in *Bull. gén. Thérap.*, 1832, **2**, 154–55.

3114 FOEDISCH. Ferdinand.
Die krankhafte Mischung des Blutes, vorzüglich bei Chlorose, Hysterie und Pneumonie, durch chemische Versuche ausgemittelt, und der Uebergang des in den Darmcanal eingebrachten Eisens. *Allg. med. Ztg*, 1832, No. 97, col. 1537.

Foedisch showed chlorotic blood to be deficient in iron. See also *Gaz. méd. Paris*, 1837, 2 sér. **5**, 7.

3115 NASSE, Hermann. 1807–1892
Das Blut in mehrfacher Beziehung physiologisch und pathologisch untersucht. Bonn, *T. Habicht*, 1836.

Nasse gave the first clear description of anaemia in pregnancy; he also noticed erythrocyte sedimentation in certain pathological conditions.

3116 CHANNING, Walter. 1786–1876
Notes on anhaemia, principally in its connections with the puerperal state, and with functional disease of the uterus: with cases. *New Engl. quart. J. Med. Surg.*, 1842, **1**, 157–88.

First description of pernicious anaemia of pregnancy.

3117 BENNETT, H. N.
Puerperal anaemia; or a peculiar anaemic condition, occurring in gestating and lactating females. *N.Y. J. Med.*, 1847, **9**, 45–48, 197–98.

Bennett described the anaemia of pregnancy and defined it as resulting from the process of reproduction.

3118 ADDISON, Thomas. 1793–1860
Anaemia: disease of the supra-renal capsules. *Lond. med. Gaz.*, 1849, **43**, 517–18.

Addison included a classical description of pernicious (Addisonian) anaemia in his papers on the condition later known as "Addison's disease". Although preceded by Combe, his account was more important in bringing the disease to the notice of the medical profession. *See also* No. 3864.

3119 GRIESINGER, Wilhelm. 1817–1868
Ein Fall von Anaemia splenica bei einem Kinde. *Berl. klin. Wschr.*, 1866, **3**, 212–14.

First reported case of infantile splenic anaemia.

3120 DUNCAN, John. 1839–1899
The treatment of aneurism by electrolysis. Edinburgh, *Oliver & Boyd*, 1867.

Duncan called attention to the fact that the essential feature in chlorosis is a quantitative change in the haemoglobin content and not a great reduction in the number of corpuscles.

3121 VALSUANI, Emilio.
Cachessia puerperale raccolta nella clinica ginecologica dell'ospitale Maggiore di Milano. Milano, *G. Bernardoni*, 1870.
"Valsuani's disease" – progressive pernicious anaemia in pregnant and lactating women, probably first described by H. N. Bennett (No. 3117).

3122 GUSSEROW, Adolf Ludwig Sigismund. 1836–1906
Ueber hochgradigste Anämie Schwangerer. *Arch. Gynak.*, 1871, **2,** 218–35.
An important account of pernicious anaemia of pregnancy.

3123 VANLAIR, Constant. 1839–1914, & MASIUS, Jean Baptiste Nicolas Voltaire. 1836–1912
De la microcythémie. *Bull. Acad. roy. Méd. Belg.*, 1871, 3 sér., **5,** 515–613.
Includes an accurate description of congenital haemolytic jaundice.

3124 BIERMER, Anton. 1827–1892
Form von progressiver perniciöser Anämie. *KorrespBl. schweiz. Ärz.*, 1872, **2,** 15–18.
In his account of progressive pernicious anaemia Biermer was first to describe the retinal haemorrhages. He was at one time accredited with the first description of pernicious anaemia; later it was shown that Addison had described the condition in his classical work on the suprarenals (No. 3118) and that Combe (No. 3112) had reported a case of pernicious anaemia as far back as 1822. On the Continent the condition is referred to as "Biermer's disease". Preliminary communication in *Versammlung deutscher Naturforscher und Aertze*, 1868, Tageblatt No. 8, IX Sect., p. 173.

3125 PEPPER, William. 1843–1898
Progressive pernicious anaemia, or anaematosis. *Amer. J. med. Sci.*, 1875, **70,** 313–47.
Pepper described bone-marrow changes of pernicious anaemia, though his actual description more closely resembles leukaemia.

3125.1 COHNHEIM, Julius Friedrich. 1839–1884
Erkrankung des Knochenmarkes bei perniciöser Anämie. *Virchows Arch. path. Anat.*, 1876, **68,** 291–93.
Cohnheim gave a more convincing account than Pepper of the bone-marrow changes in pernicious anaemia.

3125.2 EICHHORST, Hermann Ludwig. 1849–1921
Die progressive perniziöse Anämie. Leipzig, *Veit und Comp.*, 1878.
First comprehensive account.

3125.3 EHRLICH, Paul. 1854–1915
Über Regeneration und Degeneration der rothen Blutscheiben bei Anämien. *Berl. klin. Wschr.*, 1880, **17,** 405.

3125.4 ——. Über einige Beobachtungen am anämischen Blut. *Berl. klin. Wschr.*, 1881, **18,** 43.
In the above contributions to the knowledge of anaemia, Ehrlich dealt in the first paper with the blood cells in anaemia, and in the second gave the first description of the reticulocyte.

3126 BANTI, Guido. 1852–1925
Dell' anemia splenica. Firenze, *succ. Le Monnier*, 1882.
"Banti's disease." Banti described the pathological changes in the spleen in splenic anaemia. A later paper in *Sperimentale*, 1894, **48**, sez. biol., 407–32, gives an account of hepatic cirrhosis as the sequel of the earlier stage of splenic anaemia; this sequel has been named "Banti's syndrome". A translation of this latter paper is in *Med. Classics*, 1937, **1**, 901–27.

3127 GAUCHER, Philippe Charles Ernest. 1854–1918
De l'epithélioma primitif de la rate; hypertrophie idiopathique de la rate sans leucémie. Paris, 1882.
"Gaucher's disease" – familial splenic anaemia.

3128 LEICHTENSTERN, Otto. 1845–1900
Ueber progressive perniciöse Anämie bei Tabeskranken. *Dtsch. med. Wschr.*, 1884, **10,** 849.
First description of subacute combined degeneration of the spinal cord, which Leichtenstern termed progressive pernicious anaemia in tabetics.

3129 EHRLICH, Paul. 1854–1915
Ueber einen Fall von Anämie mit Bemerkungen über regenerative Veränderungen des Knochenmarks. *Charité-Ann.*, 1888, **13,** 300–09.
Ehrlich was first to distinguish the aplastic type of anaemia.

3130 HAYEM, Georges. 1841–1933
Du sang et de ses altérations anatomiques. Paris, *G. Masson*, 1889.
Includes (pp. 614–751) an important account of chlorosis; Hayem, by his accurate observation, placed the disease on a firm basis.

3131 JAKSCH, Rudolf von, *Ritter von Wartenhorst*. 1855–1947
Ueber Leukaemia und Leukocytose im Kindesalter. *Wien. klin. Wschr.*, 1889, **2,** 435–37, 456–58.
From this classical description of infantile pseudoleukaemic anaemia, the condition became known as "von Jaksch's disease".

3131.1 RINDFLEISCH, Georg Eduard. 1836–1908
Ueber die Fehler der Blutkörperchenbildung bei der perniciösen Anämie. *Virchows Arch. path. Anat.*, 1890, **121,** 176–81.
Rindfleisch made the first clear statement of the bone marrow changes in pernicious anaemia.

3132 BUNGE, Gustav von. 1844–1920
Ueber die Eisentherapie. *Verh. Congr. inn. Med.*, 1895, **13,** 133–47.
Bunge was father to the concept of iron-deficiency anaemia.

3133 HERRICK, James Bryan. 1861–1954
Peculiar elongated and sickle-shaped red blood corpuscles in a case of severe anemia. *Arch. intern. Med.*, 1910, **6,** 517–21; *Trans. Ass. Amer. Phys.*, 1910, **25,** 553–61.
Identification of the sickle-cell type of anaemia.

3134 FABER, Knud Helge. 1862–1956
Anämische Zustände bei der chronischen Achylia gastrica. *Berl. klin. Wschr.*, 1913, **50,** 958–62.
Simple achlorhydric (idiopathic microcytic) anaemia described. Faber advanced the view that achylia gastrica was a cause both of pernicious anaemia and of simple chlorotic anaemia.

3135 SCHMIDT, HARRY BURKE. 1882–
A clinical study of puerperal anaemia. *Surg. Gynec. Obstet.*, 1918, **27,** 596–600.

Four cases of pernicious anaemia of pregnancy treated by blood transfusion.

3136 OSLER, *Sir* WILLIAM, *Bart.* 1849–1919
Observations on the severe anaemias of pregnancy and the post-partum state. *Brit. med. J.*, 1919, **1,** 1–3.

A classical paper, with classification.

3137 EDELMANN, ADOLF. 1885–1939
Ueber Anaemia infectiosa chronica und ihre Aetiologie. *Wien. klin. Wschr.*, 1925, **38,** 268–69.

"Edelmann's disease" – a type of chronic infectious anaemia.

3138 LEDERER, MAX. 1885–
A form of acute hemolytic anemia probably of infectious origin. *Amer. J. med. Sci.*, 1925, **170,** 500–10.

"Lederer's anaemia" first described.

3139 ROBSCHEIT-ROBBINS, FRIEDA SAUR. 1893– , & WHIPPLE, GEORGE HOYT. 1878–
Blood regeneration in severe anaemia. II. Favourable influence of liver, heart and skeletal muscle in diet. *Amer. J. Physiol.*, 1925, **72,** 408–18.

These workers showed the beneficial effect of raw beef liver upon blood regeneration in anaemia. Their work paved the way for the liver diet treatment of Minot and Murphy.

3140 MINOT, GEORGE RICHARDS. 1885–1950, & MURPHY, WILLIAM PARRY. 1892–
Treatment of pernicious anemia by a special diet. *J. Amer. med. Ass.*, 1926, **87,** 470–76.

Introduction of raw liver diet in the treatment of pernicious anaemia. This treatment ranks as one of the greatest modern advances in therapy. See also the later paper in the same journal, 1927, **89,** 759–66. Reprinted in *Blood,* 1948, **3,** 8–21. Minot and Murphy shared the Nobel Prize with Whipple (No. 3139) in 1934.

3141 COOLEY, THOMAS BENTON. 1871–1945, *et al.*
Anemia in children, with splenomegaly and peculiar changes in the bones. *Amer. J. Dis. Child.*, 1927, **34,** 347–63.

"Cooley's erythroblastic anaemia." With E. R. Witwer and O. P. Lee.

3142 FANCONI, GUIDO. 1892–
Familiäre infantile perniziosaartige Anämie (perniziöses Blutbild und Konstitution). *Jb. Kinderheilk.*, 1927, **117,** 257–80.

"Fanconi's syndrome", congenital hypoplasia of bone marrow with multiple congenital defects occurring as a familial disease.

3142.1 PEABODY, FRANCIS WELD. 1881–1927
The pathology of the bone marrow in pernicious anaemia. *Amer. J. Path.*, 1927, **3,** 179–202.

Peabody studied the bone marrow in pernicious anaemia. He suggested that failure of blood formation rather than haemolysis was the main defect in the disease, and that the benefit from liver feeding was due to a factor in liver that promoted development and differentiation of mature erythrocytes.

3143 CASTLE, William Bosworth. 1897–
Observations on the etiologic relationship of achylia gastrica to pernicious anemia. I. The effect of the administration to patients with pernicious anemia of the contents of the normal human stomach recovered after the ingestion of beef muscle. *Amer. J. med. Sci.*, 1929, **178,** 748–64.

Castle showed pernicious anaemia to be due to absence from the gastric juice of a substance (Castle's intrinsic factor, haemopoietin) that reacts with an extrinsic factor present in many foodstuffs to form the anti-pernicious anaemia factor, His experimental work resulted in the introduction of stomach preparations for the treatment of pernicious anaemia. See also the same journal, 1929, **178**, 764; 1930, **180**, 305. Preliminary communication on *J. clin. Invest.*, 1928, **6**, 2.

3144 STURGIS, Cyrus Cressey. 1891–1966, & ISAACS, Raphael, 1891–
Desiccated stomach in the treatment of pernicious anemia. *J. Amer. med. Assoc.*, 1929, **93,** 747–49.

Sturgis and Isaacs showed that stomach tissue contains a factor active in the treatment of pernicious anaemia.

3144.1 GÄNSSLEN, M.
Ein hochwirksamer, injizierbarer Leberextrakt. *Klin. Wschr.*, 1930, **9,** 2099–2102.

Gänsslen introduced an injectable liver extract in the treatment of pernicious anaemia.

3145 WINTROBE, Maxwell Myer. 1901–
Classification of the anemias on the basis of differences in the size and hemoglobin content of the red corpuscles. *Proc. Soc. exp. Biol. (N.Y.)* 1930, **27,** 1071–73.

Wintrobe's classification of the anaemias.

3145.1 CASTLE, William Bosworth. 1897– , & TAYLOR, Francis Henry Laskey. 1900–1959
Intravenous use of extract of liver. *J. Amer. med. Ass.*, 1931, **96,** 1198–1201.

3146 WILLS, Lucy.
Treatment of "pernicious anaemia of pregnancy" and "tropical anaemia", with special reference to yeast extract as a curative agent. *Brit. med. J.*, 1931, **1,** 1059–64.

First observations of haemopoietic effect of folic acid.

3147 DAVIDSON, *Sir* Leybourne Stanley Patrick. 1894–
The classification and treatment of anaemia, with special reference to the nutritional factor. *Trans. med.-chir. Soc. Edinb.*, 1932, n.s., **46,** 105–56.

Davidson's classification of the anaemias.

3148 WILKINSON, John Frederick. 1897– , & ISRAËLS, Martin Cyril Gordon.
Achresthic anaemia. *Brit. med. J.*, 1935, **1,** 139–43, 194–97.

Achrestic anaemia described.

3149 WILLS, Lucy, & EVANS, Barbara Dorothy Fordyce.
Tropical macrocytic anaemia: its relation to pernicious anaemia. *Lancet*, 1938, **2,** 416–21.

3150 SPIES, TOM DOUGLAS. 1902–1960, *et al.*
Observations of the anti-anemic properties of synthetic folic acid. *Sth. med. J. (Nashville)*, 1945, **38,** 707–09.
Haemopoietic properties of folic acid reported. With C. F. Vilter, M. B. Koch, and M. H. Caldwell.

3151 ANGIER, ROBERT CRANE. 1917– , *et al.*
Structure and synthesis of liver *L. casei* factor. *Science*, 1946, **103,** 667–69.
Isolation, determination of structure, and final synthesis of folic acid.

3152 GOETSCH, ANNE CARLTON TOMPKINS. 1917– , *et al.*
Observations on the effect of massive doses of iron given intravenously to patients with hypochromic anemia. *Blood*, 1946, **1,** 129–42.
Intravenous iron therapy. With C. V. Moore and V. Minnich.

3153 NISSIM, JOSEPH ABRAHAM.
Intravenous administration of iron. *Lancet*, 1947, **2,** 49–51.

3154 WEST, RANDOLPH. 1890–
Activity of vitamin B_{12} in Addisonian pernicious anemia. *Science*, 1948, **107,** 398.
First demonstration of the effectiveness of vitamin B_{12} in pernicious anaemia.

3154.1 PAULING, LINUS CARL. 1901– , *et al.*
Sickle cell anemia, a molecular disease. *Science*, 1949, **110,** 543–48.
First recognition of a structural haemoglobin variant. With H. A. Itano, S. J. Singer, and I. C. Wells.

3155 UNGLEY, CHARLES CADY.
Vitamin B_{12} in pernicious anaemia: parenteral administration. *Brit. med. J.*, 1949, **2,** 1370–77.

History of the Study of Cardiovascular Diseases and Haematology

3155.1 ROLLESTON, *Sir* HUMPHRY DAVY, *Bart.* 1862–1944
Cardio-vascular diseases since Harvey's discovery. Cambridge, *Univ. Press*, 1928.
Harveian Oration, 1928.

3156 ——. The history of haematology. *Proc. roy. Soc. Med.*, 1934, **27,** 1161–78.
Includes history of the development of knowledge regarding the blood elements, chlorosis, anaemias, erythraemia, leukaemia, haemophilia, etc. There is an extensive bibliography.

3157 ——. The history of angina pectoris. *Glasg. med. J.*, 1937, **127,** 205–25.

3158 WILLIUS, FREDERICK ARTHUR. 1888– , & KEYS, THOMAS EDWARD. 1908–
Cardiac classics. A collection of classic works on the heart and circulation with comprehensive biographic accounts of the authors. St. Louis, *C. V. Mosby Co.*, 1941.
New edition, *Classics of cardiology*, New York, 1961.

3159 HERRICK, James Bryan. 1861–1954
A short history of cardiology. Springfield, *C. C. Thomas*, 1942.

3160 WILLIUS, Frederick Arthur. 1888– , & DRY, Thomas Jan. 1903–
A history of the heart and circulation. Philadelphia, *W. B. Saunders*, 1948.

3160.1 GRIFFENHAGEN, George Bernard. 1934– , & HUGHES, Calvin H.
The history of the mechanical heart. *Smithsonian Rep.*, 1955, 339–56 (Smithsonian Inst. Publ. 4241).

3160.2 EAST, Charles Frederice Terence. 1894–1967
The story of heart diseases. London, *Wm. Dawson*, [1957].
FitzPatrick Lectures, 1956–57.

3161 FOOTE, Robert Rowden.
Varicose veins, 3rd ed. London, *Butterworth*, 1960.
A chapter on historical landmarks in treatment occupies, pp. 14–45.

3161.1 BURCH, George Edward. 1910– , & DePASQUALE, Nicholas P.
A history of electrocardiography. Chicago, *Year Book Medical Publishers*, 1964.

3162–3342 DISEASES OF THE RESPIRATORY SYSTEM

3162 ARETAEUS, *the Cappadocian*. *circa* A.D. 81–138
On angina, or quinsey. In his *Extant works*, ed. F. Adams, London, 1856, 249–52; 404–07.

3163 ——. On pleurisy. In his *Extant works*, ed. F. Adams, London, 1856, 255–58; 410–16.

3164 VESALIUS, Andreas. 1514–1564
Pro magni, et illustr. Terraenovae Ducis fistula, ex levi axilla in thoracis concavum pervia, *etc*. In P. Ingrassia: *Quaestio de purgatione per medicamentum*, Venetiis, *sumpt. A. Patessii*, 1568.
Vesalius's *consilia* to Ingrassia, dated Madrid, 1562, in which he clearly described the operation for empyema.

3165 WILLIS, Thomas. 1621–1675
On the convulsive cough and asthma. In his: *Practice of physick*, London, *T. Dring, etc.*, 1684, Treatise VIII, pp. 92–96.
The modern treatment of asthma really begins with Willis, who considered it to be of nervous origin.

3166 FLOYER, *Sir* John. 1649–1734
A treatise of the asthma. London, *R. Wilkins*, 1698.
Floyer himself suffered ffom asthma for over 30 years. He recognized the influence of heredity in asthma. The above includes (p. 239) an important early account of emphysema.

3167 MILLAR, John. 1733–1805
Observations on the asthma and on the hooping cough. London, *T. Cadell*, 1769.
Includes Millar's original description of laryngismus stridulus ("Millar's asthma").

3167.1 BAILLIE, Matthew. 1760–1823
The morbid anatomy of some of the most important parts of the human body. 2nd ed. London, *J. Johnson & G. Nicol*, 1797, vol. 2, p. 72.
First clinical description of chronic obstructive pulmonary emphysema. The lung on which Baillie performed an autopsy before describing this condition is said to have been that of Samuel Johnson.

3168 BADHAM, Charles. 1780–1845
Observations on the inflammatory affections of the mucous membrane of the bronchiae. London, *J. Callow*, 1808.
Badham gave bronchitis its present name.

3169 VIRCHOW, Rudolf Ludwig Karl. 1821–1902
Beiträge zur Lehre von den beim Menschen vorkommenden pflanzlichen Parasiten. *Virchows Arch. path. Anat.*, 1856, **9,** 557–93.
First description of pulmonary aspergillosis.

3169.1 SALTER, Henry Hyde. 1823–1871
On asthma: its pathology and treatment. London, *J. Churchill*, 1860.
The best work on asthma to appear during the 19th century. Salter called special attention to asthma arising from animal emanations (cats, rabbits, horses, dogs, cattle, etc.).

3170 HEWETT, Frederick Charles Cresswell.
Thoracentesis: the plan of continuous aspiration. *Brit. med. J.*, 1876, **1,** 317.
Cresswell introduced a method of continuous aspiration of the thorax for empyema.

3171 ESTLANDER, Jacob August. 1831–1881
Résection des côtes dans l'empyème chronique. *Rev. mens. Méd. Chir.*, 1879, **3,** 157–70, 885–88.
Estlander advocated resection of the outer walls of empyema cavities, in order to allow the soft tissues to sink in and obliterate them.

3172 PARROT, Joseph. 1829–1883
L'organisme microscopique trouvé par M. Pasteur dans la maladie nouvelle provoquée par la salive d'un enfant mort de la rage. *Bull. Acad. Méd. Paris*, 1881, 2 sér., **10,** 379.
Probably the earliest record of the pneumococcus.

3173 STERNBERG, George Miller. 1838–1915
A fatal form of septicaemia in the rabbit, produced by the subcutaneous injection of human saliva. *Johns Hopk. Univ. Stud. biol. Lab.*, 1882, **2,** No. 2, 183–200.
In the same year as Pasteur, and independently, Sternberg discovered a pneumococcus, demonstrating its carriage in the healthy human mouth.

3174 FRIEDLÄNDER, Carl. 1847–1887
Ueber die Schizomyceten bei der acuten fibrösen Pneumonie. *Virchows Arch. path. Anat.*, 1882, **87,** 319–24.
Isolation of *Klebsiella pneumoniae* ("Friedländer bacillus") which Friedländer regarded as the causal organism in all cases of lobar pneumonia.

3174.1 KRÖNLEIN, Rudolph Ulrich. 1847–1910
Ueber Lungenchirurgie. *Berl. klin. Wschr.*, 1884, **21,** 129–32.
Resection of portion of a lobe that was invaded by sarcoma of the rib.

3175 FRAENKEL, Albert. 1848–1916
Die Mikrococcen der Pneumonie. *Z. klin. Med.*, 1886, **10,** 426–49; **11,** 437–58.
Fraenkel showed definitely that the organism found by Pasteur (No. 3172) and Sternberg (No. 3173) was a cause of pneumonia.

3176 WEICHSELBAUM, Anton. 1845–1920
Ueber die Aetiologie der acuten Lungen- und Rippenfellentzündungen. *Med. Jb.*, 1886, n.F. **1,** 483–554.
Weichselbaum definitely established that Friedländer's bacillus was responsible for pneumonia in a small percentage of cases.

3177 KÜSTER, Ernst Georg Ferdinand von. 1839–1930
Ueber die Grundsätze der Behandlung von Eiterungen in starrwandigen Höhlen, mit besonderer Berücksichtigung des Empyems der Pleura. *Dtsch. med. Wschr.*, 1889, **15,** 185–87.
First thoracotomy for empyema.

3178 KLEMPERER, Georg. 1865–1946, & KLEMPERER, Felix. 1866–1932
Versuche über Immunisirung und Heilung bei der Pneumokokkeninfection. *Berl. klin. Wschr.*, 1891, **28,** 833–35, 869–75.
Old antipneumococcal serum.

3179 FOWLER, George Ryerson. 1848–1906
A case of thoracoplasty for the removal of a large cicatricial fibrous growth from the interior of the chest, the result of an old empyema. *Med. Rec.* (*N.Y.*), 1893, **44,** 838–39.
First thoracoplasty.

3180 DELORME, Edmond. 1847–1929
Nouveau traitement des empyèmes chroniques. *Gaz. Hôp.* (*Paris*), 1894, **67,** 94–96.
The procedure of decortication of the lung for treatment of chronic empyema was introduced by Delorme. For his later work on the subject, see *Congr. franç. Chir.*, 1896, **10,** 379.

3181 THOREL, Christen. 1868–1935
Die Specksteinlunge. Ein Beitrag zur pathologischen Anatomie der Staublungen. *Beitr. path. Anat.*, 1896, **20,** 81–101.
Talcosis of lung reported.

3182 NOCARD, Edmond Isidore Etienne. 1850–1903, & ROUX, Pierre Paul Emile. 1853–1933
Le microbe de la péripneumonie. *Ann. Inst. Pasteur*, 1898, **12,** 240–62.
One of the earliest studies on the filtrable viruses in animal diseases was that made by Nocard and Roux, who discovered the causal organism in bovine pleuropneumonia.

3183 GROCCO, Pietro. 1856–1916
Triangolo paravertebrale opposto nella pleurite essudativa. *Lav. Congr. Med. int.* (1902), Roma, 1903, **12,** 190.
"Grocco's triangle." Grocco described paravertebral dullness on the opposite side in pleural effusion.

3184 EMERSON, Charles Phillips. 1872–1938
Pneumothorax; a historical, clinical, and experimental study. *Johns Hopk. Hosp. Rep.*, 1903, **11,** 1–450.

3185 SAUERBRUCH, Ernst Ferdinand. 1875–1951
Ueber die physiologischen und physikalischen Grundlagen bei intrathorakalen Eingriffen in meiner pneumatischen Operationskammer. *Verh. dtsch. Ges. Chir.*, 1904, **32,** pt. 2, 105–15.
Sauerbruch's negative pressure chamber for the prevention of pneumothorax.

3186 NOWOTNY, Franz. 1872–1925
Bronchoskopie und bronchoskopische Behandlung von Bronchialasthma. *Mschr. Ohrenheilk.*, 1907, **41,** 697–711.
Introduction of therapeutic bronchosopy, for treatment of asthma.

3187 KÖRTE, Werner. 1853–1937
Ueber Lungenresektion wegen bronchiektatischer Cavernen. *Verh. berl. med. Ges.*, (1908), 1909, **39,** 5–9.
Körte was the first successfully to remove bronchiectatic lobes.

3188 PASTEUR, William. 1856–1943
The Bradshaw Lecture on massive collapse of the lung. *Lancet*, 1908, **2,** 1351–55.
Pasteur discovered and described massive collapse of the lung.

3189 JACOBÆUS, Hans Christian. 1879–1937
Ueber die Möglichkeit die Zystoscopie bei Untersuchungen seröser Höhlungen anzuwenden. *Münch. med. Wschr.*, 1910, **57,** 2090–92.
Jacobaeus adapted the cystoscope for the study of the interior of the body; this led to the introduction of the thoracoscope.

3190 NEUFELD, Fred. 1861–1945, & HAENDEL, Ludwig. 1869–1939
Weitere Untersuchungen über Pneumokokken-Heilsera. III. Mitteilung. Über Vorkommen und Bedeutung atypischer Varietäten des Pneumokokkus. *Arb. k. GesundhAmte*, 1910, **34,** 293–304.
New antipneumococcus serum.

3191 TUFFIER, Théodore. 1857–1929
Gangrène pulmonaire ouverte dans les bronches et traitée par décollement pleuro-pariétal, et greffe d'une masse lipomateuse entre la plèvre décollée et les espaces intercostaux. *Bull. Soc. Chir. Paris*, 1910, **36,** 529–38.
Tuffier's method of extrapleural pneumolysis.

3192 ADLER, Isaac. 1849–1918
Primary malignant growths of the lungs and bronchi. New York, *Longmans*, 1912.

3192.1 DOCHEZ, Alphonse Raymond. 1882–1964, & GILLESPIE, Louis John. 1886–
A biological classification of pneumococci by means of immunity reactions. *J. Amer. med. Ass.*, 1913, **61,** 727–32.
Dochez and Gillespie differentiated four types of pneumococci.

3192.2 KRUSE, Walther. 1864–1943
Die Erreger von Husten und Schnupfen. *Münch. med. Wschr.*, 1914, **61,** 1547.
Kruse reported that colds could be produced in volunteers by intranasal instillation of bacteria-free filtrates of secretions from persons suffering from colds.

3193 CASTELLANI, Aldo. 1877–1971
Note sur la "broncho-spirochétose" et les "bronchites mycosiques." Affections simulant quelquefois la tuberculose pulmonaire. *Presse méd.*, 1917, **25,** 377–80.
"Castellani's bronchitis" (bronchospirochaetosis).

3194 JACKSON, Chevalier. 1865–1958
Endothelioma of the right bronchus removed by peroral bronchoscopy. *Amer. J. med. Sci.*, 1917, **153,** 371–75.
First reported case.

3195 SAUERBRUCH, Ernst Ferdinand. 1875–1951
Die Chirurgie der Brustorgane. 2 vols. Berlin, *J. Springer*, 1920–25.

3196 COUTARD, Henri. 1876–
Un cas d'épithélioma spino-cellulaire de la région latérale du pharynx, avec adénopathie angulo-maxillaire, guéri depuis six mois par la röntgenthérapie. *Bull. Ass. franç. Étude Cancer*, 1921, **10,** 160–68.
Carcinoma of pharynx cured by the Coutard method of Röntgen therapy.

3197 LYNAH, Henry Lowndes. 1879–1922, & STEWART, William Holmes. 1868–
Roentgenographic studies of bronchiectasis and lung abscess after direct injection of bismuth mixture through the bronchoscope. *Amer. J. Roentgenol.*, 1921, **8,** 49–61.
Important studies on bronchiectasis were carried out by Lynah and Stewart.

3198 HEIDELBERGER, Michael. 1888– , & AVERY, Oswald Theodore. 1877–1955
The soluble specific substance of pneumococcus. *J. exp. Med.*, 1923, **38,** 73–79; 1924, **40,** 301–16.
Heidelberger, Avery and their colleagues made a chemical study of the antigenic constituents of the pneumococcus, separating the polysaccharide antigens.

3199 SICARD, Jean Athanase. 1872–1929, & FORESTIER, Jacques. 1890–
L'exploration radiologique des cavités broncho-pulmonaires par les injections intra-trachéales d'huile iodée. *J. méd. franç.*, 1924, **13,** 3–9.
Bronchography was advanced by the work of Sicard and Forestier on the intratracheal introduction of lipiodol.

3200 LAUGHLEN, George Franklin. 1888–
Studies on pneumonia following naso-pharyngeal injections of oil. *Amer. J. Path.*, 1925, **1,** 407–14.
Lipoid pneumonia first described.

3201 BARNARD, William George. 1892–1956
The nature of the "oat-celled sarcoma" of the mediastinum. *J. Path. Bact.*, 1926, **29,** 241–44.
An important study of the histology of "oat-celled sarcoma" which Barnard showed to be primary carcinoma of the lung.

3202 BRUNN, HAROLD. 1874–1950
Surgical principles underlying one-stage lobectomy. *Arch. Surg.*, 1929, **18,** 490–515.
Brunn's one-stage lobectomy.

3202.1 CAMPS, PERCY WILLIAM LEOPOLD. 1877–1956
A note on the inhalation treatment of asthma. *Guy's Hosp. Rep.*, 1929, **79,** 496–98.
First use of adrenaline by the respiratory route for the treatment of bronchial asthma.

3203 NISSEN, RUDOLPH. 1896–
Exstirpation eines ganzen Lungenflügels. *Zbl. Chir.*, 1931, **58,** 3003–3006.
Removal of entire bronchiectatic lung; successful.

3203.1 CAMPBELL, JOHN MUNRO.
Acute symptoms following work with hay. *Brit. med. J.*, 1932, **2,** 1143–44.
"Farmer's lung."

3203.2 SHENSTONE, NORMAN STRAHAN. 1881– , & JANES, ROBERT MEREDITH. 1894–
Experiences in pulmonary lobectomy. *Canad. med. Ass. J.*, 1932, **27,** 138–45.
Introduction of the hilar tourniquet in pulmonary surgery.

3204 THOMSON, DAVID. 1884–1969, & THOMSON, ROBERT. 1888–
The common cold, with special reference to the part played by streptococci, pneumococci, and other organisms. London, *Baillière, Tindall & Cox*, 1932.
Annals of the Pickett–Thomson Research Lab., Vol. 8.

3205 GRAHAM, EVARTS AMBROSE. 1883–1957, & SINGER, JACOB JESSE. 1882–1954
Successful removal of entire lung for carcinoma of the bronchus. *J. Amer. med. Ass.*, 1933, **101,** 1371–74.
First reported case; April 5, 1933.

3206 KARTAGENER, MANES. 1897–
Zur Pathogenese der Bronchiektasien. I. Bronchiektasien bei Situs viscerum inversus. *Beitr. Klin. Tuberk.*, 1933, **83,** 489–501.
Bronchiectasis and sinus maldevelopment associated with transposition of viscera – "Kartagener's syndrome".

3207 LILIENTHAL, HOWARD. 1861–1946
Pneumonectomy for sarcoma of the lung in a tuberculous patient. *J. thorac. Surg.*, 1933, **2,** 600–15.
Total pneumonectomy.

3208 MAYTUM, CHARLES KORAN. 1895–
Tetany caused by functional dyspnea with hyperventilation: report of a case. *Proc. Mayo Clin.*, 1933, **8,** 282–84.
Hyperventilation syndrome.

3209 BARACH, ALVAN LEROY. 1895–
Use of helium as a new therapeutic gas. *Proc. Soc. exp. Biol.* (*N.Y.*), 1934, **32,** 462–64.

Introduction of helium in the treatment of respiratory affections. See also *Ann. intern. Med.*, 1935, **9**, 739–65.

3209.1 ABREU, MANOEL DE. 1892–1962
Röntgen-photographia. Processo e apparelho de röntgen-photographia. Tuberculose pulmonar. Cadastro social. Radiographia e radioscopia. Röntgen-photographia collectiva. *Rev. Assoc. paul. Med.*, 1936, **9,** 313–24.

Introduction of mass chest radiography.

3210 EVANS, GLADYS MARY, & GAISFORD, WILFRID FLETCHER. 1902–
Treatment of pneumonia with 2-(*p*-aminobenzenesulphonamido) pyridine. *Lancet*, 1938, **2,** 14–19.

M & B 693 (sulphapyridine) treatment of pneumonia. This followed the experimental work of L. E. H. Whitby (No. 1951).

3211 REIMANN, HOBART ANSTETH. 1897–
An acute infection of the respiratory tract with atypical pneumonia: a disease entity probably caused by a filtrable virus. *J. Amer. med. Ass.*, 1938, **111,** 2377–84.

Atypical pneumonia.

3211.1 CHURCHILL, EDWARD DELOS. 1895– , & BELSEY, RONALD HERBERT ROBERT.
Segmental pneumonectomy in bronchiectasis. The lingula segment of the left upper lobe. *Ann. Surg.*, 1939, **109,** 481–99.

3212 HEFFRON, RODERICK. 1901–
Pneumonia. With special reference to pneumococcus lobar pneumonia. London, *Oxford Univ. Press*, 1939.

3213 COMMISSION ON PNEUMONIA.
Primary atypical pneumonia, etiology unknown. *War Med.*, 1942, **2,** 330–33.

First use of the term.

3213.1 EATON, MONROE DAVIS. 1904– , *et al.*
Studies on the etiology of primary atypical pneumonia. A filterable agent transmissible to cotton rats, hamsters, and chick embryos. *J. exp. Med.*, 1944, **79,** 649–68.

The Eaton agent, isolated from primary atypical pneumonia. With G. Meiklejohn and W. van Herick.

3214 COMMISSION ON ACUTE RESPIRATORY DISEASES.
Transmission of primary atypical pneumonia to human volunteers. *J. Amer. med. Ass.*, 1945, **127,** 146–49.

3215 BROCK, RUSSELL CLAUDE, *Baron Brock of Wimbledon.* 1903–
The anatomy of the bronchial tree: with special reference to the surgery of lung abscess. London, *Oxford University Press*, 1946.

3215.1 KUROYA, Masahiko, *et al.*

Newborn virus pneumonitis (type Sendai). II. The isolation of a new virus possessing hemagglutinin activity. *Yokohama med. Bull.*, 1953, **4,** 217–33.

M. Kuroya, N. Ishida, and T. Shiratori isolated the first recognized Sendai (para-influenza) virus.

3215.2 CHANOCK, Robert Merritt. 1904–   , *et al.*

Recovery from infants with respiratory illness of a virus related to chimpanzee coryza agent (CCA). *Amer. J. Hyg.*, 1957, **66,** 281–90.

Respiratory syncytial virus. With B. Roizman and R. Myers.

3215.3 MEADE, Richard Hardaway. 1897–

A history of thoracic surgery. Springfield, *C. C. Thomas*, 1961.

3216–3243 PULMONARY TUBERCULOSIS

See also 2320–2361.1, Tuberculosis.

3216 MORTON, Richard. 1637–1698

Phthisiologia, seu exercitationes de phthisi. Londini, *imp. S. Smith*, 1689.

Morton left an excellent description of tuberculosis. He drew attention to the prevalence of the disease, noting that tubercles are often spontaneously healed, that they are a necessary antecedent of all cases of consumption, and that infection of one part of the body is associated with glandular swellings elsewhere. The book was translated into English in 1694. Chap. I included the first account of anorexia nervosa.

3217 MARTEN, Benjamin. 1704–1782

A new theory of consumptions: more especially of a phthisis, or consumption of the lungs. London, *R. Knaplock*, 1720.

Marten considered a parasitic micro-organism to be the cause of tuberculosis, thus forecasting the existence of the tubercle bacillus 162 years before its actual discovery.

3218 BAILLIE, Matthew. 1761–1823

The morbid anatomy of some of the most important parts of the human body. London, *J. Johnson & G. Nicol*, 1793.

Baillie's clear and comprehensive description of the pulmonary lesions of tuberculosis could hardly be bettered to-day. He differentiated the nodular and infiltrating types.

3219 LAENNEC, René Théophile Hyacinthe. 1781–1826

De l'auscultation médiate. 2 vols. Paris, *J. A. Brosson & J. S. Chaudé*, 1819.

Laennec is remembered for his invention of the stethoscope and for his book on auscultation. Garrison considers the latter the foundation stone of modern knowledge of diseases of the chest. Himself tuberculous, Laennec was considered the greatest teacher of his time on tuberculosis. Indeed, it was in elaboration of his investigation of the disease that he invented the stethoscope. He established the fact that all phthisis is tuberculous, described pneumothorax and distinguished pneumonia from the various kinds of bronchitis and from pleuritis.

3220 CARSON, James. 1772–1843

Essays, physiological and practical. Liverpool, *F. B. Wright*, 1822.

Carson proposed the induction of open pneumothorax for the treatment of pulmonary tuberculosis (p. 64). Later he attempted it on a patient (see his *An inquiry into the cause of respiration*, etc., 2nd ed., London, 1833, p. 50). The procedure was carried out by Forlanini (No. 3225).

3221 LOUIS, Pierre Charles Alexandre. 1787–1872
Recherches anatomico-pathologiques sur la phthisie. Paris, *Gabon & Cie.*, 1825.

Louis's researches were based on 358 dissections and 1,960 clinical cases, and included a numerical study of extra-pulmonary lesions. In the book he described the "angle of Louis", formed by the manubrium and the body of the sternum. He was an expert morbid anatomist. An English translation of the book was published by the Sydenham Society in 1843.

3222 MORTON, Samuel George. 1799–1851
Illustrations of pulmonary consumption. Philadelphia, *Key & Biddle*, 1834.

Morton published an important collection of illustrations delineating pulmonary tuberculosis which epitomized the knowledge of his time. It was also the first book on the subject to be published in the U.S.A.

3223 BODINGTON, George. 1799–1882
Essay on the treatment and cure of pulmonary consumption. London, *Longmans & Co.*, 1840.

Bodington was one of the first to advocate the sanatorium treatment of pulmonary tuberculosis, with "cold dry air for healing and closing cavities and ulcers of the lungs". His idea was much criticized and he was discouraged from pursuing it. The first sanatorium to be run on lines similar to those suggested by Bodington was that established by H. Brehmer at Görbersdorf in 1859. The book was reprinted in 1906.

3224 PARROT, Joseph. 1829–1883
Recherches sur les relations qui existent entre les lésions des poumons et celles des ganglions trachéo-bronchiques. *C. R. Soc. Biol. (Paris)*, 1876, sér. 6, **3**, 308–09.

The primary lesion in pulmonary tuberculosis in children ("Ghon's primary focus") was first described by Parrot.

3225 FORLANINI, Carlo. 1847–1918
A contribuzione della terapia chirurgica della tisi; ablazione del polmone? pneumotorace artificiale? *Gazz. Osp. Clin.*, 1882, **3**, 537, 585, 601, 609, 617, 625, 641, 657, 665, 689, 705.

Forlanini first discussed the induction of artificial pneumothorax in the above papers; he applied it in 1888. For his report on its application, see *Gazz. med. Torino*, 1894, **45**, 381, 401.

3226 CAYLEY, William. 1836–1916
A case of haemoptysis treated by the induction of pneumothorax so as to collapse the lung. *Trans. clin. Soc. Lond.*, 1885, **18**, 278–84.

Artificial pneumothorax by pleural incision in intractable haemoptysis. See also *Lancet*, 1885, **1**, 894–95.

3227 LOWSON, David. 1850–1907
A case of pneumonectomy. *Brit. med. J.*, 1893, **1**, 1152–54.

Partial lobectomy in pulmonary tuberculosis.

3228 TUFFIER, Théodore. 1857–1929
Chirurgie du poumon en particulier dans les cavernes tuberculeuses et la gangrène pulmonaire. Paris, *Masson*, 1897.

Describes (p. 31) first cure of tuberculosis by removal of lung apex.

3229 MACEWEN, *Sir* WILLIAM. 1848–1924
On some points in the surgery of the lung. *Brit. med. J.*, 1906, **2,** 1–7.
Removal of left lung for tuberculosis, April 24, 1895. The patient was alive in 1940.

3230 BRAUER, LUDOLPH. 1865–1951
Die Behandlung der einseitigen Lungenphthisis mit künstlichem Pneumothoraz (nach Murphy). *Münch. med. Wschr.*, 1906, **53,** 338–39.
Brauer's method of producing artificial pneumothorax by the injection of nitrogen.

3231 ——. Indications du traitement chirurgical de la tuberculose pulmonaire. *Congr. Ass. franç. Chir.*, 1908, **21,** 569–74.
First radical thoracoplasty.

3232 WILMS, MAX. 1867–1918
Eine neue Methode zur Verengung des Thorax bei Lungentuberkulose. *Münch. med. Wschr.*, 1911, **58,** 777–78.
Wilms operation.

3233 GHON, ANTON. 1866–1936
Der primäre Lungenherd bei der Tuberkulose der Kinder. Berlin & Wien, *Urban & Schwarzenberg*, 1912.
Ghon described the anatomical distribution and development of the lesions in pulmonary tuberculosis among children – "Ghon's primary focus". His book was translated into English in 1916. See also No. 3224.

3234 SAUERBRUCH, ERNST FERDINAND. 1875–1951
Die Beeinflüssung von Lungenerkrankungen durch künstliche Lähmung des Zwerchfells (Phrenikotomie). *Münch med. Wschr.*, 1913, **60,** 625–26.
Phrenicotomy in the treatment of pulmonary tuberculosis.

3235 JACOBÆUS, HANS CHRISTIAN. 1879–1937
Endopleurale Operationen unter der Leitung des Thorakoskops. *Beitr. Klin. Tuberk.*, 1916, **35,** 1–35.
Jacobæus introduced adhesion-section with the cautery, to secure collapse in artificial pneumothorax.

3236 VAJDA, LUDWIG.
Ob das Pneumoperitoneum in der Kollapstherapie der beiderseitigen Lungentuberkulose angewandt werden kann? *Z. Tuberk.*, 1933, **67,** 371–75.
Introduction of artificial pneumoperitoneum for the treatment of bilateral pulmonary tuberculosis.

3237 BANYAI, ANDREW LADISLAUS. 1893–
Therapeutic pneumoperitoneum. A review of 100 cases. *Amer. Rev. Tuberc.*, 1934, **29,** 603–27.
Banyai combined artificial pneumoperitoneum with phrenic nerve paralysis.

3238 FREEDLANDER, SAMUEL OSCAR. 1893–
Lobectomy in pulmonary tuberculosis. Report of a case. *J. thorac. Surg.* 1935, **5,** 132–42.
The modern era in lung resection for tuberculosis begins with the work of Freedlander. He performed the first planned lobectomy for pulmonary tuberculosis.

3239 SEMB, CARL BOYE. 1895–
Thoracoplasty with extrafascial apicolysis. *Acta chir. scand.*, 1935, Suppl. 37, pt. 2, 1–85.
"Semb's operation."

3240 KAYNE, GEORGE GREGORY. 1901–1945, PAGEL, WALTER. 1898– , & O'SHAUGHNESSY, LAURENCE. 1900–1940
Pulmonary tuberculosis. Pathology, diagnosis, management and prevention. London, *Oxford Univ. Press*, 1939.
Third edition, 1953, by W. Pagel, F. A. H. Simmonds, and N. Macdonald.

3241 LEHMANN, JÖRGEN. 1898–
Para-aminosalicylic acid in the treatment of tuberculosis. *Lancet*, 1946, **1**, 15–16.
p-Aminosalicylic acid used in pulmonary tuberculosis. See also his earlier paper in *Svenska LäkT.*, 1946, **43**, 2029–40.

History of Pulmonary Tuberculosis

See also 2354–2361.1, *History of Tuberculosis*

3242 PAGEL, WALTER. 1898–
Die Krankheitslehre der Phthise in den Phasen ihrer geschichtlichen Entwicklung. *Beitr. Klin. Tuberk.*, 1927, **66,** 66–98.

3243 BROWN, LAWRASON. 1871–1937
The story of clinical pulmonary tuberculosis. Baltimore, *Williams & Wilkins*, 1941.

3244–3326 LARYNGOLOGY: RHINOLOGY

See also 5046–5072, DIPHTHERIA.

3244 CODRONCHI, GIOVANNI BATTISTA. 1547–1628
De vitiis vocis, libri duo. Francofurti, *apud heredes A. Wecheli*, 1597.
First treatise devoted solely to diseases of the larynx. (See also No. 1718).

3244.1 HABICOT, NICHOLAS. 1550–1624
Question chirurgicale par laquelle il est demonstré que le chirurgien doit assurément practiquer l'opération de la bronchotomie, vulgairement dicte Laryngotomie ou perforation de la fluste tuyau du polmon. Paris, *J. Corrozet*, 1620.
Four successful cases. Scott Stevenson and Guthrie state that Brasavola performed laryngotomy (in 1546) and that Sanctorius also did so.

3245 SCHNEIDER, CONRAD VICTOR. 1614–1680
Liber primus de catarrhis. Wittebergae, *T. Mevii & E. Schumacheri*, 1660.
Schneider put an end to the idea that nasal mucus originated in the pituitary. As a result of his work the olfactory processes were definitely classified as cranial nerves.

3246 LOWER, RICHARD. 1631–1691
Dissertatio de origine catarrhi in qua ostenditur illum non provenire a cerebro. In his: *Tractatus de corde*. Londini, *typ. J. Redmayne*, 1670, pp. 221–39.
With Schneider, Lower overthrew the idea that nasal mucus originated in the brain. This discovery localized nasal catarrh in the air passages and put an end to the use of many recipes for "purging the brain". The *Dissertatio* was reprinted separately in 1672.

3247 COWPER, William. 1666–1709
Of the nose. In J. Drake: *Anthropologia nova*, London, 1707, vol. 2, pp. 526–49.
Report of cases of operation on the maxillary antrum.

3248 VIRGILI, Pedro. 1699–1776
Sur une bronchotomie faite avec succès. *Mém. Acad. roy. Chir.*, 1743, **1,** pt. 3, 141–45.
Virgili is said to have performed successful tracheotomy at Cadiz, for quinsy.

3249 JOURDAIN, Anselme Louis Bernard Berchillet. 1734–1816
Recherches sur les différens moyens de traiter les maladies des sinus maxillaires, et sur les avantages qu'il y a, dans certains cas, d'injecter des sinus par le nez. *J. Méd. Chir. Pharm.*, 1767, **27,** 52–71, 157–74.
Jourdain reported a method of washing out the antrum of Highmore through the natural opening.

3250 PLAIGNAUD.
Observation sur un fongus du sinus maxillaire. *J. Chir.* (*Paris*), 1791, **1.** 111–16.
First successful operation on a tumour of the maxillary sinus, 1789.

3251 DESCHAMPS, Jacques Louis, *fils*. 1740–1824
Dissertation sur les maladies des fosses nasales et de leurs sinus. Paris, *chez Mme veuve Richard*, an XII, 1804.
First important work on diseases of the nose and nasal sinuses.

3252 CHEYNE, John. 1777–1836
The pathology of the membranes of the larynx and bronchia. Edinburgh, *Mundell, Doig & Stevenson*, 1809.
Cheyne's important book deals mainly with the lesions of croup.

3253 CLOQUET, Jules Hippolyte. 1787–1840
Osphrésiologie, ou traité des odeurs, du sens et des organes de l'olfaction. 2me éd. Paris, *Méquignon-Marvis*, 1821.
An exhaustive work which discusses olfaction, diseases of the nose, membranous occlusion of the nostrils, deviations of the septum, rhinoplasty, coryza, vasomotor rhinitis, rhinorrhoea, etc.

3254 PORTER, William Henry. 1790–1861
Observations on the surgical pathology of the larynx and trachea. Dublin, *Hodges & M'Arthur*, 1826.
Porter was professor of surgery at the Royal College of Surgeons in Ireland. The above includes a description of "Porter's sign", tracheal tugging in aortic aneurysm.

3255 PHYSICK, Philip Syng. 1768–1837
Description of a forceps, employed to facilitate the extirpation of the tonsil. *Amer. J. med. Sci.*, 1828, **2,** 116–17.
Invention of the modern tonsillotome.

3256 ALBERS, Johann Friedrich Hermann. 1805–1867
Die Pathologie und Therapie der Kehlkopfkrankheiten. Leipzig, *C. Cnobloch*, 1829.

3257 LUDWIG, Wilhelm Friedrich von. 1790–1865
Ueber eine Form von Halsentzündung. *Med. Correspbl. württ. ärztl. Vereins*, 1836, **6**, 21–25.
"Ludwig's angina" first described. English translation and biographical note, *Bull. Hist. Med.*, 1939, **7**, 1115–26.

3258 TROUSSEAU, Armand. 1801–1867, & BELLOC, Hippolyte.
Traité pratique de la phthisie laryngée, de la laryngite chronique, et des maladies de la voix. Paris, *J. B. Baillière*, 1837.
A laryngological classic. English translation, 1839.

3259 MOTT, Valentine. 1785–1865
A nasal operation for the removal of a large tumour filling up the entire nostril and extending to the pharynx. *Amer. J. med. Sci.*, 1843, n.s. **5**, 87–91.
Removal of a fibrous growth from the nostril by division of the nasal and maxillary bones, July 8, 1841. Preliminary note in the same journal, 1842, **3**, 257.

3260 EHRMANN, Charles Henri. 1792–1878
Sur une opération de laryngotomie pratiquée dans un cas de polype du larynx. *C. R. Acad. Sci. (Paris)*, 1844, **18**, 593, 709.
First removal of a laryngeal polyp.

3261 GREEN, Horace. 1802–1866
A treatise on diseases of the air-passages. New York, *Wiley & Putnam*, 1846.
Green was the "father of laryngology" in America. He was first successfully to introduce medicaments into the larynx, trachea, and bronchi for local treatment. His claims in this connexion were the subject of bitter controversy in the U.S.A. It is possible that he somewhat exaggerated the efficacy of the methods he used and advocated.

3262 ——. On the surgical treatment of polypi of the larynx and oedema of the glottis. New York, *T. P. Putnam*, 1852.

3263 BUCK, Gurdon. 1807–1877
On the surgical treatment of morbid growths within the larynx, illustrated by an original case and statistical observations, elucidating their nature and forms. *Trans. Amer. med. Ass.*, 1853, **6**, 509–35.
Thyrotomy for removal of cancer of the larynx. The operation took place in May 1851, and the patient died in 1852.

3264 GROSS, Samuel David. 1805–1884
A practical treatise on foreign bodies in the air-passages. Philadelphia, *Blanchard & Lea*, 1854.
First systematic study of the subject. In this celebrated work Gross laid down principles concerning symptoms which are still fundamental, despite the advent of roentgenology.

3265 COCK, Edward. 1805–1892
Case of pharyngotomy. *Lancet*, 1856, **1**, 125–26.
First pharyngotomy in England. Fuller report in *Guy's Hosp. Rep.*, 1858, 3 ser., **4**, 217.

3266 GREEN, Horace. 1802–1866
Report on the use and effect of applications of nitrate of silver to the throat, either in local or general disease. *Trans. Amer. Med. Ass.*, 1856, **9**, 493–530.
See No. 3261.

3267 CATLIN, George. 1796–1872
The breath of life; or mal-respiration, and its effects upon the enjoyments and life of man. New York, *J. Wiley*, 1861.
Catlin, the famous explorer, was the first in America to call attention to the bad effects of mouth-breathing.

3268 BRUNS, Viktor von. 1812–1883
Die erste Ausrottung eines Polypen in der Kehlkopfshöhle durch Zerschneiden ohne blutige Eröffnung der Luftwege. Tübingen, *Laupp & Siebeck*, 1862.
First enucleation of a laryngeal polyp by the bloodless method.

3269 LEWIN, Georg Richard. 1820–1896
Beiträge zur Laryngoscopie. *Allg. med. Cent.-Ztg*, 1862, **31,** 9, 33.
Lewin was probably the first to extirpate a laryngeal growth with the aid of the laryngoscope. Bruns claimed this distinction, but may not have heard of Lewin.

3270 GERHARDT, Carl Adolph Christian Jacob. 1833–1902
Studien und Beobachtungen über Stimmbandlähmung. *Virchows Arch. path. Anat.*, 1863, **27,** 68–98, 296–321.
An important study of paralysis of the vocal cords was made by Gerhardt. He it was who diagnosed the growth in the larynx of Friedrich III, Emperor of Germany, whose eventual death from this condition was to have such disastrous effects on German history.

3271 BRUNS, Viktor von. 1812–1883
Die Laryngoskopie und die laryngoskopische Chirurgie. 1 vol. and atlas. Tübingen, *H. Laupp*, 1865.
Bruns claimed to have been the first to remove a tumour from the larynx with the aid of the laryngoscope.

3272 SANDS, Henry Berton. 1830–1888
Case of cancer of the larynx, successfully removed by laryngotomy. *N.Y. med. J.*, 1865, **1,** 110–26.
Laryngectomy for papillomata.

3273 TÜRCK, Ludwig. 1810–1868
Klinik der Krankheiten des Kehlkopfes und der Luftröhre. 1 vol. and atlas. Wien, *W. Braumüller*, 1866.
On p. 295 is a classical description of laryngitis sicca – "Türck's trachoma".

3274 SOLIS-COHEN, Jacob da Silva. 1838–1927
Removal of a fibrous polyp from the inferior anterior surface of the right vocal cord with the aid of the laryngoscope. *Amer. J. med. Sci.*, 1867, n.s., **53,** 404–07; **54,** 565–66.
First successful operation for cancer of the larynx.

3275 VOLTOLINI, Friedrich Eduard Rudolph. 1819–1889
Die Anwendung der Galvanokaustik im Innern des Kehlkopfes und Schlundkopfes. Wien, *W. Braumüller*, 1867.
Voltolini was the first to use the galvanocautery in laryngeal surgery.

3276 MEYER, Hans Wilhelm. 1825–1895
Om adenoide Vegetationer i Naesesvaelgrummet. *Hospitalstidende*, 1868, **11,** 177–81.
First clinical description of adenoid growths. For an English translation of the paper, see *Med.-chir. Trans.*, 1870, **53,** 191–215.

3277 HEBRA, HANS VON. 1847–1902
Ueber ein eigenthümliches Neugebilde an der Nase. – Rhinosclerom. *Wien. med. Wschr.*, 1870, **20,** 1–5.

3278 MACKENZIE, *Sir* MORELL. 1837–1892
Essay on growths in the larynx. London, *J. & A. Churchill,* 1871.
An analysis of 100 of Mackenzie's own cases.

3279 GERHARDT, CARL ADOLPH CHRISTIAN JACOB. 1833–1902
Ueber Diagnose und Behandlung der Stimmbandlähmung. *Samml. klin. Vortr.*, 1872, Nr. 36 (Inn. Med., Nr. 13), 271–82.
See No. 3270. Continuing his study of laryngeal paralysis, Gerhardt proposed the term "cadaveric position" to indicate the position of the vocal cord in total paralysis of the larynx.

3280 SOLIS-COHEN, JACOB DA SILVA. 1838–1927
Diseases of the throat: a guide to the diagnosis and treatment of affections of the pharynx, oesophagus, trachea, larynx, and nares. New York, *W. Wood & Co.*, 1872.
First American text-book on oto-rhino-laryngology.

3281 FRAENKEL, BERNHARD. 1836–1911
Fall von gutartiger Mycosis des Pharynx. *Berl. klin. Wschr.*, 1873, **10,** 94.
Mycosis pharyngis first reported.

3282 GUSSENBAUER, CARL. 1842–1903
Ueber die erste durch Th. Billroth am Menschen ausgeführte Kehlkopf-Exstirpation und die Anwendung eines künstlichen Kehlkopfes. *Verh. dtsch. Ges. Chir.*, 1874, **3,** Heft 2, 76–89.
The first complete excision of the larynx for cancer was performed by Billroth in 1873, and reported by Gussenbauer. Recurrence and death occurred one month after the operation. The paper was also published in *Arch. klin. Chir.*, 1874, **17,** 343–56.

3283 WENDT, HERMANN. 1838–1875
Rareficirender, trockner Katarrh der Nasenrachenhöhle und des Rachens (Atrophie). *In* H. von Ziemssen's *Handbuch der speciellen Pathologie*, Leipzig, 1874, **7,** I, 313–16.
First description of "Tornwaldt's bursitis", an inflammatory condition of the pharyngeal tonsil, so named from the latter's description of it in 1885 (see No. 3295).

3284 RIEGEL, FRANZ. 1843–1904
Ueber respiratorische Paralysen. *Samml. klin. Vortr.*, 1875, Nr. 95 (Inn. Med., Nr. 33), 761–96.
Riegel distinguished between respiratory and phonatory paralysis of the larynx.

3285 FRAENKEL, BERNHARD. 1836–1911
Rhinitis chronica. Ozaena. Stockschnupfen. Stinknase. In Ziemssen's *Handbuch der speciellen Pathologie und Therapie*, Leipzig, 1876, **4,** I, 125–34.
Fraenkel established ozaena as a clinical entity.

3286 JARVIS, WILLIAM CHAPMAN. 1855–1895
Surgical treatment of hypertrophic nasal catarrh. *Trans. Amer. laryng. Ass.*, (1880), 1881, **2,** 130–41.
Jarvis nasal snare described.

3287 MACKENZIE, *Sir* MORELL. 1837–1892
A manual of diseases of the throat and nose. 2 vols. London, *J. & A. Churchill*, 1880–84.

Mackenzie's great reputation earned him the title of Father of British Laryngology. In 1863 he founded the Golden Square Throat Hospital, London, the first hospital in the world devoted solely to diseases of the throat; he was also the founder of the *Journal of Laryngology*. He was called to attend Crown Prince Frederick, afterwards Emperor Frederick III of Germany, who suffered from, and succumbed to, a cancer of the larynx. Mackenzie was much maligned by a section of the German medical profession for refusing to agree to operation until biopsy had been performed. Three specimens proved negative and operation was delayed until too late. Mackenzie's health was affected by his arduous duties on behalf of the Emperor and he died in 1892. The *Manual* was the standard work on the subject and had an important influence on the development of laryngology.

3288 SEMON, *Sir* FELIX. 1849–1921
Clinical remarks on the proclivity of the abductor fibres of the recurrent laryngeal nerve to become affected sooner than the abductor fibres, or even exclusively, in cases of undoubted central or peripheral injury or disease of the roots or trunks of the pneumogastric, spinal accessory, or recurrent nerves. *Arch. Laryng.* (*N.Y.*), 1881, **2,** 197–222.

"Semon's law." Of German birth, Semon became one of the greatest laryngologists in Britain. He developed the modern operation of laryngo-fissure for early cancer of the larynx.

3289 INGALS, EPHRAIM FLETCHER. 1848–1918
Deflection of the septum narium. *Trans. Amer. laryng. Ass.*, 1882, **4,** 61–69.

Ingals devised the operation of partial excision of the septum for the correction of septum deflection.

3290 FRENCH, THOMAS RUSHMORE. 1849–1929
On photographing the larynx. *Trans. Amer. laryng. Ass.*, 1882, **4,** 32–35.

French was the first to obtain good photographs of the larynx.

3291 ——. On a perfected method of photographing the larynx. *N.Y. med. J.*, 1884, **40,** 653–56.

By means of a special camera of his own invention French improved the method of photographing the larynx.

3292 JELINEK, EDMUND. 1852–1928
Das Cocain als Anästheticum und Analgeticum für den Pharynx und Larynx. *Wien. med. Wschr.*, 1884, **34,** col. 1334–37, 1364–67.

Cocaine first employed in laryngology.

3293 OGSTON, *Sir* ALEXANDER. 1844–1929
Trephining the frontal sinuses for catarrhal diseases. *Med. Chron.*, 1884, **1,** 235–38.

3294 LOEWENBERG, BENJAMIN BENNO. 1836–1905
Die Natur und die Behandlung der Ozaena. *Dtsch. med. Wschr.*, 1885, **11,** 5–8, 22–24.

Loewenberg described a bacillus found in the secretions of ozaena (see No. 3307). He made the first attempt at the treatment of this condition.

3295 TORNWALDT, GUSTAV LUDWIG [THORNWALDT]. 1843–1910
Über die Bedeutung der Bursa pharyngea für die Erkennung und Behandlung gewisser Nasenrachenraum-Krankheiten. Wiesbaden, *J. F. Bergmann*, 1885.
"Tornwaldt's [Thornwaldt's] bursitis," first described by Wendt (No. 3283).

3296 FRAENKEL, BERNHARD. 1836–1911
Erste Heilung eines Larynx-Cancroids vermittelst Ausrottung per vias naturales. *Arch. klin. Chir.*, 1887, **34,** 281–86.
First successful intralaryngeal extirpation of a malignant growth.

3297 MIKULICZ-RADECKI, JOHANN VON. 1850–1905
Zur operativen Behandlung des Empyems der Highmorshöhle. *Arch. klin. Chir.*, 1887, **34,** 626–34.
Mikulicz's operation for the treatment of disease of the accessory nasal sinuses.

3298 BOSWORTH, FRANCKE HUNTINGTON. 1843–1925
A treatise on diseases of the nose and throat. 2 vols. New York, *W. Wood & Co.*, 1889–92.
Bosworth, a pioneer of American rhinology, advanced an important theory of the causation of ozaena.

3299 BRYAN, JOSEPH HAMMOND. 1856–1935
Diagnosis and treatment of abscess of the antrum. *J. Amer. med. Ass.*, 1889, **13,** 478–83.
Classical paper on sinusitis.

3300 KRIEG, ROBERT. 1848–
Beiträge zur Resection der Cartilago quadrangularis narium zur Heilung der Skoliosis septi. *Berl. klin. Wschr.*, 1889, **26,** 699–701, 717–20.
The operation of partial excision of the cartilage for the treatment of deflections of the nasal septum was perfected by Krieg.

3301 LUC, HENRY. 1855–1925
Des abscès du sinus maxillaire. Paris, *Steinheil*, 1889.
See No. 3305.

3302 VOLTOLINI, FRIEDRICH EDUARD RUDOLPH. 1819–1889
Die ersten Operationen in der Kehlkopfshöhle vom Munde aus, bei der Durchleuchtung des Kehlkopfes von aussen. *Dtsch. med. Wschr.*, 1889, **15,** 340–43.
The first laryngeal operation through the mouth with external illumination.

3303 AVELLIS, GEORG. 1864–1916
Klinische Beiträge zur halbseitigen Kehlkopflähmungen. *Berl. Klinik*, 1891, Heft 40, 1–26.
"Avellis's syndrome", recurrent paralysis of the soft palate.

3304 BOSWORTH, FRANCKE HUNTINGTON. 1843–1925
Various forms of disease of the ethmoid cells. *N.Y. med. J.*, 1891, **54,** 505–07.

3305 CALDWELL, GEORGE WALTER. 1866–1946
Diseases of the accessory sinuses of the nose, and an improved method of treatment of suppuration of the maxillary antrum. *N.Y. med. J.*, 1893, **58,** 526–28.
Caldwell–Luc operation (see also No. 3301). Scanes Spicer independently devised a similar operation (*Brit. med. J.*, 1894, **2,** 1359–60).

3306 GRÜNWALD, LUDWIG. 1863–
Die Lehre von den Naseneiterungen. München, Leipzig, *J. F. Lehmann*, 1893.
Grünwald was the first to attempt the surgical treatment of nasal suppuration and disease involving the ethmoid and sphenoid bones. English translation, 1900.

3307 LOEWENBERG, BENJAMIN BENNO. 1836–1905
Le microbe de l'ozène. *Ann. Inst. Pasteur*, 1894, **8,** 292–317.
Loewenberg found a bacillus of the Friedländer group in ozaena.

3308 WINGRAVE, VITRUVIUS HAROLD WYATT. 1858–1938
The pathological and clinical features of atrophic rhinitis. *J. Laryng.*, 1894, **8,** 96–110.
Classical paper on atrophic rhinitis (ozaena).

3308.1 PLAUT, HUGO KARL. 1858–1928
Studien zur bacteriellen Diagnostik der Diphtherie und der Anginen. *Dtsch. med. Wschr.*, 1894, **20,** 920–23.
"Plaut's angina." He noted the association of fusiform bacilli in ulcerating lesions of the tonsils. Vincent (No. 3309) gave the first comprehensive description of this condition.

3309 VINCENT, JEAN HYACINTHE. 1862–1950
Sur l'étiologie et sur les lésions anatomo-pathologiques de la pourriture d'hôpital. *Ann. Inst. Pasteur*, 1896, **10,** 488–510.
Vincent described a fusiform bacillus and a spirillum which, in association, were responsible for hospital gangrene. Later, in *Arch. int. Laryng.*, 1898, **11**, 44, he showed these two organisms to be present in "Vincent's angina".

3309.1 McBRIDE, PETER. 1854–1946
Photographs of a case of rapid destruction of the nose and face. *J. Laryng.*, 1897, **12,** 64–66.
Malignant granuloma of the nose first described.

3310 GLUCK, THEMISTOKLES. 1853–1942
Kehlkopfchirurgie und Laryngoplastik. *Therap. Gegenw.*, 1899, **40,** 169–79, 202–11.
Gluck improved the technique of laryngectomy.

3311 HAJEK, MARKUS. 1861–1941
Pathologie und Therapie der entzündlichen Erkrankungen der Nebenhöhlen der Nase. Leipzig, *F. Deuticke*, 1899.
Hajek, professor of laryngology in Vienna, particularly distinguished himself by his classical work on the accessory nasal sinuses. A 5th American edition of the book appeared in 1926.

3312 PEREZ, FERNANDO. 1863–1935
Recherches sur la bactériologie de l'ozène. *Ann. Inst. Pasteur*, 1899, **13,** 937–50.
Perez isolated an organism from the nose of patients suffering from ozaena. He named it *Cocco-bacillus foetidus ozaenae*, and considered it to be causally related to the disease.

3313 FREER, OTTO TIGER. 1857–1932
The correction of deflections of the nasal septum with a minimum of traumatism. *J. Amer. med. Assoc.*, 1902, **38,** 636–42; 1903, **41,** 1391–98.
Improvement of Ingals' operation (see No. 3289).

3314 KILLIAN, GUSTAV. 1860–1921
Die Killian'sche Radicaloperation chronischer Stirnhöhleneiterungen. *Arch. Laryng. Rh.in* (*Berl.*), 1903, **13**, 28–88.

Killian devised an operation for the treatment of pathological conditions in the nasal sinuses. It consists of excision of the anterior wall of the frontal sinus, removal of the diseased tissue, and formation of a permanent communication with the nose.

3315 ——. Die submucöse Fensterresektion der Nasenscheidewand. *Arch. Laryng. Rhin.* (*Berl.*), 1904, **16**, 362–87.

3316 KUTTNER, ARTHUR. 1862–
Die entzündlichen Nebenhöhlenerkrankungen der Nase im Röntgenbild. Berlin, Wien, *Urban & Schwarzenberg*, 1908.

The first important work on the radiology of the accessory nasal sinuses.

3317 WAUGH, GEORGE ERNEST. 1875–1940
A simple operation for the complete removal of tonsils, with notes on 900 cases. *Lancet*, 1909, **1**, 1314–15.

Waugh introduced blunt dissection tonsillectomy.

3318 WHILLIS, SAMUEL SHORT. 1870–1953, & PYBUS, FREDERICK CHARLES, 1882–1975
The enucleation of tonsils with the guillotine. *Lancet*, 1910, **2**, 875–78.

Reverse guillotine tonsillectomy.

3319 SLUDER, GREENFIELD. 1865–1928
A method of tonsillectomy by means of a guillotine and the alveolar eminence of the mandible. *J. Amer. med. Ass.*, 1911, **56**, 867–71.

Sluder introduced a tonsillectomy operation in which both the tonsil and its capsule are removed.

3320 PLUMMER, HENRY STANLEY. 1874–1937
Diffuse dilatation of the esophagus without anatomic stenosis (cardiospasm): a report of ninety-one cases. *J. Amer. med. Ass.*, 1912, **58**, 2013–15.

See No. 3321.

3321 VINSON, PORTER PAISLEY. 1890–
A case of cardiospasm with dilatation and angulation of the esophagus. *Med. Clin. N. Amer.*, 1919, **3**, 623–27.

See also his later paper in *Minnesota Med.*, 1922, **5**, 107–08. The syndrome of dysphagia, glossitis, and hypochromic anaemia has become known as the Plummer–Vinson syndrome (see No. 3320). A. Brown Kelly and D. R. Paterson drew attention to it in *J. Laryng.*, 1919, **34**, 285, 289.

3322 HOWARTH, WALTER GOLDIE. 1879–1962
Operations on the frontal sinus. *J. Laryng. Otol.*, 1921, **36**, 417–21.

Conservative treatment of sinusitis.

3323 ULLMANN, EGON VICTOR. 1894–
On the aetiology of the laryngeal papilloma. *Acta oto-laryng.* (*Stockh.*), 1923, **5**, 317–34.

In this classical paper Ullmann reported the transmission of the virus to animals.

3324 LYNCH, ROBERT CLYDE. 1880–
Technic of a pan-sinus operation. *South. med. J.*, 1924, **17**, 289–92.

Independently of Howarth (No. 3322), Lynch devised an operation for the conservative treatment of sinusitis.

3325 PROETZ, Arthur Walter. 1888–1966
Displacement irrigation of nasal sinuses; a new procedure in diagnosis and conservative treatment. *Arch. Otolaryng. (Chicago)*, 1926, **4,** 1–13.
Displacement method of treatment of nasal sinusitis; published in book form, St. Louis, 1931.

3326 THOMSON, *Sir* StClair. 1859–1943, & COLLEDGE, Lionel. 1883–1948
Cancer of the larynx. London, *Kegan Paul*, 1930.

Laryngoscopy; Bronchoscopy

3327 BABINGTON, Benjamin Guy. 1794–1866
[Description of the glottiscope.] *Lond. med. Gaz.*, 1829, **3,** 555.
Babington was responsible for the introduction of laryngoscopy. He demonstrated a crude "glottiscope" to the Hunterian Society on March 18, 1829, but his effort attracted little attention.

3328 LISTON, Robert. 1794–1847
Practical surgery. London, *J. Churchill*, 1837.
On page 350 Liston suggested the use of a mirror which could be used for viewing oedematous tumours of the larynx.

3329 GARCIA, Manuel Patricio Rodriguez. 1805–1906
Observations on the human voice. *Proc. roy. Soc. (Lond.)*, 1854–55, **7,** 399–410.
Garcia, a teacher of singing, invented the modern laryngoscope.

3330 TÜRCK, Ludwig. 1810–1868
Der Kehlkopfrachenspiegel und die Methode seines Gebrauches. *Z. k. k. Ges. Aerzte Wien*, 1858, n.F. **1,** 401–09.
Türck, at first sceptical of Garcia's laryngoscope, later adopted it and claimed from Czermak priority in its clinical employment; these two gentlemen fought one another bitterly for some years over this point.

3331 CZERMAK, Johann Nepomuk. 1828–1873
Physiologische Untersuchungen mit Garcia's Kehlkopfspiegel. *S.B. k. Akad. Wiss. Wien., math.-nat. Cl.*, 1858, **29,** 557–84.
Czermak was the first to demonstrate the utility of the laryngoscope invented by Garcia.

3332 ——. Ueber die Inspektion des Cavum pharyngo-nasale und der Nasenhöhle durch Choanen vermittelst kleiner Spiegel. *Wien. med. Wschr.*, 1859, **9,** 518–20; 1860, **10,** 257–61.
Czermak's method of exploring the nose and nasopharynx with small mirrors.

3333 TÜRCK, Ludwig. 1810–1868
Praktische Anleitung zur Laryngoscopie. Wien, *W. Braumüller*, 1860.

3334 MACKENZIE, *Sir* Morell. 1837–1892
The use of the laryngoscope in diseases of the throat; with an appendix on rhinoscopy. London, *R. Hardwicke*, 1865.

3335 KIRSTEIN, Alfred. 1863–1922
Autoskopie des Larynx und der Trachea. (Laryngoscopia directa, Euthyskopie, Besichtigung ohne Spiegel.) *Arch. Laryng. Rhin. (Berl.)*, 1895, **3,** 156–64.
First direct-vision laryngoscope.

3336 KILLIAN, GUSTAV. 1860–1921
Ueber directe Bronchoskopie. *Münch. med. Wschr.*, 1898, **45**, 844–47.
Introduction of direct bronchoscopy.

3337 JACKSON, CHEVALIER. 1865–1958
Tracheo-bronchoscopy, esophagoscopy and gastroscopy. St. Louis, *Laryngoscope Company*, 1907.
First text-book on endoscopy.

3338 KILLIAN, GUSTAV. 1860–1921
Die Schwebelaryngoscopie. *Arch. Laryng. Rhin.* (*Berl.*), 1912, **26**, 277–317.
Introduction of suspension laryngoscopy. English translation in 1914.

History of Laryngology and Rhinology

3339 CHAUVEAU, CLAUDE.
Histoire des maladies du pharynx. 5 vols. Paris, *J. B. Baillière*, 1901–06.

3340 KASSEL, KARL.
Geschichte der Nasenheilkunde von ihren Anfängen bis zum 18. Jahrhundert. Vol. 1. Würzburg, *C. Kabitsch*, 1914.

3341 WRIGHT, JONATHAN. 1860–1928
A history of laryngology and rhinology. 2nd ed. Philadelphia, *Lea & Febiger*, 1914.

3342 STEVENSON, ROBERT SCOTT. 1889–1967, & GUTHRIE, DOUGLAS JAMES. 1885–1975
A history of oto-laryngology. Edinburgh, *E. & S. Livingstone*, 1949.
From antiquity to the beginning of the 20th century.

3343–3415 OTOLOGY

3343 MERCURIALI, GERONIMO. 1530–1606
De compositione medicamentorum tractatus, tres libros complectens, eiusdem de oculorum et aurium affectionibus praelectiones. Francofurti, *apud J. Wechelum*, 1584.
The De oculorum et aurium represents the first "clinical" manual on diseases of the ear. Mercuriali was primarily concerned with treatment.

3344 BONIFACIO, GIOVANNI.
L'arte de' cenni, con quale, formandosi favella visibile, si tratta della muta eloquenza. Vicenza, *F. Grossi*, 1616.
Bonifacio's sign-language for the deaf and dumb employed almost every part of the body for conversational purposes.

3345 BONET, JUAN PABLO. 1579–1633
Reduction de las letras, y arte para enseñar a ablar los mudos. Madrid, *F. Abarca de Angulo*, 1620.
Bonet put into practice the "combined" system of teaching the deaf to speak and the dumb to communicate with others. He showed how the deaf could be taught to speak by reducing the letters to their phonetic value, and he advocated the use of finger-spelling. It is probable that he learned his system from Pedro Ponce de León (1510–84), another Spaniard, whose writings have been lost. English translation of the book, 1890.

3346 BULWER, John. *fl.* 1654
Chironomia: or, the art of manuall rhetorique. London, *T. Harper*, 1644.

3347 ——. Chirologia: or the naturall language of the hand. Composed of the speaking motions, and discoursing gestures thereof. Whereunto is added Chironomia: or, the art of manuall rhetoricke. London, *T. Harper for H. Twyford*, 1644.

Bulwer was the first Englishman to write about the teaching of deaf-mutes.

3348 WALLIS, John. 1616–1703
De loquela. London, 1652.

Wallis, a prominent teacher of deaf-mutes, classified the various sounds of the human voice. He taught by writing and gesture. He was Savilian professor of mathematics at Oxford.

3349 HOLDER, William. 1616–1698
Elements of speech, an essay of inquiry into the natural production of letters; with an appendix concerning persons deaf and dumb. London *T.N. for J. Msartyn*, 1669.

Includes a section on the education of deaf-mutes.

3350 DALGARNO, George. 1626?–1687
Didascalocophus or the deaf and dumb mans tutor, to which is added a discourse of the nature and number of double consonants: both which tracts being the first (for what the author knows) that have been published upon either of the subjects. Oxford, *T. Halton*, 1680.

Dalgarno considered that the deaf had an advantage over the blind in opportunities of learning languages. He invented an alphabet for the use of deaf-mutes.

3351 DUVERNEY, Joseph Guichard. 1648–1730
Traité de l'organe de l'ouïe, contenant la structure, les usages et les maladies de toutes les parties de l'oreille. Paris, *E. Michallet*, 1683.

First scientific account of the structure, function, and diseases of the ear. English translation, 1737.

3352 AMMAN, Johann Konraad. 1663–1730
Surdus loquens; seu, methodus, quâ qui surdus natus est loqui descere possit. Amstelaedami, 1692.

English translation, 1694.

3353 ——. Dissertatio de loquela, qua non solum vox humana, & loquendi artificium ex originibus suis eruuunter. Amstelaedami, *J. Wolters*, 1700.

Amman's method of instructing deaf-mutes. He was one of the most successful of all teachers in this sphere. English translation, London, 1873.

3354 GUYOT, Edmé Gilles. 1706–1786
[Instrument pour seringuer la trompe d'Eustache par la bouche.] *Hist. Acad. roy. Sci.*, 1724, Paris, 1726, 37.

Guyot, post-master at Versailles, was the first to attempt catheterization of the Eustachian tube. This he did by way of the mouth.

3355 CLELAND, Archibald.

Instruments proposed to remedy some kinds of deafness proceeding from obstructions in the external and internal auditory passages. *Phil. Trans.*, 1744, **41,** 848–51.

Cleland, an army surgeon, devised the method of catheterization of the Eustachian tube by way of the nose; he designed the instruments necessary for the operation.

3356 WATHEN, Jonathan.

A method proposed to restore the hearing, when injured from an obstruction of the tuba Eustachiana. *Phil. Trans.*, 1756, **49,** 213–22.

Wathen condemned Guyot's method of Eustachian catheterization and himself suggested a method of relieving catarrhal deafness by means of injections into the Eustachian tube through a catheter passed into the nose. Wathen was a surgeon practising in London.

3357 PETIT, Jean Louis. 1674–1750

Traité des maladies chirurgicales et des opérations qui leur conviennent. 3 vols. Paris, *P. F. Didot le jeune*, 1774.

Records (pp. 153, 160) the first successful operation for mastoiditis, performed by Petit in 1736.

3358 L'ÉPÉE, Charles Michel de, *Abbé*. 1712–1789

Institution des sourds et muets, par la voie des signes méthodiques. Paris, *Nyon l'aîné*, 1776.

3359 ——. La véritable manière d'instruire les sourds et muets. Paris, *Nyon l'aîné*, 1784.

The Abbé de L'Epée met two deaf girls, decided to educate them, and soon had a class of 60 devoted pupils, whom he supported and amongst whom he lived. He based his methods on those of Bonet and Amman, and was first to attach great importance to signs.

3360 GREEN, Francis.

Vox oculis. A dissertation on the . . . art of imparting speech to the naturally deaf; with a particular account of the academy of Messrs. Braidwood . . . By a parent [F. Green]. London, 1783.

Thomas Braidwood (1715–1806) founded the first British school for the deaf and dumb, in Edinburgh. His method consisted of a combination of lip-reading and signs.

3361 COOPER, *Sir* Astley Paston, *Bart.* 1768–1841

Further observations on the effects which take place from the destruction of the membrana tympani of the ear; with an account of an operation for the removal of a particular species of deafness. *Phil. Trans.*, 1801, **91,** 435–50.

Sir Astley Cooper reported 3 cases of Eustachian obstruction deafness relieved by perforation of the membrana tympani (myringotomy), an operation first performed by Eli, a quack, in 1760. Cooper's earlier paper on the subject appeared in vol. 90 of the *Phil. Trans.* For this work he received the Copley Medal.

3362 SAUNDERS, John Cunningham. 1773–1810

The anatomy of the human ear . . . with a treatise on the diseases of that organ. London, *R. Phillips*, 1806.

Saunders was the first to advise paracentesis in acute middle-ear suppuration.

3363 BOZZINI, PHILIPP. 1773–1809
Der Lichtleiter. Weimar, *Im Verlage des Landes-Industrie-Comptoirs*, 1807.

Bozzini introduced an aural speculum in which the idea of illumination and reflection by mirrors was utilized. Facsimile reproduction and English translation, *Quart. Bull. Northw. Univ. med. Sch.*, 1949, **23**, 332–54.

3364 ITARD, JEAN MARIE GASPARD. 1774–1838
Traité des maladies de l'oreille et de l'audition. 2 vols. Paris, *Méquignon Marvis*, 1821.

First of the modern text-books on diseases of the ear, this work did much to establish otology on a sound basis.

3365 SAISSY, JEAN ANTOINE. 1756–1822
Essai sur les maladies de l'oreille interne. Paris, *Baillière*, 1829.

Saissy described a Eustachian bougie; he was probably the first to use this instrument. Besides dealing with the labyrinth, his book discusses diseases of the tympanum and Eustachian tube. English translation, Baltimore, 1829.

3366 KRAMER, WILHELM. 1801–1875
Erfahrungen über die Erkenntniss und Heilung der langwierigen Schwerhörigkeit. Berlin, *Nicolai*, 1833.

Kramer's first and best work. English translation, 1837.

3367 ——. Die Erkenntniss und Heilung der Ohrenkrankheiten. Berlin, *Nicolai*, 1835.

Kramer was a pioneer German otologist.

3368 WEBER, ERNST HEINRICH. 1795–1878
De pulsu, resorptione, auditu et tactu. Lipsiae, *C. F. Koehler*, 1834.

Weber's hearing test (p. 41).

3369 WILDE, *Sir* WILLIAM ROBERT WILLS. 1815–1876
Practical observations on aural surgery and the nature and treatment of diseases of the ear. London, *J. Churchill*, 1853.

This work did more to place British otology on a sound scientific basis than anything previously published. In his own words, Wilde "laboured to rescue the treatment of ear diseases from empiricism and found it upon the well-established laws of modern pathology, practical surgery and reasonable therapeutics". He showed the middle ear to be the site of origin of most of the diseases of the ear. He is remembered for his method of treating acute mastoiditis, using "Wilde's incision". The book was bitterly attacked by Kramer – see especially *Lancet*, 1853, **2**, 446 – and also by Thomas Wakley, editor of that journal.

3370 RINNE, FRIEDRICH HEINRICH. 1819–1868
Beiträge zur Physiologie des menschlichen Ohres. *Vjschr. prakt. Heilk.*, 1855, **45**, 71–123; **46**, 45–72.

Rinne's test.

3371 FORGET, AMÉDÉE. 1811–1869
De la trépanation de l'apophyse mastoïde et des lésions morbides qui rendent cette opération nécessaire. *Union méd.*, 1860, n.s. **6**, 193–200.

Operative treatment of acute otitis by drainage through the antrum.

3372 MENIÈRE, PROSPER. 1799–1862

Mémoire sur des lésions de l'oreille interne donnant lieu à des symptomes de congestion cérébrale apoplectiforme. *Gaz. méd. Paris*, 1861, **16,** 88–89, 239–40, 379–80, 597–601.

First description of aural vertigo ("Menière's syndrome"). First appeared in summary form in *Bull. Acad. imp. Méd.*, 1860–61, **26**, 241, and in *Gaz. méd. Paris*, 1861, **16**, 29, with title: Sur une forme de surdité grave dépendant d'une lésion de l'oreille interne.

3373 TOYNBEE, JOSEPH. 1815–1866

The diseases of the ear; their nature, diagnosis, and treatment. London, *J. Churchill*, 1860.

A medical classic by the "Father of British otology". In this book Toynbee described the method of removing the temporal bone and discussed the post-mortem appearances in relation to the symptoms observed during life. He made over 2,000 disections of the ear. Toynbee died as a result of a self-experiment while trying out a method of treating tinnitus. His son Arnold Toynbee was the great social worker after whom the university settlement, Toynbee Hall, is named.

3374 TRÖLTSCH, ANTON FRIEDRICH VON. 1829–1890

Die Untersuchung des Gehörgangs und Trommelfells. Ihre Bedeutung. Kritik der bisherigen Untersuchungsmethoden und Angabe einer neuen. *Dtsch. Klinik*, 1860, **12,** 113–15, 121–23, 131–35, 143–46, 151–55.

Invention of the modern otoscope.

3375 ——. Ein Fall von Anbohrung des Warzenfortsatzes bei Otitis interna mit Bemerkungen über diese Operation. *Virchows Arch. path. Anat.*, 1861, **21,** 295–314.

The first modern mastoid operation was devised by von Tröltsch.

3376 ——. Die Krankheiten des Ohres. Würzburg, *Stahel*, 1862.

Tröltsch was professor of otology at Würzburg. He was the founder of the *Archiv für Ohrenheilkunde*. English translation, 1874.

3377 POLITZER, ADAM. 1835–1920

Ueber ein neues Heilverfahren gegen Schwerhörigkeit in Folge von Unwegsamkeit der Eustachischen Ohrtrompete. *Wien. med. Wschr.*, 1863, **13,** 84–87, 102–04, 117–19, 148–52.

Politzer's method of effecting permeability of the Eustachian tube.

3378 ——. Die Beleuchtungsbilder des Trommelfells im gesunden und kranken Zustande. Wien, *W. Braumüller*, 1865.

Politzer was the first to obtain pictures of the membrana tympani by means of illumination. English translation, New York, 1869.

3379 VOLTOLINI, FRIEDRICH EDUARD RUDOLPH. 1819–1889

Die akute Entzündung des heutigen Labyrinthes, gewöhnlich für Meningitis cerebro-spinalis gehalten. *Mschr. Ohrenheilk.*, 1867, **1,** 9–14.

First description of "Voltolini's disease" – an acute painful inflammation of the internal ear, followed by fever, delirium, and loss of consciousness. Voltolini was the founder of the *Monatsschrift*.

3380 WREDEN, ROBERT ROBERTOVICH. 1837–1893

Sechs Fälle von Myringomykosis (Aspergillus glaucus Lk.). *Arch. Ohrenheilk.*, 1867, **3,** 1–21.

Wreden, otologist to the Czar, was the first to call special attention to otomycosis.

3381 LUCAE, AUGUST. 1835–1911
Die Schalleitung durch die Kopfknochen und ihre Bedeutung für die Diagnostik der Ohrenkrankheiten. Würzburg, *Stahel*, 1870.

Lucae was the first to study the transmission of sounds through the cranial bones for the purpose of diagnosing diseases of the ear.

3382 SCHWARTZE, HERMANN HUGO RUDOLF. 1837–1910, & EYSELL, ADOLPH. 1846–
Ueber die künstliche Eröffnung des Warzenfortsatzes. *Arch. Ohrenheilk.*, 1873, n.F. **1,** 157–87.

These workers helped to revive the mastoid operation (which had fallen into disuse), placing it on a modern basis. They described the method of opening the ear by chiselling, "Schwartze's operation".

3383 CHARCOT, JEAN MARTIN. 1825–1893
Vertigo ab aure laesa. *Gaz. Hôp.* (*Paris*), 1874, **47,** 73–74.

Charcot completed the description of the syndrome first described by Menière.

3384 HINTON, JAMES. 1822–1875
Atlas of the membrana tympani. London, *H. S. King*, 1874.

3385 ——. The questions of aural surgery. London, *H. S. King*, 1874.

Hinton was one of the most eminent aural surgeons in England during the latter half of the 19th century, and the first Aural Surgeon to Guy's Hospital. In 1868 he performed the first operation for mastoiditis in England. He proved that aural polypus originated within the tympanum and that cholesteatomata might prove fatal by eroding the bone.

3386 BEZOLD, FRIEDRICH. 1842–1908
Erkrankungen des Warzentheiles. *Arch. Ohrenheilk.*, 1877, **13,** 26–68.

First clear description of mastoiditis.

3387 POLITZER, ADAM. 1835–1920
Lehrbuch der Ohrenheilkunde. 2 pts. Stuttgart, *F. Enke*, 1878–82.

Politzer was one of the greatest of all otologists. He was the first professor of otology in Vienna and his text-book was for many years the standard authority on the subject. English translation, 1883.

3388 ZAUFAL, EMANUEL. 1833–1910
Sinusthrombose in Folge von Otitis media. [Trepanation des Proc. mastoid mit Hammer und Meissel.] *Prag. med. Wschr.*, 1884, **9,** 474–475.

Improvement of the mastoid operation devised by Schwartze and Eysell.

3389 SCHWABACH, DAGOBERT. 1846–1920
Ueber den Werth des Rinne'schen Versuches für die Diagnostik der Gehörkrankheiten. *Z. Ohrenheilk.*, 1885, **14,** 61–148.

Schwabach's nystagmus test.

3390 ARNOLD, THOMAS.
Education of deaf-mutes. London, *Wertheimer, Lea & Co.*, 1888.

Includes a history of the subject.

3391 BERGMANN, ERNST VON. 1836–1907
Krankenvorstellung: Geheilter Hirnabscess. *Berl. klin. Wschr.*, 1888, **25,** 1054–56.

Radical mastoidectomy. (See No. 3392.)

3392 KÜSTER, Ernst Georg Ferdinand von. 1839–1930
Ueber die Grundsätze der Behandlung von Eiterungen in starrwandigen Höhlen, mit besonderer Berücksichtigung des Empyems der Pleura. *Dtsch. med. Wschr.*, 1889, **15,** 254–57.

Küster and von Bergmann developed the operation of radical mastoidectomy.

3393 STACKE, Ludwig. 1859–1918
Indicationen, betreffend die Excision von Hammer und Amboss. *Verh. X. int. med. Congr. Berlin*, 1890, **4,** xi Abt., 43–46.

Stacke introduced the operation of excision of the ossicles.

3394 ——. Weitere Mittheilungen über die operative Freilegung der Mittelohrräume nach Ablösung der Ohrmuschel. *Berl. klin. Wschr.*, 1892, **29,** 68–71.

Stacke did much to improve the surgery of the middle ear. He made important modifications in the radical mastoidectomy operation of Küster and von Bergmann.

3395 POLITZER, Adam. 1835–1920
On a peculiar affection of the labyrinthine capsule as a frequent cause of deafness. *Trans. 1st Panamer. med. Congr.*, (1893), 1895, pt. 3, 1607–08.

First report of otosclerosis as a separate clinical entity.

3396 BEZOLD, Friedrich. 1842–1908
Ueber die funktionelle Prüfung des menschlichen Gehörorgans. 3 vols. Wiesbaden, *J. F. Bergmann*, 1897–1909.

Bezold introduced important tests for audition.

3397 PASSOW, Adolf. 1859–1926
Verh. dtsch. otol. Ges., 1897, **6,** 143.

First attempt at improving hearing by fenestration. No title; forms part of a paper by R. Passe.

3398 GRADENIGO, Guiseppe. 1859–1926
Sulla leptomeningite circonscritta e sulla paralisi dell' abducente di origine otitica. *G. roy. Accad. Med. Torino*, 1904, 4 ser., **10,** 59–64, 361–67.

"Gradenigo's syndrome" – acute otitis media followed by abductor paralysis. Translation of the paper is in the German *Arch. Orhenheilk.*, 1904, **62,** 255–70.

3399 KELLER, Helen Adams. 1880–1968
The story of my life. New York, *Grosset & Dunlap*, 1905.

Helen Keller was born blind and deaf. Her education was a triumph of patience and skill on the part of her teacher, Anne M. Sullivan, and a demonstration of the great possibilities in the teaching of the blind-deaf. Hellen Keller studied French, German, Latin, Greek, arithmetic, algebra, geometry, history, poetry and literature.

3400 BÁRÁNY, Robert. 1876–1936
Ueber die vom Ohrlabyrinth ausgelöste Gegenrollung der Augen bei Normalhörenden. *Arch. Ohrenheilk.*, 1906, **68,** 1–30.

Bárány's caloric test for labyrinthine function.

3401 ——. Untersuchungen über den vom Vestibularapparat des Ohres reflektorisch ausgelösten rhythmischen Nystagmus und seine Begleiterscheinungen. *Mschr. Ohrenheilk.*, 1906, **40,** 193–297; 1907, **41,** 477–526.

Bárány's pointing test for the localization of circumscribed cerebellar lesions. Republished in book form, Berlin, 1906. He was awarded the Nobel Prize in 1914 for his work on the vestibular apparatus.

3402 ——. Vestibularapparat und Zentralnervensystem. *Med. Klin.*, 1911, **7,** 1818–21.

"Bárány's syndrome" – unilateral deafness, vertigo, and pain in the occipital region.

3403 JENKINS, George John. ?–1939
Otosclerosis: certain clinical features and experimental operative procedures. *17th Int. Congr. Med.*, London, 1913, Sect. **16,** 609–18.

Jenkins suggested the modern fenestration operation for otosclerosis.

3404 HOLMGREN, Gunnar. 1875–1954
Some experiences in the surgery of otosclerosis. *Acta oto-laryng.* (*Stockh.*), 1923, **5,** 460–66.

Holmgren's fenestration operation.

3405 GRAY, Albert Alexander. 1869–1936
Atlas of otology illustrating the normal and pathological anatomy of the temporal bone. 2 vols. Glasgow, *Maclehose* (*Jackson*), 1924–33.

3406 DANDY, Walter Edward. 1886–1946
Ménière's disease; its diagnosis and a method of treatment. *Arch. Surg.* (*Chicago*), 1928, **16,** 1127–52.

Dandy's operation for relief of Menière's syndrome.

3407 MAYER, Ernst Georg. 1893–
Otologische Röntgendiagnostik. Wien, *J. Springer*, 1930.

Includes a brief history of the subject.

3408 SOURDILLE, Maurice Louis Joseph Marie. 1885–
New technique in the surgical treatment of severe and progressive deafness from otosclerosis. *Bull. N.Y. Acad. Med.*, 1937, **13,** 673–91.

First successful attempt to restore hearing in otosclerosis by fenestration.

3409 HALLPIKE, Charles Skinner. 1900– , & CAIRNS, *Sir* Hugh William Bell. 1896–1952
Observations on the pathology of Ménière's syndrome. *Proc. roy. Soc. Med.*, 1938, **31,** 1317–36.

Hallpike and Cairns were first to describe the characteristic histological changes in Menière's disease. Also published in *J. Laryngol.*, 1938, **53**, 625–55.

3410 LEMPERT, Julius. 1890–
Improvements of hearing in cases of otosclerosis: a new, one-stage surgical technic. *Arch. Otolaryng.* (*Chicago*), 1938, **28,** 42–97.

Lempert's operation.

3411 KOPETZKY, Samuel Joseph. 1876–1950
History and present status of operations on the labyrinthine capsule for otosclerosis. *Surg. Gynec. Obstet.*, 1941, **72,** 466–89.

Kopetzky improved the technique of the fenestration operation. The above has a useful history of the development of this operation. See also his earlier papers in *Ann. Otol.* (*St. Louis*), 1930, **39**, 996; 1931, **40**, 157.

3412 SHAMBAUGH, George Elmer. 1903–
The surgical treatment of deafness. *Illinois med. J.*, 1942, **81**, 104–08.
Shambaugh improved the technique of the fenestration operation. See also *Ann. Otol.* (*St. Louis*), 1942, **51**, 817–25.

3412.1 ROSEN, Samuel. 1897–
Mobilization of the stapes to restore hearing in otosclerosis. *New York St. J. Med.*, 1953, **53**, 2650–53.

History of Otology

3413 POLITZER, Adam. 1835–1920
Geschichte der Ohrenheilkunde. 2 vols. Stuttgart, *F. Enke*, 1907–13.
It is fitting that Politzer should have been the greatest historian of otology. He was professor of otology in Vienna and his teaching had great influence upon the advancement of the subject. The *Geschichte* is a masterpiece of historical research.

3414 PAYNE, Arnold Hill.
Deaf and dumb. Education. *Encyclopaedia Britannica*, 11th ed., Cambridge, 1910, **7**, 887–94.
History and methods of teaching deaf-mutes and blind-deaf.

3415 STEVENSON, Robert Scott. 1889–1967, & GUTHRIE, Douglas James. 1885–1975
A history of oto-laryngology. Edinburgh, *E. & S. Livingstone*, 1949.

3416–3760 DISEASES OF THE DIGESTIVE SYSTEM

GENERAL WORKS; OESOPHAGUS; STOMACH; INTESTINES

3416–3558

3416 JOHN *of Arderne*. 1307–1380
Treatises of fistula in ano, haemorrhoids, and clysters. Edited by Sir D'Arcy Power. London, *Kegan Paul*, 1910.
John of Arderne's most important contribution to surgery was his operation for the cure of anal fistula. This was written about 1376. At one time John of Arderne practised at Newark-on-Trent; he moved to London in 1370.

3417 DONATI, Marcello [Donatus]. 1538–1602
De medica historia mirabili. Mantuae, *per Fr. Osanam*, 1586.
Lib. IV, Cap. iii page 196: First recorded case of gastric ulcer.

3418 LITTRE, Alexis. 1658–1726
Diverses observations anatomiques. *Hist. Acad. roy. Sci.* (*Paris*), (1710), 1732, 36–37.
Littre was first to suggest colostomy in intestinal obstruction – "Littre's operation."

3419 BLAIR, Patrick. 166–?–1728
An account of the dissection of a child. *Phil. Trans.*, 1717, **30**, 631–32.
First description of congenital hypertrophic pyloric stenosis.

3420 RAWLINSON, Christopher.
A preternatural perforation found in the upper part of the stomach, with the symptoms it produc'd. *Phil. Trans.*, 1727, **35**, 361–62.
First reported case of perforating gastric ulcer.

3421 STAHL, GEORG ERNST. 1660–1734
Abhandlung von der goldenen Ader. Leipzig, *C. J. Eysel*, 1729.
A classical work on haemorrhoids.

3422 CALDER, JAMES.
Two examples of children born with preternatural conformations of the guts. *Med. Essays Obs. Edinb.*, 1733, **1**, 203–06.
First description of congenital atresia of the ileum.

3423 VELSE, CORNELIUS HENRIK.
De mutuo intestinorum ingressu. Lugduni Batavorum, *J. Luzac*, 1742.
First recorded successful operation for intussusception in an adult. The paper is also included in Haller's Disputationes, vol, 1.

3424 HAMBERGER, GEORG ERHARD. 1697–1755
De ruptura intestini duodeni. Jenae, *lit. Ritterianis*, [1746].
First description of duodenal ulcer.

3424.1 KALTSCHMIED, CARL FRIEDRICH. 1706–1769
De tumore scirrhoso trium cum quadrante librarum glandulae parotidis extirpato. Jenae, *Lit. Tennemannianis*, 1752.
First description of parotid tumour.

3425 ARMSTRONG, GEORGE. 1719–1789
An account of the diseases most incident to children, from their birth till the age of puberty. London, *T. Cadell*, 1777.
Page 49: Important description of congenital hypertrophic pyloric stenosis.

3426 BEARDSLEY, HEZEKIAH. 1748–1790
Case of a scirrhus in the pylorus of an infant. *Cases Obs. med. Soc. New-Haven Co.*, 1788, 81–84.
First American case report on congenital hypertrophic pyloric stenosis. Reprinted in *Arch. Pediat.*, 1903, **20**, 355–57.

3427 BAILLIE, MATTHEW. 1761–1823
The morbid anatomy of some of the most important parts of the human body. London, *J. Johnson & G. Nicol*, 1793.
Page 87: First clear description of the morbid anatomy and symptoms of gastric ulcer.

3428 PENADA, JACOPO. 1748–1828
Saggio d'osservazioni, e memorie sopra alcuni case singolari riscontrati nell' esercizio della medicina, e della anatomia pratica. Padova, *Penada*, 1793.
Includes (pp. 33–56) an account of perforating duodenal ulcer.

3429 DURET, C.
Observation sur un enfant né sans anus, et auquel il a été fait une ouverture pour y suppléer. *Rec. périod. Soc. Méd. Paris*, 1798, **4**, 45–50.
First successful construction of artificial anus, for congenital atresia, Oct. 20, 1793.

3430 FINE, PIERRE. 1760–1814
Mémoire et observation sur l'entérotomie. *Ann. Soc. Méd. prat. Montpellier*, 1805, **6**, 34–54.
The first recorded colostomy for intestinal obstruction was performed by Fine in 1797. The patient survived 3½ months.

3431 MERREM, Daniel Carl Theodor. 1790–1859
Animadversiones quaedam chirurgicae experimentis in animalibus factis illustratae. Giessiae, *Tasché et Mueller*, 1810.
Experimental excision of the pylorus.

3432 PHYSICK, Philip Syng. 1768–1837
Account of a new mode of extracting poisonous substances from the stomach. *Eclectic Repert.*, 1812–13, **3,** 111, 381.
Physick was the first, in 1805, to use a stomach tube for gastric lavage in a case of poisoning. He acknowledged the priority of Monro *secundus* in the invention of a similar instrument in 1767. For history of the stomach tube, see R. H. Major, *Ann. med. Hist.*, 1934, N.S. **6**, 500–09.

3433 TRAVERS, Benjamin. 1783–1858
An inquiry into the process of nature in repairing injuries of the intestines. London, *Longman*, 1812.
Travers' researches on intestinal sutures recorded the first accurate knowledge on this subject.

3434 BÉCLARD, Pierre Augustin. 1785–1825
Extirpation de la parotide. *Arch. gén. Méd.*, 1824, **4,** 60–66.
First excision of the parotid, 1823.

3435 LEMBERT, Antoine. 1802–1851
Mémoire sur l'entéroraphie avec la description d'un procédé nouveau pour pratiquer cette opération chirurgicale. *Rep. gén. Anat. Physiol. path.*, 1826, **2,** 100–07.
Description of what is now known as Lembert's suture, which ensures that serous surface is applied to serous surface in suturing intestine – the foundation of all modern gastric and intestinal surgery. Dieffenbach (No. 3441) was the first successfully to employ Lembert's method.

3436 PHYSICK, Philip Syng. 1768–1837
Extracts from an account of a case in which a new and peculiar operation for artificial anus was performed. *Philad. J. med. phys. Sci.*, 1826, **13,** 199–202.
Physick's operation for artificial anus.

3437 DUPUYTREN, Guillaume, *le baron*. 1777–1835
Mémoire sur une méthode nouvelle pour traiter les anus accidentels. *Mém. Acad. roy. Méd. (Paris)*, 1828, Sect. Méd., **1,** 259–316.
Dupuytren invented an enterotome to perform his operation for artificial anus.

3438 ——. Abcès développé dans le petit bassin. *Rev. méd. franç. étrang.*, 1829, **1,** 367–68.
"Dupuytren's abscess" of the right iliac fossa.

3439 JOBERT DE LAMBALLE, Antoine Joseph. 1799–1867
Traité théorique et pratique des maladies chirurgicales du canal intestinal. 2 vols. Paris, *Mme. Auger-Méquignon*, 1829.
Jobert, famous French surgeon, made his reputation on this book. He was at one time Consulting Physician to Louis XVIII.

3440 BRODIE, *Sir* Benjamin Collins, *Bart.* 1783–1862
Lectures on diseases of the rectum. III. Preternatural contraction of the sphincter ani. *Lond. med. Gaz.*, 1835, **16,** 26–31.
"Brodie's pile." Reprinted in *Med. Classics*, 1938, **2,** 929–40.

3441 DIEFFENBACH, JOHANN FRIEDRICH. 1792–1847
Glückliche Heilung nach Ausscheidung eines Theiles des Darms und Netzes. *Wschr. ges. Heilk.*, 1836, 401–13.
First account of a resection in which Lembert's suture was successfully employed.

3442 AMUSSAT, JEAN ZULÉMA. 1796–1856
Mémoire sur la possibilité d'établir un anus artificiel dans la région lombaire sans pénétrer dans le péritoine. Paris, *G. Baillière*, 1839.
In 1839 Amussat performed the first lumbar colostomy for obstruction of the colon ("Amussat's operation"). His work established lumbar colostomy as the method of choice.

3443 PILLORE.
Opération d'anus artificiel, par la méthode de Littre, sur un homme adulte qui a survécu vingt-huit hours. In: AMUSSAT J. Z., *Mémoire sur la possibilité d'établir un anus artificiel*, Paris, 1829, pp. 85–88.
Pillore performed caecostomy in 1776, the patient surviving 28 days. Amussat went to considerable trouble to find the document describing the operation.

3444 BÉRARD, AUGUSTE. 1802–1846
Maladies de la glande parotide et de la région parotidienne. Paris, *Germer-Baillière*, 1841.
First important treatise on parotid tumours.

3445 CURLING, THOMAS BLIZARD. 1811–1888
On acute ulceration of the duodenum, in cases of burn. *Med.-chir. Trans.*, 1842, **25**, 260–81.
"Curling's ulcer." Although not first to report duodenal ulcers as a complication of burns, Curling correlated the work of previous writers on the subject and directed attention to it.

3446 GROSS, SAMUEL DAVID. 1805–1884
An experimental and critical inquiry into the nature and treatment of wounds of the intestines. Louisville, *Prentice & Weissinger*, 1843.

3447 REYBARD, JEAN FRANÇOIS. 1790–1863
Mémoire sur une tumeur cancéreuse affectant l'S iliaque du colon; ablation de la tumeur et de l'intestin; réunion directe et immédiate des deux bouts de cet organe. Guérison. *Bull. Acad. roy. Méd. (Paris)*, 1844, **9**, 1031–43.
First intestinal resection for cancer.

3448 WATSON, JOHN. 1807–1863
Practical observations on organic obstruction of the oesophagus; preceded by a case which called for oesophagotomy and subsequent opening of the trachea. *Amer. J. med. Sci.*, 1844, n.s., **8**, 309–31.
First oesophagotomy for relief of stricture of the oesophagus.

3449 BIRD, GOLDING. 1814–1854, & HILTON, JOHN. 1804–1878
Case of internal strangulation of intestine relieved by operation. *Med.-chir. Trans.*, 1847, **30**, 51–67.
Records the first operation for internal strangulation of the small intestine by Hilton at Guy's Hospital. No anaesthetic was used; the patient died nine hours afterwards.

3450 LEIDY, JOSEPH. 1823–1891
On the existence of Entophyta in healthy animals, as a natural condition. *Proc. Acad. nat. Sci. (Philad.)*, 1848–49, **4,** 225–33.
Discovery of the bacterial flora of the intestines.

3451 SÉDILLOT, CHARLES EMMANUEL. 1804–1883
De la gastrotomie fistuleuse. *C. R. Acad. Sci. (Paris)*, 1846, **23,** 222–227.
First gastrostomy.

3452 FENGER, CARL EMIL. 1814–1884
Ueber Anlegung einer künstlichen Magenöffnung am Menschen durch Gastrotomie. *Virchows Arch. path. Anat.*, 1854, **6,** 350–84.
Fenger's operation.

3453 BERGERON, ETIENNE JULES. 1817–1900
Note sur l'emploi du chlorate de potasse dans le traitement de la stomatite ulcéreuse. *Rec. Mém. Méd. mil.*, 1855, 2 sér., **16,** 1–46.
Classical description of ulcero-membranous stomatitis and its treatment.

3454 BRINTON, WILLIAM. 1823–1867
On the pathology, symptoms, and treatment of ulcer of the stomach. London, *J. Churchill*, 1857.
A comprehensive account of peptic ulcer; includes a review of the results of more than 7,000 post-mortems.

3455 MALMSTEN, PEHR HENRIK. 1811–1883
Infusorier, såsom intestinaldjur hos menniskan. *Hygiea (Stockh.)*, 1857, **19,** 491–501.
Discovery of *Balantidium coli*, the first parasitic protozoon to be discovered and recognized as such. German translation in *Allg. med. Central-Ztg*, 1858, **27,** 81–89.

3456 MIDDELDORPF, ALBRECHT THEODOR. 1824–1868
De polypis oesophagi atque de tumore ejus generis primo prospere exstirpato. Vratislavae, *apud Max & Soc.*, 1857.
First operation for tumour of the oesophagus.

3457 FORSTER, JOHN COOPER. 1824–1896
Description of the operation of gastrotomy. *Guy's Hosp. Rep.*, 1858, 3 ser., **4,** 13–18.
First gastrostomy in Britain.

3458 BRINTON, WILLIAM. 1823–1867
The diseases of the stomach. London, *J. Churchill*, 1859.
Includes (pp. 310–31) original description of linitis plastica ("Brinton's disease"). Brinton lectured on physiology and forensic medicine at St. Thomas's Hospital.

3459 MIDDELDORPF, ALBRECHT THEODOR. 1824–1868
Commentatio de fistulis ventriculi externis et chirurgica earum sanatione. Vratislaviae, *apud Max & Soc.*, 1859.
First operation for gastric fistula.

3460 LUSCHKA, HUBERT VON. 1820–1875
Ueber polypöse Vegetationen der gesammten Dickdarmschleimhaut. *Virchows Arch. path. Anat.*, 1861, **20,** 133–42.
First authentic description of polyposis of the colon.

3461 KRAUSS, JULIUS. 1841–
Das perforirende Geschwür im Duodenum. Berlin, *A. Hirschwald*, 1865.
First comprehensive study of duodenal ulcer.

3462 BRINTON, WILLIAM. 1823–1867
Intestinal obstruction. London, *J. Churchill*, 1867.

3463 KUSSMAUL, ADOLF. 1822–1902
Ueber die Behandlung der Magenerweiterung durch eine neue Methode (mittelst der Magenpumpe). *Dtsch. Arch. klin. Med.*, 1869, **6,** 455–500.
In 1867 Kussmaul used the stomach pump for gastric dilatation due to pyloric obstruction. Although his advocacy of gastric lavage established this method of treatment in medical practice, the instrument had already been used many years previously.

3464 MAURY, FRANCIS F. 1840–1879
Case of stricture of the oesophagus in which gastrotomy was performed. *Amer. J. med. Sci.*, 1870, **59,** 365–71.
First in America.

3465 BILLROTH, CHRISTIAN ALBERT THEODOR. 1829–1894
Ueber die Resection des Oesophagus. *Arch. klin. Chir.*, 1872, **13,** 65–69.
First resection of the oesophagus.

3466 HUTCHINSON, *Sir* JONATHAN. 1828–1913
A successful case of abdominal section for intussusception. *Med.-chir. Trans.*, 1874, **57,** 31–75.
In 1871 Hutchinson was the first successfully to operate in a case of intussusception in an infant.

3467 JONES, SYDNEY. 1831–1913
Gastrostomy for stricture (cancerous?) of oesophagus; death from bronchitis forty days after operation. *Lancet*, 1875, **1,** 678–79.
Successful human gastrostomy by the older (Sédillot's) method. Reported by S. Osborne.

3468 VERNEUIL, ARISTIDE AUGUST STANISLAS. 1823–1895
Observation de gastro-stomie pratiquée avec succès pour un rétrécissement cicatriciel infranchissable de l'oesophage. *Bull. Acad. Méd.* (*Paris*), 1876, 2 sér., **5,** 1023–38.
Verneuil's gastrostomy operation, a modification of Sédillot's method.

3469 LINDSTEDT, ADOLF FREDRIK. 1847–1915, & WALDENSTRÖM, JOHAN ANTON. 1839–1879
Volvulus flexurae sigmoideae coli – Laparo-colotomia – Helsa. *Upsala LäkFören. Forh.*, 1878–79, **14,** 513–27.
First recorded operation for volvulus.

3470 VOLKMANN, RICHARD VON. 1830–1889
Ueber den Mastdarmkrebs und die Exstirpatio recti. *Samml. klin. Vortr.*, 1878, Nr. 131 (Chir., Nr. 42), 1113–28.
First excision of the rectum for cancer.

3471 EWALD, CARL ANTON. 1845–1915
Klinik der Verdauungskrankheiten. 3 vols. Berlin, *A. Hirschwald*, 1879–1902.

An important work on disorders of digestion. With Boas, Ewald devised the test breakfast and he utilized intubation for exploring the contents of the stomach. English translation of vols. 1–2, 1891–92.

3472 PÉAN, JULES ÉMILE. 1830–1898
De l'ablation des tumeurs de l'estomac par la gastrectomie. *Gaz. Hôp. (Paris)*, 1879, **52,** 473–75.

First gastrectomy for carcinoma; unsuccessful.

3473 KOCHER, EMIL THEODOR. 1841–1917
Ueber Radicalheilung des Krebses. *Dtsch. Z. Chir.*, 1880, **13,** 134–66.

Kocher's operation of radical extirpation of the tongue for carcinoma.

3473.1 RYDYGIER, LUDWIK. 1850–1920
Wycięcie raka odźwiernika zołądkowego, śmierć w 12 godzinach. *Przegl. lek.*, 1880, **19,** 637–39.

First extirpation of carcinomatous pylorus. Death after 12 hours. German translation in *Dtsch. Z. Chir.*, 1881, 14, 252–60.

3474 BILLROTH, CHRISTIAN ALBERT THEODOR. 1829–1894
Offenes Schreiben an Herrn Dr. L. Wittelshöfer. *Wien. med. Wschr.*, 1881, **31,** 161–65, 1427.

First successful resection of the pylorus for cancer, the Billroth I operation.

3475 MIKULICZ-RADECKI, JOHANN VON. 1850–1905
Ueber Gastroskopie und Oesophagoskopie. *Wien med. Presse*, 1881, **22,** 1405–08, 1437–43, 1473–75, 1505–07, 1537–41, 1573–77, 1629–31.

Mikulicz was the first to use the electric oesophagoscope invented by Leiter in 1880. He was among the most distinguished of Billroth's pupils and contributed much to cancer surgery.

3476 WÖLFLER, ANTON. 1850–1917
Gastro-Enterostomie. *Zbl. Chir.*, 1881, **8,** 705–08.

Wölfler perfected the operation of gastro-enterostomy.

3477 LORETA, PIETRO. 1831–1889
Intorno alla divulsione digitale del pilore; osservazione cliniche. *Mem. reale Accad. Sci. Ist. Bologna*, 1882, 4 ser., **4,** 353–75.

First pyloroplasty, 1882. Abstract in English in *Brit. med. J.*, 1885, 1, 372–74.

3478 REICHMANN, MIKOLAJ. 1851–1918
Przypadek chorobowo wzmożonego wydzielania soku żołądkowego. *Gaz. Lek.*, 1882, 2 ser., **2,** 516–22.

First description of gastrosuccorrhoea ("Reichmann's disease"). German translation in *Berl. klin. Wschr.*, 1882, 19, 606.

3479 CLARK, HENRY EDWARD. 1845–1909
On a case of obstruction of the bowels due to volvulus, treated by abdominal section; recovery. *Lancet*, 1881, **2,** 678–80.

First successful operation in Britain for treatment of volvulus, performed Feb. 20, 1883.

3480 HAUER, ERNST.
Darmresektion und Enterorhaphieen, 1878–83. *Z. Heilk.*, 1884, **5,** 83–108.

Billroth was a pioneer in visceral surgery. Above is an account of many intestinal resections and enterorrhaphies carried out by him.

3481 FINKLER, Dittmar. 1852–1912, & PRIOR, J.
Untersuchungen über Cholera nostras. *Dtsch. med. Wschr.*, 1884, **10,** 579–82.

Finkler and Prior isolated *Vibrio proteus* from stools in a vase of acute gastroenteritis.

3482 TREVES, *Sir* Frederick, *Bart.* 1853–1923
Intestinal obstruction. London, *Cassell & Co.*, 1884.

Jacksonian Prize Essay.

3482.1 ALLCHIN, *Sir* William Henry. 1846–1912
Case of acute extensive ulceration of the colon. *Trans. path. Soc. Lond.*, 1885, **36,** 199–202.

First detailed description of ulcerative colitis.

3483 HACKER, Viktor von. 1852–1933
Zur Casuistik und Statistik der Magenresectionen und Gastroenterostomieen. *Verh. dtsch. Ges. Chir.*, 1885, **14,** Pt. II, 62–71.

Billroth II pylorectomy, reported by von Hacker. Also published in *Arch. klin. Chir.*, 1885, 32, 616–25.

3484 GLÉNARD, Frantz. 1848–1920
Application de la méthode naturelle à l'analyse de la dyspepsie nerveuse. – Détermination d'une espèce. *Lyon méd.*, 1885, **48,** 449–64, 492–505, 532–43, 563–83; **49,** 8–28.

Important description of enteroptosis and gastroptosis.

3485 ——. Enteroptose et neurasthénie. *Sem. méd. (Paris)*, 1886, **6,** 211–212.

Splanchnoptosis ("Glénard's disease").

3486 HACKER, Viktor von. 1852–1933
Ueber die Verwendung des Musculus rectus abdominis zum Verschlusse der künstlichen Magenfistel. *Wien. med. Wschr.*, 1886, **36,** 1073–77, 1110–14.

Von Hacker's method of gastrostomy.

3487 MIKULICZ-RADECKI, Johann von. 1850–1905
Ein Fall von Resection des carcinomatösen Oesophagus mit plastischem Ersatz des excidierten Stückes. *Prag. med. Wschr.*, 1886, **11,** 93–94.

Von Mikulicz was the first to make a plastic reconstruction of the oesophagus after the resection of its cervical portion for carcinoma.

3488 HALSTED, William Stewart. 1852–1922
Circular suture of the intestines; an experimental study. *Amer. J. med. Sci.*, 1887, **94,** 436–61.

3489 HIRSCHSPRUNG, Harald. 1831–1916
Stuhlträgheit Neugeborener in Folge von Dilatation und Hyper trophie des Colons. *Jb. Kinderheilk.*, 1887–88, n.F. **27,** 1–7.

Hirschsprung's disease (congenital megacolon).

3490 KRASKE, Paul. 1851–1930
Die sacrale Methode der Exstirpation von Mastdarmkrebsen und die Resectio recti. *Berl. klin. Wschr.*, 1887, **24,** 899–904.

Kraske introduced the sacral method of resection of the rectum for carcinoma.

3491 GEE, Samuel Jones. 1839–1911
On the coeliac affection. *St. Barth. Hosp. Rep.*, 1888, **24,** 17–20.
Coeliac disease (non-tropical sprue, idiopathic steatorrhoea) was first described by Gee. Later Thaysen (No. 3550) studied the disease, which acquired the eponym "Gee–Thaysen disease".

3492 MAYDL, Karel. 1853–1913
Zur Technik der Kolotomie. *Zbl. Chir.*, 1888, **15,** 433–39.
First successful colostomy.

3493 MIKULICZ-RADECKI, Johann von. 1850–1905
Zur operativen Behandlung des Prolapsus recti et coli invaginati. *Verh. dtsch. Ges. Chir.*, 1888, **17,** 294–317.
Description of Mikulicz's important operation for complete prolapse of the rectum.

3494 SENN, Nicholas. 1844–1908
Rectal insufflation of hydrogen gas an infallible test in the diagnosis of visceral injury of the gastro-intestinal canal in penetrating wounds of the abdomen. *J. Amer. med. Ass.*, 1888, **10,** 767–77.
Senn's method of detecting intestinal perforation by insufflation with hydrogen.

3495 EINHORN, Max. 1862–1953
Die Gastrodiaphanie. *N.Y. med. Mschr.*, 1889, **1,** 559.
Einhorn devised the method of exploration of the stomach by means of a tube – gastro-diaphany.

3496 BOAS, Ismar Isidor. 1858–1938
Ueber Darmsaftgewinnung beim Menschen. (Vorläufige Mittheilung.) *Zbl. klin. Med.*, 1889, **10,** 97–99.
Duodenal aspiration.

3497 ——. Diagnostik und Therapie der Magenkrankheiten. 2 pts. Leipzig, *G. Thieme*, 1890–93.
Boas, who devised the test breakfast, became the foremost gastro-enterologist in Europe. He founded the *Archiv für Verdauungskrankheiten*, the first journal devoted to the subject of gastro-enterology.

3498 CHIARI, Hans. 1851–1916
Ueber Magensyphilis. *Int. Beitr. wiss. Med.*, Festschr. R. Virchow, Berlin, 1891, **2,** 295–321.
Important study of gastric syphilis.

3499 PAUL, Frank Thomas. 1851–1941
A method of performing inguinal colotomy, with cases. *Brit. med. J.*, 1891, **2,** 118.
Paul's tube introduced.

3500 SAHLI, Hermann. 1856–1933
Ueber eine neue Untersuchungsmethode der Verdauungsorgane und einige Resultate derselben. *KorrespBl. schweiz. Aerzte*, 1891, **21,** 65–74.
Sahli's test for estimating the functional activity of the stomach.

3501 ABBE, Robert. 1851–1928
Intestinal anastomosis and suturing. *Med. Rec. (N.Y.)*, 1892, **41,** 365–70.
Abbe, a New York surgeon, introduced catgut rings for intestinal suturing. See also *Med. News (Phila.)*, 1889, **54,** 589–92.

3502 BLOCH, Oscar Thorvald. 1847–1926
Om extra-abdominal Behandlung af cancer intestinalis (rectum derfra undtaget) med en Fremstilling af de for denne Sygdom foretagne Operationer og deres Resultater. *Nord. med. Ark.*, 1892, N.F. **2,** 1 Heft, 1–76; 2 Heft, 1–10.

Bloch was first to employ the two-stage (Mikulicz) operation for cancer of the colon. (See also No. 3527.)

3503 EINHORN, Max. 1862–1953
On achylia gastrica. *Med. Rec. (N.Y.)*, 1892, **41,** 650–54.

Einhorn introduced the concept of achylia gastrica, to indicate a primary nervous functional disorder of the gastric secretion.

3504 JABOULAY, Mathieu. 1860–1913
De la gastro-duodénostomie. *Arch. prov. Chir. (Paris)*, 1892, **1,** 551–554.

Introduction of gastroduodenostomy.

3505 KRIEGE, Hermann.
Ein Fall von einem frei in die Bauchhöhle perforirten Magengeschwür; Laparotomie; Naht der Perforationsstelle; Heilung. *Berl. klin. Wschr.*, 1892, **29,** 1244–47, 1280–84.

In 1892 Ludwig Heusner (1846–1916) successfully sutured a perforated gastric ulcer, the first successful case on record. It was reported by H. Kriege.

3506 MIKULICZ-RADECKI, Johann von. 1850–1905
Ueber eine eigenartige symmetrische Erkrankung der Thränen- und Mundspeicheldrüsen. In: *Beiträge zur Chirurgie. Festschrift gewid. T. Billroth*, Stuttgart, 1892, 610–30.

First description of the syndrome of symmetrical inflammation of the lacrymal and salivary glands ("Mikulicz's disease"). English translation in *Medical Classics*, 1937, 2, 165–86.

3507 MURPHY, John Benjamin. 1857–1916
Cholecysto-intestinal, gastro-intestinal, entero-intestinal anastomosis, and approximation without sutures. *Med. Rec. (N.Y.)*, 1892, **42,** 665–76.

"Murphy's button" introduced.

3508 FRANK, Rudolf. 1862–1913
Eine neue Methode der Gastrostomie bei Carcinoma oesophagi. *Wien. klin. Wschr.*, 1893, **6,** 231–34.

See No. 3512.

3509 PÉNIÈRES, L.
De la gastrostomie par la méthode de la valvule ou du plissement de la muqueuse stomacale. *Arch. prov. Chir. (Paris)*, 1893, **2,** 284–93.

Pénières of Toulouse conceived the idea of the valvular method of gastrostomy.

3510 PERRY, *Sir* Edwin Cooper. 1856–1938, & SHAW, Lauriston Elgie. 1859–1923.
On diseases of the duodenum. *Guy's Hosp. Rep.*, 1893, **50,** 171–308.

A careful examination of the records of post-mortems carried out at Guy's Hospital, 1826–92, was made by Perry & Shaw, who showed that of 70 reports of duodenal ulcer 10 occurred in cases of severe burns.

3511 SENN, NICHOLAS. 1844–1908
Enterorrhaphy; its history, technique and present status. *J. Amer. med. Ass.*, 1893, **21,** 215–35.
Senn, professor of surgery at Chicago, was one of the first to investigate experimentally the subject of gastro-intestinal anastomosis.

3512 SSABANEJEW, J. F.
Über die Anlegung einer röhrenformigen Magenfistel bei Verengerungen der Speiseröhre. *Zbl. Chir.*, 1893, **20,** 862.
Ssabanejew and Frank independently developed a new method of gastrostomy, the Ssabanejew–Frank operation. The above is an abstract of the original, which appeared in *Khirurgitscheski Vestnik*, June, 1893.

3513 TOEPFER, GUSTAV.
Eine Methode zur titrimetrischen Bestimmung der hauptsächlichsten, Factoren der Magenacidität. *Hoppe-Seyl. Z. physiol. Chem.*, 1894 **19,** 104–22.
Toepfer's test for hydrochloric acid in gastric juice.

3514 BATTLE, WILLIAM HENRY. 1855–1936
Modified incision for removal of the vermiform appendix. *Brit. med. J.*, 1895, **2,** 1360.
"Battle's incision."

3515 PAUL, FRANK THOMAS. 1851–1941
Colectomy. *Brit. med. J.*, 1895, **1,** 1136–39.
Paul's operation of extra-abdominal resection of the colon.

3516 BECHER, WOLF. 1862–1906
Zur Anwendung des Röntgenschen Verfahrens in der Medicin. *Dtsch. med. Wschr.*, 1896, **22,** 202–03.
Becher introduced a solution of lead into the stomach of a guinea-pig, making it opaque to *x* rays; he thus showed the possibility of radiological diagnosis of gastric disease.

3517 SCHLATTER, CARL. 1864–1934
Ueber Ernährung und Verdauung nach vollständiger Entfernung des Magens, Oesophagoenterostomie, beim Menschen. *Beitr. klin. Chir.*, 1897, **19,** 757–76; 1899, **23,** 589–94.
First successful gastrectomy.

3518 BALDY, JOHN MONTGOMERY. 1860–1934
First removal of the stomach in America. *Amer. J. Surg. Gynec.*, 1897–98, **10,** 157–58.
Operation performed by Baldy in 1893. He refers to a claim in *J. Amer. med. Ass.* [Febr. 12, 1898, p. 341] giving credit for the first excision of the stomach in America to Bernays.

3519 CANNON, WALTER BRADFORD. 1871–1945
The movements of the stomach studied by means of the Roentgen rays. *Amer. J. Physiol.*, 1898, **1,** 359–82.
Cannon introduced the bismuth meal. He showed that bismuth, opaque to *x* rays, could be of great use in conjunction with roentgenology in the investigation of the digestive tract.

3520 GRASER, Ernst. 1860–1929
Ueber multiple falsche Darmdivertikel in der Flexura sigmoidea. *Münch. med. Wschr.*, 1899, **46,** 721–23.

A false diverticulum of the sigmoid flexure, described by Graser, has been given the eponym "Graser's diverticulum".

3521 KILLIAN, Gustav. 1860–1921
Ueber Magenspiegelung. *Dtsch. Z. Chir.*, 1900–01, **58,** 500–07.

Describes the first clinical use of the oesophagoscope by Kussmaul in 1867–68. The latter made only brief mention of it himself, in his paper on the stomach pump, *Dtsch. Arch. klin. Med.*, 1869, **6**, 456.

3522 MAYO, William James. 1861–1939
Malignant diseases of the stomach and pylorus. *Trans. Amer. surg. Ass.*, 1900, **18,** 97–123.

Mayo's operation of partial gastrectomy.

3523 DEPAGE, Antoine. 1862–1925
Nouveau procédé pour la gastrostomie. *J. Chir. (Brux.)*, 1901, **1,** 715–18.

Depage used a tube formed from the anterior wall of the stomach, lined with mucous membrane, in his gastrostomy operation.

3524 ROBSON, *Sir* Arthur William Mayo. 1853–1933, & MOYNIHAN, Berkeley George Andrew, 1*st Baron Moynihan of Leeds.* 1865–1936
Diseases of the stomach and their surgical treatment. London, *Baillière, Tindall & Cox*, 1901.

3525 WEIR, Robert Fulton. 1838–1927
A new use for the useless appendix, in the surgical treatment of obstinate colitis. *Med. Rec. (N.Y.)*, 1902, **62,** 201–02.

Weir's appendicostomy operation.

3526 KELLY, Howard Atwood. 1858–1943
Instruments for use through cylindrical rectal specula, with the patients in the knee-chest posture. *Ann. Surg.*, 1903, **37,** 924–27.

Various rectal and vesical specula were designed by Kelly.

3527 MIKULICZ-RADECKI, Johann von. 1850–1905
Chirurgische Erfahrungen über das Darmcarcinom. *Arch. klin. Chir.*, 1903, **69,** 28–47.

Development of Bloch's two-stage operation for resection of tumours of the rectum. English translation in *Medical Classics*, 1937, **2**, 210–29.

3528 HERTER, Christian Archibald. 1865–1910
On infantilism from chronic intestinal infection; characterized by the overgrowth and persistence of flora of the nursling period. New York, *Macmillan & Co.*, 1908.

"Herter's infantilism." Called also "Gee–Herter disease" (No. 3491).

3528.1 MILES, William Ernest. 1869–1947
A method of performing abdomino-perineal excision for carcinoma of the rectum and of the terminal portion of the pelvic colon. *Lancet*, 1908, **2,** 1812–13.

Miles devised the operation of abdomino-perineal resection.

3529 STUMPF, R.
Beitrag zur Magenchirurgie. *Beitr. klin. Chir.*, 1908, **59**, 551–641.
Report of Hofmeister's modification of the Billroth II gastro-enterostomy.

3530 GUISEZ, JEAN. 1872– , & BARCAT, JEAN JULES. 1875–
Essais de traitement de quelques cas d'épithélioma de l'oesophage par les applications locales directes de radium. *Bull. Soc. méd. Hôp. Paris*, 1909, **27**, 717–22.
Radium therapy by means of the oesophagoscope.

3531 LANE, *Sir* WILLIAM ARBUTHNOT, *Bart.* 1856–1943
The operative treatment of chronic constipation. London, *J. Nisbet*, 1909.
Lane's operation for chronic intestinal stasis ("Lane's kink") consisted in short-circuiting the intestine.

3532 BALFOUR, DONALD CHURCH. 1882–1963
A method of anastomosis between sigmoid and rectum. *Ann. Surg.*, 1910, **51**, 239–41.
Balfour's operation for resection of the sigmoid colon.

3533 HAUDEK, MARTIN. 1880–1931
Zur röntgenologischen Diagnose der Ulzerationen in der Pars media des Magens. *Münch. med. Wschr.*, 1910, **57**, 1587–91.
First demonstration of the characteristic niche in gastric ulcer.

3534 MAYO, WILLIAM JAMES. 1861–1939
Removal of the rectum for cancer: statistical report of 120 cases. *Ann. Surg.*, 1910, **51**, 854–62.
Mayo's radical operation for carcinoma of the rectum.

3535 MOYNIHAN, BERKELEY GEORGE ANDREW, 1*st Baron Moynihan of Leeds*. 1865–1936
Duodenal ulcer. Philadelphia, *W. B. Saunders Co.*, 1910.
Moynihan greatly advanced our knowledge of duodenal ulcer. He developed the concept of the so-called ulcer sequence, pain-food-ease, and he stressed the well-ordered sequence of symptoms. More than any other he established the surgical treatment of duodenal ulcer on a sound basis.

3536 FOCKENS, P.
Ein operativ geheilter Fall von kongenitaler Dünndarmatresie. *Zbl. Chir.*, 1911, **38**, 532–35.
Treatment of congenital atresia of ileum by lateral anastomosis.

3537 PÓLYA, EUGEN [JENÖ] ALEXANDER. 1876–?1944
Zur Stumpfversorgung nach Magenresektion. *Zbl. Chir.*, 1911, **38**, 892–94.
Pólya's modification of the Billroth II operation. Pólya is believed to have been murdered by a Nazi group during the siege of Budapest by the Russians, December, 1944, although his body was never recovered.

3538 HERTZ, ARTHUR FREDERICK [*afterwards* HURST]. 1879–1944
The cause and treatment of certain unfavourable after-effects of gastro-enterostomy. *Proc. roy. Soc. Med.*, 1913, **6**, Surg. Sect., 155–63.
First description of the "dumping syndrome", so named by C. L. Mix, *Surg. Clin. N. Amer.*, 1922, 2. 617–22.

3539 RAMMSTEDT, WILHELM CONRAD. 1867–1963
Zur Operation der angeborenen Pylorusstenose. *Med. Klin.*, 1912, **8,** 1702–05.
"Rammstedt's operation" for congenital pyloric stenosis.

3540 TOREK, FRANZ. 1861–1938
The first successful case of resection of the thoracic portion of the oesophagus for carcinoma. *Surg. Gynec. Obstet.*, 1913, **16,** 614–17.
See also *Arch. Surg.* (*Chicago*), 1925, **10**, 353–60, which reported that the patient was still living.

3541 SIPPY, BERTRAM WELTON. 1866–1924
Gastric and duodenal ulcer; medical cure by an efficient removal of gastric juice corrosion. *J. Amer. med. Ass.*, 1915, **64,** 1625–30.
"Sippy diet" for the treatment of peptic ulcer.

3542 ANDREWES, *Sir* FREDERICK WILLIAM. 1859–1932
Dysentery bacilli: the differentiation of the true dysentery bacilli from allied species. *Lancet*, 1918, **1,** 560–63.
Shigella alkalescens described.

3543 FINSTERER, HANS. 1877–1955
Ausgedehnte Magenresektion bei Ulcus duodeni statt der einfachen Duodenalresektion bzw. Pylorusausschaltung. *Zbl. Chir.*, 1918, **45,** 434–35.
Hofmeister–Finsterer gastro-enterostomy (see No. 3529).

3544 SCHINDLER, RUDOLF. 1888–
Probleme und Technik der Gastroskopie, mit der Beschreibung eines neuen Gastroskops. *Arch. VerdauKr.*, 1922, **30,** 133–66.
Schindler made gastroscopy a "method". See also his paper in the *Münch. med. Wschr.*, 1922, **69**, 535–37.

3545 WALTON, *Sir* ALBERT JAMES. 1881–1955
A text-book of the surgical dyspepsias. London, *E. Arnold*, 1923.

3546 KONJETZNY, GEORG ERNST. 1880–
Die Entzündungen des Magens. In F. Henke & O. Lubarsch: *Handbuch der speziellen pathologischen Anatomie und Histologie*, 1928, **4,** Heft 2, 768–1116.
Konjetzny has suggested that peptic ulceration is the sequel to a specific form of gastritis.

3547 HURST, *Sir* ARTHUR FREDERICK. 1879–1944, & STEWART, MATTHEW JOHN. 1885–1956
Gastric and duodenal ulcer. London, *Humphrey Milford*, 1929.

3548 PORGES, OTTO. 1879–
Ueber Gastrophotographie. *Wien. klin. Wschr.*, 1929, **42,** 89, 889.
Introduction of gastrophotography.

3549 SPIVACK, JULIUS LEO. 1889–
Eine neue Methode der Gastrostomie. *Beitr. klin. Chir.*, 1929, **147,** 308–18.
Introduction of tubo-valvular gastrostomy.

3550 THAYSEN, THORALD EINAR HESS. 1883–1936
The "coeliac affection" – idiopathic steatorrhoeas. *Lancet*, 1929, **1,** 1086–89.

Idiopathic steatorrhoea, first described by Gee (No. 3491) was extensively studied by Thaysen, in so far as it occurs in adults and adolescents in non-tropical countries. It also bears the name "Gee–Thaysen disease".

3551 CROHN, BURRILL BERNARD. 1884– , *et al.*
Regional ileitis. A pathologic and clinical entity. *J. Amer. med. Ass.*, 1932, **99,** 1323–29.

"Crohn's disease" – regional ileitis. With L. Ginzburg and G. D. Oppenheimer.

3552 CUSHING, HARVEY WILLIAMS. 1869–1939
Papers relating to the pituitary body, hypothalamus, and parasympathetic nervous system. Springfield, *C. C. Thomas*, 1932.

Cushing advanced the theory that the hypothalamus is responsible for the development of peptic ulcer (see p. 175 *et seq.*).

3553 SCHINDLER, RUDOLF. 1888–
Ein völlig ungefährliches, flexibles Gastroskop. *Münch. med. Wschr.*, 1932, **79,** 1268–69.

Introduction of the flexible gastroscope.

3554 WANGENSTEEN, OWEN HARDING. 1898–
The early diagnosis of acute intestinal obstruction with comments on pathology and treatment. With a report of successful decompression of three cases of mechanical bowel obstruction by nasal catheter suction siphonage. *West. J. Surg. Obstet. Gynec.*, 1932, **40,** 1–17.

Wangensteen's apparatus for relief of acute intestinal obstruction.

3555 BARCLAY, ALFRED ERNEST. 1876–1949
The digestive tract; a radiological study of its anatomy, physiology, and pathology. Cambridge, *Univ. Press*, 1933.

3556 MEULENGRACHT, EINAR. 1887–
Treatment of hematemesis and melaena with food. *Acta med. Scand.*, 1934, Suppl. **59,** 375–85.

Meulengracht diet.

3557 DRAGSTEDT, LESTER REYNOLD. 1893– , & OWENS, FREDERICK MITCHUM. 1913–
Supra-diaphragmatic section of the vagus nerves in treatment of duodenal ulcer. *Proc. Soc. exp. Biol. (N.Y.)*, 1943, **53,** 152–54.

Vagotomy for peptic ulcer.

3558 JUDD, JAMES R.
Atresia of the ileum. First successful case cured by enterostomy alone. *J. Pediat.*, 1947, **30,** 679–85.

3559–3572 APPENDICITIS

3559 AMYAND, CLAUDIUS. 168–?–1740
Of an inguinal rupture, with a pin in the appendix caeci, incrusted with stone; and some observations on wounds in the guts. *Phil. Trans.*, 1736, **39,** 329–42.

First recorded successful appendicectomy. Amyand was Serjeant-Surgeon to George II and first principal surgeon to Westminster Hospital. See also the paper in *Surg. Gynec. Obstet.*, 1953, **97**, 643–52, which reproduces part of the text.

3560 PARKINSON, John William Keys. 1785–1838
Case of diseased appendix vermiformis. *Med.-chir. Trans.*, 1812, **3,** 57–58.

First case of appendicitis reported in English, and the first in which perforation was recognized as the cause of death.

3561 LOUYER-VILLERMAY, Jean Baptiste. 1776–1837
Observations pour servir à l'histoire des inflammations de l'appendice du caecum. *Arch. gén. Med.*, 1824, **5,** 246–50.

Report of 2 cases of fatal peritonitis due to perforation of the appendix. Of this paper, H. A. Kelly says "it at once established a definite place for lesions of the appendix in the category of recognized diseases".

3562 MÉLIER, François. 1798–1866
Mémoire et observations sur quelques maladies de l'appendice cécale. *J. gén. Méd.*, 1827, **100,** 317–45.

Mélier was the first to show the existence of chronic appendicitis; he recognized the causal relationship between the chronic affection and abscesses of the right iliac fossa and was first to suggest operative intervention.

3563 HANCOCK, Henry. 1809–1880
Disease of the appendix caeci cured by operation. *Lond. med. Gaz.*, 1848, n.s. **7,** 547–50.

First recorded successful operation for peritonitis due to abscess in the appendix. Hancock was surgeon to Charing Cross Hospital, London.

3564 PARKER, Willard. 1800–1884
An operation for abcess of the appendix vermiformis caeci. *Med. Rec. (N.Y.)*, 1867, **2,** 25–27.

Parker was the first American to operate for appendicitis – in 1864. He advocated the opening of appendicular abscesses at an early stage; until his time such abscesses had been opened only when they pointed on the surface.

3565 SANDS, Henry Berton. 1830–1888
On perityphlitis. *Ann. surg. anat. Soc. (Brooklyn)*, 1880, **2,** 249–70.

Sands published an account of 26 cases, in which he had operated successfully in all but two. His later publications show that he recognized the early signs of perforation of the appendix, and he advocated and practised early operation.

3566 FENWICK, Samuel. 1821–1902
Clinical lectures on cases of difficult diagnosis; perforation of the appendix vermiformis. *Lancet*, 1884, **2,** 987–90, 1039–42.

In 1884 Fenwick advocated tying off and removal of the perforated appendix.

3567 FITZ, Reginald Heber. 1843–1913
Perforating inflammation of the vermiform appendix, with special reference to its early diagnosis and treatment. *Trans. Ass. Amer. Phys.*, 1886, **1,** 107–44.

A conclusive demonstration of the pathology and symptoms of disease of the vermiform appendix. Fitz invented the term "appendicitis"; his paper, which records 25 cases collected by himself, is reprinted in *Med. Classics*, 1938, **2,** 459–91.

3568 HALL, Richard John.
Suppurative peritonitis due to ulceration and suppuration of the vermiform appendix; laparotomy; resection of the vermiform appendix; toilette of the peritonaeum; drainage; recovery. *N.Y. med. J.*, 886, **43,** 662–63.

This is believed to be the first reported case of survival after removal of a perforated appendix.

3569 WOODBURY, Frank.

Cases of exploratory laparotomy followed by appropriate remedial operation. *Trans. Coll. Phys. Philad.*, 1887, **9,** 183.

Thomas George Morton (1835–1903) was one of the first deliberately to operate for and remove the inflamed appendix after correct diagnosis, April 1887. The patient survived. Case reported by Woodbury.

3570 McBURNEY, Charles. 1845–1913

Experience with early operative interference in cases of disease of the vermiform appendix. *N.Y. med. J.*, 1889, **50,** 676–84.

Describes (p. 678) "McBurney's point": "The seat of greatest pain, *determined by the pressure of one finger*, has been very exactly between an inch and a half and two inches from the anterior spinous process of the ilium on a straight line drawn from that process to the umbilicus." McBurney also includes a description of some successful cases of early operation for perforative appendicitis. The paper is reprinted in *Med. Classics*, 1938, 2, 506–31.

3570.1 TAIT, Robert Lawson. 1845–1899

Surgical treatment of typhilitis. *Bgham med. Rev.*, 1890, **27,** 26–34, 76–89.

Lawson Tait was the first British surgeon to diagnose acute appendicitis and to treat it by removal of the appendix (May 1880). See J. A. Shepherd, *Lancet*, 1956, 2, 1301.

3571 KELLY, Howard Atwood. 1858–1943, & HURDON, Elizabeth. 1869–1941

The vermiform appendix and its diseases. Philadelphia, *W. B. Saunders*, 1905.

3572 ASCHOFF, Karl Albert Ludwig. 1866–1942

Die Wurmfortsatzentzündung. Jena, *G. Fischer*, 1908.

Aschoff's theory of the enterogenous origin of appendicitis.

3573–3611 HERNIA

3573 FRANCO, Pierre. 1500–1561

Petit traite contenant une des parties principalles de chirurgie, laquelle les chirurgiens hernieres exercent. Lyon, *Antoine Vincent*, 1556.

Includes the first recorded description of an operation for strangulated hernia. Franco, in 1556, was first to perform suprapubic cystotomy. Poor, and largely self-taught, he greatly improved the technique of herniotomy.

3574 ——. Traité des hernies. Lyon, *T. Payan*, 1561.

3575 LITTRE, Alexis. 1658–1726

Observation sur une nouvelle espèce de hernie. *Hist. Acad. roy. Sci. (Paris)*, (1700), 1719, Mém., 300–10.

"Littre's hernia" – so named from his description of diverticulum hernia. Later Richter (No. 3578) described this condition more fully.

3576 POTT, Percivall. 1714–1788

A treatise on ruptures. London, *C. Hitch & L. Hawes*, 1756.

Pott was surgeon to St. Bartholomew's Hospital. Through a fall in the street he was confined to bed for many days, and during that period wrote his classical book on hernia. He refuted many of the old theories concerning its causation and methods of treatment based on these theories. The book includes the first description of congenital hernia.

3577 PETIT, JEAN LOUIS. 1674–1750
Traité des maladies chirurgicales, et des opérations qui leur conviennent. Paris, *T. F. Didot jeune*, 1774.
"Petit's hernia" and "triangle" described (vol. 2, pp. 256–58). A lumbar hernia had previously been described by R. J. C. de Garengeot, *Traité des opérations de chirurgie*, 1731, **1**, 369–71.

3578 RICHTER, AUGUST GOTTLIEB. 1742–1812
Abhandlung von den Brüchen. Göttingen, *J. C. Dieterich*, 1778–79.
Richter, lecturer on surgery at Göttingen, in his classical treatise on hernia, first described partial enterocele, or "Richter's hernia" (Chap. 24).

3579 GIMBERNAT, *Don* ANTONIO DE. 1734–1816
Nuevo método de operar en la hernia crural. Madrid, *vda. Ibarra*, 1793.
Description of Gimbernat's operation for strangulated femoral hernia. In the same work he also described the ligament in the crural arch named after him. Gimbernat was a pioneer in ophthalmology, vascular surgery, and urology. English translation of the book, by T. Beddoes, London, 1795. For biographical note, *see* N. M. Matheson, *Brit. med. Bull.*, 1945, **3**, 238–39.

3580 CAMPER, PIETER. 1722–1789
Icones herniarum. Editae a S. T. SOEMMERRING. Francofurti ad Moenum, *Varrentrapp & Wenner*, 1801.
Camper illustrated his own work, and was in fact one of the greatest anatomical artists. His illustrations of herniae are of great value.

3581 COOPER, *Sir* ASTLEY PASTON, *Bart.* 1768–1841
The anatomy and surgical treatment of abdominal hernia. 2 pts. London, *Longman & Co.*, 1804–07.
Cooper's treatise on hernia is the outstanding contribution to the subject during the 19th century. Cooper made a study of femoral hernia and described "Cooper's ligament". He also studied diaphragmatic hernia. The above book includes the description of "Cooper's hernia" (hernia femoralis fasciae superficialis).

3582 HESSELBACH, FRANZ KASPAR. 1759–1816
Anatomisch-chirurgische Abhandlung über den Ursprung der Leistenbrüche. Würzburg, *Baumgärtner*, 1806.
Includes description of "Hesselbach's hernia" and "triangle". He wrote a further volume on the subject in 1814.

3583 SCARPA, ANTONIO. 1747–1832
Sull' ernie. Memorie anatomico-chirurgiche. Milano, *d. reale Stamperia*, 1809.

3584 ——. Sull' ernia del perineo. Pavia, *P. Bizzoni*, 1821.
Scarpa's work on perineal hernia included a classical description of sliding hernia or hernia of the large bowel. His contribution to the subject of hernia ranks with that of Cooper, and he did much towards modernizing the knowledge of this speciality.

3585 CLOQUET, JULES GERMAIN. 1790–1883
Recherches sur les causes et l'anatomie des hernies abdominales. Paris, *Méquignon-Marvis*, 1819.

3586 KEY, CHARLES ANTON. 1793–1849
A memoir on the advantages and practicability of dividing the stricture in strangulated hernia on the outside of the sac. London, *Longman*, 1833.

3587 LAWRENCE, *Sir* WILLIAM. 1783–1867
Treatise on ruptures. 5th ed. London, *John Churchill*, 1838.
This was the standard text for many years. It first appeared in 1807 as *Treatise on hernia.*

3588 LUKE, JAMES. 1798–1881
Operation for strangulated hernia. *Lond. med. Gaz.*, 1841, **28,** 863–66.
Luke's operation for femoral hernia.

3589 TEALE, THOMAS PRIDGIN, *Snr.* 1801–1868
A practical treatise on abdominal hernia. London, *Longman*, 1846.

3590 RIEUX, LÉON.
Considérations sur l'étranglement de l'intestin dans la cavité abdominale et sur un mode d'étranglement non décrit par les auteurs. Paris, *Thèse No.* 128, 1853.
Retrocaecal hernia ("Rieux's hernia") first described.

3591 TREITZ, WENZEL. 1819–1872
Hernia retroperitonealis. Ein Beitrag zur Geschichte innerer Hernien. Prag, *F. A. Crednar*, 1857.
Treitz described retroperitoneal hernia through the duodeno-jejunal recess – "Treitz's hernia".

3592 GRUBER, WENZEL LEOPOLD. 1814–1890
Ueber einen Fall nicht incarcerierter, aber mit Incarceration des Ileum durch das Omentum complicirter Hernia interna mesogastrica. *Oest. Z. prakt. Heilk.*, 1863, **9,** 325–30, 341–45.
"Gruber's hernia" – internal mesogastric hernia.

3593 CZERNY, VINCENZ. 1842–1916
Studien zur Radikalbehandlung der Hernien. *Wien med. Wschr.*, 1877, **27,** 497–500, 527–30, 553–56, 578–81.

3594 MARCY, HENRY ORLANDO. 1837–1924
The radical cure of hernia by the antiseptic use of the carbolized catgut ligature. *Trans. Amer. med. Ass.*, 1878, **29,** 296–305.
Marcy introduced antiseptic ligatures in the radical cure of hernia.

3595 EVE, *Sir* FREDERIC SAMUEL. 1853–1916
A case of strangulated hernia into the fossa intersigmoidea. *Brit. med. J.*, 1885, **1,** 1195–97.
First definitely authenticated case of intersigmoid hernia.

3596 MACEWEN, *Sir* WILLIAM. 1848–1924
On the radical cure of oblique inguinal hernia by internal abdominal peritoneal pad, and the restoration of the valved form of the inguinal canal. *Ann. Surg.*, 1886, **4,** 89–119.
Macewen's method for the radical cure of oblique inguinal hernia. The sac was folded into a pad and used as a plug at the internal ring, the ring being closed in layers. Reprinted in *Brit. med. J.*, 1887, 2, 1263–71.

3597 LUCAS-CHAMPIONNIÈRE, JUST MARIE MARCELLIN. 1843–1913
Cure radicale des hernies. Paris, *A. Delahaye et E. Lecrosnier*, 1887.
A classical account.

3598 BASSINI, Edoardo. 1844–1924
Nuovo metodo per la cura radicale dell' ernia. *Atti Congr. Ass. Med. Ital.*, (1887), Pavia, 1889, **2,** 179–82.
Bassini's operation for the radical cure of inguinal hernia. Published in book form, Padua, 1889. Translation in *J. Hist. Med.*, 1966, **21**, 401–07.

3599 HALSTED, William Stewart. 1852–1922
The radical cure of hernia. *Johns Hopk. Hosp. Bull.*, 1889, **1,** 12–13, 112.
Simultaneously with Bassini Halsted devised the modern operation for the radical cure of inguinal hernia. Later his technique differed much from that of Bassini. See also his later paper on the subject in the same journal, 1893, **4**, 17–24, which is reprinted in *Med. Classics* 1938, **3**, 412–40.

3600 KOCHER, Emil Theodor. 1841–1917
Zur Radicalcur der Hernien. *KorrespBl. schweiz. Aerzte*, 1892, **22,** 561–76.
Kocher's hernia operation.

3601 MARCY, Henry Orlando. 1837–1924
The anatomy and surgical treatment of hernia. New York, *D. Appleton & Co.*, 1892.
Marcy wrote a great deal on hernia, describing high ligation of the sac, transplantation of the spermatic cord and careful reconstruction of the inguinal canal.

3602 BASSINI, Edoardo. 1844–1924
Nuovo metodo operativo per la cura radicale dell' ernia crurale. Padova, *Draghi*, 1893.
Bassini's operation for femoral hernia. Translation in *J. Hist. Med.*, 1966, **21**, 401–07.

3603 FRANKS, *Sir* Kendal. 1851–1920
Resection of the intestine and immediate suture in gangrenous hernia. *Brit. med. J.*, 1893, **1,** 696.
Franks finally demonstrated the advantages of primary resection for gangrenous gut in strangulated hernia.

3604 LOCKWOOD, Charles Barrett. 1856–1914
The radical cure of femoral and inguinal hernia. *Lancet*, London, 1893, **2,** 1297–1302.
Lockwood's operation for femoral hernia.

3605 LOTHEISSEN, Georg. 1868–
Zur Radikaloperation der Schenkelhernien. *Zbl. Chir.*, 1898, **25,** 548–50.
Lotheissen's operation for femoral hernia.

3606 BATTLE, William Henry. 1855–1936
Abstract of a clinical lecture on femoral hernia. *Lancet*, 1901, **1,** 302–05.
Battle's operation for femoral hernia.

3607 MAYO, William James. 1861–1939
An operation for the radical cure of umbilical hernia. *Ann. Surg.*, 1901, **34,** 276–80.
Mayo's operation for umbilical hernia.

3608 BLOODGOOD, JOSEPH COLT. 1867–1935
The transplantation of the rectus muscle in certain cases of inguinal hernia in which the conjoined tendon is obliterated. *Johns Hopk. Hosp. Bull.*, 1918, **19,** 96–100.
Bloodgood's operation for inguinal hernia. *See also Ann. Surg.*, 1919, **70,** 81–88.

3609 GALLIE, WILLIAM EDWARD. 1882–1959, & LEMESURIER, ARTHUR BAKER. 1889–
Living sutures in the treatment of hernia. *Canad. med. Ass. J.*, 1923, **13,** 469–80.
Gallie and LeMesurier used fascial sutures in their operation for inguinal hernia.

3611 HENRY, ARNOLD KIRKPATRICK. 1886–1962
Operation for femoral hernia by a midline extraperitoneal approach; with a preliminary note on the use of this route for reducible inguinal hernia. *Lancet*, 1936, **1,** 531–33.
Henry's operation for femoral hernia.

3612–3666.1 LIVER; GALL-BLADDER; PANCREAS

For DIABETES MELLITUS, see 3925–3979; for WEIL'S DISEASE, see 5330–5336.

3612 ARETAEUS, *the Cappadocian.* A.D. 81–138?
On jaundice, or icterus. In his *Extant works*, London, 1856, 324–28.

3613 BROWNE, JOHN. 1642–170–?
A remarkable account of a liver, appearing glandulous to the eye. *Phil. Trans.*, 1685, **15,** 1266–68.
First description of cirrhosis of the liver.

3614 LAENNEC, RENÉ THÉOPHILE HYACINTHE. 1781–1826
De l'auscultation médiate. Vol. 1. Paris, *J. A. Brosson & J. S. Chaudé*, 1819.
"Laennec's cirrhosis" – chronic interstitial hepatitis, is described on page 368.

3615 BRIGHT, RICHARD. 1789–1858
Cases and observations connected with disease of the pancreas and duodenum. *Med.-chir. Trans.*, 1832, **18,** 1–56.

3616 STANLEY, EDWARD. 1793–1862
Abscess of the liver, with hydatids. – Operation. *Lancet*, 1833, **1,** 189–90.
Diagnostic liver puncture.

3617 BRIGHT, RICHARD. 1789–1858
Observations on jaundice. *Guy's Hosp. Rep.*, 1836, **1,** 604–37.
Original description of acute yellow atrophy of the liver.

3618 ROKITANSKY, CARL, *Freiherr von.* 1804–1878
Handbuch der pathologischen Anatomie. 3 vols. Wien, *Braümuller u. Seidel*, 1842–46.
Vol. 3 (1842), p. 313: Rokitansky's classical description of the pathological picture of acute yellow atrophy of the liver. Rokitansky named the disease; it has also been called "Rokitansky's disease". English translation, 4 vols., London, 1849–54.

3619 BUDD, George. 1808–1882
On diseases of the liver. London, *J. Churchill*, 1845.
Budd was professor of medicine at King's College, London. Section III of the above book includes a description of that form of cirrhosis to which the name "Budd's disease" has been applied.

3620 FRERICHS, Friedrich Theodor. 1819–1885
Klinik der Leberkrankheiten. 2 vols and atlas. Braunschweig, *F. Vieweg u. Sohn*, 1858–61.
Frerichs' classical monograph on diseases of the liver summarized the existing knowledge and included his own important work on the subject. He discovered leucine and tyrosine in the liver in acute yellow atrophy (*Dtsch. Klin.*, 1855, **7**, 341–43), a condition to which he devoted much study. Frerichs was professor of pathology at Berlin and enjoyed a great reputation; more than any other man he was responsible for the development of scientific clinical teaching in Germany. English translation, London, 1860.

3621 BOBBS, John Stough. 1809–1870
Case of lithotomy of the gall-bladder. *Trans. med. Soc. Indiana*, 1868, 68–73.
First cholecystotomy for the removal of gall-stones.

3622 MURCHISON, Charles. 1830–1879
Clinical lectures on diseases of the liver. London, *Longmans Green & Co.*, 1868.

3623 HAYEM, Georges. 1841–1933
Contribution à l'étude de l'hépatite interstitielle chronique avec hypertrophie (sclérose ou cirrhose hypertrophique du foie). *Arch. Physiol. norm. path.*, 1874, 2 sér., **1**, 126–57.
Classical description of chronic interstitial hepatitis.

3624 HANOT, Victor Charles. 1844–1896
Etude sur une forme de cirrhose hypertrophique du foie (cirrhose hypertrophique avec ictère chronique). Paris, *Thèse No.* 465, 1875.
"Hanot's disease." First description of hypertrophic cirrhosis of the liver with icterus. Published in book form, Paris, 1876.

3625 SIMS, James Marion. 1813–1883
Remarks on cholecystotomy in dropsy of the gall-bladder. *Brit. med. J.*, 1878, **1**, 811–15.
Sims' operation of cholecystotomy.

3626 BALSER, W.
Ueber Fettnekrose, eine zuweilen tödliche Krankheit des Menschen. *Virchows Arch. path. Anat.*, 1882, **90**, 520–35.
First description of pancreatic necrosis, "Balser's fat necrosis".

3627 LANGENBUCH, Carl Johann August. 1846–1901
Ein Fall von Exstirpation der Gallenblase wegen chronischer Cholelithiasis; Heilung. *Berl. klin. Wschr.*, 1882, **19**, 725–27.
First successful removal of the gall-bladder.

3628 LÜRMAN, A.
Eine Icterusepidemie. *Berl. klin. Wschr.*, 1885, **22**, 20–23.
Dr. Lürman, a general practitioner in Bremen, was first to report homologous serum hepatitis.

3629 SENN, Nicholas. 1844–1908
The surgery of the pancreas, as based upon experiments and clinical researches. *Trans. Amer. surg. Ass.*, 1886, **4,** 99–232.

3630 BARD, Louis. 1857–1930, & PIC, Adrien. 1862–
Contribution à l'étude clinique et anatomo-pathologique du cancer primitif du pancréas. *Rev. Méd.*, 1888, **8,** 257–82, 363–405.
"Bard–Pic syndrome" first described.

3631 RIEDEL, Bernhard Moritz Carl Ludwig. 1846–1916
Ueber den zungenförmigen Fortsatz des rechten Leberlappens und seine pathognostische Bedeutung für die Erkrankung der Gallenblase nebst Bemerkungen über Gallensteinoperationen. *Berl. klin. Wschr.*, 1888, **25,** 577–81, 602–07.
"Riedel's lobe", a form of constriction lobe of the liver.

3632 FITZ, Reginald Heber. 1843–1913
Acute pancreatitis; a consideration of pancreatic hemorrhage, hemorrhagic suppurative, and gangrenous pancreatitis, and of disseminated fat necrosis. *Boston med. surg. J.*, 1889, **120,** 181–87, 205–07, 229–35.

3633 STADELMANN, Ernst. 1853–
Der Icterus und seine verschiedenen Formen. Stuttgart, *F. Enke*, 1891.

3634 NAUNYN, Bernhard. 1839–1925
Klinik der Cholelithiasis. Leipzig, *F. C. W. Vogel*, 1892.
Naunyn produced a classical monograph on gall-stones, devising an accurate chemical classification. He was one of Frerich's best pupils, and became Professor of Clinical Medicine successively at Dorpat, Berne, Königsberg, and Strassburg. English translation, London, 1896.

3635 LUCATELLO, Luigi. 1863–1926
Sulla puntura del fegato a scopo diagnostico. *Lav. Congr. Med. interna, Milano*, 1895, **6,** 327–29.
Liver puncture biopsy.

3636 CHAPPUIS, J., & CHAUVEL, H.
Calculs du rein. Calculs de la vésicule biliaire. *Bull. Acad. Méd. (Paris)*, 1896, **35,** 410–11.
Chappuis and Chauvel were the first to study biliary concretions by means of Roentgen rays.

3637 BOBROFF, Alexander Alexievich. 1850–1904
Ueber ein neues Operationsverfahren zur Entfernung von Echinococcus in der Leber und anderen parenchymatösen Bauchorganen. *Arch. klin. Chir.*, 1898, **56,** 810–26.
Important work on surgical treatment of hydatids of the liver. Originally appeared in Russian in *Khirurgiya*, 1898, 3, 3–9.

3638 BUXBAUM, A.
Ueber die Photographie von Gallensteinen in vivo. *Wien. med. Presse*, 1898, **39,** col. 534–38.
First *x*-ray demonstration of gall-stones.

3639 TALMA, Sape. 1847–1918
Chirurgische Oeffnung neuer Seitenbahnen für das Blut der Vena portae. *Berl. klin. Wschr.*, 1898, **35,** 833–36; 1900, **37,** 677–81; 1904, **41,** 893–97.
Talma's operation for the relief of ascites in cirrhosis of the liver.

3640 HEKTOEN, Ludvig. 1863–1951
Experimental bacillary cirrhosis of the liver. *J. Path. Bact.*, 1900–01, **7,** 214–20.
Hektoen produced experimental cirrhosis of the liver. His notable work in pathology includes the foundation of the *Archives of Pathology*.

3641 OPIE, Eugene Lindsay. 1873–1971
Disease of the pancreas; its cause and nature. Philadelphia, *J. B. Lippincott*, 1903.

3642 CAMMIDGE, Percy John. 1872–
The chemistry of the urine in diseases of the pancreas. *Lancet*, 1904, **1,** 782–87.
Test for diseases of the pancreas.

3643 BAUER, Richard.
Ueber die Assimilation von Galaktose und Milchzucker beim Gesunden und Kranken. *Wien. med. Wschr.*, 1906, **56,** 20–23.
Galactose tolerance test.

3644 LOEWI, Otto. 1873–1961
Ueber eine neue Funktion des Pankreas und ihre Beziehung zum Diabetes mellitus. *Arch. exp. Path. Pharmak.*, 198, **59,** 83–94.
Loewi's pancreatic function test.

3645 ASCHOFF, Karl Albert Ludwig. 1866–1942, & BACMEISTER, Adolf. 1882–1945
Die Cholelithiasis. Jena, *G. Fischer*, 1909.

3646 WOHLGEMUTH, Julius. 1874–
Beitrag zur funktionellen Diagnostik des Pankreas. *Berl. klin. Wschr.*, 1910, **47,** 92–95.
Wohlgemuth's pancreatic function test.

3647 HIJMANS VAN DEN BERGH, Albert Abraham. 1869–1943, & SNAPPER, J.
Die Farbstoffe des Blutserums. 1. Eine quantitative Bestimmung des Bilirubins im Blutserum. *Dtsch. Arch. klin. Med.*, 1913, **110,** 540–61.
The van den Bergh test.

3648 McNEE, *Sir* John William. 1887–
Experiments on haemolytic icterus. *J. Path. Bact.*, 1913–14, **18,** 325–42.
McNee showed that bile pigment formation is not a function of the liver cells alone, but can take place in other tissues. He thus disproved the theory propounded by Minkowski and Naunyn in 1886.

3649 MELTZER, SAMUEL JAMES. 1851–1920
The disturbance of the law of contrary innervation as a pathogenetic factor in the diseases of the bile ducts and the gall-bladder. *Amer. J. med. Sci.*, 1917, **153,** 469–77.
Non-surgical drainage of the gall-bladder was first suggested by Meltzer. See also No. 3651.

3650 REICH, ADOLPH. 1864–
Accidental injection of bile ducts with petrolatum and bismuth paste. *J. Amer. med. Ass.*, 1918, **71,** 1555.
Reich was the first to obtain cholangiograms.

3651 LYON, BETHUEL BOYD VINCENT. 1880–
Diagnosis and treatment of diseases of the gallbladder and biliary ducts. Preliminary report on a new method. *J. Amer. med. Ass.*, 1919, **73,** 980–82.
See No. 3649.

3652 GRAHAM, EVARTS AMBROSE. 1883–1957, & COLE, WARREN HENRY. 1898–
Roentgenologic examination of the gallbladder. *J. Amer. med. Ass.*, 1924, **82,** 613–14.
Introduction of cholecystography.

3653 ROSENTHAL, SANFORD MORRIS. 1897– , & WHITE, EDWIN CLAY. 1888–
Studies in hepatic function. VI. A. The pharmacological behaviour of certain dyes. B. The value of selected phthalein compounds in the estimation of hepatic function. *J. Pharmacol.*, 1924, **24,** 265–88.
Bromsulphthalein test for liver function.

3654 TAKATA, MAKI. 1892– & ARA, KIYOSHA.
Ueber eine neue kolloidchemische Liquorreaktion und ihre praktischen Ergebnisse. *Trans. 6th Congr. Far East. Ass. trop. Med.*, 1925, **1,** 667–71.
Takata–Ara reaction for the diagnosis of liver disease.

3655 EILBOTT, WILHELM. 1900–
Funktionsprüfung der Leber mittels Bilirubinbelastung. *Z. klin. Med.*, 1927, **106,** 529–60.
Bilirubin excretion test of liver function. See also his thesis, published in 1925.

3656 GIERKE, EDGAR OTTO KONRAD VON. 1877–1945
Hepato-nephromegalia glykogenika (Glykogenspeicherkrankheit der Leber und Nieren). *Beitr. path. Anat.*, 1929, **82,** 497–513.
"Von Gierke's disease," glycogen disease of hepatomegalic type. See also the review by S. van Creveld, *Medicine*, 1939, 18, 1–128.

3657 ROLLESTON, *Sir* HUMPHRY DAVY, *Bart.* 1862–1944, & McNEE, *Sir* JOHN WILLIAM. 1887–
Diseases of the liver, gall-bladder, and bile ducts. 3rd edition. London, *Macmillan & Co.*, 1929.

3658 BREUER, BÉLA.
Über ein neues Röntgensymptom der Gallensteinkrankheit. *Röntgenpraxis*, 1931, **3,** 879–81.
Gas in gall-stones.

3659 QUICK, ARMAND JAMES. 1894–
The synthesis of hippuric acid: a new test of liver function. *Amer. J. med. Sci.*, 1933, **185,** 630–35.
Quick's liver-function test.

3659.1 FANCONI, GUIDO. 1892– , *et al.*
Das Coeliakiesyndrom bei angeborener zysticher Pankreasfibromatose und Bronchiektasien. *Wien. med. Wschr.*, 1936, **86,** 753–56.
Cystic fibrosis of the pancreas described. With E. Uehlinger and C. Knauer.

3660 BRUNSCHWIG, ALEXANDER. 1901–
Resection of head of pancreas and duodenum for carcinoma – pancreatoduodenectomy. *Surg. Gynec. Obstet.*, 1937, **65,** 681–84.
See also the same journal, 1943, 77, 581–84.

3661 PATEK, ARTHUR JACKSON. 1904–
Treatment of alcoholic cirrhosis of the liver with high vitamin therapy. *Proc. Soc. exp. Biol.* (*N.Y.*), 1937, **37,** 329–30.
A pioneer paper on the dietary treatment of cirrhosis.

3662 HANGER, FRANKLIN MCCUE. 1894–
The flocculation of cephalin-cholesterol emulsions by pathological sera. *Trans. Ass. Amer. Phys.*, 1938, **53,** 148–51.
Cephalin-cholesterol liver-function test.

3663 QUICK, ARMAND JAMES. 1894– , *et al.*
Synthesis of hippuric acid in man following intravenous injection of sodium benzoate. *Proc. Soc. exp. Biol.* (*N.Y.*), 1938, **38,** 77–78.
Intravenous hippuric acid test for liver function. With H. N. Ottenstein and H. Weltchek. See also *Amer. J. Dis.*, 1939, 6, 716–17.

3664 IVERSON, POUL. 1889, & ROHOLM, KAJ.
On aspiration biopsy of the liver, with remarks on its diagnostic significance. *Acta med. Scand.*, 1939, **102,** 1–16.
Modern method of liver puncture.

3665 MACLAGAN, NOEL FRANCIS. 1904–
The serum colloidal gold reactions as a liver function test. *Brit. J. exp. Path.*, 1944, **25,** 15–20.

3666 ——. The thymol turbidity test as an indicator of liver dysfunction. *Brit. J. exp. Path.*, 1944, **25,** 234–41.

3666.1 FRANKEN, FRANZ HERMANN.
Die Leber und ihre Krankheiten. Zweihundert Jahre Hepatologie. Stuttgart, *F. Enke*, 1968.
Contains short biographies and an excellent bibliography.

3667–3705

DENTISTRY

3667 ARTZNEY BUCHLEIN.
Artzney Buchlein. [Leipzig, *Michael Blum*, 1530.]
The first book on dentistry. The writer confined himself to extracts from the works of recent writers on the subject; the book was intended for the general public. It attained 11 editions in 45 years. Reproduced in facsimile, Berlin, *Meusser*, 1921.

3668 EUSTACHI, Bartolommeo [Eustachius]. 1520–1574

Libellus de dentibus. In his *Opuscula anatomica*, Venetiis, 1564.

One of the great books in the history of dentistry. Eustachius gave the first accurate account of the anatomy of the teeth and the phenomena of first and second dentition. Sudhoff (No. 3697) gives a good account of this work.

3669 GUILLEMEAU, Jacques. 1550–1613

La chirurgie francoise recueillie des antiens medecins et chirurgiens. Paris, *N. Gilles*, 1594.

This work contains a good deal about dentistry; it describes pyorrhoea alveolaris for the first time and is also the first work to refer to inorganic materials for tooth fillings and for the construction of artificial teeth. English translation, Dort, 1597.

3670 ALLEN, Charles. *fl.* 1685

The operator for the teeth. York, *John White*, 1685.

First British book on dentistry. Editions were published in Dublin, 1686, and London, 1687. The Dublin edition was reprinted by the British Dental Association in 1924.

3671 FAUCHARD, Pierre. 1678–1761

Le chirurgien dentiste, ou traité des dents. 2 vols. Paris, *J. Mariette*, 1728.

Pierre Fauchard has been called the "Father of Dentistry"; his comprehensive and scientific account of all that concerned dentistry in the 18th century is one of the greatest books in the history of the subject. The second edition, published in 1746, contains a good description (vol. 1, pp. 275–77) of pyorrhoea alveolaris; it was translated by Dr. Lilian Lindsay and published by the British Dental Association in 1946.

3672 HURLOCK, Joseph.

A practical treatise upon dentition; or, the breeding of teeth in children. London, *C. Rimington & S. Austen, J. Hodges*, 1742.

The first English book on children's teeth.

3673 PFAFF, Philipp. 1716–1780

Abhandlung von den Zähnen des menschlichen Körpers und deren Krankheiten. Berlin, *Haude & Spener*, 1756.

Pfaff, dentist to Frederick the Great, was the first to describe the casting of models for false teeth. This book ranks in importance with the work of Fauchard and Hunter.

3674 BERDMORE, Thomas. 1740–1785

A treatise on the disorders and deformities of the teeth and gums. London, *B. White*, 1768.

Earliest English dental text-book. Berdmore was the first to mention the use of the microscope for the study of the minute structure of teeth.

3675 HUNTER, John. 1728–1793

The natural history of the human teeth. London, *J. Johnson*, 1771.

See No. 3676.

3676 ——. A practical treatise on the diseases of the teeth, intended as a supplement to the natural history of those parts. London, *J. Johnson*, 1778.

This classical work revolutionized the practice of dentistry and provided a basis for later dental research. Hunter introduced the classes cuspids, bicuspids, molars, and incisors; he also devised appliances for the correction of malocclusion. In the above work he includes instructions with regard to the operation of tooth transplantation.

3677 DUBOIS DE CHÉMANT, Nicolas. 1753–1824
Dissertation sur les avantages des nouvelles dents, et retaliers artificiels, incorruptibles et sans odeur. Paris, 1788.

Dubois de Chémant was the first dentist to manufacture porcelain teeth by a process modified from that originally invented by an apothecary named Duchâteau in 1776. As his patented teeth did not prove to be popular in France, Dubois de Chémant moved to London and took out an English patent.

3678 SKINNER, Richard Cortland. *d. c.* 1834
A treatise on the human teeth, concisely explaining their structure and cause of disease and decay. New York, *Johnson and Stryker*, 1801.

First American book on the teeth. It was intended for the lay public and was really an advertisement for the author. It is believed that editions were also published in 1794 and 1796, but no copies of these appear to exist.

3679 FOX, Joseph. 1776–1816
The natural history of the human teeth. London, *T. Cox*, 1803.

Fox's classical treatise on the teeth is the first to include explicit directions for correcting dental irregularities.

3680 HARRIS, Chapin Aaron. 1806–1860
The dental art, a practical treatise on dental surgery. Baltimore, *Armstrong & Berry*, 1839.

One of the most popular books on the subject ever published. Harris strove to provide adequate teaching of dentistry in the U.S.A.

3681 NASMYTH, Alexander. ?–1848
On the structure, physiology, and pathology, of the persistent capsular investments and pulp of the tooth. *Med.-chir. Trans.*, 1839, **22,** 310–328.

"Nasmyth's membrane", or persistent dental capsule.

3682 CARABELLI, Georg, *Edler von Lunkaszprie*. 1787–1842
Systematisches Handbuch der Zahnheilkunde. Bd. 2. Anatomie des Mundes. *Wien, Braumüller & Seidel*, 1844.

Original description (p. 107) of "Carabelli's cusp", tuberculus anomalus, sometimes found on the lingual surface of the upper permanent molars. It was illustrated on Tab. XI, Fig. 4e, and Tab. XIV, Fig. 4, of *Kupfertafeln zu v. Carabelli's Anatomie des Mundes*, Wien, 1842.

3683 TOMES, *Sir* John. 1815–1895
A course of lectures on dental physiology and surgery. London, *John W. Parker*, 1848.

Tomes's lectures were classical. He did much for dental surgery, persuaded the Royal College of Surgeons to grant a Licence, was a co-founder of the Odontological Society in 1856, and founded the (Royal) Dental Hospital in 1858. He played a leading part in the movement which led to the passing of the Dentists Act, 1878.

3684 GAINE, Charles.
On certain irregularities of the teeth with cases illustrative of a novel method of successful treatment. Bath, *C. W. Oliver*, 1858.

First work devoted exclusively to irregularities of the teeth.

3685 RIGGS, John M. 1810–1885
Suppurative inflammation of the gums, and absorption of the gums and alveolar process. *Penn. J. dent. Sci.*, 1876, **3,** 99–104.

"Riggs' disease" – pyorrhoea alveolaris. Treatment of the disease by scraping was introduced by Riggs.

3685.1 KINGSLEY, NORMAN WILLIAM. 1829–1913
A treatise on oral deformities. New York, *D. Appleton,* 1880.
A pioneer work.

3686 ANGLE, EDWARD HARTLEY. 1855–1930
Notes on orthodontia. *Trans. 9th Int. Congr. Med.*, 1887, **5,** 565–72.
The specialty orthodontics received a new impetus with the work of Angle. He organized and classified the various abnormalities of the teeth and jaws and devised many methods of treating them. His book on the treatment of malocclusion of the teeth is one of the outstanding contributions to the subject.

3687 MILLER, WILLOUGHBY DAYTON. 1853–1907
The micro-organisms of the human mouth. Philadelphia, *S. S. White Dental Mfg. Co.*, 1890.
Miller, who originated the chemo-parasitic theory of the origin of dental caries, greatly advanced the knowledge concerning dental bacteriology. His book appeared in a German edition in 1889.

3688 HARRISON, FRANK.
The "x" rays in the practice of dental surgery. *J. Brit. dent. Ass.*, 1896, **17,** 624–28.
Harrison was the first to describe a method of making dental radiographs.

3689 MORTON, WILLIAM JAMES. 1846–1920
The x-ray and its application to dentistry. *Dental Cosmos*, 1896, **38,** 478–86.
First dental radiography in America.

3690 THOMA, KURT HERMANN. 1883–
Oral roentgenology. Boston, Mass., *Ritter & Co.*, 1917.

3691 McINTOSH, JAMES, *et al.*
An investigation into the aetiology of dental caries. *Brit. J. exp Path.*, London, 1922, **3,** 138–45; 1924, **5,** 175–84.
Isolation of *L. odontolyticus I* and *II* from carious teeth; this organism is suspected of causing dental caries. With W. W. James and P. Lazarus-Barlow.

3692 RAPER, HOWARD RILEY.
A new kind of x-ray examination for preventive dentistry. *Int. J Orthodont.*, 1925, **11,** 275–79, 370–74, 470–77.
Original description of technique of making "bite-wing" radiographs.

3692.1 DEAN, HENRY TRENDLEY. –1962, *et al.*
Studies on mass control of dental caries through fluoridation of the public water supply. *Publ. Hlth Rep. (Wash.)*, 1950, 1403–08.
It has not been conclusively demonstrated whether fluoride serves a specific physiological rôle, but fluoridation of public water supplies was followed by a reduction in the incidence of dental caries. One of the first studies on mass control of dental caries was that published by Dean, F. A. Arnold, P. Jay, and J. W. Knutson.

History of Dentistry

3693 HILL, ALFRED. 1826–1922
The history of the reform movement in the dental profession in Great Britain during the last twenty years. London, *Trübner & Co.*, 1877.
The history of the beginnings of an organized dental profession in Britain.

3694 CROWLEY, C. GEORGE.
Dental bibliography: a standard reference list of books on dentistry published throughout the world from 1536 to 1885. Philadelphia, *S. S. White Dental Mfg. Co.*, 1885.

3695 GUERINI, VINCENZO. 1859–1955
A history of dentistry from the most ancient times until the end of the eighteenth century. Philadelphia, *Lea & Febiger*, 1909.

3696 PROSKAUER, CURT.
Kulturgeschichte der Zahnheilkunde. 4 pts. Berlin, *H. Meusser*, 1913–26.

3697 SUDHOFF, KARL FRIEDRICH JAKOB. 1853–1938
Geschichte der Zahnheilkunde. Leipzig, *J. A. Barth*, 1921.
Second edition, 1926.

3698 INDEX of the periodical dental literature published in the English language. Chicago, 1921– .
In progress. Retrospective from 1839. Now known as *Index to dental literature.*

3699 WEINBERGER, BERNHARD WOLF. 1885–1960
Orthodontics; an historical review of its origin and evolution, including an extensive bibliography of orthodontic literature up to the time of specialization. 2 pts. St. Louis, *C. V. Mosby*, 1926.

3700 STRÖMGREN, HEDVIG LIDFORSS. 1877–
Die Zahnheilkunde im achtzehnten Jahrhundert, Kopenhagen, *Levin & Munksgaard*, 1935.

3701 ——. Die Zahnheilkunde im neunzehnten Jahrhundert. Kopenhagen, *Levin & Munksgaard*, 1945.

3702 LUFKIN, ARTHUR WARD. 1889–
A history of dentistry. 2nd edition. Philadelphia, *Lea & Febiger*, 1948.

3703 WEINBERGER, BERNHARD WOLF. 1885–1960
An introduction to the history of dentistry. 2 vols. St. Louis, *C. V. Mosby Co.*, 1948.
The first volume covers the history to 1800; the second deals solely with American history.

3704 CAMPBELL, JOHN MENZIES. 1887–1974
A dental bibliography: British and American, 1692–1880. London, *David Low*, 1949.

3705 COLYER, *Sir* FRANK. 1866–1954
Old instruments used for extracting teeth. London, *Staples Press*, 1952.
The only history of dental instruments.

3706–3760 DEFICIENCY DISEASES

See also 1042–1092, *Nutrition*; *Vitamins.*

3706 STEPP, WILHELM OTTO. 1882– , & GYÖRGY, PAUL. 1895–
Avitaminosen und verwandte Krankheitszustände. Berlin, *J. Springer*, 1927.

3707 SEBRELL, WILLIAM HENRY. 1901– , & BUTLER, ROY EDWIN. 1902–
Riboflavin deficiency in man; a preliminary note. *Publ. Hlth Rep.* (*Wash.*), 1938, **53,** 2282–84.
Ariboflavinosis.

3708 WANG, Y. L., & HARRIS, LESLIE JULIUS. 1898–
Methods for assessing the level of nutrition of the human subject: estimation of vitamin B_1 in urine by the thiochrome test. *Biochem. J.*, 1939, **33,** 1356–69.
Wang's test for avitaminosis.

3709 BICKNELL, FRANKLIN, & PRESCOTT, FREDERICK.
The vitamins in medicine. 3rd ed. London, *W. Heinemann*, 1953.

Scurvy

3710 RONSSEUS, BALDUINUS [RONSSE, Boudewijn]. 1525–1597
De magnis Hippocratis lienibus, Pliniique stomacace, ac sceletyrbe, seu vulgo dicto scorbuto, libellus. Antverpiae, *apud viduam Martini Nutii*, 1564.
Jean de Joinville was probably the first, about 1250, to describe scurvy; Vasco da Gama noted its occurrence at sea, and Jacques Cartier mentions it. Ronsseus gave an early medical account, describing how sailors cured themselves by eating oranges and lemons as soon as they reached the coast of Spain.

3710.1 FOREEST, PETER VAN [FORESTUS]. 1522–1597
Observationum et curationum medicinalium liber xix de hepatis malis ac affectibus; et xx de lienis morbis: ubi de scorbutto. Lugduni Batavorum, *ex off. Plantiniana*, 1595.
An outstanding early work on scurvy.

3711 WOODALL, JOHN. 1556–1643
The surgions mate. London, *E. Griffin*, 1617.
Woodall knew the value of limes, lemons, and oranges, and gave them a prominent place in his account of the treatment of scurvy. He was surgeon to St. Bartholomew's Hospital and a contemporary of Harvey.

3712 ABREU, ALEXO DE. 1568–1630
Tratado de las siete enfermedades, de la inflammacion universal del higado, zirbo, pyloron, y riñones, y de la obstruction, de la satiriasi, de la terciana y febre maligna, y passion hipocondriaca. Lleva otros tres tratados, del mal de Loanda, del guzano, y de las fuentes y sedales. Lisboa, *P. Craesbeeck*, 1623.
Includes a precise clinical description of scurvy (fol. 150v. to 193). Abreu treated the disease with fresh milk and anti-scorbutic syrups, particularly rose syrup – a rich natural source of ascorbic acid.

3713 LIND, JAMES. 1716–1794
A treatise of the scurvy. Edinburgh, *Sands, Murray & Cochran*, 1753.
Lind, founder of naval hygiene in England, wrote a classical treatise on scurvy, in which he described many important experiments he had made on the disease. He urged the issue of lemon juice in the Navy, and even suggested preserved orange and lemon juice; it was due to Lind that scurvy was eventually eradicated from the British Navy. Reprinted, with notes, Edinburgh, 1953.

3714 COOK, James. 1728–1779
The method taken for preserving the health of the crew of H.M.S. the Resolution during her late voyage round the world. *Phil. Trans.*, 1776, **66,** 402–06.

Capt. Cook demonstrated that in voyages lasting several years scurvy could be prevented by the employment of certain articles in the diet, as suggested by Lind.

3715 BLANE, *Sir* Gilbert. 1749–1834
Observations on the diseases incident to seamen. London, *J. Cooper*, 1785.

Although Blane added nothing to the knowledge on scurvy, he demonstrated the value of fresh lemons, limes, and oranges; through his influence the issue of lemon juice in the British Navy was ordered in 1795, after which scurvy soon disappeared. Blane's extreme coldness of manner earned for him the nickname "Chilblain".

3716 TROTTER, Thomas. 1761–1832
Observations on the scurvy. Edinburgh, *C. Eliot & G. G. J. & J. Robinson* 1786.

3717 KREBEL, Rudolph.
Der Scorbut in geschichtlich-literarischer, pathologischer, prophylactischer und therapeutischer Beziehung. Leipzig, *E. Wartig*, 1836.

3718 MÖLLER, Julius Otto Ludwig. 1819–1887
Ueber akute Rachitis. *Königsb. med. Jb.*, 1859, **1,** 377–79.

Möller was the first to describe the acute form of rickets combined with scurvy now associated with the name of Sir Thomas Barlow.

3719 CHEADLE, Walter Butler. 1836–1910
Three cases of scurvy supervening on rickets in young children. *Lancet*, 1878, **2,** 685–87.

Infantile scurvy was confused with rickets until Cheadle differentiated between the two conditions.

3720 BARLOW, *Sir* Thomas. 1845–1945
On cases described as "acute rickets" which are probably a combination of scurvy and rickets, the scurvy being an essential, and the rickets a variable, element. *Med.-chir. Trans.*, 1883, **66,** 159–219.

Classical description of infantile scurvy ("Barlow's disease") which includes the pathology of the condition. See also his earlier paper in *Trans. int. med. Congr.*, 1881, **4**, 116–28. Reprinted, but without the coloured lithographs and detailed list of cases included in the original, in *Arch. Dis. Childh.*, 1935, **10**, 223–52.

3721 HOLST, Axel. 1861–1931
Experimental studies relating to "ship-beri-beri" and scurvy. *J. Hyg.* (*Lond.*), 1907, **7,** 619–33.

Experimental production of scurvy in guinea-pigs. Holst published further papers on the subject in the same journal, 1907, **7**, 634–71, and in *Z. Hyg.*, 1912, **72**, 1–120, both with Theodor Froelich. Their work made it possible to employ guinea-pigs for assessing the relative values of antiscorbutic foods.

3722 ASCHOFF, Karl Albert Ludwig. 1866–1942, & KOCH, Walter Karl. 1880–
Der Skorbut. Jena, *G. Fischer*, 1919.

3723 HESS, Alfred Fabian. 1875–1933
Scurvy, past and present. Philadelphia, *J. B. Lippincott*, (1920).

Includes a history and bibliography.

3724 BOAS, MARGARET AVERIL.
The effect of desiccation upon the nutritive properties of egg-white. *Biochem. J.*, 1927, **21,** 712–24.
Demonstration of the effect of deprivation of biotin.

3725 PARSONS, *Sir* LEONARD GREGORY. 1879–1950
Scurvy treated with ascorbic acid. *Proc. roy. Soc. Med.*, 1933, **26,** 1533.
First case of infantile scurvy cured by the administration of ascorbic acid.

Rickets

3727 WHISTLER, DANIEL. 1619–1684
Disputatio medica inauguralis, de morbo puerili Anglorum, quem patrio idiomate indigenae vocant The Rickets. Lugduni Batavorum, *ex off. WC. Boxii*, 1645.
In his 26th year Whistler published his graduation thesis at Leyden; this was the first description of rickets as a definite disease manifesting itself by a more or less constant association of symptoms. Still (No. 6356) gives an interesting account of Whistler, with abstracts from the above work. The book attracted little attention and the credit for the first description is usually given to Glisson.

3728 BOOTIUS, ARNOLDUS [BOATE]. ?1600–?1653
Observationes medicae de affectibus omissis. London, *T. Whitaker*, 1649.
Bootius, who spent many years in Ireland, included a full first-hand account of rickets in Chapter 12 of the above book ("De tabe pectorea"). He showed how widespread was the disease at that time. Reprinted in *Opuscula Selecta Neerlandicorum*, Fasc. 5, pp. 260–73, Amsterdam, 1926.

3729 GLISSON, FRANCIS. 1597–1677
De rachitide sive morbo puerili, qui vulgo The Rickets dicitur. Londini, *typ. G. Du-gardi*, 1650.
Although anticipated by Whistler and others in the description of infantile rickets, Glisson's account was the fullest that had till then appeared. He was first (Chap. 22) to describe infantile scurvy. An English translation appeared in 1651.

3730 SCHÜTTE, D.
Beobachtungen über den Nutzen des Berger Leberthrans (Oleum jecoris Aselli, von Gadus asellus L.). *Arch. med. Erfahr.*, 1824, **2,** 79–92.
First report of the value of cod-liver oil in the treatment of rickets.

3731 POMMER, GUSTAV. 1851–1935
Untersuchungen über Osteomalacie und Rachitis. Leipzig, *F. C. W. Vogel*, 1885.
Hess considered this the foremost contribution to the subject during the 19th century.

3732 HULDSCHINSKY, KURT. 1883–
Heilung von Rachitis durch künstliche Höhensonne. *Dtsch. med. Wschr.*, Berlin, 1919, **45,** 712–13.
Rickets cured by ultra-violet irradiation.

3733 MELLANBY, *Sir* EDWARD. 1884–1955
The part played by an "accessory factor" in the production of experimental rickets. *J. Physiol.* (*Lond.*), 1918–19, **52,** xi–xii, liii–liv.
First convincing experimental evidence that rickets is a deficiency disease, curable by correct diet.

3734 ——. An experimental investigation on rickets. *Lancet*, 1919, **1**, 407–12.

In his important experiments on rickets Mellanby both induced and controlled the disease by diet.

3735 HESS, ALFRED FABIAN. 1875–1933

Rickets, including osteomalacia and tetany. Philadelphia, *Lea & Febiger*, 1929.

Hess made numerous clinical observations on rickets and scurvy and discovered that anti-rachitic properties could be imparted to certain oils and to food by exposing them to ultra-violet rays. His book includes an important history and bibliography of the subject.

Beri-beri

3736 BONTIUS, JACOBUS. 1592–1631

De paralyseos quadam specie, quam indigenae beriberii vocant. In his: *De medicina Indorum*. Lugduni Batavorum, 1642, 115–20.

Beri-beri wsa mentioned in Chinese literature before the Christian era. The first modern scientific description was given by Bontius, who saw cases of it in the East Indies.

3737 TULP, NICOLAAS. 1593–1674

Observationes medicae. Amstelredami, *apud L. Elzevirium*, 1652.

One of the earliest accounts of beri-beri is on pp. 300–05 of this work. Tulp, notable as the demonstrator in Rembrandt's "Anatomy Lesson," was among the first, in the same book, to describe the ileo-caecal valve ("Tulp's valve").

3738 MALCOLMSON, JOHN GRANT. ?–1844

A practical essay on the history and treatment of beriberi. Madras, *Govt. Press*, 1835.

A classical account, in which the author brought together all that was known about the disease in his day.

3739 BAELZ, B.

Kakke (Beriberi). *Mitt. deutsch. Ges. Nat. u. Völkerk. Ostasiens*, 1880–1884, **3**, 301–19.

In his important account of beri-beri Baelz dealt with the Tokyo outbreak of 1881.

3740 TAKAKI, KANEHIRO, *Baron*. 1849–1915

On the cause and prevention of kak,ke. *Trans. Sei-I-Kwai*, Tokyo, 1885, **4**, 29–37.

Takaki was the first conclusively to show the dietary origin of beri-beri. Measures introduced by him resulted in its eradication from the Japanese Navy, where it had had previously been a serious problem.

3741 EIJKMAN, CHRISTIAAN. 1858–1930

Polyneuritis bij hoenders. *Geneesk. T. nederl. Indië*, 1890, **30**, 295; 1893, **32**, 353; 1896, **36**, 214.

Eijkman produced beri-beri experimentally in fowls; from this he was led to conclude that a diet of over-milled rice was the chief cause, both in fowls and humans. Thus his work was of great importance in determining the aetiology of beri-beri, and he further has the distinction of being the first to produce experimentally a disease of dietary deficiency origin. He shared a Nobel Prize with F. G. Hopkins in 1929. German translation in *Virchows Arch. path. Anat.*, 1897, **148**, 523–32.

3742 GRIJNS, Gerrit. 1865–1944

Over polyneuritis gallinarum. *Geneesk. T. nederl. Indië*, 1901, **41,** 3–110.

Grijns succeeded Eijkman as director of the Research Laboratory for Pathological Anatomy and Bacteriology in Batavia. He was first to adopt the view that beri-beri was simply a "deficiency disease", since he found it to be due to the lack of an unknown substance in the diet.

3743 FRASER, Henry. 1873–1930, & STANTON, *Sir* Ambrose Thomas. 1875–1938

An inquiry concerning the etiology of beri-beri. Singapore, *Kelly & Walsh*, 1909.

Studies from the Institute for Medical Research, F.M.S., No. 10. Careful and long-continued experiments on the aetiology of beri-beri were carried out by Fraser and Stanton in Malaya.

3744 FUNK, Casimir. 1884–1967

On the chemical nature of the substance which cures polyneuritis in birds induced by a diet of polished rice. *J. Physiol.* (*Lond.*), 1911, **43,** 395–400.

Funk determined the chemical nature of the substance in rice polishings which could cure beri-beri.

3745 VEDDER, Edward Bright. 1878–1952

Beriberi. New York, *W. Wood & Co.*, 1913.

Important studies of beri-beri are recorded in this book. Since its publication the author made many additional contributions to the literature on the subject.

3747 WENCKEBACH, Karel Frederik. 1864–1940

Das Beriberi-Herz. Berlin, *J. Springer*, 1934.

Wenckebach wrote a classical account of the heart in beri-beri.

Pellagra

3749 THIÉRRY, François [Thiéry]. 1719–?

Description d'une maladie appelée mal de la rosa. *J. Méd. Chir. Pharm.*, 1755, **2,** 337–46.

Thiérry wrote an account of pellagra from what he had seen or heard of Casal's cases. His work antedates that of Casal in date of publication but is not a first-hand description.

3750 CASAL Y JULIAN, Gaspar. 1679–1759

Historia natural, y medica de el Principado de Asturias. Madrid, *M. Martin*, 1762.

The first recognizable description of pellagra is included on pp. 327–60 of this book, which was written in 1735 but not published until 1762, after the writer's death. He called the disease *mal de la rosa*. Reprinted, Oviedo, 1900.

3751 FRAPOLLI, Francesco. ?–1773?

Animadversiones in morbum, vulgo pellagram. [Mediolani, *apud J. Galcatium*], 1771.

In Frapolli's careful description of pellagra, the disease was first given its present name. This book is also the first Italian account of the malady.

3752 STRAMBIO, Gaetano. 1752–1831

De pellagra. 3 vols. Mediolani, *J. B. Bianchi*, 1786–89.

By 1776 pellagra had attained serious proportions in Italy; Strambio was placed in charge of a hospital for the treatment of pellagrins, and he left an important account of the disease. He first pointed out that pellagra might occur without the cutaneous lesions, till then regarded as characteristic.

3753 ROUSSEL, JEAN BAPTISTE VICTOR THÉOPHILE. 1816–1903
Traité de la pellagre et des pseudo-pellagres. Paris, *J. B. Baillière*, 1866.

Roussel was awarded a prize of 5,000 francs for this work.

3754 LOMBROSO, CESARE. 1836–1909
Studii clinici ed esperimentali sulla natura, causa e terapia della pellagra. Bologna, *F. E. Garagnani*, 1869.

Lombroso upheld the maize theory of the origin of pellagra. He believed that the symptoms were caused by a toxin which developed in deteriorated maize. Reprinted from *Riv. clin. Bologna*, 1869, **8**, 289–314, 321–44.

3755 GOLDBERGER, JOSEPH. 1874–1929, *et al.*
The treatment and prevention of pellagra. *U.S. publ. Hlth Serv. Rep.*, 1914, **29**, 2821–25.

With C. H. Waring and D. G. Willets. A collection of Goldberger's most important papers with a list of his publications appeared in 1964.

3756 HARRIS, HENRY FAUNTLEROY. 1867–1926
Pellagra. New York, *Macmillan & Co.*, 1919.

3757 GOLDBERGER, JOSEPH. 1874–1929, & WHEELER, GEORGE ALEXANDER. 1885–
The experimental production of pellagra in human subjects by means of diet. *U.S. publ. Hlth Serv. Lab. Bull.*, No. 120, 1920, 7–116.

Goldberger was born in Central Europe in poor circumstances. He migrated to America, and, following attendance at a lecture by Austin Flint, decided to study medicine. He entered the U.S. Public Health Service in 1899. He was a pioneer in the study and treatment of pellagra, demonstrating its experimental production and its prevention by proper diet.

3758 ——. A further study of butter, fresh beef, and yeast as pellagra preventatives, with consideration of the relation of factor P-P of pellagra (and black tongue of dogs) to vitamin B. *Publ. Hlth Rep. (Wash.)*, 1926, **41,** 297–318.

Anti-pellagra vitamin. With G. A. Wheeler, R. D. Lillie, and L. M. Rogers.

3759 WILLIAMS, CICELY DELPHINE. 1893–
Kwashiorkor. A nutritional disease of children associated with a maize diet. *Lancet*, 1935, **2,** 1151–52.

Cicely Williams introduced the term "kwashiorkor." The first modern description of the condition was probably that of L. Normet in *Bull. Soc. Path. exot.*, 1926, 207–13.

3760 ELVEHJEM, CONRAD ARNOLD. 1901–1962, *et al.*
The isolation and identification of the anti-black tongue factor. *J. biol. Chem.*, 1938, **123,** 137–49.

Isolation of nicotine acid, the pellagra-preventing factor. With R. J. Madden F. N. Strong, and D. W. Woolley.

3761–3788 SPLEEN; LYMPHATICS

3761 ZAMBECCARI, GIUSEPPE. 1655–1728
Esperienz del Dottor Giuseppe Zambeccari intorno a diverse viscere tagliate a diversi animali viventi. Firenze, *F. Onofri*, 1680.

Proof that the spleen is not essential to life. For a translation and notes on the book, see *Bull. Hist. Med.*, 1941, **9**, 144–76, 311–31 (S. Jarcho).

3762 HODGKIN, THOMAS. 1798–1866
On some morbid appearances of the absorbent glands and spleen. *Med.-chir. Trans.*, 1832, **17**, 68–114.

First full description of lymphadenoma, which Wilks in 1865 referred to as "Hodgkin's disease". In 1666 Malpighi had vaguely outlined the condition. Hodgkin was pathologist at Guy's Hospital. The paper is reproduced in *Med. Classics*, 1937, **1**, 741–70.

3763 QUITTENBAUM, CARL FRIEDRICH. 1793–1852
Commentatio de splenis hypertrophia et historia extirpationis splenis hypertrophici cum fortuna adversa. Rostochii, *typ. Adlerianis*, [1836].

While most people in Germany still considered splenectomy beyond the bounds of possibility, Quittenbaum performed the operation in 1829, establishing it as a surgical procedure.

3764 WILKS, *Sir* SAMUEL, *Bart.* 1824–1911
Cases of a peculiar enlargement of the lymphatic glands frequently associated with disease of the spleen. *Guy's Hosp. Rep.*, 1856, 3 ser. **2,** 114–32; 1865, 3 ser. **11,** 56–67.

Wilks really put Hodgkin's disease "on the map"; the second paper for the first time attached Hodgkin's name to the disease.

3765 SIMON, GUSTAV. 1824–1876
Die Exstirpation der Milz am Menschen. Giessen, *Heyer*, 1857.

3766 GRIESINGER, WILHELM. 1817–1868
Ein Fall von Anaemia splenica bei einem Kinde. *Berl. klin. Wschr.*, 1866, **3,** 212–14.

First reported case of (infantile) splenic anaemia.

3766.1 VANLAIR, CONSTANT. 1839–1914, & MASIUS, JEAN BAPTISTE NICOLAS VOLTAIRE. 1836–1912
De la microcythémie. *Bull. Acad. roy. Méd. Belg.*, 1871, 3 sér., **5,** 515–613.

Vanlair and Masius were first to suggest the concept of haemolytic anaemia. Their paper was republished in book form, Brussels, 1871.

3767 LANGHANS, THEODOR. 1839–1915
Das maligne Lymphosarkom (Pseudoleukämie). *Virchows Arch. path. Anat.*, 1872, **54,** 509–37.

Langhans noted the presence of giant cells in the lesions of Hodgkin's disease.

3768 GREENFIELD, WILLIAM SMITH. 1846–1919
Specimens illustrative of the pathology of lymphadenoma and leucocythemia. *Trans. path. Soc. Lond.*, 1878, **29,** 272–304.

Greenfield also drew attention to the giant cells in lymphadenoma, which later became known as "Dorothy Reed's giant cells" (see No. 3780).

3769 GAUCHER, PHILIPPE CHARLES ERNEST. 1854–1918
De l'épithélioma primitif de la rate, hypertrophie idiopathique de la rate sans leucémie. Paris, *Thèse*, 1882.

Familial splenic anaemia ("Gaucher's disease").

3770 PEL, PIETER KLAZES. 1852–1919
Zur Symptomatologie der sog. Pseudo-Leukämie. *Berl. klin. Wschr.*, 1885, **22,** 3–7.

"Pel–Ebstein disease" (see also No. 3771).

3771 EBSTEIN, Wilhelm. 1836–1912
Das chronische Rückfallsfieber, eine neue Infektionskrankheit. *Berl. klin. Wschr.*, 1887, **24,** 565–68.

3772 DRESCHFELD, Julius. 1845–1907
Clinical lecture on acute Hodgkin's disease. *Brit. med. J.*, 1892, **1,** 893–96.
Dreschfeld preceded Kundrat in differentiating Hodgkin's disease and lymphosarcoma.

3773 KUNDRAT, Hans. 1845–1893
Ueber Lympho-Sarkomatosis. *Wien. klin. Wschr.*, 1893, **6,** 211–13, 234–39.
Kundrat separated lymphosarcoma ("Kundrat's disease") from other malignant tumours involving the lymphatic system.

3774 BANTI, Guido. 1852–1925
La splenomegalia con cirrosi del fegato. *Sperimentale*, 1894, **48,** Com. e riv., 447–52; Sez. biol., 407–32.
"Banti's syndrome", splenomegalic anaemia. Reprinted with translation, in *Med. Classics*, 1937, 1, 901–27. (For his earlier work on the subject, see No. 3126.)

3775 PALTAUF, Richard. 1858–1924
Lymphosarkom (Lymphosarkomatose, Pseudoleukämie, Myelom, Chlorom). *Ergebn. allg. Path. path. Anat.*, (1896), 1897, **3,** 1 Heft, 652–91.
"Paltauf–Sternberg disease" (see also No. 3776). On the Continent the name "Hodgkin–Paltauf–Sternberg disease" is in use.

3776 STERNBERG, Carl. 1872–1935
Ueber eine eigenartige, unter dem Bilde der Pseudoleukämie verlaufende Tuberkulose des lymphatischen Apparates. *Z. Heilk.*, 1898, **19,** 21–90.
In his classical description of lymphadenoma Sternberg separated it from aleukaemic leukaemia, with which it had hitherto been included.

3777 HAYEM, Georges. 1841–1933
Sur une variété particulière d'ictère chronique splénomégalique. *J. Méd. intern.*, 1898, **2,** 116–18.
"Hayem–Widal disease" – acquired haemolytic anaemia. (See also No. 3783.)

3778 CHAUFFARD, Anatole Marie Emile. 1855–1932
Des hépatites d'origine splénique. *Semaine méd.*, 1899, **19,** 177–78.
Chauffard and Minkowski (No. 3779) described familial haemolytic jaundice ("Minkowski–Chauffard disease").

3779 MINKOWSKI, Oscar. 1858–1931
Ueber eine hereditäre, unter dem Bilde eines chronischen Icterus mit Urobilinurie, Splenomegalie, und Nierensiderosis verlaufende Affection. *Verh. Kongr. inn. Med.*, 1900, **18,** 316–21.

3780 REED, Dorothy, *Mrs. Mendenhall.*
On the pathological changes in Hodgkin's disease, with especial reference to its relation to tuberculosis. *Johns Hopk. Hosp. Rep.*, 1902, **10,** 133–96.
Dorothy Reed's classical work on Hodgkin's disease included a study of the histological picture. She described the proliferation of the endothelial and reticular cells, and the formation of lymphadenoma cells – "Dorothy Reed's giant cells."

3781 CHAUFFARD, Anatole Marie Emile. 1855–1932
Pathogènie de l'ictère congénital de l'adulte. *Semaine méd.*, 1907, **27,** 25–29.

Discovery of the fragility of red cells in congenital haemolytic anaemia.

3782 WHIPPLE, George Hoyt. 1878–
A hitherto undescribed disease characterized anatomically by deposits of fat and fatty acids in the intestinal and mesenteric lymphatic tissues. *Johns Hopk. Hosp. Bull.*, 1907, **18,** 382–91.

"Whipple's disease." Whipple suggested the name "intestinal lipodystrophy" for this condition.

3783 WIDAL, Georges Fernand Isidor. 1862–1929, & ABRAMI, Pierre. 1879–1945
Ictères hémolytiques non congénitaux avec anémie. *Presse méd.*, 1907, **15,** 749.

"Widal–Abrami disease" (Hayem–Widal disease), acquired haemolytic anaemia. (See also No. 3777.)

3784 NIEMANN, Albert. 1880–1921
Ein unbekanntes Krankheitsbild. *Jb. Kinderheilk.*, 1914, **79,** 1–10.

First description of that form of xanthomatosis which Pick described more fully in 1926 (No. 3785) and to which the eponym "Niemann–Pick disease" has been applied.

3785 PICK, Ludwig. 1868–1935
Der Morbus Gaucher und die ihm ähnlichen Erkrankungen. (Die lipoidzellige Splenohepatomegalie Typus Niemann und die diabetische Lipoidzellenhyperplasie der Milz.) *Ergebn. inn. Med. Kinderheilk.*, 1926, **29,** 519–627.

"Niemann–Pick disease" – a form of xanthomatosis to which attention was first drawn by Niemann (No. 3784) in 1914. Pick's account is of greater importance.

3786 BRILL, Nathan Edwin. 1860–1925, *et al.*
Generalized giant lymph follicle hyperplasia of lymph nodes and spleen; a hitherto undescribed type. *J. Amer. med. Ass.*, 1925, **84,** 668–71.

See No. 3787. With G. Baehr and N. Rosenthal.

3787 SYMMERS, Douglas. 1879–
Follicular lymphadenopathy with splenomegaly: a newly recognized disease of the lymphatic system. *Arch. Path. Lab. Med.*, 1927, **3,** 816–20.

"Brill–Symmers disease" (see No. 3786).

3788 GILMAN, Alfred. 1908– , & PHILIPS, Frederick Stanley. 1916–
The biological actions and therapeutic applications of the β-chloroethyl amines and sulfides. *Science*, 1946, **103,** 409–15.

Introduction of nitrogen mustard in treatment of Hodgkin's disease.

3789–3911 ENDOCRINE DISORDERS

3789 PLATTER, Felix [Platerus]. 1536–1614
Observationum in hominis affectibus. Basileae, *L. König.*, 1614.

First known report of a case of death from hypertrophy of the thymus, in an infant, is reported on p. 172; it is reproduced on p. 239 of J. Ruhräh's *Pediatrics of the past*, New York, 1925.

3790 HUTCHINSON, *Sir* JONATHAN. 1828–1913
Congenital absence of hair and mammary glands with atrophic condition of the skin and its appendages in a boy whose mother had been almost wholly bald from alopecia areata from the age of six. *Med.-chir. Trans.*, 1886, **69**, 473–77.
First description of progeria.

3791 MARCHAND, FELIX JACOB. 1846–1928
Ueber eine Geschwulst der sogen. Glandula carotica oder des Nodulus caroticus. In *Festschrift Rudolf Virchow*, Berlin, *A. Hirschwald*, 1891, **1**, 547–54.
First account of the pathology of carotid body tumours.

3792 GILFORD, HASTINGS. 1861–1941
On a condition of mixed premature and immature development. *Med.-chir. Trans.*, 1897, **80**, 17–45.
Hastings Gilford gave progeria its name; it was first fully reported by him in *Practitioner*, 1904, 73, 188–217.

3793 SAJOUS, CHARLES EUCHARISTE DE MÉDICIS. 1852–1929
The internal secretions and the principles of medicine. 2 pts. Philadelphia, *F. A. Davis*, 1903–07.
Sajous, pioneer American endocrinologist, wrote the first treatise on the subject. In this work he regarded the adrenal, pituitary, and thyroid glands as controlling the immunizing mechanism of the body.

3794 BIEDL, ARTUR. 1869–1933
Innere Sekretion. Berlin, Wien, *Urban & Schwarzenberg*, 1910.
Biedl's classical work shows the rapid development of the knowledge concerning endocrinology. In 1890 there were few publications dealing with internal secretion, but Biedl, in the second edition of his book, 1913, was able to include a bibliography of 8,500 items.

3795 FALTA, WILHELM. 1875–1950
Die Erkrankungen der Blutdrüsen. Berlin, *J. Springer*, 1913.
First attempt to systematize the endocrine disorders. English translation, 1915.

3796 STEINACH, EUGEN. 1861–1944
Verjüngung durch experimentelle Neubelebung der alternden Pubertätsdrüse. Berlin, *J. Springer*, 1920.
Steinach rejuvenation operation, ligation of the vas deferens.

3797 VORONOFF, SERGE. 1866–1951
Greffes testiculaires. Paris, *O. Doin*, 1923.
Voronoff first reported his experimental rejuvenation by means of testicular transplants in 1919.

3798 BARKER, LEWELLYS FRANKLIN. 1867–1943
Endocrinology and metabolism presented in their scientific and practical clinical aspects by ninety-eight contributors. Edited by L. F. BARKER. 5 vols. New York, *D. Appleton & Co.*, 1922–24.

3799 DODDS, *Sir* EDWARD CHARLES. 1899–1973, *et al.*
The oestrogenic activity of certain synthetic compounds. *Nature* (*Lond.*), 1938, **141**, 247–48.
Introduction of stilboestrol, the first synthetic oestrogen. With L. Golberg, W. Lawson, and R. Robinson.

3800 DODDS, *Sir* Edward Charles. 1899–1973, *et al.*
Oestrogenic activity of alkylated stilboestrols. *Nature* (*Lond.*), 1938, **142,** 34.
Introduction of dienoestrol. With L. Golberg, W. Lawson, and R. Robinson.

3801 CAMPBELL, N. R., *et al.*
Oestrogenic activity of anol; a highly active phenol isolated from the by-products. *Nature* (*Lond.*), 1938, **142,** 1121.
Isolation of hexoestrol. With E. C. Dodds and W. Lawson.

3801.1 TURNER, Henry Hubert. 1892–1970
A syndrome of infantilism, congenital webbed neck, and cubitus valgus. *Endocrinology*, 1938, **23,** 566–74.
"Turner's syndrome."

3802 GOLDZIEHER, Maximilian A. 1883–
The endocrine glands. New York, *Appleton-Century*, 1939.
Goldzieher has for many years studied the subject of endocrinology, and in this work deals very fully with its history, theory, and practice. All the important references are included in the book.

3803 MACPHERSON, Archibald Ian Stewart, & ROBERTSON, Edwin Moody. 1902–
Clinical use of triphenylchlorethylene. *Lancet*, 1939, **2,** 1362–66.

3804 KLINEFELTER, Harry Fitch. 1912– , *et al.*
Syndrome characterized by gynecomastia, aspermatogenesis without A-Leydigism, and increased excretion of follicle-stimulating hormone. *J. clin. Endocr.*, 1942, **2,** 615–27.
Klinefelter syndrome. With E. C. Reifenstein and F. Albright.

3805–3855 THYROID GLAND

3805 BOMBASTUS AB HOHENHEIM, Aureolus Philippus Theophrastus [Paracelsus]. 1493–1541
De generatione stultorum. In his *Opera*, Strassburg, 1603, **2,** 174–82.
Paracelsus was first to note the coincidence of cretinism and endemic goitre. It was not until the 19th century that the possibility of the occurrence of cretinism in adults was entertained.

3806 DU LAURENS, André [Laurentius]. 1558–1609
De mirabili strumas sanandi. Parisiis, *M. Orry*, 1609.
An early historical record of goitre which du Laurens maintained was contagious. Du Laurens was at one time physician to Henri IV.

3807 PROSSER, Thomas.
An account and method of cure of the bronchocele or Derby neck. London, *W. Owen*, 1769.
Prosser gave the prescription of a powder containing calcined sponge, to be taken for the cure of goitre. This is probably the first recorded use of an iodine preparation in England.

3808 WILMER, Bradford.
Cases and remarks in surgery: to which is subjoined, an appendix, containing the method of curing the bronchocele in Coventry. London, *T. Longman*, 1779.
The "Coventry treatment" for goitre, which introduced the burnt sponge remedy into England, is mentioned on pp. 251–54.

3809 MALACARNE, Michaele Vincenzo Giacinto. 1744–1816
Sui gozzi e sulla stupidità ec. dei cretini. Torino, 1789.

Hirsch considered this the first important work on cretinism and goitre. See also Malacarne's *Lettre*, in J. P. Frank: *Delectus opusculorum medicorum*, 1789, **6**, 241–58.

3810 FODÉRÉ, François Emmanuel. 1764–1835
Essai sur le goitre et le crétinage. Turin, 1792.

Fodéré considered cretinism to be due to the concentrated air in the deep valleys, rather than to water. He also drew attention to the skeletal changes.

3811 FLAJANI, Giuseppe. 1741–1808
Sopra un tumor freddo nell'anterior parte del collo detto broncocele. In his *Collezione d'osservazione e riflessioni di chirurgia*, Roma, 1802, **3**, 270–73.

One of the earliest accounts of exophthalmic goitre. The author noted cardiac disturbances in thyroid enlargement.

3812 COINDET, Jean François. 1774–1834
Découverte d'un nouveau remède contre le goitre. *Bibliothèque universelle*, 1820, **14**, 190–98; also in *Ann. Chim. Phys.*, 1820, **15**, 49–59.

Coindet is usually regarded as the first to administer iodine in cases of goitre, with beneficial results. It had previously been prepared from seaweed by B. Courtois in 1812 (*Ann. Chim.* (*Paris*), 1813, **88**, 304–10), and both Ampère and Humphry Davy were interested in it. W. Prout, however, in his *Chemistry, meteorology, etc.*, London, 1834, p. 113, claimed that he had recommended it to John Elliotson, who had used it in 1819 at St. Thomas's Hospital. There is an English translation of his paper in *Lond. med. phys. J.*, 1820, **44**, 486–89.

3813 PARRY, Caleb Hillier. 1755–1822
Enlargement of the thyroid gland in connection with enlargement or palpitation of the heart. In: *Collections from the unpublished medical writings of C. H. Parry*, London, 1825, **2**, 111–29.

A classical account of exophthalmic goitre. Although Graves and Basedow have both been credited with the first description of the condition, giving their names to it, Osler has called attention to the priority of Parry's claim, and it is now sometimes referred to as "Parry's disease". Garrison says that Parry first noted the condition in 1786; he briefly reported it in his *Elements of pathology and therapeutics*, 1815. Reprinted in *Med. Classics*, 1940, **5**, 8–30.

3814 GREEN, Joseph Henry. 1791–1863
Removal of the right lobe of the thyroid gland. *Lancet*, 1828–29, **2**, 351–52.

To Green, of St. Thomas's Hospital, London, is accredited the first thyroidectomy, the patient succumbing 15 days later from sepsis.

3815 GRAVES, Robert James. 1796–1853
[Palpitation of the heart with enlargement of the thyroid gland.] *Lond. med. surg. J.* (*Renshaw*), 1835, **7**, 516–17.

This is considered the first accurate account of exophthalmic goitre, later known as "Parry's disease," "Graves' disease," and "Basedow's disease." An interesting fact about the *London Medical & Surgical Journal* is that after the first five volumes had been published by Renshaw and edited by M. Ryan, these two separated, each continuing to publish a separate edition of the same journal. Graves' paper appeared in the series published by Renshaw. Reprinted in *Med. Classics*, 1940, **5**, 33–36.

3816 BASEDOW, Carl Adolph von. 1799–1854
Exophthalmos durch Hypertrophie des Zellgewebes in der Augenhöhle. *Wschr. ges. Heilk.*, 1840, **6,** 197–204, 220–28.

In Europe, outside the British Isles, exophthalmic goitre, or Graves' disease, is known as "Basedow's disease." His accurate description of four cases in which he described exophthalmos, goitre, and palpitation led to the phrase "Merseburg triad," associating these conditions with the name of his own town. He also mentioned emaciation, excessive perspiration, and nervousness as additional symptoms and anticipated later methods of treatment by his advocacy of mineral waters containing iodide and bromide of sodium.

3817 CHATIN, Gaspard Adolph. 1813–1901
Existence de l'iode dans les plantes d'eau douce. Conséquences de ce fait pour la géognosie, la physiologie végétale, la thérapeutique et peut-être pour l'industrie. *C. R. Acad. Sci.* (*Paris*), 1850, **30,** 352–54.

Chatin showed that iodine could prevent endemic goitre and cretinism.

3818 CURLING, Thomas Blizard. 1811–1888
Two cases of absence of the thyroid body and symmetrical swellings of fat tissue at the sides of the neck, connected with defective cerebral development. *Med.-chir. Trans.*, 1850, **33,** 303–06.

Curling, of the London Hospital, was the first accurately to note the clinical picture of cretinism, which Ord was later to name "myxoedema". Curling was also the first to suggest deficiency of the thyroid as a cause of cretinism.

3819 SCHIFF, Moritz. 1823–1896
Untersuchungen über die Zuckerbildung in der Leber und den Einfluss des Nervensystems auf die Erzeugung des Diabetes. *Schweiz. Mschr. prakt. Med.*, 1859, **4,** 267–75.

In this paper is included Schiff's reports on his experimental thyroidectomies, which were attended with fatal results. Subsequently (*Arch. exp. Path. Pharmak.*, 1884, **18**, 25) he showed that intra-abdominal transplantation of the gland would obviate fatal results in thyroidectomy.

3820 GRAEFE, Friedrich Wilhelm Ernst Albrecht von. 1828–1870
Ueber Basedow'sche Krankheit. *Dtsch. Klinik*, 1864, **16,** 158–59.

"Graefe's sign" – the discovery by von Graefe of the failure of the eyelid to follow the eye when it is rolled downwards – diagnostic of exophthalmic goitre.

3821 SICK, Paul August. 1836–1900
Ueber die totale Exstirpation einer kropfig entarteten Schilddrüse, und über die Rückwirkung dieser Operation auf die Circulationsverhältnisse im Kopfe. *Med. CorrespBl. württemb. ärztl. Vereins,* 1867, **37,** 199–205.

Sick is credited with being the first to notice symptoms of loss of thyroid function following thyroidectomy. According to Halsted, the above is the first report of total thyroidectomy and "the first report of the condition which we now recognize as *status thyreoprivus*".

3822 FAGGE, Charles Hilton. 1838–1883
On sporadic cretinism. *Med.-chir. Trans.*, 1871, **54,** 155–70.

In this paper Fagge, nephew of John Hilton of Guy's Hospital, described sporadic cretinism as distinct from the endemic variety.

3823 GULL, *Sir* WILLIAM WITHEY. 1816–1890
On a cretinoid state supervening in adult life in women. *Trans. clin. Soc. Lond.*, 1873–74, **7,** 180–85.

Gull was among the first to point out the cause of myxoedema, of which the above paper gives a classical description. Gull was associated with Guy's Hospital, London, for most of his life; he acquired a large practice and left a fortune of £344,000 on his death.

3824 WATSON, *Sir* PATRICK HERON. 1832–1907
Excision of the thyroid gland. *Edinb. med. J.*, 1874, **19,** 252–55.

Watson was a pioneer of thyroidectomy in the treatment of goitre, although Green (No. 3814) was first to perform the operation. Also in *Brit. med. J.*, 1875, **2,** 386–88.

3825 ORD, WILLIAM MILLER. 1834–1902
On myxoedema. *Med.-chir. Trans.*, 1878, **61,** 57–78.

Ord coined the term "myxoedema" for the condition noted earlier by Curling and Gull.

3826 KOCHER, EMIL THEODOR. 1841–1917
Exstirpation einer Struma retrooesophagea. *KorrespBl. schweiz. Aerzte*, 1878, **8,** 702–05.

Kocher, a pupil of Billroth, was a pioneer of thyroidectomy for goitre. Before his time the operation was seldom performed. Garrison says that he performed this difficult operation 2,000 times, with a mortality rate of only 4½ per cent. Kocher received the Nobel Prize in 1909.

3827 ——. Ueber Kropfexstirpation und ihre Folgen. *Arch. klin. Chir.*, 1883, **29,** 254–337.

Kocher coined the term "cachexia strumipriva" to describe the myxoedema following total extirpation of the thyroid. His work on the subject led to a better understanding of the cause of myxoedema.

3828 REVERDIN, JACQUES LOUIS. 1842–1929
Accidents consécutifs à l'ablation totale du goitre. *Rev. méd. Suisse rom.*, 1882, **2,** 539.

Reverdin produced myxoedema by removal of the thyroid as a whole or in part. This confirmed the earlier work of Schiff, of which Reverdin had probably not heard. See also No. 3836.

3829 ——. Note sur vingt-deux opérations de goitre. *Rev. méd. Suisse rom.*, 1883, **3,** 169–98, 233–78, 309–64.

3830 MARIE, PIERRE. 1853–1940
Sur la nature et sur quelques-uns des symptomes de la maladie de Basedow. *Arch. Neurol. (Paris)*, 1883, **6,** 79–85.

The fourth cardinal sign in exophthalmic goitre – tremor – was first mentioned by Pierre Marie.

3831 SEMON, *Sir* FELIX. 1849–1921
A typical case of myxoedema. *Brit. med. J.*, 1883, **2,** 1072.

Semon argued that cachexia strumipriva, myxoedema, and cretinism were all due to loss of function of the thyroid. His contention, at first criticized, was later fully endorsed by the report of a committee set up by the Clinical Society of London to investigate the subject of myxoedema.

3832 WÖLFLER, ANTON. 1850–1917
Ueber die Entwickelung und den Bau des Kropfes. *Arch. klin. Chir.*, 1883, **29,** 1–97.

Important classification of thyroid tumours; foetal adenoma is described on p. 40.

3833 REHN, Ludwig. 1849–1930
Ueber die Exstirpation des Kropfs bei Morbus basedowii. *Berl. klin. Wschr.*, 1884, **21**, 163–66.

First thyroidectomy for exophthalmic goitre. The operation reported was performed in 1880.

3834 HORSLEY, *Sir* Victor Alexander Haden. 1857–1916
A recent specimen of artificial myxoedema in a monkey. *Lancet*, 1884, **2**, 827.

By experimental removal of the thyroid Horsley produced artificial myxoedema, confirming previous work by Reverdin and others. At the time his results were regarded as proof that total thyroidectomy produces operative myxoedema, but some of the symptoms he described are now known to have been due to removal of the parathyroids.

3835 ——. Functional nervous disorders due to loss of thyroid gland and pituitary body. *Lancet*, 1886, **1**, 5.

3836 REVERDIN, Jacques Louis. 1842–1929
Contribution à l'étude du myxoedème consécutif à l'extirpation totale ou partielle du corps thyroïde. *Rev. méd. Suisse rom.*, 1887, **7**, 275–91, 318–30.

3837 LANNELONGUE, Odilon Marc. 1840–1911
Transplantation du corps thyroïde sur l'homme. *Bull. méd.*, 1890, **4**, 225.

First thyroid transplantation (for treatment of cretinism).

3838 MURRAY, George Redmayne. 1865–1939
Note on the treatment of myxoedema by hypodermic injections of an extract of the thyroid gland of a sheep. *Brit. med. J.*, 1891, **2**, 796–97.

Murray injected thyroid extract subcutaneously in the treatment of myxoedema, with highly successful results.

3839 MÜLLER, Friedrich von. 1858–1941
Beiträge zur Kenntniss der Basedow'schen Krankheit. *Dtsch. Arch. klin. Med.*, 1893, **51**, 335–412.

Müller demonstrated that an increased metabolism accompanies exophthalmic goitre.

3840 MAGNUS-LEVY, Adolf. 1865–1955
Ueber den respiratorischen Gaswechsel unter dem Einfluss der Thyreoidea sowie unter verschiedenen pathologischen Zuständen. *Berl. klin. Wschr.*, 1895, **32**, 650.

Magnus-Levy demonstrated the increased metabolic rate in toxic goitre, confirming the work of Müller. His experimental investigations laid the foundation for the modern conception of thyroid function. See also *Z. klin. Med.*, 1897, **33**, 269–314.

3840.1 PENDRED, Vaughan. 1869–1946
Deaf-mutism and goitre. *Lancet*, 1896, **2**, 532.

Pendred drew attention to the association of goitre with deaf-mutism.

3841 RIEDEL, Bernhard Moritz Karl Ludwig. 1846–1916
Die chronische, zur Bildung eisenharter Tumoren führende Entzündung der Schilddrüse. *Verh. dtsch. Ges. Chir.*, 1896, **25**, 101–05.

Riedel described a type of chronic inflammation of the thyroid ("Riedel's disease").

3842 PINELES, Friedrich. 1868–1936
Ueber Thyreoaplasie (kongenitales Myxoedem und infantiles Myxoedem). *Wien. klin. Wschr.*, 1902, **15,** 1129–36.
Pineles differentiated endemic (familial) cretinism associated with goitre from sporadic cretinism.

3843 BRISSAUD, Édouard. 1852–1909
L'infantilisme vrai. *N. Iconogr. Salpêt.*, 1907, **20,** 1–17.
Brissaud described thyroid infantilism.

3844 MARINE, David. 1880– , & WILLIAMS, William Whitridge. 1875–
The relation of iodin to the structure of the thyroid gland. *Arch. intern. Med.*, 1908, **1,** 349–84.

3845 HASHIMOTO, Hakaru. 1881–1934
Zur Kenntniss der lymphomatösen Veränderung der Schilddrüse (Struma lymphomatosa). *Arch. klin. Chir.*, 1912, **97,** 219–48.
"Hashimoto's disease", struma lymphomatosa, lymphoid infiltration of the thyroid.

3846 WAGNER VON JAUREGG, Julius. 1857–1940
Myxödem und Kretinismus. Leipzig, *F. Deuticke*, 1912.

3847 McCARRISON, *Sir* Robert. 1878–1960
The pathogenesis of experimentally produced goitre. *Indian J. med. Res.*, 1914, **2,** 183–213.

3848 CANNON, Walter Bradford. 1871–1945, *et al.*
Experimental hyperthyroidism. *Amer. J. Physiol.*, 1915, **36,** 363–64.
First successful experimental production of exophthalmic goitre. With C. A. L. Binger and R. Fitz.

3849 ZONDEK, Hermann. 1887–
Das Myxödemherz. *Münch. med. Wschr.*, 1918, **65,** 1180–82.
First systematic study of the characteristic changes of the heart in myxoedema.

3850 GOETSCH, Emil. 1883–1963
Epinephrin hypersensitiveness test in the diagnosis of hyperthyroidism. *Penn. med. J.*, 1919–20, **23,** 431–37.
Goetsch devised a skin reaction for use in the diagnosis of hyperthyroidism.

3851 PLUMMER, Henry Stanley. 1874–1937, & BOOTHBY, William Meredith. 1880–1953
The value of iodine in exophthalmic goiter. *J. Iowa med. Soc.*, 1924, **14,** 66–73.
Plummer and Boothby recommended the pre-operative administration of iodine in exopthalmic goitre.

3852 JOLL, Cecil Augustus. 1885–1945
Diseases of the thyroid gland, with special reference to thyrotoxicosis. London, *W. Heinemann*, 1932.
Second edition, 1951. Joll was a pioneer in the treatment of thyrotoxicosis by means of subtotal thyroidectomy.

3853 HERTZ, Saul. 1905– , & ROBERTS, A.
Application of radioactive iodine in therapy of Graves' disease. *J. clin. Invest.*, 1942, **21,** 624.

3854 ASTWOOD, Edwin Bennett. 1909–
Treatment of hyperthyroidism with thiourea and thiouracil. *J. Amer. med. Ass.*, 1943, **122,** 78–81.

Astwood was the first to treat human cases of hyperthyroidism with thiourea and thiouracil.

3855 ——. Some observations on the use of thiobarbital as an antithyroid agent in the treatment of Graves' disease. *J. clin. Endocr.*, 1945, **5,** 345–52.

Clinical introduction of thiobarbital.

For history, see No. 3911.

3856–3863 PARATHYROID GLANDS

See also 4825–4838, Tetany.

3856 EISELSBERG, Anton von. 1860–1939
Ueber erfolgreiche Einheilung der Katzenschilddrüse in die Bauchdecke und Auftreten von Tetanie nach deren Exstirpation. *Wien. klin. Wschr.*, 1892, **5,** 81–85.

Experimental production of tetany by excision of the thyroid of a cat, previously successfully transplanted into the abdomen.

3857 VASSALE, Giulio. 1862–1912, & GENERALI, Francesco.
Sugli effeti dell' estirpazione delle ghiandole paratiroidee. *Riv. Patol. nerv. ment.*, 1896, **1,** 95–99.

Demonstration that tetany follows removal of the parathyroids. A French translation of the paper is in *Arch. ital. Biol.*, 1896, **25**, 459–64.

3858 ASKANAZY, Max. 1865–1940
Ueber Ostitis deformans ohne osteoides Gewebe. *Arb. path.-anat. Inst. Tübingen*, 1904, **4,** 398–422.

Askanazy was the first to associate osteitis fibrosa cystica with parathyroid tumours.

3859 MacCALLUM, William George. 1874–1944, & VOEGTLIN, Carl. 1879–1960
On the relation of tetany to the parathyroid glands and to calcium metabolism. *J. exp. Med.*, 1909, **11,** 118–51.

Proof that the parathyroids control calcium metabolism. MacCallum and Voegtlin were able to demonstrate the removal of post-parathyroidectomy tetany by administration of calcium.

3860 HALSTED, William Stewart. 1852–1922
Auto- and isotransplantation, in dogs, of the parathyroid glandules. *J. exp. Med.*, 1909, **11,** 175–99.

3861 COLLIP, James Bertram. 1892–1965
The extraction of a parathyroid hormone which will prevent or control parathyroid tetany and which regulates the level of blood calcium. *J. biol. Chem.*, 1925, **63,** 395–438.

Collip's "parathormone". He showed that it raises the calcium level in parathyroidectomized dogs.

3862 COLLIP, James Bertram. 1892–1965, & LEITCH, Douglas Burrows. 1888–
A case of tetany treated with parathyrin. *Canad. med. Ass. J.*, 1925, **15,** 59–60.
First use of parathyroid hormone in treatment of tetany.

3863 MANDL, Felix. 1892–1957
Therapeutischer Versuch bei Ostitis fibrosa generalisata mittels Exstirpation eines Epithelkörperchentumors. *Wien. klin. Wschr.*, 1925, **38,** 1343–44.
Mandl was the first successfully to treat generalized osteitis fibrosa by extirpation of a parathyroid tumour.

3864–3877 ADRENALS

3864 ADDISON, Thomas. 1793–1860
On the constitutional and local effects of disease of the supra-renal capsules. London, *S. Highley*, 1855.
Addison was the first to draw attention to the importance of the adrenals in clinical medicine. The above work first appeared in the *Lond. med. Gaz.*, 1849, **43**, 517–18, and was later expanded into book form. It described the conditions which later became known as "Addison's disease" and pernicious anaemia, which latter was renamed "Addisonian anaemia" by Trousseau. Reprinted in *Med. Classics*, 1937, **2**, 244–77. Facsimile reprint, 1966.

3865 FRÄNKEL, Felix.
Ein Fall von doppelseitigem, völlig latent verlaufenen Nebennierentumor und gleichzeitiger Nephritis mit Veränderungen am Circulationsapparat und Retinitis. *Virchows Arch. path. Anat.*, 1886, **103,** 244–63.
Phaeochromocytoma first described. Republished in book form.

3866 PEPPER, William. 1874–
A study of congenital sarcoma of the liver and suprarenal. With report of a case. *Amer. J. med. Sci.*, 1901, **121,** 287–99.
Pepper's type of adrenal medullary tumour.

3867 BULLOCH, William. 1868–1941, & SEQUEIRA, James Harry. 1865–1948
On the relation of the suprarenal capsules to the sex organs. *Trans. path. Soc. Lond.*, 1905, **56,** 189–208.
First recognition of the "adrenogenital syndrome." This paper showed a relationship to exist between the adrenals and the sex organs.

3868 HUTCHISON, *Sir* Robert. 1871–1960
On suprarenal sarcoma in children with metastases in the skull. *Quart. J. Med.*, 1907, **1,** 33–38.
Hutchison's tumours.

3869 ROTH, Grace M., & KVALE, Walter Frederick. 1907–
A tentative test for pheochromocytoma. *Amer. J. med. Sci.*, 1945, **210,** 653–60.
The Roth–Kvale histamine test for the diagnosis of phaeochromocytoma.

3870 ACHARD, EMILE CHARLES. 1860–1944, & THIERS, JOSEPH.
Le virilisme pilaire et son association à l'insuffisance glycolytique (Diabète des femmes à barbe). *Bull. Acad. Méd.*, 1921, 3 sér., **86,** 51–66.

"Achard–Thiers syndrome". These writers established as a definite syndrome the combination of hirsutism with diabetes.

3871 LABBÉ, ERNEST MARCEL. 1870–1939, *et al.*
Crises solaires et hypertension paroxystique en rapport avec une tumeur surrénale. *Bull. Soc. méd. Hôp. Paris*, 1922, 3 sér., **46,** 982–90.

First full description of chromaffin cell tumours of the adrenal medulla. With J. Tinel and E. Doumer.

3872 HOLMES, *Sir* GORDON MORGAN. 1876–1965
A case of virilism associated with a suprarenal tumour: recovery after its removal. *Quart. J. Med.*, 1925, **18,** 143–52.

Records the first removal (by P. Sargent) of an adrenal cortical tumour. This was followed by disappearance of the heterosexual symptoms, thus establishing the relationship of sexual abnormality and adrenal tumours.

3873 ROGOFF, JULIUS MOSES. 1883–1966, & STEWART, GEORGE NEIL. 1860–1930
Suprarenal cortical extracts in suprarenal insufficiency (Addison's disease). *J. Amer. med. Ass.*, 1929, **92,** 1569–71.

Rogoff and Stewart were the first to use adrenal cortical extract ("inter-renalin") in the treatment of adrenal insufficiency. See also No. 1148.

3874 SWINGLE, WILBUR WILLIS. 1891– , & PFIFFNER, JOSEPH JOHN. 1903–
The adrenal cortical hormone. *Medicine*, 1932, **11,** 371–433.

The cortical hormone prepared by Swingle and Pfiffner ("eschatin") was found to be very effective in the treatment of Addison's disease. Their first paper on the subject appeared in *Science*, 1930, **71**, 321.

3875 BROSTER, LENNOX ROSS. 1889–1965, & VINES, HOWARD WILLIAM COPLAND. 1893–
The adrenal cortex; a surgical and pathological study. London, *H. K. Lewis*, 1933.

Includes the demonstration, by Vines, of virilism with the aid of a new stain; cortical cells of the adrenals removed at operation stained an abnormal (red) colour – the so-called Ponceau fuchsin stain.

3876 YOUNG, HUGH HAMPTON. 1870–1945
Genital abnormalities, hermaphroditism, and related adrenal diseases. Baltimore, *Williams & Wilkins*, 1937.

3877 THORN, GEORGE WIDMER. 1906– , *et al.*
Treatment of adrenal insufficiency by means of subcutaneous implants of pellets of desoxycorticosterone acetate (a synthetic adrenal cortical hormone). *Bull. Johns Hopk. Hosp.*, 1939, **64,** 155–66.

With L. L. Engel and H. Eisenberg. For treatment of Addison's disease by the same method, see the same journal, pp. 339–65.

3877.1 CONN, JEROME W. 1907–
Primary aldosteronism, a new clinical syndrome. *J. Lab. clin. Med.*, 1955, **45,** 6–17.

Primary aldosteronism ("Conn's syndrome").

3878–3908 PITUITARY GLAND

3878 HAEN, Anton de. 1704–1776
De cranii ustione. In his: *Ratio medendi*, Viennae Austriae, 1759, **6,** 264–72.
Haen mentioned amenorrhoea in connexion with a pituitary tumour.

3879 FRANK, Johann Peter. 1745–1821
De curandis hominum morbis epitome. Liber V. Mannheim, *C. F. Schwann & C. G. Goetz*, 1794.
Frank was first to define diabetes insipidus (pp. 38–67).

3880 SAUCEROTTE, Nicolas. 1741–1812
Accroissement singulier en grosseur des os d'un homme agé de 39 ans. In his *Mélanges de chirurgie*, Paris, 1801, **1,** 407–11.
Saucerotte described before the Académie de Chirurgie in 1772 a case of what is now known to have been acromegaly. This is the first known clinical description of the disease, and is one of the 5 cases included in Pierre Marie's classical account (No. 3884).

3881 RAYER, Pierre François Olive. 1793–1867
Observations sur les maladies de l'appendice sus-sphenoïdal (glande pituitaire) du cerveau. *Arch. gén. Méd.*, 1823, **3,** 350–67.
Includes description of pituitary obesity.

3882 MOHR, Bernhard. 1809–1848
Hypertrophie der Hypophysis cerebri und dadurch bedingter Druck auf die Hirngrundfläche, insbesondere auf die Sehnerven, das Chiasma derselben und den linkseitigen Hirnschenkel. *Wschr. ges. Heilk.*, 1840, **6,** 565–71.
The first case of pituitary obesity with infantilism (Fröhlich's syndrome) was reported by Mohr. Coincidentally this appears in the same volume of the *Wochenschrift* as does Basedow's classical description of exophthalmic goitre.

3883 FANEAU DE LA COUR, Ferdinand Valère.
Du féminisme et de l'infantilisme chez les tuberculeux. Paris, *Thèse No.* 1, 1871.
In a letter prefaced to Faneau de La Cour's thesis, Paul Joseph Lorain (1827–1875) described the idiopathic arrest of growth now known as "Lorain's type". It was subsequently ascribed to hypopituitarism. The word "infantilism" first appeared in this work.

3884 MARIE, Pierre. 1853–1940
Sur deux cas d'acromégalie. Hypertrophie singulière non congénitale des extremités supérieures, inférieures et céphalique. *Rev. Méd.*, 1886, **6,** 297–333.
In this, the first complete clinical description of the condition, Marie suggested the name "acromegaly". The paper excited much interest and was translated into English and published by the New Sydenham Society, 1891.

3885 MINKOWSKI, Oscar. 1858–1931
Ueber einen Fall von Akromegalie. *Berl. klin. Wschr.*, 1887, **24,** 371–74.
Minkowski called attention to the constancy of pituitary enlargement in acromegaly; he was the first definitely to note this relationship.

3886 CATON, RICHARD. 1842–1926, & PAUL, FRANK THOMAS. 1851–1941
Notes on a case of acromegaly treated by operation. *Brit. med. J.*, 1893, **2,** 1421–23.

First attempt (unsuccessful) to treat acromegaly operatively. Decompression was performed to relieve cranial pressure.

3887 BABINSKI, JOSEPH FRANÇOIS FELIX. 1857–1932
Tumeur du corps pituitaire sans acromégalie et avec arrêt de développement des organes génitaux. *Rev. neurol. (Paris)*, 1900, **8,** 531–33.

Babinski preceded Fröhlich in describing dystrophia adiposo-genitalis.

3888 BENDA, CARL. 1857–1933
Beiträge zur normalen und pathologischen Histologie der menschlichen Hypophysis cerebri. *Berl. klin. Wschr.*, 1900, **37,** 1205–10.

Benda showed that the pituitary tumour in acromegaly consists of chromophil cells.

3889 FRÖHLICH, ALFRED. 1871–1953
Ein Fall von Tumor der Hypophysis cerebri ohne Akromegalie. *Wien. klin. Rdsch.*, 1901, **15,** 883–86, 906–08.

Fröhlich's classical description of dystrophia adiposo-genitalis, pituitary tumour, with obesity and sexual infantilism ("Fröhlich's syndrome"). Reprinted (in German) in Research Publications, Association for Nervous and Mental Disease, XX: *The hypothalamus*, Baltimore, 1940, pp. xvi–xxviii.

3890 CUSHING, HARVEY WILLIAMS. 1869–1939
Sexual infantilism with optic atrophy in cases of tumor affecting the hypophysis cerebri. *J. nerv. ment. Dis.*, 1906, **33,** 704–16.

3891 SCHLOFFER, HERMANN. 1868–1937
Zur Frage der Operationen an der Hypophyse. *Beitr. klin. Chir.*, 1906, **50,** 767–817.

Schloffer's operation for acromegaly. He was the first successfully to operate upon a pituitary tumour in man (see No. 3892).

3892 ——. Erfolgreiche Operation eines hypophysen Tumors auf nasalem Wege. *Wien. klin. Wschr.*, 1907, **20,** 621–24, 670–71, 1075–78.

Schloffer's operation by the nasal route.

3893 RÉNON, LOUIS. 1863–1922, & DELILLE, ARTHUR. 1876–
Insuffisance thyro-ovarienne et hyperactivité hypophysaire (troubles acromégaliques). *Bull. Soc. méd. Hôp. Paris*, 1908, 3 sér., **25,** 973–79.

Rénon–Delille syndrome – dyspituitarism manifested by lowered blood-pressure, tachycardia, oliguria, insomnia, hyperhidrosis, and intolerance to heat.

3894 CROWE, SAMUEL JAMES. 1883–1955, *et al.*
Experimental hypophysectomy. *Johns Hopk. Hosp. Bull.*, 1910, **21,** 127–69.

Demonstration that hypophysectomy causes genital atrophy. With Harvey Cushing and J. Homans.

3895 HIRSCH, OSKAR. 1877–
Ueber endonasale Operationsmethoden bei Hypophysis-Tumoren. *Berl. klin. Wschr.*, 1911, **48,** 1933–35.

Hirsch's endonasal method.

3896 CUSHING, Harvey Williams. 1869–1939
The pituitary body and its disorders. Philadelphia, *J. B. Lippincott,* 1912.

Cushing, outstanding neurological surgeon of the present century, added much to our knowledge of the pituitary body and its disorders. The above work includes a description of his own method of operating on the pituitary. He assumed that in diabetes insipidus the pituitary was involved.

3897 FRANK, Alfred Erich. 1884–1957
Ueber Beziehungen der Hypophyse zum Diabetes insipidus. *Berl. klin. Wschr.*, 1912, **49,** 393–97.

Frank was the first definitely to connect the posterior lobe of the pituitary with diabetes insipidus.

3898 MARK, Leonard Portal. 1855–1930
Acromegaly: a personal experience. London, *Baillière, Tindall & Cox,* 1912.

Mark, a medical practitioner, suffered from acromegaly from the age of 24. The condition was obvious to his friends but Mark was 50 before he realized the cause of the symptoms of which he had kept a record for many years. He left an interesting account of his personal experience and also drew attention to several sculptural and pictorial representations of acromegalics.

3899 SOUQUES, Achille Alexandre. 1860–1944, & CHAUVET, Stéphen. 1885–1950
Infantilisme hypophysaire. *Nouv. Iconogr. Salpêt.*, 1913, **26,** 69–80.

Classical account of pituitary infantilism.

3900 GLINSKI, L. K.
Z kazuistyki zmian anatomo-patologicznych w przysadce mózgowej. *Przegl. Lek.*, 1913, **4,** 13–14.

Glinski preceded Simmonds in this important description of post-partum necrosis of the anterior pituitary.

3901 SIMMONDS, Morris. 1855–1925
Ueber Hypophysisschwund mit tödlichem Ausgang. *Dtsch. med. Wschr.*, 1914, **40,** 322–23.

"Simmonds's disease" – pituitary cachexia. See also *Virchows Arch. path. Anat.*, 1914, **217,** 226–39.

3902 ERDHEIM, Jakob. 1874–1937
Nanosomia pituitaria. *Beitr. path. Anat.*, 1916, **62,** 302–77.

Erdheim made important studies on the pathology of the pituitary. He gave the name "nanosomia pituitaria" to describe pituitary dwarfism. See also his paper in *Ergebn. allg. Path.*, 1926, **21,** 482.

3903 ATKINSON, Frederick Richard Breeks. 1867–1939
Acromegaly. London, *John Bale,* 1932.

The most complete analytical tabulation of acromegaly so far published; 1,319 cases are reported.

3904 CUSHING, Harvey Williams. 1869–1939
The basophil adenomas of the pituitary body and their clinical manifestations (pituitary basophilism). *Bull. Johns Hopk. Hosp.*, 1932, **50,** 137–95.

"Cushing's syndrome."

3905 INGRAM, Walter Robinson. 1905– , *et al.*
Experimental diabetes insipidus in the monkey. *Arch. intern. Med.*, 1936, **57**, 1067–80.
With C. Fisher and S. W. Ranson.

3906 ASSOCIATION FOR RESEARCH IN NERVOUS & MENTAL DISEASE.
The pituitary gland; an investigation of the most recent advances. Baltimore, *Williams & Wilkins Co.*, 1938.
Vol. 17 of the Association's Monographs.

3907 BIGGART, John Henry. 1905– , & ALEXANDER, George Lionel.
Experimental diabetes insipidus. *J. Path. Bact.*, 1939, **48**, 405–25.
Production of diabetes insipidus in dogs by injury to the hypothalamus.

3907.1 SHEEHAN, Harold Leeming. 1900–
Simmonds's disease due to post-mortem necrosis of the anterior pituitary. *Quart. J. Med.*, 1939, **32**, 277–309.
Sheehan's syndrome – panhypopituitarism due to pituitary necrosis following post-partum haemorrhage.

3908 KINSELL, Laurance Wilkie. 1907– , *et al.*
Studies in growth. I. Interrelationship between pituitary growth factor and growth-promoting androgens in acromegaly and gigantism. II. Quantitative evaluation of bone and soft tissue growth in acromegaly and gigantism. *J. clin. Endocr.*, 1948, **8**, 1013–36.
L. W. Kinsell, G. D. Michaels, C. H. Li, and W. E. Larsen showed that there is an increase in growth hormone in plasma in acromegaly.

History of Endocrinology

3909 GARRISON, Fielding Hudson. 1870–1935
History of endocrine doctrine. In: *Endocrinology and metabolism . . .* ed. L. F. Barker, New York, 1924, **1**, 45–78.

3910 ROLLESTON, *Sir* Humphry Davy, *Bart.* 1862–1944
The endocrine organs in health and disease. With an historical review. London, *Oxford Univ. Press*, 1936.
As a history of the subject, this work is unsurpassed in detail and accuracy. References to all publications of importance are included.

3911 IASON, Alfred Herbert. 1891–
The thyroid gland in medical history. New York, *Froben Press*, 1946.

3912–3979 METABOLIC DISORDERS

3912 MARCET, Alexander John Gaspard. 1770–1822
Account of a singular variety of urine, which turned black soon after being discharged; with some particulars respecting its chemical properties. *Med.-chir. Trans.*, 1822–23, **12**, 37–45.
Alkaptonuria described.

3913 BOEDEKER, Carl Wilhelm.
Ueber das Alcapton; ein neuer Beitrag zur Frage: welche Stoffe des Harns können Kupferreduction bewirken? *Z. rat. Med.*, 1859, 3 R., **7**, 130–45.

Excretion of homogentisic acid (in alkaptonuria) first described.

3914 BANTING, William. 1797–1878
Letter on corpulence; address to the public. [London, *Harrison & Sons*], 1863.

Banting devised a diet low in saccharine, farinaceous, and oily matter, for the treatment of obesity. This became known as "bantingism" or the "Banting diet".

3914.1 THUDICHUM, Johann Ludwig Wilhelm. 1829–1901
On researches intended to promote an improved chemical identification of diseases. *10th Rep. Med. Offr Privy Council.* With appendix, 1867. London, 1868, pp. 152–294.

Discovery of the first porphyrin, haematoporphyrin (p. 227).

3915 TROUSSEAU, Armand. 1801–1867
Glycosurie, diabète sucré. In his *Clinique médicale de l'Hôtel-Dieu*, 2me. éd., Paris, 1865, **2**, 663–98.

First description of haemochromatosis.

3916 RECKLINGHAUSEN, Friedrich Daniel von. 1833–1910
Ueber Haemochromatose. *Berl. klin. Wschr.*, 1889, **26**, 925.

Recklinghausen gave to haemochromatosis its present name.

3917 DERCUM, Francis Xavier. 1856–1931
A subcutaneous connective tissue dystrophy of the arms and back, associated with symptoms resembling myxoedema. *Univ. med. Mag. (Philad.)*, 1888–89, **1**, 140–50.

First description of adiposis dolorosa ("Dercum's disease").

3918 SALKOWSKI, Ernst Leopold. 1844–1923
Ueber die Pentosurie, eine neue Anomalie des Stoffwechsels. *Berl. klin. Wschr.*, 1895, **32**, 364–68.

Pentosuria first described.

3919 NOORDEN, Carl Harko von. 1858–1944
Sammlung klinischer Abhandlungen über Pathologie und Therapie der Stoffwechsel- und Ernährungsstörungen. 9 pts. Berlin, 1900–10.

Noorden succeeded Nothnagel at Vienna. He made important studies of metabolism and its disorders.

3920 ——. Handbuch der Pathologie des Stoffwechsels. 2te. Aufl. 2 vols. Berlin, *A. Hirschwald*, 1906–07.

3921 GARROD, *Sir* Archibald Edward. 1857–1936
Inborn errors of metabolism. London, *H. Frowde*, 1909.

The influence of the individual's constitution on the incidence of disease has long been recognized. Garrod showed that constitutional variation in function, as well as in structure, can give rise to what he termed "chemical malformations" – alkaptonuria, cystinuria, pentosuria, etc.

3921.1 GÖPPERT, Friedrich. 1870–1927
Galaktosurie nach Milchzuckergabe bei angeborenem, familiärem, chronischem Leberleiden. *Berl. klin. Wschr.*, 1917, **54**, 473–77.

First clear account of galactosaemia (although A. von Reuss may have been describing a case in *Wien. med. Wschr.*, 1908, **58**, 799).

3922 FOLIN, OTTO KNUT OLOF. 1867–1934, & WU, HSIEN. 1893–1959
A system of blood analysis. *J. biol. Chem.*, 1919, **38,** 81–110.
Folin–Wu test for blood sugar.

3923 BENEDICT, STANLEY ROSSITER. 1884–1936
The analysis of whole blood. II. The determination of sugar and of saccharoids (non-fermentable copper-reducing substances). *J. biol. Chem.*, 1931, **92,** 141–59.
Benedict's test for blood sugar.

3924 FØLLING, IVAR ASBJØRN. 1888–1973
Utskillelse av fenylpyrodruesyre i urinen som stoffskifteanomali i forbindelse med imbecilletet. *Nord. med. T.*, 1934, **8,** 1054–59.
Phenylketonuria first observed. German translation in *Hoppe-Seyl. Z. physiol. Chem.*, 1934, **227**, 169–76.

3924.1 WALDENSTRÖM, JAN GÖSTA. 1906–
Incipient myelomatosis or "essential" hyperglobulinemia with fibrinogenopenia – a new syndrome? *Acta med. scand.*, 1944, **117,** 216–47.
"Waldenström's macroglobulinaemia."

3924.2 REFSUM, SIGVALD.
Heredopathia atactica polyneuritiformis; a familial syndrome not hitherto described. *Acta psychiat. scand.*, 1946, Suppl. 38.
"Refsum's syndrome", an inherited disorder of lipid metabolism.

3925–3979 DIABETES MELLITUS

3925 ARETAEUS, *the Cappadocian.* A.D. 81–138?
On diabetes. In his: *Extant works*, ed. F. ADAMS. London, 1856, 338–40, 485–86.
The first accurate account of diabetes, to which Aretaeus gave its present name; he insisted on the part which thirst plays in the symptomatology.

3926 WILLIS, THOMAS. 1621–1675
Pharmaceutice rationalis sive diatriba de medicamentorum operationibus in humano corpore. 2 vols. Londini, *R. Scott*, 1674–75.
Willis noted the sweetness of the urine in diabetes mellitus; he differentiated between this condition and diabetes insipidus. (Sect. IV, Chap. 3.) English translation, 1679.

3927 BRUNNER, JOHANN CONRAD À. 1653–1727
Experimenta nova circa pancreas. Amstelaedami, *apud H. Wetstenium*, 1683.
Brunner came near to discovering pancreatic diabetes. His experiments on the dog represent pioneer work on internal secretion. Following excision of the pancreas he recorded extreme thirst and polyuria. Translated extracts in *Ann. med. Hist.*, 1941, **3**, 91–100.

3928 DOBSON, MATTHEW. 1731?–1784
Experiments and observations on the urine in diabetes. *Med. Obs. Inqu.*, 1776, **5,** 298–316.
Dobson proved that the sweetish taste of diabetic urine was produced by sugar, an observation following on Willis's discovery of the sweetness of diabetic urine. He also discovered hyperglycaemia.

3929 CAWLEY, THOMAS.
A singular case of diabetes, consisting entirely in the quality of the urine; with an inquiry into the different theories of that disease. *Lond. med. J.*, 1788, **9**, 286–308.

Cawley was the first to suggest a relationship between the pancreas and diabetes, observing that the disease may follow injury to that organ.

3930 ROLLO, JOHN. ?–1809
An account of two cases of the diabetes mellitus, with remarks as they arose during the progress of the cure. London, *C. Dilly*, 1797.

Rollo reported the success of a meat diet in the treatment of diabetes. He was a pioneer in the systematic treatment of diabetes by restricted diet.

3931 CHEVREUL, MICHEL EUGÈNE. 1786–1889
Note sur le sucre de diabètes. *Ann. Chim.* (*Paris*), 1815, **95**, 319–20.

Chevreul proved that the sugar in diabetic urine is glucose.

3932 TROMMER, CARL AUGUST. 1806–1879
Unterscheidung von Gummi, Dextrin, Traubenzucker, und Rohrzucker. *Ann. Chem.* (*Heidelberg*), 1841, **39**, 360–62.

Trommer's test for glucose in urine.

3933 BERNARD, CLAUDE. 1813–1878
Chiens rendus diabétiques. *C. R. Soc. Biol.* (*Paris*), (1849), 1850, **1**, 60.

By experimental puncture (piqûre) of the fourth ventricle of the brain, Claude Bernard produced temporary glycosuria.

3934 SCHIFF, MORITZ. 1823–1896
Bericht über einige Versuche, um den Ursprung des Harnzuckers bei künstlichem Diabetes zu ermitteln. *Nachr. Georg-Aug. Univ. k. Ges. Wiss. Göttingen*, 1856, 243–47.

Schiff's important experiments on the production of artificial diabetes.

3935 PETTERS, WILHELM.
Untersuchungen über die Honigharnruhr. *Vjschr. prakt. Heilk.*, 1857, **55**, 81–94.

Petters discovered acetone in diabetic urine.

3936 PAVY, FREDERICK WILLIAM. 1829–1911
Researches on the nature and treatment of diabetes. London, *J. Churchill*, 1862.

Pavy devoted many years to the study of diabetes. He concluded that there was a definite relationship between the degree of hyperglycaemia and glycosuria.

3937 GERHARDT, CARL ADOLPH CHRISTIAN JACOB. 1833–1902
Diabetes mellitus und Aceton. *Wien. med. Presse*, 1865, **6**, 672.

Gerhard's iron-chloride reaction for aceto-acetic acid in acetonaemic urine.

3938 NOYES, HENRY DEWEY. 1832–1900
Retinitis in glycosuria. *Trans. Amer. ophthal. Soc.*, (1867–68), 1869, 71–75.

First investigation of retinitis accompanying glycosuria.

3939 KUSSMAUL, ADOLF. 1822–1902
Zur Lehre vom Diabetes mellitus. *Dtsch. Arch. klin. Med.*, 1874, **14**, 1–46.

Kussmaul explained diabetic coma as being due to acetonaemia. He described the air-hunger ("Kussmaul's respiration") present in this condition.

3940 BOUCHARDAT, Apollinaire. 1806–1886
De la glycosurie ou diabète sucré; son traitement hygiénique. Paris, *Germer-Baillière*, 1875.

Bouchardat used the fermentation test, polariscope and copper solutions for the detection of diabetes; he substituted fresh fats for carbohydrates, advised the avoidance of milk and alcohol, invented gluten bread and advocated the use of green vegetables. In fact, he devised the most rational method of treatment of diabetes up to his time.

3941 LEBER, Theodor. 1840–1917
Ueber die Erkrankungen des Auges bei Diabetes mellitus. *v. Graefe's Arch. Ophthal.*, 1875, **21**, Abt. iii, 206–337.

A record of Leber's important studies on the disorders of the eye in diabetes.

3942 BERNARD, Claude. 1813–1878
Leçons sur le diabète et la glycogenèse animale. Paris, *J. B. Baillière*, 1877.

Bernard showed that in diabetes there is primarily glycaemia followed by glycosuria.

3943 LANCEREAUX, Etienne. 1829–1910
Notes et reflexions à propos de 2 cas de diabète sucré avec altération du pancréas. *Bull. Acad. Méd.* (*Paris*), 1877, 2 sér., **6,** 1215–40.

Lancereaux was the first definitely to claim a causal relationship between lesions of the pancreas and diabetes.

3944 EBSTEIN, Wilhelm. 1836–1912
Ueber Drüsenepithelnekrosen beim Diabetes mellitus mit besonderer Berücksichtigung des diabetischen Coma. *Dtsch. Arch. klin. Med.*, 1881, **28,** 143–242.

"Ebstein's disease", hyaline degeneration and necrosis of the epithelial cells of the renal tubules, sometimes seen in diabetes mellitus.

3945 STADELMANN, Ernst. 1853–
Ueber die Ursachen der pathologischen Ammoniakausscheidung beim Diabetes mellitus und des Coma diabeticum. *Arch. exp. Path. Pharmak.*, 1883, **17**, 419–44.

Stadelmann studied ammonia excretion in diabetes and noted an acid substance in the urine, which Minkowski (No. 3947) showed to be β-oxybutyric acid. Stadelmann recognized that diabetic coma was the result of the increased formation and accumulation of acids.

3946 ARNOZAN, Charles Louis Xavier, & VAILLARD, Louis.
Contribution à l'étude du pancréas du lapin. Lésions provoquées par la ligature du canal de Wirsung. *Arch. Physiol. norm. path.*, 1884, 3 sér., **3,** 287–316.

Arnozan and Vaillard showed that blockage of the pancreatic ducts caused atrophy of the pancreas but not diabetes.

3947 MINKOWSKI, Oscar. 1858–1931
Ueber das Vorkommen von Oxybuttersäure im Harn bei Diabetes mellitus. *Arch. exp. Path. Pharmak.*, 1884, **18,** 35–48.

Discovery of β-oxybutyric acid in diabetic urine.

3948 JAKSCH, Rudolf von, *Ritter von Wartenhorst*. 1855–1947
Ueber Acetonurie und Diaceturie. Berlin, *A. Hirschwald*, 1885.

An important investigation concerning acetone in diabetic urine.

3949 MERING, JOSEPH VON. 1849–1908
Ueber experimentellen Diabetes. *Verh. Congr. inn. Med.*, 1886, **5,** 185–89.

Mering was able to produce experimental diabetes by means of phloridzin.

3950 ——, & MINKOWSKI, OSCAR. 1858–1931
Diabetes mellitus nach Pankreasextirpation. *Arch. exp. Path. Pharmak.*, 1890, **26,** 371–87.

Minkowski produced experimental diabetes by removing the pancreas of a dog. This proof of the rôle of the pancreas in diabetes was of the first importance; previous experiments on similar lines had attracted little attention.

3951 NOORDEN, CARL HARKO VON. 1858–1944
Die Zuckerkrankheit und ihre Behandlung. Berlin, *A. Hirschwald*, 1895.

Noorden's extensive studies on diabetes have much advanced our knowledge of the subject. He made many observations regarding metabolism in diabetes.

3952 NAUNYN, BERNARD. 1839–1925
Der Diabetes mellitus. Wien, *A. Hölder*, 1898.

Naunyn devoted his life to the study of metabolism in diabetes and in diseases of the liver and pancreas, the above book being his most important work. He was a co-founder of the *Archiv für experimentelle Pathologie.*

3953 MAGNUS-LEVY, ADOLF. 1865–1955
Die Oxybuttersäure und ihre Beziehungen zum Coma diabeticum. *Arch. exp. Path. Pharmak.*, 1899, **42,** 149–237.

3954 ——. Untersuchungen über die Acidosis im Diabetes melitus und die Säureintoxication im Coma diabeticum. *Arch. exp. Path. Pharmak.*, 1901, **45,** 389–434.

Magnus-Levy studied the relationship of β-oxybutyric acid and diabetic coma.

3955 OPIE, EUGENE LINDSAY. 1873–1971
On the relation of chronic interstitial pancreatitis to the islands of Langerhans and to diabetes mellitus. *J. exp. Med.*, 1900–01, **5,** 397–428.

3956 ——. The relation of diabetes mellitus to lesions of the pancreas. Hyaline degeneration of the islands of Langerhans. *J. exp. Med.*, 1900–01, **5,** 527–40.

Mering and Minkowski had focused attention upon the pancreas as the seat of diabetes. Opie's work was another important step forward; he established the association between failure of the islets of Langerhans and the occurrence of diabetes.

3957 SSOBOLEW, LEONID WASSILYEVITCH [SOBOLEFF]. 1876–1919
Zur normalen und pathologischen Morphologie der inneren Secretion der Bauchspeicheldrüse. (Die Bedeutung der Langerhans'-schen Inseln. *Virchows Arch. path. Anat.*, 1902, **168,** 91–128.

Ssobolew found that ligation of the pancreatic excretory ducts led to atrophy of the acinous tissue, the islets of Langerhans remaining intact.

3958 FROMMER, VIKTOR.
Neue Reaktion zum Nachweis von Aceton, samt Bemerkungen über Acetonurie. *Berl. klin. Wschr.*, 1905, **42,** 1008–10.

Frommer's test for acetone in urine.

3959 DE WITT, Lydia Maria. 1859–
Morphology and physiology of areas of Langerhans in some vertebrates. *J. exp. Med.*, 1906, **8,** 193–239.

Lydia De Witt ligated the pancreatic ducts and obtained extracts from the islets of Langerhans in cats, noting their glycolytic qualities.

3960 ROTHERA, Arthur Cecil Hamel. 1880–1915
Note on the sodium nitro-prusside reaction for acetone. *J. Physiol. (Lond.)*, 1908, **37,** 491–94.

Test for acetone bodies in urine.

3961 ZUELZER, Georg Ludwig. 1870–1949
Ueber Versuche einer specifischen Fermenttherapie des Diabetes. *Z. exp. Path. Therap.*, 1908, **5,** 307–18.

Zuelzer succeeded in isolating a pancreatic extract which contained what we now know as insulin; serious hypoglycaemic reactions sometimes followed its use, however, and led to its abandonment. Preliminary paper in *Berl. klin. Wschr.*, 1907, **44**, 474–75.

3962 MacCALLUM, William George. 1874–1944
On the relation of the islands of Langerhans to glycosuria. *Johns Hopk. Hosp. Bull.*, 1909, **20,** 265–68.

MacCallum suggested a relationship between lesions of the islands of Langerhans and the glycosuria of diabetes.

3963 MAGNUS-LEVY, Adolph. 1865–1955
Das Coma diabeticum und seine Behandlung. *Samml. zwangl. Abhandl. Geb. Verdauungs.- u. Stoffwechs.*, Halle, 1909, **1,** 1–54.

Magnus-Levy is remembered for his work on the treatment of diabetic coma.

3964 LUSK, Graham. 1866–1932
Metabolism in diabetes. *Harvey Lect.* (1908–09), 1910, 69–96.

3965 BARRON, Moses. 1883–
The relation of the islets of Langerhans to diabetes with special reference to cases of pancreatic lithiasis. *Surg. Gynec. Obstet.*, 1920, **31,** 437–48.

Barron confirmed the experimental work of Ssobolew. It was whilst reading the above paper that Banting first formulated the hypothesis upon which he based his successful experiments.

3966 BANTING, *Sir* Frederick Grant. 1891–1941, *et al.*
The internal secretion of the pancreas. *Amer. J. Physiol.*, 1922, **59,** 479.

A preliminary communication regarding the isolation of insulin, made to a meeting of the American Physiological Society in December 1921. With C. H. Best and J. J. R. Macleod. Banting and Macleod were awarded the Nobel Prize in 1923.

3967 ——, & BEST, Charles Herbert. 1899–
The internal secretion of the pancreas. *J. Lab. clin. Med.*, 1922, **7,** 251–66.

This paper reports the isolation of insulin. An extract from the pancreas of a dog, removed after ligation of the excretory duct, was found to exercise a reducing influence on the percentage of sugar in the blood. This extract was called "insulin" and was crystallized by Abel in 1926.

3968 ——. Pancreatic extracts in the treatment of diabetes mellitus. *Canad. med. Ass. J.*, 1922, **12,** 141–46.

First clinical application of insulin in the treatment of diabetes. Written in conjunction with C. H. Best, J. B. Collip, W. R. Campbell, and A. A. Fletcher.

3969 COLLIP, JAMES BERTRAM. 1892–1965
The original method as used for the isolation of insulin in semipure form for the treatment of the first clinical cases. *J. biol. Chem.*, 1923, **55,** xl–xli.

Collip improved insulin.

3970 BANTING, *Sir* FREDERICK GRANT. 1891–1941
Insulin. *Int. Clin.*, 1924, 34 ser., **4,** 109–16.

3971 ABEL, JOHN JACOB. 1857–1938
Crystalline insulin. *Proc. nat. Acad. Sci.* (*Wash.*), 1926, **12,** 132–36.

Crystallization of insulin.

3972 WILDER, RUSSELL MORSE. 1885–1959, *et al.*
Carcinoma of the islands of the pancreas; hyperinsulinism and hypoglycemia. *J. Amer. med. Ass.*, 1927, **89,** 348–55.

R. M. Wilder, F. N. Allan, M. H. Power, and H. E. Robertson reported the occurrence of carcinoma with hyperinsulinism.

3973 RUIZ, CELESTINO L. 1904– , *et al.*
Contribución al estudio sobre la composición quimica de la insulina. Estudio de algunos cuerpos sintéticos solfurados con acción hypoglucemiante. *Rev. Soc. argent. Biol.*, 1930, **6,** 134–41.

Discovery of the hypoglycaemic effect of certain sulphonamide derivatives. With L. L. Silva and L. Libenson.

3974 HAGEDORN, HANS CHRISTIAN. 1888– , *et al.*
Protamine insulinate. *J. Amer. med. Ass.*, 1936, **106,** 177–80.

H. C. Hagedorn, B. N. Jensen, N. B. Krarup, and I. Wodstrup introduced insulin combined with protamine to delay the absorption rate.

3975 KERR, ROBERT BEWS. 1908– , *et al.*
Protamine insulin. *Canad. med. Ass. J.*, 1936, **34,** 400–01.

R. B. Kerr, C. H. Best, W. R. Campbell, and A. A. Fletcher advocated the combination of zinc with insulin to delay its absorption rate. Later this was combined with protamine to form protamine zinc insulin.

3976 YOUNG, FRANK GEORGE. 1908–
Permanent experimental diabetes produced by pituitary (anterior lobe) injections. *Lancet*, 1937, **2,** 372–74.

Anterior pituitary diabetogenic hormone.

3977 DOHAN, FRANCIS CURTIS. 1907– , & LUKENS, FRANCIS DRING WETHERILL. 1899–
Experimental diabetes produced by the administration of glucose. *Endocrinology*, 1948, **42,** 244–62.

Experimental diabetes produced by artificially-induced hyperglycaemia.

3978 HALLAS-MØLLER, KNUD. 1914– , *et al.*
Kliniske undersøgelser med nye retarderet virkende insulin-praeparater. *Ugeskr. Læg.*, 1951, **113,** 1767–71.

First clinical trials of lente, ultralente, and semilente insulin zinc suspensions. See also *Science*, 1952, **116,** 394–98; and *J. Amer. med. Ass.*, 1952, **150,** 1667. With M. Jersild, K. Petersen, and J. Schlichtkrull.

3978.1 FRANKE, HANS. 1909–1955, & FUCHS, J.
Ein neues antidiabetisches Prinzip. Ergebnisse klinischer Untersuchungen. *Dtsch. med. Wschr.*, 1955, **80**, 1449–52.

Introduction of carbutamide (BZ55), the first of the sulphonylureas. It was followed by tolbutamide and chlorpropamide.

3978.2 WRENSHALL, GERALD ALFRED, *et al.*
The story of insulin: forty years of success against diabetes. London, *Bodley Head*, 1962.

With G. Hetenyi and W. R. Feasby.

3979 PAPASPYROS, NIKOS S.
The history of diabetes mellitus. 2nd ed. Stuttgart, *G. Thieme*, 1964.

3980–4158 DERMATOLOGY

3980–4011 GENERAL WORKS

3980 MERCURIALI, GERONIMO. 1530–1606
De morbis cutaneis, et omnibus corporis humani excrementis tractatus. Venetiis, *apud P. & A. Meietos*, 1572.

The first systematic text-book on diseases of the skin. Mercuriali enjoyed a great reputation in his day; he wrote on many medical subjects, including medical gymnastics.

3981 TURNER, DANIEL. 1667–1742
De morbis cutaneis. A treatise of diseases incident to the skin. London, *R. Bonwicke*, 1714.

Turner may be regarded as the founder of British dermatology. His book, the first English text on dermatology, gives a good idea of contemporary knowledge of the subject. Yale College conferred an honorary medical degree on Turner in 1723, this being the first medical degree given in English-speaking America.

3982 PLENCK, JOSEPH JACOB VON. 1738–1807
Doctrina de morbis cutaneis. Viennae, *R. Graeffer*, 1776.

A classification of skin diseases upon the basis of their clinical appearance. Until the time of Willan, von Plenck's book was the greatest authority on dermatology. He mentioned 115 different skin diseases, all that were known at that time, and divided them into 14 classes.

3983 LORRY, ANNE CHARLES DE. 1726–1783
Tractatus de morbis cutaneis. Parisiis, *P. G. Cavelier*, 1777.

Lorry is regarded as the founder of French dermatology. A pupil of Jean Astruc, his most important work is his *Tractatus*, in which he attempted the classification of diseases on the basis of essential relations, their physiological, pathological, and etiological similarities. It is the first modern text on the subject.

3984 JACKSON, SEGUIN HENRY. 1750–1816
Dermato-pathologia; or practical observations, from some new thoughts on the pathology and proximate cause of diseases of the true skin. London, *H. Reynell*, 1792.

An attempt to classify skin diseases upon the basis of their pathology.

3985 WILLAN, ROBERT. 1757–1812
On cutaneous diseases. Vol. 1. London, *J. Johnson*, [1796]–1808.

Modern dermatology may be said to start with Willan. His classification of skin diseases gained him the Fothergillian Medal of the Medical Society of London in 1790. He established a definite classical nomenclature which is still more or less in use to-day. His book was issued in parts under the title of "Description and treatment of cutaneous diseases," and only vol. 1 had been completed when Willan died. An excellent evaluation of the book is given in Pusey's *History of dermatology*, 1933, p. 61.

3986 ALIBERT, JEAN LOUIS MARC, *le baron*. 1768–1837
Description des maladies de la peau observées à l'hôpital Saint Louis. Paris, *Barrois*, 1806.

Contains Alibert's "family tree" of dermatoses, a classification later discarded for Willan's scheme; it is now merely a curiosity of dermatological history. The book is also notable for its illustrations, the first on the subject in a French book, and for its original description of mycosis fungoides (see No. 4019).

3987 ——. Précis théorique et pratique sur les maladies de la peau. 2 vols. Paris, *Caille & Ravier*, 1810–18.

3988 BATEMAN, THOMAS. 1778–1821
Delineations of cutaneous diseases exhibiting the characteristic appearances of the principal genera and species comprised in the classification of the late Dr. Willan; and completing the series of engravings begun by that author. London, *Longman*, 1817.

Bateman, the pupil of Willan, continued his teacher's classification of skin diseases. The above work is notable for its 72 coloured plates. Although Willan outshone Bateman, to the latter is due some credit for the foundation of modern dermatology.

3989 RAYER, PIERRE FRANÇOIS OLIVE. 1793–1867
Traité théorique et pratique des maladies de la peau. 2 vols. and atlas. Paris, *J. B. Baillière*, 1826–27.

A classical summary of dermatological literature of the period. An English translation appeared in 1835. Rayer first described adenoma sebaceum and xanthoma multiplex. He was the first to differentiate between acute and chronic eczema. English translation, 1833.

3990 CAZENAVE, PIERRE LOUIS ALPHÉE. 1795–1877, & SCHEDEL, HENRY EDWARD. ?–1856
Abrégé pratique des maladies de la peau. Paris, *Bechet jeune*, 1828.

This book, translated into English in 1832 and 1842, had an important influence on English dermatology. It contains one of the first classifications of skin diseases on an anatomical basis.

3991 HEBRA, FERDINAND VON. 1816–1880
Versuch einer auf pathologische Anatomie gegründeten Eintheilung der Hautkrankheiten. *Z. k. k.Ges. Aerzte Wien*, 1845, **2**, 34–52, 143–155, 211–31.

Hebra's classification of skin diseases was based upon their pathological anatomy.

3992 ——. Atlas der Hautkrankheiten. 10 parts. Wien, *k.k. Hof- und Staatsdr.*, 1856–76.

3993 ANDERSON, *Sir* THOMAS M'CALL. 1836–1908
On the parasitic affections of the skin. London, *J. Churchill*, 1861.

Anderson was professor of clinical medicine at Glasgow.

3994 WILSON, *Sir* William James Erasmus. 1809–1884
Lectures on dermatology. 4 vols. London, *J. & A. Churchill*, 1871–78.

Erasmus Wilson gave the original descriptions of several cutaneous diseases, and made a fine collection of dermatological preparations. He classified skin diseases on an anatomical basis. The above book consists of his lectures at the Royal College of Surgeons, at which institution he founded a chair of dermatology.

3995 KAPOSI, Moritz [Kohn, Moritz]. 1837–1902
Pathologie und Therapie der Hautkrankheiten. Wien & Leipzig, *Urban & Schwarzenberg*, 1880.

One of the most important books in dermatology. English translation by J. C. Johnston in 1895.

3996 FOX, George Henry. 1846–1937
Photographic illustrations of skin diseases. New York, *E. B. Treat*, 1880.

Fox, who was professor of dermatology in New York, produced a valuable atlas of skin diseases.

3997 HEBRA, Hans von. 1847–1902
Die krankhaften Veränderungen der Haut. Braunschweig, *F. Wreden*, 1884.

Hans von Hebra was the son of Ferdinand, whose work he continued. His text-book correlated skin diseases to diseases of the entire organism.

3998 CROCKER, Henry Radcliffe. 1845–1909
Diseases of the skin. London, *H. K. Lewis*, 1888.

3999 SABOURAUD, Raymond Jacques Adrien. 1864–1938
Les tricophyties humaines. Paris, 1894, *Thèse No.* 227.

In his extensive studies of the rôle of fungi in skin diseases, Sabouraud revived and elaborated the discoveries of Gruby, which had remained neglected for half a century. See also No. 4116.

4000 UNNA, Paul Gerson. 1850–1929
Die Histopathologie der Hautkrankheiten. Berlin, *A. Hirschwald*, 1894.

This monumental work is a landmark in dermatological history. Sir Norman Walker translated it into English in 1896. Unna, short in stature but a giant among dermatologists, initiated the study of the skin by means of diascopy and gave several original descriptions of affections of the skin. The acne bacillus is for the first time described on p. 357. English translation, 1896.

4001 KAPOSI, Moritz. 1837–1902
Handatlas der Hautkrankheiten. 3 pts. Wien & Leipzig, *W. Braumüller*, 1898–1900.

An extensive and valuable collection of illustrations in dermatology.

4002 FINSEN, Niels Ryberg. 1860–1904
La photothérapie. Les rayons chimiques et la variole. La lumière comme agent d'excitabilité. Traitement du lupus vulgaire par des rayons chimiques concentrés. Paris, *G. Carré & C. Naud*, 1899.

Finsen was a pioneer in the treatment of lupus by means of light. English translation, 1901.

4003 DANLOS, Henri Alexandre. 1844–1912, & BLOCH, P.
Note sur le traitement du lupus érythémateux par des applications de radium. *Bull. Soc. franç. Derm. Syph.*, 1901, **12,** 438–40.

First application of radium in the treatment of lupus.

4004 SABOURAUD, Raymond Jacques Adrien. 1864–1938
Sur la radiothérapie des teignes. *Ann. Derm. Syph.* (*Paris*), 1904, 4 sér., **5,** 577–87.
Sabouraud's method of radiological treatment of ringworm.

4005 DARIER, Jean. 1856–1938
Précis de dermatologie. Paris, *Masson & Cie.*, 1909.

4006 JADASSOHN, Josef. 1863–1936
Handbuch der Haut- und Geschlechtskrankheiten. Hrsg . . . von J. Jadassohn. 24 vols. [in 42]. Berlin, *J. Springer*, 1927–37.

4007 CHAOUL, Henri. 1887– , & ADAM, Albert.
Die Röntgen-Nahbestrahlung maligner Tumoren. *Strahlentherapie*, 1933, **48,** 31–50.
Chaoul therapy.

4008 COCKAYNE, Edward Alfred. 1880–1956
Inherited abnormalities of the skin and its appendages. London, *H. Milford*, 1933.

4009 DARIER, Jean. 1856–1938, *et al.*
Nouvelle pratique dermatologique. 8 vols. Paris, *Masson & Cie.*, 1936.

4010 CHARPY, Jacques. 1900–
Technique de traitement du lupus tuberculeux. *Ann. Derm. Syph.* (*Paris*), 1943, 8 sér., **3,** 331.
Introduction of calciferol in the treatment of lupus. A more extensive report, "Le traitement des tuberculoses cutanées par la vitamine D_2 à hautes doses," appeared in the same journal, 1946, 8 sér., **6**, 310–46.

4011 DOWLING, Geoffrey Barrow. 1891– , & THOMAS, Ebenezer William Prosser.
Lupus vulgaris treated with calciferol. *Proc. roy. Soc. Med.*, 1945, **39,** 96–99.
Dowling and Prosser Thomas introduced calciferol in the treatment of lupus independently of Charpy (No. 4010) whose work was unknown to them owing to the wartime isolation of France.

4011.1–4154 ORIGINAL OR IMPORTANT ACCOUNTS OF DERMATOSES

4011.1 DONATI, Marcello [Donatus]. 1538–1602
De medica historia mirabili. Mantuae, *per Fr. Osanam*, 1586.
Lib. VI. cap. iii. First description of angioneurotic oedema (Quincke's oedema, No. 4081).

4012 BONOMO, Giovanni Cosimo. ?–1697
Epistola che contiene osservazioni intorno a' pellicelli del corpo umano. Firenze, *P. Martini*, 1687.
First description of *Sarcoptes scabiei*. This book is in part translated by Richard Mead in *Phil. Trans.*, (1702–03), 1703, **23**, 1296–99; it is reproduced in facsimile, with Mead's translation, in *Arch. Derm. Syph.* (*Chicago*), 1928, **18**, 1–25.

4013 MACHIN, John. ?–1751
An uncommon case of a distempered skin. *Phil. Trans.*, (1731–32), 1733, **37,** 299–301.
First known description of ichthyosis hystrix. Machin's observations referred to the Lambert family and were followed through successive generations of the family by Baker (*Phil. Trans.*, 1755, **49,** 21–24) and by Tilesius (*Ausführliche Beschreibung . . . der beiden sog. Stachelschweinmenschen*, Altenburg, 1802).

4014 CRUSIO, Carlo [Curzio].
An account of an extraordinary disease of the skin and its cure. Extracted from the Italian of Carlo Crusio, with a letter of the Abbé Nollet to Mr. William Watson by Robert Watson. *Phil. Trans.*, 1754, **48,** 579–87.
The early history of scleroderma is confused with that of leprosy, ichthyosis, and keloid. Crusio appears to be the first to differentiate it. Gintrac in 1847 coined the term "scleroderma".

4015 UNDERWOOD, Michael. 1737–1820
Treatise on the diseases of children. London, *J. Mathews*, 1784.
First description (p. 76) of sclerema neonatorum ("Underwood's disease").

4016 WICHMANN, Johann Ernst. 1740–1802
Aetiologie der Krätze. Hannover, *Gebr. Helwing*, 1786.
Wichmann definitely established the parasitic aetiology of scabies.

4017 HOME, *Sir* Everard. 1756–1832
Observations on certain horny excrescences of the human body. *Phil. Trans.*, 1791, **81,** 95–105.
Original description of cornu cutaneum.

4018 WILLAN, Robert. 1757–1812
On cutaneous diseases. Vol. 1. London, *J. Johnson*, [1796]–1808.
Includes (pp. 73–76) original description of prurigo mitis; under the name "ichthyosis cornea" Willan quoted Crusio's case of scleroderma (see pp. 197–212); Willan also established psoriasis as a separate skin disease (pp. 152–88).

4019 ALIBERT, Jean Louis Marc, *le baron*. 1768–1837
Description des maladies de la peau. Paris, 1806, p. 157; pl. xxxvi.
First description of mycosis fungoides (pian fungoide, framboesia mycoides), one of several conditions to which the name of Alibert has been attached.

4020 STOKES, Whitley. 1763–1845
On an eruptive disease of children. *Dublin med. phys. Essays*, 1807–08, **1,** 146–53.
First description of ecthyma terebrans, "pemphigus gangrenosa".

4021 BATEMAN, Thomas. 1778–1821
A practical synopsis of cutaneous diseases. 2nd ed. London, 1813, p. 13.
First description of lichen urticatus.

4022 ——. Delineations of cutaneous diseases. London, *Longman*, 1817.
Includes (pl. lii) important description of herpes iris (erythema iris), and of the eczema due to external irritation (pl. lv–lviii, eczema solare, impetiginoides, rubrum mercuriale). Pl. lxi represents the first description of molluscum contagiosum, but according to Paterson (No. 4032) the disease was probably noticed by Tilesius about 1793. Bateman refers to Tilesius but calls his case molluscum pendulum.

4023 ALIBERT, Jean Louis Marc, *le baron*. 1768–1837
Note sur la keloide. *J. univ. Sci. méd.*, 1816, **2,** 207–16.

First accurate description of keloid ("Alibert's keloid"), although it was mentioned by Retz in 1790.

4024 ——. Description des maladies de la peau. 2me. édition. 2 vols. Paris, *A. Wahlen*, 1825.

Contains (vol. 2, p. 214) first description of sycosis barbae ("Alibert's mentagra").

4025 JACOB, Arthur. 1790–1874
Observations respecting an ulcer of peculiar character, which attacks the eyelids and other parts of the face. *Dublin Hosp. Rep.*, 1827, **4,** 232-39.

Arthur Jacob, professor of anatomy and physiology in Dublin, described "Jacob's ulcer", rodent ulcer attacking the face, especially the eyelid.

4026 HAWKINS, Caesar Henry. 1798–1884
On warty tumours in cicatrices. *Lond. med. Gaz.*, 1833–34, **13,** 481–82

"Hawkins' keloid" – a growth resembling a true keloid but due to hypertrophy of a cicatrix.

4027 RENUCCI, Simon François.
Sur la découverte de l'insecte qui produit la contagion de la gale, du prurigo et du phlyzacia. Paris, *Thèse No.* 83, 1835.

Demonstration of the human itch-mite, *Sarcoptes scabiei*. It was due to Renucci that the *Sarcoptes* was recognized as the one cause of scabies and its parasitic nature finally accepted.

4028 CAZENAVE, Pierre Louis Alphée. 1795–1877, & SCHEDEL, Henry Edward. ?–1856
Abrégé pratique des maladies de la peau. 3me. éd. Paris, *Bechet jeune*, 1838.

Laurent Théodore Biett (1781–1840), was a pupil of Alibert, Willan, and Bateman His classical description of lupus erythematoides migrans ("Biett's disease") occurs on pp. 11 and 415 of the above work.

4029 SCHÖNLEIN, Johann Lucas. 1793–1864
Zur Pathogenie der Impetigines. *Arch. Anat. Physiol. wiss. Med.*, 1839, 82.

The discovery of a fungus as the cause of favus (*Achorion schönleinii*). Schönlein communicated this important discovery in a letter of less than 200 words and one illustration. It represents the first conspicuous step in the attribution of disease to the action of minute parasites. Schönlein was the founder of modern clinical teaching in Germany.

4030 GRUBY, David. 1810–1898
Mémoire sur une végétation qui constitute la vraie teigne. *C. R. Acad. Sci. (Paris)*, 1841, **13,** 72–75.

Independently of Schönlein (No. 4029) Gruby discovered the achorion of favus, describing it definitely as the cause of the disease, a point about which Schönlein was in doubt.

4031 HENDERSON, William. 1810–1872
Notice of the molluscum contagiosum. *Edinb. med. surg. J.*, 1841, **56,** 213–18.

See next.

4032 PATERSON, Robert. 1814–1889
Cases and observations on the molluscum contagiosum of Bateman, with an account of the minute structure of the tumours. *Edinb. med. J.*, 1841, **56,** 279–88.
Henderson and Paterson described the inclusion body of molluscum contagiosum, "Henderson–Paterson body."

4033 BOECK, Carl Wilhelm. 1808–1875
Om den spedalske sygdom. Elephantiasis graecorum. *Norsk Mag. Lægevid.*, 1842, **4,** 1–73; 127–216.
Boeck, eminent Norwegian dermatologist and syphilologist, was the first to describe Norwegian itch, scabies crustosa ("Boeck's scabies").

4034 GRUBY, David. 1810–1898
Sur une espèce de mentagre contagieuse résultant du développement d'un nouveau cryptogame dans la racine des poils de la barbe de l'homme. *C. R. Acad. Sci.* (*Paris*), 1842, **15,** 512–15.
First description of *Trichophyton ectothrix,* the fungus responsible for sycosis barbae.

4035 ——. Recherches sur la nature, le siège et le développement du Porrigo decalvans ou phytoalopécie. *C. R. Acad. Sci.* (*Paris*), 1843, **17,** 301–03.
First accurate description of *Microsporon audouini*, the fungus of Willan's *Porrigo decalvans*, tinea tonsurans, "Gruby's disease".

4036 ——. Recherches sur les cryptogames qui constituent la maladie contagieuse du cuir chevelu décrite sous le nom de Teigne tondante (Mahon). Herpes tonsurans (Cazenave). *C. R. Acad. Sci.* (*Paris*), 1844, **18,** 583–85.
Gruby discovered a fungus, *Trichophyton tonsurans*, in ringworm of the scalp.

4037 CAZENAVE, Pierre Louis Alphée. 1795–1877
Pemphigus chronique, générale; forme rare de pemphigus foliacé; mort; autopsie; altération du foie. *Ann. Mal. Peau*, 1844, **1,** 208–10.
First description of pemphigus foliaceus, "Cazenave's disease". The article is unsigned.

4038 EICHSTEDT, Carl Ferdinand. 1816–1892
Ueber die Krätzmilben des Menschen, ihre Entwicklung und ihr Verhältniss zur Krätze. *N. Notiz. Geb. Nat. Heilk.*, 1846, **38,** col. 105–10; **39,** col. 265–70.

4039 ——. Pilzbildung in der Pityriasis versicolor. *N. Notiz. Geb. Nat. Heilk.*, 1846, **39,** col. 270–71.
Eichstedt discovered the *Microsporon furfur*, fungus of pityriasis versicolor ("Eichstedt's disease").

4040 CAZENAVE, Pierre Louis Alphée. 1795–1877
Des principales formes du lupus et de son traitement. *Gaz. Hôp.* (*Paris*), 1850, 3 sér., **2,** 383.
Lupus erythematosus – "Cazenave's lupus".

4041 ADDISON, THOMAS. 1793–1860, & GULL, *Sir* WILLIAM WITHEY. 1816–1890
On a certain affection of the skin, vitiligoidea: α Plana, β tuberosa. *Guy's Hosp. Rep.*, 1851, 2 ser., **7**, 265–76.

In their classical account of xanthoma multiplex, Addison and Gull believed they were describing a new disease, but Rayer was the first to mention it. (See No. 3989; see also the later paper by Gull, *Guy's Hosp. Rep.*, 1852, 2 ser., **8**, 149.)

4042 ——. On the keloid of Alibert, and on true keloid. *Med.-chir. Trans.*, 1854, **37**, 27–47.

Addison described two forms of keloid, that described by Alibert, and the "true keloid" (the skin disease morphoea, "Addison's keloid").

4043 BÄRENSPRUNG, FRIEDRICH WILHELM FELIX VON. 1822–1864
Ueber die Folge und den Verlauf epidermischer Krankheiten. Halle, *H. W. Schmidt*, 1854.

First description of tinea cruris (eczema marginatum, "Bärensprung's disease").

4044 DEVERGIE, MARIE GUILLAUME ALPHONSE. 1798–1879
Pityriasis pilaris, maladie de peau non décrite par les dermatologistes. *Gaz. hebd. Méd.*, 1856, **3**, 197–201.

Devergie is remembered for his clear description of pityriasis rubra pilaris, ("Devergie's disease"). He was first to demonstrate the presence of a fungus in eczema marginatum.

4045 HEBRA, FERDINAND VON. 1816–1880
Lichen exsudativus ruber. *Allg. Wien. med. Ztg*, 1857, **2**, 75–76.

First description of this condition ("Hebra's pityriasis").

4046 LE ROY DE MÉRICOURT, ALFRED. 1825–1901
Sur la coloration partielle en noir ou en bleu de la peau chez les femmes. *Bull. Acad. Méd.* (*Paris*), 1857–58, **23**, 1141–44; 1860–61, **26**, 773–75.

Chromidrosis first described.

4047 CARTER, HENRY VANDYKE. 1831–1897
On a new and striking form of fungus disease, principally affecting the foot, and prevailing endemically in many parts of India. *Trans. med. phys. Soc. Bombay*, (1860), 1861, n.s. **6**, 104–42.

First modern description of mycetoma of the foot – "Madura foot," "Carter's mycetoma". It was mentioned by E. Kaempfer in his *Amoenitates exoticae*, Lemgo, 1712, p. 561. Colebrook at the Madura Dispensary is said to have given it the name "Madura foot" in 1846. See also No. 4066.

4048 GIBERT, CAMILLE MELCHIOR. 1797–1866
Traité pratique des maladies de la peau. 3 éd., 2 vols. Paris, *H. Plon*, 1860.

Gibert's name is associated with pityriasis rosea, which he first established as a definite clinical entity. His complete and accurate description of this condition is on page 402 of vol. 1 of the above work.

4049 HEBRA, FERDINAND VON. 1816–1880
Das umschriebene Eczem. Eczema marginatum. In Virchow's *Handbuch der spec. Path. u. Therap.*, Erlangen, 1860, **3**, 1 Abt., 361–63.

Complete description of tinea cruris (eczema marginatum), first described by Bärensprung in 1854.

4050 LUTZ, Henri Charles.
De l'hypertrophie générale du système sébacé. Paris, *Thèse No.* 65, 1860.
First description of keratosis follicularis.

4051 BAZIN, Pierre Antoine Ernest. 1807–1878
Leçons sur la scrofule, *etc.* 2me édition. Paris, 1861, p. 145, 501.
Erythema induratum scrophulosorum ("Bazin's disease") first described.

4052 WILKS, *Sir* Samuel, *Bart.* 1824–1911
A peculiar atrophy of the skin (Lineae atrophicae). *Guy's Hosp. Rep.*, 1861, 3 ser., **7,** 197–301.
First description of lineae atrophicae.

4053 ——. Disease of the skin produced by post-mortem examinations, or verruca necrogenica. *Guy's Hosp. Rep.*, 1862, 3 ser., **8,** 263–65.
Description of dissecting-room warts (verrucae necrogenicae), the cutaneous tuberculosis of Laennec, sometimes called "Wilks' disease".

4054 WAGNER, Ernst Leberecht. 1829–1888
Fall einer selten Muskelkrankheit. *Arch. Heilk.*, 1863, **4,** 282–83.
First recorded case of dermatomyositis.

4055 FOX, William Tilbury. 1836–1879
On impetigo contagiosa or porrigo. *Brit. med. J.*, 1864, **1,** 78–79, 467–68, 495–96, 553–55, 607–09.
"Impetigo of Tilbury Fox", impetigo contagiosa, first described.

4056 WAGNER, Ernst Leberecht. 1829–1888
Das Colloid-Milium der Haut. *Arch. Heilk.*, 1866, **7,** 463–64.
Colloid degeneration of the skin ("Wagner's disease") was first described by Wagner who gave it the name "Colloid milium".

4057 NETTLESHIP, Edward. 1845–1913
Chronic urticaria leaving brown stains. *Brit. med. J.*, 1869, **2,** 323.
Urticaria pigmentosa, described by Nettleship, is named eponymically "Nettleship's disease".

4058 PAXTON, Francis Valentine. ?–1924
On a diseased condition of the hairs of the axilla, probably of parasitic origin. *J. cutan. Med.*, 1869, **3,** 133–36.
Tinea nodosa (trichorrhexis nodosa, "Paxton's disease") first described.

4059 TURNER, George Alexander. 1845–1900
Lafa Tokelau, or Tokelau ringworm. *Glasg. med. J.*, 1869–70, **2,** 510–12.
First description, tinea imbricata.

4060 RITTER VON RITTERSHAIN, Gottfried. 1820–1883
Dermatitis erysipelatosa; Gangraena; Enkephalitis. *Öst. Jb. Pädiat.*, 1870, **1,** 23–24.
First description of dermatitis exfoliativa neonatorum (Ritter's disease).

4061 WILSON, *Sir* William James Erasmus. 1809–1884
On dermatitis exfoliativa. *Med. Times Gaz.*, 1870, **1,** 118–20.
Although Hippocrates mentioned this condition, Erasmus Wilson first named it and described it as we know it to-day. It has been called "Wilson's disease", an eponym discarded since its use to describe the progressive lenticular degeneration of Kinnier Wilson.

4062 HEBRA, Ferdinand von. 1816–1880
Ueber einzelne während der Schwangerschaft, dem Wochenbette und bei Uterinalkrankheiten der Frauen zu beobachtende Hautkrankheiten. *Wien. med. Wschr.*, 1872, **22**, 1197–1201.

Hebra was the first to describe impetigo herpetiformis, more fully dealt with by Kaposi, his son-in-law.

4063 KAPOSI, Moritz. 1837–1902
Idiopathisches multiples Pigmentsarkom der Haut. *Arch. Derm. Syph.* (*Prag.*), 1872, **4**, 265–73.

First description of "Kaposi's multiple idiopathic haemorrhagic sarcoma".

4064 BAKER, William Morrant. 1839–1896
Erythema serpens. *St. Barth. Hosp. Rep.*, 1873, **9**, 198–211.

First description of erythema serpens, usually called "erysipeloid of Rosenbach", following the latter's paper in *Arch. klin. Chir.*, 1887, **36**, 346.

4065 FOX, William Tilbury. 1836–1879
On dysidrosis (an undescribed eruption). *Brit. med. J.*, 1873, **2**, 365–66.

Original description of dysidrosis (pompholyx).

4066 CARTER, Henry Vandyke. 1831–1897
On mycetoma, or the fungus disease of India. London, *J. & A. Churchill*, 1874.

See No. 4047.

4067 HUTCHINSON, *Sir* Jonathan. 1828–1913
Illustrations of clinical surgery. Vol. 1. London, *J. Churchill*, 1875–1878.

Pp. 49–52: Hutchinson's classical description of cheiropompholyx, dysidrosis ("Hutchinson's disease"). The first description and illustration of sarcoidosis is on p. 42.

4068 NEUMANN, Isidor, *Edler von Heilwart*. 1832–1906
Ueber eine noch wenig gekannte Hautkrankheit (Dermatitis circumscripta herpetiformis). *Vjschr. Derm.*, 1875, **2**, 41–52.

First description of porokeratosis (Mibelli).

4069 TAYLOR, Robert William. 1842–1906
On a rare case of idiopathic localized or partial atrophy of the skin. *Arch. Derm.* (*N.Y.*), 1875–76, **2**, 114–21.

First description of the condition called by Herxheimer and Hartmann in 1902 "acrodermatitis chronica atrophicans", and known eponymically as "Taylor's disease".

4070 MILTON, John Laws. 1820–1898
On giant urticaria. *Edinb. med. J.*, 1876–77, **22**, 513–26.

Although Quincke described angioneurotic oedema with great precision and has given his name to it ("Quincke's disease", "Quincke's oedema") Milton first noted it, calling it "giant urticaria".

4071 COTTLE, Wyndham. ?–1919
Warty growths. *St. George's Hosp. Rep.*, (1877–78), 1879, **9**, 753–62.

Original description of angiokeratoma ("Mibelli's disease" – so named from the latter's description of it in 1891; see No. 4105).

4073 FOX, William Tilbury. 1836–1879, & CROCKER, Henry Radcliffe. 1845–1909
The minute anatomy of dysidrosis. *Trans. path. Soc. Lond.*, 1877–78, **29,** 264–68.

4074 HUTCHINSON, *Sir* Jonathan. 1828–1913
Summer prurigo, prurigo aestivalis, seu prurigo adolescentium, seu acne-prurigo. *Med. times Gaz.*, 1878, **1,** 161–63.
Hutchinson's summer prurigo.

4075 ——. Lectures on clinical surgery. Pt. 2. London, *J. & A. Churchill,* 1879.
On p. 298 is the first description of hydradenitis destruens suppurativa, later named "Pollitzer's disease" from the latter's important description of it in *J. cutan. gen.-urin. Dis.*, 1892, **10**, 9–24.

4076 HARDAWAY, William Augustus. 1850–1923
A case of multiple tumors of the skin accompanied by intense pruritus. *Arch. Derm.* (*Philad.*), 1879, **5,** 385; 1880, **6,** 129–32.
First description of prurigo nodularis. In 1909 J. N. Hyde (*Diseases of the skin,* Philadelphia, p. 174) was responsible for its present name and for the eponym "Hyde's disease".

4077 FOX, William Tilbury. 1836–1879
Notes on unusual or rare forms of skin disease. Congenital ulceration of skin (two cases) with pemphigus eruption and arrest of development generally. *Lancet*, 1879, **1,** 766–67.
First description of epidermolysis bullosa, sometimes referred to as "Goldscheider's disease" (see No. 4079).

4078 ——. A clinical study of hydroa. *Arch. Derm.* (*Philad.*), 1880, **6,** 16–52.
First description of dermatitis herpetiformis ("Duhring's disease"; see No. 4083).

4079 GOLDSCHEIDER, Johannes Karl August Eugen Alfred. 1858–1935
Hereditäre Neigung zur Blasenbildung. *Mh. prakt. Derm.*, 1882, **1,** 163–64.
Epidermolysis bullosa, "Goldscheider's disease", previously described by Tilbury Fox (No. 4077).

4080 KAPOSI, Moritz. 1837–1902
Xeroderma pigmentosum. *Med. Jb.*, 1882, 619–33.
Excellent pathological study of this condition ("Kaposi's disease"), which he first described in Virchow's *Handbuch der speziellen Pathologie und Therapie,* 1876, **2,** 182.

4081 QUINCKE, Heinrich Irenaeus. 1842–1922
Ueber akutes umschriebenes Hautödem. *Mh. prakt. Derm.*, 1882, **1,** 129–31.
Angioneurotic oedema is also known as Quincke's oedema, from the latter's excellent description of it, but he was preceded by several other writers, including Donati (No. 4011.1) and Milton (No. 4070). It is also called "Bannister's disease".

4082 RECKLINGHAUSEN, FRIEDRICH DANIEL VON. 1833–1910
Ueber die multiplen Fibrome der Haut und ihre Beziehung zu den multiplen Neuromen. Berlin, *Hirschwald*, 1882.

One of Virchow's most distinguished pupils, von Recklinghausen gave a classical description of neurofibromatosis, adding much to the knowledge of the condition, which later became known as "von Recklinghausen's disease". The article first appeared as a contribution to the Virchow Festschrift, also published in 1882.

4083 DUHRING, LOUIS ADOLPHUS. 1845–1913
Dermatitis herpetiformis. *J. Amer. med. Ass.*, 1884, **3,** 225–29.

Duhring's best work in dermatology. He brought together, under the name of "dermatitis herpetiformis" ("Duhring's disease") the group of eruptions which morphologically lay between urticaria and the toxic erythemas on the one hand and pemphigus on the other. Duhring wrote the first American text-book on dermatology.

4084 ROBINSON, ANDREW ROSE. 1845–1924
Hidrocystoma. *Trans. Amer. derm. Ass.*, 1884, 14–16; *J. cutan. gen.-urin. Dis.*, 1893, **11,** 293–303.

Robinson wrote an excellent text-book on dermatology in 1884, the year in which he published the first description of hydrocystoma ("Robinson's disease").

4085 KAPOSI, MORITZ. 1837–1902
Ueber eine neue Form von Hautkrankheit, "Lymphodermia perniciosa". *Med. Jb.*, 1885, 129–47.

First description of lymphoderma perniciosa, premycotic or leukaemic erythrodermia.

4086 ——. Lichen ruber moniliformis – Korallen schnurartiger Lichen ruber. *Vjschr. Derm.*, 1886, **13,** 571–82.

Kaposi is credited with the first description of this condition, sometimes called "Kaposi's disease", and probably a rare variety of lichen planus.

4087 NEUMANN, ISIDOR, *Edler von Heilwart*. 1832–1906
Ueber Pemphigus vegetans (frambösioides). *Vjschr. Derm.*, 1886, **13,** 157–78.

"Neumann's disease" – pemphigus vegetans. This was first described by Alibert. English translation (New Sydenham Society), 1897.

4088 VIDAL, JEAN BAPTISTE EMILE. 1825–1893
Du lichen (lichen, prurigo, strophulus). *Ann. Derm. Syph.* (*Paris*) 1886, 2 sér., **7,** 133–54.

"Vidal's disease" – neurodermatitis.

4089 BOCKHART, MAX.
Ueber die Aetiologie und Therapie der Impetigo, des Furunkels und der Sykosis. *Mh. prakt. Derm.*, 1887, **6,** 450–71.

First description of impetigo circumpilaris infantilis ("Bockhart's impetigo").

4090 GIOVANNINI, SEBASTIANO. 1851–1920
Ueber die normale Entwicklung und über einige Veränderungen der menschlichen Haare. *Vjschr. Derm. Syph.*, 1887, **14,** 1049–75.

"Giovannini's disease." He described a rare nodular disease of the hair, produced by a fungus.

4091 KAPOSI, MORITZ. 1837–1902
Impetigo herpetiformis. *Vjschr. Derm.*, 1887, **14,** 273–96.

Although not the first to describe this condition, Kaposi established its status.

4092 UNNA, Paul Gerson. 1850–1929

Das seborrhoische Ekzem. *Mh. prakt. Derm.*, 1887, **6,** 827–46.

Unna's seborrhoeic eczema.

4093 WHITE, James Clarke. 1833–1916

Dermatitis venenata: An account of the action of external irritants upon the skin. Boston, *Cupples & Hurd*, 1887.

White, a pupil of Hebra, was an outstanding personality in American dermatology; he held the first chair in that subject in the U.S.A. His most important work (above) is the first comprehensive account of the subject. The eponym "White's disease" refers to his description of keratosis follicularis in *J. cutan. gen.-urin. Dis.*, 1889, 7, 201–09, a condition described earlier by Lutz and later by Darier.

4094 QUINQUAUD, Charles Eugène. 1841–1894

Folliculite épilante décalvante. *Réunions clin. Hôp. St. Louis, C. R.* (*Paris*), 1888–89, **9,** 17.

Folliculitis decalvans of Quinquaud first described. At about the same time P. A. Robert described it independently in his thesis, Paris, 1889.

4095 BESNIER, Ernest. 1831–1909

Lupus pernio de la face; synovites fongueuses (scrofulo-tuberculeuses) symétriques des extrémités supérieures. *Ann. Derm. Syph.* (*Paris*), 1889, 2 sér., **10,** 333–36.

Besnier–Boeck–Schaumann disease, Boeck's sarcoid. Boeck (No. 4128) wrote a classical paper on the subject and later Schaumann's paper (No. 4149) resulted in a triple eponym. (See No. 4067.)

4096 BURY, Judson Sykes. 1852–1944

A case of erythema with remarkable nodular thickening and induration of skin, associated with intermittent albuminuria. *Illustr. med. News*, 1889, **3,** 145–48.

Erythema elevatum diutinum ("Bury's disease").

4096.1 CHAUFFARD, Anatole Marie Emile. 1855–1932

Xanthélasma disséminé et symétrique, sans insuffisance hépatique. *Bull. Mém. Soc. méd. Hôp. Paris*, 1889, 3 sér., **6,** 412–19.

In 1889 Chauffard gave an important description of pseudoxanthoma elasticum. Further reports on his patient were published by Besnier and Doyon, Darier, and Hallopeau and Laffitte, the last in *Ann. Derm. Syph.* (*Paris*), 1903, **4**, 595.

4097 DARIER, Jean. 1856–1938

De la psorospermose folliculaire végétante. *Ann. Derm. Syph.* (*Paris*), 1889, **10,** 597–612.

Dyskeratosis follicularis was so well described by Darier that it is universally known as "Darier's disease". J. C. White also described it (see No. 4093) and the first description is accredited to H. C. Lutz (No. 4050).

4098 HUTCHINSON, *Sir* Jonathan. 1828–1913

A rare form of lupus (marginatus). *Arch. Surg.* (*Lond.*), 1889–90, **1,** Plates 13–14.

"Hilliard's lupus." Hutchinson made an innovation in terminology when he named the disease after the patient instead of the physician describing it. The *Archives*, which ran to 11 volumes, were written entirely by Hutchinson. See also *Polyclinic*, 1900, 2, 104–09, for a fuller description of this patient.

4099 JACQUET, Lucien. 1860–1915

Des érythèmes papuleux fessiers post-érosifs. *Rev. Mal. Enf.*, 1889, **4,** 208–18.

"Jacquet's disease", "Jacquet's dermatitis", papulo-lenticular erythema of the napkin area.

4100 TAENZER, Paul. 1858–1919
Ueber das Ulerythema ophryogenes, eine noch nicht beschriebene Hautkrankheit. *Mh. prakt. Derm.*, 1889, **8,** 197–208.
Ulerythema ophryogenes ("Taenzer's disease") first described.

4101 HALLOPEAU, François Henri. 1842–1919
Sur une nouvelle forme de dermatite pustuleuse chronique en foyer à progression excentrique. *Congr. int. Derm. Syph., C. R.*, 1889, Paris, 1890, 344.
Pyodermite végétante. Hallopeau described a suppurative form of Neumann's pemphigus vegetans.

4102 POLLITZER, Sigmund. 1859–1937, & JANOVSKY, Viktor. 1847–1925
Acanthesis nigricans. In: *Int. Atlas seltener Hautkrankheiten*, Hamburg, 1890, Heft 4, plates x–xi.
First description of acanthosis nigricans.

4103 PRINGLE, John James. 1855–1922
Ueber einen Fall von kongenitalem Adenoma sebaceum. *Mh. prakt. Derm.*, 1890, **10,** 197–211.
Sebaceous adenoma, type Pringle.

4104 HUTCHINSON, *Sir* Jonathan. 1828–1913
Infective angeioma or naevus-lupus. *Arch. Surg.* (*Lond.*), 1891–92, **3,** 166–68.
Angioma serpiginosum.

4105 MIBELLI, Vittorio. 1860–1910
L'angiocheratoma. *G. ital. Mal. vener.*, 1891, **26,** 159–80, 260–76.
Mibelli gave the name to angiokeratoma although it had already been described by Cottle in 1877. It is also called "Mibelli's disease".

4106 NONNE, Max. 1861–
Vier Fälle von Elephantiasis congenita hereditaria. *Virchows Arch. path. Anat.*, 1891, **125,** 189–96.
First description of hereditary oedema of the legs, generally known as "Milroy's disease" or as "Meige's disease" (No. 4129).

4107 BESNIER, Ernest. 1831–1909
Première note et observations préliminaires pour servir d'introduction à l'étude des prurigos diathésiques (dermatites multiformes prurigineuses chroniques exacerbantes et paroxystiques, du type du prurigo de Hebra). *Ann. Derm. Syph.* (*Paris*), 1892, 3 sér., **3,** 634–48.
"Besnier's prurigo."

4108 JADASSOHN, Josef. 1863–1936
Ueber eine eigenartige Form von Atrophia maculosa cutis. *Verh. dtsch derm. Ges.*, 1890–92, **2–3,** 342–58.
"Jadassohn's disease" – maculo-papular erythrodermia; Anetoderma erythematosum of Jadassohn.

4109 MILROY, William Forsyth. 1855–1942
An undescribed variety of hereditary oedema. *N.Y. med. J.*, 1892, **56,** 505–08.
Independently of Nonne (No. 4106) Milroy described congenital oedema of the legs; it has been given the eponym "Milroy's disease".

4110 UNNA, PAUL GERSON. 1850–1929
Drei Favusarten. *Mh. prakt. Derm.*, 1892, **14,** 1–16.
Unna described the different fungi of favus. He founded the above-mentioned journal, and he is one of the most eminent figures in modern dermatology.

4111 POSADAS, ALEJANDRO. 1870–1902
Un nuovo caso de micosis fungoidea con psorospermias. *An. Circ. med. argent.*, 1892, **15,** 585–97.
See No. 4112.

4112 WERNICKE, ROBERT JOHANN. 1873–
Pentastomas. *Rev. Asoc. med. argent.*, 1892, **1,** 186–89.
Posadas (No. 4111) and Wernicke were the first to report cases of coccidioidomycosis. German translation of Wernicke's paper in *Zbl. Bakt.*, 1892, **12,** 859–61.

4113 DARIER, JEAN. 1856–1938
Dystrophie papillaire et pigmentaire. *Ann. Derm. Syph.* (*Paris*), 1893, 3 sér., **4,** 865–75.
Acanthosis nigricans.

4114 MIBELLI, VITTORIO. 1860–1910
Contributo allo studio della ipercheratosi dei canali sudoriferi (porokeratosis). *G. ital. Mal. vener.*, 1893, **28,** 313–55.
Mibelli is sometimes credited with the original description of porokeratosis ("Mibelli's disease"), but Neumann described it in 1875 under the name of "dermatitis circumscripta herpetiformis".

4115 RESPIGHI, EMILIO.
Di una ipercheratosi non ancora descritta. *G. ital. Mal. vener.*, Milano, 1893, **28,** 356–86.
First description of hyperkeratosis excentrica, porokeratosis.

4116 SABOURAUD, RAYMOND JACQUES ADRIEN. 1864–1938
La teigne trichophytique et la teigne spéciale de Gruby. Paris, *Rueff et Cie.*, 1894.

4117 VINCENT, JEAN HYACINTHE. 1862–1950
Etude sur le parasite du "pied de Madura". *Ann. Inst. Pasteur*, 1894, **8,** 129–51.
Isolation of *Streptothrix* (*Actinomyces*) *madurae.*

4118 BUSSE, OTTO. 1867–1922
Ueber parasitäre Zelleinschlüsse und ihre Züchtung. *Dtsch. med. Wschr.*, Berlin, 1895, **21,** Vereins-Beilage, 14.
"Busse–Buschke's disease" – blastomycosis of the skin, due to *Cryptococcus neoformans.* See also No. 4119. Busse first described it it *Zbl. Bakt.*, 1894, **16,** 175–80.

4119 BUSCHKE, ABRAHAM. 1868–1943
Ueber eine durch Coccidien hervorgerufene Krankheit des Menschen. *Dtsch. med. Wschr.*, 1895, **21,** Vereins-Beilage, 14.

4120 KAPOSI, MORITZ. 1837–1902
Lichen ruber acuminatus und Lichen ruber planus. *Arch. Derm. Syph.* (*Wien*), 1895, **31,** 1–32.

4121 OSLER, *Sir* WILLIAM, *Bart.* 1849–1919
On the visceral complications of erythema exudativum multiforme. *Amer. J. med. Sci.*, 1895, **110,** 629–46.

4122 DARIER, JEAN. 1856–1938
Des "tuberculides" cutanées. *Ann. Derm. Syph. (Paris)*, 1896, 3 sér., **7,** 1431–36.
Darier grouped together, under the heading "tuberculides", the skin eruptions associated with tuberculosis.

4123 FORDYCE, JOHN ADDISON. 1858–1925
A peculiar affection of the mucous membrane of the lips and the oral cavity. *J. cutan. gen.-urin. Dis.*, 1896, **14,** 413–19.
Fordyce, remembered for the description of "Fox-Fordyce disease", also described a pseudocolloid of the buccal mucosa, which is known as "Fordyce's disease".

4124 GILCHRIST, THOMAS CASPAR. 1862–1927
A case of blastomycetic dermatitis in man. *Johns Hopk. Hosp. Rep.*, 1896, **1,** 269–83.
Gilchrist's description of blastomycosis ("Gilchrist's disease", "Busse–Buschke disease") is one of the most important contributions to the knowledge of the infectious granulomata involving the skin.

4125 MAJOCCHI, DOMENICO. 1849–1929
Sopra una dermatosi telangettode non ancora descritta "Purpura annularis" "Telangectasia follicularis annulata" studio clinico. *G. ital. Mal. vener.*, 1896, **31,** 242–43.
Purpura annularis telangiectodes (Majocchi) first described.

4126 SABOURAUD, RAYMOND JACQUES ADRIEN. 1864–1938
La séborrhée grasse et la pelade. *Ann. Inst. Pasteur*, 1897, **11,** 134–59.
Acne bacillus first cultivated.

4127 SCHENCK, BENJAMIN ROBINSON. 1873–1920
On refractory subcutaneous abscesses caused by a fungus possibly related to the sporotricha. *Johns Hopk. Hosp. Bull.*, 1898, **9,** 286–90.
Schenck first described a form of sporotrichosis, due to a pathogenic fungus, which later became known as *Sporotrichum beurmanni*, after more thorough studies upon it by de Beurmann in 1903.

4128 BOECK, CAESAR PETER MŒLLER. 1845–1917
Multipelt benignt hud-sarcoid. *Norsk Mag. Lægevid*, 1899, 4 r., **14,** 1321–34.
The syndrome of benign sarcoid ("Boeck's sarcoid") was first established by Boeck. English translation in *J. cutan. gen.-urin. Dis.*, 1899, **17,** 543–50. In 1940 Danbolt (*Schweiz. med. Wschr.*, 1947, **77,** 1149–50) re-examined Boeck's original patient, then aged 80.

4129 MEIGE, HENRY. 1866–1940
Le trophoedème chronique héréditaire. *N. Iconogr. Salpêtr.*, 1899, **12,** 453–80; 1901, **14,** 465–72.
"Meige's disease" – first described by Nonne (No.4106).

4130 SABOURAUD, RAYMOND JACQUES ADRIEN. 1864–1938
Essai critique sur l'étiologie de l'eczéma. *Ann. Derm. Syph. (Paris)*, 1899, 3 sér., **10,** 305–24.

4131 KROMPECHER, EDMUND. 1870–1926
Der drüsenartige Oberflächenepithelkrebs. *Beitr. path. Anat.*, 1900, **28,** 1–41.
"Krompecher's tumour" – rodent ulcer.

4131.1 SEEBER, GUILLERMO RUDOLFO.
Un nuevo esporozoario parasíto del hombre. Dos casos encontrados en pólipos nasales. *Tesis*, Univ. Nac. de Buenos Aires, 1900.
Rhinosporidiosis first described.

4132 EHLERS, EDVARD. 1863–1937
Cutis laxa. Neigung zu Haemorrhagien in der Haut, Lockerung mehrerer Artikulationen. *Derm. Z.*, 1901, **8,** 173–74.
First description of the syndrome to which the name "Ehlers–Danlos syndrome" was later attached (see also No. 4144).

4133 JADASSOHN, JOSEF. 1863–1936
Ueber eine eigenartige Erkrankung der Nasenhaut bei Kindern ("Granulosis rubra nasi"). *Arch. Derm. Syph.* (*Wien*), 1901, **58,** 145–158.
In his important paper on granulosis rubra nasi, Jadassohn gave the condition its present name. Previously Pringle, 1894, and Luithlen, 1900, had described probable cases.

4134 SCHAMBERG, JAY FRANK. 1870–1934
A peculiar progressive pigmentary disease of the skin. *Brit. J. Derm.* 1901, **13,** 1–5.
Schamberg's progressive pigmentary dermatosis; first description.

4135 BROCQ, LOUIS ANNE JEAN. 1856–1928
Les parapsoriasis. *Ann. Derm. Syph.* (*Paris*), 1902, 4 sér., **3,** 313–15, 433–68.
"Brocq's disease"; he proposed the term "parapsoriasis" for the condition which had previously been described under various names and often mistaken for other dermatoses.

4136 ENGMAN, MARTIN FEENEY. 1869–1953
An infectious form of an eczematoid dermatitis. *Amer. Med.*, 1902, **4,** 769–73.
"Engman's disease" – infectious eczematoid dermatitis.

4137 FOX, GEORGE HENRY. 1846–1937, & FORDYCE, JOHN ADDISON. 1858–1925
Two cases of a rare papular disease affecting the axillary region. *J. cutan. gen.-urin. Dis.*, 1902, **20,** 1–5.
"Fox-Fordyce disease." These writers described a papular, itchy eruption, confined to the axillae, nipples and pubes, and considered to be due to a dysfunction of the apocrine glands.

4138 HERXHEIMER, KARL. 1861–1944, & HARTMANN, KUNO.
Ueber Acrodermatitis chronica atrophicans. *Arch. Derm. Syph.* (*Wien*), 1902, **61,** 57–76.
Taylor described the condition in 1876 (No. 4069) and Herxheimer and Hartmann named it, separating it from other atrophies which had been called by a number of different names.

4139 SABOURAUD, RAYMOND JACQUES ADRIEN. 1864–1938
Pityriasis et alopécies pelliculaires. Paris, *Masson & Cie.*, 1904.
Classical account of the different varieties of *Trichophyton.*

4140 JULIUSBERG, MAX. 1874–
Zur Kenntnis des Virus des Molluscum contagiosum des Menschen. *Dtsch. med. Wschr.*, 1905, **31,** 1598–99.
Juliusberg showed that the virus of molluscum contagiosum passed a Chamberland filter.

4141 JACOBI, EDUARD. 1862–1915
Fall zur Diagnose (Poikilodermia vascularis atrophicans). *Verh. dtsch. derm. Ges.*, (1906), Berlin, 1907, **9,** 321–23.
First description.

4142 CIUFFO, GIUSEPPE.
Innesto positivo con filtrato de verruca volgare. *G. ital. Mal. vener.*, 1907, **42,** 12–17.
Ciuffo showed the aetiological agent in common warts to be filterable.

4143 PINKUS, FELIX. 1868–1947
Ueber eine neue knötchenförmige Hauteruption; Lichen nitidus. *Arch. Derm. Syph.* (*Wien*), 1907, **85,** 11–36.
Original description of lichen nitidus, "Pinkus's disease". Pinkus first showed a case before the Berlin Dermatological Society on Dec. 3, 1901, and himself gave the name "lichen nitidus".

4144 DANLOS, HENRI ALEXANDRE. 1844–1937
Un cas de cutis laxa avec tumeurs par contusion chronique des coudes et des genoux. *Bull. Soc. franç. Derm. Syph.*, 1908, **19,** 70–72.
Ehlers–Danlos syndrome (see also No. 4132). Danlos noted the subcutaneous tumours that may occur in this condition.

4145 LEINER, KARL. 1871–1930
Ueber Erythrodermia desquamativa, eine eigenartige universelle Dermatose der Brustkinder. *Arch. Derm. Syph.* (*Wien*), 1908, **89,** 65–76, 163–90.
Desquamative erythroderma of nurslings (Leiner); apparently a toxic eruption peculiar to bresat-fed children suffering from enteritis.

4145.1 LUTZ, ADOLFO. 1855–1940
Uma mycose pseudococcidica localisada na bocca e observada no Brazil. Contribuição ao conhocimento das hyphoblastomycoses americanas. *Brazil-méd.*, 1908, **22,** 121–24, 141–44.
South American blastomycosis.

4146 QUEYRAT, AUGUSTE. 1872–
Érythroplasie du gland. *Bull. Soc. franç. Derm. Syph.*, 1911, **22,** 378–382.
Erythroplasia of Queyrat, a condition similar to the precancerous dermatosis described by Bowen (No. 4148).

4147 BEURMANN, CHARLES LUCIEN DE. 1851–1923, & GOUGEROT, HENRI. 1881–1955
Les sporotrichoses. Paris, *F. Alcan*, 1912.
First complete description of sporotrichosis ("de Beurmann–Gougerot disease").

4148 BOWEN, JOHN TEMPLETON. 1857–1941
Precancerous dermatoses. A study of two cases of chronic atypical epithelial proliferation. *J. cutan. gen.-urin. Dis.*, 1912, **30,** 241–55.
Bowen, a Boston dermatologist, first described a precancerous dermatosis ("Bowen's disease"), which is now considered to be a variant of an intra-epidermal basal-cell epithelioma.

4149 SCHAUMANN, Jörgen Nilsen. 1879–1953
Étude sur le lupus pernio et ses rapports avec les sarcoides et la tuberculose. *Ann. Derm. Syph. (Paris)*, 1917, 5 sér., **6,** 357–73.
"Besnier–Boeck–Schaumann disease" (see also Nos. 4095, 4128). Through Schaumann's paper the systemic nature of sarcoidosis came to be recognized.

4150 STEVENS, Albert Mason. 1884–1945, & JOHNSON, F. C.
A new eruptive fever associated with stomatitis and ophthalmia; report of two cases in children. *Amer. J. Dis. Child.*, 1922, **24,** 526–33.
"Stevens–Johnson syndrome", a generalized eruption, continued fever, inflamed buccal mucosa, and severe purulent conjunctivitis. B. A. Thomas (*Brit. med. J.*, 1950, **1**, 1393) believes this to be merely a severe form of Hebra's erythema multiforme exudativum (No. 4049, p. 198).

4151 WEBER, Frederick Parkes. 1863–1962
A case of relapsing non-suppurative nodular panniculitis, showing phagocytosis of subcutaneous fat-cells by macrophages. *Brit. J. Derm.*, 1925, **37,** 301–11.
Weber–Christian disease (see No. 4152).

4152 CHRISTIAN, Henry Asbury. 1876–1951
Relapsing febrile nodular nonsuppurative panniculitis. *Arch. intern. Med.*, 1928, **42,** 338–51.
See No. 4151.

4153 KVEIM, Morten Ansgar. 1892–
En ny og spesifikk kutan-reaksjon ved Boecks sarcoid. En foreløbig meddelelse. *Nord Med.*, 1941, **9,** 169–72.
Kveim's test for sarcoidosis.

4154 CUTTINO, John Tindal. 1912– , & McCABE, Anne M.
Pure granulomatous nocardiosis: a new fungus disease distinguished by intracellular parasitism. A description of a new disease in man due to a hitherto undescribed organism, *Nocardia intracellularis*, n.sp., including a study of the biologic and pathogenic properties of this species. *Amer. J. Path.*, 1949, **25,** 1–48.
Nocardiosis described.

History of Dermatology

4155 RICHTER, Paul Caesar. 1865–1938
Geschichte der Dermatologie. In: J. Jadassohn's *Handbuch der Haut- und Geschlechtskrankheiten*, Berlin, **14,** pt. 2, pp. 1–252, 1928.

4156 PUSEY, William Allen. 1865–1940
The history of dermatology. Springfield, *C. C. Thomas*, 1933.

4157 FRIEDMAN, Reuben. 1892–1956
The story of scabies. Vol. 1. New York, *Froben*, 1947.
Reprinted from *Med. Life*, 1934, **41**, 381–424, 426–76; 1935, **42**, 217–72.

4158 SHELLEY, Walter Brown. 1917– , & CRISSEY, John Thorne. 1924–
Classics in clinical dermatology. With biographical sketches. Springfield, *C. C. Thomas*, 1953.
Contains 143 classical descriptions of cutaneous diseases by 93 writers. Many portraits are also included.

4159–4298 DISEASES OF THE GENITO-URINARY SYSTEM

See also 5195–5227, VENEREAL DISEASES; 6008–6135, GYNAECOLOGY.

4159 LAGUNA, ANDRÉS [LACUNA]. 1499–1560

Methodus cognoscendi extirpandique excrescentes in vesicae collo carunculas. [1551.]

Laguna, "the Spanish Galen", wrote several important books, among them the above, a method of excising vesical caruncles. Laguna was among the first to suggest this method.

4160 DIAZ, FRANCISCO. *fl.* 1580

Tratado de todas las enfermedades de los riñones, vexiga, y carnosidades de la verga, y urina. Madrid, *Fr. Sanchez*, 1588.

First treatise on diseases of urinary tract. Also describes the high operation for stone. Diaz is sometimes called the "Father of Urology."

4161 DEKKERS, FREDERIK [DECKERS]. 1648–1720

Exercitationes medicae practicae circa medendi methodum. Lugduni Batavorum et Amstelodami, *apud D. Abrahamum et Adrianum à Gaesbeck*, 1673.

Albuminuria was first described by Dekkers (Chapter V). A translation of this chapter is in R. H. Major: *Classic descriptions of disease*, 3rd ed., 1945, p. 528.

4162 BELLINI, LORENZO. 1643–1704

De urinis et pulsibus, de missione sanguinis, de febribus, de morbis capitis, et pectoris. Bononiae, 1683.

Bellini realized the value of the urine as an aid to diagnosis and insisted on its chemical analysis in pathological conditions.

4163 LA PEYRONIE, FRANÇOIS DE. 1678–1747

Mémoire sur quelques obstacles qui s'opposent à l'éjaculation naturelle de la semence. *Mém. Acad. roy. Chir. (Paris)*, 1743, **1**, 425–34.

"Peyronie's disease", plastic induration of the penis.

4164 POTT, PERCIVALL. 1714–1788

Practical remarks on the hydrocele or watry rupture. London, *C. Hitch & L. Hawes*, 1762.

Classical description of hydrocele.

4165 ——. Chirurgical observations relative to the cataract, the polypus of the nose, the cancer of the scrotum, *etc.* London, *T. J. Carnegy*, 1775.

Includes the first description of occupational cancer. By describing chimney-sweeps' cancer of the scrotum, Pott was the first to trace the origin of a type of cancer to a specific external cause. The above work also includes his description of senile gangrene, sometimes referred to as "Pott's gangrene".

4166 COOPER, *Sir* ASTLEY PASTON, *Bart.* 1768–1841

Observations on the structure and diseases of the testis. London, *Longmans*, 1830.

4167 GUTHRIE, GEORGE JAMES. 1785–1856

On the anatomy and diseases of the neck of the bladder and of the urethra. London, *Burgess & Hill*, 1834.

Guthrie was the first to describe non-prostatic obstruction at the neck of the bladder. On p. 252 of the above work is an account of Guthrie's prostatic catheter for use in trans-urethral prostatectomy.

4168 MAISONNEUVE, JACQUES GILLES THOMAS. 1809–1877
Mémoire sur un moyen très simple et très sur de pratiquer le cathétérisme dans les cas même les plus difficiles. *C. R. Acad. Sci.* (*Paris*), 1845, **20,** 70–72.

Maisonneuve introduced a hair catheter.

4169 PARKER, WILLARD. 1800–1884
Cystitis; lateral operation on the bladder, death; tuberculous kidney. *N.Y. J. Med.*, 1851, n.s. **7,** 83–86.

First cystotomy for inflammation and rupture of the bladder.

4169.1 SIMON, *Sir* JOHN. 1816–1904
Ectropia vesicae (absence of the anterior walls of the bladder and pubic abdominal parietes); operation for directing the orifices of the ureters into the rectum; temporary success; subsequent death; autopsy. *Lancet*, 1852, **2,** 568–70.

First uretero-intestinal anastomosis.

4170 PANCOAST, JOSEPH. 1805–1882
[Plastic operation for exstrophy of the bladder in the male; reported by S. D. Gross.] *N. Amer. med.-chir. Rev.*, 1859, **3,** 710–11.

Pancoast performed the first successful operation for exstrophy of the bladder (ectopia vesicae).

4171 HARLEY, GEORGE. 1829–1896
On intermittent haematuria; with remarks upon its pathology and treatment. *Med.-chir. Trans.*, 1865, **48,** 161–73.

Harley's classical description of paroxysmal haemoglobinuria, "Harley's disease".

4172 DESORMEAUX, ANTONIN JEAN. ?–1894
De l'endoscope et de ses applications au diagnostic et au traitement des affections de l'urèthre et de la vessie. Paris, *J. B. Baillière*, 1865.

Desormeaux was a pioneer of endoscopy.

4173 THOMPSON, *Sir* HENRY, *Bart.* 1820–1904
Clinical lectures on diseases of the urinary organs. London, *J. Churchill*, 1868.

Thompson was professor of clinical surgery at University College, London, and an eminent genito-urinary surgeon. He performed the operation of lithotrity upon Leopold I and Napoleon III; he also developed the two-glass urine test in gonorrhoea. *The versatile Victorian*, a biography of Thompson, was published by Sir Zachary Cope in 1951.

4174 GUSSENBAUER, CARL. 1842–1903
Exstirpation eines Harnblasenmyoms nach vorausgehendem tiefen und hohen Blasenschnitt. Heilung. *Arch. klin. Chir.*, 1875, **18,** 411–423.

First abdominal resection of a tumour of the bladder. The operation was performed by Billroth.

4175 NITZE, MAX. 1848–1906
Eine neue Beobachtungs- und Untersuchungsmethode für Harnröhre, Harnblase und Rectum. *Wien. med. Wschr.*, 1879, **29,** 649–52, 713–16, 776–82, 806–10.

Nitze devised an electrically lighted cytoscope in 1877, which made possible great improvements in the surgery of the bladder.

4176 FLEISCHER, RICHARD. 1848–
Ueber eine neue Form von Haemoglobinurie beim Menschen. *Berl. klin. Wschr.*, 1881, **18,** 691–94.
First description of "march haemoglobinuria" – the condition in which physical exertion gives rise to the passage of red urine containing haemoglobin in solution.

4177 GUYON, JEAN CASIMIR FÉLIX. 1831–1920
Leçons cliniques sur les maladies des voies urinaires. Paris, *J. B. Baillière*, 1881.
Guyon was the outstanding French urologist of his day, an operator of great skill and a brilliant lithotomist.

4178 SENATOR, HERMANN. 1834–1911
Die Albuminurie im gesunden und kranken Zustande. Berlin, *A. Hirschwald*, 1882.

4179 OTIS, FESSENDEN NOTT. 1825–1900
The hydrochlorate of cocaine in genito-urinary procedures. *N.Y. med. J.*, 1884, **40,** 635–37.
Local anaesthesia first employed in urology.

4180 THOMPSON, *Sir* HENRY, *Bart.* 1820–1904
On tumours of the bladder. London, *J. & A. Churchill*, 1884.
Includes description of Thompson's operation for tumours of the bladder.

4181 PAVY, FREDERICK WILLIAM. 1829–1911
On cyclic albuminuria (albuminuria in the apparently healthy). *Brit. med. J.*, 1885, **2,** 789–91.
"Pavy's disease" – recurrent albuminuria.

4182 MACCORMAC, *Sir* WILLIAM. 1836–1901
Some observations on rupture of the urinary bladder, with an account of two cases of intra-peritoneal rupture successfully treated by abdominal section and subsequent suture of the vesical rent. *Lancet*, 1886, **2,** 1118–22.
MacCormac introduced an operation for the treatment of intraperitoneal rupture of the bladder.

4183 GUYON, JEAN CASIMIR FÉLIX. 1831–1920
Leçons cliniques sur les affections chirurgicales de la vessie et de la prostate. Paris, *J. B. Baillière*, 1888.
Guyon was professor of genito-urinary surgery at Paris, and a great teacher (see also No. 4177).

4184 NITZE, MAX. 1848–1906
Lehrbuch der Kystoskopie. Wiesbaden, *J. F. Bergmann*, 1889.
Nitze introduced the cystoscope in 1877 (see No. 4175) and in 1889 published his important monograph on cystoscopy.

4185 ALBARRAN Y DOMINGUEZ, JOAQUIN MARIA. 1860–1912
Les tumeurs de la vessie. Paris, *G. Steinheil*, 1892.
Includes description of "Albarran's glands", subtrigonal glands in the bladder. See also No. 4195.

4185.1 BROWN, JAMES. 1854–1895
Catheterization of the male ureters. A preliminary report. *Johns Hopk. Hosp. Bull.*, 1893, **4,** 73–74.
First catheterization of male ureters.

4186 VAN HOOK, WELLER. 1862–1933
The surgery of the ureters. A clinical, literary, and experimental research. *J. Amer. med. Ass.*, 1893, **21**, 911–16, 965–73.

Uretero-ureterostomy. Van Hook originated modern methods of ureteral repair.

4187 KELLY, HOWARD ATWOOD. 1858–1943
The examination of the female bladder and the catheterization of the ureters under direct inspection. *Johns Hopk. Hosp. Bull.*, 1893, **4**, 101–02.

Kelly introduced aeroscopic examination of the bladder and catherization of the ureters. See also *Ann. Surg.*, 1898, **27**, 475–86.

4188 ——. Uretero-ureteral anastomosis; uretero-ureterostomy. *Ann Surg.*, 1894, **19**, 70–77.

Kelly's method of uretero-ureteral anastomosis included the use of the catheter as a temporary ureteral splint.

4189 PÉAN, JULES ÉMILE. 1830–1898
Vessie et urètre surnuméraires. *Bull. Acad. Méd.* (*Paris*), 1895, 3 sér., **33**, 542–45.

Péan was first to operate on diverticula of the bladder.

4190 NITZE, MAX. 1848–1906
Eine neue Modifikation des Harnleiterkatheters. *Zbl. Krankh. Harn.- u. SexOrg.*, 1897, **8**, 8–13.

With Nitze's operative cystoscope it became possible to excise bladder tumours *in situ*.

4191 BEVAN, ARTHUR DEAN. 1860–1943
Operation for undescended testicle and congenital inguinal hernia. *J. Amer. med. Ass.*, 1899, **33**, 773–77.

Bevan's operation for undescended testicle.

4192 VOELCKER, FRIEDRICH. 1872– , & LICHTENBERG, ALEXANDER VON. 1880–1949
Die Gestalt der menschlichen Harnblase im Röntgenbilde. *Münch. med. Wschr.*, 1905, **52**, 1576–78.

First cystograms.

4194 HAGNER, FRANCIS RANDALL. 1873–
The operative treatment of acute gonorrheal epididymitis. *Med. Rec.* (*N.Y.*), 1906, **70**, 565–68; 1909, **76**, 944–46.

Hagner devised the open operation for the relief of acute epididymitis.

4194.1 GRAY, ALFRED LEFTWICH. 1873–1932
The treatment of malignant diseases of the bladder through suprapubic incision, with report of a case. *Amer. Quart. Roentgenol.*, 1906–07, **1**, 53–56.

Radiotherapy for carcinoma of bladder.

4195 ALBARRAN Y DOMINGUEZ, JOAQUIN MARIA. 1860–1912
Médecine opératoire des voies urinaires. Paris, *Masson & Cie.*, 1909.

Albarran, a Cuban, became a teacher of the highest rank and attained a professorship at Paris in 1892. He was the first surgeon in France to perform perineal prostatectomy.

4195.1 BUERGER, Leo. 1879–1943
A new direct irrigating observation and double catheterizing cystoscope. *Ann. Surg.*, 1909, **49,** 225–37.
Brown–Buerger cystoscope.

4196 TOREK, Franz. 1861–1938
The technique of orcheopexy. *N.Y. med. J.*, 1909, **90,** 948–53.
Torek's operation for undescended testicle.

4196.1 COFFEY, Robert Calvin. 1869–1933
Physiologic implantation of the severed ureter or common bile-duct into the intestine. *J. Amer. med. Ass.*, 1911, **56,** 397–403.
The modern method of uretero-intestinal anastomosis followed the experimental work of Coffey.

4197 KAPPIS, Max. 1881–1938
Ueber Leitungsanästhesie bei Nierenoperationen und Thorakoplastiken überhaupt bei Operationen am Rumpf. *Zbl. Chir.*, 1912, **39,** 249–52.
Paravertebral anaesthesia in urology.

4198 YOUNG, Hugh Hampton. 1870–1945, & WATERS, Charles Alexander. 1885–
X-ray studies of the seminal vesicles and vasa deferentia after urethroscopic injection of the ejaculatory ducts with thorium – a new diagnostic method. *Amer. J. Roentgenol.*, 1920, n.s. **7,** 16–22.
Vesiculography first demonstrated.

4198.1 McCARTHY, Joseph Francis. 1874–
A new type of observation and operating cysto-urethroscope. *J. Urol.*, 1923, **10,** 519–23.
McCarthy foroblique pan-endoscope.

4199 OSBORNE, Earl Dorland. 1895–1960, *et al.*
Roentgenography of the urinary tract during excretion of sodium iodid. *J. Amer. med. Ass.*, 1923, **80,** 368–73.
Sodium iodide was first used in uretero-pyelography by E. D. Osborne, C. G. Sutherland, A. J. Scholl, and L. G. Rowntree.

4200 YOUNG, Hugh Hampton. 1870–1945, & DAVIS, David Melvin. 1886–
Practice of urology. 2 vols. Philadelphia, *Saunders* (1926).

4201 ——, & WATERS, Charles Alexander. 1885–
Urological röntgenology. New York, *P. B. Hoeber*, 1928.

4202 ROSENHEIM, Max Leonard, *Lord Rosenheim.* 1908–1972
Mandelic acid in the treatment of urinary infections. *Lancet*, 1935, **1,** 1032–37.
Introduction of mandelic acid in the treatment of urinary infections.

4203 CABOT, Hugh. 1872–1945
Modern urology in original contributions by American authors. 3rd ed. 2 vols. Philadelphia, *Lea & Febiger*, 1936.

4204–4257.1 KIDNEY

4204 SALICETO, Gulielmus de [Salicetti; William of Salicet]. *circa* 1210–1280
Liber in scientia medicinali. [Placentiae, *Johannes Petrus de Ferratis*, 1476.]

Contains (Cap. cxl) his classical account of renal dropsy: De duritie in renibus, an English translation of which is in R. H. Major: *Classic descriptions of disease*, 3rd ed., 1945, p. 527.

4205 WELLS, William Charles. 1757–1817
On the presence of the red matter and serum of blood in the urine of dropsy, which has not originated from scarlet fever. *Trans. Soc. Improve. med. chir. Knowl.*, 1812, **3**, 194–240.

Wells was the first to notice the presence of blood and albumin in dropsical urine. He also established the fact that the dropsy occurred in the upper parts of the body, and he described the uraemic seizures to which such cases are liable.

4206 BRIGHT, Richard. 1789–1858
Reports of medical cases selected with a view of illustrating the symptoms and cure of diseases by a reference to morbid anatomy. 2 vols. London, *Longman*, 1827–31.

Bright's classical description of chronic nephritis has led to its designation as "Bright's disease", one of the best known and most permanent of medical eponyms. Bright distinguished renal from cardiac dropsy. He was the first clearly to recognize the association of dropsy, coagulable urine, and disease of the kidney.

4207 ——. Cases and observations, illustrative of renal disease accompanied with the secretion of albuminous urine. *Guy's Hosp. Rep.*, 1836, **1**, 338–400.

As a result of greater experience on renal disease Bright rounded off his work on the subject with the above paper, wherein he recorded his extended observations; by this time he had come to more definite conclusions, especially with regard to the treatment of the condition. Bright's papers on the subject were reprinted, London, 1937, edited by A. A. Osman.

4208 RAYER, Pierre François Olive. 1793–1867
Traité des maladies des reins. 3 vols. and atlas. Paris, *J. B. Baillière*, 1839–41.

Rayer insisted on the exhaustive analysis of the urine as an aid to the diagnosis of lesions. His great treatise on diseases of the kidney is a milestone in the history of the subject.

4209 FRERICHS, Friedrich Theodor. 1819–1885
Die Bright'sche Nierenkrankheit. Braunschweig, *F. Vieweg u. Sohn*, 1851.

4210 STODDARD, Charles L.
Case of encephaloid disease of the kidney; removal, etc. *Med. Surg. Reporter (Philad.)*, 1861, **7**, 126–27.

Erastus Bradley Wolcott (1804–80) was first to excise the kidney (for renal tumour). The operation was recorded by C. L. Stoddard.

4211 DIETL, JOSEF. 1804–1878
Wandernde Nieren und deren Einklemmung. *Wien. med. Wschr.*, 1864, **14**, 563–66, 579–81, 593–95.

"Dietl's crisis." Dietl described the sudden severe attacks of nephralgic or gastric pain, chills, fever, nausea and vomiting, and general collapse, ascribing them to partial turning of the kidney upon its pedicle. First published in *Przeglad Lekarski*, 1864, **3**, 225, 233, 241.

4212 KLEBS, THEODOR ALBRECHT EDWIN. 1834–1913
Handbuch der pathologischen Anatomie. I. Abt. Berlin, *A. Hirschwald*, 1870.

A classical description of glomerulo-nephritis ("Kleb's disease") is on pp. 644–48.

4213 SIMON, GUSTAV. 1824–1876
Exstirpation einer Niere am Menschen. *Dtsch. Klin.*, 1870, **22**, 137–138.

First deliberate excision of the kidney.

4214 ——. Chirurgie der Nieren. Theil 1–2. Erlangen, *F. Enke*, 1871–76.

Simon was professor of surgery at Rostock and Heidelberg. He was a pioneer in the surgery of the kidney, being the first in Europe to excise that organ.

4215 GULL, *Sir* WILLIAM WITHEY. 1816–1890, & SUTTON, HENRY GAWEN. 1837–1891
On the pathology of the morbid state commonly called chronic Bright's disease with contracted kidney ("arterio-capillary fibrosis"). *Med.-chir. Trans.*, 1872, **55**, 273–326.

First clear description of arteriolosclerotic atrophy of the kidney ("Gull–Sutton disease").

4216 GOWERS, *Sir* WILLIAM RICHARD. 1845–1915
The state of the arteries in Bright's disease. *Brit. med. J.*, 1876, **2**, 743–45.

Gowers' important account of the changes in the retinal vessels in Bright's disease is reproduced in F. A. Willius & T. E. Keys: *Cardiac classics*, 1941, pp. 605–11.

4217 WEIGERT, CARL. 1845–1904
Die Bright'sche Nierenerkrankung vom pathologisch-anatomischen Standpunkte. *Samml. klin. Vortr.*, 1879, Nr. 162–63 (Inn. Med., Nr. 55), 1411–60.

Classical study of the pathological anatomy of Bright's disease.

4218 HAHN, EUGEN. 1841–1902
Die operative Behandlung der beweglichen Niere durch Fixation. *Zbl. Chir.*, 1881, **8**, 449–52.

Hahn devised the operation of nephropexy (nephrorrhaphy) for the relief of movable kidney.

4219 BASSINI, EDOARDO. 1844–1924
Un caso di rene mobile fissato col mezzo dell'operazione cruenta. *Ann. Univ. Med. (Milano)*, 1882, **261**, 281–86.

Important modification of Hahn's operation of nephropexy

4220 GRAWITZ, Paul Albert. 1850–1932
Die Entstehung von Nierentumoren aus Nebennierengewebe. *Verh. dtsch. Ges. Chir.*, 1884, **13,** pt. 2, 28–38.

An important investigation of the origin of hypernephroma ("Grawitz tumour"). See also *Arch. klin. Chir.*, 1884, **30**, 824–34.

4221 BOZEMAN, Nathan. 1825–1905
Chronic pyelitis, successfully treated by kolpo-uretero-cystotomy. *Amer. J. med. Sci.*, 1888, **95,** 255–65, 368–76.

Bozeman treated vesical and faecal fistulae in women, dealing with the complication of pyelitis by catheterization of the ureter through a vesico-vaginal opening.

4222 TRENDELENBURG, Friedrich. 1844–1924
Ueber Blasenscheidenfisteloperationen und über Beckenhochlagerung bei Operationen in der Bauchhöhle. *Samml. klin. Vortr.*, 1890, Nr. 355 (Chir., Nr. 109), 3373–92.

Includes an account of his attempt, 1886, to cure hydronephrosis by a plastic operation – the first recorded surgical intervention for the relief of this condition.

4223 KÜSTER, Ernst Georg Ferdinand von. 1839–1930
Ein Fall von Resektion des Harnleiters. *Zbl. Chir.*, 1892, **19,** Suppl., 110–11.

First successful plastic operation for the relief of hydronephrosis.

4224 EDEBOHLS, George Michael. 1853–1908
Movable kidney; with a report of twelve cases treated by nephrorrhaphy. *Amer. J. med. Sci.*, 1893, **105,** 247–59, 417–32.

In his nephropexy operation Edebohls utilized flaps of the capsule of the kidney. He believed that decapsulation improved the renal blood supply.

4225 FENGER, Christian. 1840–1902
Operation for the relief of valve formation and stricture of the ureter in hydro- or pyo-nephrosis. *J. Amer. med. Ass.*, 1894, **22,** 335–43.

Fenger's operation for stenosis of the uretero-pelvic junction.

4226 KORÁNYI, Sándor, *Baron*. 1866–1944
A vizelet fagypontjának diagnostikus érteke. [The diagnostic value of the freezing point of urine.] *Budapesti k. orvosegy*, 1894–iki évokönyve, 1895, 74–77.

Korányi established cryoscopy of the urine as a kidney function test. See also his later papers in *Z. klin. Med.*, 1897, **33**, 1–54; 1898, **34**, 1–52. Previously H. Dreser had made experiments on this subject; for these see *Arch. exp. Path.*, 1892, **29**, 303–19.

4227 WILMS, Max. 1867–1918
Die Mischgeschwülste. I. Die Mischgeschwülste der Niere. Leipzig, *A. Georgi*, 1899.

Embryoma of the kidney ("Wilms' tumour").

4228 EDEBOHLS, George Michael. 1853–1908
Chronic nephritis affecting a movable kidney as an indication for nephropexy. *Med. News* (*N.Y.*), 1899, **74,** 481–83.

First operation on the kidneys for the relief of Bright's disease.

4229 ——. The cure of chronic Bright's disease by operation. *Med. Rec.* (*N.Y.*), 1901, **60,** 961–70.

Edebohls introduced the operation of renal decortication for the treatment of chronic nephritis.

4230 VOELCKER, FRIEDRICH. 1872– , & JOSEPH, EUGEN. 1879– Funktionelle Nierendiagnostik ohne Ureterenkatheter. *Münch. med. Wschr.*, 1903, **50,** 2081–89.

Voelcker's kidney-function test.

4231 ——, & LICHTENBERG, ALEXANDER VON. 1880–1949 Pyelographie (Roentgenographie des Nierenbeckens nach Kollargolfüllung). *Münch. med. Wschr.*, 1906, **53,** 105–07.

Introduction of pyelography.

4232 ALBARRAN Y DOMINGUEZ, JOAQUIN MARIA. 1860–1912 Exploration des fonctions rénales. Paris, *Masson & Cie.*, 1905.

Albarran's polyuria test for renal inadequacy.

4233 ——. Technique de la néphropexie. *Presse méd.*, 1906, **14,** 253–56.

"Albarran's operation" – nephropexy.

4234 LÖHLEIN, MAX HERMANN FRIEDRICH. 1877–1921 Ueber die entzündlichen Veränderungen der Glomeruli der menschlichen Nieren und ihre Bedeutung für die Nephritis. Leipzig, *S. Hirzel*, 1907.

"Focal nephritis." Löhlein established the importance of the initial inflammatory reaction in the glomerular capillaries in glomerulo-nephritis. Forms Heft 4 of *Arb. path. Inst. Leipzig.*

4235 CARREL, ALEXIS. 1873–1944 Transplantation in mass of the kidneys. *J. exp. Med.*, 1908, **10,** 98–140.

Carrel, Nobel Prize winner in 1912, revolutionized vascular surgery. He succeeded in transplanting the kidney from one animal to another, an operation which was later carried out successfully in man.

4236 ROWNTREE, LEONARD GEORGE. 1883– , & GERAGHTY, JOHN TIMOTHY. 1876–1924 An experimental and clinical study of the functional activity of the kidneys by means of phenolsulphonephthalein. *J. Pharmacol.*, 1910, **1,** 579–661.

The phenolsulphonephthalein kidney-function test.

4237 MUNK, FRITZ. 1879– Klinische Diagnostik der degenerativen Nierenerkrankungen. *Z. klin. Med.*, 1913, **78,** 1–52.

Munk introduced the term "lipoid nephrosis". He found that urine in such cases contained anisotropic lipoid droplets.

4238 VOLHARD, FRANZ. 1872–1950, & FAHR, KARL THEODOR. 1877–1945 Die Bright'sche Nierenkrankheit. Berlin, *J. Springer*, 1914.

First full description of pure nephrosis, relating clinical features to morbid anatomy.

4238.1 HINMAN, FRANK. 1880–1961 Experimental hydronephrosis; repair following ureterocysto-neostomy in white rats with complete ureteral obstruction. *Trans. Sect. Genito-urin. Dis. Amer. med. Ass.*, 1918, **69,** 103–17; *J. Urol.*, 1919, **3,** 147–74.

Commencement of Hinman's classical work on treatment of hydronephrosis.

4239 LEATHES, JOHN BERESFORD. 1864–1956
Renal efficiency tests in nephritis, and the reaction of the urine. *Brit. med. J.*, 1919, **2,** 165–67.
Alkaline tide of urine.

4240 MACLEAN, HUGH. 1879–1957, & DE WESSELOW, OWEN LAMBERT VAUGHAN. 1883–1959
On the testing of renal efficiency, with observations on the "urea coefficient". *Brit. J. exp. Path.*, 1920, **1,** 53–65.
Urea concentration test.

4241 CARELLI, HUMBERTO HORATIO. 1882–1962, & SORDELLI, ALFREDO. 1891–1967
Un nuevo procedimiento para explorar al rinón. *Rev. Asoc. méd. argent.*, 1921, **34,** 424.
Perirenal insufflation of oxygen, for the roentgenological study of the kidney.

4242 GANTER, G.
Ueber die Beseitigung giftiger Stoffe aus dem Blute durch Dialyse. *Münch. med. Wschr.*, 1923, **70,** 1478–80.
First description of the clinical use of peritoneal dialysis in uraemia.

4243 MINAMI, SEIGO.
Ueber Nierenveränderungen nach Verschüttung. *Virchows Arch. path. Anat.*, 1923, **245,** 247–67.
Crush syndrome.

4244 ANDREWES, *Sir* CHRISTOPHER HOWARD. 1896–
An unexplained diazo-colour-reaction in uraemic sera. *Lancet*, 1924, **1,** 590–91.
Diazo-colour test of renal function.

4245 DE WESSELOW, OWEN LAMBERT VAUGHAN. 1883–1959
The excretion of chlorides by the healthy and diseased kidney. *Quart. J. Med.*, 1925, **19,** 53–73.

4245.1 IBUKA, KENJI.
Function of the autogenous kidney transplant. *Amer. J. med. Sci.*, 1926, **171,** 407–20.
Ibuka and Williamson (No. 4245.2) developed the modern operative technique for kidney transplantation.

4245.2 WILLIAMSON, CARL S. 1885–
Further studies on the transplantation of the kidney. *J. Urol. (Baltimore)*, 1926, **16,** 231–53.

4246 MÖLLER, EGGERT HUGO HEIBERG, *et al.*
Studies of urea excretion. *J. clin. Invest.*, 1928–29, **6,** 427–504.
Blood urea clearance test. With J. F. McIntosh and D. D. Van Slyke.

4247 LICHTENBERG, ALEXANDER VON. 1880–1949, & SWICK, M.
Klinische Prüfung des Uroselectans. *Klin. Wschr.*, 1929, **8,** 2089–91.
Introduction of uroselectan.

4248 FANCONI, GUIDO. 1892–
Die nicht diabetischen Glykosurien und Hyperglykämien des älteren Kindes. *Jb. Kinderheilk.*, 1931, **133,** 257–300.
"Fanconi's syndrome", dysfunction of the renal tubules with hypophosphataemia, renal glycosuria and metabolic disturbances.

4249 FISHBERG, ARTHUR MAURICE. 1898–
Hypertension and nephritis. Philadelphia, *Lea & Febiger*, 1931.
Fourth edition, 1939.

4250 MASUGI, MATAZO.
Über das Wesen der spezifischen Veränderungen der Niere und der Leber durch das Nephrotoxin bzw. das Hepatotoxin. *Beitr. path. Anat.*, 1933, **91,** 82–112.
Experimental production of acute glomerulo-nephritis. For Masugi's later work, see the same journal, 1933–34, **92**, 429, and *Klin. Wschr.*, 1935, **14**, 373.

4250.1 FOLEY, FREDERIC EUGENE BASIL. 1891–
A new plastic operation for stricture at the uretero-pelvic junction: report of 20 operations. *J. Urol.*, 1937, **38,** 643–72.
Foley's operation for hydronephrosis.

4251 ALVING, ALF SVEN. 1902– , & MILLER, BENJAMIN FRANK. 1907–
A practical method for the measurement of glomerular filtration rate (inulin clearance) with an evaluation of the clinical significance of this determination. *Arch. intern. Med.*, 1940, **66,** 306–18.
Inulin clearance test.

4252 BYWATERS, ERIC GEORGE LAPTHORNE. 1910– , BEALL, DESMOND.
Crush injuries with impairment of renal function. *Brit. med. J.*, 1941, **1,** 427–32.
Bywaters and Beall encountered cases of the "crush syndrome" among victims of the London air-raids of 1940–41.

4253 KOLFF, WILLEM JOHAN. 1911– , *et al.*
The artificial kidney: dialyser with great area. *Acta med. scand.*, 1944, **117,** 121–34.
The Kolff artificial kidney. With H. T. J. Berk and others. See also No. 1976.

4254 FINE, JACOB. 1900– , *et al.*
The treatment of acute renal failure by peritoneal irrigation. *Ann. Surg.*, 1946, **124,** 857–78.
With H. A. Frank and A. M. Seligman.

4255 WILSON, CLIFFORD. 1906– , & BYROM, FRANK BURNET.
The vicious circle in chronic Bright's disease. Experimental evidence from the hypertensive rat. *Quart. J. Med.*, 1941, **10,** 65–93.

4256 ELLIS, *Sir* ARTHUR WILLIAM MICKLE. 1883–1966
Natural history of Bright's disease. Clinical, histological and experimental observations. *Lancet*, 1942, **1,** 1–7, 34–36, 72–76.
Ellis classification of nephritis.

4257 MERRILL, JOHN PUTNAM. 1917– , *et al.*
Successful homotransplantation of the human kidney between identical twins. *J. Amer. med. Ass.*, 1955, **160,** 277–82.
The patient, both of whose own kidneys had been removed, was alive 11 months after the transplant. With J. E. Murray, J. H. Harrison, and W. R. Guild.

4257.1 KOLFF, Willem Johan. 1911– , & WATSCHINGER, B.
Further developments of a coil kidney. Disposable artificial kidney, *J. Lab. clin. Med.*, 1956, **47**, 969–77.
Disposable twin coil kidney.

4258–4277 PROSTATE

4258 LANGSTAFF, George. 1780–1846
Cases of Fungus haematodes, with observations. *Med.-chir. Trans.*, 1817, **8**, 272–305.
Prostatic carcinoma first reported (p. 279).

4259 STAFFORD, Richard Anthony. 1801–1854
A case of enlargement from melanoid tumour of the prostate gland, in a child of five years of age. *Med.-chir. Trans.*, 1839, **22**, 218–21.
Sarcoma of the prostate was first recorded by Stafford.

4260 ADAMS, John. 1806–1877
The anatomy and diseases of the prostate gland. London, *Longman*, 1851.
Adams was the first to distinguish between hypertrophy and carcinoma of the prostate.

4261 BOTTINI, Enrico. 1837–1903
Di un nuovo cauterizzatore ed incisore termo-galvanico contro le iscurie da ipertrofia prostatica. *Galvani* (*Bologna*), 1874, **2**, 437–52.
Bottini's galvano-cautery for relief of prostatic obstruction.

4262 ——. Ueber radicale Behandlung der auf Hypertrophie der Prostata beruhenden Ischurie. *Verh.* X. *int. med. Congr.*, 1890, Berlin, 1891, **3**, 7 Abt., 90–97.
Bottini's operation for hypertrophy of the prostate.

4263 FULLER, Eugene. 1858–1930
Six successful and successive cases of prostatectomy. *J. cutan. gen.-urin. Dis.*, 1895, **13**, 229–39.
Fuller was first to accomplish the removal of both intra-vesical and intra-urethral enlargements of the prostate by the process of suprapubic enucleation.

4264 FREYER, *Sir* Peter Johnston. 1851–1921
A clinical lecture on total extirpation of the prostate for medical cure of enlargement of the organ. *Brit. med. J.*, 1901, **2**, 125–29.
Freyer claimed priority over Fuller (No. 4263) in originating the recto-vesical method of prostatectomy. Although mistaken in this claim, Freyer certainly popularized the operation. Regarding the controversy, see *Brit. med. J.*, 1907, **1**, 551.

4265 YOUNG, Hugh Hampton. 1870–1945
Conservative perineal prostatectomy. *J. Amer. med. Ass.*, 1903, **41**, 999–1009.
Young's operation of perineal prostatectomy.

4266 WATSON, Francis Sedgwick. 1853–1942
Some anatomical points connected with the performance of prostatectomy. With remarks upon the operative treatment of prostatic hypertrophy. *Ann. Surg.*, 1905, **41**, 507–19.
Watson first performed median perineal prostatectomy in 1889.

4266.1 YOUNG, Hugh Hampton. 1870–1945
Early diagnosis and radical cure of carcinoma of the prostate. Being a study of 40 cases and presentation of a radical operation which was carried out in four cases. *Johns Hopk. Hosp. Bull.*, 1905, **16,** 315–21.
First radical operation for carcinoma of the prostate.

4267 BRIGGS, James Emmons. 1869–1942
A method of controlling the bleeding after suprapubic prostatectomy. *New Engl. med. Gaz.*, 1906, **41,** 391–93.
The distensible bag for controlling haemorrhage after suprapubic prostatectomy was introduced by Briggs in 1905.

4268 BEER, Edwin. 1876–1938
Removal of neoplasms of the urinary bladder. A new method of employing high-frequency (Oudin) current through a catheterizing cystoscope. *J. Amer. med. Ass.*, 1910, **54,** 1768–69.
Beer's method of transurethral fulguration of bladder tumours, from which arose the operation of transurethral prostatectomy.

4269 SQUIER, John Bentley. 1873–1948
Suprapubic intra-urethral enucleation of the prostate. *Boston med. surg. J.*, 1911, **164,** 911–17.
Squier modified the operation of total suprapubic prostatectomy.

4270 YOUNG, Hugh Hampton. 1870–1945
A new procedure (punch operation) for small prostatic bars and contracture of the prostatic orifice. *J. Amer. med. Ass.*, 1913, **60,** 253–57.
Young's punch prostatectomy operation.

4271 CAULK, John Roberts. 1881–
Infiltration anesthesia of the internal vesical orifice for the removal of minor obstructions: presentation of a cautery punch. *J. Urol.* (*Baltimore*), 1920, **4,** 399–408.
Caulk's cautery punch.

4272 GERAGHTY, John Timothy. 1876–1924
A new method of perineal prostatectomy which insures more perfect functional results. *J. Urol.* (*Baltimore*), 1922, **7,** 339–51.
Geraghty's modification of Young's perineal prostatectomy.

4273 STERN, Maximilian. 1877–
Minor surgery of the prostate gland; a new cystoscopic instrument employing a cutting current capable of operation in a water medium. *Int. J. Med. Surg.*, 1926, **39,** 72–77.
Stern's resectoscope.

4274 RANDALL, Alexander. 1885–
Surgical pathology of prostatic obstructions. Baltimore, *Williams & Wilkins*, 1931.

4275 HARRIS, Samuel Henry. 1880–1937
Suprapubic prostatectomy with closure. *Aust. N.Z. J. Surg.*, 1934–1935, **4,** 226–44.
Harris's operation, first described by him on March 26, 1927, and briefly reported in *Med. J. Aust.*, 1927, **1,** 460.

4276 HUGGINS, CHARLES BRENTON. 1901– , & HODGES, CLARENCE VERNARD. 1914–

Studies on prostatic cancer. I. The effect of castration, of estrogen, and of androgen injection on serum phosphatases in metastatic carcinoma of the prostate. *Cancer Res.*, 1941, **1**, 293–97.

Treatment of prostatic cancer with stilboestrol. For his work on hormone-dependent tumours Huggins shared the Nobel Prize with F. Peyton Rous (No. 2637) in 1966.

4277 MILLIN, TERENCE JOHN.

Retropubic prostatectomy. A new extravesical technique. *Lancet*, 1945, **2**, 693–96.

Retropubic prostatectomy.

4278–4296 URINARY CALCULI

4278 MARIANO SANTO DI BARLETTA. 1490–1550

De lapide renum. Venetiis, *per Petrum de Nicolinis da Sabio*, 1535.

Marianus Sanctus Barolitanus popularized the operation of lithotomy introduced by the father of John Vigo of Rapallo. This method passed on to Giovanni di Romani and from him to Marianus. It became known as the "Marian operation" and was the forerunner of the more modern lateral lithotomy.

4279 FRANCO, PIERRE. 1500–1561

Petit traite contenant une des parties principalles de chirurgie, laquelle les chirurgiens hernieres exercent. Lyon, *Antoine Vincent*, 1556.

Clifford Allbutt considered Franco the best lithotomist of the 16th century. His skill in extracting the stone by the perineal route was of a high order; in 1556 he introduced the operation of suprapubic cystotomy in operating for stone, which is recorded in the above.

4280 GROENVELDT, JAN [GREENFIELD, JOHN]. ?1647–1710

A compleat treatise of the stone and gravel. London, *R. Smith*, 1710.

Groenveldt was a famous lithotomist, using the suprapubic technique. He changed his name to Greenfield when he came to England from Holland.

4281 DOUGLAS, JOHN. ?–1759

Lithotomia Douglassiana, or; an account of a new method of making the high operation, in order to extract the stone out of the bladder. London, *T. Woodward*, 1720.

Douglas accused Cheselden of plagiarizing his work, although the latter had acknowledged his indebtedness to Douglas. It is possible that this was the reason which prompted Cheselden to drop the high operation in favour of lateral lithotomy.

4282 CHESELDEN, WILLIAM. 1688–1752

A treatise on the high operation for the stone. London, *J. Osborn*, 1723.

Cheselden was surgeon to St. Thomas's Hospital and an outstanding figure in British surgery in the first half of the 18th century. The above work describes his method of performing suprapubic lithotomy, a method which he abandoned in 1727 for the lateral operation. Biography of Cheselden by Sir Zachary Cope, 1953.

4282.1 COLOT, FRANÇOIS. 1630–1706

Traité de l'opération de la taille. Paris, *J. Vincent*, 1727.

François Colot was the last and best known member of the Colot family, itinerant lithotomists.

4283 LE DRAN, HENRI FRANÇOIS. 1685–1770
Parallèle des différentes manières de tirer la pierre hors de la vessie. Paris, *C. Osmont*, 1730.
Le Dran, famous French lithotomist, improved the operation of lithotomy. He was one of Haller's teachers.

4284 REID, ALEXANDER.
A remarkable case of a person cut for the stone in the new way, commonly called the lateral; by William Cheselden. *Phil. Trans.*, (1746), 1748, **44,** 33–35.
Cheselden's lateral lithotomy first described.

4285 BASEILHAC, JEAN, *Frère Côme*. 1703–1781
Nouvelle méthode d'extraire la pierre de la vessie urinaire. Paris, *D. Houry*, 1779.
Frère Côme devised several new instruments for use in suprapubic lithotomy. This operation, placed in retirement when Cheselden adopted the lateral approach, was once more brought to the fore by Frère Côme.

4286 CAMPER, PIETER. 1722–1789
Observationes circa mutationes quas subeunt calculi in vesica. Pestini, *sumpt. J. M. Weingand*, 1784.

4287 WOLLASTON, WILLIAM HYDE. 1766–1828
On gouty and urinary concretions. *Phil. Trans.*, 1797, **87,** 386–400.
Wollaston showed that, in addition to stones consisting of uric acid, renal calculi might also consist of calcium phosphate, magnesium ammonium phosphate, and calcium oxalate, or a mixture of these.

4288 CARPUE, JOSEPH CONSTANTINE. 1764–1846
A history of the high operation for the stone, by incision above the pubis; with observations on the advantages attending it; and an account of the various methods of lithotomy, from the earliest periods to the present time. London, *Longman*, 1819.
Carpue popularized suprapubic lithotomy, a procedure not often previously carried out.

4289 CIVIALE, JEAN. 1792–1867
Sur la lithotritie. Paris, 1826.
Civiale invented a "lithontriptic" for crushing stones inside the bladder and was responsible for putting the operation of lithotrity upon a sound basis. His claim to have introduced the operation was opposed by Leroy d'Etoilles and other contemporaries.

4290 HEURTELOUP, CHARLES LOUIS STANISLAS. 1793–1864
Lithotripsie. Mémoires sur la lithotripsie par percussion. Paris, *Béchet*, 1833.
Heurteloup designed the best lithotrite of the time. He was one of several claimants to the distinction of having introduced modern lithotrity.

4291 HELLER, JOHANN FLORIAN. 1813–1871
Die Harnconcretionen. Wien, *Tendler u. Comp.*, 1860.
Heller introduced several urine tests and wrote (above) an important work on urinary calculi.

4292 BIGELOW, HENRY JACOB. 1818–1890
Lithotrity by a single operation. *Amer. J. med. Sci.*, 1878, **75,** 117–34.
Introduction of litholapaxy at one sitting.

4292.1 MORRIS, *Sir* HENRY. 1844–1926
A case of nephro-lithotomy; or the extraction of a calculus from an undilated kidney. *Trans. clin. Soc. Lond.*, 1880–81, **14,** 30–44.
Nephrolithotomy; removal of a renal calculus by an incision through the lion.

4293 MACINTYRE, JOHN. 1857–1928
Roentgen rays. Photography of renal calculus. *Lancet*, 1896, **2,** 118.
First radiogram of renal calculus.

4294 ILLYÉS, GÉZA VON. 1870–
Uretercatheterezés és radiographia. *Orvosi hetilap*, 1901, **45,** 659–62.
Géza von Illyés showed that ureteral calculi could be accurately demonstrated by *x* rays with the help of an indwelling opaque catheter. German translation in *Dtsch. Z. Chir.*, 1901, **62**, 132–40.

4295 KELLY, HOWARD ATWOOD. 1858–1943
Scratch-marks on the wax-tipped catheter as a means of determining the presence of stone in the kidney and in the ureter. *Amer. J. Obstet. Dis. Wom.*, 1901, **44,** 441–54.
Kelly tipped the catheter with wax, so that it registered clearly any pressure from sharp stones. This became an important means of diagnosing calculi.

4296 McCARRISON, *Sir* ROBERT. 1878–1960
The experimental production of stone-in-the-bladder. *Indian J. med. Res.*, 1927, **14,** 895–99; 1927–28, **15,** 197–205, 485–88, 801–06.
McCarrison's experiments showed that urinary calculi could follow a diet probably deficient in vitamin A.

History of Urology

4297 DESNOS, ERNEST. 1852–1925
Histoire de l'urologie. In: Pousson, A. & Desnos, E.: *Encyclopédie française d'urologie*, Paris, 1914, **1,** 1–294.

4298 BALLENGER, EDGAR GARRISON. 1877–1945
History of urology. Prepared under the auspices of the American Urological Association. Editorial committee: Edgar G. Ballenger, William A. Frontz, Homer G. Hamer, and Bransford Lewis. 2 vols. Baltimore, *Williams & Wilkins*, 1933.
Every aspect of the subject is covered exhaustively by the various contributors to this collective work; valuable bibliographies are included.

DISEASES OF BONES AND JOINTS; ORTHOPAEDICS

4298.1–4509.1

See also 4730–4771, MYOPATHIES; 6253–6266, PELVIC ANOMALIES.

4298.1 CONNOR [O'CONNOR], BERNARD. 1666–1698
Lettre écrite à Monsieur le Chevalier Guillaume de Waldegrave . . . contenant une dissertation physique sur la continuité de plusieurs os, à l'occasion d'une fabrique surprenante d'un tronc de squelette humain, *etc*. Paris, *Jean Cusson*, 1693.
First description of ankylosing spondylitis. See *J. Hist. Med.*, 1958, **13,** 349–366.

4299 MALPIGHI, MARCELLO. 1628–1694
Opera posthuma. Amstelodami, *G. Gallet*, 1700.
Page 68: first description of leontiasis ossea.

4300 PETIT, JEAN LOUIS. 1674–1750
L'art de guérir les maladies des os. Paris, *L. d'Houry*, 1705.
New edition entitled *Traité des maladies des os*, 2 vols., 1723; English translation of latter, 1726. Petit was the first director of the Académie de Chirurgie, Paris, and the most eminent French surgeon of his day. He is particularly remembered for his work on bone diseases. He invented the screw tourniquet, gave the first account of osteomalacia, and was first to open the mastoid process.

4301 ANDRÉ, NICOLAS [ANDRY]. 1658–1742
L'orthopédie ou l'art de prévenir et de corriger dans les enfans, les difformités du corps. 3 vols. Paris, *la veuve Alix*, 1741.
The first book on orthopaedics, which term André himself introduced. He advised attention to proper posture in the prevention and correction of spinal curvature; he had a practical knowledge of body mechanics. This is also the first book on diseases of children to include mention of chlorosis. English translation, 1743, reproduced in facsimile, Philadelphia, 1961.

4302 PLATNER, JOHANN ZACHARIAS. 1694–1747
De iis, qui ex tuberculis gibberosi fiunt. Lipsiae, *ex off. Langenhemiana*, 1744.
Platner affirmed the tuberculous nature of humpback, which had earlier been surmised by Hippocrates and confirmed by Galen.

4302.1 MORAND, SAUVEUR-FRANÇOIS. 1697–1773
Sur un enfant auquel il manquoit les deux clavicules, le sternum et les cartilages, qui dans l'état naturel l'attachent aux côtes. *Hist. Acad. roy. Sci. (Paris)*, (1760), 1766, 47–48.
First description of cleido-cranial dysostosis.

4303 DAVID, JEAN PIERRE. 1737–1784
Dissertation sur les effets du mouvement et du repos dans les maladies chirurgicales. Paris, *Vve. Vallet-La-Chapelle*, 1779.
Includes a description of Pott's disease, with post-mortem findings, better than Pott's own account. This is an important early work on the effect of movement and of rest in the treatment of joint conditions. English translation, 1790.

4304 POTT, PERCIVALL. 1714–1788
Remarks on that kind of palsy of the lower limbs, which is frequently found to accompany a curvature of the spine. London, *J. Johnson*, 1779.
"Pott's disease." Percival Pott, surgeon to St. Bartholomew's Hospital for more than 40 years, left a classical description of spinal curvature due to tuberculous caries and causing paralysis of the lower limbs. He did not, however, recognize its tuberculous nature. Pott published a further book on the subject in 1782. Reprinted in *Med. Classics*, 1936, **1**, 281–328.

4304.1 EKMAN, OLAUS JACOB.
Dissertatio medica descriptionem et casus aliquot osteomalaciae sistens. Upsaliae, *J. Edman*, [1788].
In his doctorial thesis Ekman gave an account of osteogenesis imperfecta in three generations. For extensive translation see Seedorff, K. S., *Osteogenesis imperfecta*, Copenhagen, 1949 (No. 4404.1).

4305 VENEL, JEAN ANDRÉ. 1740–1791
Description de plusieurs nouveaux moyens mécaniques propres à prevénir, borner et même corriger dans certains cas les courbures latérales et la torsion de l'épine du dos. Lausanne, 1788.

Venel stressed the necessity for prolonged periods of recumbency, rather than exercise, in the correction of spinal curvature. He invented several orthopaedic appliances; in 1790 he founded at Orbe, Switzerland, the first orthopaedic hospital.

4306 SOEMMERING, SAMUEL THOMAS. 1755–1830
Abbildungen und Beschreibungen einiger Misgeburten. Mainz, *Universitätsbuchhandlung*, 1791.

Achondroplasia is first described on page 30 and pictured on plate 11.

4307 RUSSELL, JAMES. 1755–1836
A practical essay on a certain disease of the bones termed necrosis. Edinburgh, *Bell & Bradfute*, 1794.

One of the first attempts at a complete and detailed description. Russell was the first professor of clinical surgery at Edinburgh.

4308 SCARPA, ANTONIO. 1747–1832
Memoria chirurgica sui piedi torti congenita dei fanciulli, Pavia, *G. Comini*, 1803.

First accurate description of the pathological anatomy of congenital club-foot. English translation, Edinburgh, 1818.

4309 BAYNTON, THOMAS. 1761–1820
An account of a successful method of treating diseases of the spine. London, *Longman*, 1813.

By his advocacy of absolute rest in the horizontal position without the aid of caustics and setons, Baynton can be said to have introduced the modern treatment of spinal caries in England. The book is dedicated to Edward Jenner.

4310 ROMBERG, MORITZ HEINRICH. 1795–1873
De rachitide congenita. Berolini, *typ. C. A. Plateni*, 1817.

Classical description of achondroplasia. Romberg's graduation thesis. English translation (Sydenham Society), 1853.

4311 BRODIE, *Sir* BENJAMIN COLLINS, *Bart.* 1783–1862
Pathological and surgical observations on the diseases of the joints. London, *Longman*, 1818.

Brodie's best work. It includes his description of hysterical pseudo-fracture of the spine. The fifth edition, 1850, gives (p. 77) a description of "Brodie's disease" – chronic synovitis with a pulpy degeneration of the affected parts.

4312 DELPECH, JACQUES MATHIEU. 1777–1832
Considérations sur la difformité appelée pied-bots. In his *Chirurgie clinique de Montpellier*, Paris, 1823, **1**, 147–231.

Delpech described (pp. 184–92) the beneficial effect of section of the tendo Achillis for club-foot; he performed the operation on May 9, 1816, and although not first to do so, he was the first to demonstrate the value of tenotomy in the correction of contracture deformities of the extremities.

4313 SMITH, NATHAN. 1762–1829
Observations on the pathology and treatment of necrosis. *Philad. month. J. Med.*, 1827, **1**, 11–19, 66–75.

Classical early account of osteomyelitis. Smith trephined for bone necrosis. Reproduced in *Med. classics*, 1937, **1**, 820–38.

4314 BRODIE, *Sir* BENJAMIN COLLINS, *Bart.* 1783–1862
On trephining the tibia. *Lond. med. Gaz.*, 1828, **2**, 70–74.

"Brodie's abscess." The patient was first seen in 1824. Brodie published an account of some further cases in *Med.-chir. Trans.*, 1832, **17**, 239–49, which paper is reprinted in *Med. Classics*, 1938, **2**, 900–06.

4315 DELPECH, JACQUES MATHIEU. 1777–1832
De l'orthomorphie. 2 vols. and atlas. Paris, *Gabon*, 1828.

Delpech, professor of surgery at Montpellier, published a comprehensive treatise on deformities of the bones and joints. He established the tuberculous nature of Pott's disease. Delpech did more than any other man towards the development of orthopaedics in France.

4316 RANDOLPH, JACOB. 1796–1848
Some remarks on morbus coxarius, with an account of Dr. P. S. Physick's method of treating this disease. *Amer. J. med. Sci.*, 1830, **7**, 299–308.

4317 DUPUYTREN, GUILLAUME, *le baron.* 1777–1835
De la rétraction des doigts par suite d'une affection de l'aponévrose palmaire, opération chirurgicale qui convient dans ce cas. *J. univ. hebd. Méd. Chir. prat.*, 1831, 2 sér., **5**, 352–65.

Dupuytren devised an operation for the treatment of retraction of the fingers from affection of the palmar aponeurosis ("Dupuytren's contracture"). Reprinted, with translation, in *Med. Classics*, 1939, **4**, 127–50. The condition was first mentioned by Platter in his *Observationum* (No. 3789), liber 1, 140.

4318 LOBSTEIN, JEAN GEORGES CHRÉTIEN FRÉDÉRIC MARTIN. 1777–1835
De la fragilité des os, ou de l'ostéopsathyrose. In his *Traité de l'anatomie pathologique*, Paris, 1833, **2**, 204–12.

Osteopsathyrosis ("Lobstein's disease"), osteogenesis imperfecta, earlier described by Ekman (No. 4304.1).

4319 RUST, JOHANN NEPOMUK. 1775–1840
Aufsätze und Abhandlungen aus dem Gebiete der Medizin, Chirurgie und Staatsarzneikunde. Berlin, *T. C. F. Enslin*, 1834, **1**, 196.

First description of "Rust's disease" – tuberculous spondylitis of the cervical vertebrae.

4320 STROMEYER, GEORG FRIEDRICH LUDWIG. 1804–1876
Die Durchschneidung der Achillessehne, als Heilmethode des Klumpfusses, durch zwei Fälle erläutert. *Mag. ges. Heilk.*, 1833, **39**, 195–218.

Successful tenotomy for club-foot established the reputation of Stromeyer as an orthopaedic surgeon.

4321 ——. Beiträge zur operativen Orthopädik. Hannover, *Helwing*, 1838.

Stromeyer is the founder of modern surgery of the locomotor system. He advocated and practised subcutaneous tenotomy for all deformities of the body arising from muscular defects.

4322 DUPUYTREN, GUILLAUME, *le baron.* 1777–1835
Leçons orales de clinique chirurgicale. 2me. éd. Tom. 3. Paris, *Germer-Baillière*, 1839.

Pp. 455–61: Dupuytren was the first to treat wry neck by subcutaneous section of the sternomastoid muscle. This he did on Jan. 16, 1822. The operation was first reported in C. Averill: *Short treatise on operative surgery*, London, 1823, 61–64.

4323 DIEFFENBACH. JOHANN FRIEDRICH. 1792–1847
Ueber die Durchschneidung der Sehnen und Muskeln. Berlin, *A. Förster*, 1841.
Report on 140 cases of tenotomy for treatment of club-foot.

4323.1 FERGUSSON, *Sir* WILLIAM. 1808 1877
Excision of a portion of the scapula. *Lancet*, 1842–43, **1,** 917–18.
First description of operation for partial excision of scapula.

4324 BUCK, GURDON. 1807–1877
The knee-joint anchylosed at a right angle – restored nearly to a straight position after the excision of a wedge-shaped portion of bone, consisting of the patella, condyles and articular surface of the tibia. *Amer. J. Med. Sci.*, 1845, n.s. **10,** 277–84.
Buck's operation. The paper is reprinted in *Med. Classics*, 1939, **3**, 791–99.

4325 DURLACHER, LEWIS. 1792–1864
A treatise on corns, bunions, the diseases of nails, and the general management of the feet. London, *Simpkin, Marshall, & Co.*, 1845.
Durlacher, surgeon chiropodist to Queen Victoria, gave the first description of anterior metatarsalgia (p. 52), to which the name "Morton's metatarsalgia" has been given (see No. 4341).

4325.1 DALRYMPLE, JOHN. 1804–1852
On the microscopical character of mollities ossium. *Dublin Quart. J. med. Sci.*, 1846, **2,** 85–95.
Report of the histological examination of bone material from the patient described by Macintyre (No. 4327).

4326 JONES, HENRY BENCE. 1814–1873
On a new substance occurring in the urine of a patient with mollities ossium. *Phil. Trans.*, 1848, **138,** 55–62.
Bence Jones described the myelopathic albumosuria (Bence Jones proteinuria) seen in Macintyre's patient (No. 4327). Preliminary notes in *Lancet*, 1847, **2**, 88 and *Proc. roy. Soc. Lond.*, 1847, **5**, 673.

4326.1 LANGENBECK, BERNHARD RUDOLPH CONRAD VON. 1810–1887
Grosses Enchondrom (Gallertknorpel-Geschwulst) des Schulterblattes; Exstirpation des ganzen Schulterblattes mit Ausnahme des *Processus coracoides* am 6 Febr.; Tod am 7 Febr. *Dtsch. Klinik*, 1850, **2,** 73–76.
Complete excision of the scapula.

4327 MACINTYRE, WILLIAM.
Case of mollities and fragilitas ossium. *Med.-chir. Trans.*, 1850, **33,** 211–32.
Multiple myeloma first described.

4328 MATHIJSEN, ANTHONIUS. 1805–1878
Nieuwe wijze van aanwending van het gips-verband by beenbreuken. Eene bijdrage tot de militaire chirurgie. Haarlem, *van Loghem*, 1852.
Introduction of the modern plaster-of-Paris bandage. Mathijsen published a French account, Liège, 1854. Facsimiles of both editions were published, with an introduction by G. J. Bremer, in 1962.

4329 LITTLE, William John. 1810–1894
On the nature and treatment of the deformities of the human frame. London, *Longman*, 1853.

Little was the first eminent orthopaedic surgeon in the British Isles. He studied under Stromeyer and, in 1838, he founded the (Royal) Orthopaedic Hospital, London. The above work is an elaboration of lectures delivered in 1843.

4330 BREITHAUPT.
Zur Pathologie des menschlichen Fusses. *Med. Zeitung*, 1855, **24,** 169, 175.

First description of osteoperiostitis of the metatarsal bones, named "Busquet's disease" after the latter's description of it in *Rev. Chir.* (*Paris*), 1897, **17** 1065.

4331 SAYRE, Lewis Albert. 1820–1900
Exsection of the head of the femur and removal of the upper rim of the acetabulum, for morbus coxarius, with perfect recovery. *N.Y. J. med.*, 1855, n.s. **14,** 70–82.

Resection of the hip for ankylosis.

4332 EULENBURG, Moritz Michael. 1811–1877
Hochgradige Dislocation der Scapula. *Arch. klin. Chir.*, 1863, **4,** 304–11.

First description of congenital high-scapula ("Sprengel's deformity"; see also No. 4359).

4333 HENKE, Philipp Jakob Wilhelm. 1834–1896
Contractur des Metatarsus. *Z. rat. Med.*, 1863, 3 R., **17,** 188–94.

Congenital metatarsus varus described.

4334 BAUER, Louis. 1814–1898
Lectures on orthopaedic surgery. Philadelphia, *Lindsay & Blakiston*, 1864.

Before emigrating to America, Bauer studied under Stromeyer. Hugh Owen Thomas considered him "the first exponent of American orthopaedics".

4335 ENGEL, Gerhard.
Ueber einen Fall von cystoider Entartung des ganzen Skelettes. Giessen, *F. C. Pietsch*, 1864.

First description of osteitis fibrosa cystica.

4336 PRICE, Peter Charles. 1832–1864
A description of the diseased conditions of the knee-joint which require amputation of the limb, and those conditions which are favourable to excision of the joint. London, *J. Churchill*, 1865.

A valuable contribution to the knowledge and surgical treatment of diseases of the knee-joint.

4337 CHARCOT, Jean Martin. 1825–1893
Sur quelques arthropathies qui paraissent dépendre d'une lésion du cerveau ou de la moëlle épinière. *Arch. Physiol. norm. path.*, 1868, **1,** 161–78.

Charcot called attention to tabetic arthropathy, a condition which has since borne his name, while the tabetic joints he so well described are now known as "Charcot's joints".

4338 WILKS, *Sir* SAMUEL, *Bart.* 1824–1911
Case of osteoporosis, or spongy hypertrophy of the bones (calvaria, clavicle, os femoris, and rib). *Trans. path. Soc. Lond.*, 1868–69, **20,** 273–77.

A classical account of osteitis deformans. Wilks was associated with Guy's Hospital all his life. A kindly, charming man, he was described by Osler as one of the handsomest men in London in his time, even until the age of 70.

4339 WEGNER, FRIEDRICH RUDOLPH GEORG. 1843–1917
Ueber hereditäre Knochensyphilis bei jungen Kindern. *Virchows Arch. path. Anat.*, 1870, **50,** 305–22.

"Wegner's disease" – osteochondritic separation of the epiphyses in congenital syphilis.

4339.1 HOOD, WHARTON PETER. 1833–1916
On bone setting (so-called), and its relation to the treatment of joints crippled by injury, rheumatism, inflammation, etc. London, *Macmillan & Co.*, 1871.

First work on manipulation written by a physician.

4340 THOMAS, HUGH OWEN. 1834–1891
Diseases of the hip, knee and ankle joints, with their deformities, treated by a new and efficient method. Liverpool, *T. Dobb & Co.*, 1875.

Thomas splint.

4341 MORTON, THOMAS GEORGE. 1835–1903
A peculiar and painful affection of the fourth metatarso-phalangeal articulation. *Amer. J. med. Sci.*, Philadelphia, 1876, **71,** 37–45.

First complete description of anterior metatarsalgia ("Morton's disease"). See also No. 4325.

4342 BAKER, WILLIAM MORRANT. 1839–1896
On the formation of synovial cysts in the leg in connection with disease of the knee joint. *St. Barth. Hosp. Rep.*, 1877, **13,** 245–61; 1885, **21,** 177–90.

"Baker's cysts" of the knee-joint. Reprinted in *Med. Classics,* 1941, **5**, 785–820.

4343 PAGET, *Sir* JAMES, *Bart.* 1814–1899
On a form of chronic inflammation of bones (osteitis deformans). *Med.-chir. Trans.*, 1877, **60,** 37–64; 1882, **65,** 225–36.

Paget was at one time Serjeant Surgeon to Queen Victoria. His classical description of osteitis deformans led that condition to be called "Paget's disease". Reprinted in *Med. Classics*, 1936, **1**, 29–71.

4344 SAYRE, LEWIS ALBERT. 1820–1900
Treatment of fractured ribs by extension and expansion of the thorax, and retention by plaster-of-paris bandage. *Trans. Amer. med. Ass.*, 1877, **28,** 541–49.

Sayre was the first to use plaster-of-Paris as a support for the spinal column in scoliosis and Pott's disease.

4345 MADELUNG, OTTO WILHELM. 1846–1926
Die spontane Subluxation der Hand nach vorne. *Verh. dtsch. Ges. Chir.*, 1878, **7,** pt. 2, 259–76.

"Madelung's deformity."

4346 GROSS, Samuel Weissel. 1837–1889
Sarcoma of the long bones; based upon a study of one hundred and sixty-five cases. *Amer. J. med. Sci.*, 1879, n.s. **78,** 17–57, 338–77.
First comprehensive work on bone sarcoma.

4346.1 HELFERICH, Heinrich. 1851–1945
Ein Fall von sogenannter Myositis ossificans progressiver. *Aerztl. Intelligenz-Bl.*, 1879, **26,** 485–89.
Helferich described the association of microdactyly with myositis ossificans progressiva.

4347 ALBERT, Eduard. 1841–1900
Einige Fälle von kunstlicher Ankylosenbildung an paralytischen Gliedmassen. *Wien. med. Presse*, 1882, **23,** 725–28.
Surgical induction of arthrodesis.

4348 THOMAS, Hugh Owen. 1834–1891
Contributions to surgery and medicine. 8 pts. London, *H. K. Lewis*, 1883–90.
Thomas was the veritable founder of modern orthopaedics in the British Isles. The conservative methods introduced by him were developed by Sir Robert Jones. Thomas is remembered eponymically by the "Thomas splint".

4349 STRÜMPELL, Ernst Adolph Gustav Gottfried. 1853–1925
Lehrbuch der speciellen Pathologie und Therapie der innern Krankheiten. Bd. 2, ii. Leipzig, *F. C. W. Vogel*, 1884.
Strümpell gave an excellent description of ankylosing spondylitis ("Strümpell's disease", the "spondylose rhizomélique" of Pierre Marie, No. 4368) on p. 152 of his *Lehrbuch.* He published an important paper on the subject in *Dtsch. Z. Nervenheilk.*, 1897, **11**, 338–42.

4350 KÖNIG, Franz. 1832–1910
Ueber freie Körper in den Gelenken. *Dtsch. Z. Chir.*, 1888, **27,** 90–109.
König of Göttingen was the first to use the term "osteochondritis dissecans".

4351 KAHLER, Otto. 1849–1893
Zur Symptomatologie des multiplen Myeloms. *Prag. med. Wschr.*, 1889, **14,** 33–35, 44–49.
"Kahler's disease" – multiple myelomata.

4352 OLLIER, Louis Xavier Edouard Leopold. 1830–1900
Exostoses multiples. *Mém. C. R. Soc. Sci. méd. Lyon*, (1889), 1890, **29,** 2, 12.
"Ollier's disease." He described a form of dyschondroplasia.

4353 BRADFORD, Edward Hickling. 1848–1926, & LOVETT, Robert Williamson. 1859–1924
Treatise on orthopedic surgery. New York, *W. Wood & Co.*, 1890.
Includes a description of the "Bradford frame".

4354 MARIE, Pierre. 1853–1940
De l'ostéo-arthropathie hypertrophiante pneumonique. *Rev. Méd.*, 1890, **10,** 1–36.
Original description of hypertrophic osteoarthropathy, sometimes called "Bamberger–Marie disease".

4355 HOFFA, ALBERT. 1859–1908
Zur operativen Behandlung der angeborenen Hüftgelenksverrenkungen. *Verh. dtsch. Ges. Chir.*, 1890, **19,** 44–53.
Hoffa's method of operative treatment of congenital dislocation of the hip-joint.

4356 ——. Lehrbuch der orthopädischen Chirurgie. Stuttgart, *F. Enke*, 1891.
Hoffa, a leading German orthopaedist, made important contributions to the subject and founded the *Zeitschrift für orthopädische Chirurgie.*

4357 KÜMMELL, HERMANN. 1852–1937
Traumatische rarefizierende Ostitis. *Verh. Ges. Dtsch. Naturf. Aerzte*, (1891), 1892, 282–85.
"Kümmell's disease." He described a form of traumatic spondylitis.

4358 RECKLINGHAUSEN, FRIEDRICH DANIEL VON. 1833–1910
Die fibröse oder deformirende Ostitis, die Osteomalacie und die osteoplastische Carcinose in ihren gegenseitigen Beziehungen. In: *Festschrift R. Virchow*, Berlin, *G. Reimer*, 1891.
Recklinghausen gave an important description of generalized osteitis fibrosa. His reference to the earlier case reported by Engel (see No. 4335) has led to this condition being sometimes referred to as "Engel–Recklinghausen disease".

4359 SPRENGEL, OTTO GERHARD KARL. 1852–1915
Die angeborene Verschiebung des Schulterblattes nach oben. *Arch. klin. Chir.*, 1891, **42,** 545–49.
Classical description of "Sprengel's deformity", a congenital upward displacement of the scapula (see also No. 4332).

4360 BECHTEREV, VLADIMIR MICHAILOVICH [BEKHTEREV]. 1857–1927
Oderevenĭelost pozvonochnika s iskrivleniyem yevo, kak osobaya forma zabolĭevaniya. [Ankylosis of the spine with curvature as a special form of disease.] *Vrach*, 1892, **13,** 899–903.
Bechterev's disease – ankylosing spondylitis, previously described by Strümpell. A German translation of the paper is in *Neurol. Zbl.*, 1893, **12,** 426–34.

4361 KAUFMANN, EDUARD. 1860–1931
Untersuchungen über die sogennante foetale Rachitis (Chondrodystrophia foetalis). Berlin, *Reimer*, 1892.
First study of the cartilage changes in achondroplasia.

4362 KLIPPEL, MAURICE. 1858–1942
De la pseudo-paralysie générale arthritique. *Rev. Méd.*, 1892, **12,** 280–85.
First description of "Klippel's disease", arthritic general pseudo-paralysis.

4363 PARRISH, B. F.
A new operation for paralytic talipes valgus, and the enunciation of a new surgical principle. *N.Y. med. J.*, 1892, **56,** 402–03.
First successful tendon transplantation.

4364 ALBERT, EDUARD. 1841–1900
Achillodynie. *Wien. med. Presse*, 1893, **34,** 41–43.
Achillobursitis, "Albert's disease".

4365 LORENZ, ADOLF. 1854–1946
The operative treatment of congenital dislocation of the hip-joint. *Trans. Amer. orthop. Ass.*, (1894), 1895, **7,** 99–103.
Lorenz suggested a bloodless method for closed reduction of congenital dislocation of the hip-joint – the "Hoffa–Lorenz" method.

4365.1 MARFAN, BERNARD JEAN ANTONIN. 1858–1942
Un cas de déformation congénitale des quatre membres, plus prononcée aux extrémités, charactérisée par l'allongement des os avec un certain degré d'amincissement. *Bull. Mém. Soc. méd. Hôp. Paris*, 1896, 3 sér., **13,** 220–26.
"Marfan syndrome." Marfan described only the skeletal deformities. He called the condition *dolichostenomelia.* Later writers recorded bilateral ectopia lentis and cardiovascular complications in this syndrome.

4366 TUBBY, ALFRED HERBERT. 1862–1930
Deformities; a treatise on orthopaedic surgery. London, *Macmillan & Co.*, 1896.
Includes a valuable discussion of congenital anomalies of the bones and joints from the orthopaedic point of view.

4367 BRUCK, ALFRED. 1865–
Ueber eine seltene Form von Erkrankung der Knochen und Gelenke. *Dtsch. med. Wschr.*, 1897, **23,** 152–55.
"Bruck's disease" – deformity of bones, multiple fractures, ankylosis of joints, and muscular atrophy.

4368 MARIE, PIERRE. 1853–1940
Sur la spondylose rhizomélique. *Rev. Méd.*, 1898, **18,** 285–315.
Marie described as "spondylose rhizomélique" the spondylitis deformans originally reported by Strümpell and called variously "Strümpell's disease", "Bechterev's disease", "Marie's disease".

4369 ——, & SAINTON, PAUL. 1868–1958
Sur la dysostose cléido-crânienne héréditaire. *Rev. neurol. (Paris)*, 1898, **6,** 835–38.
In their important description of cleido-cranial dysostosis Marie and Sainton gave to it its present name. It was first described by Morand (No. 4302.1) in 1760.

4370 KIENBÖCK, ROBERT. 1871–1953
Ueber acute Knochenatrophie bei Entzündungsprocessen an den Extremitäten (fälschlich sogenannte Inactivitätsatrophie der Knochen) und ihre Diagnose nach dem Röntgen-Bilde. *Wien. med. Wschr.*, 1901, **51,** 1346–48.
"Kienböck's atrophy" – acute atrophy of bone in inflammatory conditions of the extremities.

4371 MOSETIG-MOORHOF, ALBERT VON. 1838–1907
Die Jodoformknochenplombe. *Zbl. Chir.*, 1903, **30,** 433–38.
Use of iodoform to plug bone defects.

4372 ALBERS-SCHÖNBERG, HEINRICH ERNST. 1865–1921
Projektions-Röntgenbilder einer seltenen Knochenerkrankung. *Fortschr. Röntgenstr.*, 1903–04, **7,** 158–59.
First description of osteosclerosis fragilis, marble bones ("Albers–Schönberg disease").

4373 OSGOOD, Robert Bayley. 1873–1956
Lesions of the tibial tubercle occurring during adolescence. *Boston med. surg. J.*, 1903, **148,** 114–17.
Osgood was the first to draw attention to a condition of the tibial tuberosity; this is now referred to as "Osgood–Schlatter disease" (see also No. 4374).

4374 SCHLATTER, Carl. 1864–1934
Verletzungen des schnabelförmigen Fortsatzes der oberen Tibiaepiphyse. *Beitr. klin. Chir.*, 1903, **38,** 874–87.
"Osgood–Schlatter disease." A further description of the painful affection of the tibial tuberosity first noted by Osgood.

4375 NAU, Pierre.
Les scolioses congénitales. Paris, *Thèse No.* 446, 1904.
First description of platyspondylia.

4376 BÜDINGER, Konrad. 1867–
Ueber Ablösung von Gelenkteilen und verwandte Prozesse. *Dtsch. Z. Chir.*, 1906, **84,** 311–65.
Büdinger was first to describe pathological fracture of the cartilage of the patella. See also his later paper in the same journal, 1908, **92**, 510–36. Later descriptions by Karl Ludloff, *Verh. dtsch. Ges. Chir.*, 1910, 223–25, and by Arthur Laewen, *Beitr. klin. Chir.*, 1925, **134**, 265–307, led to the eponym "Büdinger-Ludloff–Laewen disease".

4376.1 LOOSER, Emile.
Ueber Osteogenesis imperfecta tarda. *Verh. Dtsch. path. Ges.* (1905), 1906, 239–42.
Looser's syndrome.

4377 KÖHLER, Alban. 1874–1947
Ueber eine häufige, bisher anscheinend unbekannte Erkrankung einzelner kindlicher Knochen. *Münch. med. Wschr.*, 1908, **55,** 1923–1925.
"Köhler's disease" of the scaphoid bone of the foot in children.

4378 KIRSCHNER, Martin. 1879–1942
Ueber Nagelextension. *Beitr. klin. Chir.*, 1909, **64,** 266–79.
Kirschner wire, for skeletal traction.

4379 KIENBÖCK, Robert. 1871–1953
Über Luxationen im Bereiche der Handwurzel. *Fortschr. Röntgenstr.*, 1910–11, **16,** 103–15.
First description of a slowly progressive chronic osteitis involving the semilunar bone ("Kienböck's disease").

4380 LEGG, Arthur Thornton. 1874–1939
An obscure affection of the hip-joint. *Boston med. surg. J.*, 1910, **162,** 202–04.
First description of juvenile osteochondritis deformans ("Calvé–Legg–Perthes disease"; see also the two following entries).

4381 CALVÉ, Jacques. 1875–1954
Sur une forme particulière de pseudo-coxalgie greffée sur des déformations caractéristiques de l'extremité supérieure du fémur. *Rev. Chir. (Paris)*, 1910, **42,** 54–84.

4382 PERTHES, GEORG CLEMENS. 1869–1927
Ueber Arthritis deformans juvenilis. *Dtsch. Z. Chir.*, 1910, **107,** 111–59.

4383 GOLDTHWAIT, JOEL ERNEST. 1866–
The lumbo-sacral articulation. An explanation of many cases of "lumbago", "sciatica" and paraplegia. *Boston med. surg. J.*, 1911, **164,** 365–72.

Goldthwait suggested that lumbago and sciatica might be due to intervertebral disk injury.

4384 MIDDLETON, GEORGE STEVENSON. 1853–1928, & TEACHER, JOHN HAMMOND. 1869–1930
Injury of the spinal cord due to rupture of an intervertebral disc during muscular effort. *Glasg. med. J.*, 1911, **76,** 1–6.

Report of a case of "sciatica" due to rupture of an intervertebral disk.

4385 CROUZON, OCTAVE. 1874–1938
Dysostose cranio-faciale héréditaire. *Bull. Soc. méd. Hôp. Paris,* 1912, 3 sér., **33,** 545–55.

First description of cranio-facial dysostosis, hypertelorism.

4386 KLIPPEL, MAURICE. 1858–1942, & FEIL, ANDRÉ. 1884–
Un cas d'absence des vertèbres cervicales avec cage thoracique remontant jusqu'à la base du crane (cage thoracique cervicale). *Nouv. Iconogr. Salpêtr.*, 1912, **25,** 223–50.

"Klippel–Feil syndrome" – absence or incomplete development of cervical vertebrae.

4386.1 ALBERS-SCHÖNBERG, HEINRICH ERNST. 1869–1921
Eine seltene, bisher nicht bekannte Strukturanomalie des Skelettes. *Fortschr. Röntgenstr.*, 1915, **23,** 174–75.

First definitive description of osteopoikilosis.

4387 KÖHLER, ALBAN. 1874–1947
Eine typische Erkrankung des 2. Metatarsophalangealgelenkes. *Münch. med. Wschr.*, 1920, **67,** 1289–90.

"Köhler's disease" – juvenile deforming metatarsophalangeal osteochondritis. English translation in *Amer. J. Roentgenol.*, 1923, **10,** 705–10.

4388 EWING, JAMES. 1866–1943
Diffuse endothelioma of bone. *Proc. N.Y. path. Soc.*, 1921, n.s., **21,** 17–24.

Ewing described a form of bone sarcoma ("Ewing's sarcoma"), usually involving the shaft of long bones.

4388.1 LÉRI, ANDRÉ. 1875–1930
Une maladie congénitale et héréditaire de l'ossification: la pléonostéose familiale. *Bull. Mém. Soc. méd. Hôp. Paris,* 1921, 3 sér., **45,** 1228–30.

"Léri's pleonosteosis" first described.

4389 SCHEUERMANN, HOLGER WERFEL. 1877–
Kyphosis dorsalis juvenilis. *Z. orthop. Chir.*, 1921, **41,** 305–17.

"Scheuermann's disease" – necrosis of the epiphyses of the vertebrae, causing kyphosis.

4390 APERT, Eugène. 1868–1940, *et al.*
Nouvelle observation d'acrocéphalosyndactylie. *Bull. Soc. méd. Hôp. Paris*, 1923, 3 sér., **47**, 1672–75.
"Apert's syndrome." With Tixier, Huc, and Kermorgant.

4391 JONES, *Sir* Robert. 1858–1933, & LOVETT, Robert Williamson. 1859–1924
Orthopaedic surgery. London, *H. Frowde*, 1923.
Jones was a pupil of Hugh Owen Thomas and a pioneer of active surgical intervention in orthopaedics. He advocated tendon transplantation, bone grafting, and other conservative and restorative procedures. He did much valuable work during the war of 1914–18, and he is one of the greatest figures in British orthopaedics.

4392 GREIG, David Middleton. 1864–1936
Hypertelorism. A hitherto undifferentiated congenital cranio-facial deformity. *Edinb. med. J.*, 1924, **31**, 560–93.
First description of hypertelorism as a separate entity.

4393 CODMAN, Ernest Amory. 1869–1940
Bone sarcoma, an interpretation of the nomenclature used by the Committee on the Registry of Bone Sarcoma of the American College of Surgeons. New York, *P. B. Hoeber*, 1925.

4394 KOLODNY, Anatole. 1892–
Bone sarcoma. *Surg. Gynec. Obstet.*, 1927, **44**, Suppl., 1–214.

4395 JANSEN, Murk. 1863–1935
Dissociation of bone growth. (Exostoses and enchondromata, or Ollier's dyschondroplasia and associated phenomena.) In *The Robert Jones Birthday Volume*, London, *Oxford Univ. Press*, 1928, 43–72.
Jansen's theory of dissociation of bone growth.

4395.1 ENGELMANN, Guido. 1876–
Ein Fall von Osteopathia hyperostotica (sclerotisans) multiplex infantilis. *Fortschr. Röntgenstr.*, 1929, **39**, 1101–06.
"Engelmann's disease", a rare bone dystrophy causing osteosclerosis.

4396 MAXWELL, John Preston. 1871–1961
Further studies in osteomalacia. *Proc. roy. Soc. Med.*, 1929–30, **23**, 639–52.
Maxwell showed osteomalacia to be due to lack of vitamin D.

4397 MORQUIO, Luis. 1867–1935
Sur une forme de dystrophie osseuse familiale. *Arch. Méd. Enf.*, 1929, **32**, 129–40; *Bull. Soc. Pédiat. Paris*, 1929, **27**, 145–52.
"Morquio's disease", eccentro-osteochondrodysplasia.

4397.1 BRAILSFORD, James Frederick. 1888–1961
Chondro-osteo-dystrophy. Roentgenographic and clinical features of a child with dislocation of vertebrae. *Amer. J. Surg.*, 1929, **7**, 404–10.
Morquio–Brailsford disease (see No. 4397).

4398 MILKMAN, Louis Arthur. 1895–1951
Pseudofractures (hunger osteopathy, late rickets, osteomalacia): report of a case. *Amer. J. Roentgenol.*, 1930, **24**, 29–37.
"Milkman's syndrome."

4399 BAER, William Stevenson. 1872–1931
The treatment of chronic osteomyelitis with the maggot (larva of the blow fly). *J. Bone Jt Surg.*, 1931, **13,** 438–75.
Larrey observed the therapeutic effect of maggots on wounds; W. S. Baer inaugurated the method of treating osteomyelitis by this means ("Baer therapy").

4400 GESCHICKTER, Charles Freeborn. 1901– , & COPELAND, Murray Marcus. 1902–
Tumors of bone. New York, *Amer. J. Cancer*, 1931.

4401 ALBRIGHT, Fuller. 1900– , *et al.*
Syndrome characterized by osteitis fibrosa disseminata, areas of pigmentation and endocrine dysfunction, with precocious puberty in females. Report of five cases. *New Engl. J. Med.*, 1937, **216,** 727–46.
"Albright's syndrome." With A. M. Butler, A. O. Hampton, and P. Smith.

4402 VENABLE, Charles Scott. 1877– , *et al.*
The effects on bone of the presence of metals; based upon electrolysis. An experimental study. *Ann. Surg.*, 1937, **105,** 917–38.
Introduction of vitallium. With W. Stuck and A. Beach.

4403 SMITH-PETERSEN, Marius Nygaard. 1886–1953
Arthroplasty of the hip. A new method. *J. Bone Jt Surg.*, 1939, **21,** 269–88.
Vitallium cup arthroplasty.

4404 MØRCH, Ernst Trier. 1908–
Chondrodystrophic dwarfs in Denmark (supplemented with investigations from Sweden and Norway) with special reference to the inheritance of chondrodystrophy. Copenhagen, *E. Munksgaard*, 1941.
Mørch established the fact that chondrodystrophy may be inherited.

4404.1 SEEDORFF, Knud Stakemann.
Osteogenesis imperfecta. A study of clinical features and heredity based on 55 Danish families comprising 180 affected members. Århus, *Universitetsforlaget*, 1949.
Includes a translation of Ekman's thesis (No. 4304.1). Also gives a case reported in 1678.

4405 JUDET, Jean. 1905– , & JUDET, Robert Louis. 1909–
The use of an artificial femoral head for arthroplasty of the hip joint. *J. Bone Jt Surg.*, 1950, **32B,** 166–73.
Judet acrylic prosthesis.

4406–4435 FRACTURES AND DISLOCATIONS

4406 HIPPOCRATES. 460–375 b.c.
Fractures, joints, instruments of reduction. In his: *Works*. Ed. W. H. S. Jones and E. T. Withington, London, 1927, **3,** 83–449.

4407 WHITE, Charles. 1728–1813
An account of a new method of reducing shoulders (without the use of an ambe) which have been several months dislocated, in cases where the common methods have proved inefficient. *Med. Obs. Inqu.*, 1762, **2,** 373–81.
White's method of reducing shoulder by means of the heel in the axilla.

4408 POTT, PERCIVALL. 1714–1788
Some few general remarks on fractures and dislocations. London, *L. Hawes, W. Clarke, R. Collins*, 1765.

The methods outlined by Pott in his classical work on fractures and dislocations were eventually adopted all over the world. He described (pp. 57–64) "Pott's fracture" in this book, and he stressed the necessity for the immediate setting of a fracture and the need for relaxation of the muscles in order that the setting should be carried out successfully. Reprinted in *Med. Classics*, 1936, **1**, 332–37.

4409 CAMPER, PIETER. 1722–1789
Dissertatio de fractura patellae et olecrani. Hagae Comitum, *I. van Cleef*, 1789.

4410 COLLES, ABRAHAM. 1773–1843
On the fracture of the carpal extremity of the radius. *Edinb. med. surg. J.*, 1814, **10**, 182–86.

Colles' description of fracture of the carpal end of the radius led that type of fracture to be named "Colles' fracture". He was professor of surgery at Dublin for more than 30 years. The above paper is reprinted in *Med. Classics*, 1940, **4**, 1038–42.

4411 DUPUYTREN, GUILLAUME, *le baron*. 1777–1835
Mémoire sur la fracture de l'extrémité inférieure du péroné, les luxations et les accidens qui en sont la suite. *Annu. méd.-chir. Hôp. Paris*, 1819, **1**, 1–212.

"Dupuytren's fracture."

4412 PHYSICK, PHILIP SYNG. 1768–1837
A case of fracture of the bone of the under jaw, successfully treated with a seton. *Philad. J. med. phys. Sci.*, 1822, **5**, 116–18.

Physick introduced the use of the seton for the treatment of ununited fractures.

4413 DUPUYTREN, GUILLAUME, *le baron*. 1777–1835
Mémoire sur un déplacement originel ou congénital de la tête des fémurs. *Répert. gén. Anat. Physiol. path.*, 1826, **2**, 82–93.

First clear pathological description of congenital dislocation of the hip-joint.

4414 RODGERS, JOHN KEARNY. 1793–1851
Case of un-united fracture of the os brachii, successfully treated. *N.Y. med. phys. J.*, 1827, **6**, 521–23.

Successful wiring of ununited fracture of humerus.

4415 BARTON, JOHN RHEA. 1794–1871
Views and treatment of an important injury of the wrist. *Med. Examiner*, 1838, **1**, 365–68.

"Barton's fracture" of the radius.

4416 HEINE, JACOB VON. 1799–1879
Ueber spontane und congenitale Luxationen. Stuttgart, *Ebner & Seubert*, 1842.

4417 MALGAIGNE, JOSEPH FRANÇOIS. 1806–1865
Traité des fractures et des luxations. 2 vols. Paris, *Chez l'auteur, J. B. Baillière*, 1847–55.

This was Malgaigne's greatest work. His description of bilateral vertical fracture of the pelvis ("Malgaigne's fracture") is in vol. 1, pp. 650–56. English translation, Philadelphia, 1859.

4418 REID, William W. 1799–1866
Dislocation of the femur on the dorsum ilii, reducible without pulleys or any other mechanical power. *Buffalo med. J.*, 1851–52, **7,** 129–43.
Reduction of dislocation without manipulation.

4419 BUCK, Gurdon. 1807–1877
New treatment for fractures of femur. *Bull. N.Y. Acad. Med.*, 1860–62, **1,** 181–88.
Buck's extension apparatus, an improved method of treating fractures of the femur. Reprinted in *Med. Classics*, 1939, **3**, 764–82.

4420 HAMILTON, Frank Hastings. 1813–1886
A practical treatise on fractures and dislocations. Philadelphia, *Blanchard & Lea*, 1860.

4421 PERRIN, Maurice. 1826–1889
Luxation traumatique suivie de luxation volontaire du fémur droit. *Bull. Soc. Chir. Paris*, (1859), 1860, **10,** 12–21.
"Perrin–Ferraton disease" of the hip, later more fully dealt with by L. Ferraton, *Rev. Orthop.* (*Paris*), 1905, 2 sér. **6**, 45–51.

4422 SMITH, Nathan Ryno. 1797–1877
A new instrument for the treatment of fractures of the lower extremity. *Maryland & Virginia med. surg. J.*, 1860, **14,** 1, 177.
Smith devised an anterior splint for use in the treatment of fractures of the femur.

4423 ——. Treatment of fractures of the lower extremity, by use of the anterior suspensory apparatus. Baltimore, *Kelly & Piet*, 1867.

4424 BIGELOW, Henry Jacob. 1818–1890
The mechanism of dislocation and fracture of the hip. With the reduction of the dislocations by the flexion method. Philadelphia, *H. C. Lea*, 1869.
Bigelow was the first to describe in detail the mechanism of the ilio-femoral (Bigelow's) ligament, and to show its importance in the reduction of dislocation by the flexion method.

4425 KOCHER, Emil Theodor. 1841–1917
Eine neue Reductionsmethode für Schulterverrenkung. *Berl. klin. Wschr.*, 1870, **7,** 101–05.
Kocher was professor of surgery at Berne, and among the greatest surgeons of his day. He is remembered, among other things, for his method of reduction of subluxation of the shoulder-joint.

4426 BENNETT, Edward Hallaran. 1837–1907
Fractures of the metacarpal bones. *Dublin J. med. Sci.*, 1882, **73,** 72–75.
"Bennett's fracture" of the first metacarpal. He was professor of surgery at Trinity College, Dublin.

4426.1 ANNANDALE, Thomas. 1839–1908
An operation for displaced semilunar cartilage. *Brit. med. J.*, 1885, **1,** 779.
The first deliberate and planned operation for the relief of internal derangement of the knee-joint caused by a displaced cartilage. Annandale succeeded Lister as professor of clinical surgery at Edinburgh in 1877.

4427 SPRENGEL, OTTO GERHARD KARL. 1852–1915
Die angeborene Verschiebung des Schulterblattes nach oben. *Arch. klin. Chir.*, 1891, **42,** 545–49.
"Sprengel's deformity" – congenital dislocation of the shoulder-joint.

4428 TRENDELENBURG, FRIEDRICH. 1844–1924
Ueber den Gang bei angeborener Hüftgelenksluxation. *Dtsch. med. Wschr.*, 1895, **21,** 21–24.
"Trendelenburg's sign" of congenital dislocation of the hip-joint.

4429 LANE, *Sir* WILLIAM ARBUTHNOT. 1856–1943
A method of treating simple oblique fractures of the tibia and fibula more efficient than those in common use. *Trans. clin. Soc. Lond.*, 1894, **27,** 167–75.
Lane's method of "osteo-synthesis" in the treatment of fractures – the perfect re-apposition of the affected parts by means of operative intervention.

4430 ——. Clinical observations in the operative treatment of fractures. *Brit. med. J.*, 1907, **1,** 1037–38.
Lane's plates and screws for union of fractures.

4431 STEINMANN, FRITZ. 1872–1932
Eine neue Extensionsmethode in der Frakturenbehandlung. *Zbl. Chir.*, 1907, **34,** 938–42.
Steinmann nail.

4432 BANKART, ARTHUR SYDNEY BLUNDELL. 1879–1951
Recurrent or habitual dislocation of the shoulder-joint. *Brit. med. J.*, 1923, **2,** 1132–33.
Blundell Bankart's operation.

4433 BÖHLER, LORENZ. 1885–1973
Technik der Knochenbruchbehandlung. Wien, *W. Maudrich*, 1929.
Böhler has introduced several new methods and has devised new apparatus for the treatment of fractures. His clinic in Vienna has become world-famous. 12–13th ed., 1951.

4434 SMITH-PETERSEN, MARIUS NYGAARD. 1886–1953, *et al.*
Intracapsular fractures of the neck of the femur. Treatment by internal fixation. *Arch. Surg.* (*Chicago*), 1931, **23,** 715–59.
Smith-Petersen nail. With E. F. Cave and G. W. Van Gorder.

4435 MIXTER, WILLIAM JASON. 1880–1958, & BARR, JOSEPH SEATON. 1901–1963
Rupture of the intervertebral disc with involvement of the spinal canal. *New Engl. J. Med.*, 1934, **211,** 210–15.
Demonstration of the causal rôle of intervertebral disc herniation in sciatica.

4436–4478 AMPUTATIONS; EXCISIONS; RESECTIONS

4436 YONGE, JAMES. 1646–1721
Currus triumphalis, è terebinthô . . . wherein also, the common methods, and medicaments, used to restrain hemorrhagies, are examined. London, *J. Martyn*, 1679.
Includes an account of the first flap amputation.

4437 WHITE, CHARLES. 1728–1813
An account of a case in which the upper head of the os humeri was sawed off, a large portion of the bone afterwards exfoliated, and yet the entire motion of the limb was preserved. *Phil. Trans.*, (1769), 1770, **59,** 39–46.

First recorded excision of the head of the humerus.

4438 PARK, HENRY. 1744–1831
An account of a new method of treating diseases of the joints of the knee and elbow. London, *J. Johnson,* 1733 [1783].

This was originally a letter to Pott. Park became famous for his operation of excision and arthrodesis as a treatment for destructive joint disease. The title page is misprinted "MDCCXXXIII"; the letter is dated 1783.

4439 FOURCROY, ANTOINE FRANÇOIS. 1755–1809
La médecine éclairée par les sciences physiques. Tom. 4. Paris, *chez Buisson,* 1792.

Contains (pp. 85–88) the first description of Chopart's method of partial amputation of the foot. This is in the form of a note by Lafiteau: "Observation sur une amputation partielle du pied." Lafiteau also named "Chopart's joint," the astragalo-scaphoid and calcaneo-cuboid articulation. François Chopart was born in 1743 and died in 1795.

4440 MOREAU, P. F.
Observations pratiques relatives à la résection des articulations affectées de carie. Paris, *Farge,* an XI [1803].

Excision and arthrodesis in joint disease. Moreau was the first to excise the elbow.

4441 WACHTER, GEORG HEINRICH. 1790–1864
Diss. de articulis exstirpandis, imprimis de genu exstirpato. Groningae, *T. Spoormaker,* [1810].

4442 LARREY, DOMINIQUE JEAN, *le baron.* 1766–1842
Mémoires de chirurgie militaire. Paris, *J. Smith,* 1812, **2,** 180–95.

Successful amputation at the hip-joint. Larrey was one of the first to perform this operation, with at least two successful cases.

4443 LISFRANC, JACQUES. 1790–1847
Nouvelle méthode opératoire pour l'amputation partielle du pied dans son articulation tarso-métatarsienne. Paris, *Gabon,* 1815.

"Lisfranc's amputation" of the foot.

4444 DUPUYTREN, GUILLAUME, *le baron.* 1777–1835
Observation sur une résection de la mâchoire inférieure. *J. univ. Sci. méd.,* 1820, **19,** 77–98.

Dupuytren was the first successfully to excise the lower jaw, in 1812, as recorded in his *Leçons orales,* 1829, 2, 421–53. The above paper deals with a later operation of the same type.

4445 GUTHRIE, GEORGE JAMES. 1785–1856
A treatise on gun-shot wounds. 2nd ed. London, *Longman,* 1820, 332–40.

Successful amputation at the hip-joint, after the battle of Waterloo, July 7, 1815.

4446 JAMESON, HORATIO GATES. 1788–1855
Case of tumour of the superior jaw. *Amer. med. Recorder,* 1821, **4,** 222–30.

First excision of the superior maxilla, Nov. 11, 1820.

4447 MOTT, VALENTINE. 1785–1865
Case of osteo-sarcoma in which the right side of the lower jaw was removed successfully after tying the carotid artery. *N.Y. med. phys. J.*, 1822, **1,** 385–93.

4448 DEADRICK, WILLIAM H. 1773–1858
Successful case of removal of a portion of the lower maxillary bone. *Amer. Med. Recorder*, 1823, **6,** 516.

4449 ROGERS, DAVID L.
Case of osteo-sarcoma of the superior maxillary bone, with the operation for its removal. *N.Y. med. phys. J.*, 1824, **3,** 301–03.
Operation performed in 1810.

4450 SMITH, NATHAN. 1762–1829
On the amputation of the knee-joint. *Amer. med. Rev. J.*, 1825, **2,** 370.
Smith amputated the knee-joint in 1824, being the first in America to do so.

4451 BARTON, JOHN RHEA. 1794–1871
On the treatment of anchylosis by the formation of artificial joints. *N. Amer. med. surg. J.*, 1826, **3,** 279–92.
Barton was the originator of the operation of osteotomy for ankylosis.

4452 MOTT, VALENTINE. 1785–1865
An account of a case of osteo-sarcoma of the left clavicle, in which exsection of that bone was successfully performed. *Amer. J. med. Sci.*, 1828, **3,** 100–08.
Valentine Mott was an outstanding figure in American surgery during the first half of the 19th century. A pupil of Astley Cooper, he particularly distinguished himself in vascular surgery and in operations involving the bones and joints.

4453 SYME, JAMES. 1799–1870
Case of osteo-sarcoma of the lower jaw. *Edinb. med. surg. J.*, 1828, **30,** 286–90.
Syme's operation of excision of the lower jaw for osteosarcoma.

4454 ——. Three cases in which the elbow-joint was successfully excised. *Edinb. med. surg. J.*, 1829, **31,** 256–66.

4455 HUTCHINSON, ALEXANDER COPLAND.
Removal of the arm, scapula and clavicle. *Lond. med. Gaz.*, 1829–30, **5,** 273.
Records the first interscapulo-thoracic amputation, performed by Ralph Cuming (d. 1808), a naval surgeon, in 1808.

4456 ROUX, PHILIBERT JOSEPH. 1780–1854
Résection des os. *Rev. Méd. franç. étrang.*, 1830, **37,** 8–13.
Among the French surgeons of the 19th century, Roux was second in importance only to Dupuytren. He performed staphylorrhaphy in 1819 and sutured the ruptured female peritoneum in 1832; he is also remembered on account of his method of resection of bone.

4457 SYME, James. 1799–1870
Treatise on the excision of diseased joints. Edinburgh, *A. Black*, 1831.

Syme, teacher and father-in-law of Lister, was one of the greatest of the Scottish surgeons. He is remembered for his method of amputation at the ankle, for his speedy adoption of anaesthesia and antisepsis, and for the above book, which showed that excision of joints is usually preferable to amputation – a principle soon generally adopted.

4458 WHITE, Anthony. 1782–1849
[Excision of the head of the femur for disease of the hip-joint.] In: S. Cooper: *A dictionary of practical surgery*. 7th ed. London, 1838, 272–73.

White was the first to perform this operation, April 1821.

4459 SYME, James. 1799–1870
Amputation at the ankle-joint. *Lond. Edinb. month. J. med. Sci.*, 1843, **3**, 93–96.

"Syme's amputation" at the ankle-joint, an operation first successfully performed by him on Sept. 8, 1842.

4460 MACKENZIE, Richard James. 1821–1854
On amputation at the ankle-joint by internal lateral flap. *Monthly J. med. Sci.*, 1849, **9**, 951–54.

"Mackenzie's operation", a modification of Syme's amputation (No. 4459). Mackenzie volunteered for service in the Crimean War and died of Asiatic cholera near Sebastopol.

4461 BIGELOW, Henry Jacob. 1818–1890
Resection of the head of the femur. *Amer. J. med. Sci.*, 1852, **24**, 90.

First excision at the hip-joint in America.

4462 BRASHEAR, Walter. 1776–1860
[First case of amputation at the hip-joint in the United States.] *Trans. Kentucky med. Soc.* (1852), 1853, **2**, 265.

The first successful amputation of the hip-joint was performed by Brashear in 1806 at Bardstown, Kentucky; he first amputated the thigh through its middle third, and tied off the bleeding vessels; then he made a long incision on the outside of the limb, exposing the remainder of the bone, which was disarticulated at its socket.

4463 McCREARY, Charles. 1785–1826
Exsection of the clavicle. *Trans. Kentucky med. Soc.* (1852), 1853, **2**, 276–77.

For osteosarcoma; operation performed 1813. J. H. Johnson (*New Orleans med. surg. J.*, 1850, **6**, 474–76) gives the date as May 4, 1811.

4464 HEYFELDER, Johann Ferdinand Martin. 1798–1869
Ueber Resectionen und Amputationen. Breslau, Bonn, *E. Weber*, 1854.

4465 PIROGOV, Nikolai Ivanovich. 1810–1881
Kostno-plasticheskoye udlineniye kosteĭ goleni pri vilushtshenii stopi. [Osteoplastic elongation of the bones of the leg in amputation of the foot.] *Voyenno-med. J.*, 1854, **63**, 2 sect., 83–100.

Pirogov's method of complete osteoplastic amputation of the foot. German translation, Leipzig, 1854.

4466 GRITTI, Rocco. 1828–1920
Dell'amputazione del femore al terzo inferiore e della disarticulazione del ginocchio. *Ann. univ. Med.* (*Milano*), 1857, **161,** 5–32.
Gritti's amputation of the thigh was later improved by Stokes (see No. 4470).

4467 TEALE, Thomas Pridgin, *snr.* 1801–1868
On amputation by a long and a short rectangular flap. London, *J. Churchill,* 1858.
Teale's method of amputation.

4468 CARDEN, Henry Douglas. ?–1872
On amputation by single flap. *Brit. med. J.*, 1864, **1,** 416–21.
Carden devised a single flap operation, cutting through the femur just above the knee-joint. He published a book on the subject in 1864.

4469 LISTER, Joseph, 1*st Baron Lister.* 1827–1912
On excision of the wrist for caries. *Lancet*, 1865, **1,** 308–12, 335–38, 362–64.

4470 STOKES, *Sir* William. 1839–1900
On supra-condyloid amputation of the thigh. *Med.-chir. Trans.*, 1870, **53,** 175–86.
Gritti–Stokes amputation (see also No. 4466).

4471 BERGER, Paul. 1845–1908
Amputation du membre supérieur dans la contiguïté du tronc (désarticulation de l'omoplate). *Bull. Soc. Chir. Paris*, 1883, **9,** 656.
"Berger's operation", interscapulothoracic amputation. See also his monograph, Paris, *Masson*, 1887.

4472 JABOULAY, Mathieu. 1860–1913
La désarticulation interilio-abdominale. *Lyon méd.*, 1894, **75,** 507–10.
Interilio-abdominal amputation first described.

4473 GIRARD, Charles. 1850–1916
Désarticulation de l'os iliaque pour sarcome. *Congr. franç. Chir.*, 1895, **9,** 823–27.
First successful hind-quarter amputation.

4474 VANGHETTI, Giuliano. 1861–1940
Amputazione, disarticulazione et protesi. Firenze, 1898.
Vanghetti was the first to suggest the use of the musculature remaining above the amputation stump to form a motor unit for artificial limbs – "kinematization of stumps".

4475 CECI, Antonio. 1852–1920
Tecnica generale della amputazioni mucosi. Amputazioni plastico-ortopediche con metodo proprio secundo la proposta del Vanghetti. Dimonstrazioni pratiche. *Arch. Atti Soc. ital. Chir.*, 1906, **18.**
Ceci was the first to operate on the lines suggested by Vanghetti.

4476 KRUKENBERG, Hermann. 1863–
Eine neue osteoplastische Amputationsmethode des Oberschenkels. *Zbl. Chir.*, 1917, **44,** 578.

4477 PUTTI, Vittorio. 1880–1940
The utilization of the muscles of a stump to actuate artificial limbs: cinematic amputations. *Brit. med. J.*, 1918, **1,** 635–38.
Putti developed and improved kineplastic surgery.

4478 GORDON-TAYLOR, *Sir* GORDON. 1878–1960, & WILES, PHILIP. 1899–1967
Interinnomino-abdominal (hind-quarter) amputation. *Brit. J. Surg.*, 1935, **22**, 671–95.
One-stage operation.

History of Orthopaedic Surgery

4479 KEITH, *Sir* ARTHUR. 1866–1955
Menders of the maimed. London, *H. Frowde*, 1919.
Gives details of the work of John Hunter, John Hilton, Hugh Owen Thomas, Little, Stromeyer, Marshall Hall, Arbuthnot Lane, Syme, Julius Wolff, etc., in the development of modern orthopaedics. Second edition, 1925. Facsimile reprint of first edition, 1952.

4480 OSGOOD, ROBERT BAYLEY. 1873–1956
The evolution of orthopaedic surgery. St. Louis, *C. V. Mosby*, [1925].

4481 BLENCKE, AUGUST. 1869–1937, & GOCHT, HERMANN. 1869–1938
Die orthopädische Weltliteratur 1903–30. Herausg. von A. BLENCKE und H. GOCHT. (Ergänzungsband 1931–35, hrsg. von E. WITTE.) 3 vols. Stuttgart, *F. Enke*, 1936–38.

4482 BICK, EDGAR MILTON. 1902–
Source book of orthopaedics. Baltimore, *Williams & Wilkins*, 1948.
A history of orthopaedic surgery from the earliest times. Includes a useful bibliography.

4483 ORR, HIRAM WINNETT. 1877–1956
On the contributions of Hugh Owen Thomas of Liverpool, Sir Robert Jones of Liverpool and London, John Ridlon, M.D., of New York and Chicago, to modern orthopedic surgery. Springfield, *C. C. Thomas*, 1949.

4483.1 VALENTIN, BRUNO. 1885–
Geschichte der Orthopädie. Stuttgart, *Georg Thieme*, 1961.

4484–4509.1 RHEUMATISM AND GOUT

4484 ARETAEUS, *the Cappadocian*. A.D. 81–138?
On arthritis and schiatica. In his: *Extant works*, transl. by F. ADAMS, London, 1856, 362–65, 492–93.

4485 BAILLOU, GUILLAUME DE [BALLONIUS]. 1538–1616
Liber de rheumatismo et pleuritide dorsale. Parisiis, *J. Quesnel*, 1642.
De Baillou introduced the term "rheumatism". He was court physician in Paris at the time of Henri IV. His book, the first on rheumatism, was translated into English by C. C. Barnard in *Brit. J. Rheum.*, London, 1940, 2, 141–62.

4485.1 LA MARTINIÈRE, PIERRE MARTIN DE. 1634–1690
Traitté de la maladie vénérienne, de ses causes et des accidens provenans du mercure, ou vif-argent. Paris, *L'autheur*, 1664.
First to describe gonococcal arthritis.

4486 SYDENHAM, THOMAS. 1624–1689
Tractatus de podagra et hydrope. Londini, *G. Kettilby*, 1683.
Of the many great works of Sydenham, this is considered his masterpiece. He clearly differentiated gout from rheumatism. For an English translation, see his *Works*, published by the Sydenham Society, 1850, 2, 123–84.

4487 CHEYNE, GEORGE. 1671–1743
Observations concerning the nature and due method of treating the gout. London, *G. Strahan, W. Mears*, 1720.

4488 SWIETEN, GERARD L. B. VAN. 1700–1772
Podagra. In his *Commentaria in Hermanni Boerhaave aphorismos de cognoscendis et curandis morbis.* Lugduni Batavorum, *J. & H. Verbeek*, 1764, **4,** 287–393.

4489 CADOGAN, WILLIAM. 1711–1797
A dissertation on the gout, and all chronic diseases, jointly considered, as proceeding from the same causes; what those causes are; and a rational and natural method of cure proposed. London, *J. Dodsley*, 1771.
This book excited great attention and ran through 8 editions in one year. Cadogan's advice on moderate exercise and moderation in drinking as a cure for gout caused much criticism. Indirectly through this work Cadogan became a friend of David Garrick, at whose death he was present. A reprint of the 10th edition of this essay appears in *Ann. med. Hist.*, 1925, 7, 67–90.

4490 LANDRÉ-BEAUVAIS, AUGUSTIN JACOB. 1772–1840
Doit-on admettre une nouvelle espèce de goutte sous la dénomination de goutte asthénique primitive? Paris, an VIII [1800].
Landré-Beauvais gave the first reasonably accurate description of rheumatoid arthritis.

4491 HEBERDEN, WILLIAM, *Snr.* 1710–1801
De nodis digitorum. In his *Commentarii de morborum historia.* Londini, *T. Payne*, 1802, p. 130.
Heberden described a form of rheumatic gout in which nodules ("Heberden's nodes") appeared at the interphalangeal joints of the fingers.

4492 HAYGARTH, JOHN. 1740–1827
A clinical history of diseases. Part first: being 1. A clinical history of the acute rheumatism. 2. A clinical history of the nodosity of the joints. London, *Cadell & Davies*, 1805.
Haygarth was a pioneer epidemiologist in England. He demonstrated the uselessness of Elisha Perkins' metallic tractors by obtaining the same results with wooden ones. His little book on acute rheumatism is classical.

4493 MITCHELL, JOHN KEARSLEY. 1793–1858
On a new practice in acute and chronic rheumatism. *Amer. J. med. Sci.*, 1831, **8,** 55–64.
First description of the neurotic spinal arthropathies.

4494 BOUILLAUD, JEAN BAPTISTE. 1796–1881
Traité clinique du rhumatisme articulaire. Paris, *J. B. Baillière*, 1840.
Extension of Bouillaud's work on the coincidence of heart disease and acute rheumatism. He regarded fever as the effect of endocarditis (see also No. 2749).

4495 GARROD, *Sir* ALFRED BARING. 1819–1907
Observations on certain pathological conditions of the blood and urine in gout, rheumatism and Bright's disease. *Med.-chir. Trans.*, 1848, **31,** 83–97; 1854, **37,** 49–59.
The "thread test" in gout was introduced by Garrod. Later he wrote more fully on gout and rheumatism (see No. 4497).

4496 ADAMS, ROBERT. 1791–1875
A treatise on rheumatic gout, or chronic rheumatic arthritis, of all the joints. London, *J. Churchill*, 1857.
This excellent description of chronic rheumatic arthritis includes some fine illustrations.

4497 GARROD, *Sir* ALFRED BARING. 1819–1907
The nature and treatment of gout and rheumatic gout. London, *Walton & Maberly*, 1859.
Garrod was the leading authority of his time on gout; his book gives an excellent account of contemporary knowledge of the disease.

4498 CHARCOT, JEAN MARTIN. 1825–1893, & CORNIL, ANDRÉ VICTOR. 1837–1898
Contributions à l'étude des altérations anatomiques de la goutte. *C. R. Soc. Biol.* (*Mémoires*) (1863), 1864, 3 sér., **5,** 139–63.
Charcot and Cornil gave an important description of the renal lesions in gout.

4499 CORNIL, ANDRÉ VICTOR. 1837–1898
Mémoire sur les coincidences pathologiques du rhumatisme articulaire chronique. *C. R. Soc. Biol.* (*Paris*), (*Mémoires*), 1864, 4 sér., **1,** 3–25.
First description of chronic arthritis in childhood.

4499.1 MEYNET, P.
Rhumatisme articulaire subaigu avec production de tumeurs multiples dans les tissus fibreux périarticulaires et sur le périoste d'un grand nombre d'os. *Lyon méd.*, 1875, **20,** 495–99.
Meynet was the first to draw special attention to the subcutaneous fibroid nodules in rheumatism.

4500 BESNIER, ERNEST. 1831–1909
Rhumatisme. *Dict. encyclopéd. Sci. méd.*, Paris, 1876, 3 sér., **4,** 446–819.
Besnier wrote an important description of rheumatism.

4501 MACLAGAN, THOMAS JOHN. 1838–1903
The treatment of acute rheumatism by salicin. *Lancet*, 1876, **1,** 342–343, 383–84.
Introduction of salicylates in the treatment of rheumatism.

4501.1 FOWLER, *Sir* JAMES KINGSTON. 1852–1934
On the association of affections of the throat with acute rheumatism. *Lancet*, 1880, **2,** 933–34.
Fowler drew attention to the association of throat infection with acute rheumatism.

4502 EBSTEIN, WILHELM. 1836–1912
Das Regimen bei der Gicht. Wiesbaden, *J. F. Bergmann*, 1885.
A pupil of Frerichs, Virchow, and Romberg, Ebstein became professor of medicine at Göttingen.

4502.1 HÖCK, HEINRICH.
Ein Beitrag zur Arthritis blennorrhoica. *Wien. klin. Wschr.*, 1893, **6,** 736–38.
Gonococci isolated from an arthritic joint.

4503 STILL, *Sir* GEORGE FREDERIC. 1868–1941
On a form of chronic joint disease in children. *Med.-chir. Trans.*, 1896–97, **80,** 47–59.
"Still's disease", chronic articular rheumatism in children. See also No. 4499.

4504 PONCET, ANTONIN. 1849–1913
Polyarthrite tuberculeuse simulant des lésions rhumatismales chroniques déformantes. *Gaz. Hôp.* (*Paris*), 1897, **70,** 1219.
Tuberculous rheumatism ("Poncet's disease"). See also his later paper in *Bull. Acad. Méd.* (*Paris*), 1902, 3 sér. **48**, 97–114.

4504.1 TRIBOULET, HENRI. 1864–1920, & COYON, AMAND. 1871–1928
Bactériologie du rhumatisme articulaire. Endocardite végétante mitrale provoquée chez le lapin par inoculation intra-veineuse d'un cocco-bacille en points doubles extraits du sang du rhumatisme articulaire aigu de l'homme. *C. R. Soc. Biol.*, 1898, **50,** 124–28.
Isolation of streptococci from patients with acute rheumatism reported.

4505 POYNTON, FREDERICK JOHN. 1869–1943, & PAINE, ALEXANDER.
The etiology of rheumatic fever. *Lancet*, 1900, **2,** 861–69, 932–35.
After extensive bacteriological researches Poynton and Paine considered that a diplococcus was the cause of rheumatic fever.

4505.1 NICOLAIER, ARTHUR. 1862– , & DOHRN, MAX.
Ueber die Wirkung von Chinolincarbonsäuren und ihrer Derivate auf die Ausscheidung der Harnsäure. *Dtsch. Arch. klin. Med.*, 1908, **93,** 331–55.
Introduction of cinchophen in the treatment of gout.

4506 FELTY, AUGUSTUS ROI. 1895–
Chronic arthritis in the adult, associated with splenomegaly and leucopenia. *Johns Hopk. Hosp. Bull.*, 1924, **35,** 16–20.
"Felty syndrome."

4507 SCHLESINGER, BERNARD. 1896–
The relationship of throat infection to acute rheumatism in childhood. *Arch. Dis. Childh.*, 1930, **5,** 411–30.
Schlesinger showed that haemolytic streptococcal infection was a cause of acute rheumatism in children.

4508 HENCH, PHILIP SHOWALTER. 1896–1965, *et al.*
The effect of a hormone of the adrenal cortex (17-hydroxy-11-dehydrocorticosterone: compound E) and of pituitary adrenocorticotropic hormone on rheumatoid arthritis. *Proc. Mayo Clin.*, 1949, **24,** 181–97.
Introduction of cortisone and A.C.T.H. in treatment of rheumatoid arthritis. With E. C. Kendall, C. H. Slocumb, and H. F. Polley. Hench and Kendall shared a Nobel Prize with T. Reichstein (No. 1153) in 1950.

4509 ——. The effects of the adrenal cortical hormone 17-hydroxy-11-dehydrocorticosterone (compound E) on the acute phase of rheumatic fever: preliminary report. *Proc. Mayo Clin.*, 1949, **24,** 277–97.
Compound E (cortisone) introduced in the treatment of rheumatic fever. With C. H. Slocumb, A. R. Barnes, H. L. Smith, H. F. Polley, and E. C. Kendall.

4509.1 COPEMAN, WILLIAM SYDNEY CHARLES. 1900–
A short history of the gout and the rheumatic diseases. Berkeley, *University of California Press*, 1964.

4510–5019.8 DISEASES OF THE NERVOUS SYSTEM

4510 ARETAEUS, *the Cappadocian*. A.D. ?81–138
On paralysis. In his: *Extant works*, transl. by F. ADAMS, London, 1856, 305–09.

4511 GALEN. A.D. 130–200
De tremore, palpitatione, convulsione, et rigore. In his *Opera*, ed. C. G. KÜHN, Lipsiae, 1824, **7**, 584–642.

4511.1 PLATTER, FELIX [PLATER]. 1536–1614
Observationum in hominis affectibus. Basileae, *L. König*, 1614.
On p. 13 is recorded an account of a meningioma.

4512 FEHR, JOHANNES MICHAEL. 1610–1688, & SCHMIDT, ELIAS.
Naturae genius, medicorum Celsus, Jason Argonautarum, Bauschius occubuit. *Misc. Cur. med.-phys. Acad. nat. cur.*, Jenae, 1671, **2.**
First authentic case of trigeminal neuralgia. It concerned J. L. Bausch, who died from the condition in 1665. The account is to be found in the unpaged part of the volume, starting at sig. *d*3 and occupying the two following pages.

4513 WILLIS, THOMAS. 1621–1675
Of the headach. In his: *Practice of physick*, London, *T. Dring*, 1684, Treatise XI, pp. 105–25.

4514 SYDENHAM, THOMAS. 1624–1689
Schedula monitoria de novae febris ingressu. Londini, *G. Kettilby*, 1686.
Includes (pp. 25–28) his classical description of chorea minor ("Sydenham's chorea"). Reprinted in *Med. Classics*, 1939, **4**, 327–53. In the Sydenham Society translation (see No. 64) the passage occurs in vol. 2, pp. 198–99.

4515 COTUGNO, DOMENICO. 1736–1822
De ischiade nervosa commentarius. Neapoli, *apud frat. Simonios*, 1764.
Cotugno published a classical description of sciatica, which is useful even to-day. He recognized two types – arthritic and nervous; the latter has been called "Cotugno's disease", and his book is confined to that type. The book, which also describes a case of acute nephritis, appeared in English in 1775.

4516 FOTHERGILL, JOHN. 1712–1780
On a painful affection of the face. *Med. Obs. Inqu.*, 1776, **5**, 129–42.
Original description of facial neuralgia. Reprinted in *Med. Classics*, 1940, **5**, 100–06.

4517 ——. Remarks on that complaint commonly known under the name of the sick headach. *Med. Obs. & Inqu.*, London, 1777–84, **6**, 103–37.
First accurate description of migraine.

4518 FRANK, JOHANN PETER. 1745–1821
De vertebralis columnae in morbis dignitate. In his: *Delectus opusculorum medicorum*, Ticini, 1792, **11**, 1–50.
Frank, best remembered for his great services to public health, was the first physician to emphasize the gravity of diseases of the spinal cord.

4519 FRIEDREICH, NICOLAUS ANTON. 1761–1836
De paralysi musculorum faciei rheumatici. Wirceburgi, 1797.
Facial paralysis first described.

4520 BELL, *Sir* CHARLES. 1774–1842
On the nerves; giving an account of some experiments on their structure and functions, which lead to a new arrangement of the system. *Phil. Trans.*, 1821, **111,** 398–424.
"Bell's palsy." The facial paralysis ensuing upon lesion of the motor nerve of the face is here for the first time described. See also his later paper, with more detailed description in the same journal, 1829, **119**, 317–30. Reprinted in *Med. Classics*, 1936, **1**, 152–69.

4521 JACKSON, JAMES. 1777–1867
On a peculiar disease resulting from the use of ardent spirits. *New Engl. J. Med. Surg.*, 1822, **2,** 351–53.
Jackson drew attention to alcoholic neuritis – arthrodynia *a potu*. Jackson was professor at Boston Medical School.

4522 PARRY, CALEB HILLIER. 1755–1822
Facial hemiatrophy. In *Collections from the unpublished writings . . .* London, 1825, **1,** 478–80.
Parry was the first to record cases of facial hemiatrophy.

4523 WOOD, WILLIAM. 1774–1857
Observations on neuroma. *Trans. med.-chir. Soc. Edinb.*, 1828–29, **3,** 367–433.
Neuroma first described.

4524 ADDISON, THOMAS. 1793–1860
On the influence of electricity, as a remedy in certain convulsive and spasmodic diseases. *Guy's Hosp. Rep.*, 1837, **2,** 493–507.
First therapeutic employment of static electricity.

4525 STANLEY, EDWARD. 1793–1862
A case of disease in the posterior columns of the spinal cord. *Med.-chir. Trans.*, 1839–40, **23,** 80–84.
Stanley was the first to describe disease of the posterior columns of the spinal cord.

4526 VALLEIX, FRANÇOIS LOUIS ISIDORE. 1807–1855
Traité des névralgies ou affections douloureuses des nerfs. Paris, *J. B. Baillière*, 1841.
Includes (p. 40 *et seq.*) description of "Valleix's points", tender points on the course of certain nerves in neuralgia.

4527 ROMBERG, MORITZ HEINRICH. 1795–1873
Klinische Ergebnisse. Berlin, *A. Förstner*, 1846.
P. 75: Classical description of facial hemiatrophy – "Romberg's disease".

4528 ——. Lehrbuch der Nervenkrankheiten des Menschen. Bd. 1. Berlin, *A. Duncker*, 1846.
Romberg inaugurated the modern era in the study of diseases of the nervous system. His *Lehrbuch* is the first formal treatise in this field. On p. 795 is to be found the original description of "Romberg's sign", pathognomonic of tabes dorsalis. English translation, 1853.

4529 SMITH, Robert William. 1807–1873
A treatise on the pathology, diagnosis, and treatment of neuroma. Dublin, *Hodges & Smith*, 1849.

Includes a full description of generalized neurofibromatosis ("Recklinghausen's disease" (see No. 4566).

4530 BROWN-SÉQUARD, Charles Edouard. 1817–1894
De la transmission croisée des impressions sensitives par la moelle épinière. *C. R. Soc. Biol.* (*Paris*), (1850), 1851, **2,** 33–34.

"Brown-Séquard's paralysis." Lesion of one lateral half of the spinal cord causes paralysis of motion on one side and of sensation on the other. See also the writer's later paper on pp. 70–73 of the same volume.

4531 GUBLER, Adolphe. 1821–1897
De l'hémiplégie alterne envisagée comme signe de lésion de la protubérance annulaire et comme preuve de la décussation des nerfs faciaux. *Gaz. hebd. Méd. Chir.*, 1856, **3,** 749–54, 789–92, 811–16.

"Gubler's paralysis" – crossed hemiplegia.

4532 GULL, *Sir* William Withey. 1816–1890
Cases of paraplegia [with autopsies of ataxic cases, showing lesions in the posterior columns of the spinal cord]. *Guy's Hosp. Rep.*, 1856, 3 ser., **2,** 143–90; 1858, 3 ser., **4,** 169–216.

Gull showed the lesions of tabes dorsalis to be located in the posterior columns of the spinal cord.

4533 FOVILLE, Achille Louis François. 1799–1878
Note sur une paralysie peu connue des certains muscles de l'oeil, et sa liaison avec quelques points de l'anatomie et la physiologie de la protubérance annulaire. *Bull. Soc. Anat. Paris*, 1858, **33,** 393–414.

"Foville's syndrome" – crossed paralysis of the limbs on one side of the body and of the face on the other side, together with loss of ability to rotate the eyes to that side.

4534 REMAK, Robert. 1815–1865
Galvanotherapie der Nerven- und Muskelkrankheiten. Berlin, *A. Hirschwald*, 1858.

Remak was a pioneer of galvanotherapy.

4535 BOUCHUT, Eugène. 1818–1891
De l'état nerveux aigu et chronique ou nervosisme. Paris, *J. B. Baillière*, 1860.

First adequate description of neurasthenia.

4536 GRAEFE, Friedrich Wilhelm Ernst Albrecht von. 1828–1870
Ueber Complication von Sehnervenentzündung mit Gehirnkrankheiten. *v. Graefes Arch. Ophthal.*, 1860, **7,** 2 Abt., 58–71.

Graefe showed that most cases of blindness and impaired vision connected with cerebral disorders can be traced to optic neuritis rather than to paralysis of the optic nerve.

4537 JACKSON, John Hughlings. 1835–1911
Observations on defects of sight in brain disease. *Ophthal. Hosp. Rep.*, 1863–65, **4,** 10–19, 389–446; 1865–66, **5,** 51–78, 251–306.

In this work Jackson showed the importance of the ophthalmoscope in the investigation of diseases of the nervous system. Reprinted in *Med. Classics*, 1939, **3,** 918–26.

4538 WEBER, *Sir* HERMANN DAVID. 1823–1918
A contribution to the pathology of the crura cerebri. *Med.-chir. Trans.*, 1863, **46,** 121–39.
"Weber's syndrome" or "Weber–Gubler syndrome" – hemiplegia associated with disease of the crura cerebri; first described by Gubler (No. 4531).

4539 WILKS, *Sir* SAMUEL, *Bart.* 1824–1911
Drunkard's or alcoholic paraplegia. *Med. Times Gaz.*, 1868, **2,** 470.
Classical account of alcoholic paraplegia.

4540 ROBERTSON, DOUGLAS MORAY COOPER LAMB ARGYLL. 1837–1909
On an interesting series of eye symptoms in a case of spinal disease, with remarks on the action of belladonna on the iris. *Edinb. med. J.*, 1869, **14,** 696–708.
"Argyll Robertson pupil" first described. See also his later paper in the same journal, 1869, **15**, 487–93. Reprinted in *Med. Classics*, 1937, **1**, 851–76.

4541 BRUNS, PAUL VON. 1846–1916
Das Rankenneurom. Tübingen, *H. Laupp*, 1870.
Original description of plexiform neurofibroma.

4542 HAMMOND, WILLIAM ALEXANDER. 1828–1900
Athetosis. In his *Treatise on diseases of the nervous system.* New York, *D. Appleton & Co.*, (1871), pp. 654–62.
First description of athetosis, sometimes called "Hammond's disease".

4543 DUCHENNE DE BOULOGNE, GUILLAUME BENJAMIN AMAND. 1806–1875
De l'électrisation localisée et de son application à la pathologie et à la thérapeutique. 3me. éd. Paris, *J. B. Baillière*, 1872.
First description, page 357, of partial brachial plexus paralysis, upper type, ("Duchenne–Erb palsy": see No. 4548).

4544 MITCHELL, SILAS WEIR. 1829–1914
Injuries of nerves and their consequences. Philadelphia, *J. B. Lippincott & Co.*, 1872.
Includes the first description of ascending neuritis, and also of the treatment of neuritis by cold and splint rests. The book was written as a result of Mitchell's experiences in the American Civil War.

4545 ——. Clinical lecture on certain painful affections of the feet. *Philad. med. Times*, 1872, **3,** 81–82, 113–15.
Mitchell suggested the name "erythromelalgia" for this condition, which is also known as "Mitchell's disease" and "Weir Mitchell's disease". He records four earlier writers on the subject, the first being Graves in 1848. See also his paper in *Amer. J. med. Sci.*, 1878, **76**, 17–36.

4546 CHARCOT, JEAN MARTIN. 1825–1893
Leçons sur les maladies du système nerveux faites à La Salpêtrière. 3 vols. Paris, *A. Delahaye*, 1872–87.
An excellent idea of Charcot's work is gained by perusal of his *Leçons*, dealing with his teaching on nervous disorders. In the second volume, pp. 1–72, is a classical account of the anomalies of tabes dorsalis. Charcot became one of the greatest of all neurologists. English translation, 1877–89.

4547 JACKSON, John Hughlings. 1835–1911
On a case of paralysis of the tongue from haemorrhage in the medulla oblongata. *Lancet*, 1872, **2**, 770–73.

Jackson here described the syndrome consisting of paralysis of half the tongue, the same half of the palate, and of one vocal cord – "Jackson's syndrome".

4548 ERB, Wilhelm Heinrich. 1840–1921
Ueber eine eigenthümliche Localisation von Lähmungen im Plexus brachialis. *Verh. nat.-med. Vereins. Heidelb.*, 1873–77, n.F. **1**, 130–36.

"Erb's palsy", first described by Smellie in 1763 and later by Duchenne (No. 4543).

4549 LIVEING, Edward. 1832–1919
On megrim, sick-headache, and some allied disorders. London, *J. & A. Churchill*, 1873.

Liveing's classical account of migraine showed the close association of this condition with tetany, asthma, and false angina pectoris with epilepsy and the alternation of all these conditions in the same subject or the transference permanently from one to another.

4550 LEYDEN, Ernst von. 1832–1910
Klinik der Rückenmarks-Krankheiten. 2 vols. Berlin, *A. Hirschwald*, 1874–75.

One of Leyden's best works. He was professor of medicine at Berlin, Königsberg, and Strassburg. In vol. 2, p. 65, of the above is given an account of "Leyden's paralysis", a form of hemiplegia probably first described in 1856 by Gubler (see No. 4531).

4551 MITCHELL, Silas Weir. 1829–1914
Headaches, from heat-stroke, from fevers, after meningitis, from overuse of brain, from eyestrain. *Med. surg. Reporter*, 1874, **31**, 67–71.

Mitchell drew attention to the importance of eyestrain as a cause of headache.

4552 ——. Post-paralytic chorea. *Amer. J. med. Sci.*, 1874, **68**, 342–52.

First description.

4553 ——. On rest in the treatment of nervous disease. New York, *G. P. Putnam's Sons*, 1875.

First account of the "Weir Mitchell treatment".

4554 ——. Fat and blood and how to make them. Philadelphia, *J. B. Lippincott & Co.*, 1877.

Includes full account of Weir Mitchell's rest cure for nervous disorders.

4555 ——. The relation of pain to weather, being a study of the natural history of a case of traumatic neuralgia. *Amer. J. med. Sci.*, 1877, **73**, 305–29.

First study of the subject.

4556 ERB, Wilhelm Heinrich. 1840–1921
Ueber einen wenig bekannten spinalen Symptomencomplex. *Berl. klin. Wschr.*, 1875, **12**, 357–59.

"Erb–Charcot disease" (spastic spinal paralysis).

4557 ——. Handbuch der Krankheiten des Nervensystems. 2 vols. Leipzig, *F. C. W. Vogel*, 1876–78.

Erb was professor of neurology at Heidelberg. He gave the original descriptions of several nervous disorders, especially the muscular dystrophies, and was a pioneer in the use of electrotherapy.

4558 CHARCOT, JEAN MARTIN. 1825–1893
Leçons sur les localisations dans les maladies du cerveau. Paris, *Progrès Médical*, 1876.

Charcot is especially notable for his important study of the localization of functions in diseases of the brain. English translation (New Sydenham Society), 1883.

4559 BERNHARDT, MARTIN. 1844–1915
Neuropathologische Beobachtungen. *Dtsch. Arch. klin. Med.*, 1878, **22,** 362–93.

Bernhardt drew attention to meralgia paraesthetica in the leg ("Bernhardt's disease") due to disease of the external cutaneous nerve of the thigh.

4560 NOTHNAGEL, CARL WILHELM HERMANN. 1841–1905
Topische Diagnostik der Gehirnkrankheiten. Berlin, *A. Hirschwald*, 1879.

On p. 220 is the description of unilateral oculomotor paralysis combined with cerebellar ataxia, "Nothnagel's syndrome".

4561 GÉLINEAU, JEAN BAPTISTE EDOUARD. 1859–
De la narcolepsie. *Gaz. Hôp.* (*Paris*), 1880, **53,** 626–28, 635–37.

Narcolepsy first fully described.

4562 GOWERS, *Sir* WILLIAM RICHARD. 1845–1915
The diagnosis of diseases of the spinal cord. London, *J. & A. Churchill*, 1880.

Includes description of "Gowers's tract".

4563 FORST, J. J.
Contribution à l'étude clinique de la sciatique. Paris, *Thèse No.* 33, 1881.

"Lasègue's sign" in sciatica. Although discovered by E. C. Lasègue, it was first reported by his pupil Forst.

4564 FRIEDREICH, NIKOLAUS. 1825–1882
Paramyoklonus multiplex. *Virchows Arch. path. Anat.*, 1881, **86,** 421–30.

First description of paramyoclonus multiplex, "Friedreich's disease".

4565 BRAMWELL, *Sir* BYROM. 1847–1931
The diseases of the spinal cord. Edinburgh, *Maclachlan & Stewart*, 1882.

4566 RECKLINGHAUSEN, FRIEDRICH DANIEL VON. 1833–1910
Ueber die multiplen Fibrome der Haut und ihre Beziehung zu den multiplen Neuromen. Berlin, *Hirschwald*, 1882.

"Recklinghausen's disease" (see No. 4082).

4567 MÖBIUS, PAUL JULIUS. 1853–1907
Ueber periodisch wiederkehrende Oculomotoriuslähmung. *Berl. klin. Wschr.*, 1884, **21,** 604–08.

"Möbius's disease" – ophthalmoplegic migraine.

4568 GOWERS, *Sir* WILLIAM RICHARD. 1845–1915
Lectures on the diagnosis of diseases of the brain. London, *J. & A. Churchill*, 1885.

4569 ——. A manual of diseases of the nervous system. 2 vols. London, *J. & A. Churchill*, 1886–88.

Gowers was physician and professor of clinical medicine at University College, London. He especially distinguished himself in the field of neurology, and the above book is his greatest work. Gowers was interested in stenography, advised his students to take down his lectures in shorthand, and founded the Society of Medical Phonographers. Biography by Macdonald Critchley, London, 1949.

4570 BASTIAN, Henry Charlton. 1837–1915
Paralyses, cerebral, bulbar and spinal. London, *H. K. Lewis*, 1886.

Bastian was one of the founders of English neurology. He is remembered for "Bastian's law" (see No. 4577).

4571 MACKENZIE, *Sir* Stephen. 1844–1909
Two cases of associated paralysis of the tongue, soft palate, and vocal cord on the same side. *Trans. clin. Soc. Lond.*, 1886, **19,** 317–19.

"Mackenzie's syndrome."

4572 PANAS, Photinos. 1832–1903
D'un nouveau procédé opératoire applicable au ptosis congénital et au ptosis paralytique. *Arch. Ophthal.*, 1886, **6,** 1–14.

An operation for congenital and paralytic ptosis was introduced by Panas.

4573 BLOCQ, Paul. 1860–1896
Sur une affection caractérisée par de l'astasie et de l'abasie. *Arch. Neurol. (Paris)*, 1888, **15,** 24–51, 187–211.

"Blocq's disease" – astasia-abasia.

4574 BRAMWELL, *Sir* Byrom. 1847–1931
Intracranial tumours. Edinburgh, *Y. J. Pentland*, 1888.

4575 NOUVELLE Iconographie de la Salpêtrière. 28 vols. Paris, 1888–1918.

Henry Meige, Richer, and other pupils of Charcot published many valuable studies of the constitutional aspects of nervous diseases in the above work, an album unique in the history of medicine and of great value for the study of nervous diseases.

4576 BENEDIKT, Moritz. 1835–1920
Tremblement avec paralysie croisée du moteur oculaire commun. *Bull. méd. (Paris)*, 1889, **3,** 547–48.

"Benedikt's syndrome" – paralysis of the oculomotor nerve on one side with intensive trembling of the other side.

4577 BASTIAN, Henry Charlton. 1837–1915
On the symptomatology of total transverse lesions of the spinal cord, with special reference to the condition of the various reflexes. *Med.-chir. Trans.*, 1890, **73,** 151–217.

"Bastian's law", transverse lesion of the cord above the lumbar enlargement results in the abolition of the tendon reflexes of the lower extremities.

4578 SCHMIDT, Adolf. 1865–1918
Casuistische Beiträge zur Nervenpathologie. II. Doppelseitige Accessoriuslähmung bei Syringomyelie. *Dtsch. med. Wschr.*, 1892, **18,** 606–08.

"Schmidt's syndrome" – a hemiplegia affecting the vocal cord, palate, trapezius, and sternocleidomastoid muscles, due to lesion of the nucleus ambiguus and nucleus accessorius.

4579 WESTPHAL, CARL FRIEDRICH OTTO. 1833–1890
Gesammelte Abhandlungen. 2 vols. Berlin, 1892.

4580 DEJERINE, JOSEPH JULES. 1849–1917, & SOTTAS, JULES. 1866–
Sur la névrite interstitielle hypertrophique et progressive de l'enfance. *C. R. Soc. Biol.* (*Paris*), 1893, **45,** 63–96.
First description of hypertrophic progressive interstitial neuritis. "Dejerine–Sottas disease."

4581 HEAD, *Sir* HENRY. 1861–1940
On disturbances of sensation with especial reference to the pain of visceral disease. *Brain,* 1893, **16,** 1–133; 1894, **17,** 339–480; 1896, **19,** 153–276.
"Head's areas", zones of hyperalgesia of skin, associated with visceral disease.

4582 OPPENHEIM, HERMANN. 1858–1919
Lehrbuch der Nervenkrankheiten. Berlin, *S. Karger,* 1894.
English translation of 5th ed., 1911.

4583 BABINSKI, JOSEPH FRANÇOIS FÉLIX. 1857–1932
Sur le réflexe cutané plantaire dans certains affections organiques du système nerveux central. *C. R. Soc. Biol.* (*Paris*), 1896, **48,** 207–08.
"Babinski's reflex."

4584 BARKER, LEWELLYS FRANKLIN. 1867–1943
A case of circumscribed unilateral, and elective sensory paralysis. *J. exp. Med.,* 1896, **1,** 348–60.

4585 HILL, *Sir* LEONARD ERSKINE. 1866–1952
The physiology and pathology of the cerebral circulation. London, *J. & A. Churchill,* 1896.

4586 JACKSON, JOHN HUGHLINGS. 1835–1911
Remarks on the relations of different divisions of the central nervous system to one another and to parts of the body. *Brit. med. J.,* 1898, **1,** 65–69.

4587 REMAK, ERNST JULIUS. 1848–1911, & FLATAU, EDWARD. 1869–1932
Neuritis und Polyneuritis. 2 pts. Wien, *A. Hölder,* 1899–1900.
In Nothnagel's *Handbuch der speziellen Pathologie und Therapie,* XI, Bd. 3, Abt. 3–4.

4588 LIEPMANN, HUGO KARL. 1863–1925
Das Krankheitsbild der Apraxie (motorischen Asymbolie) auf Grund eines Falles von einseitiger Apraxie. *Mschr. Psychiat. Neurol.,* 1900, **8,** 15–44, 102–32, 182–97.
First adequate description of apraxia.

4589 BABINSKI, JOSEPH FRANCOIS FÉLIX. 1857–1932, & NAGEOTTE, JEAN. 1866–
Hémiasynergie, latéropulsion et myosis bulbaires avec hémianesthésie et hémiplégie croisées. *Rev. neurol.* (*Paris*), 1902, **10,** 358–65.
"Babinski–Nageotte syndrome."

4590 DEJERINE, JOSEPH JULES. 1849–1917, & THOMAS, ANDRÉ. 1867–
Traité des maladies de la moëlle épinière. Paris, *J. B. Baillière*, 1902.

4591 KIENBÖCK, ROBERT. 1871–1953
Kritik der sogenannten "traumatischen Syringomyelie". *Jb. Psychiat.*, 1902, **21,** 50–210.

Traumatic cavity formation in the spinal cord, so well described by Kienböck, is known as "Kienböck's disease".

4592 CESTAN, RAYMOND. 1872–1934, & CHENAIS, LOUIS JEAN. 1872–
Du myosis dans certaines lésions bulbaires en foyer (hémiplégie du type Avellis associée au syndrome oculaire sympathique). *Gaz. Hôp. (Paris)*, 1903, **76,** 1229–33.

"Cestan–Chenais syndrome."

4593 VERGER, HENRI. 1873–1930
Essai de classification de quelques névralgies faciales par les injections de cocaine loco dolenti. *Rev. Médecine*, 1904, **24,** 34–63, 134–64.

Classification of the neuralgias.

4594 GARCIA TAPIA, ANTONIO. 1875–1950
Un caso de parálisis del lado derecho de la laringe y de la lengua, con parálisis del esterno-cleido-mastoidea y trapecio del mismo lado; accompañado de hemiplejia total temporal del lado izquierdo del cuerpo. *Siglo méd.*, 1905, **52,** 211–13.

"Tapia's syndrome" – palato-pharyngo-laryngeal hemiplegia.

4594.1 FRIEDMANN, MAX.
Ueber die nicht epileptischen Absencen oder kurzen narkoleptischen Anfälle. *Dtsch. Z. Nervenheilk.*, 1906, **30,** 462–92.

First description of pyknolepsy.

4595 SLUDER, GREENFIELD. 1865–1928
The syndrome of sphenopalatine-ganglion neurosis. *Amer. J. med. Sci.*, 1910, **140,** 868–78.

"Sluder's neuralgia" first described.

4596 MESTREZAT, WILLIAM. 1883–1928
Le liquide céphalo-rachidien normal et pathologique, valeur clinique de l'examen chimique. Montpellier, *Thèse No.* 17, 1911.

Mestrezat gave the first exact description of the chemical constitution of the cerebrospinal fluid. Also published at Paris, *Maloine*, 1912.

4597 DANDY, WALTER EDWARD. 1886–1946, & BLACKFAN, KENNETH DANIEL. 1883–1941
Internal hydrocephalus. *Amer. J. Dis. Child.*, 1914, **8,** 406–82; 1917, **14,** 424–43.

Experimental production of hydrocephalus.

4598 DEJERINE, JOSEPH JULES. 1849–1917
Sémiologie des affections du système nerveux. Paris, *Masson & Cie.*, 1914.

4599 JELLIFFE, SMITH ELY. 1866–1945, & WHITE, WILLIAM ALANSON. 1870–
Diseases of the nervous system. Philadelphia, *Lea & Febiger*, 1915.

Sixth edition, 1935.

4600 QUECKENSTEDT, Hans Heinrich Georg. 1876–1918
Zur Diagnose der Rückenmarkskompression. *Dtsch. Z. Nervenheilk.*, 1916, **55**, 325–33.
"Queckenstedt's test" for determining patency of the spinal subarachnoid space.

4601 CUSHING, Harvey Williams. 1869–1939
Tumors of the nervus acusticus and the syndrome of the cerebello-pontile angle. Philadelphia, *W. B. Saunders*, 1917.
Reprinted 1963.

4602 DANDY, Walter Edward. 1886–1946
Ventriculography following the injection of air into the cerebral ventricles. *Ann. Surg.*, 1918, **68**, 5–11; also *Amer. J. Roentgenol.*, 1919, n.s. **6**, 26–36.
Dandy was responsible for the introduction of ventriculography.

4603 ——. Röntgenography of the brain after the injection of air into the spinal canal. *Ann. Surg.*, 1919, **70**, 397–403.
Introduction of pneumoencephalography.

4604 FOERSTER, Otfrid. 1873–1941
Zur Analyse und Pathophysiologie der striären Bewegungsstörungen. *Z. ges. Neurol. Psychiat.*, 1921, **73**, 1–169.
Foerster made a most important contribution to the literature on extrapyramidal diseases.

4605 SICARD, Jean Athanase. 1872–1929, & FORESTIER, Jacques. 1890–
Méthode radiographique d'exploration de la cavité épidurale par la lipiodol. *Rev. neurol. (Paris)*, 1921, **28**, 1264–66.

4606 WILSON, Samuel Alexander Kinnier. 1878–1937
Some problems in neurology. No. 2. Pathological laughing and crying. *J. Neurol. Psychopath.*, 1924, **4**, 299–333.
An important paper on the pathology of facial movements.

4607 ADIE, William John. 1886–1935
Idiopathic narcolepsy: a disease sui generis; with remarks on the mechanism of sleep. *Brain*, 1926, **49**, 257–306.
Adie's description of narcolepsy is called "maladie d'Adie" by some French writers.

4608 BAILEY, Percival. 1892– , & CUSHING, Harvey Williams. 1869–1939
A classification of the tumors of the glioma group on a histogenetic basis with a correlated study of prognosis. Philadelphia, *J. B. Lippincott*, 1926.
German translation, 1930.

4609 SCHAFFER, Károly. 1864–1939
Über das morphologische Wesen und die Histopathologie der hereditaer-systematischen Nervenkrankheiten. Berlin, *J. Springer*, 1926.
Schaffer was a pioneer Hungarian neuropathologist. He laid down a triad of criteria for judging whether or not a neurological disease is hereditary.

4610 EGAS MONIZ, Antonio Caetano de. 1874–1955
L'encéphalographie artérielle, son importance dans la localisation des tumeurs cérébrales. *Rev. neurol.* (*Paris*), 1927, **2,** 72–90.
Introduction of arterial encephalography. See also *Presse méd.*, 1928, **36**, 689–93. English translation in *J. Neurosurg.*, 1964, **21**, 145–56.

4611 ADIE, William John. 1886–1935
Pseudo-Argyll Robertson pupils with absent tendon reflexes; a benign disorder simulating tabes dorsalis. *Brit. med. J.*, 1931, **1,** 928–930.
"Adie's syndrome"; see also his later paper in *Brain*, 1932, **55**, 98–113. It was earlier reported by J. Strasburger, by A. Saenger and by M. Nonne in *Neurol Zbl.*, 1902, **21**, 738, 837, and 1000. See also No. 5950.

4611.1 LYSHOLM, Erik. 1891–1947
Apparatus and technique for roentgen examination of the skull. *Acta radiol., Stockh.*, 1931, Suppl. 12.
Lysholm–Schönander skull table, allowing precise radiography of the skull.

4612 CUSHING, Harvey Williams. 1869–1939, & EISENHARDT, Louise Charlotte. 1891–
Meningiomas. Their classification, regional behaviour, life history, and surgical end results. Springfield, *C. C. Thomas*, 1938.

4613 BUMKE, Oswald. 1877–1950, & FOERSTER, Otfrid. 1873–1941
Handbuch der Neurologie. 17 vols. [in 18]. Berlin, *J. Springer*, 1935–37.

4614 WILSON, Samuel Alexander Kinnier. 1878–1937
Neurology. Edited by A. N. Bruce. 2 pts. London, *E. Arnold & Co.*, (1940).
Wilson died before this monumental work was completed, and it was edited by A. N. Bruce. It includes a vast amount of history and hundreds of references. Second edition, 1954.

4615 STEINHAUSEN, Theodore Behn. 1914– , *et al.*
Iodinated organic compounds as contrast media for radiographic diagnoses. III. Experimental and clinical myelography with ethyl iodophenylundecylate (pantopaque). *Radiology*, 1944, **43,** 230–35.
Introduction of "pantopaque" for diagnosis of cerebral tumours. With C. E. Dungan, J. B. Furst, J. T. Plati, S. W. Smith, A. P. Darling, and E. C. Wolcott.

4616–4633 APHASIA, ETC.

4616 LINNÉ, Carl [Linnaeus]. 1707–1778
Glömska af alla substantiva och i synnerhet namn. *K. Swenska Wetensk. Acad. Handl.*, 1745, **6,** 116–17.
Aphasia first described. Facsimile reproduction and English translation by H. R. Viets, *Bull. Hist. Med.*, 1943, **13**, 328–33.

4617 BUXTORF, Johann Ludwig.
Lethargus cum impotentia loquelae, tandem convulsivus et lethalis. *Acta helv.*, 1758, **3,** 397–400.

4618 BOUILLAUD, Jean Baptiste. 1796–1881
Recherches cliniques propres à démontrer que la perte de la parole correspond à la lésion des lobules antérieurs du cerveau. *Arch. gén. Méd.*, 1825, **8**, 25–45.

Classical account of aphasia. Bouillaud was first to suggest that injuries of the frontal lobe were a cause of aphasia.

4619 BROCA, Pierre Paul. 1824–1880
Perte de la parole; ramollissement chronique et destruction partielle du lobe antérieur gauche du cerveau. *Bull. Soc. Anthrop. Paris*, 1861, **2**, 235–38.

Broca localized the speech centre in the left frontal lobe. He asserted that aphasia was associated with a lesion on the left third frontal convolution of the brain – "Broca's centre". He was preceded in this discovery by Marc Dax, a student who recorded in his unpublished thesis submitted to the Faculty of Medicine in Montpellier in 1836 his observations that the left hemisphere was usually found damaged in aphasics. See also No. 1400. English translation in *J. Neurosurg.*, 1964, **21**, 426–27.

4620 JACKSON, John Hughlings. 1835–1911
Loss of speech: its association with valvular disease of the heart, and with hemiplegia on the right side. Defects of smell. Defects of speech in chorea. Arterial regions in epilepsy. *Clin. Lect. Rep. Lond. Hosp.*, 1864, **1**, 388–471.

Jackson studied aphasia for 30 years. He emphasized its psychological aspects and laid the foundation for present knowledge of the condition, but he was ahead of his time and the value of his work was not for many years recognized.

4621 ——. Notes on the physiology and pathology of language. *Med. Times Gaz.*, 1866, **1**, 659–62.

4622 BASTIAN, Henry Charlton. 1837–1915
On the various forms of loss of speech in cerebral disease. *Brit. for. med.-chir. Rev.*, 1869, **43**, 209–36.

Bastian's first important paper on aphasia. His axiom "We think in words" explains his whole work on the subject. See also his later paper on pp. 470–92 of the same volume.

4623 WERNICKE, Carl. 1848–1905
Der aphasische Symptomencomplex. Breslau, *M. Cohn & Weigert*, 1874.

Sensory aphasia ("Wernicke's aphasia"). Wernicke did important work on the localization of aphasia; he included in his book accounts of alexia and agraphia.

4624 KUSSMAUL, Adolf. 1822–1902
Die Störungen der Sprache. Leipzig, *F. C. W. Vogel*, 1877.

Kussmaul's best work. He termed aphasia "word-blindness". The book was issued as a supplement to vol. 12 of Ziemssen's *Handbuch der speciellen Pathologie und Therapie.*

4625 PITRES, Jean Albert. 1848–1928
Considérations sur l'agraphie à propos d'une observation nouvelle d'agraphie motrice pure. *Rev. Médecine*, 1884, **4**, 855–73.

Classical account of agraphia.

4626 LICHTHEIM, Ludwig. 1845–1928
Ueber Aphasie. *Dtsch. Arch. klin. Med.*, 1885, **36,** 204–68.
"Lichtheim's disease" – subcortical sensory aphasia. Lichtheim noted that although the patient cannot speak, he is able to indicate with his fingers the number of syllables in the word of which he is thinking ("Lichtheim's sign"). The paper is translated into English in *Brain*, 1885, **7**, 433–84.

4627 BERLIN, Rudolf. 1833–1897
Eine besondere Art der Wortblindheit. Wiesbaden, *J. F. Bergmann*, 1887.
Berlin first suggested the term "dyslexia".

4628 PITRES, Jean Albert. 1848–1928
Étude sur l'aphasie chez les polyglottes. *Rev. Médecine*, 1895, **15,** 873–99.
Important account of paraphrasia.

4629 BASTIAN, Henry Charlton. 1837–1915
A treatise on aphasia and other speech defects. London, *H. K. Lewis*, 1898.
Bastian localized the auditory and visual centres, and he described word-blindness and word-deafness. (See also No. 4622.)

4630 MARIE, Pierre. 1853–1940
Revision de la question de l'aphasie; la troisième circonvolution frontale gauche ne joue aucun rôle spécial dans la fonction du langage. *Sem. méd.* (*Paris*), 1906, **26,** 241–47.
Marie disputed Broca's claim that the third left frontal convolution of the brain is the speech centre. He classified aphasia into three groups: anarthria (defects of articulation), Broca's (motor) aphasia, and Wernicke's (sensory) aphasia.

4631 HINSELWOOD, James. 1859–1919
Congenital word-blindness. London, *H. K. Lewis*, 1917.

4632 HENSCHEN, Salomon Eberhard. 1847–1930
Klinische und anatomische Beiträge zur Pathologie des Gehirns. V–VII. Upsala, *Almquist & Wiksell*, 1920–22.
An important summary of the knowledge concerning aphasia.

4633 HEAD, *Sir* Henry. 1861–1940
Aphasia and kindred disorders of speech. 2 vols. Cambridge, *Univ. Press*, 1926.
The most important work on the subject in the English language. Head's theory of aphasia conceived the condition as being "a disorder of symbolic formulation and expression". Reprinted 1963.

For history, see No. 5019.8

4634–4689.1 INFLAMMATORY CONDITIONS

4634 WHYTT, Robert. 1714–1766
Observations on the dropsy in the brain. Edinburgh, *J. Balfour*, 1768.
First account of the clinical course of tuberculous meningitis in children. This work is notable for its fullness of detail and its accuracy. Whytt divided the disease into 3 stages, according to the character of the pulse, and he attributed its various manifestations to the presence of a serous exudate in the brain.

4635 CHEYNE, John. 1777–1836
An essay on hydrocephalus acutus, or dropsy in the brain. Edinburgh, *Mundell, Doig & Stevenson*, 1808.
Acute hydrocephalus first described.

4636 GERHARD, William Wood. 1809–1872
Cerebral affections of children. *Amer. J. med. Sci.*, 1834, **13,** 313–59; **14,** 99–111.
Accurate clinical description of tuberculous meningitis.

4637 DUBINI, Angelo. 1813–1902
Primi cenni sulla corea elettrica. *Ann. univ. Med.* (*Milano*), 1846, **117,** 5–50.
First description of electric chorea, "Dubini's chorea", the myoclonic form of epidemic encephalitis.

4638 LEBERT, Hermann. 1813–1878
Ueber Gehirnabscesse. *Virchows Arch. path. Anat.*, 1856, **10,** 78–109, 352–400, 426–48.
First systematic account of brain abscess.

4639 LANDRY, Jean Baptiste Octave. 1826–1865
Note sur la paralysie ascendante aiguë. *Gaz. hebd. Méd. Chir.*, 1859, **6,** 472–74, 486–88.
"Landry's paralysis" – acute infective polyneuritis. It is difficult to assess the claim of Landry as first to record this condition, since Adolf Kussmaul reported two cases in the same year (*Zwei Fälle von Paraplegie*, Erlangen).

4640 BÄRENSPRUNG, Friedrich Wilhelm Felix von. 1822–1864
Die Gürtelkrankheit. *Ann. Charité-Krankenh. Berlin*, 1861, **9,** 2 Heft, 40–128; 1862, **10,** 1 Heft, 37–53; 1863, **11,** 2 Heft, 96–116.
Herpes zoster first ascribed to a lesion of the spinal ganglia.

4641 GAYET, Charles Jules Alphonse. 1833–1904
Affection encéphalique (encéphalite diffuse probable) localisée aux étages supérieurs des pédoncules cérébraux et aux couches optiques. *Arch. Physiol. norm. path.*, 1875, 2 sér., **2,** 341–51.
First description of acute superior haemorrhagic polioencephalitis. Called also "Wernicke's disease", following the latter's description in his *Lehrbuch der Gehirnkrankheiten*, Kassel, 1881, **2,** 229–42.

4642 LANDOUZY, Louis Théophile Joseph. 1845–1917
Fièvre zoster et exanthèmes zostériformes. *J. Conn. méd. prat. Pharm.*, 1884, 3 sér., **6,** 19, 26, 37, 44, 52.
Landouzy first suggested the infective nature of herpes.

4643 STRÜMPELL, Ernst Adolf Gustav Gottfried. 1853–1925
Ueber die akute Encephalitis der Kinder (Polioencephalitis acuta, cerebrale Kinderlähmung). *Jb. Kinderheilk.*, 1885, **22,** 173–78.
"Strümpell's disease" – polioencephalomyelitis.

4644 HEAD, *Sir* Henry. 1861–1940, & CAMPBELL, Alfred Walter. 1868–1937
The pathology of herpes zoster and its bearing on sensory localisation. *Brain*, 1900, **23,** 353–523.
Head and Campbell showed herpes zoster to be a haemorrhagic inflammation of the posterior nerve roots and the homologous spinal ganglia.

4645 FROIN, Georges. 1874–
Inflammations meningées avec réactions chromatique, fibrineuse et cytologique du liquide cephalo-rachidien. *Gaz. Hôp.* (*Paris*), 1903, **76,** 1005–06.
"Froin's syndrome" – a coagulation of the cerebrospinal fluid.

4646 SCHILDER, Paul Ferdinand. 1886–1940
Zur Kenntnis der sogenannten diffusen Sklerose (über Encephalitis periaxialis diffusa). *Z. ges. Neurol.*, 1912, **10,** Orig., 1–60.
"Schilder's disease" – encephalitis periaxialis diffusa.

4647 GUILLAIN, Georges. 1876–1961, *et al.*
Sur un syndrome de radiculo-névrite avec hyperalbuminose du liquide céphalo-rachidien sans reaction cellulaire. Remarques sur les caractères cliniques et graphiques des réflexes tendineux. *Bull. Soc. méd. Hôp. Paris*, 1916, **40,** 1462–70.
"Guillain–Barré syndrome", acute infective polyneuritis. With J. A. Barré and A. Strohl.

4648 CLELAND, *Sir* John Burton. 1878–1971, & CAMPBELL, Alfred Walter. 1868–1937
The Australian epidemics of an acute polio-encephalomyelitis (X disease). *Rep. Director-Gen. publ. Hlth, New S. Wales*, 1917, 150–280.
Murray Valley encephalitis (Australian X disease). Cleland and Campbell isolated a virus from the cerebral tissue of 3 patients.

4649 CRUCHET, Jean René. 1875– , *et al.*
Quarante cas d'encéphalo-myélite subaiguë. *Bull. Soc. méd. Hôp. Paris*, 1917, 3 sér., **41,** 614–16.
Cruchet's account of epidemic encephalitis was given on April 27, 1917, preceding that of Economo by 13 days. With Moutier and Calmettes.

4650 ECONOMO, Constantin, *Freiherr von San Serff*. 1876–1931
Encephalitis lethargica. *Wien. klin. Wschr.*, 1917, **30,** 581–85.
Economo's classical description of epidemic encephalitis ("von Economo's disease") was published on May 10, 1917; see No. 4649.

4651 LOEWE, Leo. 1896– , & STRAUSS, Israel. 1873–
Etiology of epidemic (lethargic) encephalitis. Preliminary note. *J. Amer. med. Assoc.*, Chicago, 1919, **73,** 1056–57.
Experimental transmission of encephalitis lethargica.

4652 KUNDRATITZ, Karl.
Experimentelle Übertragung von Herpes zoster auf den Menschen und die Beziehungen von Herpes zoster zu Varicellen. *Mschr. Kinderheilk.*, 1925, **29,** 516–23.
First demonstration of the infectivity of herpes.

4653 BALÓ, József. 1896–
A leukoenkephalitis periaxialis concentricaról. *Magy. orv. Arch.*, 1927, **28,** 108–24.
"Baló's disease" – encephalitis periaxialis concentrica. Translation in *Arch. Neurol. Psychiat.* (*Chicago*), 1928, **19,** 242–64.

4654 KANEKO, RENJIRO. 1886– , & AOKI, Y.
Ueber die Encephalitis epidemica in Japan. *Ergebn. inn. Med. Kinderheilk.*, 1928, **34**, 342–456.
Japanese encephalitis distinguished from encephalitis lethargica.

4655 FOTHERGILL, LEROY DRYDEN. 1901– , *et al.*
Human encephalitis caused by the virus of the Eastern variety of equine encephalomyelitis. *New Engl. J. med.*, 1933, **219**, 411.
Isolation of the virus of Eastern equine encephalitis from man. With J. H. Dingle, S. Farber, and M. L. Connerley.

4656 MUCKENFUSS, RALPH S., *et al.*
Encephalitis: studies on experimental transmission. *Publ. Hlth Rep. (Wash.)*, 1933, **48**, 1341–43.
Isolation of the St. Louis encephalitis virus. With C. Armstrong and H. A. McCordock.

4657 HAYASHI, MICHITOMO.
Übertragung des Virus von Encephalitis epidemica auf Affen. *Proc. imp. Acad. Japan*, 1934, **10**, 41–44.
Experimental transmission of Japanese B encephalitis.

4658 SABIN, ALBERT BRUCE. 1906– , & WRIGHT, ARTHUR M.
Acute ascending myelitis following a monkey bite, with the isolation of a virus capable of reproducing the disease. *J. exp. Med.*, 1934, **59**, 115–36.
Herpesvirus simiae (B virus) infection; isolation of the virus.

4659 TANIGUCHI, TENJI. 1889–1961, *et al.*
A virus isolated in 1935 epidemic of summer encephalitis of Japan. *Jap. J. exp. Med.*, 1936, **14**, 185–96.
T. Taniguchi, M. Hosokawa, and S. Kuga established a virus aetiology for Japanese B encephalitis.

4660 HOWITT, BEATRICE FAY. 1891–
Recovery of the virus of equine encephalomyelitis from the brain of a child. *Science*, 1938, **88**, 455–56.
Western equine encephalitis virus recovered from man.

4660.1 ZIL'BER, L. A.
Vesennij (vesenne-letnij) endemičeskij kleščevoj encefalit. [Vernal (verno-aestival) endemic tick-borne encephalitis.] *Arkh. biol. Nauk.*, 1939, **56**, No. 2, 9–37.
Isolation of the virus of spring-summer (Russian Far East) encephalitis.

4661 DURAND, PAUL. 1895–
Virus filtrant pathogène pour l'homme et les animaux de laboratoire, et à affinités meningée et pulmonaire. *Arch. Inst. Pasteur Tunis*, 1940, **29**, 179–227.
"Durand's disease" – D virus infection. Durand isolated the virus from his own blood. See also the paper by G. M. Findlay, *Trans. roy. Soc. trop. Med.*, 1942, **35**, 303–18.

4661.1 JUNGEBLUT, Claus W. 1897– , & SANDERS, Murray. 1910–
Studies of a murine strain of poliomyelitis virus in cotton rats and white mice. *J. exp. Med.*, 1940, **72,** 407–36.
Isolation of encephalomyocarditis virus.

4661.2 LUMSDEN, Leslie Leon. 1875–1946
St. Louis encephalitis in 1933; observations on epidemiological features. *Publ. Hlth Rep.* (*Wash.*), 1958, **73,** 340–53.
In a report to the Surgeon General in 1933, Lumsden concluded that the *Culex* mosquito was the vector of the St. Louis encephalitis virus. His report was not published until 1958.

Poliomyelitis

4662 UNDERWOOD, Michael. 1737–1820
Debility of the lower extremities. In his *Treatise on the diseases of children.* New ed., London, *J. Mathews*, 1789, **2,** 53–57.
First description of infantile paralysis.

4663 BADHAM, John.
Paralysis in childhood. Four remarkable cases of suddenly induced paralysis in the extremities, occurring in children, without any apparent cerebral or cerebro-spinal lesion. *Lond. med. Gaz.*, 1835–36, **17,** 215–18.
Important clinical description.

4664 HEINE, Jacob von. 1799–1879
Beobachtungen über Lähmungszustände der untern Extremitäten und deren Behandlung. Stuttgart, *F. H. Köhler*, 1840.
First description of acute anterior poliomyelitis, which Heine separated from other forms of paralysis; he described the deformities arising from the disease. He also called attention to congenital spastic paraplegia which, following Little's classical description (No. 4691.1), was termed "Little's disease".

4665 CHARCOT, Jean Martin. 1825–1893, & JOFFROY, Alex. 1844–1908
Une observation de paralysie infantile s'accompagnant d'une altération des cornes antérieures de la substance grise de la moelle. *C. R. Soc. Biol.* (*Paris*), (1869), 1870, 5 sér., **1,** 312–15.
First demonstration of the atrophy of the anterior horns of the spinal cord in infantile paralysis, confirming earlier suggestions of von Heine and Duchenne.

4665.1 ERB, Wilhelm Heinrich. 1840–1921
Ueber acute Spinallähmung (Poliomyelitis anterior acuta) bei Erwachsenen und über verwandte spinale Erkrankungen. *Arch. Psychiat. Nervenkr.*, 1875, **5,** 758–91.
Erb was first to use the term "acute anterior poliomyelitis".

4666 LEYDEN, Ernst von. 1832–1910
Ueber Poliomyelitis und Neuritis. *Z. klin. Med.*, 1879–80, **1,** 387–434.
Leyden enjoyed a great reputation as a neurologist, and his paper on poliomyelitis and neuritis is one of his best works. He was one of the founders of the journal in which it appeared.

4667 MEDIN, Oscar. 1847–1927
En epidemi af infantil paralysi. *Hygiea*, Stockholm, 1890, **52,** 657–668.

The epidemic character of poliomyelitis was first noted by Medin. The disease is also known as "Heine–Medin disease" from the descriptions given by these two writers (see also No. 4664).

4668 WICKMAN, Otto Ivar. 1872–1914
Studien über Poliomyelitis acuta. *Arb. path. Inst. Univ. Helsingfors*, 1905, **1,** 109–293.

Wickman was the first to produce evidence confirming the infectious nature of poliomyelitis.

4669 LANDSTEINER, Karl. 1868–1943, & POPPER, Erwin.
Uebertragung der Poliomyelitis acuta auf Affen. *Z. ImmunForsch.*, 1909, **2,** 1 Teil, 377–90.

Landsteiner and Popper were the first to transmit poliomyelitis to monkeys.

4670 FLEXNER, Simon. 1863–1946, & LEWIS, Paul A. 1879–1929
The transmission of acute poliomyelitis to monkeys. *J. Amer. med. Ass.*, 1909, **53,** 1639, 1913.

Monkeys inoculated with the twentieth generation of a filterable virus cultivated by Flexner and Lewis developed poliomyelitis.

4670.1 GAY, Frederick Parker. 1874–1939, & LUCAS, William Palmer. 1880–1960
Anterior poliomyelitis. Methods of diagnosis from spinal fluid and blood in monkeys and in human beings. *Arch. intern. Med.*, 1910, **6,** 330–38.

Gay and Lucas were the first to make accurate cell counts of the spinal fluid in poliomyelitis.

4671 KENNY, Elizabeth. 1886–1952
Infantile paralysis and cerebral diplegia: methods used for the restoration of function. Sydney, *Angus & Robertson*, 1937.

4671.1 ENDERS, John Franklin. 1897– , *et al.*
Cultivation of the Lansing strain of poliomyelitis virus in cultures of various human embryonic tissues. *Science*, 1949, **109,** 85–87.

J. F. Enders, T. H. Weller, and F. C. Robbins grew the poliomyelitis virus in cultures of different tissues. Their method proved of great value in virus research. They shared a Nobel Prize in 1954.

4672 HAMMON, William McDowell. 1904– , *et al.*
Evaluation of Red Cross gamma globulin as a prophylactic agent for poliomyelitis. *J. Amer. med. Ass.*, 1952, **150,** 739–60.

Trial of gamma globulin in the prophylaxis of poliomyelitis. With L. L. Coriell, J. Stokes, P. F. Wehrle, and C. R. Klimt.

4672.1 KOPROWSKI, Hilary. 1916– , *et al.*
Immune responses in human volunteers upon oral administration of a rodent-adapted strain of poliomyelitis virus. *Amer. J. Hyg.*, 1952, **55,** 108–26.

Successful immunization against poliomyelitis with a living attenuated virus vaccine. With G. A. Jervis and T. W. Norton.

4672.2 SALK, JONAS EDWARD. 1914–
Principles of immunization as applied to poliomyelitis and influenza. *Amer. J. publ. Hlth*, 1953, **43**, 1384–98.
Killed-virus vaccine.

4672.3 SABIN, ALBERT BRUCE. 1906–
Characteristics and genetic potentialities of experimentally produced and naturally occurring variants of poliomyelitis virus. *Ann. N.Y. Acad. Sci.*, 1955, **61**, 924–38.
Sabin's live attenuated poliomyelitis virus vaccine.

For bibliography, see No. 5016

Cerebrospinal Meningitis

4673 WILLIS, THOMAS. 1621–1675
A description of an epidemical fever . . . 1661. In his *Practice of physick*, London, *T. Dring*, 1684, Treatise VIII, pp. 46–54.
Willis was probably the first to report an epidemic of cerebrospinal fever.

4674 VIEUSSEUX, GASPARD. 1746–1814
Mémoire sur la maladie qui a régné à Genève au printemps de 1805. *J. Méd. Chir. Pharm.*, 1805, **11**, 163–82.
First definite description of cerebrospinal meningitis.

4675 STRONG, NATHAN. 1781–1837
An inaugural dissertation on the disease termed petechial, or spotted fever. Hartford, *P. B. Gleason*, 1810.
This graduation dissertation was the first published brochure on cerebrospinal meningitis.

4676 NORTH, ELISHA. 1771–1843
A treatise on a malignant epidemic, commonly called spotted fever. New York, *T. & J. Swords*, 1811.
First book on cerebrospinal meningitis; in it North recommended the use of the clinical thermometer, not in general use until the time of Wunderlich. For more information on this book, see the article by F. L. Pleadwell in *Ann. med. Hist.*, 1924, **6**, 245–57.

4677 KERNIG, VLADIMIR MIKHAILOVICH. 1840–1917
Ein Krankheitssymptom der acuten Meningitis. *St. Petersb. med. Wschr.*, 1882, **7**, 398.
Kernig drew attention to a flexor contracture of the leg on attempting to extend it on the thigh ("Kernig's sign"), almost always present in cerebrospinal meningitis and an important diagnostic sign. A fuller description is in *Z. klin. Med.*, 1907 **64**, 19–69.

4678 WEICHSELBAUM, ANTON. 1845–1920
Ueber die Aetiologie der akuten Meningitis cerebro-spinalis. *Fortschr. Med.*, 1887, **5**, 573–83, 620–26.
Weichselbaum discovered the meningococcus, *Neisseria meningitidis*, causative agent of cerebrospinal meningitis.

4679 VOELCKER, ARTHUR FRANCIS. 1861–1946
Middx Hosp. Rep. med. surg. path. Registrars, (1894), 1895, 278.
First description of the Waterhouse–Friderichsen syndrome (Nos. 4685–86). Abstract of a post-mortem report; no title.

4680 HEUBNER, JOHANN OTTO LEONHARD. 1843–1926
Beobachtungen und Versuche über den Meningokokkus intracellularis (Weichselbaum-Jaeger). *Jb. Kinderheilk.*, 1896, **43**, 1–22.
Heubner was the first to isolate meningococci from the cerebrospinal fluid of living beings.

4681 SLAWYK.
Ein Fall von Allgemeininfection mit Influenzabacillen. *Z. Hyg. InfektKr.*, 1899, **32**, 443–48.
First description of influenzal meningitis.

4682 JOCHMANN, GEORG. 1874–1915
Versuche zur Serodiagnostik und Serotherapie der epidemischen Genickstarre. *Dtsch. med. Wschr.*, 1906, **32**, 788–93.
First attempts at the serum treatment of cerebrospinal meningitis.

4683 FLEXNER, SIMON. 1863–1946
Concerning a serum therapy for experimental infection with Diplococcus intracellularis. *J. exp. Med.*, 1907, **9**, 168–85.
Flexner prepared an antiserum for use in cerebrospinal meningitis.

4684 ——, & JOBLING, JAMES WESLEY. 1876–
Serum treatment of epidemic cerebro-spinal meningitis. *J. exp. Med.*, 1908, **10**, 141–203.

4685 WATERHOUSE, RUPERT. 1873–1958
A case of suprarenal apoplexy. *Lancet*, 1911, **1**, 577–78.
Waterhouse–Friderichsen syndrome (see also Nos. 4679, 4686).

4686 FRIDERICHSEN, CARL. 1886–
Nebennierenapoplexie bei kleinen Kindern. *Jb. Kinderheilk.*, 1918, **87**, 109–25.
See No. 4685.

4687 WALLGREN, ARVID JOHAN. 1889–
Une nouvelle maladie infectieuse du système nerveux central? *Acta paediat.* (*Stockh.*), 1924, **4**, 158–82.
Acute lymphocytic choriomeningitis (aseptic meningitis syndrome) first described.

4688 ARMSTRONG, CHARLES. 1886– , & LILLIE, RALPH DOUGALL. 1896–
Experimental lymphocytic choriomeningitis of monkeys and mice produced by a virus encountered in studies of the 1933 St. Louis encephalitis epidemic. *Publ. Hlth Rep.* (*Wash.*), 1934, **49**, 1019–27.
Isolation of the virus of benign lymphocytic chriomeningitis.

4689 SCHWENTKER, FRANCIS FREDERIC. 1904– , *et al.*
The treatment of meningococcic meningitis with sulfanilamide. *J. Amer. med. Ass.*, 1937, **108**, 1407–08.
With S. Gelman and P. H. Long.

4689.1 ROSENBERG, DAVID HARRY. 1903– , & ARLING, PHILIP ARTHUR. 1908–
Penicillin in the treatment of meningitis. *J. Amer. med. Ass.*, 1944, **125**, 1011–17.

4690–4771 DEGENERATIVE DISORDERS

4690 PARKINSON, JAMES. 1755–1824
An essay on the shaking palsy. London, *Whittingham & Rowland*, 1817.
"Parkinson's disease"—paralysis agitans. Reprinted in *Med. Classics*, 1938, **2**, 964–97. Facsimile reproduction, 1959.

4691 DUNGLISON, ROBLEY. 1798–1869
Practice of medicine. Vol. 2. Philadelphia, *Lea & Blanchard*, 1842.
A case of chronic hereditary chorea in adults ("Huntington's chorea", see No. 4699) is described on pp. 321–23. This is in the form of a letter from Charles Oscar Waters (1816–1892).

4691.1 LITTLE, WILLIAM JOHN. 1810–1894
Course of lectures on the deformities of the human frame. Lecture IX. *Lancet*, 1843–44, **1**, 350–54.
Little's description of congenital cerebral spastic diplegia resulted in the condition being named "Little's disease".

4692 FRERICHS, FRIEDRICH THEODOR. 1819–1885
Ueber Hirnsklerose. *Arch. ges. Med.*, 1849, **10**, 334–50.
First important account of disseminated sclerosis. Carswell (No. 2291) and Cruveilhier (No. 2286) both gave illustrations of the disease; the latter is also accredited with the first description.

4693 ——. Klinik der Leberkrankheiten. Bd. 2. Braunschweig, *F. Vieweg u. Sohn*, 1861.
Pp. 62–64: First description of progressive familial hepatolenticular degeneration ("Kinnier Wilson's disease"; see No. 4717).

4695 GULL, *Sir* WILLIAM WITHEY. 1816–1890
Case of progressive atrophy of the muscles of the hands: enlargement of the ventricle of the cord in the cervical region, with atrophy of the gray matter. *Guy's Hosp. Rep.*, 1862, **8**, 244–50.
First description of syringomyelia.

4696 FRIEDREICH, NIKOLAUS. 1825–1882
Ueber degenerative Atrophie der spinalen Hinterstränge. *Virchows Arch. path. Anat.*, 1863, **26**, 391–419, 433–59; **27**, 1–26; 1876, **68**, 145–245; 1877, **70**, 140–52.
Friedreich was the first to describe a form of ataxia ("Friedreich's ataxia"), hereditary, attended with impairment of speech, lateral curvature of the spine, and with paralysis of the muscles of the lower limbs. The titles of the last two papers vary.

4697 CLARKE, JACOB AUGUSTUS LOCKHART. 1817–1880, & JACKSON, JOHN HUGHLINGS. 1835–1911
On a case of muscular atrophy, with disease of the spinal cord and medulla oblongata. *Med.-chir. Trans.*, 1867, **50**, 489–96.
First important account of syringomyelia.

4698 CHARCOT, JEAN MARTIN. 1825–1893
Histologie de la sclérose en plaques. *Gaz. Hop. (Paris)*, 1868, **41**, 554–55, 557–58, 566.
An important description of disseminated sclerosis.

4699 HUNTINGTON, George. 1850–1916
On chorea. *Med. surg. Reporter*, 1872, **26,** 317–21.

The classical description by Huntington of the chronic degenerative hereditary type of chorea led to the eponym "Huntington's chorea". The writer appears to have been ignorant of the earlier accounts of Waters (No. 4691) and I. W. Lyon (*Amer. med. Times*, 1863, 7, 289–90).

4700 BOURNEVILLE, Désiré Magloire. 1840–1909
Contribution à l'étude de l'idiotie. *Arch. Neurol.* (*Paris*), 1880, **1,** 69–91.

"Bourneville's disease", tuberous sclerosis, epiloia (p. 81).

4701 MORVAN, Augustin Marie. 1819–1897
De la parésie analgésique à panaris des extrémités supérieures ou paréso-analgésie des extrémités supérieures. *Gaz. hebd. Méd.*, 1883, n.s., **20,** 580–83, 590–94, 624–26, 721–22.

First description of "Morvan's disease" – a form of syringomyelia.

4702 WESTPHAL. Carl Friedrich Otto. 1833–1890
Ueber eine dem Bilde der cerebrospinalen grauen Degeneration ähnliche Erkrankung des centralen Nervensystems ohne anatomischen Befund, nebst einigen Bemerkungen über paradoxe Contraction. *Arch. Psychiat. Nervenkr.*, 1883, **14,** 87–134.

"Westphal's pseudosclerosis." Later Strümpells' description of this condition (No. 4709) led to the eponym "Westphal – Strümpell disease".

4703 PELIZAEUS, Friedrich. 1850–
Über eine eigentümliche Form spastischer Lähmung mit Cerebralerscheinungen auf hereditärer Grundlage. (Multiple Sklerose.) *Arch. Psychiat. Nervenkr.*, 1885, **16,** 698–710.

"Pelizaeus–Merzbacher disease" (see No. 4715).

4704 STRÜMPELL, Ernst Adolf Gustav Gottfried. 1853–1925
Ueber eine bestimmte Form der primären combinirten Systemerkrankungen des Rückenmarks. *Arch. Psychiat. Nervenkr.*, 1886, **17,** 217–38.

"Strümpell's disease" – hereditary spastic spinal paralysis, previously described by Erb and by Charcot.

4705 SACHS, Bernard. 1858–1944
On arrested cerebral development, with special reference to its cortical pathology. *J. nerv. ment. Dis.*, 1887, **14,** 541–53.

Sachs described the cerebral changes in amaurotic familial idiocy. Earlier, Tay (No. 5918) had recorded the ocular manifestations of this condition, which became known as "Tay–Sachs disease". Two further papers on the subject by Sachs are in the same journal, 1892, **17**, 603–07; 1986, **21**, 475–79.

4706 KAHLER, Otto. 1849–1893
Ueber die Diagnose der Syringomyelie. *Prag. med. Wschr.*, 1888, **13,** 45, 63.

First complete description of syringomyelia.

4707 PICK, Arnold. 1851–1924
Ueber die Beziehungen der senilen Hirnatrophie zur Aphasie. *Prag. med. Wschr.*, 1892, **17,** 165–67.

"Pick's disease" – circumscribed atrophy of the brain with the development of aphasia presenile dementia.

4708 PUTNAM, JAMES WRIGHT.
A case of complete athetosis with post-mortem. *J. nerv. ment. Dis.*, 1892, n.s. **17,** 124–26.
One of the earliest accounts of bilateral athetosis ("Vogt syndrome").

4708.1 FREUD, SIGMUND. 1856–1939
Die infantile Cerebrallähmung. Wien, *A. Hölder*, 1897.
Freud gave an excellent description of the various forms of cerebral palsy, with precise classification of the different spastic symptoms; he also mentioned the extra-pyramidal symptoms. Forms Bd. IX, II Theil, II Abt. of H. Nothnagel's *Specielle Pathologie und Therapie.*

4709 STRÜMPELL, ERNST ADOLF GUSTAV GOTTFRIED. 1853–1925
Ueber die Westphal'sche Pseudosklerose und über diffuse Hirnsklerose, insbesondere bei Kindern. *Dtsch. Z. Nervenheilk.*, 1898, **12,** 115–49.
"Westphal–Strümpell disease" – pseudosclerosis of the brain. (See also No. 4702.) Probably cases of Kinnier Wilson's disease.

4710 RUSSELL, JAMES SAMUEL RISIEN. 1863–1939, *et al.*
Subacute combined degeneration of the spinal cord. *Brain*, 1900, **23,** 39–110.
First full description. With F. E. Batten and J. S. Collier.

4711 MILLS, CHARLES KARSNER. 1845–1931
A case of unilateral progressive ascending paralysis, probably representing a new form of degenerative disease. *J. nerv. ment. Dis.*, 1900, **27,** 195–200.
First description of unilateral progressive ascending paralysis ("Mills' disease").

4712 BATTEN, FREDERICK EUSTACE. 1865–1918
Cerebral degeneration with symmetrical changes in the maculae in two members of a family. *Trans. ophthal. Soc. U.K.*, 1903, **23,** 386–90.
See No. 4713.

4713 MAYOU, MARMADUKE STEPHEN. 1876–1934
Cerebral degeneration, with symmetrical changes in the maculae, in three members of a family. *Trans. ophthal. Soc. U.K.*, 1904, **24,** 142–145.
"Batten–Mayou disease", juvenile amaurotic idiocy (see also No. 4712).

4714 MILLS, CHARLES KARSNER. 1845–1931
Unilateral ascending paralysis and unilateral descending paralysis. *J. Amer. med. Ass.*, 1906, **47,** 1638–45.
First description of unilateral descending paralysis.

4715 MERZBACHER, LUDWIG. 1875–
Weitere Mitteilungen über eine eigenartige hereditär-familiäre Erkrankung des Zentralnervensystems. *Med. Klin.*, 1908, **4,** 1952–55.
"Pelizaeus–Merzbacher disease", familial centrolobar sclerosis (see also No. 4703).

4716 SCHWALBE, MARCUS WALTER. 1883–
Eine eigentümliche tonische Krampfform mit hysterischen Symptomen. *Inaug. Diss.*, Berlin, 1907.
First description of torsion-spasm, dystonia musculorum deformans; also called "Ziehen–Oppenheim disease" following reports of cases by these writers in *Neurol. Zbl.*, 1911, **30**, 109, 1090.

4717 WILSON, SAMUEL ALEXANDER KINNIER. 1878–1937
Progressive lenticular degeneration, a familial nervous disease associated with cirrhosis of the liver. *Brain*, 1912, **34,** 295–509.
Classical description of progressive familial hepatolenticular degeneration ("Wilson's disease"), first described by Frerichs in 1861 (see No. 4693), now considered to be a disorder of copper metabolism.

4718 DAWSON, JAMES WALKER. 1870–1927
The histology of disseminated sclerosis. *Trans. roy. Soc. Edinb.* (1913–14), 1916, **50,** 517–740.
A classical monograph on the pathology of disseminated sclerosis.

4719 VILLARET, MAURICE. 1877–1946
Le syndrome nerveux de l'espace rétro-parotidien postérieur. *Rev. neurol. (Paris)*, 1916, **23,** pt. 1, 188–90.
"Villaret's syndrome."

4720 VOGT, CECILE. 1875– , & VOGT, OSKAR. 1870–1959
Zur Lehre der Erkrankungen des striären Systems. *J. Psychol. Neurol. (Lpz.)*, 1920, **25,** Ergänzht iii, 627–846.
"Vogt syndrome", disease of the corpora striata.

4721 FOIX, CHARLES. 1882–1927
Les lésions anatomiques de la maladie de Parkinson. *Rev. neurol. (Paris)*, 1921, **28,** 593–600.
Foix and his colleagues showed that the specific lesion in Parkinson's disease is in the substantia nigra of the mid-brain.

4722 JAKOB, ALFONS MARIA. 1884–1931
Ueber eigenartige Erkrankungen der Zentralnervensystems mit bemerkenswertem anatomischem Befunde. *Z. ges. Neurol. Psychiat.*, 1921, **64,** Orig., 147–228.
"Creutzfeldt–Jakob disease", spastic pseudosclerosis. See also the same journal, 1920, **57,** 1–18.

4723 SOUQUES, ACHILLE ALEXANDRE. 1860–1944
Rapport sur les syndromes parkinsoniens. *Rev. neurol. (Paris)*, 1921, **28,** 534–73.
Souques recognized the importance of encephalitis lethargica as a cause of parkinsonism; more than any other neurologist he was responsible for unifying its diverse manifestations.

4724 HALLERVORDEN, JULIUS. 1882– , & SPATZ, HUGO. 1888–
Eigenartige Erkrankung im extrapyramidalen System mit besonderer Beteiligung des Globus pallidus und der Substantia nigra. *Z. ges. Neurol.*, 1922, **79,** 254–302.
The (extrapyramidal) syndrome of Hallervorden and Spatz.

4725 VINCENT, CLOVIS. 1879–1947, & BOGAERT, LUDO VAN. 1897–
Contribution à l'étude des syndromes du globe pâle. La dégénérescence progressive du globe pâle et de la portion réticulée de la substance noire (maladie d'Hallervorden-Spatz). *Rev. neurol. (Paris)*, 1936, **65,** 921–59.
Clovis Vincent, a pioneer French neurosurgeon, contributed a valuable study of Hallervorden–Spatz disease.

4726 GRÜNTHAL, Ernst.
Ueber Parpanit, einen neuen extrapyramidal-motorische Störungen beeinflussenden Stoff. *Schweiz. med. Wschr.*, 1946, **76,** 1286–89.
Introduction of caramiphen ("parpanit") in the treatment of Parkinson's disease.

4727 SIGWALD, Jean. 1903– , *et al.*
Le traitement de la maladie de Parkinson par le chlorhydrate de diéthylaminoéthyl-N-thiodiphénylamine (2987 R.P.). Premiers résultats. *Rev. neurol.* (*Paris*), 1946, **78,** 581–84.
Introduction of "diparcol" in the treatment of Parkinson's disease. With D. Bovet and G. Dumont.

4728 ——. Un nouveau médicament symptomatique des syndromes parkinsoniens: le chlorhydrate de [(diéthylamino-2'-méthyl-2') éthyl-1-'] N-dibenzoparathiazine. *Presse méd.*, 1949, **57,** 819–20.
Introduction of ethopropazine ("lysivane") in the treatment of Parkinson's disease.

4729 CORBIN, Kendall Brooks. 1907–
Trihexyphenidyl. Evaluation of the new agent in the treatment of parkinsonism. *J. Amer. med. Ass.*, 1949, **141,** 377–82.
Clinical introduction of benzhexol ("artane") in Parkinson's disease.

Myopathies

4730 WILLIS, Thomas. 1621–1675
The London practice of physick. London, *T. Basset,* 1685.
A probable description of myasthenia gravis is on p. 431.

4731 FREKE, John. 1688–1756
A case of extraordinary exostoses on the back of a boy. *Phil. Trans.*, 1740, **41,** 369–70.
Probably the earliest description of myositis ossificans progressiva. Freke was a friend of Fielding, who mentioned him in *Tom Jones.*

4732 DUCHENNE DE BOULOGNE, Guillaume Benjamin Amand. 1806–1875
Recherches faites à l'aide du galvanisme sur l'état de la contractilité et de la sensibilité électro-musculaires dans les paralysies des membres supérieurs. *C. R. Acad. Sci.* (*Paris*), 1849, **29,** 667–70.
"Aran–Duchenne disease," progressive muscular atrophy, with which the name of Cruveilhier is also associated. A fuller account is included in Duchenne's *Electrisation localisée*, 1861, 437–547.

4733 ARAN, François Amilcar. 1817–1861
Recherches sur une maladie non encore décrite du système musculaire. (Atrophie musculaire progressive). *Arch. gén. Méd.*, 1850, 4 sér., **24,** 4–35, 172–214.
"Aran–Duchenne disease" (see No. 4732).

4734 CRUVEILHIER, Jean. 1791–1874
Sur la paralysie musculaire, progressive, atrophique. *Bull. Acad. Méd.* (*Paris*), 1852–53, **18,** 490–502, 546–83.
"Cruveilhier's palsy", the progressive muscular atrophy already described by Duchenne and Aran. The slimness of the anterior roots was first noticed by Cruveilhier and was thought to be the essential lesion until Luys (No. 4737) reported degeneration of the anterior horn cells.

4735 LITTLE, William John. 1810–1894
On the nature and treatment of the deformities of the human frame. London, *Longman*, 1853.
Early description of progressive muscular atrophy (p. 14).

4736 DUCHENNE DE BOULOGNE, Guillaume Benjamin Amand. 1806–1875
Paralysie musculaire progressive de la langue, du voile du palais et des lèvres; affection non encore décrite comme espèce morbide distincte. *Arch. gén. Méd.*, 1860, 5 sér., **16,** 283–96, 431–45.
First description of chronic progressive bulbar paralysis ("Duchenne's paralysis").

4737 LUYS, Jules Bernard. 1828–1897
Atrophie musculaire progressive. Lésions histologiques de la substance grise de la moelle épinière. *Gaz. méd. Paris,* 1860, 3 sér., **15,** 505.
Luys was the first to note the degeneration of the anterior horn cells in progressive muscular atrophy.

4738 GRIESINGER, Wilhelm. 1817–1868
Ueber Muskelhypertrophie. *Arch. Heilk.*, 1865, **6,** 1–13.
Progressive muscular atrophy with pseudo-hypertrophy. From the description given later by Duchenne (No. 4739) the condition has been named "Duchenne–Griesinger disease".

4739 DUCHENNE DE BOULOGNE, Guillaume Benjamin Amand. 1806–1875
Recherches sur la paralysie musculaire pseudo-hypertrophique, ou paralysie myo-sclérosique. *Arch. gén. Méd.*, 1868, 6 sér., **11,** 5–25, 179–209, 305–21, 421–43, 552–88.
(See No. 4738.)

4740 CHARCOT, Jean Martin. 1825–1893, & JOFFROY, Alex. 1844–1908
Deux cas d'atrophie musculaire progressive avec lésions de la sub-sistance grise et des faisceaux antéro-latéraux de la moelle épinière. *Arch. Physiol. norm. path.*, 1869, **2,** 744–60.
Description of the lesions of the spinal cord in muscular atrophy.

4741 MÜNCHMEYER, Ernst. 1846–1880
Ueber Myositis ossificans progressiva. *Z. rat. Med.*, 1869, 3 R., **34,** 9–41.
Münchmeyer described a form of progressive ossifying myositis ("Münchmeyer's disease").

4742 CHARCOT, Jean Martin. 1825–1893
Des amyotrophies spinales chroniques. *Progr. méd.*, 1874, **2,** 573–74.
Charcot differentiated between the ordinary (Aran–Duchenne) type of muscular atrophy and the rarer amyotrophic lateral sclerosis, at one time called "Charcot's disease".

4743 LEYDEN, Ernst von. 1832–1910
Klinik der Rückenmarks-Krankheiten. Bd. 2. Berlin, *A. Hirschwald,* 1786.
First description of myotonia congenita (p. 550).

4744 THOMSEN, ASMUS JULIUS THOMAS. 1815–1896
Tonische Krämpfe in willkürlich beweglichen Muskeln in Folge von ererbter psychischer Disposition (Ataxia muscularis?). *Arch. Psychiat. Nervenkr.*, 1876, **6**, 702–18.

Thomsen, himself a sufferer from myotonia congenita, gave the first full description of the condition, which later became known as "Thomsen's disease".

4745 WILKS, *Sir* SAMUEL, *Bart.* 1824–1911
On cerebritis, hysteria, and bulbar paralysis, as illustrative of arrest of function of the cerebro-spinal centres. *Guy's Hosp. Rep.*, 1877, 3 ser., **22**, 7–55.

The case of "bulbar paralysis" (pp. 45–55) is believed to be the first definite record of myasthenia gravis.

4746 ERB, WILHELM HEINRICH. 1840–1921
Ueber einen eigenthümlichen bulbären (?) Symptomenkomplex. *Arch. Psychiat. Nervenkr.*, 1879, **9**, 172–73.

Myasthenia gravis ("Erb–Goldflam disease"; see also No. 4757). A further paper on the subject by Erb appears in the above volume, pp. 325–50.

4747 ——. Ueber die juvenile Form der progressiven Muskelatrophie und ihre Beziehungen zur sogenannten Pseudohypertrophie der Muskeln. *Dtsch. Arch. klin. Med.*, 1884, **34**, 467–519.

Progressive muscular dystrophy ("Erb's muscular atrophy"). Erb did much to establish the modern conception of the muscular dystrophies.

4748 DEJERINE-KLUMPKE, AUGUSTA. 1859–1927
Contribution à l'étude des paralysies radiculaires du plexus brachial. *Rev. Méd.*, 1885, **5**, 591–616, 739–90.

First description of atrophic paralysis of the muscles of the hand following lesion of the brachial plexus and eighth cervical and first dorsal nerves ("Klumpke's paralysis").

4749 CHARCOT, JEAN MARTIN. 1825–1893, & MARIE, PIERRE. 1853–1940
Saur une forme particulière d'atrophie musculaire progressive souvent familiale débutant par les pieds et les jambes et atteignant plus tard les mains. *Rev. Méd.*, 1886, **6**, 97–138.

First description of the peroneal form of muscular atrophy, the so-called Charcot–Marie–Tooth type.

4750 TOOTH, HOWARD HENRY. 1856–1925
The peroneal type of progressive muscular atrophy. London, *H. K. Lewis*, 1886.

Tooth described peroneal muscular atrophy independently of, and in the same year as, Charcot and Marie.

4751 GOWERS, *Sir* WILLIAM RICHARD. 1845–1915
A manual of diseases of the nervous system. Vol. 1. London, *J. & A. Churchill*, 1886.

Page 365: first description of local panatrophy. See also *Rev. Neurol. Psychiat. (Edinb.)*, 1903, **1**, 3–4.

4752 LANDOUZY, LOUIS THÉOPHILE JOSEPH. 1845–1917, & DEJERINE, JOSEPH JULES. 1849–1917
Contribution à l'étude de la myopathie atrophique progressive (myopathie atrophique progressive, à type scapulo-huméral). *C. R. Soc. Biol. (Paris)*, 1886, 8 sér., **3**, 478–81.

"Landouzy–Dejerine type" of progressive muscular dystrophy.

4753 DANA, CHARLES LOOMIS. 1852–1935
An atypical case of Thomsen's disease (myotonia congenita). *Med. Rec.* (*N.Y.*), 1888, **33**, 433–35.
Dana described a combination of myotonia and muscular atrophy.

4754 DÉLÉAGE, FRANCISQUE. 1862–
Étude clinique sur la maladie de Thomsen (myotonie congénitale). Paris, *Thèse No.* 385, 1890; *O. Doin*, 1890.
First description of dystrophia myotonica ("Déléage's disease").

4755 WERDNIG, GUIDO. 1862–
Zwei frühinfantile hereditäre Fälle von progressiver Muskelatrophie unter dem Bilde der Dystrophie, aber auf neurotischer Grundlage. *Arch. Psychiat. Nervenkr.*, 1891, **22**, 437–80.
"Werdnig–Hoffmann muscular atrophy," an infantile familial form of progressive muscular atrophy. Hoffmann independently described it (see No. 4756).

4756 HOFFMANN, JOHANN. 1857–1919
Ueber chronische spinale Muskelatrophie im Kindesalter, auf familiärer Basis. *Dtsch. Z. Nervenheilk.*, 1891, **1**, 95–120; 1893, **3**, 427–70.
"Hoffmann's muscular atrophy" – independently described by Werdnig (No. 4755).

4757 GOLDFLAM, SAMUEL VULFOVICH. 1852–1932
Ueber einen scheinbar heilbaren bulbärparalytischen Symptomencomplex mit Betheiligung der Extremitäten. *Dtsch. Z. Nervenheilk.*, 1893, **4**, 312–52.
Myasthenia pseudoparalytica (Erb–Goldflam symptom complex). See No. 4746.

4758 CHARCOT, JEAN BAPTISTE AUGUSTE ÉTIENNE. 1867–1936
Contribution à l'étude de l'atrophie musculaire progressive type Duchenne-Aran. Paris, *Thèse No.* 313, 1895.

4759 MARIE, PIERRE. 1853–1940
Existe-t-il une atrophie musculaire progressive Aran-Duchenne? *Rev. neurol.* (*Paris*), 1897, **5**, 686–90.
Marie disbelieved in the Aran–Duchenne type of muscular progressive atrophy.

4760 OPPENHEIM, HERMANN. 1858–1919
Ueber allgemeine und localisierte Atonie der Muskulatur (Myatonie) im frühen Kindesalter. *Mschr. Psychiat. Neurol.*, 1900, **8**, 232–33.
First description of "Oppenheim's disease" – amyotonia congenita.

4761 WEIGERT, CARL. 1845–1904
Pathologisch-anatomischer Beitrag zur Erb'schen Krankheit (Myasthenia gravis). *Neurol. Zbl.*, 1901, **20**, 597–601.
Weigert noted the connexion of myasthenia gravis with hypertrophy of the thymus.

4762 GOWERS, *Sir* WILLIAM RICHARD. 1845–1915
On myopathy and a distal form. *Brit. med. J.*, 1902, **2**, 89–92.
"Distal myopathy of Gowers", a form of progressive muscular dystrophy.

4763 CRUCHET, JEAN RENÉ. 1875–
Traité des torticolis spasmodiques. Paris, *Masson*, 1907.
In this classical monograph, 357 cases of torticollis are recorded.

4764 SAUERBRUCH, Ernst Ferdinand. 1875–1951
Thymektomie bei einem Fall von Morbus Basedowi mit Myasthenie. *Mitt. Grenzgeb. Med. Chir.*, 1912–13, **25**, 746–65.
Thymectomy for myasthenia gravis. Reported by C. H. Schumacher and –. Roth.

4765 EDGEWORTH, Harriet Isabel. 1892–
A report of progress on the use of ephedrine in a case of myasthenia gravis. *J. Amer. med. Ass.*, 1930, **94**, 1136.
Harriet Edgeworth discovered by accident the beneficial effect of ephedrine in myasthenia gravis.

4766 BOOTHBY, Walter Meredith. 1880–1953
Myasthenia gravis: a preliminary report on the effect of treatment with glycine. *Proc. Mayo Clin.*, 1932, **7**, 557–62.
Introduction of glycine (glycocoll) in the treatment of myasthenia gravis.

4767 REMEN, Lazar. 1907–
Zur Pathogenese und Therapie der Myasthenie gravis pseudoparalytica. *Dtsch. Z. Nervenheilk.*, 1932, **128**, 66–78.
Introduction of prostigmine in the treatment of myasthenia gravis.

4768 WALKER, Mary Broadfoot. 1888–1974
Treatment of myasthenia gravis with physostigmine. *Lancet*, 1934, **1**, 1200–01.
Introduction of physostigmine in treatment of myasthenia gravis.

4769 LAURENT, Louis Philippe Eugene, & WALTHER, William Werner.
The influence of large doses of potassium chloride on myasthenia gravis. *Lancet*, 1935, **1**, 1434–35.
Potassium salts first used in treatment of myasthenia gravis.

4770 MINOT, Ann Stone. 1894– , *et al.*
The response of the myasthenic state to guanidine hydrochloride. *Science*, 1938, **87**, 348–50.
Guanidine first used in treatment of myasthenia gravis. With K. Dodd and S. S. Riven.

4771 BLALOCK, Alfred. 1899–1964, *et al.*
Myasthenia gravis and tumors of the thymic region. Report of a case in which the tumor was removed. *Ann. Surg.*, 1939, **110**, 544–61.
First deliberate treatment of myasthenia gravis by thymectomy. With M. F. Mason, H. J. Morgan, and S. S. Riven.

4772–4806 NEUROSYPHILIS

4772 LOEWENHARDT, Sigismund Eduard. 1796–1875
De myelophthisi chronica vera et notha. Berolini, *typ. Haynianis*, [1817].
First important account of tabes dorsalis.

4773 HORN, Wilhelm von. 1803–1871
De tabe dorsuali praelusio. Berolini, *formis Krausianis*, [1827].
Gives the views of his father, Ernst Horn [1744–1848], on tabes.

4774 DUCHENNE DE BOULOGNE, GUILLAUME BENJAMIN AMAND. 1806–1875
De l'ataxie locomotrice progressive. *Arch. gén. Méd.*, 1858, 5 sér., **12,** 641–52; 1859, **13,** 36–62, 158–81, 417–51.
Although far from being the first to describes tabes dorsalis, Duchenne gave a classical account of the condition, earning the eponym "Duchenne's disease".

4775 CHARCOT, JEAN MARTIN. 1825–1893, & BOUCHARD, ABEL. 1833–1899
Douleurs fulgurantes de l'ataxie sans incoordination des mouvements; sclérose commençante des cordons postérieurs de la moelle épinière. *Gaz. méd. Paris,* 1866, 3 sér., **21,** 122–24.
First clinical description of the electric pains in tabes.

4776 DELAMARRE, GEORGES.
Des troubles gastriques dans l'ataxie locomotrice progressive. Paris, *Thèse No.* 250, 1866.
Tabetic gastric crises first described.

4777 CHARCOT, JEAN MARTIN. 1825–1893
Sur quelques arthropathies qui paraissent dépendre d'une lésion du cerveau ou de la moëlle épinière. *Arch. Physiol. norm. path.*, 1868, **1,** 161–78.
Charcot called attention to tabetic arthropathy, which has since then borne his name, while the tabetic joints he so well described are known as "Charcot's joints".

4778 ALLBUTT, *Sir* THOMAS CLIFFORD. 1836–1925
Case of cerebral disease in a syphilitic patient. *St George's Hosp. Rep.*, 1868, **3,** 55–65.
Syphilitic endarteritis of cerebral arteries described.

4779 ——. Remarks on a case of locomotor ataxy with hydrarthrosis. *St George's Hosp. Rep.*, 1869, **4,** 259–60.
An early description of the joint symptoms in tabes dorsalis.

4780 ERB, WILHELM HEINRICH. 1840–1921
Ueber Sehnenreflexe bei Gesunden und bei Rückenmarkskranken. *Arch. Psychiat. Nervenkr.*, 1875, **5,** 792–802.
Knee-jerk first used as diagnostic measure in tabes dorsalis.

4781 WESTPHAL, CARL FRIEDRICH OTTO. 1833–1890
Ueber einige durch mechanische Einwirkung auf Sehnen und Muskeln hervorgebrachte Bewegungs-Erscheinungen. *Arch. Psychiat. Nervenkr.*, 1875, **5,** 803–34.
Westphal discovered the diagnostic value of the knee-jerk simultaneously with Erb.

4782 FOURNIER, JEAN ALFRED. 1832–1914
De l'ataxie locomotrice d'origine syphilitique. Paris, *G. Masson,* 1876.
Fournier advanced the doctrine of the syphilitic origin of tabes, a hypothesis which was opposed for a time.

4783 LEICHTENSTERN, OTTO MICHAEL. 1845–1900
Ueber progressive perniciöse Anämie bei Tabeskranken. *Dtsch. med. Wschr.*, 1884, **10** 849.
First description of subacute combined degeneration of the spinal cord.

4784 DEJERINE, JOSEPH JULES. 1849–1917
Sur un cas de paraplégie par névrites périphériques, chez un ataxique morphiomane. *C. R. Soc. Biol.* (*Paris*), 1887, 8 sér., **4,** 137–43.
First description of peripheral neuritis, "Dejerine's neurotabes".

4785 ——. Sur l'atrophie musculaire des ataxiques. Paris, *F. Alcan*, 1889.
Dejerine ranks high in French neurology. He became clinical chief at the Salpêtrière. He separated peripheral from medullary tabes, wrote on the tabetic muscular atrophies, on the parietal lobe syndrome, and made many other contributions to neurological literature.

4786 FRENKEL, HEINRICH. 1860–1931
Die Therapie atactischer Bewegungsstörungen. *Münch. med. Wschr.*, 1890, **37,** 917–20.
Frenkel devised certain muscular exercises for use in the treatment of tabes dorsalis.

4787 LEYDEN, ERNST VON. 1832–1910
Ueber acute Ataxie. *Z. klin. Med.*, 1891, **18,** 576–87.
"Leyden's (acute) ataxia."

4788 ERB, WILHELM HEINRICH. 1840–1921
Ueber syphilitische Spinalparalyse. *Neurol. Zbl.*, 1892, **11,** 161–68.
Erb's classical description of syphilitic spinal paralysis, sometimes called "Erb's disease".

4789 ——. Die Aetiologie der Tabes. *Samml. klin. Vortr.*, 1892, N.F., Nr. 53. (Inn. Med. Nr. 18), 515–42.
English translation, 1900.

4790 MARIE, PIERRE. 1853–1940
Sur l'hérédo-ataxie cérébelleuse. *Sem. méd.* (*Paris*), 1893, **13,** 444–47.
Original description of hereditary cerebellar ataxia.

4791 PEL, PIETER KLUZES. 1852–1919
Augenkrisen bei Tabes dorsalis. *Berl. klin. Wschr.*, 1898, **35,** 25–27.
"Pel's crises" – the ocular crises in tabes.

4792 NONNE, MAX. 1861–
Syphilis und Nervensystem. Berlin, *S. Karger*, 1902.

General Paralysis

4793 WILLIS, THOMAS. 1621–1675
De anima brutorum. Oxonii, *R. Davis*, 1672.
Part 2, chap. IX includes a description of general paralysis, probably the first definite recognition of the condition. English translation in his *Practice of physick*, London, 1684, Treatise XI, pp. 161–78.

4794 HASLAM, JOHN. 1764–1844
Observations on insanity. *F. & C. Rivington*, 1798.
Haslam was among the first to describe general paralysis; he recorded 3 cases (pp. 64, 67, 92, 120).

4795 BAYLE, ANTOINE LAURENT JESSÉ. 1799–1858
Recherches sur l'arachnitis chronique. Paris, *Thèse No.* 247, 1822.
Bayle was a most distinguished physician and pathologist. His classical description of dementia paralytica, the first clear delineation of general paralysis, led to the eponym "Bayle's disease". English translation in *Arch. Neurol. Psychiat.* (*Chicago*), 1934, **32,** 84.

4796 DELAYE, J. B.

Considérations sur une espèce de paralysie qui affecte particulièrement les aliénés. Paris, *Thèse No.* 224, 1824.

Delaye, a pupil of Esquirol, selected for his thesis the subject of "incomplete general paralysis of the insane", which he differentiated from other forms of paralysis. He recorded the early signs of the disease, emphasizing the speech disturbance.

4797 CALMEIL, Louis Florentin. 1798–1895

De la paralysie considérée chez les aliénés. Paris, *J. B. Baillière*, 1826.

Classical description of general paralysis.

4798 ESQUIROL, Jean Etienne Dominique. 1772–1840

Des maladies mentales. Tom. 2. Paris, *J. B. Baillière*, 1838.

Contains, p. 264, a classical description of paresis. Esquirol regarded general paralysis as a complication of various forms of mental disorder.

4799 CLOUSTON, *Sir* Thomas Smith. 1841–1915

A case of general paralysis at the age of sixteen. *J. ment. Sci.*, 1877, **23,** 419–20.

Clouston, eminent English psychiatrist, was the first definitely to recognize the relationship between paresis and congenital syphilis and to report a case. This paper is also of interest as being the only recorded case of juvenile paresis at the time Ibsen wrote *Ghosts*, with its excellent portrayal of the condition in the person of Oswald Alving.

4800 FOURNIER, Jean Alfred. 1832–1914

Les affections parasyphilitiques. Paris, *Rueff & Cie.*, 1894.

Fournier, great French venereologist, introduced the concept of "parasyphilis". He showed statistically the causal relationship of syphilis to paresis and tabes.

4801 RAECKE, Julius. 1872–1930

Paralyse und Tabes bei Eheleuten. Ein Beitrag zur Aetiologie beider Krankheiten. *Mschr. Psychiat. Neurol.*, 1899, **6,** 266–86.

4802 STORCH, Ernst. 1866–

Ueber einige Fälle atypischer progressiver Paralyse. Nach einem hinterlassenen Manuscript Dr. H. Lissauer's. *Mschr. Psychiat. Neurol.*, 1901, **9,** 401–34.

"Lissauer's atypical general paralysis" first described. Heinrich Lissauer was born in 1861, and died in 1891.

4803 NISSL, Franz. 1860–191,

Histologische und histopathologische Arbeiten über die Grosshirnrinde. Vol. 1. Jena, *G. Fischer*, 1904.

Pages 315–494 contain Nissl's classical account of the histopathology of general paresis.

4804 WASSERMANN, August von. 1866–1925, & PLAUT, Felix. 1877–

Ueber das Vorhandensein syphilitischer Antistoffe in der Cerebrospinalflüssigkeit von Paralytikern. *Dtsch. med. Wschr.*, 1906, **32,** 1769–72.

Wassermann applied his test (No. 2402) to the cerebrospinal fluid and, in paretics, obtained positive results in over 90% of cases. The test greatly facilitated the diagnosis of general paralysis.

4805 NOGUCHI, Hideyo. 1876–1928, & MOORE, Joseph Waldron. 1879–
A demonstration of Treponema pallidum in the brain in cases of general paralysis. *J. exp. Med.*, 1913, **17,** 232–38.
A pure culture of *Trep. pallidum* was obtained from a case of dementia paralytica.

4806 WAGNER VON JAUREGG, Julius. 1857–1940
Ueber die Einwirkung der Malaria auf die progressive Paralyse. *Psychiat.-neurol. Wschr.*, 1918–19, **20,** 132–34, 251–55.
In 1917 Wagner von Jauregg returned to the idea of the inoculation of paretics with malaria to induce pyrexia, first proposed by him in 1887 (Ueber die Einwirkung fieberhafter Erkrankungen auf Psychosen, *Jb. Psychiat.*, 7, 94–131). He was awarded the Nobel Prize in 1927.

4807–4824 EPILEPSY

4807 HIPPOCRATES. 460–375 B.C.
The sacred disease. In his *Works . . . edited by W. H. S. Jones and E. T. Withington*, London, 1923, **2,** 127–83.
This includes the first mention of epilepsy in children. Hippocrates grouped all convulsive attacks together as *ἱερα νοῦσος*, the sacred disease. He did not employ the word *ἐπίληψις* (which seems first to have been used in the 10th century by Avicenna) but the terms *ἱερόν νόσημα, παθος παῖδειον,* and *νοσημα παιδειον.* The English text is also reprinted in *Med. Classics*, 1938, 3, 355–69. Above is Greek and English text.

4808 ARETAEUS, *the Cappadocian. circa* A.D. 81–138
On epilepsy. In his *Extant works, translated by F. Adams*, London, 1856, 243, 296, 399, 468.
Aretaeus was well acquainted with hemi-epilepsy from local injury in the opposite half of the brain; partly from this knowledge he formulated the "decussation in the form of the letter X" of the motor path. He first described epilepsy resulting from a depressed fracture of the skull. In his excellent description he made the first mention of the aura.

4809 KELLIE, George. ?1770–1830
Reflections on the pathology of the brain. *Trans. med.-chir. Soc. Edinb.*, 1824, **1,** 123–69.

4810 BRAVAIS, Louis François.
Recherches sur les symptômes et le traitement de l'épilepsie hémiplégique. Paris, *Thèse No.* 118, 1827.
First description of hemiplegic epilepsy so well depicted by Jackson (No. 4816) and referred to by Charcot as "Bravais–Jacksonian épilepsie".

4811 BRIGHT, Richard. 1789–1858
Fatal epilepsy, from suppuration between the dura mater and arachnoid, in consequence of blood having been effused in that situation. *Guy's Hosp. Rep.*, 1836, **1,** 36–40.
Bright was the first to describe unilateral ("Jacksonian") epilepsy.

4812 HALL, Marshall. 1790–1857
Synopsis of cerebral and spinal seizures of inorganic origin and of paroxysmal form as a class; and of their pathology as involved in the structures and actions of the neck. London, *J. Mallett*, [1851].
Hall was first to suggest that the paroxysmal nervous discharges in epilepsy were produced by the spinal nervous system, first to notice the connexion of anaemia with epilepsy, and first to deduce that epilepsy was produced by anaemia of the medulla.

4813 BROWN-SÉQUARD, CHARLES ÉDOUARD. 1817–1894
Recherches expérimentales sur la production d'une affection convulsive épileptiforme, à la suite de lésions de la moelle épinière. *Arch. gén. Méd.*, 1856, 5 sér., **7**, 143–49.

Experimental epilepsy (section of sciatic nerve). See also *Arch. Physiol. norm. path.*, 1869, **2**, 211–20, 422–38, 496–503; 1870, **3**, 153–60.

4813.1 LOCOCK, *Sir* CHARLES, *Bart.* 1799–1875
[Contribution to discussion on paper by E. H. Sieveking.] *Lancet*, 1857, **1**, 528.

Locock, physician accoucheur to Queen Victoria, recommended bromide of potassium in the treatment of epilepsy.

4814 O'CONNOR, WILLIAM. ?–1880
Cases of epilepsy, associated with amenorrhoea and vicarious menstruation, successfully treated with the iodide of potassium. *Lancet*, 1857, **1**, 525.

O'Connor was apparently the first to use potassium iodide for the treatment of epilepsy.

4815 SCHROEDER VAN DER KOLK, JACOB LUDWIG CONRAD. 1797–1862
Bau und Functionen der Medulla spinalis und oblongata, und nächste Ursache und rationelle Behandlung der Epilepsie. Braunschweig, *F. Vieweg u. Sohn*, 1859.

The work of Schroeder van der Kolk brought histological examination to the forefront in connexion with theories on the localization of function. His careful microscopical studies confirmed the medulla as being the ultimate seat of epilepsy. The book was translated into English for the New Sydenham Society in the same year.

4816 JACKSON, JOHN HUGHLINGS. 1835–1911
Unilateral epileptiform seizures, attended by temporary defect of sight. *Med. Times Gaz.*, 1863, **1**, 588–89.

"Jacksonian epilepsy" is so called from the excellent account of unilateral epilepsy with spasm given by Jackson. Actually Bravais (No. 4810) was first to note the condition.

4817 ——. Case of hemikinesis. *Brit. med. J.*, 1875, **1**, 773.

4818 GOWERS, *Sir* WILLIAM RICHARD. 1845–1915
Epilepsy and other chronic convulsive diseases. London, *J. & A. Churchill*, 1881.

Gowers left a classical account of epilepsy, a book which to-day is still one of the most important on the subject. He was first to note the tetanic nature of the epileptic convulsion.

4819 UNVERRICHT, HEINRICH. 1853–1912
Die Myoclonie. Wien, *F. Deuticke*, 1891.

First description of "Unverricht's disease" – familial myoclonus epilepsy.

4820 KOZHEVNIKOV, ALEKSIEI YAKOVLEVICH. 1836–1902
Eine besonderer Form von corticaler Epilepsie. *Neurol. Zbl.*, 1895, **14**, 47–48.

"Kozhevnikov's epilepsy", an atypical form of cortical origin. First published by him in *Med. Obozrenie (Moskva)*, 1894, **42**, 94–118.

4821 GOWERS, *Sir* WILLIAM RICHARD. 1845–1915
The border-land of epilepsy. London, *J. & A. Churchill*, 1907.

4822 DAVENPORT, CHARLES BENEDICT. 1866–1944, & WEEKS, DAVID FAIRCHILD. 1874–1929
A first study of inheritance of epilepsy. *J. nerv. ment. Dis.*, 1911, **38,** 641–70.

Davenport and Weeks produced strong evidence in support of the hereditary origin of epilepsy.

4823 HAUPTMANN, ALFRED. 1881–1948
Luminal bei Epilepsie. *Münch. med. Wschr.*, 1912, **59,** 1907–09.

Introduction of phenobarbitone in the treatment of epilepsy.

4824 GOLLA, FREDERICK LUCIEN. 1878–1968, *et al.*
The electro-encephalogram in epilepsy. *J. ment. Sci.*, 1937, **83,** 137–55.

Demonstration of the changes in the electro-encephalogram in epilepsy. With S. Graham and W. Grey Walter.

For history, see Nos. 5011, 5015.

4825–4838 TETANY

See also 3856–3863, PARATHYROID GLAND.

4825 CLARKE, JOHN. 1761–1815
Commentaries on some of the most important diseases of children. Part the first. London, *Longman, etc.*, 1815.

First account of infantile tetany is given on pp. 86–97.

4826 KELLIE, GEORGE. ?1770–1830
Notes on the swelling of the tops of the hands and feet, and on a spasmodic affection of the thumbs and toes, which very commonly attends it. *Edinb. med. surg. J.*, 1816, **12,** 448–52.

In his early account of chronic tetany, Kellie referred to carpo-pedal spasm and spasms of the glottis as part of the syndrome.

4827 STEINHEIM, SALOMON LEVI. 1789–1866
Zwei seltene Formen von hitzigem Rheumatismus. *Litt. Ann. ges. Heilk.*, 1830, **17,** 22–30.

German writers usually credit Steinheim with the first description of parathyroid tetany.

4828 DANCE, JEAN BAPTISTE HIPPOLYTE. 1797–1832
Observations sur une espèce de tétanos intermittent. *Arch. gén. Méd.*, 1831, **26,** 190–205.

Dance's important early description of parathyroid tetany followed closely on that of Steinheim.

4829 CORVISART, FRANÇOIS RÉMY LUCIEN. 1824–1882
De la contracture des extrémités ou tétanie. Paris, *Thèse No.* 223, 1852.

In his graduation thesis, Lucien Corvisart, nephew of the more famous Baron Corvisart, introduced the term "tétanie".

4830 TROUSSEAU, ARMAND. 1801–1867
Clinique médicale de l'Hôtel-Dieu de Paris. Tom. 2. Paris, *J. B. Baillière*, 1861.

On pp. 112–14 Trousseau described the phenomenon in tetany which now bears his name. This is produced by pressure upon the arm sufficient to stop the circulation; the result is a sudden contraction of the fingers and hand into the so-called "obstetrical position".

4831 KUSSMAUL, ADOLF. 1822–1902
Zur Lehre von der Tetanie. *Berl. klin. Wschr.*, 1872, **9,** 441–44.

Important observations on gastric tetany were made by Kussmaul. He called attention to the convulsions sometimes accompanying dilatation of the stomach. He first mentioned "gastric tetany" in 1869 in his paper on gastric lavage (No. 3463).

4832 ERB, WILHELM HEINRICH. 1840–1921
Zur Lehre von der Tetanie nebst Bemerkungen über die Prüfung der electrischen Erregbarkeit motorischer Nerven. *Arch. Psychiat. Nervenkr.*, 1873–74, **4,** 271–316.

"Erb's sign."

4833 CHVOSTEK, FRANTIŠEK. 1835–1884
Beitrag zur Tetanie. *Wien. med. Presse*, 1876, **17,** 1201–03, 1225–27, 1253–58, 1313–16.

"Chvostek's sign," a reliable diagnostic sign in latent tetany in small children.

4834 FRANKL-HOCHWART, LOTHAR VON. 1862–1915
Die Tetanie. Berlin, *A. Hirschwald*, 1891.

4835 ESCHERICH, THEODOR. 1857–1911
Die Tetanie der Kinder. Wien, *A. Hölder*, 1909.

4836 HULDSCHINSKY, KURT. 1883
Die Beeinflussung der Tetanie durch Ultraviolettlicht. *Z. Kinderheilk.*, 1920, **26,** 207–14.

Treatment of tetany with ultra-violet light.

4837 COLLIP, JAMES BERTRAM. 1892–1965, & LEITCH, DOUGLAS BURROWS. 1888–
A case of tetany treated with parathyrin. *Canad. med. Ass. J.*, 1925, **15,** 59–60.

First use of parathyroid hormone in the treatment of tetany.

4838 HOLTZ, FRIEDRICH.
Die Behandlung der postoperativen Tetanie. *Arch. klin. Chir.*, 1933, **177,** 32–34.

Introduction of A.T. 10 ("Antitetanisches Präparat Nr. 10"), dihydrotachysterol, in the treatment of tetany.

4839–4850 NEUROSES AND PSYCHONEUROSES

4839 WILLIS, THOMAS. 1621–1675
Affectionum quae dicuntur hystericae e hypochondriacae pathologia spasmodica vindicata. Lugduni Batavorum, *Driehuysen & Lopez*, 1671.

Classical description of hysteria.

4840 CHEYNE, GEORGE. 1671–1743
The English malady; or, a treatise of nervous diseases of all kinds. London, *G. Strahan*, 1733.
Cheyne attributed hypochondria ("Cheyne's disease") to the moisture of the air and variability of the weather in the British Isles.

4841 WHYTT, ROBERT. 1714–1766
Observations on the nature, causes, and cure of those disorders which have been commonly called nervous hypochondriac, or hysteric, to which are prefixed some remarks on the sympathy of the nerves. Edinburgh, *printed for T. Becket and P. Du Hondt, London, and J. Balfour, Edinburgh*, 1765.
"First important English work on neurology after Willis" (Garrison).

4842 BRIQUET, PAUL. 1796–1881
Traité clinique et thérapeutique de l'hystérie. Paris, *J. B. Baillière*, 1859.
Includes, p. 297, first description of ataxia analgica hysterica ("Briquet's ataxia") and, p. 475, hysterical paralysis of the diaphragm with dyspnoea and aphonia ("Briquet's syndrome").

4843 BEARD, GEORGE MILLER. 1839–1883
Neurasthenia, or nervous exhaustion. *Boston med. surg. J.*, 1869, **80**, 217–21.
"Beard's disease" (neurasthenia) first described. See also No. 4846.

4844 WESTPHAL, CARL FRIEDRICH OTTO. 1833–1890
Die Agoraphobie, eine neuropathische Erscheinung. *Arch. Psychiat. Nervenkr.*, 1871–72, **3**, 138–61.
First description of agoraphobia.

4845 GULL, *Sir* WILLIAM WITHEY. 1816–1890
Anorexia nervosa (apepsia hysterica, anorexia hysterica). *Trans. clin. Soc. Lond.*, 1874, **7**, 22–28.
Classical description of anorexia nervosa.

4846 BEARD, GEORGE MILLER. 1839–1883
A practical treatise on nervous exhaustion (neurasthenia). New York, *W. Wood & Co.*, 1880.

4847 ALLBUTT, *Sir* THOMAS CLIFFORD. 1836–1925
On visceral neuroses. London, *J. & A. Churchill*, 1884.
Gulstonian Lectures.

4848 GILLES DE LA TOURETTE, GEORGES. 1857–1904
Jumping, latah, myriachit. *Arch. Neurol. (Paris)*, 1884, **8**, 68–74.
Latah, motor incoordination associated with echolalia and coprolalia, is named "Gilles de la Tourette's disease" after the latter's classical description of it.

4849 GANSER, SIGBERT JOSEPH MARIA. 1853–1931
Ueber einen eigenartigen hysterischen Dämmerzustand. *Arch. Psychiat. Nervenkr.*, 1898, **30**, 633–40.
"Ganser's syndrome" – an acute hallucinatory mania.

4850 FREUD, SIGMUND. 1856–1939
Sammlung kleiner Schriften zur Neurosenlehre. Leipzig, Wien, *F. Deuticke*, 1906.

4851–4914 NEUROSURGERY

4851 MORAND, Sauveur François. 1697–1773
Opuscules de chirurgie. Pt. 1. Paris, *G. Desprez et P. A. Le Prieur*, 1768.

Records, p. 161, a successful operation for temporo-sphenoidal abscess, 1752. The patient, a monk, had otorrhoea followed by a mastoid abscess, which Morand opened.

4852 NOTT, Josiah Clark. 1804–1873
Extirpation of the os coccygis for neuralgia. *New Orleans med. surg. J.*, 1844–45, **1**, 58–60.

4853 DETMOLD, William. 1808–1894
Abscess in the substance of the brain; the lateral ventricles opened by an operation. *Amer. J. med. Sci.*, 1850, n.s., **19**, 86–95.

Lateral ventricles of the brain first opened for the treatment of cerebral abscess.

4854 CARNOCHAN, John Murray. 1817–1887
Exsection of the trunk of the second branch of the fifth pair of nerves, beyond the ganglion of Meckel, for severe neuralgia of the face; with three cases. *Amer. J. med. Sci.*, 1858, n.s., **35**, 134–43.

First excision of the superior maxillary nerve for the treatment of facial neuralgia.

4855 PANCOAST, Joseph. 1805–1882
New operation for the relief of persistent facial neuralgia. *Philad. med. Times*, 1871–72, **2**, 285–87.

Pancoast devised the operative procedure of sectioning the second and third branches of the fifth pair of nerves as they emerge from the base of the brain. Reported by F. Woodbury.

4856 MACEWEN, *Sir* William. 1848–1924
Tumour of the dura mater – convulsions – removal of tumour by trephining – recovery. *Glasg. med. J.*, 1879, **12**, 210–13.

4857 MEARS, James Ewing. 1838–1919
Study of the pathological changes occurring in trifacial neuralgia, with the report of a case in which three inches of the inferior dental nerve were excised. *Med. News (Philad.)*, 1884, **45**, 58–63.

Mears first suggested Gasserian ganglionectomy for trigeminal neuralgia.

4858 BENNETT, Alexander Hughes. 1848–1901, & GODLEE, *Sir* Rickman John. 1849–1925
Case of cerebral tumour. *Med.-chir. Trans.*, 1885, **68**, 243–75.

First instance of diagnosis, accurate clinical localization, and operative removal of a tumour of the brain, November 25, 1884. The patient survived for one month. Preliminary report in *Lancet*, 1884, **2**, 1090–91.

4859 BERGMANN, Ernst von. 1836–1907
Die chirurgische Behandlung von Hirnkrankheiten. Berlin, *A. Hirschwald*, 1888.

Bergmann greatly improved the surgical treatment of diseases of the brain.

4860 GOWERS, *Sir* William Richard. 1845–1915, & HORSLEY, *Sir* Victor Alexander Haden. 1857–1916
A case of tumour of the spinal cord. Removal; recovery. *Med.-chir. Trans.*, 1888, **71**, 377–430.

Horsley was the founder of neurosurgery in England. The above paper records the first successful operation for the removal of an extramedullary tumour of the spinal cord.

4860.1 ABBE, Robert. 1851–1928
A contribution to the surgery of the spine. *Med. Rec.*, 1889, **35,** 149–52.
Posterior rhizotomy.

4861 ALEXANDER, William. 1844–1919
The treatment of epilepsy. Edinburgh, *Y. J. Pentland*, 1889.
Alexander was the first to attempt the treatment of epilepsy by surgical means. He removed the superior cervical sympathetic ganglia.

4861.1 BENNETT, *Sir* William Henry. 1852–1931
A case in which acute spasmodic pain in the left lower extremity was completely relieved by sub-dural division of the posterior roots of certain spinal nerves, all other treatment having proved useless. Death from sudden collapse and cerebral haemorrhage on the twelfth day after the operation, at the commencement of apparent convalescence. *Med.-chir. Trans.*, 1889, **72,** 329–48.
Posterior rhizotomy.

4862 WAGNER, Wilhelm. 1848–1900
Die temporäre Resektion der Schädeldaches an Stelle der Trepanation. *Zbl. Chir.*, 1889, **16,** 833–38.
Osteoplastic flap operation. Wagner's method of opening the skull made a large area of the brain more easily accessible than by trephining. Translation in *J. Neurosurg.*, 1962, **19**, 1099.

4863 ROSE, William. 1847–1910
Removal of the gasserian ganglion for severe neuralgia. *Lancet*, 1890, **2,** 914–15.
Gasserian ganglionectomy for trigeminal neuralgia; the patient lived for at least two years.

4864 BURCKHARDT, G.
Ueber Rindenexcisionen, als Beitrag zur operativen Therapie der Psychosen. *Allg. Z. Psychiat.*, 1891, **47,** 463–548.
Burckhardt, physician at a Swiss mental hospital, performed frontal lobotomy on four patients in 1890, with good results in some cases.

4865 HORSLEY, *Sir* Victor Alexander Haden. 1857–1916, *et al.*
Remarks on the various surgical procedures devised for the relief or cure of trigeminal neuralgia (tic douloureux). *Brit. med. J.*, 1891, **2,** 1139–43, 1191–93, 1249–52.
Horsley, with J. Taylor and W. S. Coleman, devised an operation for treatment of trigeminal neuralgia in which the Gasserian ganglion was removed by a temporal approach.

4866 KEEN, William Williams. 1837–1932
Linear craniotomy. Philadelphia, *Lea Bros. & Co.*, 1891.
Keen was a pioneer in linear craniotomy and one of the first successfully to operate for meningioma. He was professor of surgery at Jefferson Medical College.

4867 ——. A new operation for spasmodic wry neck, namely, division or exsection of the nerves supplying the posterior rotator muscles of the head. *Ann. Surg.*, 1891, **13,** 44–47.
Spastic torticollis treated by division of spinal accessory nerve and posterior roots of first, second, and third spinal nerves.

4868 WYNTER, Walter Essex. 1860–1945
Four cases of tubercular meningitis in which paracentesis of the theca vertebralis was performed for the relief of fluid pressure. *Lancet*, 1891, **1**, 981–82.

Lumbar puncture. Reprinted in *Middx Hosp. J.*, 1951, **51**, 147.

4869 QUINCKE, Heinrich Irenaeus. 1842–1922
Die Lumbalpunction des Hydrocephalus. *Berl. klin. Wschr.*, 1891, **28**, 929–33, 965–68.

Quincke popularized lumbar puncture which he had introduced independently of Wynter and others. He used it both for diagnostic and therapeutic purposes. He first presented his method at the German Congress of Internal Medicine (*Verh. Congr. inn. Med.*, 1891, **10**, 321–31).

4870 HARTLEY, Frank. 1856–1913
Intracranial neurectomy of the second and third divisions of the fifth nerve. *N.Y. med. J.*, 1892, **55**, 317–19.

Hartley originated the operation of intracranial neurectomy for facial neuralgia.

4871 KRAUSE, Fedor. 1856–1937
Resection des Trigeminus innerhalb der Schädelhöhle. *Arch. klin. Chir.*, 1892, **44**, 821–32.

Hartley–Krause operation for relief of facial neuralgia (see also No. 4870).

4872 MACEWEN, *Sir* William. 1848–1924
Pyogenic infective diseases of the brain and spinal cord. Glasgow. *J. Maclehose & Sons*, 1893.

Macewen's greatest work was in connexion with the surgery of the brain. In the above book he included extensive case reports of 65 patients under his care, with details of operative procedures. A biography of Macewen was written by A. K. Bowman, London, 1942.

4873 FÜRBRINGER, Paul. 1849–1930
Zur klinischen Bedeutung der spinalen Punction. *Berl. klin. Wschr.*, 1895, **32**, 272–77.

Fürbringer demonstrated the diagnostic value of spinal puncture.

4874 GIGLI, Leonardo. 1863–1908
Zur Technik der temporären Schädelresektion mit meiner Drahtsäge. *Zbl. Chir.*, 1898, **25**, 425–28.

Gigli's saw adapted for craniotomy. Translation in *J. Neurosurg.*, 1962, **19**, 1103.

4875 CUSHING, Harvey Williams. 1869–1939
A method of total extirpation of the Gasserian ganglion for trigeminal neuralgia, by a route through the temporal fossa and beneath the middle meningeal artery. *J. Amer. med. Ass.*, 1900, **34**, 1035–41.

4876 SPILLER, William Gibson. 1863–1940, & FRAZIER, Charles Harrison. 1870–1936
The division of the sensory root of the trigeminus for the relief of tic douloureux; an experimental, pathological, and clinical study, with a preliminary report of one surgically successful case. *Univ. Penn. med. Bull.*, 1901, **14**, 342–52.

Introduction of intracranial trigeminal neurotomy, using a modification of the techniques of Horsley (No. 4865) and Krause (No. 4871). Also published in *Philad. med. J.*, 1901, **8**, 1039–49.

4877 ABADIE, JOSEPH LOUIS IRÉNEE JEAN. 1873–
Névralgie faciale; présentation de malade. *Mém. Bull. Soc. Méd. Chir. Bordeaux*, (1902), 1903, 59–63.
Alcohol injection of the Gasserian ganglion for treatment of trigeminal neuralgia. See also pp. 91–96 of the same volume.

4878 CUSHING, HARVEY WILLIAMS. 1869–1939
Concerning surgical intervention for the intracranial hemorrhages of the new-born. *Amer. J. med. Sci.*, 1905, **130,** 563–81.
Successful operative intervention in intracranial haemorrhage of the new-born.

4879 ——. The establishment of cerebral hernia as a decompressive measure for inaccessible brain tumors. *Surg. Gynec. Obstet.*, 1905, **1,** 297–314.

4879.1 HORSLEY, *Sir* VICTOR ALEXANDER HADEN. 1857–1916, & CLARKE, ROBERT HENRY. 1850–1926
The structure and functions of the cerebellum examined by a new method. *Brain*, 1908, **31,** 45–124.
The apparatus devised by Horsley and Clarke opened the way to stereotactic surgery of the brain.

4880 FOERSTER, OTFRID. 1873–1941
Ueber eine neue operative Methode der Behandlung spastischer Lähmungen mittels Resektion hinterer Rückenmarkswurzeln. *Z. orthop. Chir.*, 1908, **22,** 203–23.
Foerster's operation of rhizotomy for spastic paralysis.

4881 ——, & KÜTTNER, HERMANN. 1870–1932
Ueber operative Behandlung gastrischer Krisen durch Resektion der 7.–10. hinteren Dorsalwurzel. *Beitr. klin. Chir.*, 1909, **63,** 245–56.
Foerster's operation for tabes.

4882 HORSLEY, *Sir* VICTOR ALEXANDER HADEN. 1857–1916
The Linacre Lecture on the function of the so-called motor area of the brain. *Brit. med. J.*, 1909, **2,** 125–32.
Horsley demonstrated that removal of the precentral cortex in man abolished athetosis.

4883 SPILLER, WILLIAM GIBSON. 1863–1940, & MARTIN, EDWARD. 1859–1938
The treatment of persistent pain of organic origin in the lower part of the body by division of the anterolateral column of the spinal cord. *J. Amer. med. Ass.*, 1912, **58,** 1489–90.
Cordotomy for the relief of intractable pain.

4884 LUCKETT, WILLIAM HENRY. 1872–
Air in the ventricles of the brain, following a fracture of the skull. *Surg. Gynec. Obstet.*, 1913, **17,** 237–40.
Luckett's finding of air in the ventricles gave Dandy (No. 4602) the idea for ventriculography.

4884.1 OPPENHEIM, HERMANN. 1858–1919, & KRAUSE, FEDOR. 1856–1937
Operative Erfolge bei Geschwülsten der Sehhügel- und Vierhügelgegend. *Berl. klin. Wschr.*, 1913, **50,** 2316–22.
Successful removal of pineal tumour.

4885 LERICHE, René. 1879–1955
De la causalgie envisagée comme une névrite du sympathique et de son traitement par la dénudation et l'excision des plexus nerveux périartériels. *Presse méd.*, 1916, **24,** 178–80.
Periarterial sympathectomy.

4886 MOSHER, Harris Peyton. 1867–
The wire gauze brain drain. *Surg. Gynec. Obstet.*, 1916, **23,** 740–41.
Mosher initiated the modern method of trephining and draining inflammatory processes of the brain.

4887 TINEL, Jules. 1879–1952
Les blessures des nerfs. Paris, *Masson & Cie.*, 1916.
A study of the effect of gunshot wounds on nerves.

4888 DANDY, Walter Edward. 1886–1946
Extirpation of the choroid plexus of the lateral ventricles in communicating hydrocephalus. *Ann. Surg.*, 1918, **68,** 569–79.

4888.1 PEET, Max Minor. 1885–1949
Tic douloureux and its treatment, with a review of the cases operated upon at the University Hospital in 1917. *J. Mich. St. med. Ass.*, 1918, **17,** 91–99.
Trigeminal nerve resection with conservation of the motor root, for treatment of trigeminal neuralgia.

4889 BALLANCE, *Sir* Charles Alfred. 1856–1926, & GREEN, Charles David.
Essays on the surgery of the temporal bone. 2 vols. London, *Macmillan*, 1919.

4890 AYER, James Bourne. 1882–
Puncture of the cisterna magna. *Arch. Neurol. Psychiat.* (*Chicago*) 1920, **4,** 529–41.
Introduction of cisternal puncture.

4891 BIANCHI, Leonardo. 1848–1919
La meccanica del cervello e la funzione dei lobi frontale. Torino, *Bocca*, 1920.
Bianchi showed that bilateral destruction of the frontal lobes caused character changes, a finding put to practical use by Egas Moniz and others.

4892 SICARD, R., & ROBINEAU, I.
Algie vélo-pharyngée essentielle. Traitement chirurgical. *Rev. neurol.*, 1920, **27,** 256–57.
Idiopathic glossopharyngeal neuralgia described and treated.

4893 HUNTER, John Irvine. 1898–1924
The influence of the sympathetic nervous system in the genesis of the rigidity of striated muscle in a spastic paralysis. *Surg. Gynec. Obstet.*, 1924, **39,** 721–43.
Hunter believed in the sympathetic innervation of skeletal muscle and on this assumption devised the technique of sympathetic ramisection carried out by Royle (No. 4894).

4894 ROYLE, Norman Dawson. ?–1944
A new operative procedure in the treatment of spastic paralysis and its experimental basis. *Med. J. Aust.*, 1924, **1,** 77–86.
Sympathetic ramisection. See also *Surg. Gynec. Obstet.*, 1924, **39**, 701–20.

4895 COTTE, Gaston. 1879–1951
La sympathectomie hypogastrique a-t-elle sa place dans la thérapeutique gynécologique? *Presse méd.*, 1925, **33,** 98–99.
Presacral neurectomy.

4896 DANDY, Walter Edward. 1886–1946
Section of the sensory root of the trigeminal nerve at the pons. Preliminary report of the operative procedure. *Bull. Johns Hopk. Hosp.*, 1925, **36,** 105–06.
Intracranial section for glossopharyngeal neuralgia. For a more detailed account see his paper in *Arch. Surg.* (*Chicago*), 1929, **18**, 687–734.

4897 PUUSEPP, Lyudvig Martinovich. 1875–1942
Die Operationstechnik der Hirntumoren (nach eigenen Erfahrungen). *Folia neuropath. eston.*, 1926, **6,** 127–49.
Puusepp was a great neurosurgeon, particularly notable for his method of removing cerebral tumours. The above journal was founded and edited by him, and vol. 16 (1935) is a *Festschrift* in his honour.

4897.1 CUSHING, Harvey Williams. 1869–1939
Electro-surgery as an aid to the removal of intracranial tumors. With a preliminary note on a new surgical-current generator by W. T. Bovie. *Surg. Gynec. Obstet.*, 1928, **47,** 751–84.
Introduction of electrocoagulation in neurosurgery.

4898 DOGLIOTTI, Achile Mario. 1897–1966
Traitement des syndromes douloureux de la périphérie par l'alcoolisation sub-arachnoïdienne des racines postérieures à leur émergence de la moelle épinière. *Presse méd.*, 1931, **39,** 1249–52.
Subarachnoid injection of alcohol for the relief of pain.

4899 BALLANCE, *Sir* Charles Alfred. 1856–1936, & DUEL, Arthur Baldwin. 1870–1936
The operative treatment of facial palsy by the introduction of nerve grafts into the Fallopian canal and by other intratemporal methods. *Arch. Otolaryng.* (*Chicago*), 1932, **15,** 1–70.
A classical paper which includes some history of the surgical treatment of facial palsy.

4900 CUSHING, Harvey Williams. 1869–1939
Intracranial tumours. Springfield, *C. C. Thomas*, 1932.
Cushing developed a technique for operating upon intracranial tumours which made him an outstanding neurosurgeon of the 20th century.

4901 DOTT, Norman McOmish. 1897–
Intracranial aneurysms: cerebral arterioradiography: surgical treatment. *Trans. med.-chir. Soc. Edinb.*, 1932–33, N.S. **47,** 219–34.
First planned intracranial operation for aneurysm.

4902 LERICHE, René. 1879–1955, & FONTAINE, René.
Techniques des diverses sympathectomies lombaires. *Presse méd.*, 1933, **41,** 1819–22.
Lumbar sympathectomy by the antero-lateral extraperitoneal approach.

4903 PUTNAM, Tracy Jackson. 1894–
Treatment of hydrocephalus by endoscopic coagulation of the choroid plexus. Description of a new instrument and preliminary report of results. *New Engl. J. Med.*, 1934, **210,** 1373–76.

4904 LIVINGSTON, William Kenneth. 1892–
The clinical aspects of visceral neurology with special reference to the surgery of the sympathetic nervous system. Springfield, *C. C. Thomas*, 1935.

4904.1 BERGSTRAND, Karl Joseph Hilding. 1886– , OLIVECRONA, Herbert. 1891– , & TÖNNIS, Wilhelm.
Gefässmissbildungen und Gefässgeschwülste des Gehirns. Leipzig, *G. Thieme*, 1936.

Olivecrona first successfully removed an intracranial aneurysm in 1932.

4905 EGAS MONIZ, Antonio Caetano de. 1874–1955
Essai d'un traitement chirurgical de certaines psychoses. *Bull. Acad. Méd. (Paris)*, 1936, 3 sér., **115,** 385–92.

Prefrontal leucotomy. Translation in *J. Neurosurg.*, 1964, **21**, 1110–14. See also his book *Tentatives opératoires dans le traitement de certaines psychoses*, Paris, 1936. Egas Moniz shared the Nobel Prize with Hess in 1949 for his work in this field.

4906 FREEMAN, Walter. 1895– , & WATTS, James Winston. 1904–
Prefrontal lobotomy in agitated depression. Report of a case. *Med. Ann. Distr. Columbia*, 1936, **5,** 326–28.

See also the book by the same authors, *Psychosurgery: Intelligence, emotion, and social behavior following prefrontal lobotomy for mental disorders.* 2nd ed., Springfield, 1951.

4907 WALTER, William Grey. 1911–
The location of cerebral tumours by electro-encephalography. *Lancet*, 1936, **2,** 305–08.

4908 SJÖQVIST, Carl Olof. 1901–
Eine neue Operationsmethode bei Trigeminusneuralgie: Durchschneidung des Tractus spinalis trigemini. *Zbl. Neurochir.*, 1937, **2,** 274–81.

Trigeminal tractotomy. See also *Acta psychiat. neurol. (Kbh.)*, 1938, Suppl. 17 1–139.

4909 DOGLIOTTI, Achile Mario. 1897–1966
First surgical sections, in man, of the lemniscus lateralis (pain-temperature path) at the brain stem, for the treatment of diffused rebellious pain. *Curr. Res. Anesth.*, 1938, **17,** 143–45.

4909.1 TORKILDSEN, Arne.
A new palliative operation in cases of inoperable occlusion of the Sylvian aqueduct. *Acta chir. scand.*, 1939, **82,** 117–24.

Ventriculocisternostomy for the relief of obstructive hydrocephalus.

4910 ELSBERG, Charles Albert. 1871–1948
Surgical diseases of the spinal cord, membranes, and nerve roots. New York, *P. B. Hoeber*, (1941).

Elsberg, American pioneer in neurosurgery, made valuable contributions to the surgery of the spinal cord. His first book on the subject appeared in 1916, and another on tumours of the cord in 1925.

4911 SEDDON, *Sir* Herbert John. 1903–
Three types of nerve injury. *Brain*, 1943, **66**, 237–88.
Seddon's classification of nerve injuries.

4912 TARLOV, Isadore Max. 1905– , & BENJAMIN, Bernard. 1903–
Plasma clot and silk suture of nerves. 1. An experimental study of comparative tissue reaction. *Surg. Gynec. Obstet.*, 1943, **76**, 366–74.
Plasma clot nerve suture. Preliminary communication in *Science*, 1942, **95**, 258.

4912.1 SPIEGEL, Ernest Adolf. 1895– , *et al.*
Stereotaxic apparatus for operations on the human brain. *Science*, 1947, **106**, 349–50.
Stereotactic surgery performed on humans. With H. T. Wycis, M. Marks, and A. J. Lee.

4913 MOORE, George Eugene. 1920– , *et al.*
Clinical use of fluorescein in neurosurgery; localization of brain tumors. *J. Neurosurg.*, 1948, **5**, 392–98.
Tumour localization by radio-isotopes. With W. T. Peyton, L. A. French, and W. W. Walker.

4914 BECK, Claude Schaeffer. 1894–1971, *et al.*
Revascularization of the brain through establishment of a cervical arteriovenous fistula. Effects in children with mental retardation and convulsive disorders. *J. Pediat.*, 1949, **35**, 317–29.
With C. F. McKhann and W. D. Belnap.

For history, see Nos. 5008, 5017–18

4915–4962.2

PSYCHIATRY

4915 ARETAEUS, *the Cappadocian. circa* A.D. 81–138
On melancholy. In his *Extant works*, ed. F. Adams, London, 1856, 298–300, 473–78.
Aretaeus advised bleeding to relieve the liver in melancholia, purging with aloes, and natural hot baths during convalescence (on account of their sulphur and bitumen content). He regarded melancholia as a modification of mania.

4916 ——. On madness. *Extant works*, ed. F. Adams, London, 1856, 301–04.
Aretaeus was probably the first to interest himself in the so-called prepsychotic personality. He distinguished mania from senile disorders of the mind.

4917 WEYER, Johann [Wierus]. 1515–1588
De praestigiis daemonum. Basileae, *per J. Oporinum*, 1563.
The founder of medical psychiatry, Weyer "was the first clinical and the first descriptive psychiatrist to leave succeeding generations a heritage which was accepted . . . He reduced the clinical problems of psychopathology to simple terms of everyday life and everyday, human, inner experiences" (Zilboorg).

4918 WILLIS, Thomas. 1621–1675
Of the lethargy. In his *Practice of physick*, London, *T. Dring*, 1684, Treatise XI, pp. 125–33.

4919 ——. Of stupidity, or foolishness. In his *Practice of physick*, London, *T. Dring*, 1684, Treatise XI, pp. 209–14.

4919.1 BATTIE, WILLIAM. 1703–1776

Treatise on madness. London, *J. Whiston & B. White*, 1758.

Battie was active in his efforts to bring about reforms in the management of the insane. He was among the first to teach psychiatry and to publish a text-book on the subject.

4920 LORRY, ANNE CHARLES DE. 1726–1783

De melancholia et morbis melancholicis. 2 vols. Lutetiae Parisiorum, *P. G. Cavelier*, 1765.

Lorry was a versatile physician; besides the above work he is remembered for his important classification of skin diseases and for his experiments which concluded that vital functions are located in the medulla.

4921 CHIARUGI, VINCENZO. 1739–1820

Della pazzia in genere, e in specie. 3 vols. Firenze, *L. Carlieri*, 1793.

Chiarugi was the first in Europe to abandon chains and fetters in a mental hospital. He encouraged the patients to work and their attendants to practise kindness towards them. Through him also sanitary conditions in asylums were much improved and attempts were made to treat the patients. His book reviewed all that was then known regarding insanity.

4922 PINEL, PHILIPPE. 1745–1826

Traité médico-philosophique sur l'aliénation mentale ou la manie. Paris, *Richard, Caille & Ravier*, an IX [1801].

Pinel was among the first to treat the insane humanely; he dispensed with chains and placed his patients under the care of specially selected physicians. Garrison considered the above book one of the foremost medical classics, giving as it did a great impetus to the humanitarian treatment of the insane. It was submitted as a prize essay in 1792, the Revolution preventing its publication at that time. English translation, 1806.

4923 REIL, JOHANN CHRISTIAN. 1759–1813

Rhapsodieen über die Anwendung der psychischen Curmethode auf Geisteszerrüttungen. Halle, *Curt*, 1803.

The versatile Reil, physician and physiologist, was an early advocate of humane treatment for the insane. He was instrumental in the establishment of the first journal devoted to mental disease – the *Magazin für Nervenheilkunde*; he was the founder of modern psychiatry.

4924 RUSH, BENJAMIN. 1745–1813

Medical inquiries and observations upon the diseases of the mind. Philadelphia, *Kimber & Richardson*, 1812.

Of this work Hack Tuke says that had Rush written nothing else, it would have given him an enduring name in the republic of medical letters. It is the first American book on psychiatry. Considering the state of that science in Rush's time, this is one of the most noteworthy books on the subject.

4925 SUTTON, THOMAS. 1767–1835

Tracts on delirium tremens. London, *T. Underwood*, 1813.

In this early account of delirium tremens Sutton differentiated the condition from phrenitis.

4926 HEINROTH, JOHANN CHRISTIAN AUGUST. 1773–1843

Lehrbuch der Störungen des Seelenlebens. Leipzig, *F. C. W. Vogel*, 1818.

Heinroth drew his psychology from the Bible and maintained that mental health was attained only by piety and that sin engendered madness; for him repentance and a return to the fold constituted a cure.

4927 WARE, JOHN. 1795–1864
Remarks on the history and treatment of delirium tremens. *Med. Commun. Massachusetts med. Soc.*, 1830–36, **5**, 136–94; 1837–41, **6**, 175–82.

Classical description of delirium tremens. Published in book form, Boston, *N. Hale*, 1831.

4928 PRICHARD, JAMES COWLES. 1786–1848
A treatise on insanity. London, *Sherwood, Gilbert & Piper*, 1835.

Prichard, better known for his work in the field of anthropology, was the first to describe moral insanity. This first appeared in the *Cyclopaedia of practical medicine* (J. Forbes), London, 1833–35, **2**, p. 12, and was afterwards enlarged.

4929 ESQUIROL, JEAN ETIENNE DOMINIQUE. 1772–1840
Des maladies mentales. 2 vols. and atlas. Paris, *J. B. Baillière*, 1838.

Esquirol succeeded Pinel at the Salpêtrière, and was the first lecturer on psychiatry. He carried on with Pinel's good work and founded ten asylums. Above is the first modern text-book on psychiatry. English translation, Philadelphia, 1845 (reprinted 1965).

4930 GRIESINGER, WILHELM. 1817–1868
Die Pathologie und Therapie der psychischen Krankheiten. Stuttgart, *A. Krabbe*, 1845.

Griesinger put an end to the moralistic theory of insanity as advanced by Heinroth. He was the first in Germany to abandon violence in the treatment of the insane; his book remained an authority on the subject for 30 years. English translation, London, 1867.

4931 LASÈGUE, ERNEST CHARLES. 1816–1883
Du délire des persécutions. *Arch. gén. Méd.*, 1852, 4 sér., **28**, 129–50.

"Lasègue's disease" – persecution mania.

4932 FALRET, JEAN PIERRE. 1794–1870
Mémoire sur la folie circulaire. *Bull. Acad. imp. Méd. (Paris)*, 1853–1854, **19**, 382–400.

Circular (manic-depressive) insanity first described.

4933 CONOLLY, JOHN. 1794–1866
The treatment of the insane without mechanical restraints. London, *Smith, Elder & Co.*, 1856.

As early as 1839 Conolly treated the insane without any form of restraint at Hanwell Asylum. Facsimile reprint, Folkestone, *Dawsons*, 1973.

4934 BUCKNILL, *Sir* JOHN CHARLES. 1817–1897, & TUKE, DANIEL HACK. 1827–1895
A manual of psychological medicine. London, *J. Churchill*, 1858.

Bucknill and Tuke were both distinguished neurologists, and advocates of no restraint in the institutional treatment of mental patients. Their book was for many years the standard English work on psychological medicine. Reprinted 1968.

4935 DOWN, JOHN LANGDON HAYDON. 1828–1896
Marriages of consanguinity in relation to degeneration of race. *Lond. Hosp. clin. Lect. Rep.*, 1866, **3**, 224–36.

4936 DOWN, John Langdon Haydon. 1828–1896
Observations on the ethnic classification of idiots. *Lond. Hosp. clin. Lect. Rep.*, 1866, **3**, 259–62.

Langdon Down suggested that the physiognomical features of certain defectives enabled them to be arranged in ethnic groups; of these he differentiated Mongolian, Ethiopian, Caucasian, and American Indian. Such an ethnic classification has been abandoned but the term "mongolism" has been used to describe one important variety of ament, although recently giving way to "Down's disease."

4936.1 SÉGUIN, Édouard. 1812–1880
Idiocy: and its treatment by the physiological method. New York, *William Wood & Co.*, 1866.

Séguin was the first to attain real success in the treatment of idiots. A pupil of Itard and Esquirol he subsequently worked in America.

4937 SANDER, Wilhelm. 1838–1922
Ueber eine spezielle Form der primären Verrücktheit. *Arch. Psychiat. Nervenkr.*, 1868–69, **1**, 387–419.

"Sander's disease" – a form of paranoia.

4938 KAHLBAUM, Karl. 1828–1899
Die Katatonie. Berlin, *A. Hirschwald*, 1874.

In 1869 Kahlbaum suggested catatonia as a separate disease process, and in 1874 appeared his classical monograph elaborating previous descriptions of this condition.

4939 LOMBROSO, Cesare. 1836–1909
L'uomo delinquente, studiato in rapporto alla antropologia, alla medicina legale ed alle discipline carcerarie. Milano, *U. Hoepli*, 1876.

4940 KRAFFT-EBING, Richard von. 1840–1902
Lehrbuch der Psychiatrie auf klinischer Grundlage. Stuttgart, *F. Enke*, 1879.

4941 KRAEPELIN, Emil. 1856–1926
Compendium der Psychiatrie. Leipzig, *A. Abel*, 1883.

Later editions of this book were called *Lehrbuch.* The sixth edition is notable in that in it manic-depressive psychoses were first mentioned as such. Ninth edition in 1927. Kraepelin, professor of psychiatry successively at Dorpat, Heidelberg, and Munich, was one of the greatest of all psychiatrists and a pioneer of experimental psychiatry.

4942 MEYNERT, Theodor Hermann. 1833–1892
Psychiatrie. Klinik der Erkrankungen des Vorderhirns. Wien, *W. Braumüller*, 1884.

Meynert, professor of neurology at Vienna, is by some regarded as the Father of the architectonics of the brain. English translation, 1886.

4943 RIBOT, Théodule Armand. 1839–1916
Les maladies de la personnalité. Paris, *Germer-Baillière*, 1885.

4944 KRAFFT-EBING, Richard von. 1840–1902
Psychopathia sexualis. Stuttgart, *F. Enke*, 1886.

4945 KORSAKOV, Sergei Sergeivich. 1853–1900
Ob alkogolnom paralichie. [Paralysis alcoholica, paraplegia alcoholica.] Moskva, *I. N. Kushnerev & Ko.*, 1887.

"Korsakov's syndrome" – alcoholic polyneuritis and psychosis with loss and falsification of memory. English translation in *Neurology*, 1955, **5**, 394–406.

4946 WAGNER VON JAUREGG, JULIUS. 1857–1940
Ueber die Einwirkung fieberhafter Erkrankungen auf Psychosen. *Jb. Psychiat.*, 1887, **7**, 94–134.

Wagner von Jauregg's first studies of the effect of fevers upon psychotic conditions. See also No. 4806.

4947 TUKE, DANIEL HACK. 1827–1895
A dictionary of psychological medicine. 2 vols. London, *J. & A. Churchill*, 1892.

4948 WESTPHAL, CARL FRIEDRICH OTTO. 1833–1890
Psychiatrische Abhandlungen. Berlin, *A. Hirschwald*, 1892.

Westphal was professor of psychiatry at Berlin. The above forms vol. 1 of his *Gesammelte Abhandlungen.*

4949 WERNICKE, CARL. 1848–1905
Grundriss der Psychiatrie in klinischen Vorlesungen. Leipzig, *G. Thieme*, 1894–1900.

Wernicke made valuable contributions to the subject of sensory aphasia, mind-blindness, and apraxia. He correlated all psychic action with the function of speech, each perversion being interpreted as showing a minus or plus activity.

4950 KRAEPELIN, EMIL. 1856–1926
Der psychologische Versuch in der Psychiatrie. *Psychol. Arb.*, 1896, **1,** 1–91.

4951 SOMMER, ROBERT. 1864–1937
Lehrbuch der psychopathologischen Untersuchungsmethoden. Berlin Wien, *Urban & Schwarzenberg*, 1899.

Sommer introduced new methods in psychopathological investigation.

4952 KRAEPELIN, EMIL. 1856–1926
Einführung in die psychiatrische Klinik. Leipzig, *J. A. Barth*, 1901.

Kraepelin evolved a new classification of insanity. He introduced the concepts "dementia praecox" and "manic-depressive insanity". (Regarding the latter, see also No. 4932.)

4953 FOREL, AUGUSTE HENRI. 1848–1931
Hygiene der Nerven und des Geistes im gesunden und kranken Zustande. Sutttgart, *E. H. Moritz*, [1903].

4954 JANET, PIERRE MARIE FÉLIX. 1859–1947
Les obsessions et la psychasthénie. Paris, *F. Alcan*, 1903.

Janet was the first to describe psychasthenia.

4955 ALZHEIMER, ALOIS. 1864–1915
Ueber eine eigenartige Erkrankung der Hirnrinde. *Allg. Z. Psychiat.*, 1907, **64,** 146–48.

"Alzheimer's disease" – presenile dementia. Preliminary note in *Neurol. Zbl.* 1906, **25**, 1134.

4956 MUCH, HANS. 1880–1932, & HOLZMANN, W.
Eine Reaktion im Blute von Geisteskrankheiten. Vorläufige Mitteilung. *Münch. med. Wschr.*, 1909, **56,** 1001–03.

Much–Holzmann reaction for diagnosis of dementia praecox and manic-depressive insanity.

4957 BLEULER, PAUL EUGEN. 1857–1939
Dementia praecox oder die Gruppe der Schizophrenien. Leipzig, Wien, *F. Deuticke*, 1911.
Bleuler introduced the concept of schizophrenia. He showed that Kraepelin's "dementia praecox" (No. 4952) should include all the schizophrenic disorders.

4958 BROUSSEAU, KATE.
Mongolism. A study of the physical and mental characteristics of mongolian imbeciles. Revised by H. G. Brainerd. Baltimore, *Williams & Wilkins*, 1928.

4959 SEN, GANNETH, & BOSE, KATRICK CHANDRA.
Rauwolfia serpentina, a new Indian drug for insanity and high blood pressure. *Indian med. Wld*, 1931, **2,** 194–201.
Rauwolfia first used in the treatment of psychoses.

4960 SAKEL, MANFRED JOSHUA. 1900–1957
Schizophreniebehandlung mittels Insulin-Hypoglykämie sowie hypoglykämischer Schocks. *Wien. med. Wschr.*, 1934, **84,** 1211–14.
Insulin shock therapy of schizophrenia. Sakel wrote several subsequent papers on this subject in the same journal. English version in *Amer. J. Psychiat.*, 1937, 93, 829–41.

4961 MEDUNA, LADISLAUS JOSEPH. 1896–1965
Versuche über die biologische Beeinflussung des Ablaufes der Schizophrenie. 1. Campher- und Cardiazolkrämpfe. *Z. ges. Neurol. Psychiat.*, 1935, **152,** 235–62.
Cardiazol (metrazol) convulsion therapy of schizophrenia was introduced by Meduna in 1934.

4962 CERLETTI, UGO. 1877–1963, & BINI, LUCIO. 1908–
Un nuovo metodo di shockterapia: "L'elettroshock." (Riassunto.) *Boll. R. Accad. Med. Roma*, 1938, **64,** 136–38.
Introduction of electric convulsion therapy.

4962.1 DELAY, JEAN. 1907– , & DENIKER, PIERRE.
Trente-huit cas de psychoses traitées par la cure prolongée et continue de 4560 R.P. *C. R. Congr. Alien. et Neurol. de Langue Franç.*, Paris, *Masson et Cie.*, 1952.
Introduction of chlorpromazine in the treatment of psychosis.

4962.2 BERGER, FRANK MILAN. 1913–
The pharmacological properties of 2-methyl-2-*m*-propyl-1, 3-propanediol dicarbamate (Miltown), a new interneuronal blocking agent. *J. Pharmacol.*, 1954, **112,** 413–23.
Introduction of meprobamate, later used for the treatment of anxiety.

For history, see Nos. 5003–7, 5010, 5012, 5019.3, 5019.4, 5019.7

4963–5000 MEDICAL PSYCHOLOGY

4963 ARISTOTLE. 384–322 B.C.
De Anima. In his *Works . . . translated into English.* Edited by J. A. SMITH and W. D. ROSS, Oxford, 1931, **3,** 402a–35b.
Artistotle, regarded as the founder of psychology, meant by *anima* or psyche the living principle which characterizes living substance.

4964 HUARTE Y NAVARRO, JUAN DE DIOS [HUARTE DE SAN JUAN]. *Circa* 1530–1592

Examen de ingenios para las ciencias. Baerca, 1575.

Huarte y Navarro was a distinguished Spanish physician and psychologist. His *Examen*, which gained for him a European reputation, was the first attempt to show the connexion between psychology and physiology. There were English editions in 1594, 1616, and 1698, and Lessing translated the book into German.

4965 DESCARTES, RENÉ. 1596–1650

Des passions de l'âme. Amsterdam, 1649.

Descartes believed the soul to be a definite entity, giving rise to thoughts, feelings, and acts of volition. He was one of the first to regard the brain as an organ integrating the functions of mind and body.

4966 WILLIS, THOMAS. 1621–1675

De anima brutorum. Oxonii, *R. Davis*, 1672.

English translation in his *Practice of physick*, London, 1684, Treatise IX.

4967 LOCKE, JOHN. 1632–1704

An essay concerning humane understanding. London, *by Eliz. Holt, for Thomas Basset*, 1690.

Locke laid the foundation of modern psychology. For two centuries the principles laid down by him were unquestioned. The writing of the *Essay* occupied him on and off for twenty years. Reprinted in 1910. Also published in Kennedy, G.: *Francis Bacon*, etc., Garden City, N.Y., 1937, pp. 203–385.

4968 BONNOT DE CONDILLAC, ÉTIENNE. 1715–1780

Traité des sensations. 2 vols. Londres, Paris, 1754.

Condillac considered that we perceive only what our senses supply in the form of sensations: the "real being" of things is beyond us.

4969 KANT, IMMANUEL. 1724–1804

Anthropologie in pragmatischer Hinsicht abgefasst. Königsberg, *F. Nicolovius*, 1798.

Kant, the greatest philosopher of the 18th century, attempted a classification of mental diseases.

4970 LOTZE, RUDOLPH HERMANN. 1817–1881

Medicinische Psychologie, oder Physiologie der Seele. Leipzig, *Weidmann*, 1852.

Lotze was a pioneer in the investigation of unconscious and subconscious states.

4971 KUSSMAUL, ADOLF. 1822–1902

Untersuchungen über das Seelenleben des neugeborenen Menschen. Leipzig, Heidelberg, *C. F. Winter*, 1859.

An investigation of the psychic life of the newborn. During his life Kussmaul studied and wrote on a wide variety of medical subjects.

4972 FECHNER, GUSTAV THEODOR. 1801–1887

Elemente der Psychophysik. 2 vols. Leipzig, *Breitkopf u. Härtel*, 1860.

The first treatise on the subject. Fechner applied the laws of mathematical physics to the physiology of sensation. He discussed the functional relations of the dependence between mind and body and investigated the cutaneous and muscular senses.

4973 DUCHENNE DE BOULOGNE, GUILLAUME BENJAMIN AMAND. 1806–1875
Mécanisme de la physionomie humaine. 1 vol. and atlas. Paris, *Vve. J. Renouard*, 1862.

Duchenne studied the mechanism of facial expression during emotion; his atlas of photographs is a most important contribution to the subject of physiognomy.

4974 DONDERS, FRANS CORNELIS. 1818–1889
Die Schnelligkeit psychischer Prozesse. *Arch. Anat. Physiol. wiss. Med.*, 1868, 657–81.

Donders was the first to measure the reaction-time of a psychical process.

4975 DARWIN, CHARLES ROBERT. 1809–1882
The expression of the emotions in man and animals. London, *John Murray*, 1872.

Darwin examined the causes, physiological and psychological, of all the fundamental emotions in man and animals. He concluded that "the chief expressive actions exhibited by man and by the lower animals are now innate or inherited," and that most of the movements of expression must have been gradually acquired. Reprinted, New York, 1955.

4976 WUNDT, WILHELM MAX. 1832–1920
Grundzüge der physiologischen Psychologie. 2 pts. Leipzig, *W. Engelmann*, 1873–74.

Wundt made experimental investigations of normal individual reactions, reflex responses, and general behaviour, and interpreted them in terms of neural mechanisms. He is the founder of experimental psychology and his book remains the most important on the subject.

4977 RIBOT, THEODULE ARMAND. 1839–1916
Psychologie de l'attention. Paris, 1889.

4978 BREUER, JOSEF. 1842–1925, & FREUD, SIGMUND. 1856–1939
Studien über Hysterie. Leipzig, Wien, *F. Deuticke*, 1895.

The revelation of the "unconscious mind". English translation 1936.

4979 PORTER, WILLIAM TOWNSEND. 1862–1949
The physical basis of precocity and dulness. *Trans. Acad. Sci. St. Louis*, 1893, **6,** 160–81.

4980 ANTON, GABRIEL. 1858–1933
Ueber den Ausdruck der Gemüthsbewegung beim gesunden und kranken Menschen. *Psychiat. Wschr.*, 1900, **2,** 165–69.

4981 ELLIS, HENRY HAVELOCK. 1859–1939
Studies in the psychology of sex. 7 vols. Philadelphia, *F. A. Davis*, 1900–28.

Ellis has probably done more than any other person to free discussion of sex from the conspiracy of silence which once surrounded it. His *Studies* represent a lifetime devoted to the subject, at first in the face of bitter opposition.

4982 FREUD, SIGMUND. 1856–1939
Zur Psychopathologie des Alltagslebens. Berlin, *S. Karger*, 1904.

English translation, 1914.

4983 ——. Drei Abhandlungen zur Sexualtheorie. Leipzig, *F. Deuticke*, 1905.

Freud opened up a new territory for exploration – the unconscious mind. His studies of the sexual instinct explained the reasons for, and suggested the treatment of, various perversions and neurotic conditions. English translation, 1910.

4984 ADLER, ALFRED. 1870–1937
Studie über Minderwertigkeit von Organen. Berlin, Wien, *Urban & Schwarzenberg*, 1907.

Adler, a disciple of Freud, introduced the concept of the inferiority complex and the method of compensation needed to overcome it.

4985 BINET, ALFRED. 1857–1911, & SIMON, THEODORE. 1873–
La mesure du développement de l'intelligence chez les jeunes enfants Paris, *A. Coneslant*, 1911.

Binet–Simon intelligence tests. As early as 1895 Binet had published a plan for studying intelligence. English translation, 1912.

4985.1 ADLER, ALFRED. 1870–1937
Über die nervösen Charakter. Wiesbaden, *J. F. Bergmann*, 1912.

Alder seceded from Freud's psycho-analytical group and founded the school of individual psychology. English translation of above, 1917. See also his *Practice and theory of individual psychology*, 1924.

4985.2 JUNG, CARL GUSTAV. 1875–1961
Wandlungen und Symbole der Libido. Beiträge zur Entwicklungsgeschichte des Denkens. *Jb. psycho-analyst. psychopath. Forsch.*, 1911, **3**, 120–227; 1912, **4**, 162–464.

Reprinted in book form, Leipzig, *F. Deuticke*, 1912. Jung was among the first to support Freud's views on psycho-analysis but in 1913 he broke away and founded the school of analytical psychology. His most notable work was his study of the unconscious mind. English translation, *Psychology of the unconscious*, 1916.

4986 TERMAN, LEWIS MADISON. 1877–1957, *et al.*
The Stanford revision and extension of the Binet-Simon scale for measuring intelligence. Baltimore, *Warwick & York*, 1917.

4987 WATSON, JOHN BROADUS. 1878–1958
Psychology from the standpoint of a behaviorist. Philadelphia, *J. B. Lippincott*, 1919.

Watson was the principal exponent of behaviourist psychology.

4988 KRETSCHMER, ERNST. 1888–1964
Körperbau und Charakter. Berlin, *J. Springer*, 1921.

Kretschmer has attempted to correlate body build and constitution with character and mentality.

4988.1 RORSCHACH, HERMANN. 1884–1922
Psychodiagnostik. Bern, *Bircher*, 1921.

Rorschach test. 2nd ed., Bern, 1932. English translation, Bern, *Huber*, 1942. See the biography of Rorschach in *Bull. Menninger Clin.*, 1954, **18**, 173–219.

4989 FREUD, SIGMUND. 1856–1939
Introductory lectures on psycho-analysis. London, *Allen & Unwin*, [1922].

4990 JANET, PIERRE MARIE FÉLIX. 1859–1947
La médecine psychologique. Paris, *E. Flammarion*, 1923.

4991 KÖHLER, WOLFGANG. 1887–1967
Gestalt psychology. New York, *Liveright Publ. Co.*, 1929.

Psychotherapy; Hypnotism

4992 MESMER, Franz Anton. 1734–1815
Mémoire sur la découverte du magnétisme animal. Genève, Paris, *P. F. Didot le jeune*, 1779.

Mesmer's work served as a basis for the more scientific development of suggestion in treatment, which has been termed after him "mesmerism". He did not realize that his clinic in Paris was being used as the meeting-place of all sorts of perverts. Following an enquiry instituted by Louis XVI, his career came to an abrupt end. English translation by Gilbert Frankau, 1948.

4993 BRAID, James. 1795–1860
Neurypnology, or, the rationale of nervous sleep. London, *J. Churchill*, 1843.

Braid inaugurated modern hypnotism, the word itself being introduced by him. His theories were adopted by Broca, Charcot, Liébeault, and Bernheim; thus he founded the French School.

4994 ELLIOTSON, John. 1791–1868
Numerous cases of surgical operations without pain in the mesmeric state. London, *H. Baillière*, 1843.

Elliotson was one of the first to perform surgical operations with the aid of hypnotism. He was a great friend of Dickens and Thackeray, but his views on hypnotism were bitterly opposed by Thomas Wakley, editor of the *Lancet*, whose onslaughts eventually led to his downfall.

4995 ESDAILE, James. 1808–1859
Mesmerism in India, and its practical application in surgery and medicine. London, *Longman, etc.*, 1846.

Esdaile performed a variety of surgical operations on Hindus, upon many of whom he appears successfully to have induced hypnotic anaesthesia. However, his similar attempts with Europeans were not so successful.

4996 FOREL, Auguste Henri. 1848–1931
Der Hypnotismus und die suggestive Psychotherapie. Stuttgart, *F. Enke*, 1888.

4997 LIÉBEAULT, Ambroise Auguste. 1823–1904
Le sommeil provoqué et les états analogues. Paris, *O. Doin*, 1889.

The substitution of psychotherapy for hypnotic suggestion starts with the work of Liébeault.

4998 ——. Thérapeutique suggestive. Paris, *O. Doin*, 1891.

4999 BERNHEIM, Hippolyte Marie. 1840–1919
Hypnotisme, suggestion, psychothérapie. Paris, *O. Doin*, 1891.

Like Liébeault, Bernheim studied the scientific applications of hypnotism and substituted verbal for sensory stimuli; he interpreted hypnotism and its consequent phenomena as being the result of suggestion.

5000 CAMUS, Jean. 1872–1924, & PAGNIEZ, Philippe.
Isolement et psychothérapie. Paris, *F. Alcan*, 1904.

For history, see Nos. 5002, 5013, 5019.5

History of Neurology and Psychiatry

5001 BUCKNILL, *Sir* John Charles. 1817–1897
The mad folk of Shakespeare. 2nd ed. London, *Macmillan*, 1867.

5002 PREYER, THIERRY WILHELM. 1841–1897
Die Entdeckung des Hypnotismus. Berlin, *Gebrüder Paetel*, 1881.
A history of hypnotism.

5003 TUKE, DANIEL HACK. 1827–1895
Chapters in the history of the insane in the British Isles. London, *Kegan Paul*, 1882.

5004 LAEHR, HANS HEINRICH. 1820–1905
Gedenktage der Psychiatrie. 4te. Aufl. Berlin, *G. Reimer*, 1893.
A history of the subject, arranged in calendar form.

5005 ——. Die Literatur der Psychiatrie, Neurologie und Psychologie von 1459–1799. 3 vols. Berlin, *G. Reimer*, 1900.

5006 HURD, HENRY MILLS. 1843–1927
The institutional care of the insane in the United States and Canada. 4 vols. Baltimore, *Johns Hopkins Press*, 1916–17.
Hurd, who edited the above, was professor of psychiatry at Johns Hopkins University. The work includes his history of American psychiatry.

5007 KRAEPELIN, EMIL. 1856–1926
Hundert Jahre Psychiatrie. *Z. ges. Neurol.*, 1918, **38**, 161–275.
English translation, New York, 1962.

5008 BALLANCE, *Sir* CHARLES ALFRED. 1856–1936
A glimpse into the history of the surgery of the brain. London, *Macmillan & Co.*, 1922.
Thomas Vicary Lecture. First published in *Lancet*, 1922, **1**, 111–6, 165–72.

5009 GARRISON, FIELDING HUDSON. 1870–1935
History of neurology. In DANA, C. L., *Text-book of nervous diseases*. 10th ed., New York, *W. Wood*, 1925, xv–lvi.
Revised edition, Springfield, 1969.

5010 LAIGNEL-LAVASTINE, MAXIME PAUL MARIE. 1875–1953, & VINCHON, JEAN.
Les maladies de l'esprit et leurs médecine du XVIe au XIXe siècle. Les étapes des connaissances psychiatriques de la Renaissance à Pinel. Paris, *Maloine*, 1930.

5011 VON STORCH, THEODOR JOSEPH CONSTANT. 1905–1965
An essay on the history of epilepsy. *Ann. med. Hist.*, 1930, n.s., **2**, 614–50.

5012 LEWIS, NOLAN DON CARPENTIER. 1889–
A short history of psychiatric achievement. New York, *W. W. Norton*, (1941).

5013 ZILBOORG, GREGORY. 1890–1959, & HENRY, GEORGE WILLIAM. 1889–
A history of medical psychology. New York, *W. W. Norton*, 1941.

5014 WARTENBERG, ROBERT. 1887–1956
Studies in reflexes. History, physiology, synthesis and nomenclature. *Arch. Neurol. Psychiat.*, 1944, **51**, 113–33, 414; **52**, 341–58, 359–82.

5015 TEMKIN, Owsei, 1902–
The falling sickness: a history of epilepsy from the Greeks to the beginnings of modern neurology. Baltimore, *Johns Hopkins Press*, 1945.
Publications of the Institute of the History of Medicine, 1st series, Monographs, vol. IV. 2nd ed., 1971.

5016 FISHBEIN, Morris. 1889– , *et al.*
A bibliography of infantile paralysis 1789–1949. With selected abstracts and annotations. Edited by M. Fishbein and Ella M. Salmonsen, with L. Hektoen. 2nd edition. Philadelphia, *Lippincott*, 1951.
An exhaustive list of books and papers.

5017 WALKER, Arthur Earl. 1907–
A history of neurological surgery. Edited by A. Earl Walker. Baltimore, *Williams & Wilkins*, 1951.
The most exhaustive account of the subject available; there is a bibliography of nearly 2,400 references.

5018 HORRAX, Gilbert. 1887–1957
Neurosurgery. An historical sketch. Springfield, *C. C. Thomas*, 1952.
A short but fully documented and illustrated history.

5019 HAYMAKER, Webb Edward. 1902–
The founders of neurology. One hundred and thirty-three biographical sketches. Springfield, *C. C. Thomas*, 1953.

5019.1 KOLLE, Kurt, 1898–
Grosse Nervenärzte. 3 vols. Stuttgart, *G. Thieme*, 1956–63.

5019.2 RIESE, Walther. 1890–
A history of neurology. New York, *M.D. Publications*, [1959].

5019.3 LEIGH, Denis.
The historical development of British psychiatry. Vol. 1– . Oxford, *Pergamon Press*, 1961– .

5019.4 HUNTER, Richard Alfred, & MACALPINE, Ida.
Three hundred years of psychiatry, 1535–1860; a history presented in selected English texts. London, *Oxford University Press*, 1963.

5019.5 KIELL, Norman. 1916–
Psychoanalysis, psychology and literature: a bibliography. Madison, *University of Wisconsin Press*, 1963.
Contains 4,460 references.

5019.6 GANDOLFI, Mario.
Storia della sciatica. Rocca San Casciano, *F. Cappelli*, 1965.

5019.7 ALEXANDER, Franz. 1891–1964, & SELESNICK, Sheldon Theodore. 1925–
The history of psychiatry: an evaluation of psychiatric thought and practice from prehistoric times to the present. New York, *Harper & Row*, 1966.

5019.8 ELDRIDGE, Margaret.
A history of the treatment of speech disorders. Edinburgh, *E. & S. Livingstone*, 1968.

5020–5546.4 COMMUNICABLE DISEASES

5020–5045 ENTERIC FEVER

5020 WILLIS, Thomas. 1621–1675
Diatribae duae medico-philosophicae, quarum prior agit de fermentatione sive de motu intestino particularum in quovis corpore, altera de febribus sive de motu earundum in sanguine animalium. Londini, *T. Roycroft*, 1659.

Includes (De febribus, cap. X, XIV) first description of epidemic typhoid. English translation in his *Practice of physick*, 1684, Treatise II, 83–98, 1111–8.

5021 ROEDERER, Johann Georg. 1727–1763, & WAGLER, Carl Gottlieb. ?–1778
De morbo mucoso. Gottingae, *V. Bossiegel*, 1762.

An exhaustive study of typhoid, which the writers confused with dysentery and relapsing fever.

5022 SMITH, Nathan. 1762–1829
A practical essay on typhous fever. New York, *E. Bliss & E. White*, 1842.

Nathan Smith left a classical account of typhoid; this was reprinted in *Med. Classics*, 1937, **1**, 781–819. He clearly recognized the contagious nature of the disease.

5023 LOUIS, Pierre Charles Alexandre. 1787–1872
Recherches anatomiques, pathologiques et thérapeutiques sur la maladie connue sous les noms de gastro-entérite, fièvre putride, adynamique, ataxique, typhoïde, etc. 2 vols. Paris, *J. B. Baillière*, 1829.

Louis introduced the term "typhoid fever" in reference to the disturbed mental condition of the patient; he first described the lenticular rose spots. His book established the pathological picture of the disease. English translation, Boston, 1836.

5023.1 PERRY, Robert. 1783–1848
Observations on continued fever, as it occurs in the city of Glasgow hospitals. *Edinb. med. surg. J.*, 1836, **45,** 64–70.

Perry correctly described many of the distinctions between typhus and typhoid.

5024 GERHARD, William Wood. 1809–1872
On the typhus fever, which occurred at Philadelphia in the spring and summer of 1836. *Amer. J. med. Sci.*, 1837, **19,** 289–322; **20,** 289–322.

Gerhard, a pupil of Louis, correctly differentiated between typhus and typhoid. Part of his paper is reproduced in R. H. Major, *Classic descriptions of disease*, 3rd. ed., 1945, p. 174.

5025 STEWART, ALEXANDER PATRICK. 1813–1883
Some considerations on the nature and pathology of typhus and typhoid fever, applied to the solution of the question of the identity or non-identity of the two diseases. *Edinb. med. surg. J.*, 1840, **54,** 289–339.

Typhoid and typhus were often confused. Stewart made a careful analysis of a number of cases of both fevers and clearly demonstrated that there were in Britain two distinct fevers – typhoid and typhus.

5026 RITCHIE, CHARLES. 1799–1878
Practical remarks on the continued fevers of Great Britain, and on the generic distinctions between enteric fever and typhus. *Monthly J. med. Sci.*, 1846–47, **7,** 347–58.

Introduction of the term "enteric fever." Ritchie carefully differentiated the symptoms of typhus and typhoid.

5027 JENNER, *Sir* WILLIAM. 1815–1898
On typhoid and typhus fevers, – an attempt to determine the question of their identity or non-identity, by an analysis of the symptoms, and of the appearances found after death in 66 fatal cases observed at the London Fever Hospital from Jan. 1847–Feb. 1849. *Monthly J. med. Sci.*, 1849, **9,** 663–80.

Despite Stewart's work there was still some controversy as to the identity of typhoid and typhus. Jenner's paper demonstrated that the aetiology of the two was quite different, that one did not communicate or protect against the other, and that epidemics of the two did not prevail simultaneously.

5028 BRAND, ERNST. 1827–1897
Die Hydrotherapie des Typhus. Stettin, *T. von der Nahmer*, 1861.

Brand's cold bath treatment of typhoid fever consisted in total immersion in water at 65° F. and the pouring of cold water over the neck and shoulders. The cold bath treatment of fevers was instituted by Currie (see No. 1988).

5029 BUDD, WILLIAM. 1811–1880
Typhoid fever; its nature, mode of spreading, and prevention. London, *Longmans, Green & Co.*, 1873.

Budd insisted that typhoid fever was spread by contagion and established the fact that infection with typhoid came from the dejecta of the patients; he strengthened the theory of water-borne infection. See also his earlier papers in *Lancet*, 1856, **2,** 617, 694.

5030 EBERTH, CARL JOSEPH. 1835–1926
Die Organismen in den Organen bei Typhus abdominalis. *Virchows Arch. path. Anat.*, 1880, **81,** 58–74.

Salmonella typhi, causal organism of typhoid, was discovered by Eberth. Some European writers refer to the disease as "Eberth's disease".

5031 KLEBS, THEODOR ALBRECHT EDWIN. 1834–1913
Der Bacillus des Abdominaltyphus und der typhöse Process. *Arch. exp. Path. Pharmak.*, 1881, **13,** 381–460.

Klebs probably saw the typhoid bacillus before Eberth, reporting it later.

5032 GAFFKY, GEORG. 1850–1918
Zur Aetiologie des Abdominaltyphus. *Mitt. k. GesundhAmte*, Berlin, 1884, **2,** 372–420.

Gaffky was the first to grow pure cultures of *Salmonella typhi*; he showed it to be the true activator of the disease. English translation (New Sydenham Society), 1886.

5033 ANTON, Bernhard, & FÜTTERER, Gustav. 1854–1922
Untersuchungen über Typhus abdominalis. *Münch med. Wschr.*, 1888, **35,** 315–18.

Salmonella typhi first demonstrated in the gall-bladder in cases of typhoid.

5034 CHANTEMESSE, André. 1851–1919, & WIDAL, Georges Fernand Isidor. 1862–1929.
De l'immunité contre le virus de la fièvre typhoïde conférée par des substances solubles. *Ann. Inst. Pasteur*, 1888, 2, 54–59.

Experimental antityphoid inoculation.

5035 ACHARD, Emile Charles. 1860–1944, & BENSAUDE, Raoul.
Infections paratyphoïdiques. *Bull. Soc. méd. Hôp. Paris*, 1896, 3 sér., **13,** 820–33.

Isolation of *Salmonella paratyphi B*. First use of the term "paratyphoid fever".

5036 GRUBER, Max. 1853–1927, & DURHAM, Herbert Edward. 1866–1945
Eine neue Methode zur raschen Erkennung des Choleravibrio und des Typhusbacillus. *Münch med. Wschr.*, 1896, **43,** 285–86.

The discovery of bacterial agglutination was made when Gruber and Durham found that the serum of typhoid patients had an agglutinating action on the typhoid bacillus; they realized its value as a clinical test in the identification of typhoid.

5037 WIDAL, Georges Fernand Isidor. 1862–1929, & SICARD, Arthur.
Recherches de la réaction agglutinante dans le sang et le sérum desséchés des typhiques et dans la sérosité des vésicatoires. *Bull. Soc. méd. Hop.* Paris, 1896, 3 sér., **13,** 681–82.

Widal and Sicard demonstrated specific agglutinins in the blood of typhoid patients, making possible an agglutination reaction for the diagnosis of typhoid ("Gruber–Widal test").

5038 GWYN, Norman Beechey. 1875–1952
On infection with a para-colon bacillus in a case with all the clinical features of typhoid fever. *Johns Hopk. Hosp. Bull.*, 1898, **9,** 54–56.

Isolation of *Salmonella paratyphi A*.

5039 WRIGHT, *Sir* Almroth Edward. 1861–1947, & LEISHMAN, *Sir* William Boog. 1865–1926
Remarks on the results which have been obtained by the antityphoid inoculations. *Brit. med. J.*, 1900, **1,** 122–29.

The active inoculation of man against typhoid was first performed by Wright in 1896. For a preliminary note see *Lancet*, 1896, 2, 807.

5040 KOCH, Robert. 1843–1910
Die Bekämpfung des Typhus. Berlin, *A. Hirschwald*, 1903.

The prophylactic measures for the control of typhoid suggested by Koch have been adopted almost everywhere.

5041 UHLENHUTH, Paul Theodor. 1870–1957, & HÜBENER, Erich August. 1870–
Weitere Mitteilungen über Schweinepest mit besonderer Berücksichtigung der Bakteriologie der Hogcholeragruppe. *Zbl. Bakt.*, 1 Abt., 1908, **42,** Beilage, 127–38.

First description of *Salmonella paratyphi C*.

5042 RUSSELL, FREDERICK FULLER. 1870–1960
The control of typhoid in the Army by vaccination. *N.Y. State J. Med.*, 1910, **10**, 535–48.

Russell carried out important and long-continued investigations on anti-typhoid vaccination in the U.S. Army, demonstrating beyond question its value in selected groups. The war of 1914–18 confirmed the value of the work of Wright and Russell.

5043 SAXL, PAUL. 1880–1932
Ueber die Behandlung von Typhus mit Milchinjektionen. *Wien. klin. Wschr.*, 1916, **29**, 1043–45.

5044 HIRZFELD, LUDWIK. 1884–1954
A new germ of paratyphoid. *Lancet*, 1919, **1**, 296–97.

Hirszfeld gave an important description of *Salmonella paratyphi C.* ("Hirszfeld's bacillus").

5044.1 KAUFFMANN, FRITZ.
Der heutige Stand der Paratyphusforschung. *Zbl. ges. Hyg.*, 1931, **25**, 273–311.

Kauffmann–White classification of *Salmonella* based on antigenic structure. For historical note, including the part played by P. B. White, see *J. Hyg. (Camb.)*, 1934, **34**, 335.

5045 FELIX, ARTHUR. 1887–1956, & PITT, R. MARGARET.
A new antigen of B. typhosus. Its relation to virulence and to active and passive immunisation. *Lancet*, 1934, **2**, 186–91.

Vi antigens first described.

5046–5072 DIPHTHERIA

5046 ARETAEUS, *the Cappadocian*. A.D. 81–138?
On ulcerations about the tonsils. In his: *Extant works*, ed. F. ADAMS, London, 1856, 253–55.

Aretaeus' description of ulcerations about the tonsils, which he called "ulcera Syriaca", clearly referred to diphtheria, of which it was the first unmistakable description. For his treatment of the disease, see pp. 409–10 of the same work.

5047 BAILLOU, GUILLAUME DE [BALLONIUS]. 1538–1616
Epidemiorum et ephemeridum libri duo. Paris, *J. Quensel*, 1640.

A pupil of Fernel, de Baillou was a brilliant writer and speaker. The above work includes a description of the epidemic of diphtheria in Paris, 1576. Later Baillou advocated tracheotomy, although there is no evidence that he himself performed that operation.

5048 MARTINE, GEORGE. 1702–1741
Account of the operation of bronchotome, as it was performed at St. Andrews. *Phil. Trans.*, 1730, **36**, 448–55.

Martine was the first in Britain to perform tracheotomy for diphtheria.

5049 FOTHERGILL, JOHN. 1712–1780
An account of the sore throat attended with ulcers. London, *C. Davis*, 1748.

First authoritative account of both diphtheria and scarlatinal angina, although the writer failed to differentiate between the two conditions. Reprinted in *Med. Classics*, 1940, **5**, 58–99.

5050 HUXHAM, John. 1692–1768
A dissertation on the malignant, ulcerous sore-throat. London, *J. Hinton*, 1757.
Huxham's reputation rests mainly on his *Essay on fevers*, but he also left an excellent account of diphtheria. Although he failed to differentiate the disease from scarlatinal angina, he was the first to observe the paralysis of the soft palate.

5051 HOME, Francis. 1719–1813
An enquiry into the nature, cause, and cure of the croup. Edinburgh, *Kincaid & Bell*, 1765.
First clear and complete clinical description of diphtheria.

5052 BARD, Samuel. 1742–1821
An enquiry into the nature, cause and cure, of the angina suffocativa, or, sore throat distemper, as it is commonly called by the inhabitants of this city and colony. New York, *S. Inslee, & A. Car*, 1771.
One of the earliest accurate descriptions of diphtheria. Osler considered the book "an American classic of the first rank".

5053 BRETONNEAU, Pierre Fidèle. 1778–1862
Des inflammations spéciales du tissu muqueux et en particulier de la diphthérite, ou inflammation pelliculaire. Paris, *Crevot*, 1826.
Bretonneau showed that croup, malignant angina, and "scorbutic gangrene of the gums" were all the same disease, for which he suggested the term "diphtheritis," later substituting "diphthérie". He performed (pp. 300–08) what is believed to be the first successful tracheotomy for croup.

5054 TROUSSEAU, Armand. 1801–1867
Mémoire sur un cas de trachéotomie pratiquée dans la période extrème de croup. *J. Connaiss. méd.-chir.*, 1833, **1**, 5, 41.
Trousseau popularized tracheotomy.

5055 KLEBS, Theodor Albrecht Edwin. 1834–1913
Ueber Diphtherie. *Verh. Congr. inn. Med.*, 1883, **2**, 139–54.
First account of *Corynebacterium diphtheriae* (Klebs-Loeffler bacillus), causal organism in diphtheria, discovered by Klebs.

5056 LOEFFLER, Friedrich. 1852–1915
Untersuchungen über die Bedeutung der Mikroorganismen für die Entstehung der Diphtherie beim Menschen, bei der Taube und beim Kalbe. *Mitt. k. GesundhAmte*, 1884, **2**, 421–99.
Loeffler succeeded in cultivating *C. diphtheriae*; he reproduced the characteristic membrane by swabbing the mucous membranes of various animals with pure cultures of the bacillus.

5057 O'DWYER, Joseph P. 1841–1898
Intubation of the larynx. *N.Y. med. J.*, 1885, **42**, 145–47.
O'Dwyer perfected the operation of laryngeal intubation in croup.

5058 ——. Analysis of fifty cases of croup treated by intubation of the larynx. *N.Y. med. J.*, 1888, **47**, 33–37.

5059 ROUX, Pierre Paul Emile. 1853–1933, & YERSIN, Alexandre Emil Jean. 1863–1943
Contribution à l'étude de la diphtérie. *Ann. Inst. Pasteur,* 1888, **2,** 629–61; 1889, **3,** 273–88; 1890, **4,** 385–426.
Confirmation of the work of Loeffler and demonstration of the exotoxin. This work is the starting point of the development of an immunizing serum.

5060 BEHRING, EMIL ADOLF VON. 1854–1917, & KITASATO, SHIBASABURO, *Baron*. 1856–1931
Ueber das Zustandekommen der Diphtherie-Immunität und der Tetanus-Immunität bei Thieren. *Dtsch. med. Wschr.*, 1890, **16**, 1113–1114, 1145–48.

Antitoxins and their immunizing powers were discovered when Behring and Kitasato published their paper dealing with immunity to tetanus and diphtheria. This work laid the foundation of all future treatment with antitoxins. The paper was reprinted in the same journal, 1940, **66**, 1348–49. Part 2, which deals with diphtheria, is by Behring alone.

5060.1 FRAENKEL, CARL. 1861–1915
Immunisirungsversuche bei Diphtherie. *Berl. klin. Wschr.*, 1890, **27**, 1133–35.

Artificial immunity to diphtheria produced in guinea-pigs by injection of attenuated cultures of the bacillus.

5061 WELCH, WILLIAM HENRY. 1850–1934, & FLEXNER, SIMON. 1863–1946
The histological changes in experimental diphtheria. *Johns Hopk. Hosp. Bull.*, 1891, **2**, 107–10; 1892, **3**, 17–18.

An account of the pathological changes brought about by experimental inoculation of diphtheria toxins.

5062 BEHRING, EMIL ADOLF VON. 1854–1917
Die Behandlung der Diphtherie mit Diphtherieheilserum. *Dtsch. med. Wschr.*, 1893, **19**, 543–47; 1894, **20**, 645–46.

In 1890 Behring and Kitasato discovered the diphtheria and tetanus antitoxins (See No. 5060). The above papers deal more fully with the use of the diphtheria antitoxin.

5063 ROUX, PIERRE PAUL EMILE. 1853–1933, & MARTIN, ANDRÉ LOUIS FRANÇOIS JUSTIN. 1853–1921
Contribution à l'étude de la diphtérie (serum thérapie). *Ann. Inst. Pasteur*, 1894, **8**, 609–39.

Roux and Martin demonstrated the value of Behring's specific antitoxin in the treatment of human diphtheria, and showed how it could be produced on a large scale.

5064 EHRLICH, PAUL. 1854–1915
Die Wertbestimmung des Diphtherieheilserums. *Klin. Jb.*, 1897, **6**, 299–326.

Ehrlich improved Behring's diphtheria antitoxin and established an international standard for this and other antitoxins. The first exposition of his side-chain theory also appeared in this paper.

5065 SCHICK, BELA. 1877–1967
Kutanreaktion bei Impfung mit Diphtherietoxin. *Münch. med. Wschr.*, 1908, **55**, 504–06.

The Schick test for the determination of susceptibility to diphtheria.

5066 ——. Die Diphtherietoxin – Hautreaktion des Menschen als Vorprobe der prophylaktischen Diphtherieheilseruminjektion. *Münch. med. Wschr.*, 1913, **60**, 2608–10.

Schick developed his test for use as an indication as to whether or not prophylactic injections of antitoxin are necessary in children already exposed to diphtheria.

5067 BEHRING, EMIL ADOLF VON. 1854–1917
Ueber ein neues Diphtherieschutzmittel. *Dtsch. med. Wschr.*, 1913, **39,** 873–76; 1914, **40,** 1139.
Toxin-antitoxin for immunization against diphtheria.

5068 PARK, WILLIAM HALLOCK. 1863–1939, *et al.*
Active immunization in diphtheria and treatment by toxin-antitoxin. *J. Amer. med. Ass.*, 1914, **63,** 859–61.
With A. Zingher and M. H. Serota. Park was an early advocate of diphtheria immunization with toxin-antitoxin. A second paper is in the same journal, 1915, **65**, 2216–20.

5069 KASSOWITZ, KARL ERHARD. 1886–
Ueber cutane Hautreaktion mittels Diphtherie-Toxin zum Nachweis der Diphterie-Immunität. *Klin. Wschr.*, 1924, **3,** 1317–18.
The "scratch test", a cutaneous reaction for determination of susceptibility to diphtheria.

5070 RAMON, GASTON LÉON. 1886–1963
L'anatoxine diphtérique. Ses propriétés – ses applications. *Ann. Inst. Pasteur*, 1928, **42,** 959–1009.
In 1923 Ramon so modified the diphtheria toxin with formaldehyde that it lost its toxic properties while retaining its antigenic virtues. This modified "anatoxin" (toxoid) superseded toxin-antitoxin as an immunizing agent against diphtheria. Preliminary paper in *C. R. Soc. Biol.* (*Paris*), 1923, **89**, 2–4.

5071 GLENNY, ALEXANDER THOMAS. 1882–
Insoluble precipitates in diphtheria and tetanus immunization. *Brit. med. J.*, 1930, **2,** 244–45.
Alum-precipitated toxoid for active immunization.

5072 ANDERSON, JAMES STIRLING. 1891– , *et al.*
On the existence of two forms of diphtheria bacillus – *B. diphtheriae gravis* and *B. diphtheriae mitis*. *J. Path. Bact.*, 1931, **34,** 667–81.
J. S. Anderson, F. C. Happold, J. W. McLeod, and J. G. Thomson were the first to distinguish the *gravis*, *mitis*, and intermediate types of *C. diphtheriae*.

5073–5084 SCARLET FEVER

5073 INGRASSIA, GIOVANNI FILIPPO. 1510–1580
De tumoribus praeter naturam. Neapoli, 1553.
Includes (p. 194) the first known description of an epidemic disease resembling scarlet fever. This was a prevalent malady in Italy, and was commonly called *rossania* or *rossalia.*

5074 SENNERT, DANIEL. 1572–1637
De febribus libri IV. Venetiis, *F. Baba*, 1641.
Sennert gave the first scientific description of scarlet fever. He was the first to mention the scarlatinal desquamation, the early arthritis, and post-scarlatinal dropsy, but made no mention of sore throat.

5075 SYDENHAM, THOMAS. 1624–1689
Febris scarlatina. In his : *Observationes medicae*, London, 1676, p. 387.
The reputation of Sydenham, "the English Hippocrates" rests to-day on his excellent accounts of diseases, of which the description of scarlet fever is one of the best. He first clearly differentiated scarlatina from measles, giving it its present name. Translation in his *Works*, London, 1850, **2**, 242.

5076 DOUGLASS, WILLIAM. 1691–1752
The practical history of a new epidemical eruptive miliary fever, with an angina ulcusculosa, which prevailed in Boston New England in the years 1735 and 1736. Boston, N.E., *T. Fleet*, 1736.
Douglass left an excellent account of the first cases of scarlet fever in New England; he called it angina ulcusculosa.

5077 FOTHERGILL, JOHN. 1712–1780
An account of the sore throat attended with ulcers. London, *C. Davis*, 1748.
First authoritative account of both diphtheria and scarlatinal angina, although failing to differentiate between the two conditions. Reprinted in *Med. Classics*, 1940, **5**, 58–99.

5078 PLENCISZ, MARC ANTON VON. 1705–1786
Opera medico-physica . . . tertius de scarlatina. 4 pts. Viennae Austriae, *J. T. Trattner*, 1762.
Plencisz was the first clearly to grasp the significance of Leeuwenhoek's *animalculae* for the aetiology of contagious disease; this idea he advanced in his book on scarlatina.

5079 WITHERING, WILLIAM. 1741–1799
An account of the scarlet fever and sore throat, or scarlatina anginosa; particularly as it appeared at Birmingham in the year 1778. London, *T. Cadell*, 1779.
Withering, best remembered for his book on the foxglove, described the epidemics of scarlet fever which occurred in England in 1771 and 1778.

5080 KLEIN, EDWARD EMANUEL. 1844–1925
Report on a disease of cows prevailing at a farm from which scarlatina had been distributed along with the milk of cows. *15th Ann. Rep. Local Govt Bd., Suppl. containing Report of the Medical Officer for 1885*, London, 1886, pp. 90–110.
Contains the first suggestion of the streptococcal origin of scarlet fever.

5080.1 BERGÉ, ANDRÉ.
Sur la pathogénie de la scarlatine. *C. R. Soc. Biol. (Paris)*, 1893, **45,** 1012–14.
Bergé stated all the essential facts concerning the aetiology of scarlet fever, and definitely attributed its cause to a streptococcus. He published a thesis on the subject in 1895.

5081 SCHULTZ, WERNER. 1878–1947, & CHARLTON, WILLY. 1889–
Serologische Beobachtungen am Scharlachexanthem. *Z. Kinderheilk.*, 1918, Orig., **17,** 328–33.
Schultz–Charlton reaction.

5082 DICK, GEORGE FREDERICK. 1881– , & DICK, GLADYS ROWENA HENRY. 1881–
A skin test for susceptibility to scarlet fever. *J. Amer. med. Ass.*, 1924, **82,** 265–66.
The "Dick test" for the determination of individual susceptibility to scarlet fever.

5082.1 ——. The etiology of scarlet fever. *J. Amer. med. Ass.*, 1924, **82,** 301–02.
Proof that streptococcus is the cause of scarlet fever.

5083 ——. A scarlet fever antitoxin. *J. Amer. med. Ass.*, 1924, **82,** 1246–1247.

Following their successful attempts to establish individual susceptibility to scarlet fever, these workers prepared an antitoxin for immunization.

5084 DOCHEZ, ALPHONSE RAYMOND. 1882–1964, & SHERMAN, LILLIAN.

The significance of Streptococcus hemolyticus in scarlet fever and the preparation of a specific anti-scarlatinal serum by immunization of the horse to Streptococcus hemolyticus-scarlatinae. *J. Amer. med. Ass.*, 1924, **82,** 542–44.

Dochez and Sherman immunized a horse by repeated injections of scarlet fever toxin. A serum obtained from the horse blanched a scarlet fever rash and, when injected subcutaneously, caused marked amelioration of the early symptoms. They also confirmed the relation of streptococci to scarlet fever.

5085–5088 WHOOPING COUGH

5085 BAILLOU, GUILLAUME DE [BALLONIUS]. 1538–1616

Quinta. In his *Epidemiorum et ephemeridum libri duo.* Paris, *J. Quesnel*, 1640, p. 237.

First description of whooping cough. This was originally written in 1578. Baillou called it "tussis quintana". For translation see R. H. Major, *Classic descriptions of disease*, 3rd ed., 1945, p. 210.

5086 WILLIS, THOMAS. 1621–1675

Pharmaceutice rationalis sive diatriba de medicamentorum operationibus in humano corpore. Pars secunda. [Oxonii], *e Theatro Sheldoniano*, 1675.

Contains (p. 99) a description of "puerorum tussis convulsiva, chincough dicta" – a clear account of whooping cough (Treatise IX, pt. 2, p. 38 of his *Practice of physick*, 1684).

5086.1 WATT, ROBERT. 1774–1819

Treatise on the history, nature, and treatment of chincough: including a variety of cases and dissections. Glasgow, *J. Smith & Son*, 1813.

Probably the first book on the subject. Watt was the compiler of the monumental *Bibliotheca Britannica* (1819–24) which includes many medical items.

5087 BORDET, JULES JEAN BAPTISTE VINCENT. 1870–1961, & GENGOU, OCTAVE. 1875–1959

Le microbe de la coqueluche. *Ann. Inst. Pasteur*, 1906, **20,** 731–41; 1907, **21,** 720–26.

The cocco-bacillus *Haemophilus pertussis*, commonly regarded as the causal organism of whooping cough, was at first named "Bordet–Gengou bacillus" after its discoverers. It has recently been renamed *Bordetella pertussis.*

5087.1 LESLIE, PATRICK HOLT, & GARDNER, ARTHUR DUNCAN. 1884–

The phases of *Haemophilus pertussis. J. Hyg.* (*Camb.*), 1931, **31,** 423–434.

Leslie and Gardner classified *H. pertussis* cultures into four types and established an experimental basis for the development of an effective vaccine.

5088 STICKER, GEORG. 1860–1960

Der Keuchhusten. Wien, *A. Hölder*, 1896.

An important history of whooping cough.

BACILLARY DYSENTERY

See also 5180.1–5194.1, AMOEBIASIS.

5089 ARETAEUS, *the Cappadocian*. A.D. 81–138?
On dysentery. In his: *Extant works*, ed. F. ADAMS, London, 1856, 353–57.

Prior to Lösch's discovery of *E. histolytica*, all forms of dysentery were differentiated only on clinical grounds.

5090 ZIMMERMANN, JOHANN GEORG. 1728–1795
Von der Ruhr unter dem Volke im Jahr 1765. Zürich, *Fuessli & Co.*, 1767.

First important monograph on bacillary dysentery. English translation, London, 1771.

5090.1 CHANTEMESSE, ANDRÉ. 1851–1919, & WIDAL, GEORGES FERNAND ISIDOR. 1862–1929
Sur les microbes de la dysentérie épidémique. *Bull. Acad. Méd. (Paris)*, 1888, **19,** 522–29.

The dysentery bacillus was isolated by Chantemesse and Widal although they failed to establish its aetological relationship to the disease.

5091 SHIGA, KIYOSHI. 1870–1957
Ueber den Dysenteriebacillus (Bacillus dysenteriae). *Zbl. Bakt.*, 1898, 1 Abt., **24,** 817–28, 870–74.

Discovery of the dysentery bacillus, *Shigella*. Preliminary paper in the same journal, 1898, 23, 599–600.

5092 KRUSE, WALTHER. 1864–1943
Ueber die Ruhr als Volkskrankheit und ihren Erreger. *Dtsch. med. Wschr.*, 1900, **26,** 637–39.

Further work on dysentery by Kruse led to the coupling of his name with Shiga to designate both the "Shiga–Kruse bacillus" and "Shiga–Kruse disease".

5093 FLEXNER, SIMON. 1863–1946
On the etiology of tropical dysentery. *Johns Hopk. Hosp. Bull.*, 1900, **11,** 231–42.

The organism isolated by Flexner was at first thought to be identical with Shiga's bacillus. Later Martini and Lentz, *Z. Hyg.*, 1902, **41**, 540, showed it to be different; it was named *Bact. flexneri*, and later *Shigella flexneri*.

5094 SONNE, CARL OLAF. 1882–1948
Ueber die Bakteriologie der giftarmen Dysenteriebacillen (Paradysenteriebacillen). *Zbl. Bakt.*, 1915, 1 Abt., **75,** Orig., 408–56.

Sonne's bacillus (*Shigella sonnei*) was probably described earlier by others, but it was Sonne who first drew serious attention to it. First published as inaugural dissertation, 1914.

5095 SCHMITZ, KARL EITEL FRIEDRICH. 1889–
Eine neuer Typus aus der Gruppe der Ruhrbazillen als Erreger einer grösseren Epidemie. *Z. Hyg. InfektKr.*, 1917, **84,** 449–516.

Schmitz's bacillus – *Bact. ambiguum* (*Shigella schmitzii*), a cause of dysentery.

5096 MARSHALL, ELI KENNERLEY. 1889–1966, *et al.*
Sulfanilylguanidine in the treatment of acute bacillary dysentery in children. *Johns Hopk. Hosp. Bull.*, 1941, **68,** 94–111.

E. K. Marshall, A. C. Bratton, L. B. Edwards, and E. L. Walker were the first to use sulphaguanidine in the treatment of bacillary dysentery.

5097–5103

BRUCELLOSIS

5097 MARSTON, JEFFERY ALLEN. 1831–1911
Report on fever (Malta). *Army med. Dept. statist. Rep.* (*Lond.*), (1861), 1863, **3**, 486–521.

Marston wrote the first description of Malta fever as a distinct disease. He contracted the disease while serving in the Mediterranean area and described his own case.

5098 BRUCE, *Sir* DAVID. 1855–1931
Note on the discovery of a microorganism in Malta fever. *Practitioner*, 1887, **39**, 161–70.

Malta fever was shown by Bruce to be due to *Micrococcus* (*Brucella*) *melitensis.*

5099 BANG, BERNHARD LAURITS FREDERIK. 1848–1932
Die Aetiologie des seuchenhaften ("infectiösen") Verwerfens. *Z. Thiermed.*, 1897, **1**, 241–78.

Discovery of *Brucella abortus.*

5100 HUGHES, MATTHEW LOUIS. 1867–1899
Mediterranean, Malta, or undulant fever. London, *Macmillan & Co.*, 1897.

An authoritative summary of current knowledge of Malta fever.

5101 WRIGHT, *Sir* ALMROTH EDWARD. 1861–1947, & SMITH, FREDERICK.
On the application of the serum test to the differential diagnosis of typhoid and Malta fever. *Lancet*, 1897, **1**, 656–59.

Agglutination test for the diagnosis of undulant fever.

5102 REPORTS of the Commission appointed by the Admiralty, the War Office, and the Civil Government of Malta, for the investigation of Mediterranean fever, under the supervision of an advisory committee of the Royal Society. **7 pts.** London, *Harrison & Sons*, 1905–07.

The important findings of the Mediterranean Fever Commission are summarized in Topley & Wilson's *Bacteriology*, 1955, p. 1899; probably the most valuable was that of T. Zammit, who showed goat's milk to be the main source of infection (pt. 4, p. 97).

5103 EVANS, ALICE CATHERINE. 1881–
Studies on Brucella (Alkaligenes) melitensis. Washington, *Govt. Printing Office*, 1925.

Forms Bulletin No. 143 of the U.S. Public Health Service Hygienic Laboratory. Alice Evans showed that the causal organism of Malta fever was closely related to *Brucella abortus*, responsible for contagious abortion in cattle. See also her earlier paper in *J. infect. Dis.*, 1918, **22**, 580–93.

5104–5112.1

CHOLERA

5104 GARCIA D'ORTA. 1501–1568
Colloquios dos simples, e drogas he causas mediçinais da India. Goa, *Joannes*, 1563.

Includes a classical description of Asiatic cholera, the first account of the disease by a European in modern times (see also No. 1815).

5104.1 SONNERAT, Pierre. 1749–1814

Voyage aux Indes Orientales et à la Chine, fait par ordre du Roi, depuis 1774 jusqu'en 1781. 2 vols. Paris, *L'Auteur*, 1782.

Vol. 1, pp. 113–16: "No author before the time of Sonnerat gives us so distinct an account of the epidemic prevalence of cholera, so full a description of its varieties, or has attributed it so positively to the physical misery of the natives of the country" (Macpherson, No. 5111.2). English translation, 1788–89.

5105 PARKIN, John. 1801–1886

Suggestions respecting the cause, nature, and treatment of cholera. *Lond. med. surg. J.*, 1832, n.s. **2,** 151–53.

Parkin suggested the water-borne character of cholera and the use of charcoal filters for water purification.

5106 SNOW, John. 1813–1858

On the pathology and mode of communication of the cholera. *Lond. med. Gaz.*, 1849, **44**, 730–32, 745–52, 923–29.

The water-borne character of cholera was demonstrated by Snow, who collected data regarding a large number of outbreaks and correlated them with water supplies. His book *On the mode of communication of cholera* appeared in the same year, and its second edition (1855), which included the story of the Broad Street pump, was reprinted in 1936 (New York).

5107 PETTENKOFER, Max Josef von. 1818–1901

Untersuchungen und Beobachtungen über die Verbreitungsart der Cholera. München, *J. G. Cotta*, 1855.

Pettenkofer gave much attention to the aetiology of cholera. He postulated the theory that a specific germ, certain local conditions, certain seasonal conditions, and certain individual conditions are all necessary for an epidemic to occur (the Boden theory).

5108 KOCH, Robert. 1843–1910

Ueber die Cholerabakterien. *Dtsch. med. Wschr.*, 1884, **10,** 725–28.

Discovery of the cholera vibrio and of its transmission by drinking water, food, and clothing.

5109 HAFFKINE, Waldemar Mordecai Wolff. 1860–1930

Le choléra asiatique chez le cobaye. *C. R. Soc. Biol.* (*Paris*), 1892, **44,** 635–37, 671.

Haffkine's vaccine against cholera was the first to meet with any success.

5110 PFEIFFER, Richard Friedrich Johannes. 1858–1945, & ISAYEV, Vasiliy Isayevich. 1854–1911

Ueber die specifische Bedeutung der Choleraimmunität (Bakteriolyse). *Z. Hyg. InfektKr.*, 1894, **17,** 355–400; **18,** 1–16.

Pfeiffer and Isayev recorded the occurrence of bacteriolysis in cholera vibrios under certain conditions ("Pfeiffer's phenomenon").

5111 KOLLE, Wilhelm. 1868–1935

Zur aktiven Immunisierung des Menschen gegen Cholera. *Zbl. Bakt.*, Abt. I, 1896, **19,** 97–104.

Kolle introduced the killed cholera vaccine.

5111.1 GOTSCHLICH, Felix. 1874–

Über Cholera- und choleraähnliche Vibrionen unter den aus Mekka zurückkehrenden Pilgern. *Z. Hyg. InfektKr.*, 1906, **53,** 281–304.

Isolation of El Tor vibrio.

5111.2 MACPHERSON, John. 1817–1890
Annals of cholera: from the earliest periods to the year 1817. London, *Ranken & Co.*, 1872.

5111.3 MACNAMARA, Nottidge Charles. 1832–1918
A history of Asiatic cholera. London, *Macmillan*, 1876.

5111.4 POLLITZER, Robert.
Cholera. Geneva, *World Health Organization*, 1959.
Includes a section on the history of cholera. *WHO Monograph Series*, No. 43.

5112 STICKER, Georg. 1860–1960
Abhandlungen aus der Seuchengeschichte und Seuchenlehre. II. Die Cholera. Giessen, *A. Töpelmann*, 1912.

5112.1 LONGMATE, Norman. 1925–
King Cholera. The biography of a disease. London, *Hamish Hamilton*, [1966].

5113–5145 PLAGUE

5113 VALESCUS DE TARANTA. 1382–1417
Tractatus de epidemia et peste. [Argentorati, *M. Flack*, c. 1470.]
One of the earliest printed medical books.

5114 STEINHÖWEL, Heinrich. 1420–1482
Buchlein der Ordnung der Pestilenz. Ulm, *Johann Zainer*, 1473.
This was a famous book and was often reprinted. It is reproduced in facsimile in A. C. Klebs: *Die ersten gedruckten Pestschriften*, 1936.

5115 JACOBI, Johannes [Jacques; Jasme]. ?–1384
A litil boke the whiche traytied and reherced many gode thinges necessaries for the . . . Pestilence. [London, *Willelmus de Machlinia*, 1485?].
First medical book printed in England. It was written about 1357, Jacobi being the papal physician and a friend of Guy de Chauliac. It was the most popular plague tract of the 15th century; a facsimile reproduction, from the copy in the John Rylands Library, Manchester, was published in 1910.

5117 DIEMERBROECK, Ysbrand van. 1609–1674
De peste libri quatuor, truculentissimi morbi historiam ratione et experientiâ confirmatum exhibentes. Arenaci, *ex off. J. Jacobi*, 1646.
Important early account of plague. English translation, 1722.

5118 KIRCHER, Athanasius. 1602–1680
Scrutinium physico-medicum contagiosae luis, quae pestis dicitur. Romae, *typ. Mascardi*, 1658.
Kircher was probably the first to employ the microscope in investigating the cause of disease. He mentioned that the blood of plague patients was filled with a "countless brood of worms not perceptible to the naked eye, but to be seen in all putrefying matter through the microscope" (Garrison). He could not have seen the plague bacillus with his low-power microscope, but he probably saw the larger micro-organisms. He was the first to state explicitly the theory of contagion by animalculae as the cause of infectious diseases.

5119 LONDON.

London's dreadful visitation, or, a collection of all the Bills of Mortality for the present year: beginning the 27th of December 1664, and ending the 19th of December following . . . By the Company of Parish Clerks of London. London, *E. Cotes*, 1665.

This is a valuable record of the great plague of 1665. (No. 6052 in the *Bibliotheca Osleriana.*)

5120 BOGHURST, William. 1631–1685

Loimographia. An account of the great plague of London in the year 1665. By William Boghurst. Now first printed from the British Museum Sloane Ms. 349, for the Epidemiological Society of London. Edited by J. F. Payne. London, *Shaw & Sons*, 1894.

This work was written in 1666 and first published as above. Boghurst, an apothecary, did good work during the great plague; in his book he differentiated plague from typhus. Payne's introduction to the book contains some valuable historical data.

5121 HODGES, Nathaniel. 1629–1688

Λοιμολογία sive pestis nuperae apud populum Londinensem grassantis narratio hisorica. Londini, *J. Nevill*, 1672.

Best medical record of the Great Plague of 1665. Hodges was physician to the City of London and the medical hero of the great epidemic. English translation by John Quincy, 1720.

5122 HASEIAH, Laurentius [Haseiac].

De postrema Melitensi lue praxis historica. Panormi, 1677.

This work, recording the epidemic of plague in Malta in 1675, is of interest as being the first medical work to be published by a Maltese.

5123 MEAD, Richard. 1673–1754

A short discourse concerning pestilential contagion, and the methods to be used to prevent it. London, *S. Buckley*, 1720.

The great Mead was asked for advice concerning the plague, and replied with the above tract. It was afterwards expanded into a book and is almost a prophecy of what was to develop as the English public health system.

5124 WESZPRÉMI, Stefan. 1723–1799

Tentamen de inoculandi peste. Londini, *J. Tuach*, 1755.

Weszprémi proposed preventive inoculation against plague.

5125 YERSIN, Alexandre Emile Jean. 1863–1943

La peste bubonique à Hong-Kong. *Ann. Inst. Pasteur*, 1894, **8**, 662–667.

Yersin discovered the plague bacillus *Pasteurella pestis* on July 30, 1894, isolating it from excised buboes. He published the first account of this organism. Preliminary note in *C. R. Acad. Sci.* (*Paris*), 1894, **119**, 356.

5126 RENNIE, Alexander. 1859–1940

The plague in the East. *Brit. med. J.*, 1894, **2**, 615–16.

Rennie appears to be the first seriously to support the theory of transmission of the plague bacillus by rats and to present evidence in support of that theory.

5127 YERSIN, Alexandre Emile Jean. 1863–1943, *et al.*

La peste bubonique. *Ann. Inst. Pasteur*, 1895, **9**, 589–92.

Successful inoculation of animals with anti-plague vaccine. With **L. C. A.** Calmette and A. Borrel.

5128 OGATA, MASANORI.
Ueber die Pestepidemie in Formosa. *Zbl. Bakt.*, 1897, Abt. I, **21**, 769–77.
To Ogata belongs the credit of first proving that the flea (principally *Xenopsylla cheopis*) is the principal, if not the sole, vector of bubonic plague infection.

5129 HAFFKINE, WALDEMAR MORDECAI WOLFF. 1860–1930
Les inoculations antipesteuses. *Bull. Inst. Pasteur*, 1906, **4**, 825–40.
Haffkine developed an anti-bubonic plague vaccine (killed bouillon cultures), for use in man.

5129.1 BACOT, ARTHUR WILLIAM. 1866–1922, & MARTIN, *Sir* CHARLES JAMES. 1866–1955
Observations on the mechanism of the transmission of plague by fleas. *J. Hyg.* (*Camb.*), 1914, Plague Suppl. 3, 423–39.
Bacot and Martin demonstrated the method by which the rat-flea transmitted the plague bacillus from rat to man.

5130 WU LIEN-TEH. 1879–1959
A treatise on pneumonic plague. Geneva, *League of Nations*, 1926.
Publication of the League of Nations, III. Health III, 13.

5131 POLLITZER, ROBERT.
Plague. Geneva, *World Health Organization*, 1954.
Includes a section on the history of plague. *WHO Monograph Series*, No. 22.

History of Plague

5132 PFEIFFER, LUDWIG. 1842–1921, & RULAND, C.
Pestilentia in nummis. Tübingen, *H. Laupp*, 1882.
A study of medals and tokens relating to epidemics of plague and other infectious diseases.

5133 GASQUET, FRANCIS AIDAN, *Cardinal*. 1846–1929
The Black Death of 1348 and 1349. London, *G. Bell*, 1893.

5134 FLETCHER, ROBERT. 1823–1912
A tragedy of the great plague in Milan in 1630. *Johns Hopk. Hosp. Bull.*, 1898, **9**, 175–80.
Fletcher tells of the torture of two innocent Milanese accused of spreading the plague; his account gives a vivid picture of the ignorance, superstitions, and cruelty of the people 300 years ago.

5135 HEITZ, PAUL.
Pestblätter des XV. Jahrhunderts. Hrsg. von P. HEITZ, mit einleitendem Text von W. L. SCHREIBER. Strassburg, *Heitz u. Mündel*, 1901.

5136 STICKER, GEORG. 1860–1960
Abhandlungen aus der Seuchengeschichte und Seuchenlehre. I. Die Pest. Giessen, *A. Töpelmann*, 1908.
Exhaustive history of the subject by a prominent epidemiologist.

5137 GAFFAREL, PAUL. 1843–?, & DURANTY, *Marquis de*.
La peste de 1720 à Marseille et en France d'après des documents inédits. Paris, *Perrin & Cie.*, 1911.

5138 CRAWFURD, *Sir* RAYMOND HENRY PAYNE. 1865–1938
Plague and pestilence in literature and art. Oxford, *Clarendon Press,* 1914.
Deals with the subject up to the end of the 18th century.

5139 BELL, WALTER GEORGE. *d.* 1942
The great plague in London in 1665. London, *John Lane*, 1924.

5140 KLEBS, ARNOLD CARL. 1870–1943, & DROZ, EUGÉNIE.
Remèdes contre la peste. Fac-similés, notes et liste bibliographique des incunables sur la peste. Paris, *Droz*, 1925.
Includes facsimile reproduction of "La regime de l'epidemie et remede contre icelle" of Jean Jasme (Johannes Jacobi), [1476?], together with the "Remede tresutile contre fièvre pestilencieuse" by the same writer.

5141 ——, & SUDHOFF, KARL FRIEDRICH JAKOB. 1853–1938
Die ersten gedruckten Pestschriften. München, *Verlag der Münchener Druck*, 1926.
Includes descriptions of 130 incunabula.

5142 NOHL, JOHANNES.
The Black Death, a chronicle of the plague. Compiled . . . from contemporary sources. Translated by C. H. CLARKE. London, *Allen & Unwin*, (1926).
German edition 1924.

5143 WILSON, FREDERICK PERERA. 1876–1926
The plague in Shakespeare's London. Oxford, *Clarendon Press*, 1927.

5144 CAMPBELL, ANNA MONTGOMERY. 1888–
The Black Death and men of learning. New York, *Columbia University Press,* 1931.

5145 HIRST, LEONARD FABIAN. 1882–
Conquest of plague. A study of the evolution of epidemiology. Oxford, *Clarendon Press*, 1953.

5146–5151 TETANUS

5146 ARETAEUS, *the Cappadocian. circa* A.D. 81–138
On tetanus. In his *Extant works,* ed. F. ADAMS, London, 1856, pp. 246–49, 400–04.
Aretaeus left a full account of tetanus.

5147 CARLE, ANTONIO. 1854–1927, & RATTONE, GIORGIO.
Studio experimentale sull' eziologia del tetano. *G. r. Accad. Med. Torino*, 1884, 3 ser., **32,** 174–80.
Demonstration of the transmissibility of tetanus by inoculation into rabbits of pus from a human case.

5148 NICOLAIER, ARTHUR. 1862–
Ueber infectiösen Tetanus. *Dtsch. med. Wschr.*, 1884, **10,** 842–44.
The discovery of the tetanus bacillus is attributed to Nicolaier; he was, however, unable to isolate the organism in pure culture.

5149 KITASATO, SHIBASABURO, *Baron.* 1856–1931
Ueber den Tetanusbacillus. *Z. Hyg. InfektKr.*, 1889, **7,** 225–34.
Kitasato obtained a pure culture of the tetanus bacillus, *Cl. tetani.*

5150 BEHRING, Emil Adolf von. 1854–1917, & KITASATO, Shibasaburo, *Baron.* 1856–1931
Ueber das Zustandekommen der Diphtherie-Immunität und der Tetanus-Immunität bei Thieren. *Dtsch. med. Wschr.*, 1890, **16,** 1113–1114, 1145–48.
Discovery of antitoxins and their immunizing powers (see also No. 5060).

5151 RAMON, Gaston Léon. 1886–1963, & ZOELLER, Christian. 1888–1934
Sur la valeur et la durée de l'immunité conférée par l'anatoxine tétanique dans la vaccination de l'homme contre le tétanos. *C.R. Soc. Biol.* (*Paris*), 1933, **112,** 347–50.
Tetanus toxoid first employed in the immunization of humans.

5152–5159 GLANDERS; MELIOIDOSIS

5152 CHABERT, Philibert. 1737–1814
Mémoire sur la morve. *Hist. Soc. roy. Méd.* (*Paris*), (1779), 1782, **3,** pt. 2, 361–91.
Chabert, the most celebrated veterinarian of his time, left a fine account of glanders.

5153 ELLIOTSON, John. 1791–1868
On the glanders in the human subject. *Med.-chir. Trans.*, 1830, **16,** 171–218; 1833, **18,** 201–07.
Proof that glanders in the horse is communicable to man.

5154 RAYER, Pierre François Olive. 1793–1867
De la morve et du farcin chez l'homme. *Mém. Acad. roy. Méd.* (*Paris*), 1837, **6,** 625–873.
A classical contribution to the knowledge of glanders and farcy in man. Rayer showed that glanders is contagious but is not a form of tuberculosis. This work is a landmark in the history of bacteriology.

5155 CHAUVEAU, Jean Baptiste Auguste. 1827–1917
Nature des virus. Détermination expérimentale des éléments qui constituent le principe virulent dans le pus varioleux et le pus morveux. *C. R. Acad. Sci.* (*Paris*), 1868, **66,** 359–63.
Demonstration of the particulate nature of the glanders bacillus.

5156 LOEFFLER, Friedrich. 1852–1915
Die Aetiologie der Rotzkrankheit. *Arb. k. GesundhAmte,* 1886, **1,** 141–98.
Discovery of *Pfeifferella mallei,* causative organism of glanders. Preliminary notice in *Dtsch. med. Wschr.*, 1882, **8,** 707.

5157 STRAUS, Isidore. 1845–1896
Sur un moyen de diagnostic rapide de la morve. *Arch. Méd. exp. Anat. path.*, 1889, **1,** 460–62.
Straus reaction for the diagnosis of glanders.

5158 BABÉS, Victor. 1854–1926
Observations sur la morve. *Arch. Méd. exp. Anat. path.*, 1891, **3,** 619–45.
Mallein reaction for the diagnosis of glanders.

5159 WHITMORE, Alfred. 1876–1946, & KRISHNASWAMI, C. S.
An account of the discovery of a hitherto undescribed infective disease occurring among the population of Rangoon. *Indian med. Gaz.*, 1912, **47,** 262–67.
First description of melioidosis. The organism isolated was subsequently named *Pfeifferella whitmori* by Stanton and Fletcher.

5160–5172.1 ANTHRAX

5160 HARTMAN, Hartmannus.
Thesis de carbunculo. Lugduni Batavorum, *ex off. F. Moyardi*, 1653.

5161 FRISCHMUTH, Johann.
Epistola . . . qua simul de anthrace, carbunculo, bubone et altauna, philologice disseritur. Jenae, *typ. vid. Krebsianae*, 1681.

5162 CHABERT, Philibert. 1737–1814
Description et traitement du charbon dans les animaux. Paris, *Imp. Royale*, 1780.
First important clinical description of anthrax. For some time after the appearance of Chabert's little book, the condition was known as "Chabert's disease".

5163 RAYER, Pierre François Olive. 1793–1867
Inoculation du sang de rate. *C. R. Soc. Biol.* (*Paris*), 1850, **2,** 141–44.
Rayer inoculated sheep with blood of other sheep dead of anthrax. Microscopically he saw the anthrax bacillus in the blood of the inoculated sheep. Rayer was associated with Davaine who later, in *Bull. Acad. Méd.*, 1875, 2 sér., **4**, 581–84, said that he had written the above account and had sent it to Rayer for publication.

5164 POLLENDER, Franz Aloys Antoine. 1800–1879
Mikroskopische und mikrochemische Untersuchung des Milzbrandblutes sowie über Wesen und Kur des Milzbrandes. *Vjschr. gerichtl. öff. Med.*, 1855, **8,** 103–14.
Pollender discovered the *B. anthracis* in 1849, but did not record this fact until 1855. He gave a more exact account of the organism than did Rayer (No. 5163).

5165 DAVAINE, Casimir Joseph. 1812–1882
Recherches sur les infusoires du sang dans la maladie connue sous le nom de sang de rate. *C. R. Acad. Sci.* (*Paris*), 1863, **57,** 220–23, 351–353.
Davaine showed that anthrax could be transmitted to sheep, horses, cattle, guinea-pigs, and mice, and that in such animals the bacilli did not appear in the blood until 4–5 hours before death.

5166 ——. Recherches sur la nature et la constitution anatomique de la pustule maligne. *C. R. Acad. Sci.* (*Paris*), 1865, **60,** 1296–99.
Davaine was the first conclusively to prove that a definite disease (anthrax) was due to a definite micro-organism (*B. anthracis*), and was thus one of the first to prove the germ theory of disease. He showed that the virulence of anthrax was in proportion to the number of bacteria present.

5167 KOCH, Robert. 1843–1910
Die Aetiologie der Milzbrand-Krankheit, begründet auf die Entwicklungsgeschichte des Bacillus anthracis. *Beitr. Biol. Pflanzen*, 1876, **2,** 277–310.

In 1876 Koch first obtained pure cultures of *B. anthracis* and described its complete life history. With Davaine (No. 5165–66) he did much to prove that infectious diseases are caused by living reproductive micro-organisms. The postulates expounded by Koch on this occasion had fundamental importance and have become the bases on which bacteriology largely rests. The paper also marks the beginning of exact knowledge of bacterial infectious diseases. It is reproduced with translation in *Med. Classics*, 1938, 2, 745–820.

5168 PASTEUR, Louis. 1822–1895, & JOUBERT, Jules François.
Etude sur la maladie charbonneuse. *C. R. Acad. Sci.* (*Paris*), 1877, **84,** 900–06.

Pasteur confirmed Koch's results regarding anthrax; with Joubert he carried the bacillus through 100 generations and succeeded in producing anthrax from the last, thus disposing of the idea of a separate virus.

5169 ——, CHAMBERLAND, Charles. 1851–1898, & ROUX, Pierre Paul Emile. 1853–1933
Sur l'étiologie du charbon. *C. R. Acad. Sci.* (*Paris*), 1880, **91,** 86–94.

First use of attenuated bacterial virus for therapeutic purposes. See also the same journal, 1881, **92,** 1378–83.

5170 SCLAVO, Achille. 1861–1930
Sulla preparazione del siero anti-carbonchioso. *Riv. Ig. San. pubbl.*, 1895, **6,** 841–43.

Specific anti-anthrax serum. German translation in *Zbl. Bakt.*, 1895, 1 Abt., **18** 744–45.

5171 ASCOLI, Alberto. 1877–1957
La precipitina nella diagnosi del carbonchio ematico. *Clin. vet.* (*Milano*), 1911, **34,** 2–20.

Ascoli's thermoprecipitin reaction for the diagnosis of anthrax. German translation in *Zbl. Bakt.*, 1911, 1 Abt., **58,** Orig., 63–70. Preliminary note in *Pathologica* 1910, **3,** 101.

5172 BECKER, Georg.
Die bakteriologische Blutuntersuchung beim Milzbrand des Menschen. *Dtsch. Z. Chir.*, 1911, **112,** 265–83.

Salvarsan first used in the treatment of anthrax.

5172.1 STERNE, Max.
The use of anthrax vaccines prepared from avirulent (uncapsulated) variants of *Bacillus anthracis*. *Onderstepoort J. vet. Sci.*, 1939, **13,** 307–12.

Nonencapsulated spore vaccine.

5173–5180 TULARAEMIA

5173 McCOY, George Walter. 1876–1952
A plague-like disease of rodents. *Publ. Hlth Bull.* (*Wash.*), 1911, **43,** 53–71.

Tularaemia first recorded (in rodents).

5174 McCOY, George Walter. 1876–1952, & CHAPIN, Charles Willard. 1877–
Further observations on a plague-like disease of rodents with a preliminary note on the causative agent, Bacterium tularense. *J. infect. Dis.*, 1912, **10,** 61–72.

Isolation of *Pasteurella tularensis*, causal organism in tularaemia.

5175 WHERRY, William Buchanan. 1875–1936, & LAMB, Benjamin Harrison. 1889–
Infection of man with Bacterium tularense. *J. infect. Dis.*, 1914, **15,** 331–40.

Wherry and Lamb were first to isolate *P. tularensis* from lesions in man.

5176 FRANCIS, Edward. 1872–1957
Tularemia. *J. Amer. med. Ass.*, 1925, **84,** 1243–50.

The important work of Francis on tularaemia, summarized in the above paper, included his demonstration of its transmission to man from rodents through insects, particularly the deerfly. He gave the disease its present name; it is also called "Francis' disease" by some writers.

5177 OHARA, Hachiro.
Ueber Identität von "Yato-Byo" (Ohara's disease) und "Tularämie", sowie ihren Erreger. *Zbl. Bakt.*, 1930, Abt. 1, **117,** 440–50.

In Japan tularaemia is known as "Ohara's disease".

5178 FOSHAY, Lee. 1896–1960
Tularemia: accurate and earlier diagnosis by means of the intradermal reaction. *J. infect. Dis.*, 1932, **51,** 286–91.

Skin test for the diagnosis of tularaemia.

5179 ——. Serum treatment of tularemia. *J. Amer. med. Ass.*, 1932, **98,** 552; 1933, **101,** 1047–49.

Foshay devised a serum for the treatment of tularaemia.

5180 ——, & PASTERNACK, A. Bernard. 1916–
Streptomycin treatment of tularemia. *J. Amer. med. Ass.*, 1946, **130,** 393–98.

5180.1–5194.1 AMOEBIASIS

See also 5089–5096, Bacillary Dysentery.

5180.1 ABREU, Alexo de. 1568–1630
Tratado de las siete enfermedades, *etc.* Lisboa, *P. Craesbeeck*, 1623.

An account of amoebiasis is given on fol. 1–42v., 61–72v., and 117v–150. For full title of the book, see No. 2262.1.

5181 KNEUSSEL, Christoph Friedrich.
De ipecacuanha novo Gallorum antidysenterico. Gissae-Hassorum, *typ. Mülleri*, 1698.

There is evidence that amoebic dysentery was known to Hippocrates. The history of its treatment begins with the use of ipecacuanha, first mentioned as a remedy in Purchas's *Pilgrimes*, 1625. Ipecacuanha was used as a secret remedy against dysentery in Paris about 1680, and was bought by the French Government for 20,000 francs in 1688.

5182 MAGENDIE, François. 1783–1855, & PELLETIER, Pierre Joseph. 1788–1842
Mémoire sur l'émétine, et sur les trois espèces d'ipecacuanha. *J. gén. Méd. Chir. Pharm.*, 1817, **59,** 223–31.
Isolation of emetine. It was not until a century later that Vedder demonstrated its value in the treatment of amoebiasis.

5183 BARDSLEY, *Sir* James Lomax. 1801–1876
Hospital facts and observations. London, *Burgess & Hill*, 1830.
First record (p. 149) of the use of emetine in the treatment of amoebiasis.

5183.1 GROS, G.
Fragments d'helminthologie et de physiologie microscopique. *Bull. Soc. imp. Nat. Moscou*, 1849, **22,** 549–73.
First observations of entozoic amoebae.

5183.2 JIMENEZ, Miguel F.
Clínica médica. Abcesos del higado. México, *M. Murguia*, 1856.
Jimenez gave a classical account of liver abscess in amoebiasis.

5184 LÖSCH, Friedrich.
Massenhafte Entwickelung von Amöben im Dickdarm. *Virchows Arch. path. Anat.*, 1875, **65,** 196–211.
Lösch discovered *Entamoeba histolytica* as the infective agent in amoebic dysentery. Before this time distinction between the different forms of dysentery had been made on purely clinical grounds.

5185 WOODWARD, Joseph Janvier. 1833–1884
Diarrhoea and dysentery. In: U.S. War Dept.: *Medical and surgical history of the War of the Rebellion*, 1879, pt. 2, **1,** 1–869.
Garrison considers this the greatest single monograph on dysentery. Woodward saw the Lösch amoeba, but without recognizing its significance; he was part author of the *Medical and surgical history of the War of the Rebellion.*

5186 KARTULIS, Stephanos. 1852–1920
Zur Aetiologie der Dysenterie in Aegypten. *Virchows Arch. path. Anat.*, 1886, **105,** 521–31.
Kartulis discovered amoebae in liver abscess. It was principally through the work of Kartulis that amoebae came to be considered the cause of dysentery in man.

5186.1 HLAVA, Jaroslav. 1855–1924
O úplavici. Předběžné sdělení. *Cas. Lék. ces.*, 1887, **26,** 70.
Hlava induced experimental amoebiasis in cats by intrarectal inoculation of stools. In an abstract of this paper Kartulis confused the author's name with that of the title, a mistake copied by writers for many years; see C. Dobell, *Parasitology*, 1938, **30,** 239–41.

5187 COUNCILMAN, William Thomas. 1854–1933, & LAFLEUR, Henri Amedée. 1863–1939
Amoebic dysentery. *Johns Hopk. Hosp. Rep.*, 1890–91, **2,** 395–548.
These workers introduced the term "amoebic dysentery" in their important investigation of the condition.

5188 QUINCKE, Heinrich Irenaeus. 1842–1922, & ROOS, Ernst. 1866–
Ueber Amöben-Enteritis. *Berl. klin. Wschr.*, 1893, **30,** 1089–94.
Entamoeba histolytica distinguished from *Bact. coli.*

5189 VEDDER, Edward Bright. 1878–1952
Experiments undertaken to test the efficacy of the ipecac treatment of dysentery. *Bull. Manila med. Soc.*, 1911, **3,** 48–53.
Vedder demonstrated the amoebicidal action of emetine; his work led to the general adoption of emetine in the treatment of amoebic dysentery.

5190 ROGERS, *Sir* Leonard. 1868–1962
The rapid cure of amoebic dysentery and hepatitis by hypodermic injections of soluble salts of emetine. *Brit. med. J.*, 1912, **1,** 1424–25.
Following up the work of Vedder, Rogers showed that the soluble salts of emetine could be safely injected subcutaneously. The general use of emetine, introduced by Rogers, diminished the incidence of liver abscess – a grave sequel.

5191 WALKER, Ernest Linwood. 1870– , & SELLARDS, Andrew Watson. 1884–
Experimental entamoebic dysentery. *Philipp. J. Sci.*, 1913, B, **8,** 253–331.
Walker and Sellards have made important additions to our knowledge of amoebiasis, including the determination of the incubation period and the demonstration that *E. tetragena* and *E. minuta* are identical with *E. histolytica.*

5192 MÜHLENS, Peter. 1874–1943, & MENK, W.
Ueber Behandlungsversuche der chronischen Amoebenruhr mit Yatren. *Münch. med. Wschr.*, 1921, **68,** 802–03.
Introduction of Yatren.

5193 MARCHOUX, Emile. 1862–1943
Le stovarsol guérit rapidement la dysenterie amibienne. *Bull. Soc. Path. exot.*, 1923, **16,** 79–81.
Introduction of stovarsol (oxyaminophenylarsenic acid) in the treatment of amoebiasis.

5194 BOECK, William Charles. 1894– , & DRBOHLAV, Jaroslav.
The cultivation of Endamoeba histolytica. *Proc. nat. Acad. Sci. (Wash.)*, 1925, **11,** 235–38.
Pure cultivation of *Entamoeba histolytica* was first accomplished by D. W. Cutler (*J. Path. Bact.*, 1918, **22,** 22), but Boeck and Drbohlav evolved the first media upon which amoebae could be cultivated for indefinite periods.

5194.1 REED, Alfred Cummings. 1884–1951, *et al.*
Carbarsone in the treatment of amebiasis. *J. Amer. med. Ass.*, 1932, **98,** 189–94.
With H. H. Anderson, N. A. David, and C. D. Leake.

5195–5227 VENEREAL DISEASES

See also 2362–2432.1, Syphilis; 4772–4806, Neurosyphilis.

5195 ASTRUC, Jean. 1684–1766
De morbis venereis libri sex. Lutetiae Parisiorum, *G. Cavelier,* 1736.
Considering the period in which it was written, this is an admirable and comprehensive book on the subject. It includes a careful review of the existing literature. Of syphilis, Astruc says that it made its appearance in Europe in 1493. The book was translated into English in 1737.

5196 BALFOUR, Francis. ?–1812
De gonorrhoea virulenta. Edinburgh, *Balfour, Auld & Smellie,* 1767.
Balfour is said to have been the first to re-affirm the duality of gonorrhoea and syphilis.

5197 HUNTER, John. 1728–1793
A treatise on the venereal disease. London, 1786.

In Hunter's day the venereal diseases were thought to be due to a single poison. In order to test this point Hunter inoculated himself with matter taken from a gonorrhoeal patient who, unknown to Hunter, also had syphilis. Hunter contracted the latter disease and maintained that gonorrhoea and syphilis were caused by a single pathogen. Backed by the weight of Hunter's authority, this experiment held back for many years the development of knowledge regarding gonorrhoea and syphilis. The hard ("Hunterian") chancre eponymizes Hunter; his book also contains the first suggestion that lymphogranuloma venereum is a separate disease.

5198 NISBET, William. 1759–1822
First lines of theory and practice in venereal diseases. Edinburgh, *C. Elliot*, 1787.

First complete description of lymphatic chancre – "Nisbet's chancre".

5199 GIRTANNER, Christoph. 1760–1800
Abhandlung über die venerische Krankheit. 3 vols. Göttingen, *J. C. Dieterich*, 1788–89.

Girtanner's important text-book on the venereal diseases contains some history.

5200 BELL, Benjamin. 1749–1806
A treatise on gonorrhoea virulenta, and lues venerea. 2 vols. Edinburgh, *J. Watson & G. Mudie*, 1793.

Bell was the first to differentiate between gonorrhoea and syphilis.

5201 COLLES, Abraham. 1773–1843
Practical observations on the venereal disease, and on the use of mercury. London, *Sherwood, Gilbert & Piper*, 1837.

See No. 2380.

5202 RICORD, Philippe. 1800–1889
Traité pratique des maladies vénériennes. Paris, *De Just Rouvier & E. Le Bouvier*, 1838.

Repeating Hunter's experiment, Ricord proved that syphilis and gonorrhoea were separate diseases. After Hunter, he was the greatest authority on venereal disease. See also No. 2381. The first of several English translations appeared in 1842.

5203 BASSEREAU, Léon. 1811–1888
Traité des affections de la peau symptomatiques de la syphilis. Paris, *J. B. Baillière*, 1852.

Bassereau defined chancroid clearly for the first time.

5204 ROLLET, Joseph Pierre. 1824–1894
Coincidence du chancre syphilitique primitif avec la gale, la blénorrhagie, le chancre simple et la vaccine. *Gaz. méd. Lyon*, 1866, **18**, 160–63.

Rollet recognized the possibility of mixed infection of one sore with syphilis and chancroid, thus establishing the dualist theory of venereal infection. The mixed chancre is named "Rollet's disease".

5204.1 MACLEOD, Kenneth. 1840–1922
Precis of operations performed in the wards of the first surgeon, Medical College Hospital, during the year 1881. *Indian med. Gaz.*, 1882, **17**, 113–23.

MacLeod was first to draw attention to granuloma inguinale.

5205 DUCREY, AUGUSTO. 1860–1940
Il virus dell' ulcera venerea. *Gazz. int. Sci. med.*, 1889, **11,** 44.

Announcement of the discovery of *Haemophilus ducreyi* (Ducrey's bacillus), causal organism in chancroid.

5205.1 CONYERS, JAMES SALTERS. 1841–1896, & DANIELS, CHARLES WILBERFORCE. 1862–1927
The lupoid form of the so-called "groin ulceration" of this colony. *Brit. Guiana med. Annu.*, 1896, **8,** 13–29.

Granuloma inguinale distinguished from other similar lesions in the genital region.

5206 JADASSOHN, JOSEF. 1863–1936
Handbuch der Haut- und Geschlechtskrankheiten. Hrsg. . . . von J. JADASSOHN. 24 vols. [in 42]. Berlin, *J. Springer*, 1927–37.

Gonorrhoea and Trichomonas Infection

5207 DONNÉ, ALFRED. 1801–1878
Animalcules observés dans les matières purulentes et le produit des sécrétions des organes génitaux de l'homme et de la femme. *C. R. Acad. Sci.* (*Paris*), 1836, **3,** 385–86.

First description of *Trichomonas vaginalis*, which Donné at first believed to be the pernicious agent in gonorrhoea. He later admitted the organism to be a normal inhabitant of the female genital tract. Donné was, by this work, the first to describe living organisms in pathological conditions, as observed by modern methods.

5208 NEISSER, ALBERT LUDWIG SIEGMUND. 1855–1916
Ueber eine der Gonorrhoe eigentümliche Micrococcusform. *Zbl. med. Wiss.*, 1879, **17,** 497–500.

Discovery of the gonococcus – causal organism in gonorrhoea.

5209 LEISTIKOW, LEO. 1847–1917
Ueber Bacterien bei den venerischen Krankheiten. *Charité-Ann.*, 1880 (1882), **7,** 750–72.

Leistikow was first to report the cultivation of the gonococcus.

5210 BUMM, ERNST VON. 1858–1925
Der Mikro-Organismus der gonorrhoischen Schleimhaut-Erkrankungen, Gonococcus-Neisser. *Dtsch. med. Wschr.*, 1885, **11,** 508–09.

Bumm cultured the gonococcus. By human inoculations he demonstrated its pathogenicity in pure culture.

5210.1 FRAENKEL, EUGEN. 1853–1925
Bericht über eine bei Kindern beobachtete Endemie infectiöser Colpitis. *Virchows Arch. path. Anat.*, 1885, **99,** 251–76.

The gonococcus shown to be the cause of vulvovaginitis in children.

5211 FINGER, ERNST ANTON FRANZ. 1856–1939
Die Blenorrhoë der Sexualorgane und ihre Complicationen. Leipzig, Wien, *F. Deuticke*, 1888.

5212 THAYER, WILLIAM SYDNEY. 1864–1932, & BLUMER, GEORGE ALBERT. 1858–1940
Ulcerative endocarditis due to the gonococcus; gonorrheal septicemia. *Johns Hopk. Hosp. Bull.*, 1896, **7,** 57–63.

Thayer and Blumer found the gonococcus in cases of gonorrhoeal endocarditis.

5213 MÜLLER, Rudolf. 1877– , & OPPENHEIM, Moritz. 1876–
Ueber den Nachweis von Antikörpern im Serum eines an Arthritis gonorrhoica Erkrankten mittels Komplementablenkung. *Wien. klin. Wschr.*, 1906, **19,** 894–95.

"Müller–Oppenheim reaction" – a complement fixation test for the diagnosis of gonorrhoea.

5213.1 LEVADITI, Constantin. 1874–1953, & VAISMAN, A.
La toxi-infection gonococcique expérimentale et son traitement chimiothérapique. *Presse méd.*, 1937, **45,** 1371–73.

Levaditi and Vaisman showed that sulphanilamide protected mice against gonococcal infection.

5214 DEES, John Essary. 1910– , & COLSTON, John Archibald Campbell. 1886–
The use of sulfanilamide in gonococcic infections. Preliminary report. *J. Amer. med. Ass.*, 1937, **108,** 1855–58.

5214.1 HERRELL, Wallace Edgar. 1909– , *et al.*
Use of penicillin in sulfonamide resistant gonorrheal infections. *J. Amer. med. Ass.*, 1943, **122,** 289–92.

With E. N. Cook and L. Thompson.

Lymphogranuloma Venereum

5215 WALLACE, William. 1791–1837
A treatise on the venereal disease and its varieties. London, *Burgess & Hill*, 1833.

On page 371 commences the first description of lymphogranuloma venereum, which Wallace called "indolent primary syphilitic bubo".

5216 HUGUIER, Pierre Charles. 1804–1873
Mémoire sur l'esthiomène, ou dartre rongeante de la région vulvo-anale. *Mém. Acad. nat. Méd.* (*Paris*), 1849, **14,** 501–96.

Huguier gave the name esthiomène to the characteristic induration and discoloration of the affected parts in lymphogranuloma venereum.

5217 DURAND, Joseph. 1876– , NICOLAS, Joseph. 1868–1960, & FAVRE, Maurice. 1876–1955
Lymphogranulomatose inguinale subaiguë d'origine génitale probable, peut-être vénérienne. *Bull. Soc. méd. Hôp. Paris*, 1913, 3 sér., **35,** 274–88.

First important description. Sometimes called "Nicolas–Favre disease" and "Nicolas–Durand–Favre disease".

5218 FREI, Wilhelm Siegmund. 1885–1943
Eine neue Hautreaktion bei "Lymphogranuloma inguinale". *Klin. Wschr.*, 1925, **4,** 2148–49.

The Frei skin test for the diagnosis of lymphogranuloma venereum.

5219 GAY PRIETO, José Antonio. 1905–
Contribución al estudio de la linfogranulomatosis inguinal subaguda o úlcera venérea adenógena de Nicolás y Favre. *Act. dermo-sifiliogr.* (*Madr.*), 1927, **20,** 122–75.

Gay Prieto was the first actually to see the virus of lymphogranuloma venereum.

5220 HELLERSTRÖM, SVEN CURT ALFRED. 1901, & WASSÉN, ERIK. Meningo-enzephalitische Veränderungen bei Affen nach intra-cerebraler Impfung mit Lymphogranuloma inguinale. *VIIIe Congr. int. Derm. Syph.*, Copenhague, 1930, *C. R. Séances*, 1931, 1147–49.

Proof that the aetiological agent of lymphogranuloma venereum is a virus. See also *C. R. Soc. Biol. (Paris)*, 1931, **106**, 802–03.

5221 STANNUS, HUGH STANNUS. 1877–1957
A sixth venereal disease. Climatic bubo, lymphogranuloma inguinale, esthiomène, chronic ulcer and elephantiasis of the genito-ano-rectal region, inflammatory stricture of the rectum. London, *Baillière, Tindall & Cox*, 1933.

In this exhaustive review of the literature the writer shows that all the above-named conditions are only different manifestations of one and the same infection – the virus of lymphogranuloma venereum. Includes historical summary and full bibliography.

5222 TAMURA, JOSEPH TAKAO. 1903–
Cultivation of the virus of lymphogranuloma inguinale and its use in therapeutic inoculation. Preliminary report. *J. Amer. med. Ass.*, 1934, **103,** 408–09.

5223 McKEE, CLARA M., *et al.*
Complement-fixation test in lymphogranuloma venereum. *Proc. Soc. exp. Biol. (N.Y.)*, 1940, **44,** 410–13.

Diagnosis of lymphogranuloma venereum by complement-fixation test. With G. W. Rake and M. F. Shaffer.

5224 OTTOLINA, CARLOS.
The vesicular test. Diagnostic method of infection by poradenic (lymphogranuloma inguinale) virus. *Amer. J. trop. Med.*, 1941, **21,** 597–602.

Vesicular test for diagnosis of lymphogranuloma venereum.

5225 BEDSON, *Sir* SAMUEL PHILLIPS. 1886–1969, *et al.*
The laboratory diagnosis of lymphogranuloma venereum. *J. clin. Path.*, 1949, **2,** 241–49.

Skin-test antigen. With C. F. Barwell, E. J. King, and L. W. J. Bishop.

History of Venereal Diseases

See also 2420–2432.1, *History of Syphilis*.

5226 PROKSCH, JOHANN KARL. 1840–1923
Die Litteratur über die venerischen Krankheiten von den ersten Schriften über Syphilis aus dem Ende des fünfzehnten Jahrhunderts bis zum Jahre 1889. (Supplement Band I. Enthält die Litteratur von 1889–99 und Nachträge aus früherer Zeit.) 5 vols. Bonn, *P. Hanstein*, 1889–1900.

5227 ——. Die Geschichte der venerischen Krankheiten. 2 vols. Bonn, *P. Hanstein*, 1895 (–1900).

Vol. 1. Alterthum und Mittelalter. Vol. 11. Neuzeit.

5228–5264.3 MALARIA

5228 HIPPOCRATES, 460–375 B.C.
Fevers at Thasos. In: *Hippocrates*, with an English translation. By W. H. S. Jones and E. T. Withington, London, 1923, **1,** 147–211.

5229 SPIEGHEL, Adriaan van den [Spigelius]. 1578–1625
De semitertiana libri quatuor. Francofurti, *apud haered. J. T. de Bry*, 1624.
First extensive account of malaria.

5230 BARBA, Pedro.
Vera praxis ad curationem tertianae. Hispali, 1642.
The first publication on cinchona bark and its use in the treatment of malaria. Barba was professor of medicine at Valladolid and physician to Philip IV.

5231 TORTI, Francesco. 1658–1741
Therapeutice specialis, ad febres quasdam perniciosas, inopinato, ac repente lethales, una vera china china, peculiare methodo ministrata, sanabiles. Mutinae, *typ. B. Soliani*, 1712.
This work is notable in that it brought about the general use of cinchona bark in Italian practice. Torti is said to have introduced the term *mal aria*.

5232 LANCISI, Giovanni Maria. 1654–1720
De noxiis paludum effluviis, eorumque remediis. Romae, *typ. J. M. Salvioni*, 1717.
Lancisi suggested that since malaria disappears after drainage it was due to some sort of poison emanating from marshes and possibly transmitted by mosquitoes. He planned a drainage scheme for marshy regions.

5233 PELLETIER, Pierre Joseph. 1788–1842, & CAVENTOU, Joseph Bienaimé. 1795–1877
Recherches chimiques sur les quinquinas. *Ann. Chim. Phys. (Paris)*, 1820, **15,** 289–318, 337–65.
Isolation of quinine.

5234 MITCHELL, John Kearsley. 1793–1858
On the cryptogamous origin of malarious and epidemic fevers. Philadelphia, *Lea & Blanchard*, 1849.
Although Hensinger in 1844 had suggested a parasite as the cause of malaria, Mitchell was the first to approach this theory in a scientific spirit. He was professor of medicine at Jefferson College, and the father of S. Weir Mitchell.

5235 BERENGER-FÉRAUD, Laurent Jean Baptiste. 1832–1901
De la fièvre bilieuse mélanurique des pays chauds comparée avec la fièvre jaune. Paris, *A. Delahaye*, 1874.
An important description of blackwater fever. Berenger-Féraud had experience of the disease in French West Africa.

5236 LAVERAN. Charles Louis Alphonse. 1845–1922
Un nouveau parasite trouvé dans le sang de plusieurs malades atteints de fièvre palustre. *Bull. Soc. méd. Hôp. Paris, (Mém.)*, 1881, 2 sér., **17,** 158–64.
Laveran first saw the malaria parasite on October 20, 1880; he at once grasped its significance. He named it *Oscillaria malariae*. He was awarded the Nobel Prize in 1907.

5237 KING, ALBERT FREEMAN AFRICANUS. 1841–1914
Insects and disease; mosquitoes and malaria. *Pop. Sci. Monthly, (N.Y.)*, 1882, **23,** 644–58.
The first reasoned argument in support of the belief of transmission of malaria by mosquitoes. Reproduced in part in R. H. Major, *Classic descriptions of disease*, 3rd ed., 1945, p. 104.

5238 MARCHIAFAVA, ETTORE. 1847–1935, & CELLI, ANGELO. 1857–1914
Weitere Untersuchungen über die Malariainfection. *Fortschr. Med.*, 1885, **3,** 787–806.
First accurate description of the malaria *Plasmodium*, discovered by Laveran in 1880. These writers were the first to adopt the name *P. malariae.*

5239 GOLGI, CAMILLO. 1844–1926
Sull' infezione malarica. *Arch. Sci. med. (Torino)*, 1886, **10,** 109–35.
Description of the development of the parasite of quartan malaria. Golgi differentiated the tertian and quartan parasites by the periods of their respective developments.

5240 ——. Sul ciclo evolutivo dei parassiti malarica nella febbre terzana. *Arch. Sci. med. (Torino)*, 1889, **13,** 173–96.
Golgi showed that the parasite of quartan differs from that of tertian malarial fever.

5241 GRASSI, GIOVANNI BATTISTA. 1854–1925, & FELETTI, RAIMONDO. 1851–1928
Malariaparasiten in den Vöǧeln. *Zbl. Bakt.*, 1891, **9,** 403–09, 429–33, 461–67.
Confirmation of the work of Laveran.

5242 ROMANOVSKY, DMITRIY LEONIDOVICH. 1861–1921
K voprosu o parazitologii i terapii bolotnoi likhoradki. [Parasitology and treatment of malarial fever.] St. Petersburg, *I. N. Skovokhodoff*, 1891.
Romanovsky made important studies of the malaria parasite and introduced a special stain for its demonstration.

5243 GOLGI, CAMILLO. 1844–1926
Azione della chinina sui parasite malarici e sui corrispondente accessi febbrili. *Gazz. med. Pavia*, 1892, **1,** 34, 79, 106.
French translation in *Arch. ital. Biol.*, 1892, **17,** 456–71.

5244 MARCHIAFAVA, ETTORE. 1847–1935, & BIGNAMI, AMICO. 1862–1929
Sulle febbre malariche estivo-autumnali. Roma, *E. Loescher*, 1892.
A summary of the Italian work on malaria. English translation, 1894.

5245 MANSON, *Sir* PATRICK. 1844–1922
On the nature and significance of the crescentic and flagellated bodies in malarial blood. *Brit. med. J.*, 1894, **2,** 1306–08.
Manson's mosquito-malaria hypothesis.

5246 MACCALLUM, WILLIAM GEORGE. 1874–1944
On the flagellated form of the malarial parasite. *Lancet*, 1897, **2,** 1240–41.
MacCallum reported at a meeting of the British Association his observation of the mode of fertilization of the malarial parasite of birds; two months later he announced that he had found the same to hold good for the human parasite.

5247 ROSS, *Sir* RONALD. 1857–1932
On some peculiar pigmented cells found in two mosquitos fed on malarial blood. *Brit. med. J.*, 1897, **2,** 1786–88.

Ross proved that the mosquito was responsible for the transmission of malaria. On August 20, 1897, he found Laveran's *Plasmodium* in the stomach of the *Anopheles* mosquito after it had fed on the blood of malaria patients. See also the earlier paper in the same journal, 1897, **1**, 251–55.

5248 LAVERAN, CHARLES LOUIS ALPHONSE. 1845–1922
Traité de paludisme. Paris, *Masson & Cie.*, 1898.

5249 OPIE, EUGENE LINDSAY. 1873–1971
On the haemocytozoa of birds. *J. exp. Med.*, 1898, **3,** 79–101.

Demonstration of sexual conjugation in the malaria parasite. See also the following entry.

5250 MACCALLUM, WILLIAM GEORGE. 1874–1944
Notes on the pathological changes in the organs of birds infected with haemocytozoa. *J. exp. Med.*, 1898, **3,** 103–16, 117–36.

5251 ROSS, *Sir* RONALD. 1857–1932
The rôle of the mosquito in the evolution of the malarial parasite. *Lancet*, 1898, **2,** 488–89.

On July 9, 1898, Ross provided the last link in the chain demonstrating the complete life cycle of the parasite of bird malaria. He found that mosquitoes which had fed on malaria-infected birds, and which had allowed the parasites to develop and lodge in their salivary glands, could then infect healthy birds, which in turn became malarious. Ross was awarded the Nobel Prize for Medicine in 1902.

5252 GRASSI, GIOVANNI BATTISTA. 1854–1925, & BIGNAMI, AMICO. 1862–1929
Ciclo evolutivo della semilune nell' Anopheles claviger. *Ann. Ig. sper.*, 1899, n.s., **9,** 258–64.

Grassi and Bignami showed that the *Plasmodium* undergoes its sexual phase only in the *Anopheles* mosquito.

5252.1 GRASSI, GIOVANNI BATTISTA. 1854–1925
Studi di uno zoologo sulla malaria. Roma, *V. Salviucci*, 1900.

Includes the best illustrations of the various stages of the malaria parasite published up to that time.

5252.2 MANSON, *Sir* PATRICK. 1844–1922
Experimental proof of the mosquito-malaria theory. *Brit. med. J.*, 1900, **2,** 949–51.

In a classical demonstration Manson allowed infected mosquitoes from Rome to bite a volunteer (his son) in London, who developed malaria 15 days later, with tertian parasites in the blood and who was cured by quinine.

5253 LEISHMAN, *Sir* WILLIAM BOOG. 1865–1926
Note on a simple and rapid method of producing Romanowsky staining in malarial and other blood films. *Brit. med. J.*, 1901, **2,** 757–758.

"Leishman's stain", a modification of that introduced by Romanovsky in 1891.

5254 SCHAUDINN, FRITZ RICHARD. 1871–1906
Studien über krankheitserregende Protozoen. II. Plasmodium vivax (Grassi & Feletti), der Erreger des Tertianfiebers beim Menschen. *Arb. k. GesundhAmte*, 1903, **19,** 169–250.

Confirmation of the work of Ross and of Grassi.

5255 CRAIG, CHARLES FRANKLIN. 1872–1950
Intracorpuscular conjugation in the malarial plasmodia and its significance. *Amer. Med.*, 1905, **10,** 982–86, 1029–32.
Demonstration of the existence of malaria carriers.

5255.1 BASS, CHARLES CASSEDY. 1875– , & JOHNS, FOSTER MATTHEW. 1889–
The cultivation of malaria plasmodia (*Plasmodium vivax* and *Plasmodium falciparum*) in vitro. *J. exp. Med.*, 1912, **16,** 567–79.
Cultivation of the malaria parasite.

5255.2 STEPHENS, JOHN WILLIAM WATSON. 1865–1946
A new malaria parasite of man. *Ann. trop. Med. Parasit.*, 1922, **16,** 383–88.
Plasmodium ovale described.

5256 ROEHL, WILHELM. *d.* 1929
Die Wirkung des Plasmochins auf die Vogelmalaria. *Arch. Schiffs- u. Tropenhyg.*, 1926, **30,** Beihefte, 311–18; 1927, **31,** Beihefte, 48–58.
Introduction of plasmoquine (pamaquin) in the treatment of malaria.

5256.1 SINTON, JOHN ALEXANDER. 1884–1956, & BIRD, WILLIAM.
Studies in malaria, with special reference to treatment. Part IX Plasmoquine in the treatment of malaria. *Indian J. med. Res.*, 1928, **16,** 159–77.
Clinical trials of pamaquin.

5257 KIKUTH, WALTHER. 1896–1968
Zur Weiterentwicklung synthetisch dargestellter Malariamittel. I. Ueber die chemotherapeutische Wirkung des Atebrin. *Dtsch. med. Wschr.*, 1932, **58,** 530–31.
Introduction of atebrin (mepacrine).

5257.1 PETER, F. M.
Über die Wirkung des Atebrin gegen natürliche Malariainfektion. *Dtsch. med. Wschr.*, 1932, **58,** 533–35.

5258 JAMES, SYBIL P., & TAIT, P.
Newer knowledge of the life cycle of malaria parasites. *Nature (Lond.)*, 1937, **139,** 545.
Description of the exo-erythrocytic cycle in *P. gallinaceum.*

5259 MUDROW, LILI. 1908–1957
Klinische und parasitologische Befunde und chemotherapeutische Ergebnisse bei der Hühnermalaria. *Arch. Schiffs- u. Tropenhyg.*, 1940, **44,** 257–75.
Discovery of the developmental forms of *P. gallinaceum* in the incubation period.

5259.1 SHORTT, HENRY EDWARD. 1887– , *et al.*
The form of *Plasmodium gallinaceum* present in the incubation period of the infection. *Indian J. med. Res.*, 1940, **28,** 273–76.
Independently of Mudrow, H. E. Shortt, K. P. Menon, and P. V. Seetharama Iyer found pre-erythrocytic forms of *P. gallinaceum* in the tissues.

5260 CURD, Francis Henry Swinton. 1909–1948, *et al.*
Studies on synthetic antimalarial drugs. *Ann. trop. Med. Parasit.*, 1945, **39,** 139–64, 208–16.
F. H. S. Curd, D. G. Davey, and F. L. Rose synthesized proguanil ("paludrine") and first tested it in avian malaria.

5261 ADAMS, Alfred Robert Davies, *et al.*
Studies on synthetic antimalarial drugs. XIII. Results of a preliminary investigation of the therapeutic action of 4888 (paludrine) on acute attacks of benign tertian malaria. *Ann. trop. Med. Parasit.*, 1945, **39,** 225–31.
First use of proguanil in human malaria. With B. G. Maegraith, J. D. King, R. H. Townsend, T. H. Davey, and R. E. Havard.

5261.1 MOST, Harry. 1907– , *et al.*
Chloroquine for treatment of acute attacks of *vivax* malaria. *J. Amer. med. Ass.*, 1946, **131,** 963–67.
Clinical trials of chloroquine. With I. M. London, C. A. Kane, P. H. Lavietes, E. F. Schroeder, and J. M. Hayman. See also *J. Amer. med. Ass.*, 1946, **130**, 1069.

5261.2 ALVING, Alf Sven. 1902– , *et al.*
Pentaquine (Sn-13,276), a therapeutic agent effective in reducing the relapse rate in *vivax* malaria. *J. clin. Invest.*, 1948, **27,** No. 3, pt. 2, 25–33.
Clinical trials of pentaquine. With B. Craige, R. Jones, C. M. Whorton, T. N. Pullman, and L. Eichelberger.

5262 SHORTT, Henry Edward. 1887– , *et al.*
The pre-erythrocytic stage of mammalian malaria. *Brit. med. J.*, 1948, **1,** 192–94.
Demonstration of the pre-erythrocytic stage of *P. cynomolgi* in the monkey. With P. C. C. Garnham and B. Malamos. Preliminary communication in *Nature* (*Lond.*), 1948, **161**, 126. Subsequently these workers demonstrated the pre-erythrocytic forms of *P. vivax* (*Brit. med. J.*, 1948, **1**, 547) and of *P. falciparum* (*Brit. med. J.*, 1949, **2**, 1006–08) in man.

5262.1 EDGCOMB, John Harold. 1924– , *et al.*
Primaquine, S.N. 13,272, a new curative agent in vivax malaria: a preliminary report. *J. nat. Malaria Soc.*, 1950, **9**, 288–372.
Introduction of primaquine.

History of Malaria

5263 JONES, William Henry Samuel. 1876–1963
Malaria and Greek history. To which is added The history of Greek therapeutics and the malaria theory, by E. T. Withington. Manchester, *Univ. Press*, 1909.
The view is put forward by the writer that malarial infection was the cause of the decadence of the Greeks.

5264 CELLI, Angelo. 1857–1914
The history of malaria in the Roman Campagna from ancient times. Edited and enlarged by Anna Celli-Fraentzel. London, *John Bale*, 1933.

5264.1 STEPHENS, John William Watson. 1865–1946
Blackwater fever, a historical survey and summary of observations made over a century. Liverpool, *University Press*, 1937.

5264.2 JARAMILLO-ARANGO, Jaime. 1897–1962
The conquest of malaria. London, *William Heinemann*, 1950.

5264.3 RUSSELL, Paul Farr. 1894–
Man's mastery of malaria. London, *Oxford University Press*, 1955.
Heath Clark Lectures, 1953.

5265–5289 TRYPANOSOMIASIS

5265 ATKINS, John. 1685–1757
The sleepy distemper. In his: *The navy surgeon*, London, 1734, pp. 364–67.
First English description of African trypanosomiasis.

5266 WINTERBOTTOM, Thomas Masterman. 1765–1859
An account of the native Africans in the neighbourhood of Sierra Leone. Vol. 2. London, *J. Hatchard & J. Mawman*, 1803.
In his travels in Africa Winterbottom saw sleeping sickness, which he described (pp. 29–31) as a species of lethargy. He also noticed that slave-dealers would not buy slaves whose neck glands showed signs of enlargement.

5267 CLARKE, Robert.
Observations on the disease lethargus: with cases and pathology. *Lond. med. Gaz.*, 1840, **26,** 970–76.
Clarke left a detailed account of African trypanosomiasis; he saw cases of the disease whilst a colonial surgeon at Sierra Leone and named it "narcoleptic dropsy".

5267.1 VALENTIN, Gabriel Gustav. 1810–1883
Ueber ein Entozoon im Blute von Salmo fario. *Arch. Anat. Physiol. wiss. Med.*, 1841, 435–36.
Valentin was the first to discover a trypanosome; this was in a salmon.

5268 GRUBY, David. 1810–1898
Recherches et observations sur une nouvelle espèce d'hématozoaire, Trypanosoma sanguinis. *C. R. Acad. Sci.* (*Paris*), 1843, **17,** 1134–36.
Gruby discovered trypanosomes in the frog. He it was who first suggested the name "trypanosome" to describe the parasite.

5269 LIVINGSTONE, David. 1813–1873
Missionary travels and researches in South Africa. London, *John Murray*, 1857.
Livingstone gave an accurate account of the tsetse fly *Glossina morsitans* and of the disease in cattle following its bite (see pp. 80–83; picture of the tsetse fly on p. 571). In his time the bite of the fly was thought to be (and perhaps was) harmless to man.

5270 ——. Arsenic as a remedy for the tsetse bite. *Brit. med. J.*, 1858, 360–61.
Livingstone was probably the first to administer arsenic for the treatment of "nagana," a disease of horses caused by trypanosomes. This followed a suggestion by James Braid.

5270.1 LEWIS, Timothy Richards. 1841–1886
The microscopic organisms found in the blood of man and animals, and their relation to disease. *Ann. rep. sanit. Comm. India* (1877), 1878, **14,** Appendix B, 157–208.
First description of a trypanosome (*T. lewisi*) in a mammal.

5271 EVANS, Griffith. 1835–1935
On a horse disease in India known as "surra", probably due to a haematozoon. *Vet. J.*, 1881, **13,** 1–10, 82–88, 180–200, 326–33.
While serving in India as a veterinary surgeon, Evans discovered parasites in the blood of horses suffering from surra; this was the first pathogenic trypanosome to be described.

5272 NEPVEU, Gustave. 1841–1903
Étude sur les parasites du sang chez les paludiques. *C. R. Soc. Biol. (Paris)*, 1891, **43,** 39–50.
Nepveu, whilst in Algeria, was the first to see trypanosomes in human blood.

5273 BRUCE, *Sir* David. 1855–1931
Preliminary report on the tsetse fly disease or nagana, in Zululand. Durban, *Bennett & Davis,* 1895.
In 1895 Bruce found that *nagana,* the tsetse fly disease of Zululand, was due to a trypanosome (*T. brucei*).

5274 FORDE, Robert Michael. 1861–1948
Some clinical notes on a European patient in whose blood a trypanosoma was observed. *J. trop. Med. Hyg.*, 1902, **5,** 261–63.
In 1901 Forde saw (but did not at first recognize as such) trypanosomes in the blood of a patient in Gambia. (See No. 5275.)

5275 DUTTON, Joseph Everett. 1876–1905
Preliminary note upon a trypanosome occurring in the blood of man. *Thompson Yates Lab. Rep.*, 1902, **4,** 455–68.
Dutton was the first to recognize human trypanosomiasis. He saw Forde's patient (see No. 5274) and named the trypanosome *T. gambiense.* Sleeping sickness itself has been referred to as "Dutton's disease".

5276 CASTELLANI, Aldo. 1877–1971
On the discovery of a species of trypanosoma in the cerebrospinal fluid of cases of sleeping sickness. *Proc. roy. Soc.*, 1903, **71,** 501–08.
Whilst in Uganda, Castellani discovered *T. gambiense* in human cerebrospinal fluid.

5277 ROYAL SOCIETY, LONDON.
Reports of the Sleeping Sickness Commission of the Royal Society. 17 pts. London, 1903–19.
Bruce and Nabarro were sent to Africa by the Royal Society to study sleeping sickness, and in their report they showed that the tsetse fly was the vector of trypanosomiasis. They also found that Gambia fever and sleeping sickness were two stages of the same infection.

5278 LAVERAN, Charles Louis Alphonse. 1845–1922, & MESNIL, Félix. 1868–1938
Trypanosomes et trypanosomiases. Paris, *Masson & Cie.*, 1904.
Laveran and Mesnil discovered that trypanosomes could be maintained indefinitely in rats and mice by serial passage.

5279 THOMAS, Harold Wolferstan, & BREINL, Anton.
Report on trypanosomes, trypanosomiasis, and sleeping sickness, being an experimental investigation into their pathology and treatment. London, *Williams & Norgate,* 1905.

Thomas and Breinl discovered that atoxyl, an organic derivative of arsenic acid, was more potent in the treatment of laboratory trypanosomiasis than arsenic in inorganic form. The above is Memoir XVI of the Liverpool School of Tropical Medicine.

5280 NICOLLE, Maurice. 1862–1932, & MESNIL, Félix. 1868–1938
Traitement des trypanosomiases par les "couleurs de benzidine". *Ann. Inst. Pasteur,* 1906, **20**, 417–48, 513–38.

Introduction of trypan-blue in the treatment of trypanosomiasis. Second paper by Mesnil and Nicolle.

5281 EHRLICH, Paul. 1854–1915
Chemotherapeutische Trypanosomen-Studien. *Berl. klin. Wschr.,* 1907, **44,** 233–36, 280–83, 310–14, 341–44.

Includes an account of "Trypanrot," by which Ehrlich succeeded in curing experimental trypanosomiasis. It was his work on this subject which led Ehrlich eventually to the production of salvarsan. He shared the Nobel Prize for Medicine with Metchnikoff in 1908.

5282 PLIMMER, Henry George. 1856–1918, & THOMSON, John D.
Further results of the experimental treatment of trypanosomiasis in rats. *Proc. roy. Soc. B.,* 1908, **80,** 1–12.

Trial of antimony in the treatment of trypanosomiasis.

5283 CHAGAS, Carlos Justiniano Ribeiro. 1879–1934
Neue Trypanosomen. *Arch. Schiffs- u. Tropenhyg.,* 1909, **13,** 120–22.

Chagas discovered *T. cruzi,* the causal organism in American trypanosomiasis ("Chagas's disease").

5284 LEVADITI, Constantin. 1874–1953
Le mécanisme d'action des dérivés arsenicaux dans les trypanosomiases. *Ann. Inst. Pasteur,* 1909, **23,** 604–43.

A study of the action of atoxyl and arsacétine.

5285 STEPHENS, John William Watson. 1865–1946, & FANTHAM, Harold Benjamin. 1875–1937
On the peculiar morphology of a trypanosome from a case of sleeping sickness and the possibility of its being a new species (T. rhodesiense). *Proc. roy. Soc. B,* 1910, **83,** 28–33.

T. rhodesiense discovered.

5285.1 VIANNA, Gaspar Oliveira de. 1885–1914
Contribuição para o estudo da anatomia patalojica da "molestia de Carlos Chagas". *Mem. Inst. Osw. Cruz,* 1911, **3,** 276–94.

Demonstration of the mode of reproduction of *T. cruzi.* Text in Portuguese and German. See also the paper by Chagas in pp. 219–75 of the same journal.

5285.2 KINGHORN, Allan. *d.* 1955, & YORKE, Warrington. 1883–1943
On the transmission of human trypanosomes by *Glossina morsitans,* Westw.; and on the occurrence of human trypanosomes in game. *Ann. trop. Med. Parasit.,* 1912, **6,** 1–23.

Glossina morsitans shown to be the transmitting fly of *T. rhodesiense.*

5286 HAENDEL, Ludwig. 1869–1939, & JOETTEN, Karl Wilhelm. 1886–
Ueber chemotherapeutische Versuche mit "205 Bayer", einem neuen trypanoziden Mittel von besonderer Wirkung. *Berl. klin. Wschr.*, 1920, **57,** 821–23.
Introduction of "Bayer 205" (germanin, suramin, naphuride).

5287 PEARCE, Louise. 1886–1959
Studies on the treatment of human trypanosomiasis with tryparsamide (the sodium salt of N-phenylglycineamide-*p*-arsonic acid). *J. exp. Med.*, 1921, **34,** Suppl., 1–104.
Introduction of tryparsamide in the treatment of trypanosomiasis.

5288 FOURNEAU, Ernest. 1872–1949
Chimiothérapie des trypanosomiases. *Paris méd.*, 1923, **49,** 501–08.
Introduction of moranyl ("Fourneau 309").

5289 LEVADITI, Constantin. 1847–1953, *et al.*
Essai de prophylaxie des trypanosomiases par des dérivés phénylarsiniques administrés *per os*. *Bull. Soc. Path. exot.*, 1926, **19**, 737–46.
First attempt to induce prophylaxis by chemical means in trypanosomiasis. With S. Nicolau and I. Galloway.

5290–5302

LEISHMANIASIS

5290 RUSSELL, Alexander. 1715?–1768
Natural history of Aleppo. London, *A. Millar*, 1856 [1756].
Includes (Chap. iv) a good account of "Aleppo boil", which Russell found to be endemic in Aleppo.

5291 ALIBERT, Jean Louis Marc, *le baron*. 1768–1837
Sur la pyrophlyctide endémique, ou pustule d'Aleppo. *Rev. méd. franç. étrang.*, 1829, n.s., **3,** 62–71.
Important description of "Aleppo boil", furunculosis orientalis.

5292 CLARKE, John James. 1827–1895
Kala azar, the black disease. *Ann. sanit. Rep. Prov. Assam*, 1882, Appendix A.
Earliest definite description of kala-azar.

5293 CUNNINGHAM, David Douglas. 1843–1914
On the presence of peculiar parasitic organisms in the tissue of a specimen of Delhi boil. *Sci. Mem. med. Off. Army India*, [1884], 1885, **1,** 21–31.
Cunningham saw and described bodies in Delhi boil; these were almost certainly Leishman–Donovan bodies.

5294 BOROVSKY, Petr Fokich. 1863–1932
[On sart sore.] *Voenno med. Zhur.*, 1898, **76,** 925–41.
First description of the protozoon later named *Leishmania tropica*. The paper is in Russian; for a translation, see C. A. Hoare, in *Trans. roy. Soc. trop. Med. Hyg.*, 1938, **32**, 78–90.

5295 LEISHMAN, *Sir* WILLIAM BOOG. 1865–1926
On the possibility of the occurrence of trypanosomiasis in India. *Brit. med. J.*, 1903, **1,** 1252–54; **2,** 1376–77.

An organism found by Leishman in 1900 was later described by him as possibly a trypanosome. C. Donovan found the same organism in blood in July 1903. The name *Leishmania donovani* (Leishman–Donovan bodies) was later attached to these organisms.

5296 DONOVAN, CHARLES. 1863–1951
On the possibility of the occurrence of trypanosomiasis in India. *Brit. med. J.*, 1903, **2,** 79.

See previous entry.

5297 WRIGHT, JAMES HOMER. 1870–1928
Protozoa in a case of tropical ulcer (Delhi sore). *J. med. Res.*, 1903, **10,** 472–82.

Wright found *Leishmania tropica* in Delhi sore.

5298 LEISHMAN, *Sir* WILLIAM BOOG. 1865–1926
Note on the nature of the parasitic bodies found in tropical splenomegaly. *Brit. med. J.*, 1904, **1,** 303.

5299 ROGERS, *Sir* LEONARD. 1868–1962
Note on the occurrence of Leishman–Donovan bodies in "cachexial fevers" including kala-azar. *Brit. med. J.*, 1904, **1,** 1249–51.

Rogers demonstrated the Leishman–Donovan bodies in kala-azar. See also the same journal, 1904, 2, 645–50. At about the same time Bentley reported similar findings in India.

5300 NICOLLE, CHARLES JULES HENRI. 1866–1936
Le kala azar infantile. *Ann. Inst. Pasteur*, 1909, **23,** 361–401, 441–71.

Nicolle considered infantile kala-azar to be caused by a distinct species of *Leishmania*; to this he gave the name *L. infantum.*

5301 VIANNA, GASPAR OLIVEIRA DE. 1885–1914
Sobre o tratemento da leishmaniose tegumentar. *Ann. paulist. Med. Cir.*, 1914, **2,** 167–69.

Vianna introduced tartar emetic in the treatment of S. American leishmaniasis. His preliminary announcement on this form of treatment was made to the Brazilian Dermatological Society and appears in *Arch. brasil. Med.*, 1912, 2, 426–28.

5302 SWAMINATH, C. S., *et al.*
Transmission of Indian kala-azar to man by the bites of *Phlebotomus argentipes*, Ann. and Brun. *Indian J. med. Res.*, 1942, **30,** 473–77.

Successful transmission of kala-azar to man by the bite of *Phlebotomus argentipes* reported, showing it to be the vector of *Leishmania.* With H. E. Shortt and L. A. P. Anderson.

5303–5308.2 YAWS

5303 PISO, WILLEM [LE POIS (GUILLAUME)]. 1611–1678
De lue Indica. In his *Historia naturalis Brasiliae*, (De medica Brasiliensi, p. 35), Lugduni Batavorum, *apud F. Hackium*, 1648.

Piso was the first to separate yaws from syphilis.

5304 BANCROFT, EDWARD. 1774–1821
Essay on the natural history of Guiana, in South America. London, *T. Becket*, 1769.
Bancroft was an English physician who lived for many years in America. He noted the transmission of yaws by flies (p. 385 of his book).

5305 BREDA, ACHILLE. 1850–1933
Beitrag zum klinischen und bacteriologischen Studium der brasilianischen Framboesie oder "Boubas". *Arch. Dermat. Syph.* (*Wien*), 1895, **33**, 3–28.
"Breda's disease" – Brazilian yaws. English translation (New Sydenham Society), 1897.

5306 CASTELLANI, ALDO. 1877–1971
On the presence of spirochaetes in two cases of ulcerated parangi (yaws). *Brit. med. J.*, 1905, **2**, 1280, 1330–31, 1430.
Castellani demonstrated in scrapings of yaws tissue a spirochaete, *T. pertenue*, later found to be the causal organism. He thus finally established it as a distinct organism from the syphilis spirochaete. Preliminary note in *J. Ceylon Br. Brit. med. Ass.*, 1905, **2**, pt. 1, 54.

5307 WELLMANN, FREDERICK CREIGHTON. 1871–1960
On a spirochaete found in yaws papules. *J. trop. Med. Hyg.*, 1905, **8**, 345.
Independently of Castellani (No. 5306) Wellmann discovered *Treponema pertenue.*

5308 NICHOLS, HENRY JAMES. 1877–1927
Experimental yaws in the monkey and rabbit. *J. exp. Med.*, 1910, **12**, 616–22; 1911, **14**, 196–216.

5308.1 SAENZ, BRAULIO, *et al.*
Demonstración de un treponema en el borde activo de un caso de pinto de las manos y pies y en la linfa de ganglios superficiales (reporte preliminar). *Arch. Med. interna*, 1938, **4**, 112–17.
B. Saenz, J. Grau Triana, and J. Alfonso Armenteros indicated that pinta is caused by a treponeme, *T. carateum.*

5308.2 WORLD HEALTH ORGANIZATION.
Bibliography on yaws, 1905–62. Genève, *World Health Organization*, 1963.
Over 1,700 items.

5309–5321 RELAPSING FEVERS

5309 RUTTY, JOHN. 1698–1775
A chronological history of the weather and seasons and of the prevailing diseases in Dublin. London, *Robinson & Roberts*, 1770.
Rutty kept continuous records of weather and diseases in Dublin from 1724–64. On page 75 of the above book is given the first clear description of relapsing fever.

5310 CORMACK, *Sir* JOHN ROSE. 1815–1882
Natural history, pathology and treatment of the epidemic fever at present prevailing in Edinburgh and other towns. London, *J. Churchill*, 1843.
The epidemic of relapsing fever in Edinburgh in 1843 was well described by Cormack. He was first editor of the *Association Medical Journal* which later became the *British Medical Journal.*

5311 CRAIGIE, DAVID. 1793–1866
Notice of a febrile disorder which has prevailed at Edinburgh during the summer of 1843. *Edinb. med. surg. J.*, 1843, **60,** 410–18.
Relapsing fever was given its name by Craigie, in his description of the Edinburgh epidemic.

5311.1 HENDERSON, WILLIAM. 1810–1872
On some of the characters which distinguish the fever at present epidemic from typhus fever. *Edinb. med. surg. J.*, 1844, **61,** 201–25.
Henderson, professor of pathology at Edinburgh, gave a good account of relapsing fever seen during the epidemic in 1843. He was one of the first to differentiate it from typhus.

5312 SILLIAU, PIERRE MARIE.
Fièvre à rechutes. Paris, *Thèse No.* 205, 1869.
Silliau gave a good account of the epidemic of relapsing fever at Réunion, 1865. He showed the contagious nature of the disease.

5313 PARRY, JOHN S. 1843–1876
Observations on relapsing fever, as it occurred in Philadelphia in the winter of 1869 and 1870. *Amer. J. med. Sci.*, 1870, n.s., **60,** 336–58.
Parry called attention to infection from articles of clothing worn by victims of the epidemic of relapsing fever in Philadelphia in 1869.

5314 OBERMEIER, OTTO HUGO FRANZ. 1843–1873
Vorkommen feinster, eine Eigenbewegung zeigender Fäden im Blute von Recurrenskranken. *Zbl. med. Wiss.*, 1873, **11,** 145–47.
Discovery (in 1868) of *Borrelia recurrentis*, causative agent in relapsing fever.

5315 MOCZUTKOWSKY, OSHIP OSIPOVICH [MOSCHUTKOWSKY]. 1845–1903
Materialien zur Pathologie und Therapie des Rückfallstyphus. *Dtsch. Arch. klin. Med.*, 1879, **24,** 80–97.
By inoculating healthy subjects with the blood of patients suffering from relapsing fever, and producing the fever in the former, Moczutkowsky demonstrated not only the communicability of the disease but also the specific pathogenic significance of the spirochaete.

5316 CARTER, HENRY VANDYKE. 1831–1897
Spirillum fever. London, *J. & A. Churchill*, 1882.
Asiatic relapsing fever; original work on this disease by Carter is remembered by the eponym "Carter's fever" and the name *Trep. carteri.* He reproduced the disease in the monkey.

5317 ROSS, PHILIP HEDGELAND. 1876–1929, & MILNE, ARTHUR DAWSON. ?–1932
"Tick fever." *Brit. med. J.*, 1904, **2,** 1453–54.
Ross and Milne discovered the causative agent in the African variety of relapsing (tick) fever.

5318 DUTTON, JOSEPH EVERETT. 1877–1905, & TODD, JOHN LANCELOT. 1876–1949
The nature of tick fever in the eastern part of the Congo Free State. *Brit. med. J.*, 1905, **2,** 1259–60.
Independently of Ross and Milne, Dutton and Todd demonstrated relapsing fever in monkeys conveyed by infected ticks, *Ornithodorus moubata.* The organism was named *Sp. duttoni.*

5319 NORRIS, CHARLES. 1867–1935, *et al.*
Study of a spirochete obtained from a case of relapsing fever in man, with notes on morphology, animal reactions, and attempts at cultivation. *J. infect. Dis.*, 1906, **3,** 266–90.

Spirochaete causing the American variety of relapsing fever first isolated. With A. W. Pappenheimer and T. Flournoy.

5320 NOVY, FREDERICK GEORGE. 1864–1957, & KNAPP, RICHARD EDWARD. 1884–
Studies in *Spirillum obermeieri* and related organisms. *J. infect. Dis.*, 1906, **3,** 291–393.

Novy and Knapp made important observations on the spirochaete isolated by Norris *et al.* from a case of (American) relapsing fever, proving it to be different from *Sp. obermeieri.* The organism is sometimes referred to as "Novy's bacillus", *Trep. novyi.* The above paper includes work on the immunology of the disease.

5321 MACKIE, FREDERICK PERCIVAL. 1875–1944
The part played by Pediculus corporis in the transmission of relapsing fever. *Brit. med. J.*, 1907, **2,** 1706–09.

Proof that relapsing fever is conveyed by the body louse, *Pediculus corporis.*

5322–5329 RAT-BITE FEVER

5322 WILCOX, WHITMAN.
Violent symptoms from the bite of a rat. *Amer. J. med. Sci.*, 1840, **26,** 245–46.

First report of rat-bite fever to appear in a medical journal.

5323 CARTER, HENRY VANDYKE. 1831–1897
Note on the occurrence of a minute blood-spirillum in an Indian rat. *Sci. Mem. med. Off. Army India,* (1887), 1888, **3,** 45–48.

Demonstration of *Spirillum minus,* later shown to be a cause of rat-bite fever. (See also No. 5327.)

5324 HATA, SAHACHIRO. 1873–1938
Salvarsantherapie der Rattenbisskrankheit in Japan. *Münch. med. Wschr.*, 1912, **59,** 854–57.

Salvarsan first used in the treatment of rat-bite fever.

5325 SCHOTTMÜLLER, HUGO. 1867–1936
Zur Aetiologie und Klinik der Bisskrankheit. *Derm. Wschr.*, 1914, **58,** Suppl., 77–103.

Isolation of *Streptothrix* (*Actinomyces*) *muris ratti* from human patients bitten by rats.

5326 FUTAKI, KENZŌ. 1873– , *et al.*
The cause of rat-bite fever. *J. exp. Med.*, 1916, **23,** 249–50; 1917, **25,** 33–44.

K. Futaki, I. Takaki, T. Taniguchi, and S. Osumi found a spirillum (*Sp. morsus muris*) in the lymphatic glands and blood stream in cases of rat-bite fever (sodoku).

5327 ROBERTSON, ANDREW.
Observations on the causal organism of rat-bite fever in man. *Ann. trop. Med. Parasit.*, 1924, **16,** 157–75

Robertson proved one of the causal organisms of rat-bite fever to be *Sp. morsus muris.* He re-named it *Spirillum minus* Carter, 1887, identifying it as the first spiral micro-organism to be described from a rodent.

5328 PLACE, Edwin Hemphill. 1880– , *et al.*
Erythema arthriticum epidemicum; preliminary report. *Boston med. surg. J.*, 1926, **194,** 285–87.

"Haverhill fever" first reported. The writers isolated an organism, later found to be identical with *Streptothrix muris ratti* and *Streptobacillus moniliformis.* With L. E. Sutton and O. Willner.

5329 LEMIERRE, Andre. 1875– . *et al.*
Sur une nouvelle fièvre par morsure de rat. *Bull. Acad. Méd.* (*Paris*), 1937, 3 sér., **117,** 705–13.

A. Lemierre, J. Reilly, A. Laporte, and M. Morin isolated *Streptobacillus moniliformis* from a case of rat-bite fever.

5330–5336 LEPTOSPIROSES

5330 MARSTON, Jeffery Allen. 1831–1911
Report on fever (Malta). *Army med. Dept. statist. sanit. Rep.* (1861), 1863, **3,** 486–521.

Marston was apparently the first to describe "Weil's disease" (p. 513).

5331 LANDOUZY, Louis Théophile Joseph. 1845–1917
Fièvre bilieuse ou hépatique. *Gaz. Hôp.* (*Paris*), 1883, **56,** 809–10, 913–14.

An early account of "Weil's disease", Leptospirosis icterohaemorrhagica.

5332 WEIL, Adolf. 1848–1916
Ueber eine eigenthümliche, mit Milztumor, Icterus und Nephritis einhergehende, acute Infectionskrankheit. *Dtsch. Arch. klin. Med.*, 1886, **39,** 209–32.

In his classical description of Leptospirosis icterohaemorrhagica Weil differentiated the disease from other types of acute jaundice. It is better known as "Weil's disease".

5333 STIMSON, Arthur Marston. 1876–
Note on an organism found in yellow-fever tissue. *Publ. Hlth Rep.* (*Wash.*), 1907, **22,** 541.

Stimson discovered a spirochaete in the organs of persons dying of (?) yellow fever. He called it *Sp. interrogans*, but it was almost certainly *Leptospira icterohaemorrhagiae*, the spirochaete of infective jaundice.

5334 INADA, Ryukichi. 1874–1950, *et al.*
The etiology, mode of infection, and specific therapy of Weil's disease (Spirochaetosis icterohaemorrhagica). *J. exp. Med.*, 1916, **23,** 377–402.

R. Inada, Y. Ido, R. Hoki, R. Kaneko, and H. Ito proved that *Sp.* (*Leptospira*) *icterohaemorrhagiae* is the causal organism in infective jaundice. Preliminary report (in Japanese) in *Tokyo Ijishinshi*, 1915, No. 1908.

5334.1 IDO, Yutaka, *et al.*
The rat as a carrier of Spirochaeta icterohaemorrhagiae, the causative agent in Weil's disease (spirochaetosis icterohaemorrhagica). *J. exp. Med.*, 1917, **26,** 341–53.

Rats shown to be the carriers of *Leptospira.* With R. Hoki, H. Ito, and H. Wani.

5334.2 ——. Spirochaeta hebdomadis, the causative agent of seven-day fever (nanukayami). *J. exp. Med.*, 1918, **28,** 435–48.

Discovery of *Leptospira hebdomadis*, carried by a mouse. With H. Ito and H. Wani.

5335 KLARENBEEK, Arie. 1888– , & SCHÜFFNER, Wilhelm August Paul. 1867–1949
Het voorkomen van een afwijkend Leptospira-ras in Nederland. *Ned. T. Geneesk.*, 1933, **77,** 4271–76.
Leptospira canicola first isolated (1931) from the urine of a dog.

5336 DHONT, C. M., *et al.*
De leptospiroses bij den hond, en de beteekenis der *Leptospira canicola. Ned. T. Geneesk.*, 1934, **78,** 5197–209.
First reported cases of human infection with *L. canicola.* With A. Klarenbeek, W. A. P. Schüffner, and J. Voet.

DISEASES DUE TO METAZOAN PARASITES

5336.1–5369.1

5336.1 WELSCH, Georg Hieronymus. 1624–1677
Exercitatio de vena Medinensi. Augustae Vindelicorum. *T. Goebel,* 1674.
An exhaustive survey of dracontiasis.

5336.2 CHISHOLM, Colin. 1755–1825
An essay on the malignant pestilential fever introduced into the West Indian Islands from Boullam, on the coast of Guinea, as it appeared in 1793 and 1794. London, *C. Dilly,* 1795.
Chisholm was apparently the first to observe the mode of transmission of the Guinea worm, *Dracunculus medinensis.*

5336.3 TIEDEMANN, Friedrich. 1781–1861
Notiz. a. d. Geb. d. Natur- u. Heilk., Weimar, 1821, **1,** col. 64.
Description of the calcified cysts of trichinosis in human muscle. No title.

5336.4 HILTON, John. 1804–1878
Notes of a peculiar appearance observed in human muscle, probably depending upon the formation of very small cysticerci. *Lond. med. Gaz.*, 1833, **11,** 605.
Hilton described *Trichinella spiralis* and suggested its parasitic nature.

5337 OWEN, *Sir* Richard. 1804–1892
Description of a microscopic entozoon (Trichina spiralis) infesting the muscles of the human body. *Lond. med. Gaz.*, 1834–35, **16,** 125–127; *Trans. zool. Soc. Lond.*, 1835, **1,** 315–24.
Trichinella spiralis was seen by Paget while still a student; he took specimens to Owen, who published an account.

5338 LEIDY, Joseph. 1823–1891
Trichina spiralis in hogs. *Proc. Acad. nat. Sci. Phila.*, 1846, **3,** 107.
First description of trichinosis in the pig.

5339 BILHARZ, Theodor Maximilian. 1825–1862
Ein Beitrag zur Helminthographia humana aus brieflichen Mittheilungen des Dr. Bilharz in Cairo, nebst Bemerkungen von C. T. v Siebold. *Z. wiss. Zool.*, 1852, **4,** 53–76.
Discovery, in 1851, of *Schistosoma haematobium,* the parasite of bilharziasis. Bilharz was professor of zoology at Cairo.

5340 SIEBOLD, Carl Theodor Ernst von. 1804–1885
Ueber die Band- und Blasenwürmer. Leipzig, *W. Engelmann*, 1854.

Siebold succeeded in infecting dogs with *Taenia echinococcus*. Translation by T. H. Huxley (Sydenham Society), London, 1857.

5341 KÜCHENMEISTER, Gottlob Friedrich Heinrich. 1821–1890
Die in und an dem Körper des lebenden Menschen vorkommenden Parasiten. 2 vols. Leipzig, *B. G. Teubner*, 1855.

5342 ZENKER, Friedrich Albert. 1825–1898
Ueber die Trichinen-Krankheit des Menschen. *Virchows Arch. path. Anat.*, 1860, 561–72.

The intestinal and muscular forms of trichinosis were first noted by Zenker, who established their connexion with the disease.

5343 LEUCKART, Karl Georg Friedrich Rudolf. 1823–1898
Untersuchungen über Trichina spiralis. Leipzig, *C. F. Winter*, 1860.

Leuckart provided an accurate and detailed description of *Trichinella spiralis*.

5344 ——. Die menschlichen Parasiten und die von ihnen herrührenden Krankheiten. 2 vols. Leipzig, *C. F. Winter*, 1863–76.

Includes the first complete and accurate account of the life history and morphology of *Taenia echinococcus*. Leuckart proved the relationship between hydatid cysts and minute tape-worms in dogs.

5344.1 DEMARQUAY, Jean Nicolas. 1811–1875
Note sur une tumeur des bourses contenant un liquide laiteux (galactocèle de Vidal) et renfermant de petits êtres vermiformes que l'on peut considérer comme les helminthes hématoïdes à l'état d'embryon. *Gaz. méd. Paris*, 1863, **33**, 665–67.

Description of the embryonic stage of *Wuchereria bancrofti* in hydrocele fluid.

5344.2 COBBOLD, Thomas Spencer. 1828–1886
Entozoa. London, *Groombridge & Sons*, 1864.

Cobbold suggested (p. 36) that a mollusc was the intermediate host in bilharziasis.

5344.3 HARLEY, John. 1833–1921
On the endemic haematuria of the Cape of Good Hope. *Med.-chir. Trans.*, 1864, **47**, 55–74.

Like Cobbold, Harley expressed the view that a mollusc was the intermediate host in bilharziasis.

5344.4 WUCHERER, Otto Eduard Heinrich. 1820–1873
Noticiar preliminar sobre vermes de uma especie ainda não descripta, encontrados na urina de doentes de hematuria intertropical no Brazil. *Gaz. med. Bahia*, 1868, **3**, 97–99.

In 1866 Wucherer saw the embryo form of the filaria worm. Later the name *Wuchereria bancrofti* was applied to it.

5344.5 FEDCHENKO, Aleksiei Pavlovich. 1844–1873
[On the structure and reproduction of *Filaria medinensis* L.] *Izvest. imp. Obsh. Liub. Estes. (Mosk.)*, 1869–70, **8**, 71–82.

Fedchenko elucidated the life cycle of *Dracunculus medinensis*, the parasite of dracontiasis. English translation in *Amer. J. trop. Med.*, 1971, **20**, 511–23.

5344.6 LEWIS, Timothy Richards. 1841–1886
On a haematozoon inhabiting human blood. Its relation to chyluria and other diseases. *Ann. Rep. sanit. Comm. India* (1871), **8,** Appendix E, 241–60.
Independently of Demarquay (No. 5344.1) and Wucherer (No. 5344.4), Lewis found microfilariae in the urine and blood in chyluria. He was first to use the term *Filaria sanguinis hominis* for the parasite.

5345 MANSON, *Sir* Patrick. 1844–1922
Further observations on Filaria sanguinis hominis. *Med. Rep. Imperial Maritime Customs, China*, 1877, **14,** 1–26.
Manson showed that *Wuchereria bancrofti*, the cause of filarial elephantiasis in man, develops in, and is transmitted by, the Culex mosquito. This was the first proof that infective diseases are spread by animal vectors. See also his later paper in *J. Linnean Soc.*, 1879, (Zool.), **14**, 304–11.

5346 BANCROFT, Joseph. 1836–1894
Cases of filarious disease. *Trans. path. Soc. Lond.*, 1878, **29,** 406–19.
Discovery (1876) of *Wuchereria bancrofti*. See also *Lancet*, 1877, 2, 70.

5347 THOMAS, John Davies. 1844–1893
Notes upon the experimental breeding of *Taenia echinococcus* in the dog from the echinococci of man. *Proc. roy. Soc. Lond.*, 1885, **38,** 449–57.
Thomas succeeded in transmitting *Taenia echinococcus* to the dog from human sources.

5348 BROWN, Thomas Richardson. 1872–1950
Studies on trichinosis, with especial reference to the increase of the eosinophilic cells in the blood and muscle, the origin of these cells and their diagnostic importance. *J. exp. Med.*, 1898, **3,** 315–47.
Brown pointed out the occurrence of eosinophilia in trichinosis. A preliminary communication upon the subject, by W. S. Thayer, was published in *C. R. XII Congr. int. Med.*, Moscou, 1897, 126–31.

5349 LOW, George Carmichael. 1872–1952
A recent observation on *Filaria nocturna* in *Culex*: probable mode of infection of man. *Brit. med. J.*, 1900, **1,** 1456–57.
Demonstration of the complete chain of filarial infection from man-to-mosquito-to-man.

5350 FLEIG, Charles Auguste. 1883–1912, & LISBONNE, Marcel. 1883–
Recherches sur un séro-diagnostic du kyste hydatique par la méthode des précipitines. *C. R. Soc. Biol. (Paris)*, 1907, **62,** 1198–1201.
Precipitin reaction for the diagnosis of hydatid disease.

5350.1 FUJINAMI, Akira. 1870–1934, & NAKAMURA, Hachitaro.
Ueber den Wohnort von *Schistosomum japonicum*. [Japanese text.] *Kyoto Igaku Zassi*, 1907, **4,** No. 4.
Fujinami and Nakamura identified the intermediate host of *S. japonicum*. Abstract in *Arch. Schiffs- u. Tropenhyg.*, 1908, **12**, 471.

5350.2 MIYAIRI, K., & SUZUKI, Minoru
Der Zwischenwirt des *Schistosomum japonicum* Katsurada. *Mitt. med. Fak. Univ. Kyushu*, 1914, **1,** 187–97.
Miyairi and Suzuki found snails to be the intermediate host of *Schistosoma japonicum*.

5350.3 LEIPER, Robert Thomson. 1881–1969.
Report of the results of the bilharzia mission in Egypt, 1915. *J. roy. Army med. Cps*, 1915, **25,** 1–55, 147–92, 253–67; 1916, **27,** 171–90; 1918, **30,** 235–60.

Leiper identified the snail responsible for the transmission of *Schistosoma mansoni* and *S. haematobium.*

5350.4 CHRISTOPHERSON, John Brian. 1868–1955
The successful use of antimony in bilharziosis. *Lancet*, 1918, **2,** 325–27.

Introduction of tartar emetic (antimony) in the treatment of schistosomiasis.

5351 DEW, *Sir* Harold Robert. 1891–
Hydatid disease. Its pathology, diagnosis and treatment. Sydney, *Australasian Med. Publ. Co.*, 1928.

5351.1 AUGUSTINE, Donald Leslie. 1895– , & THEILER, Hans. 1894–
Precipitin and skin tests as aids in diagnosing trichinosis. *Parasitology*, 1932, **24,** 60–86.

Intradermal test for trichinosis.

5351.2 HEWITT, Redginal Irving. 1911– , *et al.*
Experimental chemotherapy of filariasis. III. Effect of l-diethylcarbamyl-4-methyl-piperazine hydrochloride against naturally acquired filarial infections in cotton rats and dogs. *J. Lab. clin. Med.*, 1947, **32,** 1314–29.

Proof of antifilarial action of diethylcarbamazine citrate (hetrazan). With S. Kushner, H. W. Stewart, E. White, W. S. Wallace, and Y. SubbaRow.

5352 KHALIL, Mohamed.
The bibliography of schistosomiasis (bilharziasis). Cairo, *Egyptian University*, 1931.

5352.1 BOUILLON, Albert.
Bibliographie des schistosomes et des schistosomiases (bilharzioses) humaines et animales de 1931 à 1948. *Mémoires, Institut Royal Colonial Belge, Section des Sciences Naturelles et Médicales*, 1949, **18,** fasc. 5.

Continues and supplements No. 5352.

5352.2 WORLD HEALTH ORGANIZATION.
Bibliography of bilharziasis, 1949–1958. Genève, *World Health Organization*, 1960.

Continues and supplements Nos. 5352 and 5352.1.

Hookworm Disease

5353 DUBINI, Angelo. 1813–1902
Nuovo verme intestinale umano (Agchylostoma duodenale), costituente un sesto genere dei nematoidei proprii dell' uomo. *Ann. univ. Med.* (*Milano*), 1843, **106**, 5–51.

Dubini first found the hookworm of ankylostomiasis in 1838. His account of 1843, describing it, named it *Agchylostoma duodenale*, a name etymologically erroneous.

5354 SIEBOLD, Carl Theodor Ernst von. 1804–1885
Bericht über die Leistungen im Gebiete der Helminthologie während des Jahres 1843 und 1844. *Arch. Naturgesch.*, 1845, **2,** 202–55.
(Pp. 220–21.) Siebold classified the hookworm as belonging to the *Strongyloidae.*

5355 GRIESINGER, Wilhelm. 1817–1868
Klinische und anatomische Beobachtungen über die Krankheiten von Aegypten. *Arch. physiol. Heilk.*, 1854, **13,** 528–75.
Griesinger connected the worm of ankylostomiasis with Egyptian chlorosis, a condition in which the worm had previously been noted without its being considered the causal agent (pp. 555–61). Apparently Bilharz in 1853 came to the same conclusion. The disease was for a time called "Griesinger's disease".

5356 WUCHERER, Otto Eduard Heinrich. 1820–1873
Estudos sobre a hypoemia intertropical. *Gaz. med. Bahia*, 1866, **1,** 27.
Wucherer corroborated the work of Griesinger. He showed that the Brazilian disease known as hypohemia intertropicalis, or "oppilação," was due to hookworm infestation. See also the same journal, 1869, **3,** 170–72, 183–84, 198–200, and, for a German translation, *Dtsch. Arch. klin. Med.*, 1872, **10,** 379–400.

5357 GRASSI, Giovanni Battista. 1854–1925, *et al.*
Intorno all' Anchilostoma duodenale (Dubini). *Gazz. med. lombardia*, 1878, 7 ser. **5,** 193–96.
Faecal diagnosis of hookworm disease. Before this time hookworm had been diagnosed only post mortem. With C. Parona and E. Parona.

5358 BOZZOLO, Camillo. 1845–1920
L'anchilostomiasi e l'anemia che ne conseguita (anchilostomanemia). *G. int. Sci. med.*, 1879, n.s., **1,** 1054–69, 1245–53.
Introduction of thymol as a hookworm vermifuge.

5359 LEIDY, Joseph. 1823–1891
Remarks on parasites and scorpions. *Trans. Coll. Phys. Philad.*, 1886, 3 ser., **8,** 441–43.
Leidy found the hookworm in the cat and suggested that it might also be found in man as a cause of pernicious anaemia.

5360 BLICKHAHN, Walter L.
A case of ankylostomiasis. *Med. News* (*Philad.*), 1893, **63,** 662–63.
First recognition of ankylostomiasis in America. It had previously been reported and described under various names.

5361 ASHFORD, Bailey Kelly. 1873–1934
Ankylostomiasis in Puerto Rico. *N. Y. med. J.*, 1900, **71,** 552–56.
Ashford found that nearly one-third of the deaths in Puerto Rico were due to hookworm infestation and the consequent anaemia. His work drew attention to the disease in Puerto Rico and led to a campaign for its extermination.

5362 LOOSS, Arthur. 1861–1923
Ueber das Eindringen der Ankylostomalarven in die menschliche Haut. *Zbl. Bakt.*, Abt. 1, 1901, **29,** Orig. 733–39.
Looss discovered that hookworms can penetrate the skin; he himself became infected when hookworm culture accidentally spilled on his hands.

5363 STILES, Charles Wardell. 1867–1941
A new species of hookworm (Uncinaria americana) parasitic in man. *Amer. Med.*, 1902, **3,** 777–78.
Discovery of the American species of hookworm, afterwards re-named *Necator americanus.* It was later believed to have originated in Africa, being brought over by slaves.

5364 STILES, CHARLES WARDELL. 1867–1941.
Report upon the prevalence and geographical distribution of hookworm disease (*uncinariasis or anchylostomiasis*) in the United States. Washington, *Govt. Printing Office*, 1903.

Bull. No. 10, U.S. Marine Hospital Service Hygienic Laboratory.

5365 LOOSS, ARTHUR. 1861–1923
The anatomy and life history of Agchylostoma duodenale Dub. A monograph. 2 pts. Cairo, *National Printing Office*, 1905–11.

Vols. 3 & 4 of *Records of the School of Medicine, Cairo.* In 1898 Looss discovered that hookworm larvae can penetrate the skin. His monograph epitomized all knowledge of the condition to 1911.

5366 PERRONCITO, EDOARDO. 1847–1936
La malattia dei minatori dal S. Gottardo al Sempione. Torino, *C. Pasta*, 1910.

Includes reprints of Perroncito's earlier papers. He insisted on the parasitic origin of the disease as it occurred among the St. Gotthard tunnellers in 1880, and he introduced *Felix mas* as a vermifuge against hookworm.

5367 SCHÜFFNER, WILHELM. 1867–1949, & VERVOORT, HERMAN.
Das Oleum chenopodii anthelmintici gegen Ankylostomiasis im Vergleich zu anderen Wurmmitteln. *Trans. int. Congr. Hyg. Demogr.*, 1912, Washington, 1913, **1**, 734–39.

Schüffner and Vervoort introduced oil of chenopodium for the treatment of ankylostomiasis as early as 1900.

5368 HALL, MAURICE CROWTHER. 1881–1938
The use of carbon tetrachloride for the removal of hook worms. *J. Amer. med. Ass.*, 1921, **77**, 1641–43.

Introduction of the carbon tetrachloride treatment of ankylostomiasis.

5369 ROCKEFELLER FOUNDATION.
Bibliography of hookworm disease. New York, *Rockefeller Foundation*, 1922.

Contains 5,680 references to all aspects of hookworm disease, prefaced by a short history.

5369.1 WORLD HEALTH ORGANIZATION.
Bibliography of hookworm disease (ancylostomiasis) 1920–62. Genève, *World Health Organization*, 1965.

5370–5403 RICKETTSIAL INFECTIONS

5370 CARDANO, GIROLAMO [CARDANUS (HIERONYMUS)]. 1501–1576.
De malo recentiorum medicorum medendi usu libellus. Venetiis, *apud O. Scotum*, 1536.

Includes (cap. XXXVI) an early account of typhus, *morbus pulicaris.* This chapter is available in English translation in R. H. Major, *Classic descriptions of disease*, 3rd ed., Springfield, 1945, p. 163.

5371 FRACASTORO, GIROLAMO [FRACASTORIUS]. 1478–1553
De sympathia et antipathia rerum liber unus. De contagione et contagiosis morbis et curatione. Venetiis, *apud heredes L. Iuntae*, 1546.

This book, which contains one of the first authentic accounts of typhus, marks an epoch in the history of medicine, since Fracastorius enunciated in it, perhaps for the first time, the modern doctrine of the specific characters and infectious nature of fevers. He is remembered for his poem on syphilis, but he was also eminent as physicist, geologist, astronomer and pathologist.

5372 BRAVO, Francisco.
Tavardete. In his *Opera medicinalia*, Mexico, *P. Ocharte*, 1570, ff. 1–90.
Original description of tabardillo (Spanish or Mexican typhus). The *Opera* was the first medical book published in the New World; it includes references to native drugs and to parturition and its complications.

5372.1 COYTTARUS, Joannes. *d.* 1590
De febre purpura epidemiali et contagiosa libri duo. Parisiis, *apud M. Juvenem*, 1578.
Coyttarus distinguished between petechial typhus and typhoid.

5373 COBER, Tobias. ? –1625
Observationum medicarum Castrensium Hungaricarum. Helmstadii, *F. Lüderwald*, 1685.
Pp. 49–51: Cober, a German physician, reported the relationship between typhus and pediculosis.

5374 PRINGLE, *Sir* John. 1707–1782
Observations on the nature and cure of hospital and jayl-fevers. London, *A. Millar & D. Wilson*, 1750.
Pringle was a strong advocate of better ventilation in prisons and hospitals as a means of preventing typhus, which he showed to be identical with "hospital fever".

5375 HILDENBRAND, Johann Valentin von. 1763–1818
Ueber den ansteckenden Typhus. Wien, 1810.
Hildenbrand gave a classical description of typhus. The French literature sometimes refers to the condition as "Hildenbrand's disease". English translation by S. D. Gross, 1829.

5376 VIRCHOW, Rudolf Ludwig Karl. 1821–1902
Ueber den Hungertyphus. Berlin, *A. Hirschwald*, 1868.
English translation, 1868.

5376.1 BAELZ, Erwin. 1849–1913, & KAWAKAMI.
Das japanische Fluss- oder Ueberschwemmings-fieber, eine acute Infectionskrankheit. *Virchows Arch. path. Anat.*, 1879, **78,** 373–420, 528–30.
Early scientific account of tsutsugamushi fever.

5377 MAXEY, Edward Ernest. 1867–1934
Some observations on the so-called spotted fever of Idaho. *Med. Sentinel* (*Portland, Ore.*), 1899, **7,** 433–38.
Rocky Mountain spotted fever first described.

5378 RICKETTS, Howard Taylor. 1871–1910
The transmission of Rocky Mountain spotted fever by the bite of the wood-tick (*Dermacentor occidentalis*). *J. Amer. med. Ass.*, 1906, **47,** 358.
Ricketts (who himself died of typhus) demonstrated that the wood tick *Dermacentor andersoni* is a vector of Rocky Mountain spotted fever.

5379 ——. A micro-organism which apparently has a specific relationship to Rocky Mountain spotted fever. A preliminary report. *J. Amer. med. Ass.*, 1909, **52,** 379–80.
Description of the causal organism, in blood smears.

5380 RICKETTS, Howard Taylor. 1871–1910, & WILDER, Russell Morse. 1885–
The relation of typhus fever (tabardillo) to Rocky Mountain spotted fever. *Arch. intern. Med.*, 1910, **5,** 361–70.
Ricketts and Wilder differentiated Rocky Mountain spotted fever and typhus.

5380.1 ——. The etiology of the typhus fever (tabardillo) of Mexico City. A further preliminary report. *J. Amer. med. Ass.*, 1910, **54,** 1373–75.
Demonstration of the causal organism or typhus.

5381 WILSON, William James. 1879–1954
On heterologous agglutinins more particularly those present in the blood serum of cerebro-spinal fever and typhus fever cases. *J. Hyg. (Camb.)*, 1909, **9,** 316–40.
The reaction described by Wilson was later developed by Weil and Felix and named after them (see No. 5390). See also the paper by Wilson in *J. Hyg.*, 1920, **19,** 115–30.

5382 BRILL, Nathan Edwin. 1860–1925
An acute infectious disease of unknown origin. A clinical study based on 221 cases. *Amer. J. med. Sci.*, 1910, **139,** 484–502.
"Brill's disease" – recrudescent typhus; first description.

5383 CONOR, Alfred Leon Joseph. 1870–1914, & BRUCH, A.
Une fièvre éruptive observée en Tunisie. *Bull. Soc. Path. exot.*, 1910, **3,** 492–96.
First description of fièvre boutonneuse, a form of tick-borne typhus found in Tunisia.

5384 NICOLLE, Charles Jules Henri. 1866–1936
Recherches expérimentales sur le typhus exanthématique. *Ann. Inst. Pasteur*, 1910, **24,** 243–75; 1911, **25,** 97–144; 1912, **26,** 250–80, 332–50.
Nicolle demonstrated the transmission of typhus by the body louse *Pediculus corporis*. He also produced the disease in monkeys and guinea-pigs by the injection of infected blood. He was awarded the Nobel Prize in 1928. Preliminary communication in *C. R. Acad. Sci. (Paris)*, 1909, **149,** 486–89.

5384.1 PROWAZEK, Stanislaus Joseph Matthias von. 1875–1915
Ätiologische Untersuchungen über den Flecktyphus in Serbien 1913 und in Hamburg 1914. *Beitr. Klin. InfektKr.*, 1915, **4,** 5–31.
Prowazek, like Ricketts and Wilder, demonstrated the specific causal agent in typhus. Like Ricketts he died of the disease.

5385 GRAHAM, John Henry Porteus. ?1869–1957
A note on a relapsing febrile illness of unknown origin. *Lancet*, 1915, **2,** 703–04.
First reported case of "trench fever".

5386 HUNT, George Herbert. 1884–1926, & RANKIN, Allan Coats. 1877–1959
Intermittent fever of obscure origin, occurring among British soldiers in France. The so-called "trench fever". *Lancet*, 1915, **2,** 1133–36.
In this paper trench fever is so named for the first time.

5387 HIS, Wilhelm, *Jnr.* 1863–1934
Ueber eine neue periodische Fiebererkrankung (Febris Wolhynica). *Berl. klin. Wschr.*, 1916, **53,** 322–23.
His encountered a form of "trench fever" in Volhynia, Russia, and named it after that district.

5388 ROCHA-LIMA, HENRIQUE DA. 1879–1956
Zur Aetiologie des Fleckfiebers. *Berl. klin. Wschr.*, 1916, **53,** 567–69.
Rickettsia prowazeki, cause of typhus, was first isolated by da Rocha-Lima, who named it after Ricketts and Prowazek, both of whom died of the disease.

5389 TÖPFER, HANS WILLI. 1876–
Zur Ursache und Uebertragung des Wolhynischen Fiebers. *Münch. med. Wschr.*, 1916, **63,** 1495–96.
Isolation of *Rickettsia quintana* from lice found on patients suffering from trench fever.

5390 WEIL, EDMUND. 1880–1922, & FELIX, ARTHUR. 1887–1956
Zur serologischen Diagnose des Fleckfiebers. *Wien. klin. Wschr.*, 1916, **29,** 33–35.
Weil–Felix reaction for the diagnosis of typhus. See also the later paper in the same journal, 1916, **29,** 974–78.

5391 WOLBACH, SIMEON BURT. 1880–1954
Studies on Rocky Mountain spotted fever. *J. med. Res.*, 1919, **41,** 1–197.
In his important aetiological and pathological studies of Rocky Mountain spotted fever Wolbach named the causal agent *Dermacentroxenus rickettsi.*

5392 LOEWE, LEO. 1896– , *et al.*
Cultivation of rickettsia-like bodies in typhus fever. *J. Amer. med. Ass.*, 1921, **77,** 1967–69.
Isolation of *Rickettsia prowazeki* from the blood. With S. A. Ritter and G. Baehr.

5393 WOLBACH, SIMEON BURT. 1880–1954, *et al.*
The etiology and pathology of typhus. Cambridge, *Harvard Univ. Press*, 1922.
The carefully controlled experiments of Wolbach, J. L. Todd, and F. W. Palfrey eliminated all doubt that *R. prowazeki* was the causal agent in typhus.

5394 FLETCHER, WILLIAM. –1938, & LESSLAR, J. E.
Tropical typhus in the Federated Malay States, with a compilation on epidemic typhus. London, *John Bale*, 1925.
Bull. Inst. med. Res., F.M.S., 1925, No. 2.

5395 ——. The Weil-Felix reaction in sporadic tropical typhus. London, *John Bale*, 1926.
Bull. Inst. Med. Res., F.M.S., 1926, No. 1. Demonstration that scrub-typhus patients developed agglutinins against the OX-K strain of *B. proteus* but not the OX-19 strain.

5396 MAXCY, KENNETH FULLER. 1889–
Clinical observations on endemic typhus (Brill's disease) in Southern United States. *Publ. Hlth Rep.* (*Wash.*), 1926, **41,** 1213–20, 2967–95.
Maxcy described murine (flea-borne) typhus ("Maxcy's disease").

5396.1 MOOSER, HERMANN. 1891–
Experiments relating to the pathology and the etiology of Mexican typhus (tabardillo). *J. infect. Dis.*, 1928, **43,** 241–72.
Mooser differentiated murine from epidemic typhus. The causative organism was later named *Rickettsia mooseri.*

5396.2 DYER, ROLLO EUGENE. 1886– , *et al.*
Typhus fever. A virus of the typhus type derived from fleas collected from wild rats. *Publ. Hlth Rep.* (*Wash.*), 1931, **46,** 334–38.
Murine typhus shown to be caused by an organism later named *Rickettsia mooseri*, transmitted by fleas from rats to man. With A. Rumreich and L. F. Badger.

5396.3 OGATA, NORIO.
Aetiologie der *Tsutsugamushi*-Krankheit: *Rickettsia tsutsugamushi. Zbl. Bakt.*, I Abt. Orig., 1931, **122,** 249–53.
Ogata isolated the causal agent of tsutsugamushi disease in 1927.

5396.4 ZINSSER, HANS. 1878–1940
Varieties of typhus virus and the epidemiology of the American form of European typhus fever (Brill's disease). *Amer. J. Hyg.*, 1934, **20,** 513–32.
Zinsser advanced the theory that Brill's disease is a recrudescence of epidemic typhus in persons who have contracted typhus some time previously. The condition has subsequently been renamed "Brill–Zinsser disease".

5397 DERRICK, EDWARD HOLBROOK. 1898–
"Q" fever, a new fever entity: clinical features and laboratory investigation. *Med. J. Aust.*, 1937, **2,** 281–99.
First account of "Q" (= query) fever. See also No. 5398.

5398 BURNET, *Sir* FRANK MACFARLANE. 1899– , & FREEMAN, MAVIS.
Experimental studies on the virus of "Q" fever. *Med. J. Aust.*, 1937, **2,** 299–305.
Discovery of *Rickettsia burneti*, causal agent in Q fever.

5398.1 SUSSMAN, LEON NATHANIEL. 1907–
Kew Gardens' spotted fever. *New York Med.*, 1946, **2,** No. 15, 27–28.
Rickettsialpox described.

5399 STOKER, MICHAEL GEORGE PARKE. 1918–
Serological evidence of Q fever in Great Britain. *Lancet*, 1949, **1,** 178–79.
Relationship of primary atypical pneumonia and Q fever.

5400 YEOMANS, ANDREW. 1907– , *et al.*
The therapeutic effect of para-aminobenzoic acid in louse-borne typhus fever. *J. Amer. med. Ass.*, 1944, **126,** 349–56.
With J. C. Snyder, E. S. Murray, C. J. D. Zarafonetis, and R. S. Ecke.

5401 FULTON, FORREST. 1913– , & JOYNER, L.
Cultivation of *Rickettsia tsutsugamushi* in lungs of rodents. Preparation of a scrub-typhus vaccine. *Lancet*, 1945, **2,** 729–34.
Scrub-typhus vaccine.

5401.1 HUEBNER, ROBERT JOSEPH. 1914– , *et al.*
Rickettsialpox. A newly recognized rickettsial disease. IV. Isolation of a rickettsia apparently identical with the causative agent of rickettsialpox from *Allodermanyssus sanguineus*, a rodent mite. *Publ. Hlth Rep.* (*Wash.*), 1946, **61,** 1677–82.
Isolation of *Rickettsia akari*, aetiologic agent of rickettsialpox. With W. L. Jellison and C. Pomerantz.

5402 SMADEL, Joseph Edwin. 1907–1963, & JACKSON, Elizabeth B. Chloromycetin, an antibiotic with chemotherapeutic activity in experimental rickettsial and viral infections. *Science*, 1947, **106**, 418–419.

Chloramphenicol used in treatment of typhus.

5403 ZINSSER, Hans. 1878–1940
Rats, lice and history: being a study in biography, which, after 12 preliminary chapters indispensable for the preparation of the lay reader, deals with the life history of typhus fever. Boston, *Little, Brown & Co.*, 1935.

5404–5436.1 SMALLPOX; VACCINATION

5404 RHAZES, Abu Bakr Muhammad ibn Zakarīyā al-Razi. ?850–?923
De variolis et morbillis commentarius. Londini, *G. Bowyer*, 1766.

The first medical description of smallpox was written by Rhazes, about the year 910. It is the only work of Rhazes to be printed in Arabic (in the above edition, which includes a parallel Latin translation by John Channing), and is considered his most important work. For an English translation see *Med. Classics*, 1939, **4**, 22–84. An English translation was also published by the Sydenham Society in 1848.

5405 VOLLGNAD, Heinrich. 1634–1682
Globus vitulinus. *Misc. Curiosa sive Ephem. nat. cur.*, Jenae, 1671, **2,** 181–82.

First authentic report on variolation.

5406 THACHER, Thomas. 1620–1678
A brief rule to guide the common-people of New-England how to order themselves and theirs in the small pocks, or measels. Boston, *J. Foster*, 1677 [i.e., 1678].

Broadside. The first medical publication of North America and the only one to appear in the 17th century. The sheet was reprinted, with a bibliographical and biographical study, in *Bibliotheca Medica Americana*, Vol. 1, Baltimore, 1937.

5407 SYDENHAM, Thomas. 1624–1689
Observationes medicae circa morborum acutorum historiam et curationem. Ed. quarta. Londini, *G. Kettilby*, 1685.

Contains (Book 3, Cap. 2; Book 5, Cap. 4) an important account of smallpox, particularly the epidemics of 1667–69 and 1674–75. Sydenham attributed smallpox to a specific inflammation of the blood; he clearly distinguished it from measles. His treatment of fevers with fresh air and cooling drinks was an improvement on the sweating methods previously employed. English translation in his *Works*, ed. R. G. Latham, London, 1848, **1**, 123, 219.

5408 PYLARINI, Giacomo. 1659–1718
Nova et tuta variolas excitandi per transplantationem methodus; nuper inventa et in usum tracta. Venetiis, *apud J. G. Hertz*, 1715.

Inoculation was practised in ancient times. Pylarini in 1701 inoculated 3 children at Constantinople with smallpox virus. He is accredited with the "medical" discovery of variolation, and is thus the first immunologist. His book records his many researches on the subject.

5409 TIMONI, Emanuel. *d.* 1718
An account, or history, of the procuring of the smallpox by incision or inoculation, as it has for some time been practised at Constantinople. *Phil. Trans.*, 1714–16, **29,** 72–82.

A letter from Timoni of Constantinople to John Woodward described the practice in that city of inoculation against smallpox. The letter aroused interest in inoculation in England. Timoni was the first to write on this subject for western physicians, although Pylarini's researches had commenced in 1701.

5410 PYLARINI, Giacomo. 1659–1718
Nova & tuta variolas excitandi per transplantationem methodus, nuper inventa & in usum tracta. *Phil. Trans.*, 1714–16, **29,** 393–99.

This appeared in the same volume as Timoni's paper. Both were republished in Latin: Pylarini, G.: *Tractatus bini de nova variolas per transplantationem excitandi methodo*, Leyden, 1721.

5411 COLMAN, Benjamin. 1673–1747
Some observations on the new method of receiving the smallpox by ingrafting or inoculating. Boston, *B. Green, for S. Gerrish*, 1721.

Earliest N. American book dealing with inoculation.

5412 DOUGLASS, William. 1691–1752
Inoculation of the small pox as practised in Boston. Boston, *J. Franklin*, 1722.

5413 ——. The abuses and scandals of some late pamphlets in favour of inoculation of the small-pox. Boston, *J. Franklin*, 1722.

Douglass at first opposed inoculation for smallpox, but by 1730 he had changed his views and had become an advocate of inoculation.

5414 MATHER, Cotton. 1663–1728
An account of the method and success of inoculating the small pox in Boston in New England. London, 1722.

Mather republished reports of earlier writers on inoculation. It was he who persuaded Boylston to adopt the practice, and he supported Boylston during a period of great opposition to inoculation.

5415 BOYLSTON, Zabdiel. 1680–1766
An historical account of the small-pox inoculated in New England. London, *S. Chandler*, 1726.

Boylston was the first in America to inoculate for the smallpox, at Boston on June 26, 1721.

5416 KIRKPATRICK, James [Killpatrick]. *d.* 1770
An essay on inoculation, occasioned by the small-pox being brought into South Carolina in the year 1738. London, *J. Huggonson*, 1743.

After its initial popularity, inoculation fell into disuse in England. Kirkpatrick, who became a prominent inoculator in England after experience in America, helped considerably in reviving its popularity. He attempted the attenuation of the virus by his arm-to-arm method of inoculation.

5417 MEAD, Richard. 1673–1754
De variolis et morbillis liber. Londini, *J. Brindley*, 1747.

Includes a Latin translation of Rhazes' commentary. Mead favoured inoculation, and his great authority and influence helped towards a more general acceptance of this measure. English translation of the book in 1747.

5418 THOMSON, ADAM. ?–1767
A discourse on the preparation of the body for the small-pox; and the manner of receiving the infection. Philadelphia, *B. Franklin & D. Hall*, 1750.

Thomson was the originator of the American method of inoculation against smallpox.

5419 FRANKLIN, BENJAMIN. 1706–1790
Some account of the success of inoculation for the small-pox in England and America. London, *W. Strahan*, 1759.

5420 DIMSDALE, THOMAS, *Baron Dimsdale*. 1712–1800
The present method of inoculating for the small-pox. London, *W. Owen*, 1767.

Dimsdale is notable as having inoculated Catherine of Russia and her son. For this he received a fee of £10,000 and a life pension. His reputation and the exalted rank of his patient helped in popularizing the measure in England. Dimsdale used material from the inoculated site of another patient.

5421 HUNTER, JOHN. 1728–1793
Account of a woman who had the smallpox during pregnancy, and who seemed to have communicated the same disease to the foetus. *Phil. Trans.*, 1780, **70,** 128–42.

5422 RUSH, BENJAMIN. 1745–1813
The new method in inoculating for the small pox. Philadelphia, *C. Cist*, 1781.

5423 JENNER, EDWARD. 1749–1823
An inquiry into the causes and effects of the variolae vaccinae. London, *S. Low*, 1798.

Jenner established the fact that a "vaccination" or inoculation with vaccinia (cowpox) lymph matter protects against smallpox. He performed his first vaccination on May 14, 1796. The above work, describing 23 successful vaccinations, announced to the world one of the greatest triumphs in the history of medicine. Jennerian vaccination soon superseded the protective inoculation of material from human cases of smallpox, which had previously been in vogue. What is probably the first mention of anaphylaxis appears on p. 13 of the book. A *Bio-bibliography of Edward Jenner*, 1749–1823, by W. R. LeFanu, was published in 1951. Facsimile reproductions of the *Inquiry* appeared in 1923 (Milan), 1949 (Denver), and 1966 (London).

5424 WATERHOUSE, BENJAMIN. 1754–1846
A prospect of exterminating the small-pox. 2 pts. Boston, *W. Hilliard*, (Cambridge [Mass.], *Univ. Press*), 1800–02.

Jennerian vaccination was introduced into N. America by Waterhouse. See J. B. Blake, *Benjamin Waterhouse and the introduction of vaccination. A reappraisal.* Philadelphia, 1957.

5425 COXE, JOHN REDMAN. 1773–1864
Practical observations on vaccination: or inoculation for the cow pock. Philadelphia, *J. Humphreys*, 1802.

Coxe did much to destroy ignorant prejudice against vaccination; he was the first in Philadelphia to practise it.

5426 WEIGERT, CARL. 1845–1904
Anatomische Beiträge zur Lehre von den Pocken. 2 pts. Breslau, *M. Cohn u. Weigert*, 1874–75.

In the course of his important studies on smallpox Weigert carried out the first successful staining of bacteria (see No. 2482). His fine description of the destructive effect of the smallpox virus on the skin led to the coining of the term "coagulation necrosis" as a name for the process causing the development of the lesions.

5427 BUIST, JOHN BROWN. 1846–1915
The life-history of the micro-organisms associated with variola and vaccinia. An abstract of results obtained from a study of smallpox and vaccination in the surgical laboratory of the University of Edinburgh. *Proc. roy. Soc. Edinb.*, 1886, **13**, 603–20.

The "Paschen elementary bodies" (No. 5430) were first recognized and demonstrated by Buist. Republished as an appendix to his *Vaccinia and variola*, London, 1887.

5428 GUARNIERI, GUISEPPE. 1856–1918
Ricerche sulla patogenesi ed etiologia dell' infezione vaccinica e vaiolosa. *Arch. Sci. med.*, 1893, **16**, 403–24.

Guarnieri described bodies found in the specific lesions of smallpox, *Cytorrhyctes variolae guarnieri*, which he believed to be the causative organism of the disease.

5429 COPEMAN, SYDNEY ARTHUR MONCKTON. 1862–1947
Vaccination, its natural history and pathology. London, *Macmillan & Co.*, 1899.

Milroy Lectures, Royal College of Physicians, 1898. Copeman's bacteriological studies permanently determined the validity of vaccination as a preventive of smallpox.

5429.1 MAGRATH, GEORGE BURGESS. 1870–1938, & BRINCKERHOFF, WALTER REMSEN. 1875–1911
On experimental variola in the monkey. *J. med. Res.*, 1904, **11**, 230–46.

Inoculation of smallpox into the monkey. An earlier report of successful inoculation by W. Zuelzer (*Zbl. med. Wiss.*, 1874, **12**, 82) is not generally accepted.

5430 PASCHEN, ENRIQUE. 1860–1936
Was wissen wir über den Vakzineerreger? *Münch. med. Wschr.*, 1906, **53**, 2391–93.

"Paschen elementary bodies"; see also No. 5427.

5430.1 NOGUCHI, HIDEYO. 1876–1928
Pure cultivation in vivo of vaccine virus free from bacteria. *J. exp. Med.*, 1915, **21**, 539–70.

Noguchi obtained a pure culture of vaccinia virus.

5431 PAUL, GUSTAV. 1859–1935
Zur Differentialdiagnose der Variola und der Varicellen. Die Erscheinungen an der variolierten Hornhaut des Kaninchens und ihre frühzeitige Erkennung. *Zbl. Bakt.*, I Abt., 1915, **75**, Orig., 518–24.

Paul's test for the diagnosis of smallpox.

5432 GORDON, MERVYN HENRY. 1872–1953
Studies of the viruses of vaccinia and variola. London, *H.M. Stationery Office*, 1925.

Medical Research Council Special Report No. 98; a summary of the more important additions to the knowledge of the subject.

5433 LEDINGHAM, *Sir* John Charles Grant. 1875–1944
Studies on variola, vaccinia, and avian molluscum. *J. State Med.*, 1926, **34,** 125–43.
Ledingham's diagnostic test.

5434 McKINNON, Neil E. 1894– , & DEFRIES, Robert Davies. 1889–
The reaction of the skin of the normal rabbit following intradermal injection of material from smallpox lesions: the specificity of this reaction and its application as a diagnostic test. *Amer. J. Hyg.*, 1928, **8,** 93–106.
McKinnon's diagnostic test.

History of Smallpox and Vaccination

5435 CROOKSHANK, Edgar March. 1858–1928
History and pathology of vaccination. 2 vols. London, *H. K. Lewis*, 1889.
This very full history of the subject caused a good deal of controversy; see the review of it in *Lancet*, 1890, **1**, 470–72. Crookshank was an opponent of vaccination.

5435.1 EDWARDES, Edward Joshua.
A concise history of small-pox and vaccination in Europe. London, *H. K. Lewis*, 1902.
A comprehensive summary, in tabular form.

5436 KLEBS, Arnold Carl. 1870–1943
The historic evolution of variolation. *Johns Hopk. Hosp. Bull.*, 1913, **24,** 69–83.

5436.1 MILLER, Genevieve. 1914–
The adoption of inoculation for smallpox in England and France. Philadelphia, *University of Pennsylvania Press*, 1957.
The appendixes contain the early histories of inoculation and a list of German doctoral dissertations on inoculation, 1720–52. There is also an excellent bibliography.

5437–5440.1

CHICKENPOX

5437 INGRASSIA, Giovanni Filippo. 1510–1580
De tumoribus praeter naturam. Neapoli, 1553.
Ingrassia was first to differentiate varicella from scarlet fever (p. 194–95).

5438 HEBERDEN, William, *Snr.* 1710–1801
On the chickenpox. *Med. Trans. Coll. Phys. Lond.*, 1768, **1,** 427–36.
In a paper read before the (Royal) College of Physicians on August 11, 1767, Heberden first definitely differentiated chickenpox from smallpox.

5439 HUTCHINSON, *Sir* Jonathan. 1828–1913
On gangrenous eruptions in connection with vaccination and chickenpox. *Med.-chir. Trans.*, 1882, **65,** 1–12.
Original description of varicella gangrenosa.

5439.1 BOKAY, JANOS. 1858–1937
Das Auftreten von Varizellen unter eigentümlichen Verhältnissen. *Magy. orv. Arch.*, 1892, (Nov. 3).
Bokay was the first to suggest an aetiological relationship between varicella and herpes zoster. See also his paper in *Wien. klin. Wschr.*, 1909, **22**, 1323–26.

5440 TYZZER, ERNEST EDWARD. 1875–1965
The histology of the skin lesions in varicella. *J. med. Res.*, 1905–06, **14**, 361–92.
Tyzzer was first to recognize inclusion bodies in varicella.

5440.1 WELLER, THOMAS HUCKLE. 1915–
Serial propagation *in vitro* of agents producing inclusion bodies derived from varicella and herpes zoster. *Proc. Soc. exp. Biol. (N.Y.)*, 1953, **83**, 340–46.
Isolation of the varicella-herpes virus.

5441–5449.3

MEASLES

5441 SYDENHAM, THOMAS. 1624–1689
Observationes medicae circa morborum acutorum historiam et curationem. Londini, *G. Kettilby*, 1676.
Includes (pp. 272–80) the most minute and careful description of measles that had so far appeared; this is reprinted in *Med. Classics*, 1939, **4**, 313–19.

5442 HOME, FRANCIS. 1719–1813
Medical facts and experiments. London, *A. Millar*, 1759.
Experimental human transmission of measles (pp. 266–88).

5443 PANUM, PETER LUDVIG. 1820–1885
Iagttagelser, anstillede under Maeslinge-Epidemien paa Faerøerne i Aaret 1846. *Bibl. Laeger*, 1847, 3 R., **1**, 270–344.
When only 26 years of age, Panum was sent by the Danish Government to investigate the epidemic of measles then raging in the Faroes. His report on the subject was a valuable contribution to medical literature. A translation of his paper is in *Med. Classics*, 1939, **3**, 829–86. It was also published in translation by the Delta Omega Society, New York, 1940.

5444 KOPLIK, HENRY. 1858–1927
The diagnosis of the invasion of measles from a study of the exanthema as it appears on the buccal mucous membrane. *Arch. Pediat.*, 1896, **13**, 918–22.
Koplik, American paediatrician, was first to note and report on "Koplik's spots" the buccal spots which are an important early diagnostic sign in measles.

5445 JOSIAS, ALBERT HENRI LOUIS. 1852–1906
Recherches expérimentales sur la transmissibilité de la rougeole animaux. *Méd. mod. (Paris)*, 1898, **9**, 153.
Measles transmitted to animals.

5446 HEKTOEN, LUDVIG. 1863–1951
Experimental measles. *J. infect. Dis.*, 1905, **2**, 238–55.
Experimental human transmission of measles.

5447 CENCI, F.
Alcune esperienze di sieroimmunizzazione e sieroterapia nel morbillo. *Riv. Clin. pediat.*, 1907, **5**, 1017–25.
First use of convalescent serum in prophylaxis against measles.

5448 ANDERSON, John F. 1873–1958, & GOLDBERGER, Joseph. 1874–1929
Experimental measles in the monkey. *Publ. Hlth Rep.* (*Wash.*), 1911, **26,** 847–48, 887–95.
Measles transmitted to monkeys.

5449 PLOTZ, Harry. 1890–1947
Culture "in vitro" du virus de la rougeole. *Bull. Acad. Méd.* (*Paris*), 1938, **119,** 598–601.
Successful cultivation of measles virus.

5449.1 ORDMAN, Charles William. 1914– , *et al.*
Chemical, clinical, and immunological studies on the products of human plasma fractionation. XII. The use of concentrated normal human serum gamma globulin (human immune serum globulin) in the prevention and attenuation of measles. *J. clin. Invest.*, 1944, **23,** 541–49.
Gamma globulin used for passive immunization against measles. With C. G. Jennings and C. A. Janeway.

5449.2 ENDERS, John Franklin. 1897– , & PEEBLES, Thomas C. 1921–
Propagation in tissue cultures of cytopathogenic agents from patients with measles. *Proc. Soc. exp. Biol.* (*N.Y.*), 1954, **86,** 277–86.
Isolation of measles virus.

5449.3 ENDERS, John Franklin. 1897– , *et al.*
Studies on attenuated measles-virus vaccine. I. Development and preparation of the vaccine: technics for assay of effects of vaccination. *New Engl. J. Med.*, 1960, **263,** 153–59.
Living virus vaccine. With S. L. Katz, M. V. Milovanović, and A. Holloway.

5449.4–5468 YELLOW FEVER

5449.4 ABREU, Alexo de. 1568–1630
Tratado de las siete enfermedades, *etc.* Lisboa, *P. Craesbeeck*, 1623.
Contains (fol. 193v.–199v.) an account of yellow fever. For full title of the book, see No. 2262.1.

5450 DU TERTRE, Jean Baptiste.
Histoire générale des Antilles habités par les Français. Tom. 1. Paris, 1667.
Du Tertre, a priest, described (pp. 81, 99, 423) the outbreaks of yellow fever at Guadeloupe in 1635, 1640, and 1648.

5451 CAREY, Mathew. 1760–1839
A short account of the malignant fever, lately prevalent in Philadelphia. Philadelphia, *The Author*, 1793.
In this little book, which passed through 4 editions in a few months, Carey left a graphic account of the great yellow fever epidemic of Philadelphia in 1793. He gave a good clinical description of the disease, mentioning the efficacy and the failure of many forms of treatment.

5452 CURRIE, William. 1754–1828
A description of the malignant, infectious fever prevailing at present in Philadelphia. Philadelphia, *T. Dobson*, 1793.

5453 RUSH, BENJAMIN. 1745–1813

An account of the bilious remitting yellow fever, as it appeared in the city of Philadelphia in the year 1793. Philadelphia, *T. Dobson*, 1794.

Benjamin Rush was the most eminent figure in Philadelphia medicine in his day. His description of the yellow fever epidemic of 1793 is classical. He did magnificent work in treating the sick during the epidemic and in proposing measures to prevent a recurrence.

5454 NOTT, JOSIAH CLARK. 1804–1873

Yellow fever contrasted with bilious fever – reasons for believing it a disease sui generis – its mode of propagation – remote cause – probable insect or animalcular origin. *New Orleans med. surg. J.*, 1848, **4**, 563–601.

Nott advanced the theory that yellow fever was caused by minute animalcula. Reproduced in part in R. H. Major, *Classic descriptions of disease*, 3rd ed., 1945, p. 122.

5454.1 BEAUPERTHUY, LOUIS DANIEL. 1807–1871

Fiebre amarilla. *Gaceta Oficial de Cumanà*, Año 4, No. 57, Mayo 23, 1854.

Beauperthuy was the first protagonist of the mosquito theory of the transmission of yellow fever. Reprinted in Beauperthuy's *La Obra*, Caracas, 1963, pp. 260–70; French translation in *Travaux scientifiques de Louis-Daniel Beauperthuy*, Bordeaux, 1891, pp. 131–42.

5455 FINLAY, CARLOS JUAN. 1833–1915

El mosquito hipoteticamente considerado como agente de transmisión de la fiebre amarilla. *Ann. r. Acad. Cienc. méd. Habana*, 1881–82, **18,** 147–69.

Finlay was the first to suggest that the mosquito carried yellow fever infection from man to man. The paper is reprinted, with translation, in *Med. Classics*, 1938, 2, 569–612.

5456 CARTER, HENRY ROSE. 1852–1925

A note on the interval between infecting and secondary cases of yellow fever from the records of yellow fever at Orwood and Taylor, Mississippi, in 1898. *New Orleans med. surg. J.*, 1900, **52,** 617–36.

Carter did important work on yellow fever. His determination of its incubation period decided the direction of Reed's later researches, which in turn ended in the discovery of the mode of transmission of the yellow fever virus.

5457 REED, WALTER. 1851–1902, CARROLL, JAMES. 1854–1907, AGRAMONTE Y SIMONI, ARISTIDE. 1868–1931, & LAZEAR, JESSE WILLIAM. 1866–1900

The etiology of yellow fever. *Philad. med. J.*, 1900, **6,** 790–96.

First definite proof that the organism causing yellow fever is transmitted to man by the mosquito *Aëdes aegypti*. During the period spent by these workers in the investigation of the disease, Lazear died from yellow fever after having been accidentally bitten by a mosquito. Reproduced in part in R. H. Major, *Classic descriptions of disease*, 3rd ed., 1945, p. 131.

5459 MARCHOUX, EMILE. 1862–1943, *et al.*

La fièvre jaune. *Ann. Inst. Pasteur*, 1903, **17,** 665–731.

Yellow fever convalescent serum employed. With A. T. Salimbeni and P. L. Simond.

5460 GORGAS, WILLIAM CRAWFORD. 1854–1920
Sanitation of the tropics with special reference to malaria and yellow fever. *J. Amer. med. Ass.*, 1909, **52,** 1075–77.

In 1901 Gorgas was sent to Havana to undertake a special campaign against the yellow fever mosquito *Aëdes aegypti.* His methods of sanitation were so successful that in 3 months yellow fever was practically eradicated from Havana. Gorgas outlined the main principles of his methods in the above paper.

5461 HINDLE, EDWARD. 1886–
A yellow fever vaccine. *Brit. med. J.*, 1928, **1,** 976–77.

First vaccine for immunization against yellow fever. Hindle devised a method for the transportation of frozen infected material from West Africa to London, making it possible to carry on experimental work in the latter place.

5462 STOKES, ADRIAN. 1887–1927, *et al.*
Experimental transmission of yellow fever to laboratory animals. *Amer. J. trop. Med.*, 1928, **8,** 103–64.

Experimental infection of the monkey, *Macacus rhesus*, with the yellow fever virus. Stokes succumbed to yellow fever while investigating the disease. With J. H. Bauer and N. P. Hudson.

5463 THEILER, MAX. 1899–
Studies on the action of yellow fever virus in mice. *Ann. trop. Med. Parasit.*, 1930, **24,** 249–72.

The intracerebral protection test in mice, a test for the diagnosis of yellow fever and for the determination of its past existence in a community, was made possible by Theiler's discovery that white mice are susceptible to the intracerebral inoculation of the virus. He was awarded the Nobel Prize in 1951.

5464 SAWYER, WILBUR AUGUSTUS. 1879–1951, & LLOYD, WRAY DEVERE MARR. 1902–1936
The use of mice in tests of immunity against yellow fever. *J. exp. Med.*, 1931, **54,** 533–35.

Intraperitoneal protection test.

5465 ——, *et al.*
Vaccination against yellow fever with immune serum and virus fixed for mice. *J. exp. Med.*, 1932, **55,** 945–69.

These workers devised an immune serum for prophylactic inoculation against yellow fever. With S. F. Kitchen and W. D. M. Lloyd.

5465.1 HAAGEN, EUGEN, & THEILER, MAX. 1899–
Untersuchungen über das Verhalten des Gelbfiebervirus in der Gewebekultur. Mit besonderer Berücksichtigung seiner Kultivierbarkeit. *Zbl. Bakt.*, I Abt. Orig., 1932, **125,** 145–58.

Yellow fever virus grown in tissue culture.

5466 THEILER, MAX. 1899–
A yellow fever protection test in mice by intracerebral injection. *Ann. trop. Med. Hyg.*, 1933, **27,** 57–77.

Intracerebral protection test.

5467 ——, & SMITH, HUGH HOLLINGSWORTH. 1902–
The use of yellow fever virus modified by *in vitro* cultivation for human immunization. *J. exp. Med.*, 1937, **65,** 787–800.

Immunization without the use of immune serum.

5468 CARTER, Henry Rose. 1852–1925
Yellow fever: an epidemiological and historical study of its place of origin. Edited by Laura Armistead Carter and Wade Hampton Frost. Baltimore, *Williams & Wilkins*, 1931.

5469–5475.1 DENGUE

5469 BYLON, David.
Korte aantekening wegens eene algemeene ziekte, doorgaans genaamd knokkel-koorts. *Verh. Batav. Genootsch. Kunst en Wet.*, Batavia, 1780, **2,** 17–30.

Bylon described an epidemic of dengue which appeared in the Dutch East Indies in 1779, the first definite description of the disease. O. H. P. Pepper has published a photographic reproduction of the article in *Ann. med. Hist.*, 1941, 3rd ser., **3,** 363–68.

5470 RUSH, Benjamin. 1745–1813
An account of the bilious remitting fever. In his *Medical inquiries and observations*, Philadelphia, 1789, **1,** 104–21.

One of the first important accounts of dengue ("breakbone fever"). Rush described the Philadelphia outbreak of 1780.

5471 DICKSON, Samuel Henry. 1798–1872
On dengue; its history, pathology, and treatment. Philadelphia, *Haswell, Barrington & Haswell*, 1839.

5472 BANCROFT, Thomas Lane. 1860–1933
On the etiology of dengue fever. *Aust. med. Gaz.*, 1906, **25,** 17–18.

Bancroft was the first to produce evidence that *Aëdes aegypti* is a vector of dengue.

5473 ASHBURN, Percy Moreau. 1872–1940, & CRAIG, Charles Franklin. 1872–1950
Experimental investigations regarding the aetiology of dengue fever, with a general consideration regarding the disease. *Philipp. J. Sci. B.*, 1907, **2,** 93–152.

Proof that the causal organism of dengue is a filterable virus. Published also in *J. infect. Dis.*, 1907, **4,** 440–75.

5474 CLELAND, *Sir* John Burton. 1878–1971, *et al.*
On the transmission of Australian dengue by the mosquito Stegomyia fasciata. *Med. J. Aust.*, 1916, **2,** 179–84, 200–05.

These workers proved that *Aëdes aegypti* (*Stegomyia fasciata*) is capable of transmitting dengue fever. See also *J. Hyg.* (*Camb.*), 1918, **16,** 317–418. With C. H. B. Bradley and W. McDonald.

5475 SIMMONS, James Stevens. 1890–1954, *et al.*
Experimental studies of dengue. *Philipp. J. Sci.*, 1931, **44,** 1–251.

Proof that *Aëdes albopictus* is a vector of dengue. See also the earlier paper in the same journal, 1930, **41,** 215–29. With J. H. St. John and F. H. K. Reynolds.

5475.1 SABIN, Albert Bruce. 1906– , & SCHLESINGER, Robert Walter. 1913–
Production of immunity to dengue with virus modified propagation in mice. *Science*, 1945, **101,** 640–42.

Successful propagation of dengue in mice and production of a vaccine.

5476–5480 PHLEBOTOMUS (PAPPATACI) FEVER

5476 PICK, Alois. 1859–1945
Zur Pathologie und Therapie einer eigenthümlichen endemischen Krankheitsform. *Wien. med. Wschr.*, 1886, **36,** 1141–45, 1168–71.
This is generally regarded as the first description of pappataci fever.

5477 DOERR, Robert. 1871–1952
Ueber ein neues invisibles Virus. *Berl. klin. Wschr.*, 1908, **45,** 1847–1849.
Doerr showed the relation of phlebotomus fever to the sandfly, *Phlebotomus.*

5478 ——, & RUSS, Viktor Karl. 1879–
Weitere Untersuchungen über das Pappatacifieber. *Arch. Schiffs- u. Tropenhyg.*, 1909, **13,** 693–706.
Doerr and Russ suggested that the virus of phlebotomus fever may be transmitted from one generation of infected *Phlebotomus papatasii* to another.

5479 DOERR, Robert. 1871–1952, *et al.*
Das Pappatacifieber. Leipzig, Wien, *F. Deuticke*, 1909.
An Austrian military commission consisting of R. Doerr, K. Franz, and S. Taussig proved that the causal organism of pappataci fever was a virus and that *Phlebotomus papatasii* was the vector.

5480 SHORTT, Henry Edward. 1887– , *et al.*
Cultivation of the viruses of sandfly fever and dengue fever on the chorio-allantoic membrane of the chick-embryo. *Indian J. Med. Research*, Calcutta, 1936, **23,** 865–70.
Cultivation of the virus of phlebotomus fever. With R. S. Rao and C. S. Swaminath.

5481–5484.3 RABIES

5481 ZINKE, Georg Gottfried.
Neue Ansichten der Handswuth, ihrer Ursachen und Folgen, nebst einer sichern Behandlungsart der von tollen Thieren gebissenen Menschen. Jena, *C. E. Gabler*, 1804.
Zinke transmitted rabies from a rabid dog to a normal one by injection of saliva and proved the disease to be infectious.

5481.1 KRÜGELSTEIN, Franz Christian Karl. 1779–1864
Die Geschichte der Hundswuth und der Wasserscheu und deren Behandlung. Gotha, *In der Hennings'schen Buchhandlung*, 1826.
A full account of rabies, summarizing current knowledge, with a bibliography of about 300 items.

5481.2 PASTEUR, Louis. 1822–1895, *et al.*
Sur la rage. *C. R. Acad. Sci. (Paris)*, 1881, **92,** 1259–60.
This paper marks the beginning of Pasteur's studies on rabies. With C. Chamberland, P. P. E. Roux, and T. Thuillier.

5482 ——. Nouvelle communication sur la rage. *C. R. Acad. Sci. (Paris)*, 1884, **98,** 457–63, 1229–31.
Demonstration in the blood of the rabies virus. With C. Chamberland and P. P. E. Roux.

5483 PASTEUR, Louis. 1822-1895.
Méthode pour prévenir la rage après morsure. *C. R. Acad. Sci. (Paris)*, 1885, **101,** 765–74.
Pasteur's specific vaccine treatment of rabies (see also No. 2541).

5484 NEGRI, Adelchi. 1876–1912
Contributo allo studio dell' eziologia della rabia. *Boll. Soc. med.-chir. Pavia*, 1903, 88, 229; 1904, 22; 1905, 321.
Discovery of the "Negri bodies" in rabies, making possible prompt microscopic diagnosis. German translation in *Z. Hyg. InfektKr.*, 1903, **43**, 507–28.

5484.1 FERMI, Claudio. 1862–
Über die Immunisierung gegen Wutkrankheit. *Z. Hyg. InfektKr.*, 1908, **58,** 233–76.
Fermi was the first to use chemical treatment of tissue suspensions of fixed rabies virus for the preparation of vaccine (Fermi vaccine). He introduced the use of carbolic acid for this purpose.

5484.2 WEBSTER, Leslie Tillotson. 1894–1943, & CLOW, Anna D.
Propagation of rabies virus in tissue culture and the successful use of culture virus as an antirabic vaccine. *Science*, 1936, **84,** 487–88.
Webster and Clow succeeded in growing rabies virus in tissue culture.

5484.3 DAWSON, James Robertson. 1908–
Infection of chicks and chick embryos with rabies. *Science*, 1939, **89,** 300–01.
Cultivation of rabies virus in the chick embryo. Soon afterwards I. J. Kligler and H. Bernkopf, *Nature*, 1939, **143**, 899, made a similar report.

5485–5487

GLANDULAR FEVER

5485 FILATOV, Nil Feodorovich. 1847–1902
Lektsii ob ostrikh infektsionnîkh bolieznyakh u dietei. [Lectures on acute infectious diseases of children.] 2 vols. Moskva, *A. Lang*, 1885–87.
Glandular fever (infectious mononucleosis) was first described by Filatov under the name of idiopathic adenitis ("Filatov's disease"). A German translation of his book appeared in 1895–97.

5486 PFEIFFER, Emil. 1846–1921
Drüsenfieber. *Jb. Kinderheilk.*, 1889, **29,** 257–64.
"Pfeiffer's disease." He is by some accredited with the original description of infectious mononucleosis, ascribed to Filatov. Pfeiffer's paper is a most comprehensive discussion of the clinical aspects of the disease.

5487 PAUL, John Rodman. 1893–1971, & BUNNELL, Walls Willard. 1902–
The presence of heterophile antibodies in infectious mononucleosis. *Amer. J. med. Sci.*, 1932, **183,** 90–104.
The Paul–Bunnell test for the diagnosis of infectious mononucleosis.

5488–5500

INFLUENZA

5488 SAILLANT, Charles Jacques. 1747–1804
Tableau historique et raisonné des épidémies catharrales vulgairement dites la grippe; depuis 1510 jusques et y compris celle de 1780. Paris, *Didot*, 1780.

5489 THOMPSON, THEOPHILUS. 1807–1860
Annals of influenza or epidemic catarrhal fever in Great Britain from 1510 to 1837. London, *Sydenham Society*, 1852.

5490 PFEIFFER, RICHARD FRIEDRICH JOHANNES. 1858–1945
Vorläufige Mittheilungen über die Erreger der Influenza. *Dtsch. med. Wschr.*, 1892, **18,** 28.
Pfeiffer discovered a bacillus, *Haemophilus influenzae*, "Pfeiffer's bacillus", which he believed to be the causal organism of influenza.

5491 LEICHTENSTERN, OTTO. 1845–1900
Influenza und Dengue. Wien, *A. Hölder*, 1896.
Forms Bd. IV, Teil I of Nothnagel's *Specielle Pathologie und Therapie.*

5492 GREAT BRITAIN. *Ministry of Health.*
Report on the pandemic of influenza 1918–19. London, H.M. *Stationery Office*, 1920.
Reports on Public Health and Medical Subjects, No. 4. The most widespread and serious pandemic of influenza occurred in 1918–19. It spread throughout Europe, Russia, Canada, S. America, New Zealand, Australia, Africa, India, China, and Japan. About 21,000,000 people died from the disease (2,000,000 in Europe alone).

5493 SHOPE, RICHARD EDWIN. 1901–1966
Swine influenza. III. Filtration experiments and etiology. *J. exp. Med.*, 1931, **54,** 373–85.
Shope's important work on the aetiology of influenza included the isolation of the Shope virus.

5494 SMITH, WILSON. 1897– , *et al.*
A virus obtained from influenza patients. *Lancet*, 1933, **2,** 66–68.
W. Smith, C. H. Andrewes, and P. P. Laidlaw successfully infected ferrets with filtered throat-washings from influenzal patients by intranasal instillation (influenza A virus).

5495 THOMSON, DAVID. 1884–1969, & THOMSON, ROBERT. 1888–
Influenza. 2 vols. London, *Baillière, Tindall & Cox*, 1933–34.
Annals of the Pickett Thomson Research Lab., Monograph 16.

5496 BURNET, *Sir* FRANK MACFARLANE. 1899–
Propagation of the virus of epidemic influenza on the developing egg. *Med. J. Aust.*, 1935, **2,** 687–89.
Cultivation of the influenza virus.

5497 SMITH, WILSON. 1897– , & STUART-HARRIS, CHARLES HERBERT. 1909–
Influenza infection of man from the ferret. *Lancet*, 1936, **2,** 121–23.
First record of successful passage of influenza from animal to man. The ferret had previously been infected with a virus from a case of influenza.

5498 FRANCIS, THOMAS. 1900–
A new type of virus from epidemic influenza. *Science*, 1940, **92,** 405–408.
Recovery of influenza B virus.

5499 MAGILL, THOMAS PLEINES. 1903–
A virus from cases of influenza-like upper-respiratory infection. *Proc. Soc. exp. Biol. (N.Y.)*, 1940, **45,** 162–64.
Recovery of influenza B virus.

5500 TAYLOR, RICHARD MORELAND. 1887–
Studies on survival of influenza virus between epidemics and antigenic variants of the virus. *Amer. J. publ. Hlth*, 1949, **39,** 171–78.
Recovery of influenza C virus.

5501–5509.2 RUBELLA AND ALLIED CONDITIONS

5501 WAGNER.
Die Rötheln, als für sich bestehende Krankheit. *Litt. Ann. ges. Heilk.*, 1829, **13,** 420–28.
Wagner separated rubella from measles and scarlet fever.

5502 VEALE, HENRY RICHARD LOBB. 1832–1908
History of an epidemic of rötheln, with observations on its pathology. *Edinb. med. J.*, 1866, **12,** 404–14.
Veale introduced the term "rubella" to describe German measles.

5503 FILATOV, NIL FEODOROVICH. 1847–1902
Lektsii ob ostrikh infektsionnîkh bolieznyakh u dietei. [Lectures on acute infectious diseases of children.] Vol. 2. Moskva, *A. Lang*, 1887.
On p. 113 is Filatov's account of a form of rubella with a scarlatiniform rash. To this he gave the name "rubeola scarlatinosa." (See also No. 5505.)

5504 TSCHAMER, ANTON.
Ueber örtliche Rötheln. *Jb. Kinderheilk.*, 1889, n.F., **29,** 372–79.
First description of acute infectious erythema, "fifth disease", called also "Sticker's disease" after the latter's description of it in *Z. prakt. Aerzte*, 1899, **8**, 353.

5505 DUKES, CLEMENT. 1845–1925
On the confusion of two different diseases under the name of rubella (rose-rash). *Lancet*, 1900, **2,** 89–94.
Dukes described a condition similar to that noted earlier by Filatov (No. 5503). Dukes called it the "fourth disease", distinguishing it from scarlet fever, measles, and rubella on the ground that an attack of any of these diseases gives no immunity. The autonomy of this disease ("Filatov–Dukes' disease") is not universally accepted.

5506 ZAHORSKY, JOHN. 1871–
Roseola infantilis. *Pediatrics (N.Y.)*, 1910, **22,** 60–64.
Roseola (exanthema) subitum first described as a distinct entity.

5506.1 HESS, ALFRED FABIAN. 1875–1933
German measles (rubella): an experimental study. *Arch. intern. Med.*, 1914, **13,** 913–16.
Experimental proof that rubella is caused by a virus.

5506.2 HIRO, Y., & TASAKA, S.
Die Röteln sind eine Viruskrankheit. *Mschr. Kinderheilk.*, 1938, **76,** 328–32.
Successful transfer of rubella to children by means of filtered nasal washings.

5507 GREGG, *Sir* NORMAN MCALISTER. 1892–1966
Congenital cataract following German measles in the mother. *Trans. ophthal. Soc. Aust.*, 1941, **3,** 35–46.
Gregg drew attention to congenital defects in infants following rubella in the mother during the early part of pregnancy.

5508 HABEL, KARL. 1908–
Transmission of rubella to *Macacus mulatta* monkeys. *Publ. Hlth Rep. (Wash.)*, 1942, **57,** 1126–39.
Successful transmission of rubella.

5509 SWAN, CHARLES SPENCER, *et al.*
Congenital defects in infants following infectious diseases during pregnancy. *Med. J. Aust.*, 1943, **2,** 201–10.
Figures demonstrating that rubella in the first or second month of pregnancy always results in an abnormal infant. With A. L. Tostevin, B. Moore, H. Mayo, and G. H. B. Black.

5509.1 WELLER, THOMAS HUCKLE. 1915– , & NEVA, FRANKLIN ALLEN. 1922–
Propagation in tissue culture of cytopathic agents from patients with rubella-like illness. *Proc. Soc. exp. Biol. (N.Y.)*, 1962, **111,** 215–25.
Isolation of rubella virus. It was simultaneously isolated by P. D. Parkman, *et al.* (No. 5509.2.)

5509.2 PARKMAN, PAUL DOUGLAS. 1932– , *et al.*
Recovery of rubella virus from army recruits. *Proc. Soc. exp. Biol. (N.Y.)*, 1962, **111,** 225–230.
With E. L. Buescher and M. S. Artenstein.

5510–5515 ACTINOMYCOSIS; NOCARDIOSIS

5510 BOLLINGER, OTTO. 1843–1909
Ueber eine neue Pilzkrankheit beim Rinde. *Zbl. med. Wiss.*, 1877, **15,** 481–85.
First effective description of *Actinomyces bovis*.

5511 ISRAEL, JAMES. 1848–1926
Neue Beobachtungen auf dem Gebiete der Mykosen des Menschen. *Virchows Arch. path. Anat.*, 1878, **74,** 15–53.
Israel contributed an important early paper on the ray fungus *Actinomyces*. He included some drawings made by Langenbeck in 1845 and was the first to describe a human case of actinomycosis.

5512 PONFICK, EMIL. 1844–1913
Ueber Actinomykose. *Berl. klin. Wschr.*, 1880, **17,** 660–61.
Ponfick recognized the causative role of *Actinomyces* in human actinomycosis; he established the identity of the human and animal forms of the disease. He published a book on the subject in 1882.

5512.1 NOCARD, EDMOND ISIDORE ETIENNE. 1850–1903
Note sur la maladie des boeufs de la Guadeloupe, connue sous le nom de farcin. *Ann. Inst. Pasteur*, 1888, **2,** 293–302.
The first pathogenic aerobic actinomycete to be described. It was later named *Nocardia farcinica* and is probably identical with *N. asteroides*.

5513 BOSTROEM, EUGEN. 1850–1928
Untersuchungen über die Aktinomykose des Menschen. *Beitr. path. Anat.*, 1890, **9,** 1–240.
Isolation of *Actinomyces graminis* from human actinomycosis, and staining method for *Actinomyces*.

5513.1 EPPINGER, HANS. 1846–1916
Ueber eine neue, pathogene Cladothrix und eine durch sie hervorgerufene Pseudotuberculosis (cladothrichica). *Beitr. path. Anat.*, 1891, **9,** 287–328.

Eppinger isolated *Cladothrix* (*Nocardia*) *asteroides* in a patient suffering from pseudo-tuberculosis with brain abscesses and meningitis.

5514 WOLFF, MAX. 1844–1923, & ISRAEL, JAMES. 1848–1926
Ueber Reincultur des Actinomyces und seine Uebertragbarkeit auf Thiere. *Virchows Arch. path. Anat.*, 1891, **126,** 11–59.

Isolation of *Actinomyces bovis.*

5515 COPE, *Sir* VINCENT ZACHARY. 1881–1974
Actinomycosis. London, *Oxford University Press*, 1938.

5516–5519 CANDIDIASIS

5516 UNDERWOOD, MICHAEL. 1737–1820
Aphthae or thrush. In his *Treatise on the diseases of children*, London, *J. Mathews*, 1784, pp. 43–52.

5517 LANGENBECK, BERNHARD RUDOLPH CONRAD VON. 1810–1887
Auffindung von Pilzen auf der Schleimhaut der Speiseröhre einer Typhus-Leiche. *Neue Notiz. Geb. Natur- u. Heilk.* (Froriep), 1839, **12,** cols. 145–47.

Discovery of *Candida albicans*, which Berg (No. 5518) showed to be the causal organism in thrush.

5518 BERG, FREDRIK THEODOR. 1806–1887
Torsk i mikroskopiskt anatomiskt hänseende. *Hygiea* (*Stockh.*), 1841, **3,** 541–50.

Discovery of *Candida albicans* in thrush.

5519 GRUBY, DAVID. 1810–1898
Recherches anatomiques sur une plante cryptogame qui constitue le vrai muguet des enfants. *C. R. Acad. Sci.* (*Paris*), 1842, **14,** 634–36.

Independently of Berg, Gruby found *Candida albicans* in thrush.

5520–5546.4 OTHER COMMUNICABLE DISEASES

5520 CORDUS, EURICIUS, 1486–1535
Ein Regiment: wie man sich vor der newen Plage der Englische Schwaisz genannt, bewaren, unnd so mann damit ergryffen wirt, darinn halten soll. Marpurg, 1529.

Euricius Cordus, father of Valerius, wrote an important account of sweating sickness. Another edition was published at Nuremberg, also in 1529. Reproduced in Gruner's *Scriptores*, 1847.

5521 SCHYLLER, JOACHIM [SCHILLER]. *fl.* 1529
De peste Brittanica commentariolus vere aureus. Basileae, *H. Petrus*, 1531.

Schyller's book on sweating sickness deals with the German epidemic of 1528–30.

5522 CAIUS, John [Kaye]. 1510–1573
A boke, or conseill against the disease commonly called the sweate, or sweatyng sicknesse. London, *Richard Grafton*, 1552.

First English book on sweating sickness, and the first devoted to a single disease to be published in England. Caius' work appeared a year after the last epidemic visit of the disease. From it we learn that the disease was febrile, the sweating merely a manifestation of the fever, and that it was accompanied by pain in the limbs, nausea, vomiting, and delirium. A facsimile edition of the book was published in New York, 1937; it also appears in C. G. Gruner: *Scriptores de sudore anglico*, 1847, pp. 310–51.

5523 HAMILTON, Robert. 1721–1793
An account of a distemper, by the common people in England vulgarly called the mumps. *Trans. roy. Soc. Edinb.*, 1790, **2**, 59–72.

First modern account of the occurrence of parotitis and orchitis complicating it. Hamilton's paper, read in 1773, by its fullness and clarity made the disease more generally known, so that within a few years many text-books included descriptions of it.

5524 GRUNER, Christian Gottfried. 1744–1815
Scriptores de sudore anglico superstites. Colliget C. G. Gruner. Post mortem auctoris adornavit et edidit H. Haeser. Jenae, *F. Mauk*, 1847.

A collection of all the important earlier writings on sweating sickness.

5525 SALAZAR, Tomas. 1830–1917
Historia de la verrugas. *Gac. méd. Lima*, 1858, **2**, 161–64, 175–78.

Verruga peruana.

5526 BOLLINGER, Otto. 1843–1909
Mycosis der Lunge beim Pferde. *Virchows Arch. path. Anat.*, 1870, **49**, 583–86.

Botriomycosis first described.

5527 RITTER, Jacob.
Beitrag zur Frage des Pneumotyphus. (Eine Hausepidemie in Uster [Schweiz] betreffend.) *Dtsch. Arch. klin. Med.*, 1879, **25**, 53–96.

First description of psittacosis in a human.

5528 PALTAUF, Arnold. 1860–1893
Mycosis mucorina. *Virchows Arch. path. Anat.*, 1885, **102**, 543–64.

First authentic case reported in man.

5529 SMITH, Theobald. 1859–1934, & KILBORNE, Frederick Lucius. 1858–1936
Investigations into the nature, causation and prevention of Texas or Southern cattle fever. Washington, *Govt. Printing Office*, 1893.

U.S. Bureau of Animal Industry, Bulletin No. 1. Discovery of the parasite of Texas cattle fever, *Pyrosoma bigeminum*, and proof that its transmission is due to the cattle tick, *Boöphilus bovis*.

5530 ODRIOZOLA, Ernesto. 1862–1921
La erupción en la enfermedad de Carrión (verruga peruana). *Monitor méd.*, 1895, **10**, 309–11.

"Carrión's disease" (Oroya fever) was so named by Odriozola, after Daniel Carrión (1859–85), a student. In order to prove or disprove the connexion between Oroya fever and verruga peruana Carrión had himself inoculated with blood from a patient suffering from verruga peruana and later died of the disease.

5530.1 LAVERAN, Charles Louis Alphonse. 1845–1922
Au sujet de l'hématozoaire endoglobulaire de *Padda oryzivora*. *C. R. Soc. Biol.* (*Paris*), 1900, **52,** 19–20.
Toxoplasma described.

5531 LIGNIÈRES, Joseph Léon Marcel. 1868–1933, & SPITZ, J.
Actinobacilosis. *Semana méd.*, 1902, **9,** 207–15.
Discovery of the actinobacillus.

5531.1 STRONG, Richard Pearson. 1872–1948
A study of some tropical ulcerations of skin with particular reference to their etiology. *Philipp. J. Sci.*, 1906, **1,** 91–116.
Strong described organisms consistent with *Histoplasma capsulatum* before Darling, although his work was overshadowed by the latter.

5532 DARLING, Samuel Taylor. 1872–1925
A protozoon general infection producing pseudotubercles in the lungs and focal necroses in the liver, spleen and lymphnodes. *J. Amer. med. Ass.*, 1906, **46,** 1283–85.
Histoplasmosis, "Darling's disease".

5533 BARTON, A. L.
Descripción de elementos endo-globulares hallados en las enfermos de fiebre verrucosa. *Crón. méd.* (*Lima*), 1909, **26,** 7–10.
The causal organism of Oroya fever and verruga peruana was named *Bartonella bacilliformis* after Barton, who was one of the first to observe it.

5534 NICOLLE, Charles Jules Henri. 1866–1936, & MANCEAUX, Louis Herbert. 1865–1943
Sur une infection à corps de Leishman (ou organismes voisins) du gondi. *C. R. Acad. Sci.* (*Paris*), 1908, **147,** 763–66.
Toxoplasma described.

5534.1 SPLENDORE, Alfonso.
Un nuovo protozoa parassito de' conigli incontrato nelle lesioni anatomiche d'una malattia che ricorda in molti punti il kala azar dell'uomo. *Rev. Soc. Sci. S. Paulo*, 1908, **3,** 109–12.
Splendore discovered *Toxoplasma* in a rabbit; it was named *T. cuniculi.*

5535 GOUGEROT, Henri. 1881– , & CARAVEN, Pierre Jean Baptiste. 1879–1958
Mycose nouvelle: l'hémisporose. Ostéite humaine primitive du tibia due à l'*Hemispora Stellata*. *C. R. Soc. Biol.* (*Paris*), 1909, **66,** 474–76.
Hemisporosis described.

5535.1 CASTELLANI, Aldo. 1877–1971
Note on certain protozoa-like bodies in a case of protracted fever with splenomegaly. *J. trop. Med.*, 1914, **17,** 113–14.
Castellani was first to suspect that toxoplasmosis could affect humans.

5536 MAGROU, Joseph Emile. 1883–
Les grains botryomycotiques. Leur signification en pathologie et en biologie générales. Laval, *L. Barnéoud*, 1914.
Thèse de Paris, No. 267, 1914. Magrou showed botriomycosis (granuloma pyogenicum) to be due to a staphylococcus.

5537 STODDARD, JAMES LEAVITT. 1889– , & CUTLER, ELLIOTT CARR. 1888–
Torula infection in man. *Monograph* 6, *Rockefeller Inst. med. Res.*, 1916.
Description of *Torula histolytica* infection in man.

5538 ZAHORSKY, JOHN. 1871–
Herpetic sore throat. *Sth. med. J.* (*Nashville*), 1920, **13,** 871–72.
First description of herpangina, an acute infection associated with Coxsackie viruses.

5538.1 ASHWORTH, JAMES HARTLEY. 1874–1936
On *Rhinosporidium seeberi* (Wernicke, 1903), with special reference to its sporulation and affinities. *Trans. roy. Soc. Edinb.*, 1923, **53,** 301–42.
Ashworth was the first to show that *Rhinosporidium* was a fungus.

5538.2 NOGUCHI, HIDEYO. 1876–1928, *et al.*
Etiology of Oroya fever. XIV. The insect vectors of Carrión's disease. *J. exp. Med.*, 1929, **49,** 993–1008.
Phlebotomus shown to be the vector of Oroya fever. With R. C. Shannon, E. B. Tilden, and J. B. Tyler.

5538.3 BECKER, FREDERICK EDWARD. 1888–
Tick-borne infections in Colorado. I. The diagnosis and management of infections transmitted by the wood tick. *Colorado Med.*, 1930, **27,** 36–44.
Becker first clearly described Colorado tick fever as a separate entity and suggested that the causal organism was transmitted by the tick, *Dermacentor andersoni.*

5539 LEVINTHAL, CLAUDE WALTER. 1886–1963
Die Ätiologie der Psittakosis. *Klin. Wschr.*, 1930, **9,** 654.
Discovery of the virus of psittacosis. Simultaneously A. C. Coles (*Lancet*, 1930, **1**, 1011–12) and R. D. Lillie (*Publ. Hlth Rep., Wash.*, 1930, **45**, 773–78) made the same discovery.

5540 SYLVEST, EJNAR OLUF SØRENSEN. 1880–
En Bornholmsk epidemi – myositis epidemica. *Ugeskr. Lag.*, 1930, **92,** 798–801.
First full description of epidemic myositis, "Bornholm disease". See also Sylvest's monograph on the subject, London, 1934.

5541 DAUBNEY, ROBERT. 1891– , & HUDSON, JOHN RICHARD.
Enzootic hepatitis or Rift Valley fever. An undescribed virus disease of sheep, cattle and man from East Africa. *J. Path. Bact.*, 1931, **34,** 545–79.
First description.

5541.1 BEDSON, *Sir* SAMUEL PHILLIPS. 1886–1969, & BLAND, J. O. W.
A morphological study of psittacosis virus, with the description of a developmental cycle. *Brit. J. exp. Path.*, 1932, **13,** 461–66.
Conclusive proof of the causal relationship of the psittacosis virus to the infection.

5541.2 HANSMANN, GEORGE HENRY. 1890– , & SCHENKEN, JOHN RUDOLPH. 1905–
A unique infection in man caused by a new yeast-like organism, a pathogenic member of the genus Sepedonium. *Amer. J. Path.*, 1934, **10,** 731–38.
Cultivation of *Histoplasma capsulatum* before DeMonbreun (No. 5542); preliminary announcement in *Science*, 1933, **77**, Suppl. 2002, p. 8.

5542 DeMONBREUN, William Andrew. 1899–
Cultivation and cultural characteristics of Darling's Histoplasma capsulatum. *Amer. J. trop. Med.*, 1934, **14,** 93–125.

5543 JOHNSON, Claud D., & GOODPASTURE, Ernest William. 1886–1960
An investigation of the etiology of mumps. *J. exp. Med.*, 1934, **59**, 1–19.
Isolation of mumps virus.

5544 RIVERS, Thomas Milton. 1888–1962, & BERRY, George Packer. 1898–
Diagnosis of psittacosis in man by means of injections of sputum into white mice. *J. exp. Med.*, 1935, **61,** 205–12.

5544.1 WOLF, Abner. 1902– , & COWEN, David. 1907–
Granulomatous encephalomyelitis due to an encephalitozoon, (encephalitozoic encephalomyelitis) a new protozoon disease of man. *Bull. neurol. Inst. N.Y.*, 1937, **6,** 306–71.
Definite recognition of human toxoplasmosis. See also their later paper in the same journal, 1938, **7**, 266–83.

5545 DALLDORF, Gilbert Julius. 1900– , & SICKLES, Grace Mary. 1898–1959
An unidentified, filtrable agent isolated from the feces of children with paralysis. *Science*, 1948, **108**, 61–62.
Isolation of the Coxsackie virus.

5546 CURNEN, Edward Charles. 1909– , *et al.*
Disease resembling nonparalytic poliomyelitis associated with a virus pathogenic for infant mice. *J. Amer. med. Ass.*, 1949, **141,** 894–901.
Isolation of the Coxsackie virus from patients with poliomyelitis. With E. W. Shaw and J. L. Melnick.

5546.1 FLORIO, Lloyd Joseph. 1910– , *et al.*
Colorado tick fever. Isolation of the virus from *Dermacentor andersoni* in nature and a laboratory study of the transmission of the virus in the tick. *J. Immunol.*, 1950, **64,** 257–63.
Isolation of the virus of Colorado tick fever. With M. S. Miller and E. R. Mugrage.

5546.2 GREER, William Edward R. 1918– , & KEEFER, Chester Scott. 1897–
Cat-scratch fever. A disease entity. *New Engl. J. Med.*, 1951, **244,** 545–48.
First description.

History of Communicable Diseases

5546.3 BLOOMFIELD, Arthur Leonard. 1888–
A bibliography of internal medicine. Communicable diseases. Chicago, *University of Chicago Press*, 1958.
An exhaustive bibliography for communicable diseases with substantial excerpts from practically every important reference made to each of thirty such diseases from about 1800 to the present.

5546.4 COCKBURN, AIDAN.
The evolution and eradication of infectious diseases. Baltimore, *John Hopkins Press*, 1963.

5547–5813.7 SURGERY

See also 3021–3047.3, CARDIOVASCULAR SURGERY; 4851–4914, NEUROSURGERY; and under organs and regions.

5547–5632 GENERAL WORKS

5547 EDWIN SMITH PAPYRUS.
The Edwin Smith Surgical Papyrus. Published in facsimile and hieroglyphic transliteration with translation and commentary by JAMES HENRY BREASTED. 2 vols. Chicago, *Univ. Press*, 1930.

Edwin Smith, pioneer Egyptologist, purchased at Luxor in 1862 the papyrus which bears his name. It is now in the possession of the New York Academy of Medicine. The original text was written about 3000 B.C. and the present manuscript is a copy dating about 1600 B.C. It is the oldest known surgical treatise and consists entirely of case reports; it describes 47 different cases of injuries and affections of the head, nose and mouth, together with methods of bandaging.

5548 HIPPOCRATES, 460–375 B.C.
Chirurgie d'Hippocrate. 2 vols. Paris, *J. B. Baillière*, 1877.

Greek-French bilingual, by J. E. Pétrequin. Hippocrates performed trephining and paracentesis; his most important successes were in the reduction of fractures and dislocations. His knowledge of surgery was limited by his ignorance of anatomy.

5549 PAUL *of Aegina*. A.D. 625–690
The seven books of Paulus Aegineta. Translated from the Greek . . . by FRANCIS ADAMS. 3 vols. London, *Sydenham Society*, 1844–47.

Book VI is entirely devoted to operative surgery. Adams himself says that it "contains the most complete system of operative surgery which has come down to us from ancient times". Book IV contains much information on surgical diseases. (See also No. 36.)

5550 ALBUCASIS [ABUL QASIM]. 936–1013
De chirurgia. Arabice et Latine cura Johannis Channing. 3 vols. *Oxonii, e typ. Clarendoniano*, 1778.

The surgical section of Albucasis' *Altasrif*. During the Middle Ages it was the leading text-book on surgery until superseded by Saliceto. Of the above translation Osler said "it was by far the most important Arabic work in medicine edited and translated by an Englishman". A French translation by L. Leclerc appeared in 1861.

5551 DAREMBERG, CHARLES VICTOR. 1817–1872
Glossulae quatuor magistrorum super chirurgiam Rogerii et Rolandi. Ed. C. DAREMBERG. Neapoli et Parisiis, *J. B. Baillière*, 1854.

In Roger of Palermo's *Practica chirurgiae*, which appeared about 1180, end-to-end suture is described, as also the value of mercurial inunction in chronic skin diseases; in his recommendation of seaweed for the treatment of goitre Roger anticipated Coindet (No. 3812). Roland of Parma was a pupil of Roger, and edited his master's books about A.D. 1230. The work was one of the most important emanating from the School of Salerno.

5551.1 THEODORIC, *Bishop of Cervia.* 1210–1298

The surgery of Theodoric ca. 1267. Translated from the Latin by ELDRIDGE CAMPBELL and JAMES COLTON. 2 vols. New York, *Appleton-Century-Crofts*, 1955–60.

Theodoric, a Dominican friar, was a pupil of Hugh of Lucca (*c.* 1160–1257) whose teachings are reflected in his writings. Allbutt considered Theodoric to be one of the most original surgeons of all time.

5552 SALICETO, GULIELMUS DE [SALICETTI; WILLIAM OF SALICET]. 1210–1280

La ciroxia vulgarmente fata. [Venice, *F. de Pietro*, 1474.]

Saliceto was professor of surgery at Bologna about 1268. He was a skilful surgeon and his book on surgery was the most important on the subject during the 13th century. It was written about 1275; the original Latin version was printed two years after the above Italian edition. Book IV contains the first known treatise on surgical anatomy. A French translation by P. Pifteau was published in Toulouse in 1898. Book IV contains the first known treatise on surgical anatomy.

5553 LANFRANCHI, *of Milan.* ?–1315

La chirurgie d'Alanfranc traduit du latin par Guillaume Yvoire. Lyon, *Jean de la Fontaine*, 1490.

Lanfranc, the founder of French surgery, was a pupil of William of Salicet. He enjoyed a great reputation for his lecturing and bedside teaching. His *Chirurgia magna* was completed in 1296. According to Hirsch and others it was first published in Venice in 1490, but no copy of this edition has been traced. Above is a French translation; an English version appeared in 1565 and the Early English Text Society published an Old English version, *Science of cirurgie*, in 1894. Lanfranc was the first surgeon to describe cerebral concussion and to distinguish between simple hypertrophy and cancer of the breast. He wrote a *Chirurgia parva* about 1295.

5554 MONDEVILLE, HENRI DE. ?1260–1320

Die Chirurgie des Heinrich de Mondeville. Hrsg. von JULIUS LEOPOLD PAGEL. Berlin, *A. Hirschwald*, 1892.

Henri de Mondeville was the teacher of Guy de Chauliac; he belonged to the School of Montpellier. His work was first printed as above; French translations by E. Nicaise, 1893, and A. Bos, 1897; the latter was reprinted in 1965.

5555 YPERMAN, JAN. 1295–1351

La chirurgie de maître Jean Yperman . . . Mise au jour et annotée par J. M. F. CAROLUS. Gand, *F. & E. Gyselynck*, 1854.

Jan Yperman, a pupil of Lanfranc, became the first authority on surgery in the Low Countries during the 14th century. His work was first printed in *Ann. Soc. Méd. Gand*, 1854, **32** and re-issued as above. Another edition was published in Paris, 1936.

5556 GUY DE CHAULIAC. ?1298–1368

La pratique en chirurgie du maistre Guidon de Chauliac. Lyon, *Barthelemy Buyer*, 1478.

Guy de Chauliac was the most eminent surgeon of his time; his authority remained for some 200 years. He distinguished the various kinds of hernia from varicocele, hydrocele, and sarcocele and described an operation for the radical cure of hernia. The book, which was originally written about 1363, includes Guy's views on fractures, and gives an excellent summary of the dentistry of that period. It is the greatest surgical text of the time. A modern French edition by E. Nicaise was published in Paris, 1890.

5557 JOHN *of Arderne*. 1306–1390?
De arte phisicale et de cirurgia. Translated by D'ARCY POWER from a transcript made by Eric Millar from the replica of the Stockholm manuscript in the Wellcome Historical Medical Museum. London, *John Bale*, 1922.

John of Arderne was the first English surgeon of note.

5558 PFOLSPEUNDT, HEINRICH VON. *fl.* 1460
Buch der Bündth-Ertznei. Hrsg. von H. HAESER und A. MIDDELDORPF. Berlin, *G. Reimer*, 1868.

Although not printed until 1868, this work was written about 1460, and is the first work of the early German surgeons. Pfolspeundt was a Bavarian army surgeon; his book includes the first allusion to the extraction of bullets, and gives an account of rhinoplasty. Some authorities have used the name "Pfolsprundt"; for an explanation of this mistake, see Muffat, in *S.B. k. bayer. Akad. Wiss. München*, 1869, 1, 564.

5559 BRUNSCHWIG, HIERONYMUS [BRAUNSCHWEIG]. 1450–1533
Dis ist das buch der Cirurgia Hantwirkckung der wundartzny von Hyeronimo brunschwig. Strassburg, [*J. Grüninger*], 1497.

First important printed surgical treatise in German. It combines a compilation of the ancient and mediaeval authorities with Brunschwig's own extensive experience. It contains the first detailed account of gunshot wounds in medical literature and is notable for its wood-cuts, some of the earliest specimens of medical illustration. It was reproduced in facsimile in 1911 (Munich) and 1923 (Milan). English translation, Southwark, 1525.

5559.1 VIGO, GIOVANNI DE. 1450–1525
Practica in arte chirurgica copiosa . . . continens novem libros. [Rome, *per S. Guillireti et H. Bononiensem*], 1514.

The first complete system of surgery after that of Guy de Chauliac. It contains an account of gunshot wounds and a section on syphilis. It was "a book which especially suited a practitioner who knew nothing of anatomy and feared or disliked to make use of the knife" (J. S. Billings). The book went through 40 editions; an English translation by B. Traheron was published in London, 1543.

5560 GERSDORFF, HANS VON [GERSSDORFF; SCHYLHANS]. *fl.* 1500
Feldtbůch der wundartzney. Strassburg, *J. Schott*, 1517.

Gersdorff performed nearly 200 amputations. He opposed Paré's abandonment of boiling oil for the cauterization of wounds. The book contains some instructive pictures of early surgical procedures and includes the first picture ever made of an amputation.

5561 PARACELSUS [BOMBASTUS AB HOHENHEIM (AUREOLIUS PHILIPPUS THEOPHRASTUS)]. 1493–1541
Die grossenn Wundartzney. Augspurg, *H. Steyner*, 1536.

Paracelsus was doctor, chemist, lecturer, and reformer. His novel doctrines gained him many followers. He disbelieved in the use of boiling oil for the purification of gunshot wounds. His *Chirurgia magna* attained many editions and translations.

5562 CHIRURGIA.
De chirurgia scriptores optimi quique veteres et recentiores, plerique in Germania antehac non editi. Tiguri, *apud A. et J. Gesnerum*, 1555.

A collection made by C. Gesner of various surgical works by M. A. Blondus, A. Bolognini, G. dei Dondus, A. Ferri, Galen, C. Gesner, J. Hollerius, J. Langius, B. Maggius, Marianus Sanctus, Oribasius, and J. Tagaultius.

5563 WÜRTZ, Felix [Wirtz]. 1518–1574
Practica der Wundartzney. Basel, 1563.

Würtz, famous surgeon in the 16th century, studied at Nuremberg. He was a friend of Gesner and an admirer of Paracelsus; his book went through many editions and was translated into English, French, and Dutch. It describes the treatment of gunshot wounds, fractures, and dislocations, but does not include operative surgery.

5564 PARÉ, Ambroise. 1510–1590
Dix livres de la chirurgie, avec le magasin des instrumens necessaires à icelle. Paris, *imp. Jean de Royer*, 1564.

Paré's first large surgical work; it includes his first description of the use of the ligature in amputations. See No. 5565.

5565 ——. Les oeuvres de M. Ambroise Paré. Paris, *G. Buon*, 1575.

Paré was the greatest of the army surgeons before Larrey. Born in poor circumstances, he became the most famous surgeon in France. He is particularly remembered for his abandonment of boiling oil and the cautery (No. 2139), for his revival of podalic version (No. 6140), his re-introduction of the ligature and his invention of many new surgical instruments. He was the first to suggest that syphilis is a cause of aneurysm. He popularized the truss, introduced artificial limbs, and (in dentistry) re-implantation of the teeth. See also No. 59. English translation by Thomas Johnson, London, 1634.

5566 FABRY, Wilhelm [Fabricius *Hildanus*]. 1560–1634
De gangraena et sphacelo. Cölln, *P. Keschedt*, 1593.

Fabricius, the "Father of German surgery" was the first to advocate amputation above the gangrenous or injured part. He is accredited with the first amputation of the thigh. In his work he makes no reference to Paré's methods; he believed in the efficacy of the "weapon-salve". See also No. 5570.

5567 LOWE, Peter. 1560–1610
A discourse on the whole art of chyrurgerie. London, *T. Purfoot*, 1596.

Lowe was the founder of the Faculty of Physicians and Surgeons of Glasgow. He studied and practised for many years in France.

5568 UFFENBACH, Peter. ?–1635
Thesaurus chirurgiae. Francofurti, *typ. N. Hoffmanni, imp. J. Fischeri*, 1610.

An anthology of 16th-century writers; a good summary of the surgical knowledge of that period.

5569 BRADWELL, Stephen.
Helps for suddain accidents endangering life. London, *T. Purfoot*, 1633.

First book on first-aid.

5570 FABRY, Wilhelm [Fabricius *Hildanus*]. 1560–1634
Observationum et curationum chirurgicarum centuriae. 6 vols. Basle, Frankfort, & Lyons, 1606–1641.

Fabricius' most important work; it was the best collection of case-records available for many years. Among other things, Fabricius used a magnet to extract an iron splinter from the eye – an idea suggested to him by his wife – and he described the first field-chest of drugs for army use. He was first to remove a gallstone from a living patient (1618).

5571 SCHULTES, JOHANN [SCULTETUS]. 1595–1645
Χειροπλοθήκη seu armamentarium chirurgicum. Ulmae Suevorum, *imp. B. Kühnen*, 1655.

Scultetus is famous for his illustrations of surgical procedures and instruments. English translation, London, 1674.

5572 MARCHETTI, PIETRO DE. 1589–1673
Observationum medico-chirurgicarum rariorum sylloge. Amstelodami, *ex off. Petri le Grand*, 1665.

Pietro de Marchetti was professor of surgery at Padua. His book contains many valuable observations in surgery.

5573 WISEMAN, RICHARD. 1622–1676
Severall chirurgicall treatises. London, *R. Royston*, 1676.

Wiseman ranks in surgery as high as does Sydenham in medicine. He made many valuable contributions to the subject; he was the first to describe tuberculosis of the joints ("tumor albus") and he gave a good account of gunshot wounds. Wiseman became surgeon to Charles II in 1672.

5574 LE CLERC, CHARLES GABRIEL. 1644–1700?
La chirurgie complète. Paris, *E. Michallet*, 1695.

This "quiz-compend" passed through eighteen editions. Among other things it mentions the use of vitriol buttons for checking haemorrhage and the mode of manual compression used at the Hôtel-Dieu.

5575 DIONIS, PIERRE. ?–1718
Cours d'opérations de chirurgie, demonstrées au Jardin Royal. Paris, *L. d'Houry*, 1707.

Dionis taught operative surgery at the Jardin-du-Roi, Paris, a famous training ground for surgeons. English translation, London, 1710.

5576 HEISTER, LORENZ. 1683–1758
Chirurgie, in welcher alles, was zur Wund-Artzney gehöret, nach der neuesten und besten Art. Nürnberg, *J. Hoffmann*, 1718.

Heister is the founder of scientific surgery in Germany. His book contains many interesting illustrations and includes an account of tourniquets used in his time; Heister introduced a spinal brace. English translation, London, 1743.

5577 POTT, PERCIVALL. 1714–1788
Observations on the nature and consequences of wounds and contusions of the head, fractures of the skull, concussions of the brain, etc. London, *C. Hitch & L. Hawes*, 1760.

This book, which showed Pott's extensive knowledge of surgical literature, systematized the treatment of head injuries. It shows what a variety of injuries of the head could be sustained even before the advent of the motor-car. Includes the first description of "Pott's puffy tumour." Pott was born in Threadneedle Street, where the Bank of England now stands; he succeeded Cheselden as the greatest surgeon of his day. The book was altered and re-published under a different title in 1768.

5578 BELL, BENJAMIN. 1749–1806
A treatise on the theory and management of ulcers. Edinburgh, *C. Elliot*, 1778.

Important classification of ulcers.

5579 ——. A system of surgery. 6 vols. Edinburgh, *C. Elliot*, 1782–87.

Bell studied under the Monros at Edinburgh. He was surgeon to the Royal Infirmary, Edinburgh, for 29 years. He improved the methods of amputation, introducing the "triple incision of Bell". Above is his best work.

5580 DESAULT, Pierre Joseph. 1744–1795
Oeuvres chirurgicales. 3 vols. Paris, *C. Ve. Desault*, an VI [1798]–1803.

Desault was a great French surgeon, one of the first professors at the Ecole Pratique de Chirurgie, Paris. He made many suggestions regarding the treatment of fractures and dislocations and is one of the founders of modern vascular surgery. He was Bichat's teacher.

5581 BELL, John. 1763–1820
The principles of surgery. 3 vols. [in 4]. Edinburgh, London, *T. Cadell & W. Davies*, 1801–08.

John Bell, the Scottish anatomist, is regarded as the founder of surgical anatomy. He was first to ligate the gluteal artery and tied the common carotid and internal iliac. His illustrations were his own work, and were of a high standard.

5582 HEY, William. 1736–1819
Practical observations in surgery. London, *T. Cadell, jun., & W. Davies*, 1803.

Hey is remembered for "Hey's saw" and "Hey's internal derangement of the knee". He was an outstanding surgeon in his day; he founded and was senior surgeon of the General Infirmary, Leeds. He devised a type of amputation of the foot ("Hey's amputation"). His book includes the description of the falciform ligament of the saphenous opening, "Hey's ligament".

5583 BELL, *Sir* Charles. 1774–1842
A system of operative surgery. 2 vols. London, *Longman*, 1807–09.

Famous as anatomist, physiologist, and neurologist, Charles Bell was also, like his brother John, an eminent surgeon. His artistic talent was even greater than that of his brother. (See No. 5588.)

5584 ABERNETHY, John. 1764–1831
Surgical observations. London, *Longman*, 1809.

A pupil of John Hunter, Abernethy became a leading surgeon in London. He was most industrious, and it is said that not even on his wedding day did he fail to give his usual daily lecture at St. Bartholomew's Hospital. His book was, in the view of D'Arcy Power, epoch-making; on pp. 234–92 is recorded the first successful ligation of the external iliac artery for aneurysm, an operation carried out by Abernethy in 1796.

5585 COOPER, Samuel. 1780–1848
A dictionary of practical surgery. London, *J. Murray*, 1809.

Cooper was surgeon on the field at Waterloo, and was later appointed to the chair of surgery at University College, London. His great dictionary went through seven editions during his lifetime and was translated into French, German and Italian.

5586 PHYSICK, Philip Syng. 1768–1837
[Buck-skin and kid ligatures]. *Eclect. Repert.*, 1816, **6**, 389.

Physick, the "Father of American surgery", graduated at Edinburgh, having been a pupil of John Hunter. He introduced several new procedures in surgery, one of which was the use of absorbable kid and buckskin ligatures.

5587 COOPER, *Sir* Astley Paston, *Bart.* 1768–1841, & TRAVERS, Benjamin. 1783–1858
Surgical essays. 2 vols. London, *Cox & Son*, 1818–19.

Cooper, the pupil and great interpreter of Hunter, was the most popular surgeon in London during the Regency. In 1802 he gained the Copley Medal of the Royal Society. Travers was surgeon to St. Thomas's Hospital, and particularly distinguished himself in vascular surgery and ophthalmology. The book includes a description of "Cooper's tumour".

5588 BELL, *Sir* Charles. 1774–1842
Illustrations of the great operations of surgery. London, *Longman*, 1821.

5589 JAMESON, Horatio Gates. 1778–1855
Observations upon traumatic haemorrhage, illustrated by experiments upon living animals. *Amer. med. Recorder*, 1827, **11**, 1–70.

Jameson was for twenty years surgeon to Baltimore Hospital. He performed some great and original operations.

5590 DUPUYTREN, Guillaume, *le baron*. 1777–1835
Leçons orales de clinique chirurgicale. 4 vols. Paris, *Germer-Baillière*, 1832–34.

Dupuytren was born in poverty and died a millionaire. He became the best surgeon of his time in France. He was "a shrewd diagnostician, an operator of unrivalled aplomb, a wonderful clinical teacher, and a good experimental physiologist and pathologist" (Garrison); his greatest contributions were in the field of surgical pathology.

5591 MALGAIGNE, Joseph François. 1806–1865
Manuel de médecine opératoire. Paris, *Germer-Baillière*, 1834.

Malgaigne was a brilliant lecturer, notable also as a historian of mediaeval surgery. His *Manuel* was an important work on operative surgery, and was translated into English, German, Italian, and Arabic.

5592 VELPEAU, Alfred Armand Louis Marie. 1795–1867
Nouveaux éléments de médecine opératoire. Bruxelles, *H. Dumont*, 1835.

In its time this was the most comprehensive work on operative surgery in France; it contains some useful historical information. English translation, New York, 1847.

5593 LISTON, Robert. 1794–1847
Practical surgery. London, *J. Churchill*, 1837.

In his day Liston was the most dexterous and resourceful surgeon in the British Isles. He was the first in the country to remove the scapula and the first – on Dec. 21, 1846 – to perform a major operation with the aid of an anaesthetic. His method of laryngoscopy is described on p. 350 of the above work.

5594 MALGAIGNE, Joseph François. 1806–1865
Traité d'anatomie chirurgicale et de chirurgie expérimentale. 2 vols. Paris, *J. B. Baillière*, 1838.

5595 AMMON, Friedrich August von. 1799–1861
Die angeborenen chirurgischen Krankheiten des Menschen in Abbildungen dargestellt. 2 vols. Berlin, *F. A. Herbig*, 1842.

5596 FERGUSSON, *Sir* William. 1808–1877
A system of practical surgery. London, *J. Churchill*, 1842.

Fergusson was the founder of conservative surgery. He was surgeon of the Royal Infirmary, Edinburgh, before being appointed to the chair of surgery at King's College Hospital, London, a position in which he was succeeded by Lister.

5597 NÉLATON, Auguste. 1807–1873
Elémens de pathologie chirurgicale. 5 vols. Paris, *Germer-Baillière*, 1844–59.

Nélaton was a great teacher and operator at the Hôpital St. Louis. He invented several surgical instruments. In vol. 2, p. 46 of the above work is to be found the description of "Nélaton's tumour" of bone, and on p. 441 "Nélaton's line".

5598 PANCOAST, JOSEPH. 1805–1882
A treatise on operative surgery. Philadelphia, *Carey & Hart*, 1844.
Pancoast was professor of anatomy and surgery at Jefferson Medical College. He was a fine operator and devised a number of new surgical operations and instruments.

5599 SYME, JAMES. 1799–1870
Contributions to the pathology and practice of surgery. Edinburgh, *Sutherland & Knox*, 1848.
Syme, one-time colleague of Liston, succeeded to the latter's extensive practice in Scotland. He came to London for a short time as professor of surgery at University College, but soon returned to Scotland. He was a popular teacher and a fine, conservative surgeon, one of the first to adopt ether anaesthesia and to welcome the antiseptic principles laid down by his son-in-law, Lister.

5600 NÉLATON, AUGUSTE. 1807–1873
De l'influence de la position dans les maladies chirurgicales. Paris, *Germer-Baillière*, 1851.

5601 PIROGOV, NIKOLAI IVANOVICH. 1810–1881
Klinische Chirurgie. 3 pts. Leipzig, *Breitkopf u. Härtel*, 1851–54.
Pirogov is considered the greatest Russian surgeon and one of the greatest military surgeons of all time. He was among the first in Europe to employ ether anaesthesia. He served in the Crimean campaign and was responsible for the introduction there of female nursing of the wounded.

5602 ERICHSEN, *Sir* JOHN ERIC. 1818–1896
The science and art of surgery. London, *Walton & Maberly*, 1853.
The most popular text-book on the subject for many years. Erichsen was surgeon to University College Hospital, London, and Lister served as his house surgeon.

5603 PRAVAZ, CHARLES GABRIEL. 1791–1853
Sur un nouveau moyen d'opérer la coagulation du sang dans les artères, applicable à la guérison des anévrismes. *C. R. Acad. Sci. (Paris)*, 1853, **36,** 88–90.
Pravaz invented the modern galvanocautery.

5604 MIDDELDORPF, ALBRECHT THEODOR. 1824–1868
Die Galvanokaustik. Breslau, *J. Max u. Co.*, 1854.
Middeldorpf improved the galvano-cautery and introduced it in major surgery.

5605 SIMS, JAMES MARION. 1813–1883
Silver sutures in surgery. New York, *S. S. & S. W. Wood*, 1858.
Sims, famous American gynaecologist, introduced a silver wire suture, in order to avoid sepsis.

5606 CHASSAIGNAC, EDOUARD PIERRE MARIE. 1804–1879
Traité pratique de la suppuration et du drainage chirurgical. 2 vols. Paris, *V. Masson*, 1859.
Chassaignac, who introduced india-rubber tubes to drain abscesses, put the whole subject of surgical drainage on a scientific and methodical footing.

5607 GROSS, SAMUEL DAVID. 1805–1884
A system of surgery. 2 vols. Philadelphia, *Blanchard & Lea*, 1859.
Gross wrote the most important surgical treatise of his time. He was a famous American surgeon, a prolific writer, and was professor of surgery at Louisville and Jefferson Medical College.

5608 BILLROTH, CHRISTIAN ALBERT THEODOR. 1829–1894
Die allgemeine chirurgische Pathologie und Therapie. Berlin, *G. Reimer*, 1863.

Billroth, professor of surgery at Zürich and Vienna, ranked high as an operator, especially in the surgery of the alimentary tract. The above work, which placed him in the front rank, was translated into several languages.

5609 HILTON, JOHN. 1804–1878
On rest and pain. London, *G. Bell*, 1863.

John Hilton was surgeon to Guy's Hospital. He suggested that symptoms are disordered reflexes and advocated complete rest in the treatment of surgical disorders of all parts of the body. His book, a surgical classic still in demand among students, is fully discussed in Sir A. Keith's *Menders of the maimed*, London, 1919, pp. 18–34. Sixth edition in 1950.

5610 RIZZOLI, FRANCESCO. 1809–1880
Collezione della memorie chirurgiche ed ostetriche. 2 vols. Bologna, *regia tipog.*, 1869.

Rizzoli was professor of surgery at Bologna and an outstanding operative surgeon. He introduced a compressor for aneurysms, a tracheotome, cystotome, lithotrite, enterotome, osteoclast, and performed acupressure as early as 1854.

5611 ESMARCH, JOHANN FRIEDRICH AUGUST VON. 1823–1908
Ueber künstliche Blutleere bei Operationen. *Samml. klin. Vortr.*, 1873, Nr. 58 (Chir., Nr. 19), 373–84.

Esmarch bandage for surgical haemostasis. English translation (New Sydenham Society), 1876.

5612 VERNEUIL, ARISTIDE AUGUSTE STANISLAS. 1823–1895
De la forcipressure. *Bull. Mém. Soc. méd. chir. Paris*, 1875, n.s., **1**, 17, 108, 273, 522, 646.

Introduction of forcipressure in the control of haemorrhage. Republished in book form, 1875.

5613 ——. Mémoires de chirurgie. 5 vols. Paris, *G. Masson*, 1877–88.

Verneuil, Paris surgeon, introduced forcipressure in haemorrhage (see No. 5612), dry bandaging, and iodoform in the treatment of abscesses. All his works are included in his *Mémoires*.

5614 PAQUELIN, CLAUDE ANDRÉ. 1836–1905
Du cautère Paquelin. *Bull. gén. Thérap.*, 1877, **93**, 145–58.

Paquelin introduced a thermocautery ("Paquelin's cautery").

5615 WELLS, *Sir* THOMAS SPENCER. 1818–1897
Remarks on forcipressure and the use of pressure-forceps in surgery. *Brit. med. J.*, 1879, **1**, 926–28; **2**, 3–4.

Spencer Wells forceps.

5616 LISTER, JOSEPH, 1*st Baron Lister*. 1827–1912
[An address on the catgut ligature]. *Trans. clin. Soc. Lond.*, 1881, **14**, pp. xliii–lxiii.

5617 VOLKMANN, RICHARD VON. 1830–1889
Die ischaemischen Muskellähmungen und Kontrakturen. *Zbl. Chir.*, 1881, **8**, 801–03.

"Volkmann's ischaemic contracture" first described.

5618 MOSETIG-MOORHOF, ALBERT VON. 1838–1907
Der Jodoform-Verband. *Samml. klin. Vortr.*, Leipzig, 1882, Nr. 211, (Chir., Nr. 68), 1811–64.
Introduction of iodoform dressing in surgery.

5619 ROSENBACH, ANTON JULIUS FRIEDRICH. 1842–1923
Mikro-Organismen bei den Wund-Infektions-Krankheiten des Menschen. Wiesbaden, *J. F. Bergmann*, 1884.
Rosenbach isolated *Strep. pyogenes* (*Strep. haemolyticus*) and gave the first full description of *Staph. pyogenes*, dividing it into *albus* and *aureus*.

5619.1 KOCHER, EMIL THEODOR. 1841–1917
Eine einfache Methode zur Erzielung sicherer Asepsis. *CorrespBl. schweiz. Aerzte*, 1888, **18,** 3–20.
Kocher introduced silk sutures.

5620 SENN, NICHOLAS. 1844–1908
Experimental surgery. Chicago, *W. T. Keener*, 1889.
Senn was one of the leading surgeons in North America. He made important experimental studies on air embolism, introduced a method of diagnosing intestinal perforation by means of insufflation of hydrogen (see No. 3494), and used Roentgen rays in the treatment of leukaemia. He was professor of surgery at Rush Medical College.

5621 WELCH, WILLIAM HENRY. 1850–1934
Conditions underlying the infection of wounds. *Trans. Congr. Amer. Phys. Surg.*, 1892, **2,** 1–28.
Discovery of *Staph. epidermidis albus* and its relation to the infection of wounds.

5622 CRILE, GEORGE WASHINGTON. 1864–1943
An experimental research into surgical shock. Philadelphia, *J. B. Lippincott*, [1899].
Crile saw and recorded elevations in systemic and portal venous pressures under experimental shock.

5623 FOWLER, GEORGE RYERSON. 1848–1906
Diffuse septic peritonitis, with special reference to a new method of treatment, namely, the elevated head and trunk posture, to facilitate drainage into the pelvis, with a report of nine consecutive cases of recovery. *Med. Rec. (N.Y.)*, 1900, **57,** 617–23, 1029–31.
First description of the "Fowler position". Reprinted in *Med. Classics*, 1940, **4,** 551–80.

5624 CRILE, GEORGE WASHINGTON. 1864–1943
An experimental and clinical research into certain problems relating to surgical operations. Philadelphia, *J. B. Lippincott Co.*, 1901.
Crile made important contributions to the knowledge regarding shock. He originated the theory that it is due to exhaustion of the vasomotor centre. (See also No. 5629.)

5625 OCHSNER, ALBERT JOHN. 1858–1925
The cause of diffuse peritonitis complicating appendicitis and its prevention. *J. Amer. med. Ass.*, 1901, **36,** 1747–54.
Ochsner was professor of clinical surgery at the University of Illinois. The above is reprinted in *Med. Classics*, 1940, **4,** 600–26.

5626 BIER, August Karl Gustav. 1861–1949
Hyperaemie als Heilmittel. Leipzig, *F. C. W. Vogel*, 1903.
Bier introduced hyperaemia, active and passive, as an adjuvant in surgical therapy.

5627 CRILE, George Washington. 1864–1943
Blood-pressure in surgery. Philadelphia, *J. B. Lippincott Co.*, 1903.

5628 ——. Hemorrhage and transfusion. New York, *D. Appleton & Co.*, 1909.

5629 ——. The kinetic theory of shock and its prevention through anoci-association (shockless operation). *Lancet*, 1913, **2,** 7–16.
Crile advanced the anoci-association concept in which local and general anaesthesia are combined in a sequence to eliminate pre-operative fear and tension.

5630 DALE, *Sir* Henry Hallett. 1875–1968, & LAIDLAW, *Sir* Patrick Playfair. 1881–1940
Histamine shock. *J. Physiol.* (*Lond.*), 1919, **52,** 355–90.
Experimental shock produced by histamine and shown to be similar to traumatic and surgical shock.

5631 BURGER, Karl. 1893–
Künstliche Scheidenbildung mittels Eihäuten. *Zbl. Gynak.*, 1937, **61,** 2437–40.
Introduction of amnioplastin.

5632 TRUETA, Joseph. 1897–
Treatment of war wounds and fractures, with special reference to the closed method as used in the war in Spain. London, *Hamish Hamilton*, 1939.
Trueta's method of treatment of wounds – application of closed plaster after packing the excised wound with sterile vaselined gauze.

5633–5645.1 ANTISEPSIS; ASEPSIS

See also 6267–6281, Puerperal Fever.

5633 LABARRAQUE, Antoine Germain. 1777–1850
De l'emploi des chlorures d'oxide de sodium et de chaux. Paris, *Mme Hazard*, 1825.
First chlorine solution for disinfecting purposes. English translation, 1826.

5634 LISTER, Joseph, 1*st Baron Lister*. 1827–1912
On a new method of treating compound fracture, abscess, etc., with observations on the conditions of suppuration. *Lancet*, 1867, **1,** 326–29, 357–59, 387–89, 507–09; **2,** 95–96.
Lister's first work on the antiseptic principle in surgery. He believed that bacteria could enter wounds and cause suppurtation and putrefaction and that it was necessary to kill the bacteria already in wounds and to apply dressings impregnated with some bactericidal substance. He finally hit on carbolic acid for this purpose. When this work was done it had not yet been proved that bacteria were the cause of disease. The above work is reprinted in *Med. Classics*, 1937, **2**, 28–71.

5635 ——. On the antiseptic principle in the practice of surgery. *Lancet*, 1867, **2,** 353–56, 668–69.
Having realized the significance of Pasteur's work on fermentation, Lister evolved the idea of the antiseptic prevention of wound infection. This and the preceding entry represent two of the most epoch-making contributions to surgery. The paper is reprinted in *Med. Classics*, 1937, **2**, 72–83.

5636 LUCAS-CHAMPIONNIÈRE, Just Marie Marcellin. 1843–1913
Chirurgie antiseptique. Paris, *J. B. Baillière*, 1876.

Lucas-Championnière, eminent French surgeon, was one of the first to adopt the principles of Listerism. He wrote the first authoritative work on antiseptic surgery and introduced antisepsis into France.

5637 NEUBER, Gustav Adolf. 1850–1932
Die aseptische Wundbehandlung in meinen chirurgischen Privat-Hospitälern. Kiel, *Lipsius u. Tischer*, 1886.

The first attempts at asepsis were made by Neuber.

5638 BERGMANN, Ernst von. 1836–1907
Zur Sublimatfrage. *Therap. Mh.*, 1887, **1**, 41–44.

Bergmann wsa a pioneer in the evolution of asepsis. His corrosive sublimate method of antisepsis was gradually merged into steam sterilization and the present-day elaborate ritual of asepsis.

5639 TARNIER, Stéphane. 1828–1897
De l'asepsie et antisepsie en obstétrique. Paris, *G. Steinheil*, 1894.

Tarnier was the first to adopt Listerism in obstetrics. In the discussion following a paper in *Trans. int. med. Congr.*, London, 1881, **4**, 390–91, he showed that he was the first to employ carbolic acid solution in obstetrics.

5640 HALSTED, William Stewart. 1852–1922
Johns Hopk. Hops. Rep., 1894, **4**, plate XII.

Depicts the use of rubber gloves during an operation by Halsted. In a later paper (*J. Amer. med. Ass.*, 1913, **60**, 1123–24) he gives some account of this, from which it appears that he was responsible for this innovation.

5641 BERGER, Paul. 1845–1908
De l'emploi du masque dans les opérations. *Bull. Soc. Chirurgiens Paris*, 1899, n.s., **25**, 187–96.

Introduction of the gauze face mask, October 1897.

5642 CARREL, Alexis. 1873–1944, *et al.*
Traitement abortif de l'infection des plaies. *Bull. Acad. Méd. (Paris)*, 1915, 3 sér., **74**, 361–68.

Carrel–Dakin treatment of wounds. With Dakin, Daufresne, Dehelly, and Dumas.

5643 DAKIN, Henry Drysdale. 1880–1952
On the use of certain antiseptic substances in the treatment of infected wounds. *Brit. med. J.*, 1915, **2**, 318–20.

"Dakin's solution" was employed by Carrel (No. 5642) in the Carrel–Dakin method of irrigation of wounds.

5644 MORISON, James Rutherford. 1853–1939
The treatment of infected suppurating war wounds. *Lancet*, 1916, **2**, 268–72.

Introduction of "Bipp" in the treatment of wounds.

5645 JENSEN, Nathan Kenneth. 1910–   , *et al.*
Local implantation of sulfanilamide in compound fractures. *Surgery*, 1939, **6**, 1–12.

Sulphonamide dressing of wounds. With L. W. Johnsrud and M. C. Nelson.

5645.1 LUFT, Rolf, & OLIVECRONA, Herbert. 1891–
Experiences with hypophysectomy in man. *J. Neurosurg.*, 1953, **10,** 301–16.

Demonstration of the beneficial effect of hypophysectomy in cancer of the breast and of the testis.

5646–5733.1 SURGICAL ANAESTHESIA

5646 DAVY, *Sir* Humphry. 1778–1829
Researches, chemical and philosophical, chiefly concerning nitrous oxide. London, *J. Johnson*, 1800.

Davy discovered the anaesthetic properties of nitrous oxide and suggested its use during surgical operations, a suggestion which was not turned to useful account until 1844. Reprinted, London, *Butterworths*, 1972.

5647 HICKMAN, Henry Hill. 1800–1830
A letter on suspended animation, containing experiments showing that it may be safely employed during operations on animals, with the view of ascertaining its probable utility in surgical operations on the human subject. Ironbridge, *W. Smith*, 1824.

Hickman was the first to prove that the pain of surgical operations could be abolished by the inhalation of a gas. He rendered animals unconscious, first through partial asphyxiation by the exclusion of air, then by inhalation of carbon dioxide. He amputated limbs without pain and with good surgical results. His work, the first in the field of surgical anaesthesia, was received with apathy, and no use was made of it. His "Letter" is re-published in the *Hickman centenary volume*, published by the Wellcome Historical Medical Museum, London, 1930.

5648 GUTHRIE, Samuel. 1782–1848
New mode of preparing a spirituous solution of chloric ether. *Amer. J. Sci. Arts*, 1832, **21,** 64–65; **22,** 105–06.

Guthrie, Liebig, and Soubeiran discovered chloroform independently of one another. Guthrie discovered the modern method of making chloroform by distilling alcohol with chlorinated lime. The second paper has title: On pure chloric ether.

5649 SOUBEIRAN, Eugène. 1793–1858
Recherches sur quelques combinaisons du chlore. *Ann. Chim. (Paris)*, 1831, **48,** 113–57.

Soubeiran, like Liebig and Guthrie, discovered chloroform; it is difficult to determine priority as each may have allowed an interval of time to elapse between discovery and publication.

5650 LIEBIG, Justus von. 1803–1873
Ueber die Verbindungen, welche durch die Einwirkung des Chlors auf Alkohol, Aether, ölbildenes Gas und Essiggeist entstehen. *Ann. Pharm. (Lemgo)*, 1832, **1,** 182–230.

Discovery, in 1831, of chloroform and chloral.

5651 BIGELOW, Henry Jacob. 1818–1890
Insensibility during surgical operations produced by inhalation. *Boston med. surg. J.*, 1846, **35,** 309–17, 379–82.

Morton used ether as an anaesthetic for the first time on October 16, 1846, and it became recognized that complete anaesthesia could be produced by the inhalation of ether vapour. Bigelow has left an excellent account in the above paper, which was read before the Boston Society of Medical Improvement on Nov. 9, 1846, an abstract having been previously read before the American Academy of Arts and Sciences on Nov. 3.

5652 MORTON, William Thomas Green. 1819–1868
Circular. Morton's Letheon. Boston, *Dutton & Wentworth*, [1846].

Unaware of Long's results with ether, Morton discovered independently its anaesthetic effects. At first he tried to patent his discovery and published the above circular, in which he called his anaesthetic by the name of "Letheon". Fortunately Bigelow had detected the nature of Morton's discovery; his paper (No. 5651) soon spread the news throughout the world.

5653 ——. Remarks on the proper mode of administering sulphuric ether by inhalation. Boston, *Dutton & Wentworth*, 1847.

Morton announced that his method of producing anaesthesia was obtained by the inhalation of sulphuric ether. He subsequently gave up a lucrative practice in order to devote himself to the study of surgical anaesthesia and the dissemination of information concerning it. He spent more than £20,000 in furthering the use of ether, and in so doing reduced himself to poverty. His sacrifice was recognized when a national subscription was organized in the U.S.A. in order to pay his debts and to assure him of comfort during the last years of his life.

5654 FLOURENS, Marie Jean Pierre. 1794–1867
Note touchant l'action de l'éther sur les centres nerveux. *C. R. Acad. Sci. (Paris)*, 1847, **24**, 340–44.

On March 8, 1847, Flourens announced that chloroform had an anaesthetic effect analogous to that of ether. Little notice seems to have been taken of his paper, but later in the year Simpson independently demonstrated the value of chloroform.

5655 PIROGOV, Nikolai Ivanovich. 1810–1881
Nouveau procédé pour produire, au moyen de la vapeur d'éther, l'insensibilité chez les individus soumis à des opérations chirurgicales. *C. R. Acad. Sci. (Paris)*, 1847, **24,** 789.

Pirogov was the first to practise rectal etherization, suggested by Roux earlier in 1847.

5656 ——. Recherches pratiques et physiologiques sur l'éthérisation. St. Pétersbourg, *Imprimerie Française,* 1847.

Pirogov, the great military surgeon, was with Syme the first in Europe to adopt ether anaesthesia, and he left an interesting account of his experiences with it.

5657 SIMPSON, *Sir* James Young. 1811–1870
Discovery of a new anaesthetic agent, more efficient than sulphuric ether. *Lond. med. Gaz.*, 1847, n.s., **5,** 934–37; *Lancet*, 1847, **2,** 549.

In an attempt to find an anaesthetic less irritating than ether, Simpson discovered the advantages of chloroform. He had previously used ether with great benefit in midwifery, but now substituted chloroform, being the first to do so. Preliminary announcement in *Lond. med. Gaz.*, 1847, n.s. **5**, 906.

5658 SNOW, John. 1813–1858
On the inhalation of the vapour of ether in surgical operations. London, *J. Churchill*, 1847.

Includes an account of Snow's regulating inhaler, the first to control the amount of ether vapour received by the patient. Snow forecast this apparatus in *Lond. med. Gaz.*, 1847, n.s. **4**, 156.

5659 SYME, James. 1799–1870
On the use of ether in the performance of surgical operations. *(Lond. Edinb.) Month. J. med. Sci.*, 1847–48, **8,** 73–76.

Syme was, with Pirogov, the first in Europe to adopt ether anaesthesia in surgical operations.

5660 WELLS, Horace. 1815–1848
A history of the discovery of the application of nitrous oxide gas, ether, and other vapours, to surgical operations. Hartford, *J. G. Wells*, 1847.

In 1844 Wells, a Hartford dentist, successfully used nitrous oxide as a dental anaesthetic. To publicise his discovery he arranged a demonstration at Harvard Medical School, but this proved a fiasco. Wells eventually committed suicide by opening a vein in his arm and at the same time inhaling ether vapour.

5661 CHANNING, Walter. 1786–1876
A treatise on etherization in childbirth. Boston, *W. D. Ticknor & Co.*, 1848.

Channing was an early advocate of anaesthesia in obstetrics. In his book, and in several earlier papers, he brought the importance of this branch of anaesthetics into the foreground.

5662 HEYFELDER, Johann Ferdinand Martin. 1798–1869
Die Versuche mit dem Schwefeläther, Salzäther und Chloroform. Erlangen, *C. Heyder*, 1848.

Introduction of ethyl chloride in anaesthesia.

5663 SNOW, John. 1813–1858
On the inhalation of chloroform and ether. With description of an apparatus. *Lancet*, 1848, **1**, 177–80.

Snow's chloroform inhaler.

5664 LONG, Crawford Williamson. 1815–1878
An account of the first use of sulphuric ether by inhalation as an anaesthetic in surgical operations. *South. med. surg. J.*, 1849, **5**, 705–713.

There is no doubt that Long was the first successfully to use ether vapour as an anaesthetic. This was on March 30, 1842, at Jefferson, Georgia. Unfortunately he did not publish his results until others, notably Morton, had independently introduced it. See also No. 5731, also the biography of Long by Frances Long Taylor, New York, 1928.

5665 SNOW, John. 1813–1858
On narcotism by the inhalation of vapours. *Lond. med. Gaz.*, 1850, n.s., **11**, 749–54; 1851, n.s., **12**, 622–27.

Snow attempted carbon dioxide absorption.

5666 ——. On chloroform and other anaesthetics: their action and administration. London, *J. Churchill*, 1858.

Snow, a pioneer anaesthetist, delivered Queen Victoria with the aid of chloroform in 1853 and 1857. His book is classical; his work put the administration of chloroform and ether on a scientific basis. Snow also investigated amylene, which he was the first to administer. Reproduced in facsimile, 1950.

5667 FISCHER, E.
Ueber die Einwirkung von Wasserstoff auf Einfach-Chlorkohlenstoff. *Jena, Z. Naturw.*, 1864, **1**, 123–24.

Discovery of trichlorethylene.

5668 JUNKER, Ferdinand Ethelbert.
Description of a new apparatus for administering narcotic vapours. *Med. Times Gaz.*, 1867, **2**, 590; 1868, **1**, 171–73.

Junker's chloroform inhaler.

5669 ANDREWS, Edmund. 1824–1904
The oxygen mixture; a new anesthetic combination. *Med. Examiner*, 1868, **9,** 656–61.
Andrews advocated the use of an oxygen-nitrous oxide mixture.

5669.1 TRENDELENBURG, Friedrich. 1844–1924
Beiträge zu den Operationen an den Luftwegen. *Arch. klin. Chir.*, 1871, **12,** 112–33.
Endotracheal anaesthesia by means of a tracheostomy.

5670 LABBÉ, Leon. 1832–1916, & GUYON, E.
Sur l'action combinée de la morphine et du chloroforme. *C. R. Acad. Sci. (Paris)*, 1872, **74,** 627–29.
Labbé and Guyon developed pre-anaesthetic medication.

5671 CLOVER, Joseph Thomas. 1825–1882
Description of a new double current inhaler for administering ether. *Brit. med. J.*, 1873, **1,** 282–83.
Clover's gas-ether inhaler.

5672 ORÉ, Pierre Cyprien.
De l'anesthésie produite chez l'homme par les injections de chloral dans les veines. *C. R. Acad. Sci. (Paris)*, 1874, **78,** 515–17, 651–54.
First successful human intravenous anaesthesia. Oré, professor of physiology at Bordeaux, reported the successful use of this method in animals in *Bull. Soc. Chir. Paris*, 1872, 3 sér., 1, 400–12. See also his monograph on the subject, Paris, 1875.

5673 BERNARD, Claude. 1813–1878
Leçons sur les anesthésiques et sur l'asphyxie. Paris, *J. B. Baillière*, 1875.
As early as 1864 Bernard discovered that chloroform anaesthesia could be prolonged and intensified by the injection of morphine. J. N. von Nussbaum also observed this.

5674 CLOVER, Joseph Thomas. 1825–1882
On an apparatus for administering nitrous oxide gas and ether, singly or combined. *Brit. med. J.*, 1876, **2,** 74–75.
Clover's ether inhaler. See also the same journal, 1877, **1**, 69. He invented an inhaler in 1862; this was described, but not by Clover, in *Med. Times Gaz.*, 1862, 2, 149.

5675 ANREP, Vasili Konstantinovich. 1852–?
Ueber die physiologische Wirkung des Cocain. *Pflügers Arch. ges. Physiol.*, 1880, **21,** 38–77.
Anrep studied the action of cocaine and, like Moréno y Maiz, suggested its use as a local anaesthetic.

5676 MACEWEN, *Sir* William. 1848–1924
Clinical observations on the introduction of tracheal tubes by the mouth instead of performing tracheotomy or laryngotomy. *Brit. med. J.*, 1880, **2,** 122–24, 163–65.
First administration of an anaesthetic (chloroform) through a metal tracheal tube introduced by the mouth (endotracheal anaesthesia).

5677 FREUND, August von. 1835–1892
Über Trimethylene. *Mh. Chem.*, 1882, **3,** 625–35.
Cyclopropane (trimethylene) first prepared.

5678 KOLLER, Carl. 1857–1944
Vorläufige Mittheilung über locale Anästhesirung am Auge. *Klin. Mbl. Augenheilk.*, 1884, **22,** Beilageheft, 60–63.

Introduction of cocaine as a local anaesthetic; this was the first local anaesthetic employed (Sept. 16, 1884). Freud is by some accredited with this innovation, but in this connection see the letter by Koller in *J. Amer. med. Ass.*, 1941, **117**, 1284. English translation in *Arch. Ophthal.* (*Chicago*), 1934, **12**, 473–74.

5679 HALSTED, William Stewart. 1852–1922
Practical comments on the use and abuse of cocaine; suggested by its invariably successful employment in more than a thousand minor surgical operations. *N.Y. med. J.*, 1885, **42,** 294–95.

The first experiments on local infiltration anaesthesia were made by Halsted, who even produced anaesthesia by the intradermal injection of water.

5680 CORNING, James Leonard. 1855–1923
Spinal anaesthesia and local medication of the cord. *N.Y. med. J.*, 1885, **42,** 483–85.

Spinal anaesthesia introduced. See also Corning's earlier paper in the same journal, 1885, **42**, 317–19.

5681 PERNICE, Ludwig.
Ueber Cocainanästhesie. *Dtsch. med. Wschr.*, 1890, **16,** 287–89.

Max Oberst's method of conduction anaesthesia was first reported by Pernice, his pupil.

5682 HEWITT, *Sir* Frederic William. 1857–1916
Anaesthetics and their administration. London, *C. Griffin & Co.*, 1893.

Hewitt, anaesthetist to Edward VII, did much to develop the use of ether, and advanced our knowledge of the pharmacology of anaesthetics. In 1892 he introduced the first practical gas and oxygen apparatus.

5683 SCHLEICH, Carl Ludwig. 1859–1922
Zur Infiltrationsanästhesie. *Ther. Mh.*, 1894, **8,** 429–36.

Infiltration anaesthesia was developed by Schleich after pioneer work by Halsted (No. 5679). Schleich published a paper in English on the subject in *Int. Clin.*, 1895, 5 ser., **2**, 177–92.

5684 BIER, August Karl Gustav. 1861–1949
Versuche über Cocainisirung des Rückenmarkes. *Dtsch. Z. Chir.*, 1899, **51,** 361–69.

Bier introduced the use of cocaine as a spinal anaesthetic.

5685 EINHORN, Alfred. 1856–1917
Ueber die Chemie der localen Anaesthetica. *Münch. med. Wschr.*, 1899, **46,** 1218–20, 1254–56.

Synthesis of procaine (novocaine).

5685.1 MEYER, Hans Horst. 1853–1939
Zur Theorie der Alkoholnarkose. Erste Mitteilung. *Arch. exp. Path. Pharmak.*, 1899, **42,** 109–18.

Meyer's theory of narcosis.

5686 CATHELIN, Fernard. 1873–
Une nouvelle voie d'injection rachidienne. Méthode des injections épidurales par le procédé du canal sacré. Applications à l'homme. *C. R. Soc. Biol.* (*Paris*), 1901, **53,** 452–53.

Caudal anaesthesia.

5687 CRILE, George Washington. 1864–1943
On the physiologic action of cocain and eucain when injected into tissues. In his *Experimental and clinical research into certain problems relating to surgical operations.* Philadelphia, 1901, 88–163.
Anaesthetic blocking of nerve trunks.

5688 OVERTON, Charles Ernest. 1865–1933
Studien über die Narkose. Jena, *G. Fischer*, 1901.
Overton developed the lipid theory of narcosis.

5689 CUSHING, Harvey Williams. 1869–1939
On the avoidance of shock in major amputations by cocainization of large nerve-trunks preliminary to their division. *Ann. Surg.*, 1902, **36,** 321–45.
W. S. Halsted was first to use infiltration anaesthesia (see No. 5679) and it was later developed by Cushing.

5690 FOURNEAU, Ernest. 1872–1949
Stovaine, anesthésique locale. *Bull. Soc. Pharmacol.* (*Paris*), 1904, **10,** 141–48.
Introduction of stovaine, 1903.

5691 BRAUN, Heinrich Friedrich Wilhelm. 1862–1934
Die Lokalanästhesie, ihre wissenschaftliche Grundlagen und praktische Anwendung. Leipzig, *J. A. Barth*, 1905.
Braun's important book on local anaesthesia greatly stimulated the development of that subject.

5692 ——. Ueber einige neue örtliche Anaesthetica (Stovain, Alypin, Novocain). *Dtsch. med. Wschr.*, 1905, **31,** 1667–71.
Procaine (novocaine), synthesized by Einhorn, was first used clinically by Braun.

5693 KUHN, Franz. 1866–1929
Perorale Tubagen mit und ohne Druck. *Dtsch. Z. Chir.*, 1905, **76,** 148–207.
Kuhn introduced the intratracheal insufflation method of anaesthetization about 1900; he used a flexible metal tube and a curved introducer. He also experimented with positive and negative pressure insufflation.

5694 MELTZER, Samuel James. 1851–1920, & AUER, John. 1875–1948
Continuous respiration without respiratory movements. *J. exp. Med.*, 1909, **11,** 622–25.
Meltzer and Auer experimented further with the intratracheal insufflation method introduced by Kuhn (No. 5693).

5695 ELSBERG, Charles Albert. 1871–1948
Zur Narkose beim Menschen mittelst der kontinuierlichen intratrachealen Insufflation von Meltzer. *Berl. klin. Wschr.*, 1910, **47,** 957–58.
The clinical introduction of Meltzer and Auer's method of intratracheal insufflation marks the beginning of modern endotracheal anaesthesia. Also reported in *Ann. Surg.*, 1910, **52**, 23–29.

5696 LEHMANN, KARL BERNHARD. 1858–1940
Experimentelle Studien über den Einfluss technisch und hygienisch wichtiger Gase und Dämpfe auf den Organismus. Die gechlorten Kohlenwasserstoffe der Fettreihe. *Arch. Hyg. (Berl.)*, 1911, **74,** 1–60.
Introduction of trichlorethylene ("trilene").

5697 McKESSON, ELMER ISAAC. 1881–
Nitrous oxid-oxygen anaesthesia. With a description of a new apparatus. *Surg. Gynec. Obstet.*, 1911, **13,** 456–62.
Intermittent gas-oxygen machine.

5698 COTTON, FREDERIC JAY. 1869–1938, & BOOTHBY, WALTER MEREDITH. 1880–1953
Nitrous oxide-oxygen-ether anesthesia: notes on administration; a perfected apparatus. *Surg. Gynec. Obstet.*, 1912, **15,** 281–89.
Boothby and Cotton's flowmeter.

5699 GWATHMEY, JAMES TAYLOR. 1865–1944
Oil-ether anaesthesia. *N.Y. med. J.*, 1913, **98,** 1101–04.
Gwathmey produced anaesthesia by injection into the rectum of liquid ether with olive oil dissolved in it (synergistic anaesthesia).

5700 BOYLE, HENRY EDMUND GASKIN. 1875–1941
Nitrous oxide-oxygen-ether outfit. *Proc. roy. Soc. Med.*, 1917–18, **11,** Sect. Anaesth., 30.
Boyle's continuous-flow anaesthetic machine.

5701 KAPPIS, MAX. 1881–1938
Zur Technik der Splanchnicusanästhesie. *Zbl. Chir.*, 1920, **47,** 98.
Splanchnic anaesthesia. See also *Dtsch. Med. Wschr.*, 1920, **46**, 535.

5702 PAGÉS MIRAVÉ, FIDEL. ?–1924
Anestesia metamérica. *Rev. Sanid. milit. (Madr.)*, 1921, **11,** 351–65, 389–96.
Introduction of peridural anaesthesia.

5703 ROWBOTHAM, EDGAR STANLEY. 1890– , & MAGILL, *Sir* IVAN WHITESIDE. 1888–
Anaesthetics in the plastic surgery of the face and jaws. *Proc. roy. Soc. Med.*, 1921, **14,** Sect. Anaesth., 17–27.
Further improvement of the endotracheal inhalation method of anaesthetization.

5704 LABAT, GASTON LOUIS. 1877–1934
Regional anesthesia: its technic and clinical application. Philadelphia, *W. B. Saunders*, 1922.

5705 LUCKHARDT, ARNO BENEDICT. 1885–1957, & CARTER, JAY BAILEY. 1898–
Physiologic effects of ethylene; a new gas anesthetic. *J. Amer. med. Ass.*, 1923, **80,** 765–70.
Introduction of ethylene.

5706 PAGE, IRVINE HEINLY. 1901–
Isoamyl ethyl barbituric acid – an anesthetic without influence on blood sugar regulation. *J. Lab. clin. Med.*, 1923, **9,** 194–96.
Sodium amytal described.

5707 HENDERSON, YANDELL. 1873–1944
A lecture on respiration in anaesthesia: control by carbon dioxide. *Brit. med. J.*, 1925, **2,** 1170–75.

Henderson's important investigations on the physiology of respiration included his demonstration of the relation of acapnia to anaesthesia and the recommendation that carbon dioxide inhalation be used to overcome collapse due to anaesthesia.

5708 EICHHOLTZ, FRITZ. 1889–
Ueber rektale Narkose mit Avertin (E 107). *Dtsch. med. Wschr.*, 1927, **53,** 710–12.

Experimental use of "avertin" (tribromethanol).

5709 BUTZENGEIGER, O.
Klinische Erfahrungen mit Avertin (E 107). *Dtsch. med. Wschr.*, 1927, **53,** 712–13.

First clinical use of "avertin".

5710 KIRSCHNER, MARTIN. 1879–1942
Eine psycheschonende und steuerbare Form der Allgemeinbetäubung. *Chirurg*, 1929, **1,** 673–82.

Intravenous use of "avertin".

5711 LUCAS, GEORGE HERBERT WILLIAM. 1894– , & HENDERSON, VELYIEN EWART. 1877–1945
A new anaesthetic gas: cyclopropane. A preliminary report. *Canad. med. Ass. J.*, 1929, **21,** 173–75.

5712 ZERFAS, LEON GROTIUS. 1897– , *et al.*
Induction of anesthesia in man by intravenous injection of sodium iso-amyl-ethyl barbiturate. *Proc. Soc. exp. Biol.* (*N.Y.*), 1929, **26,** 399–403.

Sodium amytal. With J. T. C. McCallum, H. A. Shonle, E. E. Swanson, J. B. Scott, and G. H. A. Clowes.

5712.1 FITCH, RICHARD HOMER. 1903– , *et al.*
The intravenous use of the barbituric acid hypnotics in surgery. *Amer. J. Surg.*, 1930, **9,** 110–14.

Intravenous use of pentobarbitone sodium. With R. M. Waters and A. L. Tatum.

5713 LEAKE, CHAUNCEY DEPEW. 1896– , & CHEN, MEI-YU.
The anesthetic properties of certain unsaturated ethers. *Proc. Soc. exp. Biol.* (*N.Y.*), 1930, **28,** 151–54.

Demonstration of the anaesthetic properties of divinyl ether.

5714 WEESE, HELLMUT. 1897–1954, & SCHARPFF, WALTHER.
Evipan, ein neuartiges Einschlafmittel. *Dtsch. med. Wschr.*, 1932, **58,** 1205–07.

Introduction of evipan (evipal).

5715 GELFAN, SAMUEL. 1903– , & BELL, I. R.
The anesthetic action of divinyl oxide on humans. *J. Pharmacol.*, 1933, **47,** 1–3.

Clinical application of divinyl ether.

5716 JACKSON, DENNIS EMERSON. 1878–
A study of anesthesia and analgesia, with special reference to such substances as trichlorethylene and vinesthene (divinyl ether), together with apparatus for their administration. *Curr. Res. Anesth.*, 1934, **13,** 198–203.

Experimental use of trichlorethylene as anaesthetic.

5717 STILES, JOHN ALDEN. 1905– , *et al.*
Cyclopropane as an anesthetic agent: a preliminary clinical report. *Curr. Res. Anesth.*, 1934, **13,** 56–60.

First clinical use of cyclopropane. With W. B. Neff, E. A. Rovenstine, and R. M. Waters.

5718 WATERS, RALPH MILTON. 1883– , & SCHMIDT, ERWIN RUDOLPH. 1890–
Cyclopropane anesthesia. *J. Amer. med. Ass.*, 1934, **103,** 975–83.

Closed circuit method.

5719 KING, HAROLD. 1887–1956
Curare. *Nature (Lond.)*, 1935, **135,** 469–70.

Isolation from curare of *d*-tubocurarine chloride.

5720 LUNDY, JOHN SILAS. 1894–
Intravenous anesthesia: preliminary report of the use of two new thiobarbiturates. *Proc. Mayo Clin.*, 1935, **10,** 536–43.

Introduction of thiopentone sodium.

5721 STRIKER, CECIL. 1897– , *et al.*
Clinical experiences with the use of trichlorethylene in the production of over 300 analgesias and anesthesias. *Curr. Res. Anesth.*, 1935, **14,** 68–71.

Human anaesthetization with trichlorethylene. With S. Goldblatt, I. S. Warm, and D. E. Jackson.

5722 LEMMON, WILLIAM THOMAS. 1896–
A method of continuous spinal anesthesia. A preliminary note. *Ann. Surg.*, 1940, **111,** 141–44.

Continuous spinal analgesia introduced.

5723 EPSTEIN, HANS GEORG, *et al.*
The Oxford vaporiser No. 1. *Lancet*, 1941, **2,** 62–64.

With R. R. Macintosh and K. Mendelssohn. The Oxford vaporiser No. 2 is described in the same journal, pp. 64–66, by S. L. Cowan, R. D. Scott, and S. F. Suffolk.

5724 GRIFFITH, HAROLD RANDALL. 1894– , & JOHNSON, G. ENID.
The use of curare in general anesthesia. *Anesthesiology*, 1942, **3,** 418–20.

Introduction of curare in anaesthesia.

5725 BOVET, DANIEL. 1907– , *et al.*
Propriétés curarisantes du di-iodoéthylate de *bis*-[quinoléyloxy-8'] 1.5-pentane. *C. R. Acad. Sci. (Paris)*, 1946, **223,** 597–98.

Introduction of gallamine triethiodide ("flaxedil"). With S. Courvoisier, R. Ducrot, and R. Horclois. See also the same journal, 1947, **225,** 74.

5726 PATON, William Drummond Macdonald. 1917– , & ZAIMIS Eleanor. 1915–
Curare-like action of polymethylene *bis*-quaternary ammonium salts. *Nature* (*Lond.*), 1948, **161,** 718–19.
Methonium compounds. See also the same journal, 1948, **162,** 810.

5727 ——. The pharmacological actions of polymethylene bistrimethylammonium salts. *Brit. J. Pharmacol.*, 1949, **4,** 381–400.
Introduction of hexamethonium bromide.

5728 BOVET, Daniel. 1907– , *et al.*
Proprietà farmacodinamiche di alcuni derivati della succinilcolina dotati di azione curarica. Esteri di trialchiletanolammonio di acidi bicarbossilici alifatici. *R. C. Ist. sup. Sanità*, 1949, **12,** 106–37.
Introduction of succinylcholine chloride. With F. Bovet-Nitti, S. Guarino, V. G. Longo, and M. Marotta.

5729 BRÜCKE, H., *et al.*
Bis-Cholinester von Dicarbonsäuren als Muskelrelazantien in der Narkose. *Wien. klin. Wschr.*, 1951, **63,** 464–66.
Clinical use of succinylcholine chloride. With K. H. Ginzel, H. Klupp, F. Pfaffenschlager, and G. Werner.

5729.1 RAVENTÓS, J.
The action of fluothane – a new volatile anaesthetic. *Brit. J. Pharmacol.*, 1956, **11,** 394–410.
Halothane ("fluothane") a non-inflammable and non-irritant anaesthetic, was synthesized by C. W. Suckling at the I.C.I. Laboratories in Manchester. It was introduced clinically by M. Johnstone (*Brit. J. Anaesth.*, 1956, **28**, 392–410).

History of Anaesthesia

5730 BIGELOW, Henry Jacob. 1818–1890
Ether and chloroform: a compendium of their history and discovery. Boston, *D. Clapp*, 1848.
Bigelow's speedy publication of Morton's discovery, and his subsequent advocacy of ether assured its adoption throughout the civilized world. The above work deals with the priority claims in general and with a defence of Morton's claim in particular.

5731 YOUNG, Hugh Hampton. 1870–1945
Long, the discoverer of anaesthesia. A presentation of his original documents. *Johns Hopk. Hosp. Bull.*, 1897, **8,** 174–84.
Documents presented by Young leave no doubt that C. W. Long was the first, in 1842, to use ether as an anaesthetic (see also No. 5664).

5732 KEYS, Thomas Edward. 1908–
The history of surgical anesthesia. New York, *Schuman's*, 1945.
Reprinted with corrections and additions, 1963.

5733 DUNCUM, Barabara Mary.
The development of inhalation anaesthesia, with special reference to the years 1846–1900. London, *Oxford Univ. Press*, 1947.
Publications of the Wellcome Historical Medical Museum, New series, No. 2.

5733.1 COLE, Frank. 1909–
Milestones in anesthesia. Readings in the development of surgical anesthesia, 1665–1940. Lincoln, *University of Nebraska Press*, 1965.
First-hand accounts of discoveries and advances in anaesthesia.

5734–5768 GRAFTS; PLASTIC SURGERY

5734 TAGLIACOZZI, GASPARE. 1545–1599
De curtorum chirurgia per insitionem. Venetiis, *apud G. Bindonum, jun.*, 1597.

Tagliacozzi of Bologna became famous for his work on rhinoplasty, of which he was a pioneer, but Paré and Fallopius both abused him and his work, and the Church (which regarded such operations as meddling with the work of God) exhumed his body and reburied it in unconsecrated ground. Italian translation, Bologna, 1964. Tagliacozzi first described his work in G. Mercuriali's *De decoratione*, Francofurti, 1587. Biography of Tagliacozzi by Martha T. Gnudi and J. P. Webster, New York, 1950.

5735 MEEKEREN, JOB JANSZOON VAN. 1611–1666
Heel- en geneeskonstige aanmerkkingen. Amsterdam, *C. Commelijn*, 1668.

Van Meekeren was first to record a bone graft. He states (Chap. 1) that he read a report of it in a letter received by the Rev. Engebert Sloot of Slooterdijk from John Kraanwinkel, a missionary in Russia, where the operation had been performed. It consisted of the transplantation of a piece of bone from a dog's skull into a cranial defect in a soldier. Although healing was perfect, the Church ordered the removal of the graft. German translation of the book, 1675; Latin translation, 1682.

5736 BARONIO, GIUSEPPE. 1759–1811
Degli innesti animali. Milano, *stemp. e fond. del Genio*, 1804.

Baronio was among the first to attempt transplantation and experimental surgery in animals. He successfully carried out free transplants of pieces of skin as large as 12.5 × 7.5 cm.

5737 CARPUE, JOSEPH CONSTANTINE. 1764–1846
An account of two successful operations for restoring a lost nose from the integuments of the forehead. London, *Longman, Hurst, etc.*, 1816.

Carpue revived the Hindu method of rhinoplasty, as chronicled in the Suśruta Samhita, and reported two successful cases.

5738 GRAEFE, CARL FERDINAND VON. 1787–1840
Rhinoplastik. Berlin, *G. Reimer*, 1818.

Graefe was the founder of modern plastic surgery. He developed the operations of rhinoplasty and blepharoplasty. He was professor of surgery at Berlin, 1810–40.

5739 ——. Die Gaumennath, ein neuentdecktes Mittel gegen angeborene Fehler der Sprache. *J. Chir. Augenheilk.*, 1820, **1**, 1–54.

Graefe devised an operation for the treatment of congenital cleft palate.

5739.1 STEPHENSON, JOHN. 1797–1842
Dissertatio chirurgo-medica inauguralis de velosynthesi. Edinburgi, *J. Moir*, 1820.

Stephenson, a medical student, was the first to be operated upon by Roux (No. 5741) for the repair of cleft palate. He described the operation in his graduation thesis. For translations see *J. Hist. Med.*, 1963, **18**, 209–19, and *Brit. J. plast. Surg.*, 1966, **19**, 1–14.

5740 DIEFFENBACH, JOHANN FRIEDRICH. 1792–1847
Nonnula de regeneratione et transplantatione. Herbipoli, *typ. Richterianis*, 1822.

Dieffenbach's thesis for the degree of M.D., Würzburg.

5741 ROUX, Philibert Joseph. 1780–1854
Mémoire sur la staphyloraphie, ou la suture du voille du palais. *Arch. gén. Méd.*, 1825, **7**, 516–38.

First staphylorrhaphy. Reported earlier by the patient himself (see No. 5739.1).

5742 WARREN, John Collins. 1778–1856
On an operation for the cure of natural fissure of the soft palate. *Amer. J. med. Sci.*, 1828, **3**, 1–3.

Warren introduced the operation of staphylorrhaphy for the treatment of fissure of the soft palate. It was at one of Warren's classes at Harvard Medical School that Wells was allowed to demonstrate nitrous oxide, in January 1845.

5743 DIEFFENBACH, Johann Friedrich. 1792–1847
Chirurgische Erfahrungen, besonders über die Wiederherstellung zerstörter Theile des menschlichen Körpers nach neuen Methoden. 3 vols. [in 4] and atlas. Berlin, *T. C. F. Enslin*, 1829–34.

Dieffenbach was professor of surgery in Berlin. He was a pioneer in the field of plastic and orthopaedic surgery, performing tenotomy and skin-grafting successfully.

5744 AMMON, Friedrich August von. 1799–1861
Die plastische Chirurgie. Berlin, *G. Reimer*, 1842.

5745 WARREN, Jonathan Mason. 1811–1867
Operations for fissure of the hard and soft palate. *New Engl. quart. J. Med. Surg.*, 1842–43, **1**, 538–47.

Warren devised an operation for fissure of the hard and soft palates.

5746 JOBERT DE LAMBALLE, Antoine Joseph. 1799–1867
Traité de chirurgie plastique. 2 vols. and atlas. Paris, 1849.

5747 HAMILTON, Frank Hastings. 1813–1886
Elkoplasty, or anaplasty applied to the treatment of old ulcers. New York, *Holman, Gray & Co.*, 1854.

Hamilton was among the first to treat ulcers by skin-grafting.

5748 LANGENBECK, Bernhard Rudolph Conrad von. 1810–1887
Die Uranoplastik mittelst Ablösung des mucös-periostalen Gaumenüberzuges. *Arch. klin. Chir.*, 1862, **2**, 205–87.

Langenbeck has several operations named after him, one of the most important being that for cleft palate.

5749 SIMON, Gustav. 1824–1876
Beiträge zur plastischen Chirurgie. Prag, *C. Reichendecker*, 1868.

5750 REVERDIN, Jacques Louis. 1842–1929
Greffe épidermique. Expérience faite dans le service de M. le docteur Gryon à l'hôpital Necker. *Bull. Soc. imp. Chir. Paris*, (1869), 1870, 2 sér., **10**, 511–15.

Reverdin's work on the transplantation of free skin, as contrasted with the previous method of pedunculated flaps, attracted much attention.

5751 LAWSON, George. 1831–1903
On the transplantation of portions of skin for the closure of large granulating surfaces. *Trans. clin. Soc. Lond.*, 1871, **4**, 49–53.

Lawson, surgeon to the Middlesex Hospital, London, was the first successfully to transplant sizeable areas of skin, as compared with the small grafts of Reverdin, and of whole thickness skin as well.

5752 OLLIER, Louis Xavier Edouard Léopold. 1830–1900
Greffes cutanées ou autoplastiques. *Bull. Acad. Méd.* (*Paris*), 1872, 2 sér., **1,** 243–50.
First description of intermediate thickness skin grafts. Ollier used large grafts and carried out complete excision of scar tissue and its replacement with skin.

5753 THIERSCH, Carl. 1822–1895
Ueber die feineren anatomischen Veränderungen bei Aufheilung von Haut auf Granulationen. *Verh. dtsch. Ges. Chir.*, 1874, **3,** 69–75.
Thiersch's first paper on transplantation of skin.

5754 WOLFE, John Reissberg. 1824–1904
A new method of performing plastic operations. *Brit. med. J.*, 1875, **2,** 360–61.
Wolfe insisted that in free skin grafts the subcutaneous tissue at the site of the graft must be removed, and that the graft should consist of skin only. His name is perpetuated in the "Wolfe–Krause graft rest".

5755 KRAUSE, Fedor. 1856–1937
Ueber die Transplantation grosser ungestielter Hautlappen. *Verh. dtsch. Ges. Chir.*, 1893, **22,** pt. 2, 46–51.
Krause popularized the use of whole thickness skin grafts.

5756 MORESTIN, Hippolyte. 1869–1919
De l'ablation esthétique des tumeurs bénignes du sein. *Presse med.*, 1902, **10,** 975–77.
Morestin's method of mammaplasty. He was also responsible for several of the techniques employed in maxillo-facial surgery. Reprinted, Pittsburgh, 1959.

5756.1 DAVIS, John Staige. 1872–1946
A method of splinting skin grafts. *Ann. Surg.*, 1909, **49,** 416–18.
The Davis graft was devised by Halsted but Davis popularized its use.

5756.2 GUTHRIE, Charles Claude. 1880–1963
Blood-vessel surgery and its applications. London, *E. Arnold*, 1912.
This book describes Guthrie's pioneer work in tissue and organ transplantation.

5757 ALBEE, Fred Houdlett. 1876–1945
Bone-graft surgery. Philadelphia, *W. B. Saunders Co.*, 1915.
Albee was the first to employ living bone grafts as internal splints. He used cutting machines and saws to make inlaid, perfectly fitting grafts. See especially his "Transplantation of a portion of the tibia into the spine for Pott's disease. A preliminary report," *J. Amer. med. Ass.*, 1911, **57**, 885–86.

5758 GILLIES, *Sir* Harold Delf. 1882–1960
Plastic surgery of the face. London, *H. Frowde*, 1920.
Gillies introduced the tubed pedicle flap in 1918.

5759 ——, & FRY, *Sir* William Kelsey. 1889–
A new principle in the surgical treatment of "congenital cleft palate", and its mechanical counterpart. *Brit. med. J.*, 1921, **1,** 335–38.
Gillies' operation for cleft palate.

5760 KRASKE, Hans.
Die Operation der atrophischen und hypertrophischen Hängebrust. *Munch. med. Wschr.*, 1923, **70,** 672.
Plastic operation for enlarged breasts.

5761 WARDILL, William Edward Mandall. 1894–1960
Cleft palate. *Brit. J. Surg.*, 1928, **16,** 127–48.
Wardill's operation for cleft palate.

5761.1 BLAIR, Vilray Papin. 1871–1955, & BROWN, James Barrett. 1899–
The use and uses of large split skin grafts of intermediate thickness. *Surg. Gynec. Obstet.*, 1929, **49,** 82–97.
Split-skin grafts introduced.

5762 BIESENBERGER, Hermann.
Deformitäten und kosmetische Operationen der weiblichen Brust. Wien, *W. Maudrich*, 1931.

5763 VEAU, Victor. 1871–1949
Division palatine. Paris, *Masson*, 1931.
Includes Veau's operation for cleft palate.

5763.1 PADGETT, Earl Calvin. 1893–1946
Calibrated intermediate skin grafts. *Surg. Gynec. Obstet.*, 1939, **69,** 779–93.
Padgett dermatome.

5764 INCLAN, Alberto Francis. 1916–
The use of preserved bone grafts in orthopaedic surgery. *J. Bone Jt Surg.*, 1942, **24,** 81–96.
These studies form the basis of the modern use of bone preserved by refrigeration.

5765 SANO, Machteld Elisabeth. 1903–
Skin grafting. A new method based on the principles of tissue culture. *Amer. J. Surg.*, 1943, **61,** 105–06.
First use of fibrin glue for skin grafting. See also *Surg. Gynec. Obstet.*, 1943, **77,** 510–13.

5766 THOREK, Max. 1880–1960
Plastic surgery of the breast and abdominal wall. Springfield, *C. C. Thomas*, 1942.

History of Plastic Surgery

5767 ZEIS, Eduard. 1807–1868
Die Literatur and Geschichte der plastischen Chirurgie. Leipzig, *W. Engelmann*, 1863.
Nachträge, 1864. Photographic reprint, including Nachträge, Bologna, 1963.

5768 MALTZ, Maxwell. 1899–
Evolution of plastic surgery. New York, *Froben Press*, 1946.

5769–5788 DISEASES OF THE BREAST

5769 COOPER, *Sir* Astley Paston, *Bart.* 1768–1841
Illustrations of the diseases of the breast. London, *Longman, Rees & Co.*, 1829.
Includes one of the earliest descriptions of hyperplastic cystic disease of the breast, which Cooper referred to as "hydatid disease".

5770 BRODIE, *Sir* BENJAMIN COLLINS, *Bart.* 1783–1862
Lecture on sero-cystic tumors of the breast. *Lond. med. Gaz.*, 1840, **25,** 808–14.

"Brodie's tumour." Reprinted in *Med. Classics*, 1938, **2**, 941–54.

5771 VELPEAU, ALFRED ARMAND LOUIS MARIE. 1795–1867
Traité des maladies du sein et de la région mammaire. Paris, *V. Masson*, 1854.

Velpeau was the leading French surgeon of the first half of the 19th century. His great treatise on tumours of the breast, his best work, was the most important of its time on the subject. It includes a good account of hyperplastic cystic disease of the breast. English translation, 1856.

5772 PAGET, *Sir* JAMES, *Bart.* 1814–1899
On disease of the mammary areola preceding cancer of the mammary gland. *St. Barth. Hosp. Rep.*, 1874, **10,** 87–89.

First description of "Paget's disease of the nipple" – eczema of the nipple with cancer. The paper is reprinted in *Med. Classics*, 1936, **1**, 75–78. Paget was Serjeant Surgeon to Queen Victoria, and a great surgical pathologist. He was associated with St. Bartholomew's Hospital during most of his life.

5773 BILLROTH, CHRISTIAN ALBERT THEODOR. 1829–1894
Die Krankheiten der Brustdrüsen. Stuttgart, *F. Enke*, 1880.

5774 RECLUS, PAUL. 1847–1914
La maladie kystique des mamelles. *Bull. Soc. Anat. Paris*, 1883, **58,** 428–33.

"Reclus's disease." Reclus was professor of surgery in Paris; he left a classical description of chronic cystic mastitis.

5775 SCHIMMELBUSCH, CURT. 1860–1895
Das Cystadenom der Mamma. *Arch klin. Chir.*, 1892, **44,** 117–34.

"Schimmelbusch's disease."

5776 HALSTED, WILLIAM STEWART. 1852–1922
The treatment of wounds with especial reference to the value of the blood clot in the management of dead spaces. *Johns Hopk. Hosp. Rep.*, 1890–91, **2,** 255–314.

Contains description of Halsted's method of radical mastectomy – one of the greatest contributions ever made to the treatment of mammary cancer. Halsted was one of the leading American surgeons of modern times; he was the first to operate wearing rubber gloves.

5777 ——. The results of operations for the cure of cancer of the breast performed at the Johns Hopkins Hospital from June, 1889 to January, 1894. *Johns Hopk. Hosp. Rep.*, 1894–95, **4,** 297–350.

Reprinted in *Med. Classics*, 1938, **3**, 441–509.

5778 ——. A clinical and histological study of certain adenocarcinomata of the breast, and a brief consideration of the supraclavicular operations for cancer of the breast from 1889 to 1898 at Johns Hopkins Hospital. *Trans. Amer. surg. Ass.*, 1898, **16,** 144–81.

5778.1 BEATSON, *Sir* GEORGE THOMAS. 1848–1933
On the treatment of inoperable cases of carcinoma of the mamma: suggestions for a new method of treatment, with illustrative cases. *Lancet*, 1896, **2,** 104–07, 162–65.

Öophorectomy in the treatment of breast cancer.

5779 BEATSON, *Sir* GEORGE THOMAS. 1848–1933
The treatment of cancer of the breast by oöphorectomy and thyroid extract. *Brit. med. J.*, 1901, **2,** 1145–48.

5780 BLOODGOOD, JOSEPH COLT. 1867–1935
Senile parenchymatous hypertrophy of female breast. *Surg. Gynec. Obstet.*, 1906, **3,** 721–30.

Bloodgood's theory of the causation of chronic mastitis.

5781 CORNIL, ANDRÉ VICTOR. 1837–1908
Les tumeurs du sein. Paris, *F. Alcan*, 1908.

5782 HANDLEY, WILLIAM SAMPSON. 1872–1962
Cancer of the breast and its treatment. 2nd ed. London, *J. Murray*, 1922.

Sampson Handley advanced the theory that in mammary cancer metastasis is due to extension along lymphatic vessels – "lymphatic permeation" – and not to dissemination by way of the blood stream. The book was first published in 1906.

5783 DARTIGUES, LOUIS. 1869–1940
Mammectomie totale et autogreffe libre aréolomamelonnaire; mammectomie bilatérale esthétique. *Bull. Soc. Chirurgiens Paris*, 1928, **20,** 739–44.

The modern operation of total bilateral mammectomy, with transplantation of the nipple and areola, was especially developed by Dartigues.

5784 CHEATLE, *Sir* GEORGE LENTHAL. 1865–1951, & CUTLER, MAX. 1899–
Tumours of the breast. Their pathology, symptoms, diagnosis, and treatment. London, *E. Arnold & Co.*, 1931.

5785 CUTLER, MAX. 1899–
The cause of "painful breasts" and treatment by means of ovarian residue. *J. Amer. med. Ass.*, 1931, **96,** 1201–05.

Cutler was the first to employ ovarian hormone systematically in the treatment of chronic mastitis.

5786 KEYNES, *Sir* GEOFFREY LANGDON. 1887–
The radium treatment of carcinoma of the breast. *Brit. J. Surg.*, 1932, **19,** 415–80.

5787 LACASSAGNE, ANTOINE MARCELLIN. 1884–1971
Apparition de cancers de la mamelle chez la souris mâle, soumise à des injections de folliculine. *C. R. Acad. Sci.* (*Paris*), 1932, **195,** 630–632.

Demonstration of the carcinogenic effect of ovarian hormone.

5788 ADAIR, FRANK EARL. 1887–
Plasma cell mastitis – a lesion simulating mammary carcinoma. *Arch. Surg.* (*Chicago*), 1933, **26,** 735–49.

First description of plasma-cell mastitis.

History of Surgery

5789 HALLER, ALBRECHT VON. 1708–1777
Bibliotheca chirurgica. 2 vols. Bernae & Basileae, *Haller & Schweighauser*, 1774–75.

5790 MALGAIGNE, Joseph François. 1806–1865
Histoire de la chirurgie en Occident depuis de VIe jusqu'au XVIe siècle, et histoire de la vie et des travaux d'Ambroise Paré. Paris, *J. B. Baillière,* [1840].
Billings considered Malgaigne "the greatest surgical historian and critic the world has ever seen"; Leonardo (No. 5812) says that his greatest contribution to surgery was his unique manner of evaluating surgical techniques and innovations by which the then new methods of statistical computation were conjoined with actual surgical experiments.

5791 GRÜNDER, Johann Wilhelm Ludwig. 1819–1866
Geschichte der Chirurgie von den Urzeiten bis zu Anfang des achtzehnten Jahrhunderts. Breslau, *Trewendt & Granier,* 1859.

5792 TRENDELENBERG, Friedrich. 1844–1924
De veterum Indorum chirurgia. Berolini, *G. Schade,* [1866].
Trendelenburg's graduation thesis.

5793 FERGUSSON, *Sir* William. 1808–1877
Lectures on the progress of anatomy and surgery during the present century. London, *J. Churchill & Sons,* 1867.

5794 FISCHER, Georg. 1836–1921
Chirurgie vor 100 Jahren; historische Studie. Leipzig, *F. C. W. Vogel,* 1876.

5795 GROSS, Samuel David. 1805–1884
A century of American surgery. *Amer. J. med. Sci.,* 1876, n.s., **71,** 431–84.
Full account of American surgery to 1876.

5796 ROHLFS, Heinrich. 1827–1898
Die chirurgischen Classiker Deutschlands. 2 vols. Leipzig, *C. L. Hirschfeld,* 1883–85.

5797 SOUTH, John Flint. 1797–1882
Memorials of the craft of surgery in England . . . Edited by D'Arcy Power. London, *Cassell & Co.,* 1886.
South, trained in Germany, became surgeon to St. Thomas's Hospital. Through his efforts John Hunter's body was reburied in Westminster Abbey and South himself wrote the inscription on the tablet there.

5798 YOUNG, Sidney.
The annals of the Barber-Surgeons of London, compiled from their records and other sources. London, *Blades, East & Blades,* 1890.

5799 BILLINGS, John Shaw. 1838–1913
The history and literature of surgery. In F. S. Dennis: *System of surgery,* New York, 1895, **1,** 17–144.
One of the best histories of surgery in English.

5800 GURLT, Ernst Julius. 1827–1899
Geschichte der Chirurgie und ihrer Ausübung. 3 vols. Berlin, *A. Hirschwald,* 1898.
A history of surgery to the end of the 16th century.

5801 TILLMANNS, Robert Hermann. 1844–1927
Hundert Jahre Chirurgie. *Verh. Ges. dtsch. Naturf. Aerzte*, 1898, **70,** 1 Heft, 38–60.
History of 18th-century German surgery.

5802 BUSCHAN, Georg Hermann Theodor. 1863–1942
Chirurgisches aus der Völkerkunde. Leipzig, *B. Konegen*, 1902.

5803 ALLBUTT, *Sir* Thomas Clifford. 1836–1925
The historical relations of medicine and surgery to the end of the sixteenth century. London, *Macmillan & Co.*, 1905.
Considered by Garrison the best history of mediaeval surgery in English.

5804 HELFREICH, Friedrich. 1842–1927
Geschichte der Chirurgie. In T. Puschmann's *Handbuch der Geschichte der Medizin*, Jena, 1905, **3,** 1–306.
One of the best histories of the subject.

5805 SMITH, Stephen. 1823–1922
The evolution of American surgery. In *American practice of surgery*, edited by J. D. Bryant and A. H. Buck, New York, 1906, **2,** 1–67.

5806 MILNE, John Stewart. –1913
Surgical instruments in Greek and Roman times. Aberdeen, 1907.

5807 POWER, *Sir* D'Arcy. 1855–1941
A short history of surgery. London, *John Bale*, 1933.

5808 BLANCHARD, Charles Elton. 1868–
The romance of proctology, which is the story of the history and development of this much neglected branch of surgery. Youngstown, *Medical Success Press*, 1938.

5810 GRAHAM, Harvey [Isaac Harvey Flack]. 1912–
Surgeons all. London, *Rich & Cowan*, 1939.
American edition, *The Story of Surgery*, New York.

5811 THOMPSON, Charles John Samuel. 1862–1943
The history and evolution of surgical instruments. New York, *Schuman*, 1942.

5812 LEONARDO, Richard Anthony. 1895–
History of surgery. New York, *Froben Press*, 1943.

5813 KILLIAN, Hans. 1892– , & KRÄMER, G.
Meister der Chirurgie und die Chirurgenschulen im Deutschen Raum. Stuttgart, *G. Thieme*, 1951.

5813.1 BISHOP, William John. 1903–1961
A history of surgical dressings. Chesterfield, *Robinson & Sons*, 1959.
A short account of theories and practice in regard to surgical dressings from the earliest times.

5813.2 RANDERS-PEHRSON, Justine. 1910–
The surgeon's glove. Springfield, *C. C. Thomas*, 1960.
Contains an extensive bibliography.

5813.3 ZIMMERMAN, LEO M. 1898– , & VEITH, ILZA. 1915–
Great ideas in the history of surgery. Baltimore, *Williams & Wilkins*, 1961.

5813.4 WHIPPLE, ALLEN OLDFATHER. 1881–
The story of wound healing and wound repair. Springfield, *C. C. Thomas* [1963].

5813.5 ELLIOTT, ISABELLE MARY ZENA.
A short history of surgical dressings. London, *Pharmaceutical Press*, 1964.
Based on material collected by James Rawling Elliott (1905–1958).

5813.6 COPE, *Sir* VINCENT ZACHARY. 1881–1974
A history of the acute abdomen. London, *Oxford University Press*, 1965.

5813.7 HUARD, PIERRE ALPHONSE. 1901– , & GRMEK, MIRKO DRAŽEN.
Mille ans de chirurgie en occident: Ve–XVe siècles. Paris, *Roger Dacosta*, [1966].

5814–6007 OPHTHALMOLOGY

5814 AETIUS *of Amida*. A.D. 502–575
Die Augenheilkunde. Griechisch und Deutsch hrsg. von J. HIRSCHBERG. Leipzig, *Veit & Co.*, 1899.
Aetius left an exhaustive treatise on diseases of the eye. Although he did not describe cataract, he was familiar with 61 affections of the eye. Most of his work consists of compilations of earlier writers, but he recorded his own observations on ophthalmic therapeutics.

5815 'ALI IBN-'ISA [JESU HALY]. *circa* 940–1010
Memorandum book of a tenth-century oculist for the use of modern ophthalmologists. A translation of the Tadhkirat. First edition in English by CASEY A. WOOD. Chicago, *Northwestern University*, 1936.
The *Tadhkirat al-Kahhalin* was one of the oldest and best of the medieval Arabic works on ophthalmology. It carefully described 130 diseases of the eye and became the standard work on the subject in the Middle East. German translation, 1904.

5816 GRASSI, BENVENUTO [GRAPHEUS]. *fl.* 12th cent.
De oculis eorumque egritudinibus et curis. [Ferrara, *Severinus de Ferrara*, 1474].
The earliest printed book on ophthalmology. Grassi was the most celebrated ophthalmic surgeon of the Middle Ages. English translation by Casey A. Wood, 1229.

5817 BARTISCH, GEORG. 1535–1606
'Οφθαλμοδουλεία, das ist, Augendienst. Dresden, *M. Stöckel*, 1583.
Bartisch, the founder of modern ophthalmology, was a skilful operator and the first to practise the extirpation of the bulbus in cancer of the eye. The illustrations in his book form a comprehensive picture-book of Renaissance eye-surgery; some of the woodcuts show the parts of the eye lying successively one under the other, by means of pictures superimposed on each other like the pages of a book. Facsimile reprint, 1966.

5818 GUILLEMEAU, Jacques. 1550–1612
Traité des maladies de l'oeil. Paris, *chez Charles Massé*, 1585.
Garrison considers this the best of the Renaissance books on ophthalmology. Guillemeau was a pupil of Ambroise Paré; his book was an epitome of the existing knowledge on the subject, chiefly from Greek and Arabian sources.

5819 BAYLEY, Walter [Bailey; Baley]. 1529–1592
A briefe treatise touching the preseruation of the eie sight. [London, *R. Waldegrave*], 1586.
This is the first separate work on ophthalmology printed in England.

5820 BANISTER, Richard. *fl.* 1620
A treatise of one hundred and thirteene diseases of the eyes. London, *F. Kynaston for T. Man*, 1622.
Although much of this is a translation of Guillemeau, the first 112 pages are Banister's own work, "Banister's Breviary". He was an itinerant but honest oculist; he noted the hardness of the eye ball in glaucoma.

5821 DAZA DE VALDES, Benito. ?1591–?
Uso del los antojos para todo genero de vistas, en que se enseña a conocer los grados que a cada uno le faltan de su vista, y los que tienen qualesquier antojos. Sevilla, *Diego Perez*, 1623.
The earliest scientific work dealing with spectacles. It includes sight-testing tables and points out the value of convex lenses after cataract operations.

5822 BRIGGS, William. 1642–1704
Two remarkable cases relating to vision. *Phil. Trans.*, 1684, **14,** 561–65.
Includes the first known description of nyctalopia.

5823 STAHL, Georg Ernst. 1660–1734
De fistula lachrymali. [Halae Magdeburgi], 1702.
In this work the true cause of lachrymal fistula was for the first time expounded.

5824 MAÎTRE-JAN, Antoine [Maître-jean]. 1650–1730
Traité des maladies de l'oeil. Troyes, *J. le Febure*, 1707.
Called "the Father of French ophthalmology", Maître-Jan energetically supported Brisseau's doctrine, ensuring its acceptance. As far back as 1692 Maître-Jan had proved that the opaque lens is cataract, but before Brisseau's work appeared it had been regarded as a sort of skin or pellicle immediately inside the capsule of the lens.

5825 BRISSEAU, Michel. 1676–1743
Traité de la cataracte et du glaucoma. Paris, *L. d'Houry*, 1709.
Brisseau was the first to demonstrate the true nature and location of cataract. His book was reprinted in facsimile, 1921.

5826 ANEL, Dominique. 1679–1730
Observation singulière sur la fistule lacrimale, dans la quelle l'on verra, que la matière des fistules lacrimales s'évacuë très souvent par les points lacrimaux; en même tems l'on aprendra la méthode de les guérir radicalement, *etc.* Turin, *P. J. Zappatte*, 1713.
Lachrymal duct catheterized for the first time.

5827 SAINT-YVES, Charles de. 1667–1733
Nouveau traité des maladies des yeux. Paris, *P. A. Le Mercier*, 1722.
Records the removal of a cataract "en masse" from a living subject. English edition, 1741.

5828 CHESELDEN, William. 1688–1752

An account of some observations made by a young gentleman who was born blind, or lost his sight so early, that he had no remembrance of ever having seen, and was couch'd between 13 and 14 yrs. of age. *Phil. Trans.*, (1727–28), 1729, **35,** 447–52.

The versatile Cheselden made an artificial pupil in an eye in which the products of inflammation had closed or obscured the natural pupil. This iridotomy operation was, next to Daviel's cataract operation, the most important contribution to ophthalmology during the 18th century.

5829 DAVIEL, Jacques. 1696–1762

Sur une nouvelle méthode de guérir la cataracte par l'extraction du cristalin. *Mém. Acad. roy. Chir.* (*Paris*), 1753, **5,** 369–400.

Daviel originated the modern method of cataract by extraction of the lens.

5830 SHARP, Samuel. 1700–1778

A description of a new method of opening the cornea, in order to extract the crystaline humor. *Phil. Trans.*, (1753), 1754, **48,** 161–63, 322–31.

Sharp, a pupil of Cheselden, was the first to cut the cornea with a knife in operating for cataract; his suggestion that a special instrument be designed for this purpose led to the invention of several forms of "cataract knife".

5831 HEBERDEN, William, *Sr.* 1710–1801

Of the night-blindness or nyctalopia. *Med. Trans. Coll. Phys. Lond.*, 1768, **1,** 60–63.

A classical description of nyctalopia. Report of a single case.

5832 HUDDART, Joseph. 1741–1816

An account of persons who could not distinguish colours. *Phil. Trans.*, 1777, **67,** 260–65.

First reliable record of colour blindness. Written in the form of a letter to Joseph Priestley, who communicated it to the Royal Society.

5833 HAÜY, Valentin. 1745–1822

Essai sur l'education des aveugles. Paris, *Imp. d. Enf. Aveugles*, 1786.

Haüy founded the first school for the blind. To him belongs the honour of being the first to emboss paper as a means of reading for the blind. His *Essai* originated modern methods of teaching and caring for blind persons.

5834 DALTON, John. 1766–1844

Extraordinary facts relating to the vision of colours. *Mem. lit. phil. Soc. Manch.*, 1798, **5,** pt. 1, 28–45.

First scientific description of colour-blindness, or "Daltonism". Dalton himself suffered from red-green blindness. His paper was read to the Society in 1794.

5835 SCARPA, Antonio. 1747–1832

Saggio di osservazioni e d'esperienze sulle principali malattie degli occhi. Pavia, *B. Comino*, 1801.

This beautifully illustrated work was the first text-book on the subject to be published in the Italian language. Its author has been called "the father of Italian ophthalmology".

5836 SCHMIDT, Johann Adam. 1759–1809

Ueber Nachstaar und Iritis nach Staaroperationen. *Abhandl. k. k. med.-chir. Josephs-Acad. Wien*, 1801, **2,** 209–92.

Inflammation of the iris was named iritis by Schmidt. In 1801, with Himly, he founded the first journal devoted to ophthalmology, the *Ophthalmologische Bibliothek.*

5837 LARREY, Dominique Jean, *le baron*. 1766–1842
Mémoire sur l'ophtalmie régnante en Egypte. Kaire, an IX [1802].
The great military surgeon Larrey served during the Napoleonic campaign in Egypt, where he observed trachoma; he was the first to point out the contagious nature of this disease.

5838 SCHMIDT, Johann Adam. 1759–1809
Ueber die Krankheiten des Thränenorgans. Wien, *J. Geissinger*, 1803.
Schmidt was professor of ophthalmology at Vienna.

5839 VETCH, John. 1783–1835
An account of the ophthalmia which has appeared in England since the return of the British Army from Egypt. London, *Longman*, 1807.
Vetch described trachoma.

5840 WARDROP, James. 1782–1869
Essays on the morbid anatomy of the human eye. 2 vols. Edinburgh, *G. Ramsay & Co.*, 1808–18.
Wardrop was the first to classify the various inflammations of the eye according to the structures attacked. He was also the first to use the term "keratitis".

5841 LANGENBECK, Conrad Johann Martin. 1776–1851
Prüfung der Keratonyxis, einer neuen Methode den grauen Staar durch die Hornhaut zu recliniren oder zu zerstückeln. Göttingen, *J. F. Danckwerts*, 1811.
Langenbeck's operation of iridencleisis for construction of artificial pupil. He was professor of anatomy and surgery at Göttingen.

5842 BEER, Georg Joseph. 1763–1821
Lehre von den Augenkrankheiten. 2 vols. Wien, *Camesina*; *Heubner & Volke*, 1813–17.
Beer is remembered for his text-book; the doctrines in it dominated practice for many years. He described the symptoms of glaucoma and noted the luminosity of the fundus in aniridia. He was a distinguished iridectomist. Many of his pupils became famous ophthalmic surgeons. Beer opened the first known eye hospital, in 1786, in Vienna. He was the first Jew to graduate in Austria. First published as *Lehreder Augenkrankheiten*, 2 vols., Wien, 1792. English translation, Glasgow, 1821.

5843 TRAVERS, Benjamin. 1783–1858
A synopsis of the diseases of the eye. London, *Longman*, 1820.
The earliest systematic treatise in English on diseases of the eye. The book became the authority in Europe and America. Travers, a pupil of Sir Astley Cooper, became surgeon to St. Thomas's Hospital.

5844 FRICK, George. 1793–1870
A treatise on the diseases of the eye. Baltimore, *F. Lucas jnr.*, 1823.
First important American text-book of ophthalmology.

5845 GUTHRIE, George James. 1785–1856
Lectures on the operative surgery of the eye. London, *Burgess & Hill*, 1823.
Guthrie founded the Royal Westminster Ophthalmic Hospital, London, in 1816. He was the earliest teacher of the subject in the British Isles. The above includes important work on artificial pupil.

5846 REISINGER, Franz. 1787–1855
Ophthalmologische Versuche bey Thieren mit dem Hyoscyamin und Atropin. *Med.-chir. Ztg*, 1825, **1**, 237, 253.

Hyoscyamine and atropine first used in the examination of the eye. English translation in *Edinb. med. surg. J.*, 1826, **26**, 276–79.

5847 AIRY, *Sir* George Biddell. 1801–1892
On a peculiar defect in the eye, and a mode of correcting it. *Trans. Cambr. phil. Soc.* (1825), 1827, **2**, 267–73.

Airy drew attention to astigmatism from which he himself suffered, and he fitted cylindrical lenses for its correction.

5848 MACKENZIE, William. 1791–1868
A practical treatise on diseases of the eye. London, *Longman*, 1830.

In this book Mackenzie, one of the foremost ophthalmologists of his time, included a classical description of the symptomatology of glaucoma, and was probably the first to draw attention to the increase of intra-ocular pressure as a characteristic of the condition. He introduced the term "asthenopia", and was the first to describe sympathetic ophthalmia as a distinct disease.

5849 LAWRENCE, *Sir* William. 1783–1867
A treatise on the diseases of the eye. London, *J. Churchill*, 1833.

This comprehensive work marks an epoch in ophthalmic surgery. It is based on lectures delivered by Lawrence at the London Ophthalmic Infirmary. He was surgeon to St. Bartholomew's Hospital; he succeeded Abernethy as lecturer on surgery and did much to advance the surgery of the eye.

5850 JULLIARD, Étienne François.
De l'emploi de l'excision et de la cautérisation à l'aide du nitrate d'argent fondu dans l'ophthalmie blenorrhagique. Paris, *Thèse No.* 26, 1835.

Silver nitrate for treatment of gonococcal ophthalmia.

5851 BRAILLE, Louis. 1809–1852
Procédé pour écrire au moyen des points. Paris, 1837.

Braille, himself blind, modified the system of elevated points first suggested by Charles Barbier in 1820 for enabling the blind to read. His types are to-day used throughout the world.

5852 AMMON, Friedrich August von. 1799–1861
Klinische Darstellungen der Krankheiten und Bildungsfehler des menschlichen Auges, der Augenlider und der Thränenwerkzeuge nach eigenen Beobachtungen und Untersuchungen. 4 pts. Berlin, *G. Reimer*, 1838–47.

This great atlas is probably the best summary of the knowledge of diseases of the eye prior to the introduction of the ophthalmoscope.

5853 CARRON DU VILLARDS, Charles Joseph Frédéric. 1801–1860
Guide pratique pour l'étude et le traitement des maladies des yeux. 2 vols. Paris, *Soc. encycl.*, 1838.

Carron du Villards taught ophthalmology in Paris; his book is one of the best of the period.

5854 FERRALL, Joseph Michael [*afterwards* O'Ferrall]. 1790–1860
On the anatomy and pathology of certain structures in the orbit not previously described. *Dublin J. med. Sci.*, 1841, **19**, 329–56.

Ferrall's operation for enucleation of the eyeball (p. 354).

5855 BOLTON, JAMES. 1812–1869
A treatise on strabismus, with a description of new instruments designed to improve the operation for its cure. Richmond, Va., *P. D. Bernard*, 1842.

5856 DIEFFENBACH, JOHANN FRIEDRICH. 1792–1847
Ueber das Schielen und die Heilung desselben durch eine Operation. Berlin, *A. Förstner*, 1842.

The first successful attempt at treating strabismus by myotomy. The operation was later abandoned owing to the frequently disastrous final effects. A preliminary paper appeared in *Med. Ztg*, 1839, **8**, 227.

5857 HIMLY, CARL. 1772–1837
Die Krankheiten und Missbildungen des menschlichen Auges und deren Heilung. 2 vols. Berlin, *A. Hirschwald*, 1843.

Himly was professor of ophthalmology at Jena and later at Göttingen. He introduced clinical teaching in ophthalmology.

5858 KÜCHLER, HEINRICH. 1811–1873
Schriftnummerprobe für Gesichtsleidende. Darmstadt, *J. P. Diehl*, 1843.

Küchler introduced test readings of print at a distance, for examination of patients.

5859 BRÜCKE, ERNST WILHELM VON, *Ritter*. 1819–1892
Anatomische Untersuchungen über die sogenannten leuchtenden Augen bei den Wirbelthieren. *Arch. Anat. Physiol. wiss. Med.*, 1845, 387–406.

Von Brücke studied the luminosity of the eye in animals, and, by passing a tube through a candle flame, was able to see the fundus. See also the same journal, 1847, 225–27.

5860 WALTHER, PHILIPP FRANZ VON. 1782–1849
Ueber die Hornhautflecken. *J. Chir. Augenheilk.*, 1845, **34**, 1–90.

First description of corneal opacity.

5861 CUMMING, WILLIAM. 1812–1886
On a luminous appearance of the human eye, and its application to the detection of disease of the retina and posterior part of the eye. *Med.-chir. Trans.*, 1846, **29**, 283–96.

While a student at the London Hospital, Cumming, by shading the eye of a fellow student from the light, was able to look directly into it and obtained both the retinal reflex and the white light from the entrance of the optic nerve. He made the first suggestion for the construction of a device for examining the fundus.

5862 JONES, THOMAS WHARTON. 1808–1891
A manual of the principles and practice of ophthalmic medicine and surgery. London, *J. Churchill*, 1847.

5863 DESMARRES, LOUIS AUGUSTE. 1810–1882
Traité théorique et pratique des maladies des yeux. Paris, *Germer-Baillière*, 1847.

5864 ——. Opérations qui se pratiquent sur les yeux. Paris, [1850].

5865 ARLT, Carl Ferdinand von. 1812–1887
Die Krankheiten des Auges. 3 vols. Prag, *F. A. Credner & Kleinbub*, 1851–56.

Arlt described granular conjunctivitis ("Arlt's trachoma") and an operation for transplantation of the ciliary bulbs in the treatment of distichiasis.

5866 HELMHOLTZ, Hermann Ludwig Ferdinand von. 1821–1894
Beschreibung eines Augen-Spiegels zur Untersuchung der Netzhaut im lebenden Auge. Berlin, *A. Förstner*, 1851.

Invention of the ophthalmoscope, one of the greatest events in the history of ophthalmology. English translation by T. H. Shastid, 1916.

5867 BOWMAN, *Sir* William. 1816–1892
Observations on artificial pupil, with a description of a new method of operating in certain cases. *Med. Times Gaz.*, 1852, n.s., **4,** 11–14, 33–35.

Bowman devised an operation for the formation of an artificial pupil.

5868 SICHEL, Jules. 1802–1868
Iconographie ophthalmologique. 1 vol. and atlas. Paris, *J. B. Baillière*, 1852–59.

5869 STELLWAG VON CARION, Carl. 1823–1904
Die Ophthalmologie vom naturwissenschaftlichen Standpunkte aus bearbeitet. 2 vols. [in 3]. Freiburg, Erlangen, *Herder*, *F. Enke*, 1853–58.

English translation, 1868.

5870 TÜRCK, Ludwig. 1810–1868
Ein Fall von Hämorrhagie der Netzhaut beider Augen. *Z. k. k. Ges. Aerzte Wien*, 1853, **9,** 1 Abt., 214–18.

Türck was the first to note the correlation of retinal haemorrhage with tumours of the brain.

5871 GRAEFE, Friedrich Wilhelm Ernst Albrecht von. 1828–1870
Notiz über die Behandlung der Mydriasis. *v. Graefes Arch. Ophthal.*, 1854–55, **1,** 1 Abt., 315–19.

5872 ——. Vorläufige Notiz über das Wesen des Glaucoms. *v. Graefes Arch. Ophthal.*, 1854–55, **1,** 1 Abt., 371–82.

5873 ——. Ueber die Coremorphosis als Mittel gegen chronische Iritis und Iridochorioiditis. *v. Graefes Arch. Ophthal.*, 1855–56, **2,** 2 Abt., 202–57.

Graefe introduced iridectomy in the treatment of iritis and iridochoroiditis.

5874 JONES, Thomas Wharton. 1808–1891
Report on the ophthalmoscope. *Brit. for. med.-chir. Rev.*, 1854, **14,** 549–57.

Jones reported that Charles Babbage (1792–1871), the mathematician, had produced a simple ophthalmoscope in 1847.

5875 MECKEL VON HEMSBACH, Heinrich. 1822–1856
Die pyämische Ophthalmie in Beziehung zur feinsten Organisation des Entzündungs-Produkts und zu der eigenthümlichen Struktur des Glaskorpers. *Ann. Charité-Krankenh.*, 1854, **5,** 2 Heft, 276–89.

First account of metastatic ophthalmia.

5876 BENDZ, Jacob Christian. 1802–1858
Quelques considérations sur la nature de l'ophthalmie dite militaire, par rapport à son apparition dans l'armée danoise depuis 1851. *Ann. Oculist.* (*Brux.*), 1855, **33,** 164–76.
Description of trachoma.

5877 LIEBREICH, Richard. 1830–1917
Seitliche Beleuchtung und mikroskopische Untersuchung am lebenden Auge. *v. Graefes Arch. Ophthal.*, 1855, **1,** 2 Abt., 351–56.
Liebreich introduced lateral illumination in microscopic investigation of the living eye.

5878 WILLIAMS, Henry Willard. 1821–1895
Iritis – non-mercurial treatment. *Boston med. surg. J.*, 1856, **55,** 49–55, 69–74, 92–99.
The second and third papers are entitled "On the treatment of iritis without mercury".

5879 BOWMAN, *Sir* William. 1816–1892
On the treatment of lacrymal obstructions. *Ophthal. Hosp. Rep.*, 1857–59, **1,** 10–20, 88.

5880 GRAEFE, Friedrich Wilhelm Ernst Albrecht von. 1828–1870
Beiträge zur Lehre vom Schielen und von der Schiel-Operation. *v. Graefes Arch. Ophthal.*, 1857, **3,** 1 Abt., 177–286.
Graefe's operation for strabismus.

5881 ——. Ueber die Iridectomie bei Glaucom und über den glaucomatösen Process. *v. Graefes Arch. Ophthal.*, 1857, **3,** 2 Abt., 456–560; 1858, **4,** 2 Abt., 127–61; 1862, **8,** 2 Abt., 242–313.
Iridectomy for the treatment of glaucoma was introduced by Graefe.

5882 ——. Ueber Embolie der Arteria centralis retinae als Ursache plötzlicher Erblindung. *v. Graefes Arch. Ophthal.*, 1859, **5,** 1 Abt., 136–57.
Discovery of embolism of the retinal artery as a cause of sudden blindness.

5883 GRAEFE, Alfred Carl. 1830–1899
Klinische Analyse der Motilitätsstörungen des Auges. Berlin, *H. Peters*, 1858.
Alfred Carl Graefe, cousin of Albrecht, made a careful clinical analysis of disordered movements of the eye. He also invented a special "localization ophthalmoscope", and, with Saemisch, edited the great *Handbuch der gesamten Augenheilkunde* (see No. 5944).

5884 KNAPP, Hermann Jakob. 1831–1911
Die Krümmung der Hornhaut des menschlichen Auges. Heidelberg, *J. C. B. Mohr*, 1859.
Knapp wrote valuable monographs on curvature of the cornea (above) and on intraocular tumours (see No. 5902). He became one of the leading ophthalmologists in America.

5885 DEMARQUAY, Jean Nicholas. 1811–1875
Traité des tumeurs de l'orbite. Paris, *V. Masson*, 1860.

5886 GRAEFE, Friedrich Wilhelm Ernst Albrecht von. 1828–1870
Ueber Complication von Sehnervenentzündung mit Gehirnkrankheiten. *v. Graefes Arch. Ophthal.*, 1860, **7,** 2 Abt., 58–71.

Graefe showed that most cases of blindness and impaired vision connected with cerebral disorders are a result of optic neuritis rather than to paralysis of the optic nerve.

5887 JAEGER, Eduard, *Ritter von Jaxtthal.* 1818–1884
Schriftskalen. 3te. Aufl. Wien, *L. W. Seidel*, 1860.

Jaeger first introduced his test types in 1854; Emil Fuchs improved them in 1895.

5888 MITCHELL, Silas Weir. 1829–1914
On the production of cataract in frogs by the administration of sugar. *Amer. J. med. Sci.*, 1860, n.s., **39,** 106–10.

5889 DONDERS, Frans Cornelis. 1818–1889
Astigmatisme en cilindrische glazen. Utrecht, *Post*, 1862.

Includes statement of "Donders' law" – the rotation of the eye around the line of sight is not voluntary. French and German translations, 1862.

5890 SNELLEN, Hermann. 1834–1908
Probebuchstaben zur Bestimmung der Sehschärfe. Utrecht, *P. W. van de Weijer*, 1862.

Snellen's test-types ("Optotypi") which soon gained acceptance in all civilised countries.

5891 JACOBSON, Julius. 1828–1889
Ein neues und gefahrloses Operations-Verfahren zur Heilung des grauen Staares. Berlin, *Peters*, 1863.

Jacobson used a peripheral incision in his operation for cataract.

5892 LIEBREICH, Richard. 1830–1917
Atlas der Ophthalmoscopie. Darstellung des Augengrundes im gesunden und krankhaften Zustande enthalten. Berlin, *A. Hirschwald*, 1863.

First atlas of the fundus. Text in French and German. English translation by M. R. Swanzy, 1870 and 1884. Liebreich became ophthalmic surgeon to St. Thomas's Hospital, London.

5893 DONDERS, Frans Cornelis. 1818–1889
On the anomalies of accommodation and refraction of the eye . . . Translated from the author's manuscript by W. D. Moore. London, *New Sydenham Soc.*, 1864.

This work is of the highest importance in the field of physiological optics. It contains Donders' explanation of astigmatism, his definitions of aphakia and hypermetropia, his sharp distinctions between myopia and hypermetropia, etc.

5894 AGNEW, Cornelius Rea. 1830–1888
A method of operating for divergent squint. *Trans. Amer. ophthal. Soc.*, 1865–72, **1,** 3rd Ann. Mtg, 31–34.

Agnew devised an operation for the treatment of divergent squint.

5895 WILLIAMS, Henry Willard. 1821–1895
Suture of the flap, after extraction of cataract. *Trans. Amer. ophthal. Soc.*, 1865–72, **1,** 3rd Ann. Mtg, 45–46.

A method of suturing the flap after cataract extraction was introduced by Williams.

5896 PAGENSTECHER, ALEXANDER. 1828–1879
Ueber die Extraktion des grauen Staares bei uneröffneter Kapsel durch den Scleralschnitt. In *Klinische Beobachtungen aus der Augenheilanstalt zu Wiesbaden*, hrsg. von E. H. PAGENSTECHER u. T. SAEMISCH. Heft 3, 10–46. Wiesbaden, *J. Niedner*, 1866.

Extraction of the lens in the closed capsule through a scleral incision, for the treatment of cataract.

5897 GRAEFE, FRIEDRICH WILHELM ERNST ALBRECHT VON. 1828–1870
Ueber modificirte Linearextraction. *v. Graefes Arch. Ophthal.*, 1865, **11,** 3 Abt., 1–106; 1866, **12,** 1 Abt., 150–223; 1868, **14,** 3 Abt., 106–48.

Graefe's improvement of the operation for cataract by the modified linear extraction reduced the incidence of eye loss from 10 to 2·3%.

5898 ——. Zur Lehre der sympathischen Ophthalmie. *v. Graefes Arch. Ophthal.*, 1866, **12,** 2 Abt., 149–74.

A classical contribution to the literature of sympathetic ophthalmia.

5899 ——. Symptomenlehre der Augenmuskellähmungen. Berlin, *H. Peters*, 1867.

Graefe's monograph on the symptomatology of ocular paralyses forms the basis of modern knowledge on the subject.

5900 ——. Ueber Ceratoconus. *Berl. klin. Wschr.*, 1868, **5,** 241–44, 249–254.

Classical description of conical cornea (keratoconus).

5901 JAVAL, LOUIS EMILE. 1839–1907
Sur un nouvel instrument pour la détermination de l'astigmatisme. *Ann. Oculist. (Brux.)*, 1867, **57,** 39–43.

Javal invented the astigmometer, and described it in the above paper.

5902 KNAPP, HERMANN JAKOB. 1831–1911
Die intraocularen Geschwülste nach eigenen klinischen Beobachtungen und anatomischen Untersuchungen. Carlsruhe, *C. F. Müller*, 1868.

English translation, New York, 1869.

5903 HORNER, JOHANN FRIEDRICH. 1831–1886
Ueber eine Form von Ptosis. *Klin. Mbl. Augenheilk.*, 1869, **7,** 193–98.

"Horner's syndrome" – due to lesion of the cervical sympathetic. The same syndrome was evoked in animals by du Petit in 1727 (see No. 1313). It was also described by Claude Bernard, *Leçons sur la physiologie et la pathologie du système nerveux*, 1858, **2**, 473–74, and, less impressively, by E. S. Hare, *Lond. med. Gaz.*, 1838–39, **1**, 16–18.

5904 JAEGER, EDUARD, *Ritter von Jaxtthal.* 1818–1884
Ophthalmoskopischer Hand-Atlas. Wien, 1869.

A fine atlas which was for many years unsurpassed.

5905 SAEMISCH, EDWIN THEODOR. 1833–1909
Das Ulcus corneae serpens und seine Therapie. Bonn, *M. Cohen u. Sohn*, 1870.

First description of serpiginous ulcer of the cornea and its treatment. Called also "Saemisch's ulcer".

5906 LEBER, Theodor. 1840–1917
Ueber hereditäre und congenital-angelegte Sehnervenleiden. *v. Graefes Arch. Ophthal.*, 1871, **17,** 2 Abt., 249–91.
First description of hereditary optic atrophy, "Leber's optic atrophy".

5907 BERLIN, Rudolf. 1833–1897
Zur sogenannten Commotio retinae. *Klin. Mbl. Augenheilk.*, 1873, **11,** 42–78.
Berlin, professor of ophthalmology at Rostock, described the traumatic oedema of the retina which is sometimes referred to as "Berlin's oedema".

5908 CUIGNET, Ferdinand Louis Joseph. 1823–
Kératoscopie. *Rec. Ophtal.*, 1873–74, **1,** 14–23.
Introduction of the shadow test (retinoscopy), sometimes called "Cuignet's method".

5909 MOON, William. 1818–1894
Light for the blind: a history of the origin and success of Moon's system of reading . . . for the blind. London, 1873.
Moon became totally blind at the age of 22. He taught other blind persons and devised a simplified form of roman letters, embossed on paper, for use by blind readers. This was in 1845, and two years later he published his first book in Moon type.

5910 PAGENSTECHER, Ernst Hermann. 1844–1918, & GENTH, Carl Philipp. 1844–1904
Atlas der pathologischen Anatomie des Augapfels. Wiesbaden, *C. W. Kreidel*, 1873–75.
Text in German and English; Sir W. R. Gowers was responsible for the English translation.

5911 HOLMGREN, Alarik Frithiof. 1831–1897
Om den medfödda färgblindhetens diagnostik och teori. *Nord. med. Ark.*, 1874, **6,** Nr. 24, 1–21; Nr. 28, 1–35.
Holmgren introduced the wool-skein test for the diagnosis of colour-blindness.

5912 ARLT, Carl Ferdinand von. 1812–1887
Ueber die Verletzungen des Auges mit besonderer Rücksicht auf deren gerichtsärztliche Würdigung. Wien, *W. Braumuller*, 1875.
An important work dealing with the medico-legal aspects of eye injuries. English translation by C. S. Turnbull, 1878.

5913 LAQUEUR, Ludwig. 1839–1909
Ueber eine neue therapeutische Verwendung des Physostigmin. *Zbl. med. Wiss.*, 1876, **14,** 421–22.
Introduction of physostigmine in the treament of glaucoma.

5914 SAEMISCH, Edwin Theodor. 1833–1909
Der Frühjahrskatarrh. In Graefe and Saemisch: *Handbuch der gesammten Augenheilkunde*, Leipzig, 1876, **4,** Theil 2, 25–29.
First description of vernal conjunctivitis.

5915 FÖRSTER, Carl Friedrich Richard. 1825–1902
Beziehungen der Allgemein-Leiden und Organ-Erkrankungen zu Veränderungen und Krankheiten des Sehorgans. In Graefe and Saemisch: *Handbuch der gesammten Augenheilkunde*, Leipzig, 1877, **7,** Theil 5, 59–234.
Förster was among the first to study the relationship between eye disease and general and organic disease of the body.

5916 HOLMGREN, Alarik Frithiof. 1831–1897
Om färgblindheten i dess förhållande till jernvägstrafiken och sjöväsendet. *Upsala Lakaref. Förh.*, 1876–77, **12,** 171–251, 267–358.

A serious railway accident in Sweden in 1875 was believed by Holmgren to be due to colour-blindness, and resulted in the above important paper dealing with the condition and its relation to railway and maritime traffic. Translation in *Rep. Smithsonian Inst.*, 1877, Washington, 1878, 131–200.

5917 THOMSON, William. 1833–1907
On astigmatism as a cause for persistent headache and other nervous symptoms. *Med. News (Philad.)*, 1879, **27,** 81–88.

Thomson was a pioneer in the study of refraction. He was much interested in colour-blindness and modified Holmgren's wool-skein test. Himself affected with hypermetropia, he made important investigations on this condition, and (above) on astigmatism as a cause of headache.

5918 TAY, Waren. 1843–1927
Symmetrical changes in the region of the yellow spot in each eye of an infant. *Trans. ophthal. Soc. U.K.*, 1880–81, **1,** 55–57.

Tay was the first to describe amaurotic familial idiocy, his paper dealing mainly with the ocular manifestations. The condition later became known as "Tay–Sachs' disease" (see also No. 4705).

5919 WECKER, Louis de. 1832–1906, & LANDOLT, Edmond. 1846–1926
Traité complet de l'ophtalmologie. 4 vols. Paris, *Vve. A. Delahaye et Cie.*, 1880–89.

5920 JAVAL, Louis Emile. 1839–1907, & SCHIÖTZ, Hjalmar. 1850–1927
Un ophtalmomètre pratique. *Ann. Oculist. (Brux.)*, 1881, **86,** 5–21.

Javal and Schiötz here describe an ophthalmometer invented by them.

5921 DEUTSCHMANN, Richard. 1852–1935
Ein experimenteller Beitrag zur Pathogenese der sympathischen Augen-Entzündung. *v. Graefes Arch. Ophthal.*, 1882, **28,** 2 Abt., 291–300.

Deutschmann was the chief protagonist of the infective theory of sympathetic ophthalmia.

5922 PLACIDO DA COSTA, Antonio. 1849–1916
Neue Instrumente. *Zbl. prakt. Augenheilk.*, 1882, **6,** 30–31.

Introduction of the keratoscope.

5923 KOCH, Robert. 1843–1910
Bericht über die Thätigkeit der deutschen Cholerakommission in Aegypten und Ostindien. *Wien. med. Wschr.*, 1883, **33,** 1548–51.

Koch–Weeks bacillus. Koch discovered the bacilli of two varieties of Egyptian conjunctivitis. See also No. 5930.

5924 CREDÉ, Carl Sigmund Franz. 1819–1892
Die Verhütung der Augenentzündung der Neugeborenen. Berlin, *A. Hirschwald*, 1884.

Credé introduced the practice of instilling silver nitrate into the eyes of newborn infants as a preventive measure against ophthalmia neonatorum.

5925 KOLLER, Carl. 1857–1944
Vorläufige Mittheilung über locale Anästhesirung am Auge. *Klin. Mbl. Augenheilk.*, 1884, **22**, Beilageheft, 60–63.

Koller was first to demonstrate the practical value of cocaine as a local anaesthetic in ophthalmology.

5926 FUCHS, Ernst. 1851–1930
Die periphere Atrophie des Sehnerven. *v. Graefes Arch. Ophthal.*, 1885, **31**, 1 Abt., 177–200.

Peripheral atrophy of the optic nerve was described by Fuchs and called "Fuchs' optic atrophy".

5927 HIRSCHBERG, Julius. 1843–1925
Der Electromagnet in der Augenheilkunde. Leipzig, *Veit & Co.*, 1885.

The introduction of the electromagnet into ophthalmology. Hirschberg was one of the most voluminous writers in the field of ophthalmology. Besides his dictionary (see No. 5932) he wrote a classical history of the subject (see No. 5996) which to-day remains the authoritative work of reference on ophthalmology. He founded the *Centralblatt für praktische Augenheilkunde* in 1877.

5928 MULES, Philip Henry. 1843–1905
On the surgical, physiological, and aesthetic advantages of the artificial vitreous body. *Brit. med. J.*, 1885, **2**, 1153–55.

"Mules's operation", evisceration of the eyeball with insertion of artificial vitreous.

5929 PANAS, Photinos. 1832–1903
D'un nouveau procédé opératoire applicable au ptosis congénital et au ptosis paralytique. *Arch. Ophtal.*, 1886, **6**, 1–14.

An operation for congenital and paralytic ptosis was introduced by Panas.

5930 WEEKS, John Elmer. 1853–1949
The bacillus of acute conjunctival catarrh or "pink-eye". *Arch. Ophthal. (N.Y.)*, 1886, **15**, 441–51.

In 1883 Koch discovered the bacilli of two different forms of infectious conjunctivitis (Egyptian ophthalmia); in 1886 Weeks discovered the same organism to be the cause of "pink-eye". The organism has become known as the Koch–Weeks bacillus (see also No. 5923).

5931 COHN, Hermann Ludwig. 1828–1906
Die ärztliche Ueberwachung der Schulen zur Verhütung der Verbreitung der Kurzsichtigkeit. *Arb. VII. int. Congr. Hyg. Demogr.*, Wien, 1887–88, **1**, Heft 12, 9–28.

Cohn was a pioneer in his advocacy of the routine examination of the eyes of schoolchildren.

5932 HIRSCHBERG, Julius. 1843–1925
Wörterbuch der Augenheilkunde. Leipzig, *Veit & Co.*, 1887.

5933 HIPPEL, Arthur von. 1841–1917
Eine neue Methode der Hornhauttransplantation. *v. Graefes Arch. Ophthal.*, 1888, **34**, 1 Abt., 108–30.

Modern keratoplasty is based on the technique introduced by von Hippel.

5934 FUCHS, Ernst. 1851–1930
Keratitis punctata superficialis. *Wien. klin. Wschr.*, 1889, **2**, 837–41.
Epidemic keratoconjunctivitis first described.

5935 ——. Lehrbuch der Augenheilkunde. Leipzig u. Wien, *F. Deuticke*, 1889.
Fuchs' text-book was an outstanding contribution to the literature, and was translated into many languages. The last English edition appeared in 1933.

5936 PARINAUD, Henri. 1844–1905, & GALEZOWSKI, Xavier. 1832–1907
Conjonctivite infectieuse transmise par les animaux. *Ann. Oculist.* (*Brux.*), 1889, **101**, 252.
Parinaud described an infectious tuberculous conjunctivitis transmissible from animals to man. In 1924 Gifford suggested the name "Parinaud's oculo-glandular syndrome" as a more suitable description. See also *Rec. Ophtalmologie*, 1889, 3 sér., **11**, 176–80.

5937 EDRIDGE-GREEN, Frederick William. 1863–1953
Colour-blindness and colour-perception. London, *Kegan Paul, Trench, Trübner & Co.*, 1891.
Includes (p. 262 *et seq.*) description of Edridge-Green's lantern test for colour-blindness. This was officially adopted in Great Britain in 1915 in place of the Holmgren test.

5938 AXENFELD, Karl Theodor Paul Polykarpos. 1867–1930
Ueber die eitrige metastatische Ophthalmie, besonders ihre Aetiologie und prognostische Bedeutung. *v. Graefes Arch. Ophthal.*, 1894, **40**, Abt. 3, 1–129.
Classical account of metastatic ophthalmia.

5939 PARINAUD, Henri. 1844–1905
Conjonctivite lacrymale à pneumocoques des nouveau-nés. *Ann. Oculist.* (*Paris*), 1894, **112**, 369–73.

5940 HIPPEL, Eugen von. 1867–1939
Vorstellung eines Patientin mit einem sehr ungewöhnlichen Netzhaut-, beziehungsweise Aderhautleiden. *Ber. ophthal. Ges. Heidelb.*, 1895, **24**, 269.
First description of angiomatosis of the retina – "Hippel's disease".

5941 AXENFELD, Karl Theodor Paul Polykarpos. 1867–1930
Beiträge zur Aetiologie der Bindehautentzündungen. Ueber chronische Diplobacillenconjunctivitis. *Ber. ophthal. Ges. Heidelb.*, (1896), 1897, **25**, 140–55.
Description of the diplobacillary form of chronic conjunctivitis.

5942 MORAX, Victor. 1866–1935
Note sur un diplobacille pathogène pour la conjunctiva humaine. *Ann. Inst. Pasteur*, 1896, **10**, 337–45.
Morax and Axenfeld (No. 5941) independently isolated a diplobacillus which causes a chronic conjunctivitis – the Morax–Axenfeld haemophilus.

5943 SCHMIDT-RIMPLER, HERMANN. 1838–1915
Die Erkrankungen des Auges im Zusammenhang mit anderen Krankheiten. Wien, *A. Hölder*, 1898.

Like Förster, Schmidt-Rimpler was early interested in the relationship between eye diseases and general organic diseases; like Cohn, he was an advocate of the routine examination of the eyes of schoolchildren.

5944 GRAEFE, ALFRED CARL. 1830–1899, & SAEMISCH, EDWIN THEODOR. 1833–1909
Handbuch der gesamten Augenheilkunde. 2te. Aufl. 15 vols. [in 41]. Leipzig, *W. Engelmann*, 1899–1918.

The first edition of this great collective work, of which Graefe and Saemisch were the editors, appeared between 1874–80. A third edition is in progress.

5945 GULLSTRAND, ALLVAR. 1862–1930
Allgemeine Theorie der monochromatischen Aberrationen und ihre nächsten Ergebnisse für die Ophthalmologie. Upsala, *E. Berling*, 1900.

Gullstrand was professor of ophthalmology at Upsala. He was awarded the Nobel Prize in 1911. The above work is the exposition of his general theory of monochromatic aberrations.

5946 SMITH, HENRY. 1862–1948
Extraction of cataract in the capsule. *Indian med. Gaz.*, 1900, **35,** 241–46; 1901, **36,** 220–25; 1905, **40,** 327–30.

Smith, an officer in the Indian Medical Service, had remarkable success with his method of extraction of cataract within the capsule, one of the most important contributions of recent times. He modified his operation in 1926 (*Arch. Ophthal N.Y.*, **55**, 213–24).

5947 PARSONS, *Sir* JOHN HERBERT. 1868–1957
The pathology of the eye. 4 vols. London, *Hodder & Stoughton, Henry Frowde*, 1904–08.

5948 TOTI, ADDEO. 1861–
Nuovo metodo conservatore di cura radicale delle suppurazioni croniche del sacco lacrimale (dacriocistorinostomia). *Clin. mod. (Pisa)*, 1904, **10,** 385–87.

Toti's account of dacryoscytorhinostomy, a procedure he himself introduced.

5949 HEINE, LEOPOLD. 1870–
Die Cyklodialyse, eine neue Glaukomoperation. *Dtsch. med. Wschr.*, 1905, **31,** 824–26.

Introduction of cyclodialysis in glaucoma.

5950 MARKUS, CHARLES.
Notes on a peculiar pupil phenomenon in cases of partial iridoplegia. *Trans. ophthal. Soc. U.K.*, 1906, **26,** 50–56.

Markus was among the first to describe the condition known as "Adie's syndrome" (No. 4611).

5950.1 ZIRM, EDUARD KONRAD. 1863–1944
Eine erfolgreiche totale Keratoplastik. *v. Graefes Arch. Ophthal.*, 1806, **64,** 580–93.

First successful corneal transplantation (keratoplasty).

5951 HALBERSTAEDTER, Ludwig. 1876– , & PROWAZEK, Stanislaus Joseph Matthias von. 1875–1915
Über Zelleinschlüsse parasitärer Natur beim Trachom. *Arb. k. GesundhAmte*, 1907, **26,** 44–47.
Halberstaedter and Prowazek first described the cytoplasmic inclusion bodies of trachoma.

5952 HOLTH, Sören. 1863–1937
Iridencleisis antiglaucomatosa. *Ann. Oculist.* (*Paris*), 1907, **137,** 345–75.
Introduction of iridencleisis for glaucoma.

5953 LAGRANGE, Pierre Félix. 1857–1928
Nouveau traitement du glaucome chronique; iridectomie et sclérectomie combinée. *Gaz. hebd. Sci. méd. Bordeaux*, 1907, **28,** 2–4.
Sclerectomy for the treatment of glaucoma.

5954 COATS, George. 1876–1915
Forms of retinal disease with massive exudation. *Ophthal. Hosp. Rep.*, 1908, **17,** 440–525.
"Coats' disease" (retinitis circinata).

5955 ELLIOT, Robert Henry. 1864–1936
A preliminary note on a new operative procedure for the establishment of a filtering cicatrix in the treatment of glaucoma. *Ophthalmoscope*, 1909, **7,** 804–06.
The operation of sclero-corneal trephining for glaucoma was introduced by Elliot in 1909.

5956 STARGARDT, Karl Bruno. 1875–1927
Über Epithelzellveränderungen beim Trachom und andern Conjunctivalerkrankungen. *v. Graefes Arch. Ophthal.*, 1909, **69,** 525–42.
Demonstration of the inclusion bodies in ophthalmia neonatorum.

5957 ELSCHNIG, Anton. 1863–1939
Studien zur sympathischen Ophthalmie. 1. Wirkung von Antigenen vom Augeninnern aus. *v. Graefes Arch. Ophthal.*, 1910, **75,** 459–73.
Elschnig suggested the anaphylactic theory of the pathogenesis of sympathetic ophthalmia.

5958 HERBERT, Herbert. 1865–1942
The small flap incision for glaucoma. *Trans. ophthal. Soc. U.K.*, 1910, **30,** 199–215.
Herbert's small flap sclerotomy.

5959 HULEN, Vard Houghton. 1865–1939
Vacuum fixation of the lens and flap suture in the extraction of a cataract in its capsule. *J. Amer. med. Ass.*, 1911, **57,** 188–89.
Hulen devised a vacuum method of cataract extraction.

5960 BOTTERI, Albert. 1879–1955
Klinische, experimentelle und mikroskopische Studien über Trachom, Einschlussblenorrhöe und Frühjahrskatarrh. *Klin. Mbl. Augenheilk.*, 1912, **50,** i, 653–90.
Filtration of the virus of inclusion conjunctivitis.

5961 NICOLLE, Charles Jules Henri. 1866–1936, *et al.*
Le magot animal réactif du trachôme. Filtrabilité du virus. Pouvoir infectant des larmes. *C. R. Acad. Sci.* (*Paris*), 1912, **155,** 241–43.
Filtration of the trachoma virus. With L. Blaisot and A. Cuénod.

5962 PURTSCHER, Otmar. 1852–1927
Angiopathia retinae traumatica. Lymphorrhagien des Augengrundes. *v. Graefes Arch. Ophthal.*, 1912, **82,** 347–71.
"Purtscher's disease", traumatic angiopathy of the retina, first described.

5963 STANCULEANU, Gheorghe. 1874–
Intrakapsuläre Staroperationen. *Klin. Mbl. Augenheilk.*, 1912, **50,** 527–37.
Stanculeanu's technique for cataract extraction.

5964 KNAPP, Arnold Herman. 1869–
Report of one hundred successive extractions of cataract in the capsule after subluxation with the capsule forceps. *Arch. Ophthal.*, (*N.Y.*), 1915, **44,** 1–9.
Knapp's method of extraction of cataract with forceps. See also his later paper in the same journal, 1921, **50**, 426–30.

5965 BARRAQUER, Ignacio. 1884– , & ANDUYNED.
Un procédé d'extrême douceur pour l'extraction "in toto" de la cataracte. *Clin. Ophtal.*, 1917, **22,** 328–33.
Attempts to extract cataract by suction and aspiration date from ancient times. Barraquer employed a special machine of his own invention.

5966 ISHIHARA, Shinobu. 1879–
Tests for colour-blindness. Tokio, 1917.
Ishihara's colour tests. 15th ed., 1960.

5967 TSCHERNING, Marius Hans Erik. 1854–1939
L'adaptation compensatrice de l'oeil. *Ann. Oculist.* (*Brux.*), 1922, **159,** 625–37.
Introduction of the photometric spectacle lens.

5968 URIBE TRONCOSO, Manuel. 1867–
Gonioscopy and its clinical applications. *Amer. J. Ophthal.*, 1925, **8,** 433–49.
Troncoso's gonioscope.

5969 WOODS, Alan Churchill. 1889–
Diseases of the uvea. I. Sympathetic ophthalmia: the use of uveal pigment in diagnosis and treatment. *Trans. ophthal. Soc. U.K.*, 1925, **45,** 208–51.
Intradermal pigment test in sympathetic ophthalmitis.

5970 HAMBURGER, Carl. 1870–1944
Glaukosantropfen, Glaukom und Akkommodation. *Klin. Mbl. Augenheilk.*, 1926, **76,** 400–03.
Introduction of glaucosan.

5971 LINDAU, Arvid Vilhelm. 1892–
Studien über Kleinhirncysten. Bau, Pathogenese und Beziehungen zur Angiomatosis retinae. *Acta path. microbiol. scand.*, 1926, Suppl. **1.**
Lindau's important histological study of haemangiomatosis retinae ("Lindau's disease").

5972 GONIN, Jules. 1870–1935
Nouveaux cas de guérison opératoire de décollements rétiniens. *Ann. Oculist.* (*Paris*), 1927, **164,** 817–26.
Gonin's operation of ignipuncture for treatment of detachment of the retina.

5973 NOGUCHI, Hideyo. 1876–1928
Experimental production of a trachoma-like condition in monkeys by means of a micro-organism isolated from American Indian trachoma. *J. Amer. med. Ass.*, 1927, **89,** 739–42.
Isolation of *Bact. granulosis*, believed by Noguchi to be the causal organism in trachoma. See also his monograph in *J. exp. Med.*, 1928, **48**, Suppl. 2.

5974 VERHOEFF, Frederick Herman. 1874–
A new operation for removing cataracts with their capsules. *Trans. Amer. ophthal. Soc.*, 1927, **25,** 54–64.
Verhoeff's buttonhole iridectomy.

5975 ELSCHNIG, Anton. 1863–1939
Keratoplasty. *Arch. Ophthal.* (*N.Y.*), 1930, **4,** 165–73.
Elschnig developed the method of corneal grafting introduced by von Hippel (No. 5933) and produced good results on the human eye.

5976 HEINE, Leopold. 1870–
Ueber den Ausgleich sämtlicher Brechungsfehler des Auges durch geschliffene Haftgläser (unter den Lidern getragene Schalen). *Münch. med. Wschr.*, 1930, **77,** 6–7, 271–72.
The manufacture of modern contact glasses has been made possible by the work of Heine. See also his paper in *Lancet*, 1931, **1**, 631–32. For a brief history of this subject, see *Schweiz. med. Wschr.*, 1946, **76**, 719.

5977 LARSSON, Sven.
Operative Behandlung von Netzhautabhebung mit Elektroendothermie und Trepanation; vorläufige Mitteilung. *Acta ophthal.*, (*Kbh.*), 1930, **8,** 172–83.
Superficial diathermy treatment of retinal detachment. See also *Arch. Ophthal.* (*N.Y.*), 1932, **7**, 661–80.

5978 MOORE, Robert Foster. 1878–1963
Choroidal sarcoma treated by the intra-ocular insertion of radon needles. *Brit. J. Ophthal.*, 1930, **14,** 145–52.
Foster Moore's technique for the radiation treatment of choroidal neoplasms.

5979 THOMAS, *Sir* James William Tudor. 1893–
Transplantation of cornea: a preliminary report on a series of experments on rabbits. *Trans. ophthal. Soc. U.K.*, 1930, **50,** 127–41.
See also his paper in *Brit. J. Ophthal.*, 1934, **18**, 129–42.

5980 GUIST, Gustav.
Eine neue Ablatiooperation. *Z. Augenheilk.*, 1931, **74,** 232–42.
Guist's operation for detachment of the retina (multiple trephining and chemical cauterization of the choroid).

5981 CASTROVIEJO, Ramon. 1904–
Keratoplasty. A historical and experimental study, including a new method. *Amer. J. Ophthal.*, 1932, **15,** 825–38, 905–16.
Castroviejo's method of keratoplasty.

5982 DUKE-ELDER, *Sir* WILLIAM STEWART. 1898–
Text-book of ophthalmology. Vol. 1–7. London, *H. Kimpton*, 1932–54.

5983 LÓPEZ LACARRÈRE, JULIO.
Nuestro método original de extracción total de la catarata senil: la electrodiafaquia. Primeros ensayos. *Arch. Oftal. hisp.-amer.*, 1932, **32**, 293–303.
Intracapsular extraction of cataract by diathermy with the electro-diaphake. Preliminary report in *Klin. Mbl. Augenheilk.*, 1932, **88**, 778–83.

5984 ŠAFŘ, KARL.
Behandlung der Netzhautabhebung mit Elektroden für multiple diathermische Stichelung. *Klin. Mbl. Augenheilk.*, 1932, **88**, 814.
Safr's method of treatment of retinal detachment.

5985 DALLOS, JOSEF.
Ueber Haftgläser und Kontaktschalen. *Klin. Mbl. Augenheilk.*, 1933, **91**, 640–59.
Contact lenses introduced.

5986 FILATOV, VLADIMIR PETROVICH. 1875–1956
Transplantation of the cornea. *Arch. Ophthal.* (*N.Y.*), 1935, **13**, 321–47.
Earlier papers recording the important work of Filatov on corneal transplantation appeared in Russian journals.

5987 MANN, IDA CAROLINE. 1893–
Developmental abnormalities of the eye. Cambridge, *Univ. Press*, 1937.

5988 VOGT, ALFRED. 1879–1943
Ergebnisse der Diathermiestichelung des Corpus ciliare (Zyklodiathermiestichelung) gegen Glaukom. *Klin. Mbl. Augenheilk.*, 1937, **99**, 9–15.
Vogt's operation of cyclodiathermy for glaucoma.

5989 TERRY, THEODORE LASATER. 1899–1946
Extreme prematurity and fibroblastic overgrowth of persistent vascular sheath behind each crystalline lens. I. Preliminary report. *Amer. Ophthal.*, 1942, **25**, 203–04.
Retrolental fibroplasia first described. See also the same volume, pp. 1409–23, and *Trans. Sect. Ophthal. Amer. med. Ass.*, 1942, 213–29, for later papers.

5990 SANDERS, MURRAY. 1910– , & ALEXANDER, R. C.
Epidemic keratoconjunctivitis. I. Isolation and identification of a filterable virus. *J. exp. Med.*, 1943, **77**, 71–96.

5991 RIDLEY, NICHOLAS HAROLD LLOYD. 1906–
Intra-ocular acrylic lenses after cataract extraction. *Lancet*, 1952, **1**, 118–21.

5991.1 T'ANG, FEI FAN, *et al.*
Studies on the etiology of trachoma with special reference to isolation of the virus in chick embryo. *Chinese med. J.*, 1957, **75**, 429–47.
Isolation of trachoma agents. With H. L. Chang, Y. T. Huang, and K. C. Wang.

History of Ophthalmology

5992 JUGLER, JOHANN HEINRICH. 1758–1812
Bibliothecae ophthalmicae specimen primum eruditorum examini subjicit. Hamburg, *J. P. C. Reuse*, 1783.
Believed to be the earliest bibliography and history of ophthalmology.

5993 MAGNUS, HUGO FRIEDRICH. 1842–1907
Geschichte des grauen Staares. Leipzig, *Veit & Co.*, 1876.
A good history of cataract.

5994 HIRSCH, AUGUST. 1817–1894
Geschichte der Ophthalmologie. In GRAEFE and SAEMISCH: *Handbuch der gesammten Augenheilkunde*, Leipzig, 1877, **7**, Theil 5, 235–554.
A valuable short history of ophthalmology; the first systematic history of the subject.

5995 DENEFFE, VICTOR. 1835–1908
Les oculistes gallo-romains au IIIe siècle. Anvers, *H. Caals*, 1896.

5996 HIRSCHBERG, JULIUS. 1843–1925
Geschichte der Augenheilkunde. 10 pts. Leipzig, *W. Engelmann*, 1899–1918.
This monumental work remains to-day the authoritative history of ophthalmology. Its thoroughness and critical judgment mark it as one of the greatest of all histories of scientific subjects. Forms Bde. 12–15 of Graefe–Saemisch *Handbuch der gesamten Augenheilkunde*, 2te Aufl.

5997 MAGNUS, HUGO FRIEDRICH. 1842–1907
Die Augenheilkunde der Alten. Breslau, *J. V. Kern*, 1901.
A history of ancient ophthalmology in which the writer has attempted to reconstruct the anatomical concepts of the ancient Greeks.

5998 PANSIER, PIERRE. 1864–1939
Histoire des lunettes. Paris, *A. Maloine*, 1901.

5999 ——. Histoire de l'ophtalmologie. In P. F. LAGRANGE and E. VALUDE: *Encyclopédie française d'ophtalmologie*, Paris, 1903, **1**, 1–86.

6000 BOCK, EMIL. 1857–1916
Die Brille und ihre Geschichte. Wien, *J. Šafař*, 1903.

6001 HORSTMANN, CARL. 1847–1912
Geschichte der Augenheilkunde. In PUSCHMANN, T.: *Handbuch der Geschichte de Medizin*, Jena, 1905, **3**, 489–572.

6002 HUBBELL, ALVIN ALLACE. 1846–1911
The development of ophthalmology in America, 1800 to 1870. Chicago, *Amer. Med. Assoc. Press*, 1908.

6003 GREEFF, CARL RICHARD. 1862–1938
Die Erfindung der Augengläser. Berlin, *Optische Bücherei*, 1921.

6004 JAMES, ROBERT RUTSON. 1881–1959
Studies in the history of ophthalmology in England prior to the year 1800. Cambridge, *University Press*, 1933.

6005 CHANCE, BURTON. 1868–1965
Ophthalmology. New York, *P. B. Hoeber*, 1939.
This excellent little book of 240 pages is issued in the *Clio Medica* series of primers on the history of medicine. It traces in brief the progress of ophthalmology from ancient times to the present day and presents its story in a most interesting form.

6006 SORSBY, ARNOLD. 1900–
A short history of ophthalmology. 2nd ed. London, *Staples Press*, 1948.

6007 OVIO, GIUSEPPE. 1863–1957
Storia dell' oculista. Vol. 1. Cuneo, *ed. Chibaudo*, 1950.

6008–6135 GYNAECOLOGY

6008 SORANUS *of Ephesus*. A.D. 98–138
De arte obstetricia morbisque mulierum quae supersunt. Ex apographo F. R. Dietz. Regimontii Pr., *Graef et Unzer*, 1838.
Soranus is the leading authority on the gynaecology and obstetrics of antiquity. He recognized atresia of the vagina as being congenital or acquired from inflammation. He packed the uterus for haemorrhage and performed hysterectomy for prolapse. He described podalic version. The above has a Greek text. English translation of Soranus's *Gynecology* by O. Temkin, Baltimore, 1956.

6009 ——. Die Gynäkologie, Geburtshilfe, Frauen- und Kinder-Krankheiten, Diätetik der Neugeborenen. Uebersetzt von H. Lüneberg. München, *J. F. Lehmann*, 1894.

6010 BERENGARIO DA CARPI, GIACOMO. 1470–1550
Commentaria cum amplissimis additionibus super anatomia Mundini. (Bononiae, *per H. de Benedictis*, 1521.)
On fol. ccxxv Berengario gives the first authentic report of vaginal hysterectomy for prolapse. He describes two cases, one performed by himself in 1507 and the other by his father.

6011 WOLFF, CASPAR [WOLF]. 1525–1601
Volumen gynaeciorum, hoc est, de mulierum tum aliis, tum gravidarum, parientium et puerperarum affectibus et morbis. Basileae, *per T. Guarinum*, 1566.
A celebrated collection of gynaecological classics, collected and edited by Wolff. It forms a record of contemporary gynaecological knowledge.

6012 BAUHIN, CASPAR [BAUHINUS]. 1560–1624
Gynaeciorum sive de mulierum affectibus commentarii. 4 vols. Basileae, *per T. Guarinum*, 1586–88.
An enlarged version of No. 6011, now edited by Bauhin.

6013 SPACH, ISRAEL. 1560–1610
Gynaeciorum sive de mulierum tum communibus, tum gravidarum, parientum, et puerperarum affectibus et morbis, libri. Argentinae, *sumpt. L. Zetzneri*, 1597.
Spach was the editor of this great collection of gynaecological writings. It is in effect the third edition of the collection previously issued by Wolff (No. 6011) and Bauhin (No. 6012).

6014 BAILLOU, GUILLAUME DE [BALLONIUS]. 1538–1616
De virginum et mulierum morbis liber. Parisiis, *J. Quisnel*, 1643.

6015 ROONHUYZE, HENDRIK VAN. 1622–1672
Heel-konstige aanmerkkingen betreffende de gebreeken der vrouwen. Amsterdam, *weduwe van T. Jacobsz*, 1663.

Roonhuyze's book is regarded as the first work on operative gynaecology in the modern sense. He several times successfully performed caesarean section, and he used retractors for the repair of vesico-vaginal fistulae. English edition, 1676.

6016 STAHL, GEORG ERNST. 1660–1734
Ausführliche Abhandlung von den Zufällen und Kranckheiten des Frauenzimmers. Leipzig, *J. C. Eyssel*, 1724.

6017 HOUSTOUN, ROBERT [HOUSTON]. ?–1734
An account of a dropsy of the left ovary of a woman, aged 58, cured by a large incision made in the side of the abdomen. *Phil. Trans.*, (1724–25), 1726, **33,** 8–15.

Houstoun was the first to treat ovarian dropsy by tapping the cyst, 1701.

6018 EISENMANN, GEORG HEINRICH. 1693–1768
Tabulae anatomicae quatuor uteri duplicis. Argentorati, *ex off. A. Königii*, 1752.

6019 ASTRUC, JEAN. 1684–1766
Traité des maladies des femmes. 6 vols. Paris, *P. G. Cavelier*, 1761–1765.

Mettler considers this "the most pretentious gynecologic work of the [eighteenth] century . . . chiefly useful for its historical orientation".

6020 HUNTER, WILLIAM. 1718–1783
On retroversion of the uterus. *Med. Obs. Inqu.*, 1772, **4,** 400–09; 1776, **5,** 388–93.

6021 BAILLIE, MATTHEW. 1761–1823
An account of a particular change of structure in the human ovarium. *Phil. Trans.*, 1789, **79,** 71–78.

Matthew Baillie's notable anatomico-pathological studies on dermoid cysts of the ovary. Also published in *Lond. med. J.*, 1789, **10**, 322–32.

6022 SOEMMERRING, SAMUEL THOMAS. 1755–1830
Ueber die Wirkungen der Schnürbrüste. Berlin, *Voss*, 1793.

Soemmerring enumerated the bad effects of tight corsets on the internal organs of women. His paper created much interest and resulted in a great decline in the fad of tight lacing and hoop skirts. The first edition was published at Leipzig, 1788, but is less important as it had no illustrations.

6023 McDOWELL, EPHRAIM. 1771–1830
Three cases of extirpation of diseased ovaria. *Eclect. Repert. Analyt. Rev.*, 1817, **7,** 242–44.

McDowell was a pioneer ovariotomist. Although not the first to perform this operation, he deserves credit for putting it upon a permanent basis. The above records his first ovariotomy, performed in 1809, together with two later cases. Reprinted in *Med. Classics*, 1938, **2**, 651–53.

6024 SMITH, Nathan. 1762–1829
Case of ovarian dropsy, successfully removed by a surgical operation. *Amer. Med. Recorder*, 1822, **5,** 124–26.
Smith was the first in the U.S.A. after McDowell to perform ovariotomy, for ovarian dropsy. Smith was apparently without knowledge of the previous operations of McDowell.

6025 SIEBOLD, Adam Elias von. 1775–1826
Ueber den Gebärmutterkrebs, dessen Entstehung und Verhütung. Berlin, *F. Dummler*, 1824.
Classical account of cancer of the uterus.

6026 LIZARS, John. 1794–1860
Observations on extraction of diseased ovaria. Edinburgh, *D. Lizars*, 1825.
Lizars performed the first (unsuccessful) ovariotomy in Britain. His book made generally known the practical possibility of this operation.

6027 STRACHAN, John B.
Case of successful excision of the cervix uteri in a scirrhous state. *Amer. J. med. Sci.*, 1829, **5,** 307–09.
First successful excision of the cervix in America. Reported by T. F. Gillian.

6028 BOIVIN, Marie Anne Victoire, *née Gillain*. 1773–1841, & DUGÈS, Antoine. 1798–1838
Traité pratique des maladies de l'utérus et de ses annexes. 2 vols. and atlas. Paris, *J. B. Baillière*, 1833.
Boivin and Dugès practised amputation of the cervix for chronic ulceration. On page 648 of vol. 2 is the first recorded case of cancer of the female urethra. English translation, 1834.

6029 ROUX, Philibert Joseph. 1780–1854
Mémoire sur la restauration du périnée chez la femme dans les cas de division ou de rupture complète de cette partie. *Gaz. méd. Paris*, 1834, 2 sér., **2,** 17–22.
Roux was the first to suture the ruptured female perineum.

6030 HAYWARD, George. 1791–1863
Case of vesico-vaginal fistula, successfully treated by an operation. *Amer. J. med. Sci.*, 1839, **24,** 283–88.
Hayward's successful treatment of vesico-vaginal fistula was performed after Mettauer's although reported earlier.

6031 METTAUER, John Peter. 1787–1875
Vesico-vaginal fistula. *Boston med. surg. J.*, 1840, **22,** 154–55.
The first successful operation for vesico-vaginal fistula is believed to be that performed in August 1838, by Mettauer, a Virginian gynaecologist. He introduced metallic sutures and a retention catheter.

6031.1 WILTON, William. 1809–1899
Hydatids, terminating fatally, by haemorrhage. *Lancet*, 1840, **1,** 691–693.
First report of a chorionic tumour.

6032 CLAY, CHARLES. 1801–1893
Cases of peritoneal section, for the extirpation of diseased ovaria, by the large incision from sternum to pubes, successfully treated. *Med. Times*, 1842, **7,** 43, 59, 67, 83, 99, 139, 153, 270.

Clay, pioneer ovariotomist in Great Britain, introduced the word "ovariotomy". (See also his later paper, No. 6054.)

6033 RÉCAMIER, JOSEPH CLAUDE ANTHELME. 1774–1852
Invention du spéculum plein et brisé. *Bull. Acad. Méd.* (*Paris*), 1842–43, **8,** 661–68.

Description of the speculum invented by Récamier.

6034 ATLEE, JOHN LIGHT. 1799–1885
Case of ovarian tumors – both the right and the left being removed at the same operation. *N.Y. J. Med.*, 1843, **1,** 168–70.

First successful double oöphorectomy. Communicated in a letter to the editor by J. M. Foltz.

6035 SIMPSON, *Sir* JAMES YOUNG. 1811–1870
Contributions to the pathology and treatment of disease of the uterus. *Lond. Edinb. month. J. med. Sci.*, 1843, **3,** 547–56, 701–15, 1009–27; 1844, **4,** 208–17.

Simpson introduced many important procedures into gynaecology and obstetrics; among them may be mentioned his use of the uterine sound for diagnosing retro-positions of the uterus.

6036 BENNET, JAMES HENRY. 1816–1891
A practical treatise on inflammation, ulceration, and induration of the neck of the uterus. London, *J. Churchill*, 1845.

Bennet was the first to differentiate between benign and malignant uterine tumours.

6037 SIMS, JAMES MARION. 1813–1883
On the treatment of vesico-vaginal fistula. *Amer. J. med. Sci.*, 1852, n.s., **23,** 59–82.

Original description of Sims' operation for the treatment of vesico-vaginal fistula. Reprinted in *Med. Classics*, 1938, 2, 677–712.

6038 ATLEE, WASHINGTON LEMUEL. 1808–1878
A table of all the known operations of ovariotomy. From 1701–1851. *Trans. Amer. med. Ass.*, 1851, **4,** 286–314.

Atlee is said to have performed ovariotomy 387 times; with his brother John he firmly established the operation in the U.S.A.

6039 ——. The surgical treatment of certain fibrous tumours of the uterus. Philadelphia, *T. K. & P. G. Collins*, 1853.

Atlee was among the first to study the surgical removal of uterine fibroids.

6040 BURNHAM, WALTER. 1808–1883
Extirpation of the uterus and ovaries for sarcomatous disease. *Nelson's Amer. Lancet*, 1853, **7,** 147.

First successful abdominal hysterectomy, May 25, 1853.

6041 SIMON, GUSTAV. 1824–1876
Ueber die Heilung der Blasen-Scheidenfisteln. Giessen, *E. Heinemann*, 1854.

Simon is perhaps best remembered as being the first in Europe to excise the kidney; he also wrote a fine monograph on vesico-vaginal fistula.

6042 KIMBALL, GILMAN. 1804–1892
Successful case of extirpation of the uterus. *Boston med. surg. J.*, 1855, **52,** 249–55.
First successful abdominal hysteromyomectomy (for fibromyoma), Sept. 1, 1853.

6043 FERGUSSON, *Sir* WILLIAM. 1808–1877
System of practical surgery. 4th ed. London, *J. Churchill*, 1857.
On p. 724 is described Fergusson's vaginal speculum.

6044 NOEGGERATH, EMIL. 1827–1895
On epicystomy. *N.Y. J. Med.*, 1858, 3 ser., **4,** 9–24.
Noeggerath, who devised the operation of epicystotomy, spent many years in America, where he became a leading gynaecologist and obstetrician.

6045 WAGNER, ERNST LEBERECHT. 1829–1888
Der Gebärmutterkrebs. Leipzig, *B. G. Teubner*, 1858.
In this work Wagner presented the first important contribution to the knowledge of the gross pathology of uterine cancer.

6046 AYRES, DANIEL. 1822–1892
Congenital exstrophy of the urinary bladder, complicated with prolapsus uteri following pregnancy; successfully treated by a new plastic operation. *Amer. med. Gaz.*, 1859, **10,** 81–89.
First successful plastic operation for exstrophy of the female bladder.

6047 ATLEE, WASHINGTON LEMUEL. 1808–1878
Case of successful operation for vesico-vaginal fistula. *Amer. J. med. Sci.*, 1860, n.s., **39,** 67–82.
Atlee's operation for vesico-vaginal fistula.

6048 BERNUTZ, GUSTAVE LOUIS RICHARD. 1819–1887, & GOUPIL, JEAN ERNEST. 1829–1864
Clinique médicale sur les maladies des femmes. 2 vols. Paris, *F. Chamerot*, 1860–62.
One of the most important texts on the subject during the mid-nineteenth century. English translation (New Sydenham Society), 1867.

6049 SIMS, JAMES MARION. 1813–1883
Amputation of the cervix uteri. *Trans. N.Y. med. Soc.*, 1861, 367–71.
Sims' method for amputating the cervix.

6050 ——. On vaginismus. *Trans. obstet. Soc. Lond.*, (1861), 1862, **3,** 356–67.

6051 KOEBERLÉ, EUGÈNE. 1828–1915
De l'ovariotomie. *Mém. Acad. imp. Méd. (Paris)*, 1863, **26,** 321–472.
The introduction of ovariotomy into France was in part due to Koeberlé. He made great advances in gynaecological operative technique.

6052 ——. Exstirpation de l'utérus et des ovaires. *Gaz. méd. Strasbourg*, 1863, **23,** 101.
First successful excision of uterus and ovaries for tumour.

6053 ——. Documents pour servir a l'histoire de l'extirpation des tumeurs fibreuses de la matrice par la méthode suspubienne. *Mém. Soc. de Méd. de Strasbourg*, (1863–64), 1865, **4,** 84–158.

6054 CLAY, CHARLES. 1801–1893
Observations on ovariotomy, statistical and practical. Also, a successful case of entire removal of the uterus and its appendages. *Trans. obstet. Soc. Lond.*, (1863), 1864, **5**, 58–74.

For many years Clay was the most eminent ovariotomist in Great Britain. In all, he performed 395 ovariotomies, with a mortality of 25%.

6055 EMMET, THOMAS ADDIS. 1828–1919
On the treatment of dysmenorrhoea and sterility, resulting from anteflexion of the uterus. *N.Y. med. J.*, 1865, **1**, 205–19.

Emmet was an outstanding American gynaecological surgeon, a disciple of Sims.

6056 WELLS, *Sir* THOMAS SPENCER. 1818–1897
Diseases of the ovaries. 2 vols. London, *J. Churchill*, 1865–72.

Wells was perhaps the greatest of the pioneer ovariotomists; he performed his firs ovariotomy in 1858.

6057 SIMS, JAMES MARION. 1813–1883
Clinical notes on uterine surgery. London, *R. Hardwicke*, 1866.

Includes, pp. 16–18, the description of Sims' duck-bill speculum. Sims came of poor parents, but by his great ability rose to the front rank as a surgeon and gynaecologist.

6058 EMMET, THOMAS ADDIS. 1828–1919
Vesico-vaginal fistula from parturition and other causes: with cases of recto-vaginal fistula. New York, *William Wood*, 1868.

A comprehensive and valuable account of the management of vesico-vaginal fistula based on Sims' technique.

6059 ——. Surgery of the cervix in connection with the treatment of certain uterine diseases. *Amer. J. Obstet. Dis. Wom.*, 1869, **1**, 339–62.

Surgical repair of lacerations of the cervix.

6060 THOMAS, THEODORE GAILLARD. 1831–1903
A practical treatise on diseases of women. Philadelphia, *H. C. Lea*, 1868.

In its day, Thomas's book on gynaecology was the outstanding work on the subject.

6061 ——. Vaginal ovariotomy. *Amer. J. med. Sci.*, 1870, **59**, 387–90.

First vaginal ovariotomy.

6062 BATTEY, ROBERT. 1828–1895
Normal ovariotomy. *Atlanta med. surg. J.*, 1872, **10**, 321–39; also in *Trans. med. Ass. Georgia*, 1873, **24**, 36–69.

Battey's ovariotomy operation for the treatment of non-ovarian conditions. This operation later acquired a greater significance in connexion with more modern work on endocrinology. Preliminary communication in *J. gynaec. Soc. Boston*, 1872, **7**, 331–35.

6063 EMMET, THOMAS ADDIS. 1828–1919
Chronic cystitis in the female, and mode of treatment. *Amer. Practit.*, 1872, **5**, 65–92.

Vaginal cystotomy for chronic cystitis.

6064 NOEGGERATH, EMIL. 1827–1895
Die latente Gonorrhoe im weiblichen Geschlecht. Bonn, *M. Cohen & Sohn*, 1872.

Noeggerath was the first to point out the late effects of gonorrhoea in women, particularly its role in the production of sterility.

6065 PRIESTLEY, *Sir* WILLIAM OVEREND. 1829–1901
Cases of intermenstrual or intermediate dysmenorrhoea. *Brit. med. J.*, 1872, **2**, 431–32.
First report of cases of *Mittelschmerz*.

6066 MARTIN, AUGUST EDUARD. 1847–1933
Zur Enucleation der intraparietalen Myome des Corpus uteri. *Z. Geburtsh. Frauenkr.*, 1876, **1**, 143–67.

6066.1 CHIARI, HANS. 1851–1916
Uber drei Fälle von primärem Carcinom im Fundus und Corpus des Uterus. *Med. Jb.*, 1877, 364–68.
Choriocarcinoma first reported.

6067 HEGAR, ALFRED. 1830–1914
Ueber die Exstirpation normaler und nicht zu umfänglichen Tumoren degenerirter Eierstöcke. *Zbl. Gynäk.*, 1877, **1**, 297–307; 1878, **2**, 25–39.
Hegar developed Battey's operation (No. 6062) and employed it for the treatment of various ovarian conditions.

6068 LE FORT, LÉON CLÉMENT. 1829–1893
Nouveau procédé pour la guérison du prolapsus utérin. *Bull. gén. Thérap.*, 1877, **92**, 337–44.
Le Fort's operation for prolapse.

6069 RUGE, CARL ARNOLD. 1846–1926, & VEIT, JOHANN. 1852–1917
Anatomische Bedeutung der Erosionen am Scheidentheil. *Zbl. Gynäk.*, 1877, **1**, 17–19.

6070 FREUND, WILHELM ALEXANDER. 1833–1918
Eine neue Methode der Exstirpation des ganzen Uterus. *Berl. klin. Wschr.*, 1878, **15**, 417–18.
Freund performed the first successful abdominal hysterectomy for cancer. Although removal of the uterus by the abdominal route had been carried out earlier, to Freund belongs the credit for the invention of the operation, in which he utilized Lister's antiseptic method.

6071 TAIT, ROBERT LAWSON. 1845–1899
Removal of normal ovaries. *Brit. med. J.*, 1879, **1**, 813–14.
Lawson Tait reported that he had performed Battey's operation on Aug. 1, 1872, 16 days before Battey.

6072 CZERNY, VINCENZ. 1842–1916
Ueber die Ausrottung des Gebärmutterkrebses. *Wien. med. Wschr.*, 1879, **29**, 1171–74.
First total hysterectomy by the vaginal route.

6073 ——. Ueber die Enukleation subperitonealer Fibrome der Gebärmutter durch das Scheidengewölbe; vaginale Myoniotomie. *Wien. med. Wschr.*, 1881, **31**, col. 501–05, 525–29.
The operation of enucleation of subperitoneal uterine fibroids by the vaginal route was introduced by Czerny. In the second paper the words "Fibromyome" and "Myomotomie" replace "Fibrome" and "Myoniotomie" in the title.

6074 SCHRÖDER, KARL LUDWIG ERNST. 1838–1887
Ueber die theilweise und vollständige Ausschneidung der carcinomatösen Gebärmutter. *Z. Geburtsh. Gynäk.*, 1881, **6**, 213–30.

6075 TAIT, Robert Lawson. 1845–1899
A case of removal of the uterine appendages. *Brit. med. J.*, 1881, **1,** 766–67.
Oöphorectomy, February 1881.

6076 ADAMS, James Alexander. 1857–1930
A new operation for uterine displacements. *Glasg. med. J.*, 1882, **17,** 437–46.
Adams devised an operation for retroversion of the uterus, similar to that performed by Alexander (No. 6077).

6077 ALEXANDER, William. 1844–1919
A new method of treating inveterate and troublesome displacements of the uterus. *Med. Times Gaz.*, 1882, **1,** 327–28.
Alexander's suspension operation for retroversion of the uterus, first performed by him in 1881.

6078 EMMET, Thomas Addis. 1828–1919
A study of the etiology of perineal laceration, with a new method for its proper repair. *Trans. Amer. gynec. Soc.*, (1883), 1884, **8,** 198–216.
First description of Emmet's technique for perineorrhaphy.

6079 APOSTOLI, Georges. 1847–1900
Sur la faradisation utérine double ou bipolaire. *Union méd.*, 1884, 3 sér., **38,** 709–13, 733–36.
Apostoli was the first to employ the double faradic current in the electrotherapy of uterine diseases.

6080 SCHRÖDER, Karl Ludwig Ernst. 1838–1887
Ueber die Enucleation interstitieller Myome. *Z. Geburtsh. Gynäk.*, 1884, **10,** 156–62.

6081 TAIT, Robert Lawson. 1845–1899
General summary of conclusions from one thousand cases of abdominal section. Birmingham, *R. Birbeck*, 1884.

6082 BREISKY, August. 1832–1889
Ueber Kraurosis vulvae, eine wenig beachtete Form von Hautatrophie am pudendum muliebre. *Z. Heilk.*, 1885, **6,** 69–80.
Although not the first to describe kraurosis vulvae, Breisky left an important account, and the condition became known as "Breisky's disease".

6083 OLSHAUSEN, Robert von. 1835–1915
Ueber ventrale Operation bei Prolapsus und Retroversio uteri. *Zbl. Gynäk.*, 1886, **10,** 698–701.
First account of Olshausen's operation for retroversion of the uterus.

6084 PÉAN, Jules Émile. 1830–1898
Ablation des tumeurs fibreuses ou myomes du corps de l'utérus par la voie vaginale. *Gaz. Hôp.* (*Paris*), 1886, **59,** 445–47.
Péan's method of morcellement of the uterus for the removal of tumours.

6085 BOZEMAN, Nathan. 1825–1905
The gradual preparatory treatment of the complications of urinary and faecal fistulae in women. *Trans. int. med. Congr.*, Washington, 1887, **2,** 514–58.
Pyelitis complicating vesical and faecal fistulae in women was successfully treated by Bozeman.

6086 KELLY, HOWARD ATWOOD. 1858–1943
Hysterorrhaphy. New York, *W. Wood & Co.*, 1887.

6087 TAIT, ROBERT LAWSON. 1845–1899
On the method of flap-splitting in certain plastic operations. *Brit. gynaec. J.*, 1887–88, **3**, 367–76; 1891–92, **7**, 195–214.
Tait devised a flap-splitting operation for rectocele which, with some modifications, is in use to-day.

6088 SÄNGER, MAX. 1853–1903
Die Tripperansteckung beim weiblichen Geschlechte. Leipzig, *O. Wigand*, 1889.

6089 PFANNENSTIEL, HERMANN JOHANN. 1862–1909
Ueber die Pseudomucine der cystischen Ovariengeschwülste. Leipzig, *A. T. Engelhardt*, 1890.

6090 PRICE, JOSEPH. 1853–1911
Pus in the pelvis and how to deal with it. *Trans. sth. surg. gynec. Ass.*, (1889), 1890, **2**, 102–12.

6091 TRENDELENBURG, FRIEDRICH. 1844–1924
Ueber Blasenscheidenfisteloperationen und über Beckenhochlagerung bei Operationen in der Bauchhöhle. *Samml. klin. Vortr.*, 1890, Nr. 355 (Chir., Nr. 109), 3372–92.
Includes description of the "Trendelenburg position". Reprinted, with translation, in *Med. Classics*, 1940, **4**, 936–88. The first description of Trendelenburg's elevated pelvic position was given by one of his students, W. Meyer, in *Arch. klin. Chir.*, 1885, **31**, 494–525.

6092 WILLIAMS, JOHN WHITRIDGE. 1866–1931
Contributions to the histogenesis of the papillary cystoma of the ovary. *Johns Hopk. Hosp. Bull.*, 1891, **2**, 149–57.

6093 BAER, BENJAMIN FRANKLIN. 1846–1920
Supravaginal hysterectomy without ligature of the cervix, in operation for uterine fibroids; a new method. *Amer. J. Obstet. Dis. Wom.*, 1892, **26**, 489–504.
Baer's operation.

6093.1 TAIT, ROBERT LAWSON. 1845–1899
On the occurrence of pleural effusion in association with disease of the abdomen. *Med.-chir. Trans.*, 1892, **75**, 109–18.
Lawson Tait was apparently the first to describe what is now known as Meigs's syndrome (ovarian fibroma combined with pleural effusion).

6094 SÄNGER, MAX. 1853–1903
Ueber Sarcoma uteri deciduo-cellulare und andere deciduale Geschwülste. *Arch. Gynäk.*, 1893, **44**, 89–148.
A detailed classification of "deciduomata", chorionic neoplasms, and a review of the literature.

6095 HENROTIN, FERNAND. 1847–1906
Vaginal hysterectomy in bilateral peri-uterine suppuration. *Amer. J. Obstet. Dis. Wom.*, 1892, **26**, 448–60.
Henrotin's method of removing the uterus.

6096 HENROTIN, Fernand. 1847–1906
Conservative surgical treatment of para- and peri-uterine septic diseases. *Amer. gynaec. obstet. J.*, 1895, **6,** 769–83.

6097 KAHLDEN, Clemens von. 1859–1903
Ueber eine eigenthümliche Form des Ovarialcarcinoms. *Zbl. allg. Path.*, 1895, **6,** 257–64.
Granulosa cell tumour first described.

6097.1 MARCHAND, Felix Jacob. 1846–1928
Über die sogenannten "decidualen" Geschwülste im Anschluss an normale Geburt, Abort, Blasenmole und Extrauterinschwangerschaft. *Mschr. Geburtsh.*, 1895, **1,** 419–38, 513–62.
Marchand's theory of the histogenesis of choriocarcinoma (chorionepithelioma). He considered that such tumours derived from trophoblast and not from decidua.

6098 OLSHAUSEN, Robert von. 1835–1915
Über Exstirpation der Vagina. *Zbl. Gynäk.*, 1895, **19,** 1–6.
The operation of excision of the vagina was introduced by Olshausen.

6099 WERTHEIM, Ernst. 1864–1920
Ueber Uterus-Gonorrhöe. *Verh. dtsch. Ges. Gynäk.*, 1895, **6,** 199–223.
Wertheim emphasized the importance of latent uterine gonorrhoea.

6100 WILLIAMS, John Whitridge. 1866–1931
Deciduoma malignum. *Johns Hopk. Hosp. Rep.*, 1895, **4,** 461–504.
First case of choriocarcinoma reported in N. America.

6101 KRUKENBERG, Friedrich Ernst. 1870–1946
Ueber das Fibrosarcoma ovarii mucocellulare (carcinomatodes). *Arch. Gynäk.*, 1896, **50,** 287–321.
Original description of "Krukenberg's tumour".

6102 MACKENRODT, Alwin Karl. 1859–1925
Ueber den künstlichen Ersatz der Scheide. *Zbl. Gynäk.*, 1896, **20,** 546–50.
Mackenrodt's operation for the plastic reconstruction of the vagina.

6103 WERTHEIM, Ernst. 1864–1920
Über Blasen-Gonorrhöe. *Z. Geburtsh. Gynäk*, 1896, **35,** 1–10.
Wertheim demonstrated the gonococcus in acute cystitis.

6104 WINTER, Georg. 1856–1943
Lehrbuch der gynäkologischen Diagnostik. Leipzig, *S. Hirzel*, 1896.

6105 FAURE, Jean Louis. 1863–1944
Sur un nouveau procédé d'hystérectomie abdominale totale; la section médiane de l'utérus. *Presse méd.*, 1897, **5,** ii, 237–38.

6106 MENGE, Karl. 1864–1945, & KRÖNIG, Claus Ludwig Theodor Bernhard. 1863–1918
Bakteriologie des weiblichen Genital-Kanales. 2 vols. Leipzig, *A. Georgi*, 1897.

6107 ALEXANDER, William. 1844–1919
Enucleation of uterine fibroids. *Brit. gynaec. J.*, 1898, **14,** 47–61.
An outstanding account of myomectomy.

6108 KELLY, Howard Atwood. 1858–1943
Operative gynecology. 2 vols. New York, *D. Appleton & Co.*, 1898.
Kelly, professor of gynaecology at Pennsylvania and Johns Hopkins University, was a leading gynaecologist in America.

6109 ——. The removal of pelvic inflammatory masses by the abdomen after bisection of the uterus. *Amer. J. Obstet. Dis. Wom.*, 1900, **42,** 818–39.

6109.1 ORTHMANN, Ernst Gottlob. 1858–1922
Zur Casuistik einiger seltenerer Ovarial- und Tuben-Tumoren. *Mschr. Geburtsh. Gynäk.*, 1899, **9,** 771–82.
"Brenner tumour" first described; see also No. 6118.

6110 CULLEN, Thomas Stephen. 1868–1953
Cancer of the uterus. New York, *Appleton & Co.*, 1900.
Includes first clinical and pathological study of hyperplasia of the endometrium. Cullen is remembered eponymically for "Cullen's sign", a discoloration of the skin about the umbilicus, regarded as a sign of ruptured ectopic gestation.

6111 GILLIAM, David Tod. 1844–1923
Round-ligament ventrosuspension of the uterus: a new method. *Amer. J. Obstet. Dis. Wom.*, 1900, **41,** 299–303.
Gilliam's operation for prolapse.

6112 NOBLE, George Henry. 1860–
A flap operation for atresia of the vagina. *Trans. sth. surg. gynec. Ass.*, 1900, **13,** 78–83.
Noble introduced a flap operation for atresia of the vagina.

6113 PFANNENSTIEL, Hermann Johann. 1862–1909
Ueber die Vortheile der suprasymphysären Fascienquerschnitts für die gynäkologischen Koeliotomieen. *Samml. klin. Vortr.*, Leipzig, 1900, n.F., Nr. 268 (Gynäk. Nr. 97), 1735–56.
"Pfannenstiel's incision."

6114 WERTHEIM, Ernst. 1864–1920
Zur Frage der Radicaloperation beim Uteruskrebs. *Arch. Gynäk.*, 1900, **61,** 627–68; 1902, **65,** 1–39.
Wertheim's radical operation for cancer of the uterus.

6115 EDEBOHLS, George Michael. 1853–1908
Panhysterokolpectomy; a new prolapsus operation. *Med. Rec. (N.Y.)*, 1901, **60,** 561–64.

6116 WEBSTER, John Clarence. 1863–1950
A satisfactory operation for certain cases of retroversion of the uterus. *J. Amer. med. Ass.*, 1901, **37,** 913.
"Baldy–Webster operation." Webster's method of treating retrodisplacement of the uterus was later modified by J. M. Baldy, *N.Y. med. J.*, 1903, **78,** 167–69.

6117 BALDWIN, James Fairchild. 1850–1936
The formation of an artificial vagina by intestinal transplantation. *Ann. Surg.*, 1904, **40,** 398–403.
Baldwin's operation.

6118 BRENNER, Fritz. 1877–
Das Oophoroma folliculare. *Frankf. Z. Path.*, 1907, **1,** 150–71.
"Brenner tumour", earlier described by Orthmann (No. 6109.1). See the historical note in *Cancer*, 1956, **9**, 217.

6119 DONALD, Archibald. 1860–1937
Operation in cases of complete prolapse. *J. Obstet. Gynaec. Brit. Emp.*, 1908, **13,** 195–96.
Donald's operation for prolapse.

6120 SCHAUTA, Friedrich. 1849–1919
Die erweiterte vaginale Totalexstirpation des Uterus bei Kollumkarzinom. Wien, Leipzig, *J. Šafař*, 1908.
Radical vaginal hysterectomy for carcinoma of the cervix.

6121 BELL, William Blair. 1871–1936
The principles of gynaecology. London, *Longmans, Green & Co.*, 1910.
Blair Bell was an outstanding figure in British gynaecology and one of the founders of the Royal College of Obstetricians and Gynaecologists.

6122 CARY, William Hollenback. 1883–
Note on determination of patency of Fallopian tubes by the use of collargol and x-ray shadow. *Amer. J. Obstet. Dis. Wom.*, 1914, **69,** 462–64.
Cary was first to perform salpingography.

6123 RUBIN, Isador Clinton. 1883–1958
X-ray diagnosis in gynecology with the aid of intra-uterine collargol injection. *Surg. Gynec. Obstet.*, 1915, **20,** 435–42.
Independently of Cary (No. 6122) Rubin performed salpingography. Preliminary communication in *Zbl. Gynäk.*, 1914, **38**, 658–60.

6124 FOTHERGILL, William Edward. 1865–1926
Anterior colporrhaphy and its combination with amputation of the cervix as a single operation. *J. Obstet. Gynaec. Brit. Emp.*, 1915, **27,** 146–47.
Fothergill's modification of Donald's operation for prolapse.

6125 FORSSELL, Carl Gustaf [Gösta] Abrahamsson. 1876–1950
Översikt över resultaten av kräftbehandling vid Radiumhemmet i Stockholm 1910–1915. *Hospitalstidende*, 1917, 8 R., **10,** 273–83.
The Stockholm method of radium treatment of cancer of the uterus, as carried out at the Radiumhemmet, Stockholm, follows the technique devised by Forssell.

6126 SCHROEDER, Robert. 1884–
Die Pathogenese der Meno- und besonders der Metrorrhagien. *Arch. Gynäk.*, 1919, **110,** 633–58.
First description of metropathia haemorrhagica.

6127 RUBIN, Isador Clinton. 1883–1958
Nonoperative determination of patency of Fallopian tubes in sterility. Intra-uterine inflation with oxygen, and production of an artificial pneumoperitoneum. *J. Amer. med. Ass.*, 1920, **74.** 1017; **75,** 661–67.
Tubal insufflation method for the diagnosis and treatment of sterility due to occlusion of the Fallopian tubes.

6128 SAMPSON, JOHN ALBERTSON. 1873–1946
Perforating hemorrhagic (chocolate) cysts of the ovary. *Arch. Surg.* (*Chicago*), 1921, **3**, 245–323.
The true nature of ovarian endometriomata was elucidated by Sampson.

6129 HALBAN, JOSEF VON. 1870–1937, & SEITZ, LUDWIG. 1872–
Biologie und Pathologie des Weibes. Hrsg. von J. HALBAN und L. SEITZ. 8 vols. [in 15]. Berlin, *Urban & Schwarzenberg*, 1924–29.
Second edition, 1941– ; in progress.

6130 KAUFMANN, CARL.
Die Behandlung der Amenorrhoë mit hohen Dosen der Ovarialhormone. *Klin. Wschr.*, 1933, **12**, 1557–62.
First use of oestrogenic hormone for the treatment of amenorrhoea.

6131 REGAUD, CLAUDE. 1870–1940
Considérations sur la radiothérapie des cancers cervico-uterins, d'après l'expérience et les résultats acquis à l'Institut du Radium de Paris. *Radiophysiol. et Radiothérap.*, 1933–39, **3**, 155–70.
The Paris method of radium treatment of cancer of the uterus was devised by Regaud.

6132 SCHILLER, WALTER.
Early diagnosis of carcinoma of the cervix. *Surg. Gynec. Obstet.*, 1933, **56**, 210–22.
Schiller's test for carcinoma of the cervix.

6132.1 STEIN, IRVING FREILER. 1887– , & LEVENTHAL, MICHAEL LEO. 1901–
Amenorrhea associated with bilateral polycystic ovaries. *Amer. J. Obstet. Gynec.*, 1935, **29**, 181–91.
Stein–Leventhal syndrome.

6133 McINDOE, *Sir* ARCHIBALD HECTOR. 1900–1960, & BANISTER, JOHN BRIGHT. 1880–1938
An operation for the cure of congenital absence of the vagina. *J. Obstet. Gynaec. Brit. Emp.*, 1938, **45**, 490–94.
McIndoe's operation for the construction of an artificial vagina.

6135 PAPANICOLAOU, GEORGE NICHOLAS. 1883–1962, & TRAUT, HERBERT FREDERICK. 1894–
The diagnostic value of vaginal smears in carcinoma of the uterus. *Amer. J. Obstet. Gynec.*, 1941, **42**, 193–206.
Smear diagnosis of carcinoma of the cervix. Papanicolaou first reported that he could recognize cancer cells in 1928 (Proc. Third Race Betterment Conf., p. 528) but the importance of his findings was not generally accepted and he abandoned the work for some years.

For history of gynaecology, see nos. 6287, 6293, 6296, 6297, 6300, 6301, 6302, 6303, 6305, 6306, 6308, 6309, 6310, 6311.1, 6311.2

6136–6311.3 OBSTETRICS

6136 MUSCIO [Moschion]. *fl. circa* A.D. 500
De mulierum passionibus liber. Viennae, *apud R. Gräffer*, 1793.

Muscio was a pupil of Soranus. His book is arranged in catechism form; it was first published in Caspar Wolff's *Gynaeciorum*, 1566. The above Greek-Latin bilingual text was edited by F. O. Dewez.

6137 AETIUS *of Amida*. A.D. 502–575
Geburtshülfe und Gynäkologie . . . ins Deutsche übersetzt von Max Wegscheider. Berlin, *J. Springer*, 1901.

Aetius epitomized all previous knowledge regarding obstetrics. A translation from the Latin edition of 1542, with annotations, was published by J. V. Ricci, Philadelphia, 1950.

6138 RÖSSLIN, Eucharius [Rhodion; Röslin]. ?–1526
Der swangern frawen und hebammen roszgarten. [Hagenau, *H. Gran*,] 1513.

Earliest printed text-book for midwives. It survived 40 editions, being used as late as 1730. An English translation by Richard Jonas was published in 1540, printed by Thomas Raynalde. This translation, entitled "The Byrth of Mankynde" was the first book on the subject to be printed in English. For a bibliographical study of the work, see Sir D'Arcy Power's article in *The Library*, 1927, 4 ser. **8**, 1–37, subsequently reprinted in book form. There were three editions in 1513, the last of which was reproduced in facsimile in 1910 at Munich.

6139 ——. The byrth of mankynde. London, *T. R.*, 1540.

See No. 6138. Interesting bibliographical details regarding this book are given by J. W. Ballantyne in *J. Obstet. Gynaec. Brit. Emp.*, 1906, **10**, 297–325.

6140 PARÉ, Ambroise. 1510–1590
Briefve collection de l'administration anatomique: avec la manière de conjoindre les os: et d'extraire les enfans tant mors que vivans du ventre de la mère, lors que nature de soy ne peult venir à son effect. Paris, *G. Cavellat*, 1549.

Paré's revival of podalic version repopularized the procedure, which had been described by Soranus of Ephesus.

6141 RUEFF, Jacob [Ruff; Ruoff]. 1500–1558
De conceptu et generatione hominis. Tiguri, *C. Froschoverus*, 1554.

An improved version of Rösslin's *Swangern frawen.* Rueff described smooth and toothed forceps for extraction of the dead foetus. A German version of his book, *Trostbüchle*, was published by Froschouer in the same year.

6142 RATISBON.
Ordnung eines erbarn Raths der Statt Regenspurg, die Hebammen betreffende. [Regenspurg, *H. Khol*, 1555.]

Earliest public document in the vernacular containing legislation governing midwives.

6143 LONITZER, Adam [Lonicerus]. 1528–1586
Reformation, oder Ordnung für die Hebammen. Franckfurt a. M., *getruckt bey C. Egenolffs Erben*, 1573.

Legislation governing the practice of midwifery was introduced in the city of Frankfurt in 1573.

6144 MERCURIO, Geronimo Scipione. 1550–1616
La commare o riccoglitrice. Ventia, *G. B. Ciotti*, 1596.

First Italian book on obstetrics. It is a work of importance for the study of the history of Caesarean section; in it Mercurio advocated the Caesarean operation in cases of contracted pelvis.

6145 BOURGEOIS, Louise [dite *Boursier*]. 1563–1636
Observations diverses sur la sterilite, perte de fruict, foecondite, accouchements, et maladies des femmes, et enfants nouveaux naiz. Paris, *A. Saugrain*, 1609.

Louise Bourgeois was accoucheuse to the French Court. She was one of the pioneers of scientific midwifery; her *Observations* was the vade mecum of contemporary midwives. She induced premature labour in patients with contracted pelves, an idea probably derived from Paré.

6146 HARVEY, William. 1578–1657
Exercitationes de generatione animalium. Londini, *O. Pulleyn*, 1651.

The chapter on labour ("De partu") in this book represents the first original work on obstetrics to be published by an English author. English translation, 1653.

6146.1 LA COURVÉE, Jean Claude de. 1615–1664
De nutritione foetus in utero paradoxa. Dantisci, *G. Förster*, 1655.

Page 245 contains a report of successful symphysiotomy.

6147 MAURICEAU, François. 1637–1709
Des maladies des femmes grosses et accouchées. Paris, *chez l'Auteur*, 1668.

The outstanding text-book of the time. Mauriceau, leading obstetrician of his day, introduced the practice of delivering his patients in bed instead of in the obstetrical chair. It was to Mauriceau that Hugh Chamberlen attempted to sell the secret of his forceps; Chamberlen translated the *Traité* into English in 1673. This book established obstetrics as a science.

6148 PORTAL, Paul. 1630–1703
La pratique des accouchemens soutenue d'un grand nombre d'observations. Paris, *G. Martin*, 1685.

Portal's important treatise included his demonstration that version could be done with one foot. He also taught that face presentation usually ran a normal course. English translation, 1705.

6149 SIEGEMUNDIN, Justine [Dittrichin]. 1650–1705
Die Chur-Brandenburgische Hoff-Wehe-Mutter. Cölln an der Spree, *U. Liebperten*, 1690.

With Mauriceau, Justine Siegemundin was responsible for introducing the practice of puncturing the amniotic sac to arrest haemorrhage in placenta praevia. She was midwife to the Court of the Elector of Brandenburg, and the most celebrated of the German midwives of the 17th century.

6150 MAUQUEST DE LA MOTTE, Guillaume. 1665–1737
Traité complet des accouchemens. Paris, *L. d'Houry*, 1722.

This was an important treatise in its time; it shows that Mauquest de la Motte applied podalic version to head presentations. English translation, 1746.

6151 OULD, *Sir* Fielding. 1710–1789
A treatise of midwifry. Dublin, *O. Nelson & C. Connor*, 1742.

The teaching of Ould did much towards the advancement of midwifery in the British Isles. His *Treatise* is the first text-book of obstetrics of any importance in English.

6152 LEVRET, André. 1703–1780
Observations sur les causes et les accidens de plusieurs accouchemens laborieux. Paris, *C. Osmont*, 1747.

Levret, who improved the obstetric forceps, was a famous teacher in Paris.

6153 ——. L'art des accouchemens. Paris, *Delaguette*, 1753.

Besides introducing a curved forceps (see No. 6152) Levret invented several other obstetric instruments and made fundamental observations on pelvic anomalies. His book covered the whole field of obstetrics and remained a standard work for many years.

6154 SMELLIE, William. 1697–1763
Treatise on the theory and practice of midwifery. London, *D. Wilson*, 1752.

Smellie, a dominating figure among the obstetricians of the 18th century, owed much to his association with William Hunter. In his *Treatise* he described more accurately than any previous writer the mechanism of parturition, stressing the importance of exact measurement of the pelvis. He was first to lay down safe rules regarding the use of forceps, and himself introduced the steel-lock, the curved, and the double forceps. His book was followed by two volumes of case reports, 1754 and 1764; it was re-published by the New Sydenham Society, 3 vols., 1876–78. It includes the first illustration of a rachitic pelvis. Biography by R. W. Johnstone, Edinburgh, 1952.

6155 BARD, John. 1716–1799
A case of extra-uterine foetus. *Med. Obs. Soc. Physicians Lond.*, 1764, **2**, 369–72.

In 1759 Bard successfully operated for ectopic pregnancy.

6156 HARVIE, John.
Practical directions, shewing a method of preserving the perinaeum in birth, and delivering the placenta without violence. London, *D. Wilson & G. Nicol*, 1767.

Harvie, Smellie's successor, advocated external expression of the placenta instead of traction on the cord, anticipating Credé in this connexion by almost a century (see No. 6183). Reprinted in H. Thoms: *Classic contributions to obstetrics and gynecology*, 1935, pp. 131–38.

6157 HUNTER, William. 1718–1783
Anatomia uteri humani gravidi tabulis illustrata. The anatomy of the human gravid uterus exhibited in figures. Birmingham, *John Baskerville*, 1774.

Contains 34 copper plates depicting the gravid uterus, life-size. This is William Hunter's best work and one of the finest anatomical atlases ever to be produced, "anatomically exact and artistically perfect" (Choulant). Except for J. Dalby's little book, *Virtues of cinnabar and musk against the bite of a mad dog*, 1762, it is the only medical publication to come from the famous Baskerville press. The letterpress is in both Latin and English. The Sydenham Society published a reprint of the atlas in 1851.

6158 RIGBY, Edward. 1747–1821
An essay on the uterine haemorrhage, which precedes the delivery of the full grown foetus: illustrated with cases. London, *J. Johnson*, 1775.

Rigby differentiated between premature separation of the normal placenta (accidental haemorrhage) and placenta praevia (unavoidable haemorrhage).

6160 BOËR, Lucas Johann [Boogers]. 1751–1835
Abhandlungen und Versuche geburtshilflichen Inhalts. 2 vols. Vienna, *C. F. Wappler*, 1791–1806.
Boër, a pioneer of "natural childbirth", was the founder of the Viennese school of obstetrics.

6161 MOHRENHEIM, Joseph Jacob von, *Freiherr*. *d.* 1789
Abhandlung über die Entbindungskunst. St. Petersburg, *K. Akad. d. Wiss.*, 1791.
This work was edited by order of Catherine II of Russia, to whom von Mohrenheim was accoucheur. The importance of this work lies mainly in its splendid engravings, some of which were taken from Smellie (see No. 6154). The work includes a brief literary history of obstetrics.

6162 HOME, *Sir* Everard. 1763–1832
Account of the dissection of an hermaphrodite dog. *Phil. Trans.*, 1799, **18,** 157–78.
Home records (p. 162) that John Hunter suggested artificial insemination in 1790. The actual insemination was performed by the husband with a syringe.

6163 SCHMITT, Wilhelm Joseph. 1760–1827
Drey Wahrnehmungen von Schwangerschaften ausserhalb der Gebährmutter. *Beobacht. k. k. med.-chir. Josephs Acad. Wien*, 1801, **1,** 59–96.
Interstitial pregnancy first reported.

6164 STEARNS, John. 1770–1848
Account of the pulvis parturiens, a remedy for quickening childbirth. *Med. Reposit.*, 1808, 2 Hex., **5,** 308–09.
First use of ergot in the induction of labour in America. Reprinted in H. Thoms: *Classic contributions to obstetrics and gynecology*, 1935, pp. 21–23.

6165 BOIVIN, Marie Anne Victoire, *née Gillain*. 1773–1841
Mémorial de l'art des accouchements. Paris, *Méquignon père*, 1812.
Mme Boivin was one of the most famous of the Paris midwives. She improved the speculum and wrote intelligently on hydatidiform mole.

6166 KING, John.
Case of an extra-uterine foetus, produced alive through an incision made into the vagina of the mother, who recovered after delivery, without any alarming symptoms. *Med. Reposit.*, 1817, n.s., **3,** 388–94.
First successful operation for abdominal pregnancy.

6167 ——. An analysis of the subject of extrauterine foetation and of the retroversion of the gravid uterus. Norwich, *G. Wright*, 1818.
Expansion of No. 6166. First book on the subject.

6168 WENZEL, Carl. 1769–1827
Allgemeine geburtshülfliche Betrachtungen und über die künstliche Frühgeburt. Mainz, *F. Kupferberg*, 1818.
Artificial induction of premature labour.

6169 NAEGELE, Franz Karl. 1778–1851
Ueber den Mechanismus der Geburt. *Dtsch. Arch. Physiol.*, 1819, **5,** 483–531.

6170 LA CHAPELLE, Marie Louise, *Mme.* [Dugès]. 1769–1821
Pratique des accouchemens. 3 vols. Paris, *J. B. Baillière*, 1821–25.

Mme La Chapelle was a famous midwife and a colleague of Baudelocque. She supervised 5,000 deliveries and her vast experience enabled her to write her book. She reduced the 94 theoretical presentations suggested by Baudelocque to 22; her deductions form the basis of present teaching in this respect.

6171 LEJUMEAU, Jean Alexandre, *Vicomte de Kergaradec.* 1787–1877
Mémoire sur l'auscultation appliquée à l'étude de la grossesse. Paris, *Méquignon-Marvis*, 1822.

Although not first to record the auscultation of the foetal heart sound, Lejumeau brought the importance of this diagnostic procedure to the notice of the medical profession.

6172 BOIVIN, Marie Anne Victoire, *née Gillain.* 1773–1841
Nouvelles recherches sur l'origine, la nature et le traitement de la mole vésiculaire ou grossesse hydatique. Paris, *Méquignon l'âiné père*, 1827.

Classical description of hydatidiform mole.

6173 MONTGOMERY, William Fetherston. 1797–1859
An exposition of the signs and symptoms of pregnancy. London, *Sherwood, Gilbert, & Piper*, 1837.

"Montgomery's glands", the sebaceous glands of the areola, were previously described by Morgagni. They are described, with his "tubercles" (the secondary areola seen in pregnancy) in the above work.

6174 JACQUEMIER, Jean Marie. 1806–1879
Recherches d'anatomie et de physiologie sur le système vasculaire sanguin de l'utérus humain pendant la gestation, et plus spécialement sur les vaisseaux utéro-placentaires. *Arch. gén. Méd.*, 1838, 3 sér., **3,** 165–94.

Jacquemier's sign, diagnostic of pregnancy.

6175 NAEGELE, Hermann Franz Joseph. 1810–1851
Die geburtshülfliche Auscultation. Mainz, *V. von Zabern*, 1838.

6176 LEVER, John Charles Weaver. 1811–1858
Cases of puerperal convulsions, with remarks. *Guy's Hosp. Rep.*, 1843, 2 ser., **1,** 495–517.

Lever, of Guy's Hospital, was the first to report the finding of albuminous urine in connexion with puerperal convulsions.

6177 MEIGS, Charles Delucena. 1792–1869
The heart-clot. *Med. Exam.*, 1849, **5,** 141–52.

Meigs drew attention to embolism as a cause of sudden death in childbed. Previously such deaths had been attributed to syncope.

6178 NÉLATON, Auguste. 1807–1873
Leçons sur l'hématocèle rétro-utérine. *Gaz. Hôp.* (*Paris*), 1851, 3 sér., **3,** 573, 578–79, 581; 1852, 3 sér., **4,** 45–46, 66–67.

Classical description of pelvic haematocele.

6179 DU BOIS, Paul. 1795–1871
Considérations sur l'avortement provoqué dans les cas de vomissements. *Bull. Acad. Méd.* (*Paris*), 1852, **17,** 557–83.

Classical description of hyperemesis gravidarum.

6180 TALIAFERRO, VALENTINE H. 1831–1888
Rigidity of the soft parts – delivery effected by incision in the perineum. *Stethoscope & Virginia med. Gaz.*, 1852, **2,** 382.
First episiotomy in America, December 2, 1851.

6181 DUNCAN, JAMES MATTHEWS. 1826–1890
On the displacements of the uterus. *Edinb. med. surg. J.*, 1854, **81,** 321–48.
"Duncan's folds", the peritoneal folds of the uterus. Republished in book form, Edinburgh, 1854. Duncan, a leading Edinburgh obstetrician, became lecturer on the subject at St. Bartholomew's Hospital.

6182 WRIGHT, MARMADUKE BURR. 1803–1879
Difficult labors and their treatment. Cincinnati, *Jackson, White & Co.*, 1854.
Wright was responsible for the introduction of combined cephalic version.

6183 CREDÉ, CARL SIEGMUND FRANZ. 1819–1892
De optima in partu naturali placentum amovendi ratione. Lipsiae, *A. Edelmannum*, [1860].
Credé's method of removing the placenta by external manual expression. It is first mentioned in his *Klinische Vorträge über Geburtshilfe*, Berlin, 1854, 599–603.

6184 BRAUN, GUSTAV AUGUST. 1829–1911
Ueber das technische Verfahren bei vernachlässigten Querlagen und über Decapitationsinstrumente. *Wien. med. Wschr.*, 1861, **11,** 713–16.
Braun's decapitation hook.

6185 HODGE, HUGH LENOX. 1796–1873
The principles and practice of obstetrics. Philadelphia, *Blanchard & Lea*, 1864.
Hodge wrote an important text-book of midwifery. He invented the "Hodge pessary".

6186 HICKS, JOHN BRAXTON. 1823–1897
On combined external and internal version. *Trans. obstet. Soc. Lond.* (1863), 1864, **5,** 219–67.
Introduction of combined podalic version.

6187 ——. On the condition of the uterus in obstructed labour. *Trans. obstet. Soc. Lond.*, (1867), 1868, **9,** 207–39.

6188 BRAUNE, CHRISTIAN WILHELM. 1831–1892
Die Lage des Uterus und Foetus am Ende der Schwangerschaft nach Durchschnitten an gefrornen Cadavern. Leipzig, *Veit u. Co.*, 1872.
A classical atlas of frozen sections of the uterus and foetus. Published as a supplement to No. 424.

6189 HICKS, JOHN BRAXTON. 1823–1897
On the contractions of the uterus throughout pregnancy: their physiological effects and their value in the diagnosis of pregnancy. *Trans. obstet. Soc. Lond.*, (1871), 1872, **13,** 216–31.
"Braxton Hicks' sign."

6190 BANDL, LUDWIG. 1842–1892
Ueber das Verhalten des Uterus und Cervix in der Schwangerschaft und während der Geburt. Stuttgart, *F. Enke*, 1876.
"Bandl's ring." Bandl was professor of obstetrics and gynaecology at Vienna and Prague.

6191 PARRY, JOHN S. 1843–1876
Extra-uterine pregnancy. Philadelphia, *H. C. Lea*, 1876.
Lawson Tait regarded this as the first authoritative work on the subject. Parry showed the necessity for operation in such cases and it was this book, more than anything else, which determined Tait (No. 6196) to do so.

6192 TARNIER, STÉPHANE. 1828–1897
Description de deux nouveaux forceps. Paris, *Lauwereyns*, 1877.
Tarnier invented the axis-traction forceps. See also *Ann. Gynéc.*, 1877, **7**, 241–64.

6193 PINARD, ADOLPHE. 1844–1934
Traité du palper abdominal au point de vue obstétrical. Paris, *H. Lauwereyns*, 1878.
Pinard, professor of obstetrics in Paris, showed the importance of abdominal palpation as an aid to obstetrical diagnosis. English translation, 1885.

6194 DUNCAN, JAMES MATTHEWS. 1826–1890
Clinical lecture on hepatic disease in gynaecology and obstetrics. *Med. Times Gaz.*, 1879, **1**, 57–59.
Matthews Duncan pointed out that pernicious vomiting in pregnancy may be associated with hepatic lesions.

6195 CREDÉ, CARL SIEGMUND FRANZ. 1819–1892
Die Verhütung der Augenentzündung der Neugeborenen. Berlin, *A. Hirschwald*, 1884.
Credé introduced the practice of instillation of silver nitrate into the eyes of all newborn children as a preventive measure against ophthalmia neonatorum.

6196 TAIT, ROBERT LAWSON. 1845–1899
Five cases of extra-uterine pregnancy operated upon at the time of rupture. *Brit. med. J.*, 1884, **1**, 1250–51.
The first successful operation for ruptured ectopic pregnancy was performed by Lawson Tait on March 1, 1883.

6197 WERTH, RICHARD. 1850–1918
Beiträge zur Anatomie und zur operativen Behandlung der Extrauterinschwangerschaft. Stuttgart, *F. Enke*, 1887.

6198 CHAMPETIER DE RIBES, CAMILLE LOUIS ANTOINE. 1848–1935
De l'accouchement provoqué; dilatation du canal génital (col de l'utérus, vagin et vulve) à l'aide de ballons introduits dans la cavité utérine pendant la grossesse. *Ann. Gynéc. Obstet.*, 1888, **30**, 401–38.
The "Champetier de Ribes bag".

6199 TAIT, ROBERT LAWSON. 1845–1899
Lectures on ectopic pregnancy and pelvic haematocele. Birmingham, *Journal Printing Works*, 1888.

6200 WALCHER, GUSTAV ADOLF. 1856–1935
Die Conjugata eines engen Beckens ist keine konstante Grosse, sondern lässt sich durch die Körperhaltung der Trägerin verändern. *Zbl. Gynäk.*, 1889, **13**, 892–93.
Description of the "Walcher position".

6201 BOSSI, Luigi Maria. 1859–1919
Sulla provocazione artificiale del parto e sul parto forzato col mezzo della dilatazione meccanica del collo uterino. *Ann. Ostet. Ginec.*, 1892, **14,** 881–928.
Bossi originated the method of induction of premature labour by means of forced dilatation of the cervix.

6202 BREUS, Carl. 1852–1914
Das tuberöse subchoriale Hämatom der Decidua. Eine typische Form der Molenschwangerschaft. Leipzig, Wien, *F. Deuticke*, 1892.
Tuberous ("Breus") mole first described.

6203 WEBSTER, John Clarence. 1863–1950
Tubo-peritoneal ectopic gestation. Edinburgh, *Y. J. Pentland*, 1892.

6204 GIGLI, Leonardo. 1863–1908
Über ein neues Instrument zum Durchtrennen der Knochen, die Drahtsäge. *Zbl. Chir.*, 1894, **21,** 409–11.
Gigli's saw, first used for pubiotomy.

6205 HEGAR, Alfred. 1830–1914
Diagnose der frühesten Schwangerschaftsperiode. *Dtsch. med. Wschr.*, 1895, **21,** 565–67.
Hegar's sign – softening of the lower segment of the uterus, an early diagnostic sign of pregnancy. It was first described by his assistant, C. Reinl, in *Prag. med. Wschr.*, 1884, 9, 253–54.

6206 KOUWER, Benjamin Jan. 1861–1933
Een geval van ovariaalzwangerschap (zwangerschap in een Graafschen follikel). *Ned. T. Verlosk. Gynaec.*, 1897, **8,** 157–68.
First description of ovarian pregnancy.

6207 STROGANOFF, Vasili Vasilyevich. 1857–1938
[On the treatment of eclampsia]. *Vrach*, St. Petersburg, 1900, **21,** 1137–40.
The first of Stroganoff's important papers on the pathogenesis and treatment of eclampsia.

6208 BALLANTYNE, John William. 1861–1923
Manual of antenatal pathology and hygiene. 2 vols. Edinburgh, *William Green & Sons*, 1902–04.
Ballantyne was a pioneer advocate of antenatal care. For an appreciation of his work, see F. J. Browne's *Antenatal and postnatal care*, 4th ed., 1942, 6–9.

6209 GIGLI, Leonardo. 1863–1908
Sinfisiotomia classica e taglio lateralizzato del pube. *Clin. mod.*, 1902, **8,** 302–08.
"Gigli's operation." Gigli substituted pubiotomy for symphysiotomy.

6210 STEINBÜCHEL, Richard von.
Vorläufige Mittheilung über die Anwendung von Skopolamin-Morphium-Injektionen in der Geburtshilfe. *Zbl. Gynäk.*, 1902, **26,** 1304–06.
"Twilight sleep."

6211 WILLIAMS, John Whitridge. 1866–1931
Obstetrics. New York, *D. Appleton*, 1903.
8th edition, 1941.

6212 GAUSS, Carl Joseph. 1875–1957
Geburten in künstlichem Dämmerschlaf. *Arch. Gynäk.*, 1906, **78,** 579–631.
"Twilight sleep." Gauss developed the method introduced by Steinbüchel (No. 6210).

6213 SELLHEIM, Hugo. 1871–1936
Die Mechanik der Geburt. *Samml. klin. Vortr.*, 1906, n.F., Nr. 421, (Gynäk., Nr. 156), 659–82.

6214 MOMBURG, Fritz August. 1870–1939
Die künstliche Blutleere der unteren Körperhälfte. *Zbl. Chir.*, 1908, **35,** 697–99.
Abdominal ligature in prevention of post-partum haemorrhage.

6215 BELL, William Blair. 1871–1936
The pituitary body and the therapeutic value of the infundibular extract in shock, uterine atony, and intestinal paresis. *Brit. med. J.*, 1909, **2,** 1609–13.

6216 EDLING, Lars. 1878–
Ueber die Anwendung des Roentgenverfahrens bei der Diagnose der Schwangerschaft. *Fortschr. Röntgenstr.*, 1911, **17,** 345–55.
First use of *x* rays for the diagnosis of pregnancy.

6217 DeLEE, Joseph Bolivar. 1869–1942
The principles and practice of obstetrics. Philadelphia, *W. B. Saunders*, 1913.
10th edition, 1951.

6218 LYNCH, Frank Worthington. 1871–
Eutocia by means of nitrous oxid gas analgesia; a safe substitute for the Freiburg method. *J. Amer. med. Ass.*, 1915, **64,** 1187–89.
Introduction of gas-oxygen anaesthesia in childbirth.

6219 KIELLAND, Christian. 1871–1941
Ueber die Anlegung der Zange am nicht rotierten Kopf mit Beschreibung eines neuen Zangenmodelles und einer neuen Anlegungsmethode. *Mschr. Geburtsh. Gynäk.*, 1916, **43,** 48–78.
Kielland forceps.

6220 MACKENZIE, *Sir* James. 1853–1925
Heart disease and pregnancy. London, *H. Frowde*, 1921.

6221 POTTER, Irving White. 1868–
Version. *Amer. J. Obstet. Gynec.*, 1921, **1,** 560–73.
Potter's operation of podalic version.

6222 ASCHHEIM, Selmar. 1878– , & ZONDEK, Bernhard. 1891–1966
Schwangerschaftsdiagnose aus dem Harn (durch Hormonnachweis). *Klin. Wschr.*, 1928, **7,** 8–9, 1404–11, 1453–57.
The Aschheim–Zondek test for the diagnosis of pregnancy.

6223 MENEES, Thomas Orville. 1890–1937, *et al.*
Amniography; preliminary report. *Amer. J. Roentgenol.*, 1930, **24,** 363–66.
Introduction of amniography. With J. D. Miller and L. E. Holly.

6224 FRIEDMAN, MAURICE HAROLD. 1903– , & LAPHAM, MAXWELL EDWARD. 1899–

A simple, rapid procedure for the laboratory diagnosis of early pregnancies. *Amer. J. Obstet. Gynec.*, 1931, **21,** 405–10.

Friedman test for the diagnosis of pregnancy.

6225 READ, GRANTLY DICK. 1890–1959

Natural childbirth. London, *W. Heinemann*, 1933.

Read advocated natural childbirth for many years; he demonstrated that prenatal education in methods of relaxation in many cases makes labour almost painless.

6226 BELLERBY, CHARLES WILLIAM.

A rapid test for the diagnosis of pregnancy. *Nature* (*Lond.*), 1934, **133,** 494–95.

The *Xenopus* toad test for the diagnosis of pregnancy; this preliminary note followed Hogben's demonstration that *Xenopus* responds by ovulation to the gonadotrophic hormone (*Trans. roy. Soc. S. Africa*, 1930, Ser. A, **5**, 19). For detailed history of the development of this test, see *Brit. med. J.*, 1946, **2,** 554.

6227 KAPELLER-ADLER, REGINE.

Über eine neue chemische Schwangerschaftsreaktion. *Klin. Wschr.*, 1934, **13,** 21–22.

Kapeller-Adler test for diagnosis of pregnancy.

6228 MINNITT, ROBERT JAMES. 1892–

A new technique for the self-administration of gas-air analgesia in labour. *Lancet*, 1934, **1,** 1278–79.

Introduction of the "Minnitt apparatus."

6229 SNOW, WILLIAM. 1898– , & POWELL, CLILIAN BETHANY. 1894–

Roentgen visualization of the placenta. *Amer. J. Roentgenol.*, 1934, **31,** 37–40.

Direct radiography of the placenta.

6230 DUDLEY, HAROLD WARD. 1887–1935, & MOIR, JOHN CHASSAR. 1900–

The substance responsible for the traditional clinical effect of ergot. *Brit. med. J.*, 1935, **1,** 520–23.

Isolation and introduction of ergometrine.

6231 WHITE, PRISCILLA. 1900– , *et al.*

Prediction and prevention of late pregnancy accidents in diabetes. *Amer. J. med. Sci.*, 1939, **198,** 482–92.

First report of hormone treatment. Written with R. S. Titus, E. P. Joslin, and H. Hunt.

6232 STEINER, PAUL EBY. 1902– , & LUSHBAUGH, CLARENCE CHANCELUM. 1916–

Maternal pulmonary embolism by amniotic fluid as a cause of obstetric shock and unexpected deaths in obstetrics. *J. Amer. med. Ass.*, 1941, **117,** 1245–54, 1340–45.

Amniotic fluid embolism described.

6233 O'SULLIVAN, JAMES VINCENT.

Acute inversion of the uterus. *Brit. med. J.*, 1945, **2,** 282–83.

O'Sullivan's method of replacement by intravaginal hydraulic pressure.

6234 GALLI MAININI, Carlos. 1914–1961
Reacción diagnóstica del embarazo en la que se usa el sapo macho como animal reactivo. *Sem. méd.* (*B. Aires*), 1947, **1**, 337–40.
Male toad test. An English account is in *J. clin. Endocr.*, 1947, **7**, 653–58.

6235 RAPP, Gustav William. 1917– , & RICHARDSON, Garwood Colvin. 1897–
A saliva test for prenatal sex determination. *Science*, 1952, **115**, 265.

6236–6252 CAESAREAN SECTION

6236 ROUSSET, François [Roussetus; Rossetus]. 1535–1590?
Traitte nouveau de l'hysterotomotokie, ou enfantement caesarien. Paris, *Denys du Val*, 1581.
Rousset records 15 successful Caesarean sections carried out by various persons during the preceding 80 years.

6236.1 BARLOW, James. 1767–1839
A case of the caesarean operation performed, and the life of the woman preserved. *Medical Records and Researches Selected from the Papers of a Private Medical Association*, London, *T. Cox*, 1798, pp. 154–62.
This is apparently the first Caesarean section in England from which the mother recovered. It was performed on Nov. 27, 1793. Barlow's account is reproduced by Young (No. 6307), pp. 54–58. A note on Barlow is in *Practitioner*, 1965, **195**, 103–08.

6237 OSIANDER, Friedrich Benjamin. 1759–1822
Handbuch der Entbindungskunst. 4 vols. Tübingen, *C. F. Osiander*, 1818–25.
Includes (Bd. 2, Abt. II, p. 302) description of Osiander's lower-segment Caesarean operation.

6238 RITGEN, Ferdinand August Marie Franz. 1787–1867
Geschichte eines mit ungünstigem Erfolge verrichteten Bauchscheidenschnitts und Folgerung daraus. *Heidelb. klin. Ann.*, 1825, **1**, 263–77.
Ritgen first performed gastro-elytrotomy in 1821.

6239 THOMAS, Theodore Gaillard. 1831–1903
Gastro-elytrotomy; a substitute for the Caesarean section. *Amer. J. Obstet. Dis. Wom.*, 1870, **3**, 125–39.
Thomas revived and modified Ritgen's operation.

6240 PORRO, Edoardo 1842–1902
Della amputazione utero-ovarica come complemento di taglio cesareo. *Ann. univ. Med. Chir.*, 1876, **237**, 289–350.
Caesarean section with excision of the uterus and adnexa ("Porro's operation").

6241 KEHRER, Ferdinand Adolf. 1837–1914
Ueber ein modificirtes Verfahren beim Kaiserschnitte. *Arch. Gynäk.*, 1882, **19**, 177–209.
Kehrer improved the technique of the Caesarean operation.

6242 SÄNGER, MAX. 1853–1903
Der Kaiserschnitt bei Uterusfibromen nebst vergleichender Methodik der Sectio Caesarea und der Porro-Operation. Leipzig, *W. Engelmann*, 1882.
"Sänger's operation" – the so-called "classical Caesarean section". A preliminary is in *Arch, Gynäk*, 1882, **19**, 370.

6243 CHAMPNEYS, *Sir* FRANCIS HENRY. 1848–1930
A case of Caesarean section for contracted pelvis. *Trans. obstet. Soc. Lond.*, 1889, **31,** 136–60.
Champneys' advocacy of the Sänger operation was a powerful factor in its adoption in Britain.

6244 HALBERTSMA, TJALLING. 1841–1898
Eclampsia gravidarum: eene nieuwe indicatie voor sectie caesarea. *Ned. T. Geneesk.*, 1889, 2 D., **25,** 485–91.
Halbertsma first performed Caesarean section in puerperal convulsions.

6245 TAIT, ROBERT LAWSON. 1845–1899
An address on the surgical aspect of impacted labour. *Brit. med. J.*, 1890, **1,** 657–61.
The Tait–Porro operation, by which Tait performed Caesarean section in cases of placenta praevia.

6246 DÜHRSSEN, ALFRED. 1862–1933
Über vaginalen Kaiserschnitt. *Samml. klin. Vortr.*, 1898, n.F., Nr. 232 (Gynäkol., Nr. 84), 1365–88.
The vaginal Caesarean operation was introduced by Dührssen in April, 1895.

6247 FRANK, FRITZ. 1856–1923
Die suprasymphysäre Entbindung und ihr Verhältniss zu den anderen Operationen bei engen Becken. *Arch. Gynäk.*, 1907, **81,** 46–94.
Suprasymphyseal transperitoneal Caesarean section.

6248 SELLHEIM, HUGO. 1871–1936
Die extraperitoneale Uterusschnitt. *Zbl. Gynäk.*, 1908, **32,** 133–42.
Sellheim's operation. For his three subsequent modifications, see the same journal, 319–31, 641–51, and *Mschr. Geburtsh. Gynäk.*, 1911, **34**, 34–45.

6249 LATZKO, WILHELM. 1863–
Der extraperitoneale Kaiserschnitt. Seine Geschichte, seine Technik und seine Indikationen. *Wien. klin. Wschr.*, 1909, **22,** 477–82.
Latzko's extraperitoneal lower-segment Caesarean operation. Preliminary report in the same journal, 1908, **21**, 737.

6250 DÖDERLEIN, ALBERT SIEGMUND GUSTAV. 1860–1941, & KRÖNIG BERNARD. 1863–1917
Operative Gynäkologie. 3rd ed. Leipzig, *Georg Thieme*, 1912.
Includes (p. 879) first description of Krönig's operation of transperitoneal lower-segment Caesarean section.

6251 DeLEE, JOSEPH BOLIVAR. 1869–1942
The newer methods of cesarean section. Report of 40 cases. *J. Amer. med. Ass.*, 1919, **73,** 91–95.
DeLee's low cervical operation (laparotrachelotomy).

6252 PORTES, Louis. 1891–1950
Césarienne suivie d'extériorisation temporaire de l'utérus et de réintégration secondaire dans le bassin. *Bull. Soc. Obstét. Gynéc. Paris*, 1924, **13**, 171–76.

Portes operation – the classical Caesarean section followed by temporary exteriorization of the uterus. More fully described in *Gynéc. et Obstét.*, 1924, **10**, 225–50.

For history, see No. 6307

6253–6266 PELVIS; PELVIC ANOMALIES

6253 DEVENTER, Hendrik van. 1651–1724
Operationes chirurgicae novum lumen exhibentes obstetricantibus. Lugduni Batavorum, *A. Dyckhuisen*, 1701.

This work gives the first accurate description of the female pelvis and its deformities, and the effect of the latter in complicating labour. Van Deventer was the greatest obstetrician of his time, the "father of modern midwifery".

6254 HUNTER, William. 1718–1783
A singular case of the separation of the ossa pubis. *Med. Obs. Inqu.*, 1762, **2**, 321–39, 415–18.

A case of osteomalacic pelvis was reported to Hunter by a country practitioner.

6255 BAUDELOCQUE, Jean Louis. 1746–1810
L'art des accouchemens. 2 vols. Paris, *Méquignon*, 1781.

Baudelocque invented a pelvimeter and advanced the knowledge of pelvimetry and of the mechanism of labour. The external conjugate diameter is known as "Baudelocque's diameter". English translation, London, 1790.

6256 NAEGELE, Franz Karl. 1778–1851
Das weibliche Becken. Carlsruhe, *C. F. Muller*, 1825.

6257 ——. Das schräg verengte Becken nebst einem Anhange über die wichtigsten Fehler des weiblichen Beckens überhaupt. Mainz, *V. von Zabern*, 1839.

First description of the obliquely contracted pelvis. English translation, 1939.

6258 ROKITANSKY, Carl, *Freiherr von*. 1804–1878
Beyträge zur Kenntniss der Rückgrathskrümmungen, und der mit demselben zusammentreffenden Abweichungen des Brustkorbes und Beckens. *Med. Jb. österr. Staates*, 1839, **19**, 41, 195.

Original description of spondylolisthesis.

6259 MICHAELIS, Gustav Adolf. 1798–1848
Das enge Becken: nach eigenen Beobachtungen und Untersuchungen. Leipzig, *G. Wigand*, 1851.

First important work dealing with pelvic deformities since the time of van Deventer. It is a pioneer work in the literature dealing with pelvic architecture; Michaelis was one of the first to differentiate between the non-rachitic flat pelvis and the rachitic pelvis.

6260 LITZMANN, Carl Conrad Theodor. 1815–1890
Das schräg-ovale Becken. Kiel, *Akad. Buchhandlung*, 1853.

Litzmann (see also No. 6263) described in this work the coxalgic, scoliotic and kyphoscoliotic forms of pelvis.

6261 KILIAN, HERMANN FRIEDRICH. 1800–1863
Schilderungen neuer Beckenformen und ihres Verhaltens im Leben. Mannheim, *Bassermann & Mathey*, 1854.

First description of pelvis spinosa.

6262 ——. De spondylolisthesi gravissimae pelvangustiae causa nuper detecta. Bonnae, *C. Georg*, [1854].

An important study of the spondylolisthetic pelvis, which Kilian called "pelvis obtecta".

6263 LITZMANN, CARL CONRAD THEODOR. 1815–1890
Die Formen des Beckens, insbesondere des engen weiblichen Beckens. Berlin, *G. Reimer*, 1861.

Litzmann devised a clinical classification of pelves which was for many years generally used, and he described various deformities of the female pelvis.

6264 NEUGEBAUER, FRANZ LUDWIG. 1856–1914
Neuer Beitrag zur Aetiologie und Casuistik der Spondyl-olisthesis. *Arch. Gynäk.*, 1885, **25,** 182–252.

6265 BREUS, CARL. 1852–1914, & KOLISKO, ALEXANDER. 1847–1918
Die pathologischen Beckenformen. Leipzig, *F. Deuticke*, 1900–04.

Classical description and classification of pelvic deformities.

6266 CALDWELL, WILLIAM EDGAR. 1880–1943, & MOLOY, HOWARD CARMAN. 1903–1953
Anatomical variations in the female pelvis and their effect in labor, with a suggested classification. *Amer. J. Obstet. Gynec.*, 1933, **26,** 479–505.

The modern classification of the female pelvis is based on the work of Caldwell and Moloy.

6267–6281 PUERPERAL FEVER

6267 HIPPOCRATES. 460–375 B.C.
The genuine works. Translated . . . by F. ADAMS. Vol. 1. London, 1849.

Contains, p. 373, the earliest known reference to puerperal fever; *Epidemics* Bk. 1, Case IV.

6268 BURTON, JOHN. 1697–1771
An essay towards a complete new system of midwifery, theoretical and practical. London, *J. Hodges*, 1751.

Burton was the first to suggest that puerperal fever is contagious.

6269 LEAKE, JOHN. 1729–1792
Practical observations on the child-bed fever. London, *J. Walter*, [1772].

Leake insisted on the contagious nature of puerperal fever.

6270 WHITE, CHARLES. 1728–1813
A treatise on the management of pregnant and lying-in-women. London, *E. & C. Dilly*, 1773.

White was a strong advocate of surgical cleanliness in obstetrics and his book is a pioneer work in aseptic midwifery. He was the first after Hippocrates to make any substantial contribution towards the solution of the aetiology and management of puerperal fever.

6271 ——. An inquiry into the nature and cause of that swelling, in one or both of the lower extremities, which sometimes happens to lying-in-women. Warrington, *printed by W. Eyres, for C. Dilly in the Poultry London*, 1784.

First clinical description of phlegmasia alba dolens. White ascribed it to destruction of the lymphatics due to pressure of the foetal head.

6272 GORDON, Alexander. 1752–1799
A treatise on the epidemic puerperal fever of Aberdeen. London, *G. G. & J. Robinson*, 1795.

Gordon was the first to advance as a definite hypothesis the contagious nature of puerperal fever, thus preceding Holmes and Semmelweis by half a century. He also advocated the disinfection of the clothes of the doctor and midwife.

6273 DAVIS, David Daniel. 1777–1841
An essay on the proximate cause of the disease called phlegmasia dolens. *Med.-chir. Trans.*, 1823, **12,** 419–60.

Davis was the first to state that phlegmasia alba dolens was due to inflammation of the veins. He was physician-accoucheur at the birth of Queen Victoria.

6274 HOLMES, Oliver Wendell. 1809–1894
The contagiousness of puerperal fever. *N. Engl. quart. J. Med. Surg.*, 1842–43, **1,** 503–30.

Oliver Wendell Holmes was the first definitely to establish the contagious nature of puerperal fever. His essay on the subject took a strong line against the opinions then prevailing, stirring up violent opposition among the obstetricians of Philadelphia. Reprinted in *Med. Classics*, 1936, **1**, 211–43.

6275 SEMMELWEIS, Ignaz Philipp. 1818–1865
Höchst wichtige Erfahrungen über die Aetiologie der in Gebär-anstalten epidemischen Puerperalfieber. *Z. k. k. Ges. Aerzte Wien*, 1847–48, **4,** pt. 2, 242–44; 1849, **5,** 64–65.

Semmelweis, pioneer of antisepsis in obstetrics, was the first to recognize that puerperal fever is a septicaemia. (See also his more important work, No. 6277.)

6276 HOLMES, Oliver Wendell. 1809–1894
Puerperal fever, as a private pestilence. Boston, *Ticknor & Fields*, 1855.

Holmes enlarged his famous essay on the contagiousness of puerperal fever, and in this reiteration mentioned the steps already being taken by Semmelweis. The work has been reprinted in *Med. Classics*, 1936, **1**, 245–68.

6277 SEMMELWEIS, Ignaz Philipp. 1818–1865
Die Aetiologie, der Begriff und die Prophylaxis des Kindbettfiebers. Pest, Wien & Leipzig, *C. A. Hartleben*, 1861.

One of the epoch-making books in medical literature. Semmelweis, who earlier had shown puerperal fever to be a septicaemia, strove to improve conditions in the lying-in wards of Vienna and Budapest. Misunderstood and maligned by many, he eventually published this book in support of his views on the aetiology of puerperal sepsis. He had no literary style and his book is difficult reading; it had an overwhelming mass of badly-presented statistics. Sir W. J. Sinclair, his biographer, said of him that "if he could have written like Oliver Wendell Holmes, his 'Aetiology' would have conquered Europe in 12 months." Semmelweis died in an asylum on Aug. 13, 1865. An English translation of the book, by F. P. Murphy, is in *Med. Classics*, 1941, **5**, 350–773.

6278 PASTEUR, Louis. 1822–1895
Sépticémie puerpérale. *Bull. Acad. Méd.* (*Paris*), 1879, 2 sér., **8,** 505–508.
Description of the streptococcus of puerperal sepsis.

6279 DÖDERLEIN, Albert Siegmund Gustav. 1860–1941
Das Scheidensekret und seine Bedeutung für das Puerperalfieber. Leipzig, *O. Durr.*, 1892.
A classical study of the vaginal secretion in relation to puerperal fever. Includes the first description of "Döderlein's bacillus".

6280 HALBAN, Josef von. 1870–1937, & KÖHLER, Robert. 1884–
Die pathologische Anatomie des Puerperalprozesses. Wien, Leipzig, *W. Braumüller*, 1919.

6281 COLEBROOK, Leonard. 1883–1967, & KENNY, Méave.
Treatment of human puerperal infections, and of experimental infections in mice, with prontosil. *Lancet*, 1936, **1,** 1279–86.
Chemotherapeutic treatment of puerperal sepsis.

History of Gynaecology and Obstetrics

6282 AVELING, James Hobson. 1828–1892
English midwives. London, *J. & A. Churchill*, 1872.
Reprinted with biographical sketch by J. L. Thornton, London, 1967.

6283 ——. The Chamberlens and the midwifery forceps. London, *J. & A. Churchill*, 1882.

6284 ENGELMANN, George Julius. 1847–1903
Labor among primitive peoples. St. Louis, *J. H. Chambers & Co.*, 1882.

6285 WITKOWSKI, Gustave Jules A. 1843–?
Les accouchements à la cour. Paris, *G. Steinheil*, 1887.

6286 ——. Histoire des accouchements chez tous les peuples. 2 vols. Paris, *G. Steinheil*, [1889].

6287 McKAY, William John Stewart. 1866–1948
The history of ancient gynaecology. London, *Baillière, Tindall & Cox*, 1901.

6288 SIEBOLD, Eduard Caspar Jacob von. 1801–1861
Versuch einer Geschichte der Geburtshilfe. 2te. Aufl. 2 vols. Tübingen, *F. Pietzcker*, 1901–02.
First edition, 1839–45. Continuation by R. Dohrn, for the period 1840–80, forming Bd. 3 (see No. 6289).

6289 DOHRN, Rudolf. 1836–1915
Geschichte der Geburtshülfe der Neuzeit. 2 pts. Tübingen, *F. Pietzcker*, 1903–04.
A supplement to No. 6288.

6290 MÜLLERHEIM, Robert Nathan. 1862–
Die Wochenstube in der Kunst. Stuttgart, *F. Enke*, 1904.

6291 FASBENDER, Heinrich. 1843–1914
Geschichte der Geburtshülfe. Jena, *G. Fischer*, 1906.
Probably the most valuable history of the subject.

6292 INGERSLEV, Ove Emmerik Gustav Hoegh-Guldberg. 1844–1916
Fragmenter af fødselshjaelpens historie. 2 vols. Kjøbenhavn, 1906–1907.

6293 WEINDLER, Fritz.
Geschichte der gynäkologisch-anatomischen Abbildungen. Dresden, *Zahn u. Jaensch*, 1908.

6294 LEÓN, Nicolas. 1859–1929
La ostetricia en México: notas, bibliográficas, etnicas, históricas, documentarias y criticas, de los origenes históricos hasta el año 1910. 2 pts. México, *Diaz de León*, 1910.

6295 LA TORRE, Felice. 1846–1923
L'utero attraverso i secoli da Erofilo al giorni nostri; storia, iconografia, struttura, fisiologia. Città di Castello, *Unione Arti Grafiche*, 1917.
Contains an important collection of illustrations.

6296 FISCHER, Isidor. 1868–1943
Geschichte der Gynäkologie. In J. von Halban and L. Seitz: *Biologie und Pathologie des Weibes*, Berlin, 1924, **1**, 1–202.

6297 FEHLER, Hermann Johann Karl. 1847–1925
Entwicklung der Geburtshilfe und Gynäkologie im 19. Jahrhundert. Berlin, *J. Springer*, 1925.

6298 SONDEREGGER, Albert.
Missgeburten und Wundergestalten in Einblattdrucken und Handzeichnungen des 16. Jahrhunderts. Zürich, *O. Füssli*, 1927.

6299 SPENCER, Herbert Ritchie. 1860–1941
History of British midwifery from 1650–1800. London, *John Bale*, 1927.

6300 VIANA, Odorico. 1877–1942, & VOZZA Francesco.
L'ostetricia e la ginecologia in Italia. Milano, *A. Cordani*, 1933.

6301 THOMS, Herbert. 1885–
Classic contributions to obstetrics and gynecology. Springfield, *C. C. Thomas*, 1935.

6302 JAMESON, Edwin Milton. 1902–
Gynecology and obstetrics. New York, *P. B. Hoeber*, 1936.
An excellent short history of the progress of gynaecology and obstetrics. A useful bibliography is included. *Clio Medica* series.

6303 DIEPGEN, Paul. 1878–1966
Geschichte der Frauenheilkunde. 1 Teil. Die Frauenheilkunde der alten Welt. München, *J. F. Bergmann*, 1937.
Forms Bd. 12, Teil 1, of *Handbuch der Gynäkologie*, hrsg. J. Veit u. W. Stoeckel. See also No. 6311.2.

6304 CLAYE, *Sir* ANDREW MOYNIHAN. 1896–
The evolution of obstetric analgesia. London, *Oxford University Press*, 1939.

6305 RICCI, JAMES VINCENT. 1890–
The genealogy of gynaecology. History of the development of gynaecology throughout the ages 2000 B.C.–A.D. 1800. Philadelphia, *Blakiston*, (1943).

6306 LEONARDO, RICHARD ANTHONY. 1895–
History of gynecology. New York, *Froben Press*, 1944.

6307 YOUNG, JOHN HARLEY.
Caesarean section. The history and development of the operation from earliest times. London, *H. K. Lewis*, 1944.

6308 USANDIZAGA SORALUCE, MANUEL.
Historia de la obstetricia y de la ginecología en España. Santander, *Aldus*, 1944.

6309 RICCI, JAMES VINCENT. 1890–
One hundred years of gynaecology, 1800–1900. Philadelphia, *Blakiston*, (1945).

6310 ——. The development of gynaecological surgery and instruments . . . from the Hippocratic age to the Antiseptic period. Philadelphia, *Blakiston*, 1949.

6311 RADCLIFFE, WALTER.
The secret instrument. The birth of the midwifery forceps. London, *W. Heinemann*, 1947.

6311.1 KERR, JOHN MARTIN MUNRO. 1868–1960, *et al.*
Historical review of British obstetrics and gynaecology, 1800–1950. Edinburgh, *E. & S. Livingstone*, 1954.

Edited by J. M. Munro Kerr, R. W. Johnstone, and M. H. Phillips. Supplements No. 6299.

6311.2 DIEPGEN, PAUL. 1878–1966
Frau und Frauenheilkunde in der Kultur des Mittelalters. Stuttgart, *G. Thieme*, 1963.

A continuation of No. 6303.

6311.3 RADCLIFFE, WALTER.
Milestones in midwifery. Bristol, *John Wright*, 1967.

6312–6357.1

PAEDIATRICS

6312 SORANUS, *of Ephesus*. A.D. 98–138
Die Gynäkologie, Geburtshilfe, Frauen- und Kinder-Krankheiten, Diätetik der Neugeborenen. Übersetzt von H. Lüneberg. München, *J. F. Lehmann*, 1894.

In his treatise on diseases of women, Soranus included full instructions on the care and management of infants. English translation by O. Temkin and others, Baltimore, 1956.

6313 RHAZES [ABU BAKR MUHAMMAD IBN ZAKARĪYĀ AL-RĀZĪ]. *c.* 850–923
De curis puerorum in prima aetate. In his *Opuscula*. Mediolani, *per L. Pachel et V. Scincenzeller*, 1481.

Rhazes was the first to devote an entire treatise to diseases of children. Although he lived so many years before the advent of printing, he was still regarded as an authority in the 15th century and his works were amongst the earliest medical books to be printed. Sudhoff includes the above work in his *Erstlinge der pädiatrischen Literatur*, München, 1925.

6314 LOUFFENBERG, HEINRICH VON. ? *d.* 1458
Versehung des Leibs. Augsburg, [*Erhard Ratholdt*], 1491.

Includes the first poem on paediatrics. It is written in old Swabian; its author was a monk. For details of this rare work, see J. Ruhräh, *Pediatrics of the past*, New York, 1925, pp. 465–86.

6315 BAGELLARDO, PAOLO. *d.* 1494
De egritudinibus et remediis infantium. [Patavia, *B. de Valdezoccho*, 1472].

First printed book dealing exclusively with paediatrics; this is also the first medical treatise to make its original appearance in printed form. The book is based mainly on the writings of Avicenna and Rhazes. It appears in facsimile in Sudhoff's *Erstlinge* (see No. 6355), and there is a translation by H. F. Wright in J. F. Ruhräh's *Pediatrics of the past*, 1925.

6316 METLINGER, BARTHOLOMAEUS. ? *d.* 1492
Regiment der jungen Kinder. [Augsburg, *G. Zainer*, 1473].

This work has very little originality, being derived mainly from the Arabic physicians of 500 years before, but is noteworthy as being the first book on paediatrics printed in German. It includes what is probably the first reference in medical literature to microcephaly. It was several times reprinted before 1500. Facsimile in Sudhoff's *Erstlinge* (see No. 6355). The edition of 1497 is the first printed work on paediatrics to contain an illustration.

6317 PHAER, THOMAS [PHAYER; PHAYR]. 1510–1560
The regiment of life, whereunto is added a treatise of the pestilence, with the boke of children. London, 1545.

The "boke of children" is the first work on diseases of children to be written by an Englishman. Phaer enabled Englishmen to read and think of paediatrics in their own language. He is notable also as having translated the *Aeneid*. Reprint, edited by A. V. Neale and H. R. E. Wallis, Edinburgh, 1955.

6318 VALLAMBERT, SIMON DE [VALLEMBERT].
Cinq livres, de la maniere de nourrir et gouverner les enfans des leur naissance. a Poictiers, *de Marnesz, & Bouchetz*, 1565.

This, the first work on paediatrics in French, was also the first to contain a reference to syphilis in children.

6319 WÜRTZ, FELIX [WIRTZ]. 1518–1574
Ein schönes und nützliches Kinderbůchlein. In his *Practica der Wundartzney*, Basel, *S. Henricpetri*, 1616, pp. 725–84.

First work dealing with infant surgery. English translation 1656, which is reprinted in J. Ruhräh's *Pediatrics of the past*, 1925.

6320 PEMELL, ROBERT. *d.* 1653
De morbis puerorum, or, a treatise of the diseases of children. London, *J. Legatt for P. Stevens*, 1653.

More than 100 years after the publication of Phaer's book appeared this, the second work in English on paediatrics. Pemell was a general practitioner living at Cranbrook in Kent; he was buried only 5 days after the publication of his book.

6321 HARRIS, WALTER. 1647–1732
De morbis acutis infantum. Londini, *Samuel Smith*, 1689.

Harris was physician to William and Mary. His book served for nearly a century as a standard work on paediatrics. He anticipated the modern treatment of tetany by using calcium salts in infantile convulsions. For a study of the book, see *Ann. med. Hist.*, 1919, 2, 228–40. English translations 1693, 1742.

6322 CADOGAN, WILLIAM. 1711–1797
An essay upon nursing, and the management of children, from their birth to three years of age. London, *J. Roberts*, 1748.

Cadogan's famous essay laid down rules on the nursing, feeding, and clothing of infants, and filled a great need at a time when infant welfare was much neglected through the ignorance of those concerned. As a result of this work, Cadogan was elected a physician of the Foundling Hospital in 1754. He became a friend of Garrick, and was present at that great actor's death-bed.

6323 ROSÉN VON ROSENSTEIN, NILS. 1706–1773
Underrättelser om barn-sjukdomar och deras botemedel. Stockholm, *Kongl. Wet. Acad.*, 1764.

Sir Frederic Still considered this work "the most progressive which had yet been written"; it gave an impetus to research which influenced the future course of paediatrics. Rosén was the founder of modern paediatrics and was particularly interested in infant feeding. The *Underrättelser* were originally published in the calendars of the Academy and were later collected and issued in book form in 1764. English and German translations in 1766. For a biography, bibliography, and essays on this book, see *Nils Rosen von Rosenstein and his textbook on paediatrics*, ed. B. Vahlquist and A. Wallgren. *Acta paediat.*, 1964, Suppl. 156.

6324 ARMSTRONG, GEORGE. 1719–1789
An essay on the diseases most fatal to infants. London, *T. Cadell*, 1767.

One of the best paediatric works of the period. Armstrong is noteworthy as the founder of the first children's dispensary in Europe, in 1769.

6325 ——. An account of the diseases most incident to children, from their birth till the age of puberty. London, *T. Cadell*, 1777.

An enlarged and more important (third) edition of No. 6324.

6326 UNDERWOOD, MICHAEL. 1737–1820
A treatise on the diseases of children. London, *J. Mathews*, 1784.

Underwood laid the foundation of modern paediatrics. His work was superior to anything that had previously appeared and remained the most important book on the subject for sixty years, passing through many editions. Includes (p. 76) the first description of sclerema neonatorum ("Underwood's disease"); the second edition (1789) contains a description of congenital heart disease in children, being the first paediatric treatise to do so.

6327 HEBERDEN, WILLIAM, *Jr.* 1767–1845
Morborum puerilium epitome. London, *T. Payne*, 1804.

English translation, Uttoxeter, 1805. Like his father, Heberden junior was a great clinician. It is probable that the above work was compiled from notes left by Heberden senior.

6328 CLARKE, JOHN. 1761–1815
Commentaries on some of the most important diseases of children. Part the first. London, *Longman, etc.*, 1815.

Clarke died before this work was published. In it he gave a clear description of tetany and of laryngismus stridulus.

6329 GOELIS, Leopold Anton. 1765–1827
Praktische Abhandlungen über die vorzüglicheren Krankheiten des kindlichen Alters. 2 vols. Wien, *C. Gerold*, 1815–18.

6330 DAVIS, John Bunnell. 1780–1824
A cursory inquiry into some of the principal causes of mortality among children. London, *T. & G. Underwood*, 1817.

Davis called attention to the high infant-mortality rate, especially in London. His suggestion that poor mothers should be instructed in the care of their infants resulted in a system of health-visiting by benevolent ladies. He founded a dispensary for sick and indigent children at St. Andrew's Hill, London, in 1816; this was later removed to the Waterloo Road and eventually became the Royal Waterloo Hospital for Children and Women.

6331 DEWEES, William Potts. 1768–1841
Treatise on the physical and medical treatment of children. Philadelphia, *H. C. Carey & I. Lea*, 1825.

First American text-book on paediatrics.

6332 BILLARD, Charles Michel. 1800–1832
Traité des maladies des enfans nouveau-nés à la mamelle. 1 vol. and atlas. Paris, *J. B. Baillière*, 1828.

Billard performed several hundred autopsies on infants and children and correlated the data obtained with clinical observations he had done. This pioneer work on the pathological anatomy of infants includes interesting observations on cerebral congestion, intestinal disturbances, the pulse, teething, etc. English translation of third edition, 1839.

6333 RILLIET, Frederic. 1814–1861, & BARTHEZ, Antoine Charles Ernest. 1811–1891
Traité clinique et pratique des maladies des enfants. 3 vols. Paris, *G. Baillière*, 1843.

6334 WEST, Charles. 1816–1898
Lectures on the diseases of infancy and childhood. London, *Longman*, 1848.

In its day this was the best English work on the subject, and was translated into several other languages. West was one of the founders of the Hospital for Sick Children, Gt. Ormond Street, London.

6335 BEDNAŘ, Alois. 1816–1888
Die Krankheiten der Neugebornen und Säuglinge. 4 vols. Wien, *C. Gerold*, 1850–53.

Bednař was a famous Viennese paediatrician. His description of aphthae of the palate in the newborn ("Bednař's aphthae") is in vol. 1, p. 104 of his book.

6336 HENOCH, Eduard. 1820–1910
Beiträge zur Kinderheilkunde. Berlin, *A. Hirschwald*, 1861.

6337 GERHARDT, Carl Adolph Christian Jacob. 1833–1902
Handbuch der Kinderkrankheiten. Hrsg. von C. Gerhardt. 9 vols. [in 16]. Tübingen, *H. Laupp*, 1877–93.

Gerhardt edited this great work, which was written by the foremost paediatricians of the time and which gives a close-up view of paediatric knowledge at the end of the 19th century.

6338 WINCKEL, FRANZ CARL LUDWIG VON. 1837–1911
Ueber eine bisher nicht beschriebene endemisch aufgetretene Erkrankung Neugeborener. *Dtsch. med. Wschr.*, 1879, **5**, 303–07, 415–418, 431–36, 447–50.

First description of "Winckel's disease" of the newborn, characterized by icterus, haemorrhage, haemoglobinuria, and cyanosis.

6339 HENOCH, EDUARD. 1820–1910
Vorlesungen über Kinderkrankheiten. Berlin, *A. Hirschwald*, 1881.

Henoch, whose name is remembered for his description of purpura, initiated the modern concept of paediatrics. English translation, New York, 1882.

6340 ESCHERICH, THEODOR. 1857–1911
Die Darmbakterien des Säuglings und ihre Beziehungen zur Physiologie der Verdauung. Stuttgart, *F. Enke*, 1886.

Escherich described *Bact. coli* infection. The genus *Escherichia* is named after him.

6341 SOXHLET, FRANZ VON. 1848–1926
Ueber Kindermilch und Säuglings-Ernährung. *Münch. med. Wschr.*, 1886, **33**, 253, 276.

Soxhlet wrote on the nature of milk droplets, estimated the specific gravity of milk with his lactodensimeter, described an apparatus for the sterilization of milk, and devised a test for the estimation of fats in milk.

6342 JACOBI, ABRAHAM. 1830–1919
The intestinal diseases of infancy and childhood. Detroit, *G. S. Davis*, 1887.

Jacobi was the first in the United States to specialize in the teaching of paediatrics, and in 1862 founded the first paediatric clinic there (in New York). He wrote extensively on paediatrics; the above is probably his best work.

6343 HEUBNER, JOHANN OTTO LEONARD. 1843–1926
Lehrbuch der Kinderheilkunde. 2 vols. Leipzig, *J. A. Barth*, 1903–1906.

Heubner was professor of paediatrics at Berlin. With Rubner he determined the caloric requirements of infants and did other important work on infant feeding.

6344 SELTER, PAUL. 1866–
Ueber Trophodermatoneurose. *Verh. Ges. Kinderheilk.*, 1903, **20**, 45–50.

First clear description of infantile acrodynia ("pink disease").

6345 CZERNY, ADALBERT. 1863–1941, & KELLER, ARTHUR. 1868–
Des Kindes Ernährung, Ernährungsstörungen und Ernährungs therapie. 2 vols. Leipzig, *F. Deuticke*, 1906–17.

6346 LANGSTEIN, LEOPOLD. 1877–1933, & MEYER, LUDWIG. 1879–
Säuglingsernährung und Säuglingsstoffwechsel. Wiesbaden, *J. F. Bergmann*, 1910.

6347 PFAUNDLER, MEINHARD VON. 1872–1947, & SCHLOSSMANN, ARTHUR. 1867–1932
Handbuch der Kinderheilkunde. 2te. Aufl. 6 vols. Leipzig, *F. C. W. Vogel*, 1910–12.

English translation, 1912–24.

6348 SWIFT, Harry. 1858–1937
Erythroedema. *Trans.* 10*th Australasian med. Congr.*, 1914, 547–52.
Acrodynia ("pink disease," "Swift's disease"); first full description.

6349 FEER, Emil. 1864–1955
Eine eigenartige Neurose des vegetativen Systems beim Kleinkinde. *Ergeb. inn. Med. Kinderheilk.*, 1923, **24,** 100–22.
Feer described a vegetative neurosis ("Feer's disease") affecting infants and characterized by cyanosis of the extremities, recurrent sweating, tremor, motor weakness, rapid pulse, and insomnia. It was first described by Selter (No. 6344) and later by Swift, with whose names it is sometimes associated; it is also termed infantile acrodynia and pink disease.

6350 MARRIOTT, Williams McKim. 1885–1936
The food requirements of malnourished infants with a note on the use of insulin. *J. Amer. med. Ass.*, 1924, **83,** 600–03.
Marriott introduced the insulin-fattening method of treatment of malnutrition in infants.

History of Paediatrics

6351 MEISSNER, Friedrich Ludwig. 1796–1860
Grundlage der Literatur der Pädiatrik. Leipzig, *Fest'sche Verlagsbuchhandlung*, 1850.
An extensive bibliography of paediatric literature, containing about 7,000 references.

6352 BÓKAY, János. 1858–1937
Die Geschichte der Kinderheilkunde. Berlin, *J. Springer*, 1922.

6353 GARRISON, Fielding Hudson. 1870–1935
History of pediatrics. In I. Abt, *System of pediatrics*, Philadelphia, 1923, **1,** 1–170.
Re-issued separately with an appendix on the history of paediatrics in recent times by A. F. Abt, Philadelphia, *W. B. Saunders*, 1965.

6354 RUHRÄH, John. 1872–1935
Pediatrics of the past: an anthology. New York, *P. B. Hoeber*, 1925.
Contains sketches of the lives of the more important paediatricians of the past, with a comprehensive selection of their works, translated where necessary into English. Ruhräh has thrown much light on the important contributions of long-forgotten writers, and he has carefully traced the progress of paediatrics from ancient times to the 19th century. The book includes a valuable bibliography.

6355 SUDHOFF, Karl Friedrich Jakob. 1853–1938
Erstlinge der pädiatrischen Literatur. München, *Münchener Drucke*, 1925.
Facsimile reproductions of the 3 earliest printed works on paediatrics: Bagellardo, Metlinger, and Roelants, together with a valuable prefatory essay on their importance.

6356 STILL, *Sir* George Frederic. 1868–1941
The history of paediatrics. The progress of the study of diseases of children up to the end of the XVIIIth century. London, *Oxford Univ. Press*, 1931.
This work covers the whole field of paediatrics to the end of the 18th century. It is a very readable, interesting and accurate history of the subject.

6357 LEVINSON, ABRAHAM. 1888–1955
Pioneers of pediatrics. 2nd ed. New York, *Froben Press*, 1943.

6357.1 PEIPER, ALBRECHT. 1880–
Chronik der Kinderheilkunde. 4te. Aufl. Leipzig, *G. Thieme*, 1966.

CONDITIONS AND SYNDROMES NOT CLASSIFIED ELSEWHERE

6358–6375.1

6358 DANZ, FERDINAND GEORG. 1761–1793
Von Menschen ohne Haare und Zähne. *Arch. Geburtsh.* (*Jena*), 1792, **4**, 684.

Hereditary ectodermal dysplasia first described.

6358.1 AXMANN, EDMUND.
Merkwürdige Fragilität der Knochen ohne dyskrasische Ursache als krankhafte Eigenthümlichkeit dreier Geschwister. *Ann. ges. Heilk* (*Karlsruhe*), 1831, **4**, 58–68.

Axmann of Wertheim described osteogenesis imperfecta occurring in himself and his two brothers. He referred to the occurrence of articular dislocations and blue sclerotics. See also No. 6367.

6359 SMITH, *Sir* THOMAS. 1833–1909
Skull-cap showing congenital deficiencies of bone. *Trans. path. Soc. Lond.*, 1865, **16**, 224–25.

6360 ——. Haemorrhagic periostitis of the shafts of several of the long bones, with separation of the epiphyses. *Trans. path. Soc. Lond.*, 1876, **27**, 219–22.

Craniohypophysial xanthomatosis was first reported by Sir Thomas Smith (see also No. 6359). Hand in 1893 (No. 6361), Schüller in 1915 (No. 6362), and Christian in 1919 (No. 6363) also reported cases, and the condition became known as the "Hand–Schüller–Christian syndrome".

6360.1 BALZER, FÉLIX. 1849–1929
Recherches sur les caractères anatomiques du xanthélasma. *Arch. Physiol. norm. Path.*, 1884, 3 sér., **4**, 65–80.

First description of skin changes and necropsy findings in pseudoxanthoma elasticum.

6361 HAND, ALFRED. 1868–1949
Polyuria and tuberculosis. *Proc. path. Soc. Philad.*, 1893, **16**, 282–84; *Arch. Pediat.*, 1893, **10**, 673–75.

"Hand–Schüller–Christian syndrome", which Hand called polyuria and tuberculosis.

6362 SCHÜLLER, ARTUR. 1874–1958
Ueber eigenartige Schädeldefekte im Jugendalter. *Fortschr. Röntgenstr.*, 1915–16, **23**, 12–18.

Schüller described two more cases of the condition to which his name, with those of Hand and Christian, has been attached.

6363 CHRISTIAN, HENRY ASBURY. 1876–1951
Defects in membranous bones, exophthalmos, and diabetes insipidus; an unusual syndrome of dyspituitarism; a clinical study. In *Contributions to medical and biological research, dedicated to Sir William Osler.* New York, *P. B. Hoeber*, 1919, **1**, 390–401.
"Hand–Schüller–Christian syndrome."

6364 HEERFORDT, CHRISTIAN FREDERIK. 1871–
Ueber eine "Febris uveo-parotidea subchronica", an der Glandula parotis und der Uvea des Auges lokalisiert und häufig mit Paresen cerebrospinaler Nerven kompliziert. *v. Graefes Arch. Ophthal.*, 1909, **70**, 254–73.
"Heerfordt's syndrome", uveo-parotid fever.

6365 RENDU, ROBERT. 1886–
Sur un syndrome caractérisé par l'inflammation simultanée de toutes les muqueuses externes (conjunctivale, nasale, linguale, bucco-pharyngée, anale et balano-préputiale) coexistant avec une éruption varicelliforme puis purpurique des quatres membres. *J. Prat. (Paris)*, 1916, **30**, 351.
First description of the "Stevens–Johnson syndrome" (see No. 4150).

6366 ROWLAND, RUSSELL STURGIS. 1874–
Xanthomatosis and the reticulo-endothelial system. *Arch. intern. Med.*, 1928, **42**, 611–74.
"Rowland collected 14 cases of the Hand–Schüller–Christian syndrome, and made the important generalization that it was due to xanthomatosis" (Rolleston).

6367 EDDOWES, ALFRED. 1850–1946
Dark sclerotics and fragilitas ossium. *Brit. med. J.*, 1900, **2**, 222.
"Eddowes' syndrome" – blue sclerotics and fragility of the bones, occurring as a familial syndrome; osteogenesis imperfecta. See also No. 6358.1.

6368 LAURENCE, JOHN ZACHARIAH. 1830–1874, & MOON, ROBERT CHARLES. 1844–1914
Four cases of "retinitis pigmentosa", occurring in the same family, and accompanied by general imperfections of development. *Ophthal. Rev.*, 1866, **2**, 32–41.
Laurence–Moon (–Biedl) syndrome first described. See also No. 6369.

6369 BIEDL, ARTUR. 1869–1933
Geschwisterpaar mit adiposo-genitaler Dystrophie. *Dtsch. med. Wschr.*, 1922, **48**, 1630.
Laurence–Moon–Biedl syndrome (see also No. 6368). Biedl's cases were more fully described by W. Raab, in *Wien. Arch. inn. Med.*, 1924, **7**, 443–530.

6370 FIESSINGER, NOEL. 1881–1946, & LEROY, EDGAR.
Contribution à l'étude d'une épidémie de dysenterie dans la Somme (juillet-octobre 1916). *Bull. Soc. méd. Hôp. Paris*, 1916, **40**, 2030–69.
Includes several references to the condition later known as "Reiter's syndrome" (No. 6371).

6371 REITER, HANS CONRAD JULIUS. 1881–1968
Ueber eine bisher unerkannte Spirochäteninfektion (Spirochaetosis arthritica). *Dtsch. med. Wschr.*, 1916, **42**, 1535–36.
"Reiter's syndrome", a disease of males characterized by initial diarrhoea, urethritis, conjunctivitis, and arthritis. See also No. 6370.

6371.1 HUNTER, CHARLES. 1872–1955
A rare disease in two brothers. *Proc. roy. Soc. Med.*, 1917, **10,** Sect. Dis. Child., 104–16.
First definite description of the Hurler syndrome (No. 6371.2). Hunter became professor of medicine in the University of Manitoba.

6371.2 HURLER, GERTRUD.
Ueber einen Typ multipler Abartungen, vorwiegend am Skelettsystem. *Z. Kinderheilk.*, 1919, **24,** 220–34.
Hurler syndrome (lipochondrodystrophy, gargoylism), earlier described by Hunter (No. 6371.1).

6372 LETTERER, ERICH. 1895–
Aleukämische Reticulose. (Ein Beitrag zu den proliferativen Erkrankungen des Retikuloendothelialapparates.) *Frankf. Z. Path.*, 1924, **30,** 377–94.
"Letterer–Siwe disease"; see also No. 6373.

6372.1 WEVE, HENRICUS JACOBUS MARIE. 1888–1962
Ueber Arachnodaktylie (Dystrophia mesodermalis congenita, Typus Marfan). *Arch. Augenheilk.*, 1931, **104,** 1–46.
Weve of Utrecht first clearly demonstrated the heritable nature of the Marfan syndrome (see No. 4365.1).

6373 SIWE, STURE AUGUST. 1897–
Die Reticuloendotheliose – eine neues Krankheitsbild unter den Hepatosplenomegalien. *Z. Kinderheilk.*, 1933, **55,** 212–47.
See No. 6372.

6374 BEHÇET, HULÜSI. 1889–1948
Über rezidivierende, aphthöse, durch ein Virus verursachte Geschwüre am Mund, am Auge und an den Genitalien. *Derm. Wschr.*, 1937, **105,** 1152–57.
"Behçet's syndrome", previously described by H. Planner and F. Remenovsky, *Arch. Derm. Syph. (Berlin)*, 1922, **140**, 162–88.

6375.1 ZOLLINGER, ROBERT MILTON. 1903– , & ELLISON, EDWIN HOMER. 1918–
Primary peptic ulcerations of the jejunum associated with islet cell tumors of the pancreas. *Ann. Surg.*, 1955, **142,** 709–28.
Zollinger–Ellison syndrome.

6376–6703.1 HISTORY OF MEDICINE

(Histories of special subjects will be found under these subjects.)

6376–6451.3 GENERAL

6376 CHAMPIER, SYMPHORIEN. 1472–1539
De medicinae claris scriptoribus in quinque partibus tractatus. Lyon, *J. de Campis*, 1506.
First history of medicine of any importance and the best for many years after its publication. A bibliographical study of Champier by P. A. Allut appeared from Lyons in 1859; a check-list of his writings was published by J. F. Ballard and M. Pijoan in *Bull. med. Libr. Ass.*, 1940, **28**, 182–88.

6377 DONATI, MARCELLO. 1538–1602
De medica historia mirabili libri sex. Mantuae, *per Fr. Osanam*, 1586.

6378 FREIND, JOHN. 1675–1728
The history of physick; from the time of Galen to the beginning of the sixteenth century. 2 vols. London, *J. Walthoe*, 1725–26.

Freind was the first English historian of medicine; his book is the best English work on the period of which it treats. Freind dabbled in politics and planned the above work while committed to the Tower of London on a charge of high treason, a charge of which he was innocent. Sir Robert Walpole, Prime Minister at the time, suffered much from renal calculi and called in Mead, a great friend of Freind. Mead refused to treat Walpole until Freind was released, and this was speedily arranged!

6379 LE CLERC, DANIEL. 1652–1728
Histoire de la médecine. A La Haye, *I. van der Kloot*, 1729.

The first large history of medicine. It is still consulted to-day. Le Clerc is sometimes called the "Father of the History of Medicine". The first edition of this work appeared in 1696, but later editions are more useful. English translation, 1699.

6380 MIDDLETON, PETER. *d.* 1781
A medical discourse, or an historical inquiry into the ancient and present state of medicine. New York, *H. Gaine*, 1769.

The first American contribution to medical history.

6381 LETTSOM, JOHN COAKLEY. 1744–1815
History of the origin of medicine. London, *E. & C. Dilly*, 1778.

6382 SPRENGEL, KURT POLYKARP JOACHIM. 1766–1833
Versuch einer pragmatischen Geschichte der Arzneikunde. 5 vols. Halle, *J. J. Gebauer*, 1792–1803.

A monumental work, full of important information which has been of great assistance to later historians. Includes a useful chronology. Third edition, 1821–40; fourth edition of vol. 1, 1846.

6383 HECKER, JUSTUS FRIEDRICH KARL. 1795–1850
Geschichte der Heilkunde. 2 vols. Berlin, *Enslin*, 1822–29.

An important early German work on the history of medicine.

6384 HAESER, HEINRICH. 1811–1884
Lehrbuch der Geschichte der Medicin und der Volkskrankheiten. Jena, *F. Mauke*, 1845.

The most important German work on the history of medicine and one of the most outstanding contributions. Haeser was eclipsed only by his fellow-countryman Sudhoff. A third edition of this book, in 3 volumes, appeared in 1875–82.

6385 PUCCINOTTI, FRANCESCO. 1794–1872
Storia della medicina. 3 vols. [in 4]. Livorno, *M. Wagner*, 1850–66.

6386 WUNDERLICH, CARL REINHOLD AUGUST. 1815–1877
Geschichte der Medicin. Stuttgart, *Ebner & Seubert*, 1859.

6387 DAREMBERG, CHARLES VICTOR. 1817–1872
Histoire des sciences médicales. 2 vols. Paris, *J. B. Baillière*, 1870.

Daremberg was one of the most distinguished French medical historians and held the Chair of Medical History at Paris.

6388 LITTRÉ, MAXIMILIEN PAUL EMILE. 1801–1881
Médecine et médecins. Paris, *Didier & Cie.*, 1872.

6389 BAAS, JOHANN HERMANN. 1838–1909
Grundriss der Geschichte der Medicin. Stuttgart, *F. Enke*, 1876.

Until superseded by Garrison, Baas's book was the most important one-volume text on the history of medicine. For an expert evaluation of it, see Garrison's *History*, 4th ed., p. 884. An English translation, by H. E. Handerson, was published in New York in 1889.

6390 HOLMES, OLIVER WENDELL. 1809–1894
Medical essays: 1842–1882. Boston, *Houghton Mifflin & Co.*, 1883.

"The most important American book dealing with the history of medicine up to its day" (Garrison).

6391 PUSCHMANN, THEODOR. 1844–1899
Geschichte des medizinischen Unterrichtes von den ältesten Zeiten bis zur Gegenwart. Leipzig, *Veit & Co.*, 1889.

English translation, 1891.

6392 PETERSEN, JAKOB JULIUS. 1840–1912
Hauptmomente in der älteren Geschichte der medicinischen Klinik. Kopenhagen, *A. F. Høst*, 1890.

6393 BOUCHUT, EUGENE. 1818–1891
Histoire de la médecine et des doctrines médicales. 2 vols. Paris, *Germer-Baillière*, 1873.

6394 MITCHELL, SILAS WEIR. 1829–1914
The early history of instrumental precision in medicine. New Haven, *Tuttle, Moorehouse & Taylor*, 1892.

6395 WITHINGTON, EDWARD THEODORE. 1860–1947
Medical history from the earliest times. London, *Scientific Press*, 1894.

Although it does not go beyond the early 19th century this is one of the finest short works on medical history. Reprinted 1964.

6396 PAGEL, JULIUS LEOPOLD. 1851–1912
Geschichte der Medicin. 2 vols. Berlin, *S. Karger*, 1898.

A collection of lectures. The bibliography of the revised edition of 1922, for which Sudhoff was responsible, is a great improvement upon the first edition.

6397 VIRCHOW, RUDOLF LUDWIG KARL. 1821–1902
Die neueren Fortschritte in der Wissenschaft und ihr Einfluss auf Medicin und Chirurgie. Berlin, *A. Hirschwald*, 1898.

6398 PUSCHMANN, THEODOR. 1844–1899
Handbuch der Geschichte der Medizin. Begründet von THEODOR PUSCHMANN. 3 vols. Jena, *G. Fischer*, 1902–05.

Puschmann died before the completion of this work, and it was then edited by Pagel and Neuburger. It is one of the most important books on the subject, ranking with the work of Haeser; many authorities collaborated in the writing of the histories of the various subjects treated.

6399 SUDHOFF, KARL FRIEDRICH JAKOB. 1853–1938
Iatromathematiker vornehmlich im 15. und 16. Jahrhundert. Breslau, *J. U. Kern*, 1902.

6400 ALLBUTT, *Sir* THOMAS CLIFFORD. 1836–1925
The historical relations of medicine and surgery to the end of the sixteenth century. London, *Macmillan*, 1905.

6401 NEUBURGER, MAX. 1868–1955
Geschichte der Medizin. Vol. 1–2, pt. 1. Stuttgart, *F. Enke*, 1906–1911.

An English translation was published in London between 1910–25.

6402 BOINET, EDOUARD LOUIS DÉSIRÉ. 1859–1939
Les doctrines médicales: leur évolution. Paris, *E. Flammarion*, 1907.

6403 PAGEL, JULIUS LEOPOLD. 1851–1912
Zeittafeln zur Geschichte der Medizin. Berlin, *A. Hirschwald*, 1908.

6404 FOSSEL, VIKTOR. 1846–1913
Studien zur Geschichte der Medizin. Stuttgart, *F. Enke*, 1909.

6405 EIJKMAN, PIETER HENDRIK. 1862–1914
Internationalisme médical. Amsterdam, *F. van Rossen*, 1910.

6406 VIERORDT, KARL HERMANN. 1853–1944
Medizinisches aus der Geschichte. 3te. Aufl. Tübingen, *H. Laupp*, 1910.

6407 MEUNIER, LÉON JOSEPH. 1856–1911
Histoire de la médecine depuis ses origines jusqu'à nos jours. Paris, *J. B. Baillière*, 1911.

6408 GARRISON, FIELDING HUDSON. 1870–1935
An introduction to the history of medicine. Philadelphia, London, *W. B. Saunders*, 1913.

One of the best single-volume histories of medicine. Garrison was the leading American authority on the subject and wrote many papers on various aspects of medical history. The above book, of which a fourth edition appeared in 1929, is recognized as the authoritative work on the subject in English.

6409 VIERORDT, KARL HERMANN. 1853–1944
Medizin-geschichtliches Hilfsbuch mit besonderer Berücksichtigung der Entdeckungsgeschichte und der Biographie. Tübingen, *H. Laupp*, 1916.

6410 BUCK, ALBERT HENRY. 1842–1922
The growth of medicine from the earliest times to about 1800. New Haven, *Yale Univ. Press*, 1917.

6411 SINGER, CHARLES JOSEPH. 1876–1960
Studies in the history and method of science. Edited by CHARLES SINGER. 2 vols. Oxford, *Clarendon Press*, 1917–21.

A collection of essays by several authorities.

6412 BUCK, ALBERT HENRY. 1842–1922
The dawn of modern medicine. An account of the revival of the science and art of medicine which took place in Western Europe during the latter half of the eighteenth century and the first part of the nineteenth. New Haven, *Yale Univ. Press*, 1920.

6413 MEYER-STEINEG, THEODOR. 1873–1936, & SUDHOFF, KARL FRIEDRICH JAKOB. 1853–1938
Geschichte der Medizin im Überblick. Jena, *G. Fischer*, 1921.
5th edition, 1965, under the title *Illustrierte Geschichte der Medizin.*

6414 OSLER, *Sir* WILLIAM, *Bart.* 1849–1919
The evolution of modern medicine. New Haven, *Yale Univ. Press*, 1921.
This book is based on the Silliman Lectures delivered at Yale in 1913. It is one of the most interesting short histories of medicine, written in Osler's usual charming style, and is perhaps the best book with which to commence the study of medical history. Reprinted 1972, New York, *Arno Press.*

6415 CUMSTON, CHARLES GREENE. 1868–1927
An introduction to the history of medicine from the time of the Pharaohs to the end of the XVIIIth century . . . With an essay on the relation of history and philosophy to medicine, by F. G. CROOKSHANK. London, *Kegan Paul*, 1926.

6416 DANA, CHARLES LOOMIS. 1852–1935
The peaks of medical history. An outline of the evolution of medicine for the use of medical students and practitioners. New York, *Hoeber*, 1926.

6417 NEUBURGER, MAX. 1868–1955
Die Lehre von der Heilkraft der Natur im Wandel der Zeiten. Stuttgart, *F. Enke*, 1926.
The standard work on the history of the doctrine of "the healing power of Nature". English translation, New York, 1932.

6418 CASTIGLIONI, ARTURO. 1874–1953
Storia della medicina. Milano, *Soc. Ed. Unitas*, 1927.
This work is similar in plan and scope to that of Garrison (No. 6408). Much attention is devoted to palaeopathology, while the accounts of the School of Salerno, and mediaeval and Renaissance Italian medicine are especially valuable. The bibliographies are excellent. This is one of the most accurate and comprehensive text-books on the subject. An English translation by E. B. Krumbhaar was published in 1941 and revised in 1947.

6419 SARTON, GEORGE ALFRED LÉON. 1884–1956
Introduction to the history of science. Vol. 1–3 [in 5]. Baltimore, *Williams & Wilkins*, 1927–48.
An invaluable survey to the end of the 14th century of the progress of science throughout the world.

6420 HOLLÄNDER, EUGEN. 1867–1932
Äskulap und Venus. Berlin, *Propyläen-Verlag*, 1928.

6421 SINGER, CHARLES JOSEPH. 1876–1960
A short history of medicine. Oxford, *Clarendon Press*, 1928.
An excellent outline of the subject. It is especially valuable for non-medical readers and for those who have time to deal only with the principal events of medical history. A second edition, revised by E. A. Underwood, 1962, includes an account of recent developments and an excellent bibliography.

6422 THORNDIKE, Lynn. 1882–1965
A history of magic and experimental science. 8 vols. London, *H. Milford*, 1923–58.

Vols. 1–2 deal with the first 13 centuries of the Christian era; vols. 3–4 with the 14th and 15th centuries, vols. 5–6 with the 16th century, and vols. 7–8 with the 17th century.

6423 CAMAC, Charles Nicoll Bancker. 1868–1940
Imhotep to Harvey: backgrounds of medical history. Foreword by Henry Fairfield Osborn. New York, *Hoeber*, 1931.

6424 SIGERIST, Henry Ernest. 1891–1957
Einführung in die Medizin. Leipzig, *G. Thieme*, 1931.

Traces the evolution of medicine from the stage of superstition and magic to the present time, and shows how our knowledge of the subject has developed through the study of anatomy and physiology. A useful introduction to the study of the history of medicine. An English translation ("Man and Medicine") was published in New York in 1932.

6425 GARCIA DEL REAL, Eduardo. 1870–1947
Historia contemporánea de la medicina. Madrid, *Espasa-Calpe*, 1934.

6426 LAIGNEL-LAVASTINE, Maxime Paul Marie. 1875–1953
Histoire générale de la médecine, de la pharmacie, de l'art dentaire et de l'art véterinaire. 3 vols. Paris, *Michel*, 1936–49.

This magnificent work, beautifully illustrated, was written by experts in each branch of the subject, with Laignel-Lavastine as general editor.

6427 DELAUNAY, Paul. 1878–1958
La vie médicale aux XVIe, XVIIe et XVIIIe siècles. Paris, *Editions Hippocrate*, 1935.

6428 DUMESNIL, René.
Histoire illustrée de la médecine. Paris, *Librairie Plon*, 1935.

6429 FÜLÖP-MILLER, René. 1891–
Kulturgeschichte der Heilkunde. München, *Bruckmann*, 1935–37.

6430 DAWSON, George Gordon.
Healing; pagan and Christian. London, *Society for the Promotion of Christian Knowledge*, [1935].

6431 LLOYD, Wyndham Edward Buckley.
A hundred years of medicine. London, *Duckworth*, [1936].

New edition 1968.

6432 MAJOR, Ralph Hermon. 1884–
Disease and destiny. New York, *Appleton-Century*, 1936.

6433 SHRYOCK, Richard Harrison. 1893–1972
The development of modern medicine, an interpretation of the social and scientific factors involved, Philadelphia, *University of Pennsylvania Press*, 1936.

6434 MAYRHOFER, Bernhard. 1868–1938
Kurzes Wörterbuch zur Geschichte der Medizin. Jena, *Fischer*, 1937.

6435 GALDSTON, Iago. 1895–
Progress in medicine: a critical review of the last hundred years. New York, *Knopf*, 1940.

6436 CLENDENING, LOGAN. 1884–1945
Source book of medical history. New York, *Hoeber*, 1942.

6437 NEUBURGER, MAX. 1868–1955
British medicine and the Vienna School: contacts and parallels. London, *Heinemann*, 1943.

6438 ROBINSON, VICTOR. 1886–1947
The story of medicine. New York, *New Home Library*, (1944).

6439 GUTHRIE, DOUGLAS JAMES. 1885–1975
A history of medicine. London, *Nelson*, (1945).

6440 METTLER, CECILIA CHARLOTTE. 1909–1943
History of medicine. A correlative text, arranged according to subjects. Edited by FRED A. METTLER. Philadelphia, *Blakiston Co.*, 1947.

6441 PAZZINI, ADALBERTO. 1898–
Storia della medicina. 2 vols. Milano, *Soc. Editrice Libraria*, 1947.

6443 CREUTZ, RUDOLPH, & STEUDEL, JOHANNES. 1901–
Einführung in die Geschichte der Medizin in Einzeldarstellungen. Iserlohn, *Silva Verlag*, 1948.

6444 ARTELT, WALTER. 1906–
Einführung in die Medizinhistorik. Ihr Wesen, ihre Arbeitsweise und ihre Hilfsmittel. Stuttgart, *F. Enke*, 1949.

6445 DIEPGEN, PAUL. 1878–1966
Geschichte der Medizin. Die historische Entwicklung der Heilkunde und des ärztlichen Lebens. 2 vols. [in 3]. Berlin, *W. de Gruyter*, 1949–55.

6446 BRITISH MEDICAL JOURNAL.
Fifty years of medicine. A symposium from the "British Medical Journal". London, *British Medical Association*, 1950.
A survey of medical progress, 1900–49.

6447 GOTFREDSEN, EDVARD. 1899–1963
Medicinens historie. Kjøbenhavn, *Busck*, 1950.
2nd edition, 1964.

6448 SIGERIST, HENRY ERNEST. 1891–1957
A history of medicine. Vol. 1–2. New York, *Oxford University Press*, 1951–61.

6449 SARTON, GEORGE ALFRED LÉON. 1884–1956
A guide to the history of science. A first guide for the study of the history of science. With introductory essays on science and tradition. Waltham, Mass., *Chronica Botanica Co.*, 1952.
Contains extensive bibliographies.

6450 ——. A history of science. Vol. 1– . Cambridge, Mass., *Harvard Univ. Press*, 1953– .
To be completed in eight volumes.

6451 INDEX ZUR GESCHICHTE DER MEDIZIN. Vol. 1–2. München, *Urban & Schwarzenberg*, 1953–66.

Vol. 1 contains over 10,000 and vol. 2 7,000 references to books and papers. Vol. 1 edited by W. Artelt, vol. 2 edited by J. Steudel. Covers the years 1945–48 and 1949–52.

6451.1 CURRENT WORK IN THE HISTORY OF MEDICINE. AN INTERNATIONAL BIBLIOGRAPHY. No. 1– . London, *Wellcome Institute of the History of Medicine*, 1954– .

A quarterly subject index to periodical literature on the history of medicine. Also lists new books alphabetically by author.

6451.2 MAJOR, Ralph Hermon. 1884–
A history of medicine. 1 vol. [in 2]. Springfield, *C. C. Thomas*, 1954.

6451.3 BIBLIOGRAPHY OF THE HISTORY OF MEDICINE. No. 1– . Bethesda, Md., 1965–

Annual. Published by the National Library of Medicine.

6452–6467.1 PREHISTORIC, PRIMITIVE, AND FOLK MEDICINE

6452 BLACK, William George. 1857–1932
Folk-medicine; a chapter in the history of culture. London, *E. Stock*, 1883.

Folk-Lore Society Publication No. 12. The authoritative English work on medical folk-lore.

6453 BARTELS, Maximilian Carl August. 1843–1904
Die Medicin der Naturvölker. Leipzig, *T. Grieben*, 1893.

6455 HOVORKA, Oskar von. 1866–1930, & KRONFELD, Adolf. 1861–1938
Vergleichende Volksmedizin. 2 vols. Stuttgart, *Strecker & Schröder*, 1908–09.

Most authoritative work so far available on the subject.

6456 MADDOX, John Lee. 1878–
The medicine man; a sociological study of the character and evolution of shamanism. . . . With a foreword by Professor A. G. Keller. New York, *Macmillan*, 1923.

6457 MOODIE, Roy Lee. 1880–1934
The antiquity of disease. Chicago, *University of Chicago Press*, (1923).

The writer was a leading authority on palaeopathology.

6458 JAYNE, Walter Addison. 1853–
The healing gods of ancient civilizations. New Haven, *Yale Univ. Press*, 1925.

6459 McKENZIE, Dan. 1870–1935
The infancy of medicine. An enquiry into the influence of folk-lore upon the evolution of scientific medicine. London, *Macmillan*, 1927.

6460 STONE, Eric Percy. 1892–
Medicine among the American Indians. New York, *P. B. Hoeber*, 1932.

Clio Medica series. This useful study of the subject makes available information which is otherwise hard to obtain. Although a great deal has been written on the knowledge of medicine among the American Indians, most of it is buried in periodical publications.

6461 CORLETT, William Thomas. 1854–1948
The medicine-man of the American Indian and his cultural background. Springfield, *Thomas*, 1935.

6462 KEMP, Phyllis.
Healing ritual: studies in the technique and tradition of the southern Slavs. London, *Faber*, 1935.

6463 CHAUVET, Stéphen. 1885–1950
La médecine chez les peuples primitifs. Paris, *A. Maloine*, 1936.

6464 PARDAL, Ramón. 1896–1955
Medicina aborigen americana. Buenos Aires, *Anesi*, [1937].

6465 WECK, Wolfgang. 1881–
Heilkunde und Volkstum auf Bali. Stuttgart, *Enke*, 1937.

6466 HARLEY, George Way. 1894–
Native African medicine. Cambridge, *Harvard University Press*, 1941.

6467 PAZZINI, Adalberto. 1898–
La medicina primitiva. Milano, "*Arte e Storia*", 1941.

6467.1 KRASINSKI, Cyrill Korvin.
Die tibetische Medizinphilosophie. Zürich, *Origo*, 1953.

2nd edition, 1965.

6468–6471.2 ANCIENT EGYPT

6468 ALPINO, Prospero. 1553–1617
De medicina Aegyptiorum, libri quatuor. Venetiis, *apud Fr. de Franciscis*, 1591.

First important work on the history of Egyptian medicine. Alpino became professor of botany at Padua after having spent three years in Egypt.

6469 SCHWIMMER, Ernst. 1837–1898
Die ersten Anfänge der Heilkunde und die Medizin im alten Aegypten. Eine kulturgeschichtliche Skizze. Berlin, *Habel*, 1876.

Sammlung gemeinverständlicher wissenschaftlicher Vorträge, Nr. 255.

6470 HURRY, Jamieson Boyd. 1857–1930
Imhotep: the vizier and physician of King Zoser, and afterwards the Egyptian god of medicine. Oxford, *Univ. Press*, 1926.

6471 DAWSON, Warren Royal. 1888–1968
The beginnings. Egypt and Assyria. New York, *Hoeber*, 1930.

Clio Medica series.

6471.1 LEAKE, CHAUNCEY DEPEW. 1896–
The old Egyptian medical papyri. Kansas, *University of Kansas Press*, 1952.
A guide to the chief Egyptian medical papyri, with particular attention to therapeutics.

6471.2 GRAPOW, HERMANN. 1885–1967
Grundriss der Medizin der alten Ägypter. Vol. 1– . Berlin, *Akademie-Verlag*, 1954– .
Critical studies, texts, translations.

6472–6473.1 BABYLONIA AND ASSYRIA

6472 OEFELE, FELIX, *Freiherr* VON. 1861–
Keilschriftmedicin. Breslau, *J. N. Kern*, 1902.
Cuneiform medicine.

6473 CONTENAU, GEORGES.
La médecine en Assyrie et en Babylonie. Paris, *Maloine*, 1938.

6473.1 KÖCHER, FRANZ.
Die babylonisch-assyrische Medizin in Texten und Untersuchungen. 3 vols. Berlin, *Walter de Gruyter*, 1963–64.

6474–6485.1 GREECE AND ROME

6474 DAREMBERG, CHARLES VICTOR. 1817–1872
La médecine dans Homère. Paris, *Didier et Cie.*, 1865.

6475 ——. État de la médecine entre Homère et Hippocrate. Paris, *Didier et Cie.*, 1869.

6476 WALTON, ALICE.
The cult of Asklepios. [Ithaca, N.Y.], *Ginn*, 1894.
Cornell Studies in Classical Philology, III. Reprinted, 1966.

6477 CATON, RICHARD. 1842–1926
The temples and ritual of Asklepios at Epidauros and Athens. Liverpool, *University Press*, 1900.

6478 SUDHOFF, KARL FRIEDRICH JAKOB. 1853–1938
Aerztliches aus griechischen Papyrus-Urkunden. Leipzig, *J. A. Barth*, 1907.

6479 ALLBUTT, *Sir* THOMAS CLIFFORD. 1836–1925
Greek medicine in Rome. London, *Macmillan & Co.*, 1921.
FitzPatrick Lectures, 1909–10. Allbutt was Regius Professor of Physic at Cambridge and a great literary stylist. Underwood described him as the most learned and distinguished physician of the last hundred years.

6480 SINGER, CHARLES JOSEPH. 1876–1960
Greek biology and Greek medicine. Oxford, *Clarendon Press*, 1922.

6481 TAYLOR, HENRY OSBORN. 1856–1941
Greek biology and medicine. London, *Harrap*, (1922).

6482 SUDHOFF, KARL FRIEDRICH JAKOB. 1853–1938
Kos und Knidos. München, *Münchner Drucke*, 1927.

6483 LUND, FRED BATES. 1865–1950
Greek medicine. New York, *Hoeber*, 1936.
Clio Medica series.

6484 RUIZ MORENO, ANÍBAL. 1907–1960
La medicina en la mitologia grecorromana. Buenos Aires, *Ferrari*, 1940.

6485 KERÉNYI, CHARLES.
Le médecin divin. Promenades mythologiques aux sanctuaires d'Asclépios. Basel, *Ciba*, 1948.

6485.1 SCHUMACHER, JOSEPH. 1902–
Antike Medizin. Die naturphilosophischen Grundlagen der Medizin in der griechischen Antike. 2nd ed. Berlin, *W. de Gruyter*, 1963.

6486–6491.1

INDIA

6486 SINH JEE, *Sir* BHAGVAT, *Maharajah of Gondal*. 1865–1944
A short history of Aryan medical science. London, *Macmillan & Co.*, 1890.

6487 HOERNLE, AUGUST FRIEDRICH RUDOLF. 1841–1918
Studies in the medicine of ancient India. Vol. 1. Oxford, *Clarendon Press*, 1907.

6488 MUKHOPADHYAYA, GIRANDRANATH. 1872–1935
The surgical instruments of the Hindus, with a comparative study of the surgical instruments of the Greek, Roman, Arab and the modern Eouropean [sic] surgeons. 2 vols. Calcutta, *University Press*, 1913–1914.
Vol. 2 consists of plates.

6488.1 ——. History of Indian medicine. 3 vols. Calcutta, *Univ. of Calcutta*, 1923–29.

6489 BURMA. *Public Health Department.*
Report of the Committee of Enquiry into the Indigenous System of Medicine. Rangoon, *Supdt. Govt. Printing*, 1931.

6490 MARIADASSOU, PARAMANANDA.
Médecine traditionelle de l'Inde. Conférences faites à l'Ecole de Médecine de Pondichéry . . . Préface de M. Georges Bourret. 3 vols. [in 1]. Pondichéry, *Imp. Ste. Anne*, 1934–35.

6491 ZIMMER, HENRY ROBERT. 1890–1943
Hindu medicine. Edited with a foreword and preface by LUDWIG EDELSTEIN. Baltimore, *Johns Hopkins Press*, 1948.
Publications of the Institute of the History of Medicine, Johns Hopkins University, 3rd. ser.

6491.1 KUTUMBIAH, P.
Ancient Indian medicine. Bombay, *Orient Longmans*, 1962.

6492–6495.1 CHINA

6492 CLEYER, ANDREAS. *fl.* 1650
Specimen medicinae Sinicae. Francofurti, *J. P. Zubrodt*, 1682.
Cleyer's early study of Chinese medicine includes many interesting plates dealing with Chinese anatomy and pulse-lore.

6493 WONG, K. CHIMIN, & WU LIEN-TEH. 1879–1959
History of Chinese medicine. Tientsin, *Tientsin Press*, [1932].
The writers spent 15 years in the compilation of this work, the first important contribution to the history of Chinese medicine. Beginning with demonology, plant lore and folk medicine, the writers deal with the subject from the earliest times to the present. They tell of the high standards attained by the Chinese in the 8th century B.C. of the effect of Confucianism upon the development of surgery, of the "doctrine of the pulse," of Chinese pharmacy and acupuncture, and of the establishment of Western Medicine in present-day China. Second edition, 1936.

6494 MORSE, WILLIAM REGINALD. 1874–1939
Chinese medicine. New York, *P. B. Hoeber*, 1934.
Clio Medica series. This brief history forms an excellent introduction to the larger study of the subject by Wong and Wu Lien-Teh. The author spent many years in China and writes with an intimate knowledge of Chinese medicine.

6495 HUME, EDWARD HICKS. 1876–1957
The Chinese way in medicine. Baltimore, *Johns Hopkins Press*, 1940.

6495.1 HUARD, PIERRE ALPHONSE. 1901– , & WONG, MING.
La médecine chinoise au cours des siècles. Paris, *Roger Dacosta*, [1959].
English translation by B. Fielding, London, 1968.

6496–6501.1 JEWISH; BIBLICAL

6496 BARTHOLIN, THOMAS. 1616–1680
De morbis biblicis miscellanea medica. 2nd ed. Francofurti, *D. Paulli*, 1672.
A study of the diseases mentioned in the Bible.

6497 EBSTEIN, WILHELM. 1836–1912
Die Medizin im Alten Testamente. Stuttgart, *Enke*, 1901.

6498 PREUSS, JULIUS. 1861–1913
Biblisch-talmudische Medizin. Berlin, *S. Karger*, 1911.
3rd edition, 1923.

6499 BRIM, CHARLES JACOB. 1891–
Medicine in the Bible. The Pentateuch, Torah. New York, *Froben Press*, 1936.
References to medicine in the Old Testament, with notes and definitions, and references to the Talmud.

6500 FRIEDENWALD, HARRY. 1864–1950
The Jews and medicine. 2 vols. Baltimore, *Johns Hopkins Press*, 1944.
Publications of the Institute of the History of Medicine. First series: Monographs. Vols. II and III.

6501 KAGAN, Solomon Robert. 1881–1955
Jewish medicine. Boston, *Medico-Historical Press*, 1952.

6501.1 SHORT, Arthur Rendle. 1880–1953
The Bible and modern medicine: a survey of health and healing in the Old and New Testaments. London, *Paternoster Press*, 1953.

6502–6510 ARABIA

6502 WÜSTENFELD, Heinrich Ferdinand. 1808–1899
Geschichte der arabischen Aerzte und Naturforscher. Göttingen, *Vandenhoeck & Reprecht*, 1840.

Reprinted 1963.

6503 BERTHERAND, Emile Louis.
Médecine et hygiène des Arabes. Études sur l'exercise de la médecine et de la chirurgie chez les Musulmans de l'Algérie . . . Précédées de considérations sur l'état général de la médecine chez les principales nations Mahométanes. Paris, *Baillière*, 1855.

6504 DJÉLÂL ED-DIN, Abou Soleiman Dâoud.
La médecine du Prophète. Traduit par N. Perron, Paris, *Baillière*, 1860.

First appeared in *Gaz. méd. d'Algérie*, 1859, **4**.

6505 LECLERC, Lucien. 1816–1893
Histoire de la médecine arabe. 2 vols. Paris, *E. Leroux*, 1876.

6506 OPITZ, Adolf Hermann Karl. 1877–
Die Medizin im Koran. Stuttgart, *F. Enke*, 1906.

6507 BROWNE, Edward Granville. 1862–1926
Arabian medicine. Cambridge, *Univ. Press*, 1921.

FitzPatrick Lectures, 1919–20. Browne, an eminent authority on oriental languages, became professor of Arabic in the University of Cambridge.

6508 HILTON-SIMPSON, Melville William. 1881–1938
Arab medicine and surgery. A study of the healing art in Algeria. London, *Oxford Univ. Press*, 1922.

An interesting account of medicine, surgery and pharmacology as practised among the nomadic Arabs in Algeria at the present time.

6509 CAMPBELL, Donald. –1949
Arabian medicine and its influence on the Middle Ages. 2 vols. London, *Kegan Paul*, 1926.

An important survey of the Arabian medical writings of the Eastern and Western Caliphates. The second volume includes a list of translators into Latin of Arabic works and a reconstruction of the Galenic library. The book includes a valuable bibliography.

6510 KHAIRALLAH, Amin Asad.
Outline of Arabic contributions to medicine and the allied sciences. Beirut, *American Press*, 1946.

6511–6515 PERSIA

6511 FONAHN, Adolf. 1873–1940
Zur Quellenkunde der persischen Medizin. Leipzig, *J. A. Barth*, 1910.

6512 FICHTNER, Horst. 1893–
Die Medizin im Avesta. Leipzig, 1924.

6513 NAFICY, Abbas. 1905–
La médecine en Perse des origines à nos jours. Ses fondements théoriques d'après l'Encyclopédie médicale de Gorgani. Paris, *Editions Vega*, 1933.

6514 ELGOOD, Cyril. 1892–
Medicine in Persia. New York, *P. B. Hoeber*, 1934.
Clio Medica series. Comparatively little has been written regarding the history of Persian medicine, and the above concise work is therefore of especial value.

6515 ——. A medical history of Persia and the Eastern Caliphate from the earliest times until the year A.D. 1932. Cambridge, *University Press*, 1951.
A continuous history of the art and practice of medicine in Persia and bordering countries from the earliest times.

6516–6524.2 MEDIAEVAL

6516 HECKER, Justus Friedrich Karl. 1795–1850
Die Tanzwuth, eine Volkskrankheit im Mittelalter. Berlin, *T. C. F. Enslin*, 1832.
A study of the dancing mania of the Middle Ages. An English translation (see No. 1678) appeared in 1837.

6517 ——. Kinderfahrten, eine historisch-pathologische Skizze. Berlin, *A. W. Schade*, 1845.

6518 RENZI, Salvatore de. 1801–1871
Storia documentata della scuola medica di Salerno. 2nd ed. Napoli, *Nobile*, 1857.

6519 HENSLOW, George. 1835–1925
Medical works of the fourteenth century; together with a list of plants recorded in contemporary writings, with their identification. London, *Chapman & Hall*, 1899.

6520 WALSH, James Joseph. 1865–1942
Old time makers of medicine. The story of the students and teachers of the sciences related to medicine during the Middle Ages. New York, *Fordham Univ. Press*, 1911.

6521 ——. Medieval medicine. London, *A. & C.* Black, 1920.

6522 LARSEN, Henning.
An old Icelandic medical miscellany. MS. Royal Irish Academy 23 D 43, with supplement from MS. Trinity College (Dublin) L.2.27. Oslo, *Dybwad*, 1931.

6523 RIESMAN, DAVID. 1867–1940
The story of medicine in the Middle Ages. New York, *P. B. Hoeber*, 1935.
One of the best histories of the period.

6524 MACKINNEY, LOREN CAREY. 1891–1963
Early medieval medicine with special reference to France and Chartres. The Hideyo Noguchi Lectures. Baltimore, *Johns Hopkins Press*, 1937.
Publications of the Institute of the History of Medicine, Johns Hopkins University, 3rd series, vol. 3.

6524.1 GORDON, BENJAMIN LEE. 1875–
Medieval and renaissance medicine. New York, *Philosophical Library*, 1959.

6524.2 MACKINNEY, LOREN CAREY. 1891–1963
Medical illustrations in medieval manuscripts. London, *Wellcome Historical Medical Library*, 1965.

6525–6529.1 AUSTRIA

6525 HIRSCHEL, BERNHARD. 1815–1874
Compendium der Geschichte der Medicin von den Urzeiten bis auf die Gegenwart, mit besonderer Berücksichtigung der Neuzeit und der Wiener Schule. 2te. Aufl. Wien, *Braumüller*, 1862.

6526 PUSCHMANN, THEODOR. 1844–1899
Die Medicin in Wien während der letzten 100 Jahre. Wien, *M. Perles*, 1884.

6527 NEUBURGER, MAX. 1868–1955
Die Entwicklung der Medizin in Oesterreich. Wien, *C. Fromme*, 1918.

6528 ——. Das alte medizinische Wien in zeitgenössischen Schilderungen. Wien, *M. Perles*, 1921.

6529 SCHOENBAUER, LEOPOLD. 1888–1963
Das medizinische Wien: Geschichte, Werden, Würdigung. 2nd ed. Wien, *Urban & Schwarzenberg*, 1947.

6529.1 BREITNER, BURGHARD. 1884–
Geschichte der Medizin in Österreich. Wien, *Rohrer*, 1951.
Forms Bd.226, Heft 5, of *Österr. Akad. Wiss., Sitzungsber. Phil.-hist. Kl.*

6530–6533 BELGIUM; FLANDERS; NETHERLANDS

6530 BROECKX, CORNEILLE. 1807–1869
Essai sur l'histoire de la médecine belge avant le XIXe siècle. Gand, *L. Hebbelynck*, 1837.

6531 ——. Coup d'oeil sur les institutions médicales belges, depuis les dernières années du dix-huitième siècle jusqu'à nos jours, suivie de la bibliographie de cette époque. Bruxelles, *Soc. Encyclographique des Sciences Médicales*, 1841.

6532 FAIDHERBE, ALEXANDRE JOSEPH. 1867–
Les médecins et les chirurgiens de Flandre avant 1789. Lille, *Danel*, 1892.

6533 LINT, JAN GERARD DE. 1867–1936
Geneeskundige volksprenten in de Nederlanden. Academisch Proefschrift. Gorinchem, *Noorduyn*, 1918.

6534–6550 BRITISH ISLES

6534 COCKAYNE, THOMAS OSWALD. 1807–1873
Leechdoms, wortcunning, and starcraft of early England. 3 vols. London, *Longman*, 1864–66.

One of the most important pieces of medical scholarship that has so far appeared from the pen of an English writer. Written by a clergyman, it contains a vast amount of material on Western barbarian medicine and on the Anglo-Saxon language. It contains the Herbal of Apuleius, in Anglo-Saxon English, the Leech Book of Bald, etc. Reprinted, 1961.

6535 PAYNE, JOSEPH FRANK. 1840–1910
English medicine in the Anglo-Saxon times. Oxford, *Clarendon Press*, 1904.

FitzPatrick Lectures, 1903.

6535.1 BARRETT, CHARLES RAYMOND BOOTH.
The history of the Society of Apothecaries of London. London, *Elliot Stock*, 1905.

6536 MOORE, *Sir* NORMAN. 1847–1922
The history of the study of medicine in the British Isles. Oxford, *Clarendon Press*, 1908.

FitzPatrick Lectures, 1905–06.

6537 ——. The physician in English history. Cambridge, *Univ. Press*, 1913.

Linacre Lecture, 1913.

6538 CHAPLIN, THOMAS HANCOCK ARNOLD. 1864–1944
Medicine in England during the reign of George III. London, *The Author*, 1919.

FitzPatrick Lectures, 1917–18.

6539 SINGER, CHARLES JOSEPH. 1876–1960
Early English magic and medicine. London, *H. Milford*, [1920].

Reprinted from *Proc. Brit. Acad.*, 1919–20, **9**, 341–74.

6540 POWER, *Sir* D'ARCY. 1855–1941
Medicine in the British Isles. New York, *P. B. Hoeber*, 1930.

Clio Medica series.

6541 COMRIE, JOHN DIXON. 1875–1939
History of Scottish medicine. 2nd ed. 2 vols. London, *Baillière, Tindall & Cox*, 1932.

Traces fully and accurately the history of medicine in Scotland from the earliest times.

6544 COLLIS, William Robert Fitzgerald. 1900–
The state of medicine in Ireland. Carmichael prize essay. Dublin, *Parkside Press*, 1943.

6545 FLEETWOOD, John.
History of medicine in Ireland. Dublin, *Browne & Nolan Ltd.*, 1951.

6546 GRATTAN, John Henry Grafton. 1878–1951, & SINGER, Charles Joseph. 1876–1960
Anglo-Saxon magic and medicine. London, *Oxford University Press*, 1952.

6548 JARAMILLO-ARANGO, Jaime. 1897–1962
The British contribution to medicine. Edinburgh, *E. & S. Livingstone*, 1953.

6549 BONSER, Wilfrid. 1887–1971
The medical background of Anglo-Saxon England; a study in history, psychology, and folklore. London, *Wellcome Historical Medical Library*, 1963.

6550 WALL, Cecil. 1869–1947, *et al.*
A history of the Worshipful Society of Apothecaries of London. Abstracted and arranged from the MS notes of Cecil Wall by H. Charles Cameron; revised, annotated and edited by E. Ashworth Underwood. Vol. 1: 1617–1815. London, *Wellcome Historical Medical Museum*, 1963.

6554–6556 FRANCE

6554 WICKERSHEIMER, Charles Adolphe Ernest. 1880–1965
La médecine et les médecins en France à l'époque de la Renaissance. Paris, *Maloine*, 1906.

Maloine, 1906. Wickersheimer, librarian of the University of Strasbourg, has contributed several scholarly works on the history of medicine.

6555 LAIGNEL-LAVASTINE, Maxime. 1875–1953, & MOLINÉRY, Raymond. 1876–1946
French medecine. Translated by E. B. Krumbhaar. New York, *P. B. Hoeber*, 1934.

Clio Medica series.

6556 GUIART, Jules. 1870–1945
Histoire de la médecine française: son passé, son présent, son avenir. Paris, *Editions Nagel*, 1947.

6557–6560 GERMANY

6557 ROHLFS, Heinrich. 1827–1898
Geschichte der deutschen Medicin. 4 vols. Stuttgart, *F. Enke*, 1875–77.

6558 HIRSCH, August. 1817–1894
Geschichte der medicinischen Wissenschaften in Deutschland. München, *Oldenbourg*, 1893.

6559 STICKER, GEORG. 1860–1960
Die Entwickelung der ärztlichen Kunst in Deutschland. München, *Münchner Drucke*, 1927.

6560 HABERLING, WILHELM GUSTAV MORITZ. 1871–1940
German medicine. Translated by JULES FREUND. New York, *P. B. Hoeber*, 1934.

Clio Medica series. Perusal of this little work reminds the reader especially of the wonderful era of scientific achievement in Germany from the 19th century until the present time.

6561–6565 ITALY

6561 RENZI, SALVATORE DE. 1801–1871
Storia della medicina italiana. 5 vols. Napoli, tipog. del. *Filiatre-Sebezio*, 1845–48.

6562 PITRÈ, GIUSEPPE. 1842–1916
Medicina popolare siciliana. Torino, *Clausen*, 1896.

6563 CASTIGLIONI, ARTURO. 1874–1953
Italian medicine. Translated by E. B. KRUMBHAAR. New York, *P. B. Hoeber*, 1932.

Clio Medica series.

6564 ——. The renaissance of medicine in Italy . . . The Hideyo Noguchi Lectures. Baltimore, *Johns Hopkins Press*, 1934.

Publications of the Institute of the History of Medicine. Third series. Vol. 1.

6565 PAZZINI, ADALBERTO. 1898–
Bibliografia di storia della medicine italiana. Roma, *Tosi*, 1939.

MALTA

6565.1 CASSAR, PAUL.
Medical history of Malta. London, *Wellcome Historical Medical Library*, 1964.

6566–6569 U.S.S.R.

6566 RICHTER, WILHELM MICHAEL VON. 1767–1822
Geschichte der Medicin in Russland. 3 vols. Moskwa, *N. S. Wsewolojsky*, 1813–17.

6567 GANTT, WILLIAM ANDREW HORSLEY. 1893–
Russian medicine. New York, *P. B. Hoeber*, 1937.

Clio Medica series. A valuable contribution to a little known section of medical history.

6568 RAVITCH, MICHAEL LEO. 1867–1947
The romance of Russian medicine. New York, *Liveright Pub. Corp.*, 1937.

6569 SIGERIST, HENRY ERNEST. 1891–1957
Medicine and health in the Soviet Union. New York, *Citadel Press*, 1947.

6570–6574.1 SCANDINAVIA

6570 INGERSLEV, Johan Vilhelm Christian. 1835–1918
Danmarks Læger og Lægevæsen fra de ældste Tider indtil Aar 1800. 2 vols. Kjøbenhavn, *E. Jespersen*, 1873.

6571 CARØE, Kristian Frederik. 1851–1921
Den Danske Laegestand, 1479–1900. 5 vols. København, *Gyldendal*, 1905–22.
Biographies of Danish physicians and surgeons.

6572 LENNMALM, Frithiof. 1858–1924
Svenska Läkaresällskapets historia 1808–1908. Stockholm, *I. Marcus*, 1908.
Continued (1908–38) by Gunnar Nilson, Stockholm, *General-Statens litograf. Anstalt*, 1947.

6573 LAACHE, Sören Bloch. 1854–1941
Norsk medicin i hundrede aar. Kristiania, *Steenske Bogtrykkeri*, 1911.

6574 QVIGSTAD, Just Knud. 1853–
Lappische Heilkunde. Oslo, *H. Aschehoug*, 1932.

6574.1 REICHBORN-KJENNERUD, Ingjald. 1865–1949, *et al.*
Medisinens historie i Norge. Oslo, *Grøndal*, 1936.
With F. Gron and I. Kobro.

6575–6579.1 SPAIN AND PORTUGAL

6575 CHINCHILLA Y PIQUERAS, Anastasio. 1801–1867
Anales históricos de la medicina en general, y biográfico-bibliográficos de la española en particular. 8 vols. Valencia, *Lopez, Cervera*, 1841–46.
Includes No. 6576, together with *Historia particular de las operaciones quirúrgicas*, 1841; *Historia general de la medicina*, 2 vols., 1841–43; and *Vade mecum histórico y bibliográfico*, etc., 1844. Facsimile reproduction, 1964.

6576 ——. Historia de la medicina española. 4 vols. Valencia, *Lopez, Cervera*, 1841–46.
Forms vols. 3–6 of No. 6575.

6576.1 HERNÁNDEZ MOREJÓN, Antonio. 1773–1836
Historia bibliográfica de la medicina española. 7 vols. Madrid, 1842–52.

6576.2 LA PLATA Y MARCOS, Miguel de.
Coleccion bio-bibliográfica de escritores médicos españoles. Madrid, *A. Gómez, Fuentenebro*, 1882.

6577 LEMOS, Maximiano Augusto d'Oliveira. 1860–1923
História da medicina em Portugal. 2 vols. Lisboa, *M. Gomes*, 1899.

6578 COMMENGE Y FERRER, Luis.
La medicina en Cataluña (bosquejo histórico). Barcelona, *Henrich* 1908.

6579 GARCIA DEL REAL, EDUARDO. 1870–1947
Historia de la medicina en España. Madrid, *Editorial Reus*, 1921.

6579.1 FERREIRA DE MIRA, MATIAS BOLETO. 1875–
História da medicina portuguesa. Lisboa, *Empresa Nacional de Publicidade*, 1947.

6580–6581 SWITZERLAND

6580 GAUTIER, LEON. 1853–1916
La médecine à Genève jusqu'à la fin du dix-huitième siècle. Genève, *Jullien*, 1906.

6581 BRUNNER, CONRAD. 1859–1927
Über Medizin und Krankenpflege im Mittelalter in Schweizerischen Landen. Zürich, *Füssli*, 1922.

6582–6584 CANADA

6582 CANNIFF, WILLIAM. 1830–1910
The medical profession in Upper Canada, 1783–1850. Toronto, *W. Briggs*, 1894.
Rescues from oblivion many historical facts and discusses the pioneer medical men of Canada. Biographies of many famous physicians of Canada are included.

6583 HEAGERTY, JOHN JOSEPH. 1879–
Four centuries of medical history in Canada. 2 vols. London, *Simpkin Marshall*, 1928.
The authoritative work on the history of medicine in Canada.

6584 HOWELL, WILLIAM BOYMAN. 1873–
Medicine in Canada. New York, *P. B. Hoeber*, 1933.
Clio Medica series.

6585–6596 UNITED STATES OF AMERICA

6585 TONER, JOSEPH MEREDITH. 1825–1896
Contributions to the annals of medical progress and medical education in the United States before and during the War of Independence. Washington, *Govt. Printing Office*, 1874.

6586 CLARKE, EDWARD HAMMOND, *et al.* 1820–1877
A century of American medicine 1776–1876. By EDWARD H. CLARKE, H. J. BIGELOW, S. D. GROSS, T. GAILLARD THOMAS and J. S. BILLINGS. Philadelphia, *H. C. Lea*, 1876.

6587 VIETS, HENRY ROUSE. 1890–1969
A brief history of medicine in Massachusetts. Boston, *Houghton, Mifflin, Co.*, 1930.

6588 BLANTON, WYNDHAM BOLLING. 1890–1960
Medicine in Virginia in the seventeenth century. Richmond, Va., *W. Byrd Press*, [1930].

6589 ——. Medicine in Virginia in the eighteenth century. Richmond, Va., *Garrett & Massie*, 1931.

6590 PACKARD, FRANCIS RANDOLPH. 1870–1950
History of medicine in the United States. 2nd ed. 2 vols. New York, *P. B. Hoeber*, 1931.

This is the authoritative source-book of the history of medicine in the United States. The first edition appeared in 1901. Dr. Packard edited the *Annals of Medical History*, the leading American periodical on the subject, from its commencement in 1917 until its decease in 1942.

6591 HARRIS, HENRY. 1874–
California's medical story. San Francisco, *J. W. Stacey*, 1932.

6592 SIGERIST, HENRY ERNEST. 1891–1957
Amerika und die Medizin. Leipzig, *G. Thieme*, 1933.

This is not a systematic history of American medicine, but an account of the most important landmarks in the development of medical science and teaching in the United States. An English translation, *American Medicine*, was published in New York in 1934.

6593 SHAFER, HENRY BURNELL. 1906–
The American medical profession, 1783 to 1850. New York, *Columbia Univ. Press*, 1936.

6595 SHRYOCK, RICHARD HARRISON. 1893–1972
American medical research, past and present. New York, *Commonwealth Fund*, 1947.

6596 GORDON, MAURICE BEAR. 1916–
Aesculapius comes to the Colonies. The story of the early days of medicine in the thirteen original colonies. Ventnor, N.J., *Ventnor Publishers*, 1949.

6597–6603.4 CENTRAL AND SOUTH AMERICA

6597 FLORES, FRANCISCO A.
Historia de la medicina en México desde la epoca de los Indios hasta la presente. 3 vols. México, 1886–88.

6598 SCHIAFFINO, RAFAEL. 1881–
Historia de la medicina en el Uruguay. 3 vols. Montevideo, *Imprenta Nacional, "Rosgal,"* 1927–52.

6599 RIBEIRO, LEONIDIO.
Brazilian medical contributions. Rio de Janeiro, *Livraria José Olympio*, 1939.

6600 MOLL, ARISTIDES ALCIBIADES. 1882–
Aesculapius in Latin America. Philadelphia, *Saunders*, 1944.

6601 SANTOS, LYCURGO DE CASTRO.
História da medicina no Brasil. (Do século XVI ao século XIX). 2 vols. São Paulo, *Edit. Brasiliense*, 1947.

6602 LASTRES Y QUINONES, JUAN B. 1902–1960
Historia de la medicina peruana. 3 vols. *Imprenta Santa Maria*, 1951.

6602.1 PERERA, AMBROSIO.
Historia de la medicina en Venezuela. Caracas, *Imprenta Nacional*, 1951.

6603 GUERRA, FRANCISCO. 1916–
Historiografía de la medicina colonial hispanoamericana. México, *Abastecedora de Impresos*, 1953.

6603.1 BALCÁZAR, JUAN MANUEL. 1894–
Historia de la medicina en Bolivia. La Paz, *Ediciones Juventud*, 1956.

6603.2 SOMOLINOS D'ARDOIS, GERMÁN. 1911–
Historia y medicina; figuras y hechos de la historiografía médica mexicana. México, *Imprenta Universitaria*, 1957.

6603.3 ARCHILA, RICARDO. 1909–
Historia de la medicina en Venezuela. Epoca colonial. Caracas, *Tip. Vargas*, 1961.

6603.4 PAREDES BORJA, VIRGILIO.
Historia de la medicina en el Ecuador. 2 vols. Quito, *Casa de la Cultura Ecuatoriana*, 1963.

6604–6604.2 JAPAN; PHILIPPINES

6604 WHITNEY, WILLIS NORTON.
Notes on the history of medical progress in Japan. Yokohama, *Meiklejohn*, 1885.

From *Trans. Asiatic Soc. Japan*, 1885, **12**, 245–469.

6604.1 FUJIKAWA, YU. 1865–1940
Geschichte der Medizin in Japan. Tokyo, 1911.

History of Japanese medicine from the earliest times to 1911; this work shows the influence of the Chinese upon the development of Japanese medicine, and the later effect of Portuguese and Dutch contact with Japan. In 1934 J. Ruhräh produced an abridged translation in the *Clio Medica* series, to which was added a chapter on recent Japanese medicine by K. W. Amano.

6604.2 BANTUG, JOSÉ POLICARPIO. 1884–
A short history of medicine in the Philippines during the Spanish regime. 1565–1898. Manila, *Colegio Médico-Farmacéutico de Filipinas*, 1953.

6605–6610 ART AND MEDICINE

6605 CHARCOT, JEAN MARTIN. 1825–1893, & RICHTER, PAUL MARIE LOUIS PIERRE. 1849–1933
Les démoniaques dans l'art. Paris, *A. Delahaye & E. Lecrosnier*, 1887.

Charcot was a talented artist; he collaborated with Richer, artist at La Salpêtrière, in the production of interesting books on disease and deformity as portrayed by artists, books which have put the study of medicine in relation to art upon a sound footing.

6606 ——. Les difformes et les malades dans l'art. Paris, *Lecrosnier & Babé*, 1889.

6607 RICHER, PAUL MARIE LOUIS PIERRE. 1849–1933
L'art et la médecine. Paris, *Gaultier & Cie.*, 1902.

6608 HOLLÄNDER, EUGEN. 1867–1932
Die Medizin in der klassischen Malerei. Stuttgart, *F. Enke*, 1903.
4th edition, 1950 (a re-impression of 3rd edition, 1923).

6609 ——. Plastik und Medizin. Stuttgart, *F. Enke*, 1912.

6610 VETH, CORNELIS. 1880–
De arts in de caricatuur. Amsterdam, *Van Munster*, [*c*. 1925].
German edition, Berlin, 1927.

6611–6612 COSTUME IN MEDICINE

6611 CABANÈS, AUGUSTIN. 1862–1928
Le costume du médecin en France des origines au XVIIe siècle. Paris, *Longuet*, [1921].

6612 ——. Le costume du médecin à l'étranger. Paris, *Longuet*, [*c*. 1925].

6613–6623.1 LITERATURE AND MEDICINE

6613 BARTHOLIN, THOMAS. 1616–1680
De medicis poetis dissertatio. Hafniae, *apud D. Paulli*, 1669.

6614 MENIÈRE, PROSPER. 1799–1862
Études médicales sur les poètes latins. Paris, *Baillière*, 1858.

6615 BUCKNILL, *Sir* JOHN CHARLES. 1817–1897
The medical knowledge of Shakespeare. London, *Longman*, 1860.

6616 CHÉREAU, ACHILLE. 1817–1885
Le Parnasse médical français. Paris, *A. Delahaye*, 1874.
Dictionary of French medical poets.

6617 FLETCHER, ROBERT. 1823–1912
Medical lore in the older English dramatists and poets exclusive of Shakespeare. *Johns Hopk. Hosp. Bull.*, 1895, **6**, 73–84.
Fletcher, who was born in Bristol, England, assisted J. S. Billings in the creation of the *Index-Catalogue* (No. 6763).

6618 MOYES, JOHN. 1848–1895
Medicine and kindred arts in the plays of Shakespeare. Glasgow, *J. MacLehose*, 1896.

6619 HOLLÄNDER, EUGEN. 1867–1932
Die Karikatur und Satire in der Medizin. Stuttgart, *F. Enke*, 1905.
An encyclopaedic collection of medical wit and caricature of all ages. Second edition, 1921.

6620 BLANCHARD, RAPHAEL ANATOLE ÉMILE. 1857–1919
Épigraphie médicale. 2 vols. Paris, 1909–15.

6621 PIA, Pascal.
Bouquet poëtique des médecins, chirurgiens, dentistes et apothicaires. Paris, *Coll. de l'Écritoire*, 1933.

6622 YEARSLEY, Percival Macleod. 1867–1951
Doctors in Elizabethan drama. London, *John Bale*, 1933.

6623 McDONOUGH, Mary Lou McCarthy.
Poet physicians: an anthology of medical poetry written by physicians. Springfield, *C. C. Thomas*, 1945.

6623.1 SIMPSON, Robert Ritchie.
Shakespeare and medicine. Edinburgh, *E. & S. Livingstone*, 1959.

6624–6629 MAGIC AND SUPERSTITION

6624 MAGNUS, Hugo Friedrich. 1842–1907
Der Aberglauben in der Medicin. Breslau, *M. Müller*, 1903.

6625 MERCIER, Charles Arthur. 1852–1919
Astrology in medicine. London, *Macmillan*, 1914.
FitzPatrick Lectures, 1913.

6626 SELIGMANN, Siegfried. 1870–1926
Die magischen Heil- und Schutzmittel aus der unbelebten Natur. Stuttgart, *Strecker & Schröder*, 1927.

6627 VILLIERS, Elizabeth.
Amulette und Talismane und andere geheime Dingen. München, *Drei Masken Verlag*, 1927.

6627.1 BUDGE, *Sir* Ernest Alfred Thompson Wallis. 1857–1934
Amulets and superstitions: the original texts with translations and descriptions. London, *Oxford University Press*, 1930.
Reprinted, 1961.

6628 MOON, Robert Oswald. 1865–1953
Medicine and mysticism. London, *Longmans, Green & Co.*, 1934.

6629 THOMPSON, Charles John Samuel. 1862–1943
Magic and healing. London, *Rider*, [1947].

6630–6631 MEDICAL PROFESSION

6630 RIVINGTON, Walter. 1835–1897
The medical profession. Dublin, *Fannin & Co.*, 1879.
A history of the organization of the medical profession with particular reference to Britain.

6631 BAAS, Johann Hermann. 1838–1909
Die geschichtliche Entwicklung des ärztlichen Standes. Berlin, *F. Wreden*, 1896.

6632–6633 NUMISMATICS

6632 GARRISON, Fielding Hudson. 1870–1935
Medical numismatics. *Ann. med. Hist.*, 1926, **8,** 128–35.
An excellent short paper on the subject, with references to the more important previous work.

6633 STORER, HORATIO ROBINSON. 1830–1922
Medicina in nummis. A descriptive list of the coins, medals, jetons relating to medicine, surgery and the allied sciences. Boston, *Wright & Potter Print Co.*, 1931.

This consists mainly of a catalogue of 6,000 medals collected by Storer, an eminent Boston gynaecologist. The collection is now in the Countway Medical Library, and the book, edited by M. Storer, includes some excellent reproductions, a select bibliography, and a short résumé of the subject.

6634–6639.1 NURSING

6634 HAESER, HEINRICH. 1811–1884
Geschichte christlicher Krankenpflege und Pflegerschaften. Berlin, *W. Hertz*, 1857.

6635 NUTTING, MARY ADELAIDE. 1858–1948, & DOCK, LAVINIA L. 1858–1956
A history of nursing. 4 vols. New York, *G. P. Putnam*, 1907–12.

The authoritative history of the subject. Vols. 3–4 by L. L. Dock only.

6636 SEYMER, LUCY RIDGELY.
A general history of nursing. London, *Faber & Faber*, 1932.

Second edition, 1949.

6637 JENSEN, DEBORAH MACLURG. 1900–
History of nursing. St. Louis, *C. V. Mosby Co.*, 1943.

Second edition, *History and trends of professional nursing*, 1950.

6638 SELLEW, GLADYS. 1887– , & NUESSE, CELESTINE JOSEPH. 1913–
A history of nursing. St. Louis, *C. V. Mosby*, 1946.

6639 PAVEY, AGNES ELIZABETH. 1889–
The story of the growth of nursing as an art, a vocation, and a profession. Fourth edition. London, *Faber & Faber*, 1953.

6639.1 SHRYOCK, RICHARD HARRISON. 1893–1972
The history of nursing; an interpretation of the social and medical factors involved. Philadelphia, *W. B. Saunders*, 1959.

6639.2 PHILATELY

6639.2 BISHOP, WILLIAM JOHN. 1903–1961, & MATHESON, NORMAN MURDOCH.
Medicine and science in postage stamps. London, *Harvey & Blythe*, 1948.

6640–6643.1 QUACKERY

6640 MAGNUS, HUGO FRIEDRICH. 1842–1907
Das Kurpfuscherthum. Breslau, *M. Müller*, 1903.

History of quackery in medicine.

6641 ——. Die Kurierfreiheit und das Recht auf den eigenen Körper. Ein geschichtlicher Beitrag zum Kampf gegen das Kurpfuschertum. Breslau, *M. Müller*, 1905.

6642 CORSINI, ANDREA. 1875–1961
Medici ciarlatani e ciarlatani medici. Bologna, *N. Zainichelli*, 1922.

6643 THOMPSON, CHARLES JOHN SAMUEL. 1862–1943
The quacks of old London. London, *Brentano's* (1928).

6643.1 JAMESON, ERIC.
The natural history of quackery. London, *Michael Joseph*, 1961.

6644–6649 RELIGION AND PHILOSOPHY IN RELATION TO MEDICINE

6644 ALLBUTT, *Sir* THOMAS CLIFFORD. 1836–1925
Science and mediaeval thought. London, *C. J. Clay & Sons*, 1901.
Harveian Oration, 1900.

6645 MOON, ROBERT OSWALD. 1865–1953
The relation of medicine to philosophy. London, *Longmans, Green*, 1909.

6646 CRAWFURD, *Sir* RAYMOND HENRY PAYNE. 1865–1938
The king's evil. Oxford, *Clarendon Press*, 1911.
FitzPatrick Lectures, 1911. A classical account of the history of touching for the "king's evil," scrofula, a practice of kings from ancient times until the 18th century.

6647 MOON, ROBERT OSWALD. 1865–1953
Hippocrates and his successors in relation to the philosophy of their time. London, *Longmans, Green & Co.*, 1923.
FitzPatrick Lectures, 1921–22.

6648 PAZZINI, ADALBERTO. 1898–
I santi nella storia della medicina. Roma, *Casa Ed. "Mediterranea"*, 1937.

6649 MAJOR, RALPH HERMON. 1884–
Faiths that healed. New York, *Appleton*, 1940.

6650–6650.1 WOMEN IN MEDICINE

6650 HURD-MEAD, KATE CAMPBELL. 1867–1941
A history of women in medicine from the earliest times to the beginning of the nineteenth century. Haddam, Conn., *Haddam Press*, 1938.
Most complete and authentic work so far available upon the subject.

6650.1 SCHÖNFELD, WALTHER.
Frauen in der abendländischen Heilkunde, vom klassischen Altertum bis zum Ausgang des 19. Jahrhunderts. Stuttgart, *F. Enke*, 1947.

A SELECTION OF PERIODICALS DEVOTED TO THE HISTORY OF MEDICINE 6651–6703.1

6651 ABHANDLUNGEN ZUR GESCHICHTE DER MEDICIN.
Hsg. von H. MAGNUS, MAX NEUBURGER und K. SUDHOFF. 1–18, Breslau, 1902–06.

6652 ABHANDLUNGEN ZUR GESCHICHTE DER MEDIZIN UND NATURWISSENSCHAFTEN.
1–18, Berlin, 1934–42.
Medico-historical monographs.

6653 ACTA HISTORICA SCIENTIARUM NATURALIUM ET MEDICINALIUM.
1– , København, 1942– .
Monographic series. In progress.

6653.1 ACTA MEDICAE HISTORIAE PATAVINA.
1– , Padova, 1954– .

6653.2 ACTA PHARMACIAE HISTORICA DE L'ACADÉMIE INTERNATIONALE D'HISTOIRE DE LA PHARMACIE.
No. 1– , La Haye, 1959– .

6654 ACTA PARACELSICA.
1–5, München, 1930–32.
See No. 6688.2.

6655 AESCULAPE.
Revue mensuelle illustrée. Médecine, chirurgie, pharmacie, sciences, lettres, arts, dans leurs rapports avec la médecine. 1– , Paris, 1911–
Publication suspended Aug. 1914–Dec. 1922 and June 1940–Oct. 1949. Vols. 5–12 apparently never published.

6656 ALCMEONE.
Rivista trimestrale di storia della medicina. 1– , New York, 1939– .

6656.1 ANALECTA BOERHAAVIANA.
1– , Leiden, 1959– .
Monographic series.

6656.2 ANALECTA MEDICO-HISTORICA ACADEMIAE INTERNATIONALIS HISTORIAE MEDICINAE.
1– , Oxford, 1966– .
Monographic series.

6657 ANALES CHILENOS DE HISTORIA DE LA MEDICINA.
1– , Santiago, 1959– .

6658 ANNALS OF MEDICAL HISTORY.
1–10, 1917–28; new series, 1–10, 1929–38; 3rd series, 1–4, 1939–42. New York, 1917–42.
Index (1917–42) compiled by Hilda C. Lipkin. New York, *Schuman*, 1946.

6658.1 ARBEITSGEMEINSCHAFT FÜR GESCHICHTE DER MEDIZIN.
(Deutsche Gesellschaft für die gesamte Hygiene). Mitteilungen. No. 1– , Berlin, 1967– .

6659 ARCHIV FÜR GESCHICHTE DER MEDIZIN.
Hsg. von der Puschmann-Stiftung an der Universität Leipzig unter Redaktion von K. Sudhoff. 1–36, Heft 1–2, Leipzig, 1907–43.
Continued as No. 6700.1.

6659.1 ARCHIVO IBEROAMERICANO DE HISTORIA DE LA MEDICINA.
1–15, Madrid, 1949–63.
Continued as No. 6660.2.

6660 ARCHIVOS DE HISTORIA DA MEDICINA PORTUGUEZA.
1–6; new series, 1–14, Porto, 1886–1923.

6660.1 ARCHIWUM HISTORII I FILOZOFII MEDYCYNY.
1– , Poznan, 1924– .
Suspended 1949–56. Title shortened to *Archiwum Historii Medycyny* in 1957.

6660.2 ASCLEPIO.
16– , Madrid, 1964– .
Continuation of No. 6659.1.

6661 ATTI E MEMORIE DELL'ACCADEMIA DI STORIA DELL'ARTE SANITARIA.
Ser. 11, Anno 1– , Roma, 1935–
Continuation of No. 6664.

6661.1 BASLER VERÖFFENTLICHUNGEN ZUR GESCHICHTE DER MEDIZIN UND DER BIOLOGIE.
1– , Basel, 1953– .
Monographic series.

6662 BERNER BEITRÄGE ZUR GESCHICHTE DER MEDIZIN UND DER NATURWISSENSCHAFTEN.
1– , Bern, 1942– .
Monographic series.

6663 BIJDRAGEN TOT DE GESCHIEDENIS DER GENEESKUNDE.
1—, Amsterdam, 1921—.

6663.1 BOLETÍN INFORMATIVO HISPANOAMERICANO DE HISTORIA DE LA MEDICINA.
1– , Caracas, 1864– .

6663.2 BOLETÍN DE LA SOCIEDAD ESPAÑOLA DE HISTORIA DE LA MEDICINA.
1– , Madrid, 1960– .

6664 BOLLETTINO DELL' ISTITUTO STORICO ITALIANO DELL' ARTE SANITARIA.
Anno 1–14, Roma, 1921–34.
Continued as No. 6661.

6664.1 BULLETIN OF THE HISTORY OF DENTISTRY.
1– , Chicago, 1953– .

6665 BULLETIN OF THE HISTORY OF MEDICINE.
7– , Baltimore, 1939– .
Continuation of No. 6666.

6666 BULLETIN OF THE INSTITUTE OF THE HISTORY OF MEDICINE, JOHNS HOPKINS UNIVERSITY.
1–6, Baltimore, 1933–38.
Continued as No. 6665.

6666.1 BULLETIN ET MÉMOIRES DE LA SOCIÉTÉ INTERNATIONALE D'HISTOIRE DE LA MÉDECINE.
1– , Bruxelles, 1954– .

6666.2 BULLETIN OF POLISH MEDICAL HISTORY AND SCIENCE.
1– , Chicago, 1956– .

6667 BULLETIN DE LA SOCIÉTÉ FRANÇAISE D'HISTOIRE DE LA MÉDECINE.
1–34, No. 1, Paris, 1902–40.
Continued (1945) as No. 6687.

6668 BULLETIN DE LA SOCIÉTÉ D'HISTOIRE DE LA PHARMACIE.
1–17, Paris, 1913–29.
Continued as No. 6698.

6668.1 BULLETIN OF THE SOCIETY OF MEDICAL HISTORY OF CHICAGO.
1–6, No. 1, Chicago, 1911–48.

6668.2 CAHIERS LYONNAIS D'HISTOIRE DE LA MÉDECINE.
1– , Lyon, 1955– .

6668.3 CASTALIA; RIVISTA DI STORIA DELLA MEDICINA.
1–22, Milano, 1945–66.

6669 CENTAURUS.
International magazine of the history of science and medicine.
1– , Copenhagen, 1950– .

6670 CHINESE JOURNAL OF MEDICAL HISTORY.
1– , Shanghai, 1947– .

6671 CHRONIQUE MÉDICALE.
1–45, Paris, 1894–1938.

6672 CIBA SYMPOSIA.
1–11, Summit, N.J., 1939–51.

6672.1 CIBA SYMPOSIUM.
1– , Basel, 1953– .
Continuation of No. 6673.

6673 CIBA ZEITSCHRIFT.
1–11, Basel, 1933–52.
Superseded by No. 6672.1.

6673.1 CLIO MEDICA. ACTA ACADEMIAE INTERNATIONALIS HISTORIAE MEDICINAE.
1– , Oxford, 1965– .

6673.2 COMMUNICATIONES EX BIBLIOTHECA HISTORIAE MEDICAE HUNGARICA.
1, Budapest, 1955– .

6673.3 CUADERNOS DE HISTORIA DE LA MEDICINA ESPAÑOLA.
1– , Salamanca, 1962– .

6673.4 DE HISTORIA MEDICINAE.
1– , Birmingham, Ala., 1956– .

6673.5 EPISTEME.
Rivista critica di storia delle scienze mediche e biologiche. 1– Milano, 1967– .

6673.6 FINLAY. REVISTA MEDICO-HISTORICA CUBANA.
1– , Havana, 1963– .

6674 GESNERUS.
Vierteljahrsschrift für Geschichte der Medizin und der Naturwissenschaften. 1– , Aarau, 1943– .

6675 HIPPOCRATE.
Revue d'humanisme médical. 1–7, Paris, 1933–39.

6676 HISTOIRE DE LA MÉDECINE.
1– , Paris, 1951– .

6677 HUMANA STUDIA
Bollettino bimestrale dell'Istituto di Storia della Medicina dell' Università di Roma. Ser. 11, 1–8, Roma, 1949–56.
First series published as part of *Gazzetta Internazionale di Medicina e Chirurgia*. Continued as No. 6689.2.

6677.1 INDIAN JOURNAL OF THE HISTORY OF MEDICINE.
1– , Madras, 1956– .

6678 ISIS.
1– , Wondelgem-lez-Gand, *etc.*, 1913– .
Official publication of the History of Science Society and probably the most important periodical devoted to the history of science.

6679 JANUS.
Zeitschrift für Geschichte und Literatur der Medicin. 1–3, Leipzig, etc., 1846–48.

6680 JANUS.
Central-Magazin für Geschichte und Literärgeschichte der Medizin. 1–2, Gotha, 1851–53.

6681 JANUS.
Archives internationales pour l'histoire de la médecine. 1– , Amsterdam, etc., 1896– .

6681.1 JORNAL DE HISTÓRIA DA MEDICINA.
1– , Recife, 1956– .

6682 JOURNAL OF THE HISTORY OF MEDICINE AND ALLIED SCIENCES.
1– , New Haven, 1946– .

6682.1 KOROTH. A QUARTERLY JOURNAL DEVOTED TO THE HISTORY OF MEDICINE AND SCIENCE.
1– , Jerusalem, Tel-Aviv, 1952– .

6683 KYKLOS.
Hsg. vom Institut für Geschichte der Medizin an der Universität Leipzig. 1–4, Leipzig, 1928–32.

6684 MEDICAL CLASSICS.
Compiled by EMERSON C. KELLY. 1–5, Baltimore, 1936–41.
Reprints of classical texts, with English translations where necessary. Biographical notes and full bibliographies.

6684.1 MEDICAL HISTORY.
1– , London, 1957– .

6685 MEDICAL LEAVES.
1–5, Chicago, 1937–43.
Jewish medical history.

6686 MEDICAL LIFE.
27–45, New York, 1920–38.
No more published. Previously *Mississippi Valley Medical Journal.*

6686.1 MEDICINA NEI SECOLI.
1– , Perugia, 1964– .

6686.2 MEDIZIN HISTORISCHES JOURNAL.
1– , Hildesheim, 1966– .

6687 MÉMOIRES DE LA SOCIÉTÉ FRANÇAISE D'HISTOIRE DE LA MÉDECINE.
1– , Paris, 1945– .
Continuation of No. 6667.

6687.1 MITTEILUNGEN AUS DEM INSTITUT FÜR GESCHICHTE DER MEDIZIN UND DER NATURWISSENSCHAFTEN.
1–40, Hamburg & Leipzig, 1902–42; 1– , Kiel, 1963– .
Suspended 1943–60.

6688.1 MONSPELIENSIS HIPPOCRATES.
Revue de la Société Montpelliéraine d'Histoire de la Médecine. 1– , Montpellier, 1958– .

6688.2 NOVA ACTA PARACELSICA.
Jahrbuch der Schweizerischen Paracelsus-Gesellschaft. 1–8, Basel and Einsiedeln. 1944–57.
See No. 6654.

6689 OPUSCULA SELECTA NEERLANDICORUM DE ARTE MEDICA.
1– , Amsterdam, 1907– .

6689.1 ORSZÁGOS ORVOSTÖRTÉNETI KÖNYVTÁR KÖZLEMÉNYEI.
Communicationes ex Bibliotheca Historiae Medicae Hungarica. 1– , Budapest, 1955– .

6689.2 PAGINE DI STORIA DELLA MEDICINA.
Ser. 2, 1– , Roma, 1949– .
Continuation of No. 6677.

6690 PROCEEDINGS OF THE CHARAKA CLUB.
1– , New York, 1902– .

6691 PROCEEDINGS OF THE ROYAL SOCIETY OF MEDICINE.
6– , Section of the History of Medicine, 1– , London, 1913– .

6692 PUBLICACIONES; CÁTEDRA DE HISTORIA DE LA MEDICINA.
1– , Buenos Aires, 1938– .

6693 QUELLEN UND STUDIEN ZUR GESCHICHTE DER NATURWISSENSCHAFTEN UND DER MEDIZIN.
1–8, Berlin, 1931–42.

6694 REVISTA ARGENTINA DE HISTORIA DE LA MEDICINA.
1–5, Buenos Aires, 1942–46.

6695 REVISTA BRASILEIRA DE HISTÓRIA DA MEDICINA.
1–14, Rio de Janeiro, 1949–63.

6695.1 REVISTA DE LA SOCIEDAD CUBANA DE HISTORIA DE LA MEDICINA.
1– , Habana, 1958– .

6696 REVISTA DE LA SOCIEDAD VENEZOLANA DE HISTORIA DE LA MEDICINA.
1– , Caracas, 1953– .

6696.1 REVUE D'HISTOIRE DE L'ART DENTAIRE.
1– , Paris, 1962– .

6697 REVUE D'HISTOIRE DE LA MÉDECINE HÉBRAÏQUE.
1– , Paris, 1948– .

6698 REVUE D'HISTOIRE DE LA PHARMACIE.
18– , Paris, 1930– .
Continuation of No. 6668.

6699 RIVISTA DI STORIA (CRITICA) DELLE SCIENZE MEDICHE E NATURALI.
1–47, Faenza (Siena, Firenze), 1910–56.
Continued as No. 6699.1.

6699.1 RIVISTA DI STORIA DELLA MEDICINA.
1– , Roma, 1957– .
Continuation of No. 6699.

6699.2 SALERNO.
1– , Salerno, 1967– .

6699.3 SCOTTISH SOCIETY OF THE HISTORY OF MEDICINE. REPORT OF PROCEEDINGS.
Edinburgh, 1948– .

6700 STUDIEN ZUR GESCHICHTE DER MEDIZIN.
1–23, Leipzig, 1907–34.
Heft 1–12 written mainly by Sudhoff.

6700.1 SUDHOFF'S ARCHIV FÜR GESCHICHTE DER MEDIZIN UND DER NATURWISSENSCHAFTEN. Wiesbaden.
Bd. 36, Heft 3– , Wiesbaden, 1952– .
Continuation of No. 6659.

6700.2 TÜRK TIB TARIHI ARKIVI. (ARCHIVES D'HISTOIRE DE LA MÉDECINE TURQUE.)
1– , Istanbul, 1935– .

6701 VERÖFFENTLICHUNGEN DER SCHWEIZERISCHEN GESELLSCHAFT FÜR GESCHICHTE DER MEDIZIN UND DER NATURWISSENSCHAFTEN.
1– , Zürich, Aarau, 1922– .
Monographic series.

6701.1 YPERMAN. BULLETIN DE LA SOCIÉTÉ BELGE D'HISTOIRE DE LA MÉDECINE.
1– , Louvain, 1953– .

6702 ZEITSCHRIFT FÜR GESCHICHTE DER NATURWISSENSCHAFTEN, TECHNIK UND MEDIZIN.
1– , Berlin, 1960– .

6703 ZÜRCHER MEDIZINGESCHICHTLICHE ABHANDLUNGEN
1– , Zurich, 1924.
Monographic series, devoted to the history of medicine in Switzerland.

6703.1 ZUR GESCHICHTE DER PHARMAZIE.
1– , Eutin, 1949– .

6704–6742.2 MEDICAL BIOGRAPHY

6704 ELOY, Nicolas François Joseph. 1714–1788
Dictionnaire historique de la médecine ancienne et moderne, ou mémoires disposés en ordre alphabétique pour servir à l'histoire de cette science, et à celle des medecins, anatomistes, botanistes, chirurgiens et chymistes de toutes nations. 4 vols. Mons, *H. Hoyois*, 1778.
Earliest exhaustive collection of medical biographies. The first edition of this work appeared in 1755; the above edition is the most useful.

6705 AIKIN, John. 1747–1822
Biographical memoirs of medicine in Great Britain from the revival of literature to the time of Harvey. London, *J. Johnson*, 1780.
The first collection of British medical biographies.

6706 MARINI, G.
Degli archiatri pontifici. 2 vols. Roma, 1784.
Biographies of papal physicians.

6707 HUTCHINSON, BENJAMIN.
Biographia medica; or, historical and critical memoirs of the lives and writings of the most eminent medical characters that have existed from the earliest account of time to the present period; with a catalogue of their literary productions. 2 vols. London, *J. Johnson*, 1799.

British and foreign medical biographies.

6708 DICTIONNAIRE des sciences médicales. Biographie médicale. 7 vols. Paris, *C. L. F. Panckoucke*, 1820–25.

Preface signed by A. J. L. Jourdan [1788–1848], to whom the work is by some attributed.

6709 MACMICHAEL, WILLIAM. 1784–1839
The gold-headed cane. London, *J. Murray*, 1827.

This charming "autobiography" tells of the adventures of the famous gold-headed cane, successively in the possession of Radcliffe, Mead, Askew, William and David Pitcairn, and Baillie, and then retired to a glass case in the library of the Royal College of Physicians of London. Besides good biographies of the several owners of the cane, the book gives interesting information on the condition of medicine in England in the 18th century. Several good reprints of the book are available; in particular may be mentioned that of 1915 which has an introduction by Osler and a preface by F. R. Packard, and one edited by H. S. Robinson, 1932; the latter reproduces the illustrations of the 1828 (second) edition (the first edition was not illustrated). An illustrated edition appeared in 1953.

6710 THACHER, JAMES. 1754–1844
American medical biography. 2 vols. Boston, *Richardson, etc.*, 1828.

Thacher was the first American medical historian. He was active in the American War of Independence and in 1823 he published his interesting *Medical Journal during the American Revolutionary War*. The above biography is a valuable source of information on the early medical history of the United States.

6711 PETTIGREW, THOMAS JOSEPH. 1791–1865
Medical portrait gallery. Biographical memoirs of the most celebrated physicians, surgeons, etc. etc. who have contributed to the advancement of medical science. 4 vols. London, *Fisher, Son & Co.*, *Whittaker & Co.*, [1838]–40.

6712 BAYLE, ANTOINE LAURENT JESSÉ. 1799–1858, & THILLAYE, AUGUST JEAN.
Biographie médicale par ordre chronologique. 2 vols. Paris, *A. Delahaye*, 1855.

6713 KIÆR, FRANTZ CASPER. 1835–1893
Norges Laeger i det nittende Aarhundrede (1800–1871). Christiania, 1873.

Several supplements under the same title.

6714 ALLGEMEINE DEUTSCHE BIOGRAPHIE.
56 vols. Leipzig, 1875–1912.

Continued by *Biographisches Jahrbuch und deutscher Nekrolog*, 18 vols., Berlin, 1897–1917, and by *Deutsches biographisches Jahrbuch*, 2 vols., 1925–32.

6715 MUNK, WILLIAM. 1816–1898
The roll of the Royal College of Physicians of London; comprising biographical sketches. Second edition. 3 vols. London, *The College*, 1878.

Covers the period 1518–1825. A fourth volume (1826–1925) was published in 1955, and a fifth (1926–65) in 1968.

6716 HIRSCH, August. 1817–1894
Biographisches Lexikon der hervorragenden Ärzte aller Zeiten und Völker. 6 vols. Wien, Leipzig, *Urban & Schwarzenberg*, 1884–88.
This is one of the best sources of medical biography. A revised edition was completed in 1935. Reprinted, Munich, 1962.

6717 BETTANY, George Thomas. 1850–1891
Eminent doctors: their lives and their work. Second edition. 2 vols. London, *J. Hogg*, 1885.
Deals with British doctors only.

6718 STEPHEN, *Sir* Leslie. 1832–1904
Dictionary of national biography. Edited by Leslie Stephen (and Sydney Lee). 73 vols. London, *Smith Elder & Co.*, *Oxford Univ. Press*, 1885–1959.

6719 WATSON, Irving Allison. 1849–1918
Physicians and surgeons of America. Concord, *Rep. Press Assoc.*, 1896.

6720 PAGEL, Julius Leopold. 1851–1912
Biographisches Lexikon hervorragender Aerzte des neunzehnten Jahrhunderts. Berlin, Wien, *Urban & Schwarzenberg*, 1901.

6721 RICHARDSON, *Sir* Benjamin Ward. 1828–1896
Disciples of Aesculapius. 2 vols. London, *Hutchinson & Co.*, 1900.
Biography of Richardson by Sir Arthur MacNalty, 1950.

6722 OSLER, *Sir* William, *Bart.* 1849–1919
An Alabama student, and other biographical essays. London, *Oxford Univ. Press*, 1908.

6723 JOHNSTON, William. 1843–1914
Roll of commissioned officers in the medical service of the British Army. Aberdeen, *University Press*, 1917.
Covers the period from the accession of George II in 1727 to the formation of the Royal Army Medical Corps, 1898.
Reprinted 1968 together with the complementary *List of commissioned medical officers of the Army, Charles II to accession of George II, 1660 to 1727*, by Alfred Peterkin, Aberdeen, *University Press*, 1925, as vol. 1 of *Commissioned officers in the medical services of the British Army 1660–1960*, edited by Robert Drew. London, *Wellcome Historical Medical Library*, 1968. Vol. 2 covers the period 1898–1960.

6724 GROTE, Louis Ruyter Radcliffe. 1886–
Die Medizin der Gegenwart in Selbstdarstellungen. Hrsg. von L. R. Grote. Vol. 1–8. Leipzig, *F. Meiner*, 1923–29.

6725 CAPPARONI, Pietro. 1868–1947
Profili bio-bibliografici di medici e naturalisti celebri Italiani dal sec. XVo al sec. XVIIIo. 2 vols. Roma, *Ist. Naz. Med. Farm.*, 1925–28.

6726 DICTIONARY OF AMERICAN BIOGRAPHY.
21 vols. New York, *Charles Scribners' Sons*, 1928–44.

6727 GARRISON, Fielding Hudson. 1870–1935
Available sources and future prospects of medical biography. *Bull. N.Y. Acad. Med.*, 1928, 2 ser., **4**, 586–607.
Includes a valuable bibliography of sources of medical biography.

6728 KELLY, Howard Atwood. 1858–1943, & BURRAGE, Walter Lincoln. 1860–1935
Dictionary of American medical biography. Lives of eminent physicians of the United States and Canada, from the earliest times. New York, *D. Appleton & Co.*, 1928.

6729 CRAWFORD, Dirom Grey. 1857–1942
Roll of the Indian Medical Service 1615–1930. London, *W. Thacker & Co.*, 1930.

6730 PLARR, Victor Gustave. 1863–1929
Plarr's Lives of the Fellows of the Royal College of Surgeons of England. Revised by Sir D'Arcy Power, with the assistance of W. G. Spencer and G. E. Gask. 2 vols. Bristol, *John Wright & Sons*, 1930.
Supplement, 1930–51, by Sir D'Arcy Power and W. R. LeFanu, 1953.

6731 SACKLÉN, Johan Fredric. 1763–1851, *et al.*
Sveriges läkare-historia ifran Konung Gustaf den I:s till närvarande tid. 1–4 series. Stockholm, *P. A. Nørstedt & Søner*, 1822–1935.

6732 FISCHER, Isidor. 1868–1943
Biographisches Lexikon der hervorragenden Ärzte der letzten fünfzig Jahre. 1 vol. [in 2]. Berlin & Wien, *Urban & Schwarzenberg*, 1932–33.
A supplement to the *Biographisches Lexikon* compiled by A. Hirsch (No. 6716). Reprinted, Munich, 1962.

6733 OLPP, Gottlieb. 1872–
Hervorragende Tropenärzte in Wort und Bild. München, *Otto Gmelin*, 1932.

6734 ROYAL SOCIETY, LONDON.
Obituary notices of Fellows of the Royal Society. Vol. 1–9. London, 1932–54.
Continued as *Biographical Memoirs of Fellows of the Royal Society*, vol. 1– 1955–

6735 SIGERIST, Henry Ernest. 1891–1957
Grosse Aerzte. Leipzig, *J. F. Lehmann*, 1932.
A series of biographies of the great men in medical history. English translation, New York, 1933; second (German) edition, 1954.

6736 WICKERSHEIMER, Charles Adolphe Ernest. 1880–1965
Dictionnaire biographique des médécins en France au moyen âge. 2 vols. Paris, *E. Droz*, 1936.

6737 BAILEY, Hamilton. 1894–1961, & BISHOP, William John. 1903–1961
Notable names in medicine and surgery. London, *H. K. Lewis*, 1944.
Biographical notes and portraits of men and women whose names are perpetuated in well-known medical eponyms. 3rd edition 1959.

6738 MARMELSZADT, Willard. 1919–
Musical sons of Aesculapius. New York, *Froeben Press*, 1946.

6739 DOOLIN, William. 1887–1962
Wayfarers in medicine. London, *W. Heinemann*, 1947.

6740 LEONARDO, Richard Anthony. 1895–
Lives of master surgeons. New York, *Froeben Press*, 1948–49.
One volume and supplement.

6742 MONRO, Thomas Kirkpatrick. 1865–1958
The physician as man of letters, science and action. 2nd ed. Edinburgh, *E. & S. Livingstone*, 1951.

6742.1 GILBERT, Judson Bennett. 1895–1950
Disease and destiny. A bibliography of medical references to the famous. London, *Dawsons*, 1962.

6742.2 NOBEL FOUNDATION.
Nobel lectures. Physiology or medicine. 4 vols. Amsterdam, *Elsevier*, 1964–72.
Prize lectures 1901–70, with biographies of prize-winners.

6743–6786.9 MEDICAL BIBLIOGRAPHY

See also under the histories of individual subjects

6743 GESNER, Conrad. 1516–1565
Bibliotheca universalis, sive catalogus omnium scriptorum locupletissimus, in tribus linguis, Latina, Graeca, and Hebraica. 3 vols. and appendix. Tiguri, *apud C. Froschouerum*, 1545–55.
This was one of the first attempts at a universal bibliography. Unfortunately the section on medicine (liber xxi) was never published. Osler used the *Bibliotheca universalis* as one of the models for his own *Bibliotheca Osleriana*. He placed Gesner in the most important section ("Bibliotheca prima"), and once remarked: "I am not sure that this fellow should go into 'Prima', but I love him so much that I must put him there. Besides, he is the father of Bibliography".

6743.1 LECOQ, Pascal. 1567–1632
Bibliotheca medica. Sive catalogus illorum, qui ex professo artem medicam in hunc usque annum scriptis illustrarunt. Basileae, *C. Waldkirch*, 1590.
The first systematic medical bibliography. Includes an annotated list of 1,224 authors writing in Latin, lists of French, German, and Italian writers, and other material.

6744 LINDEN, Joannes Antonides van der. 1609–1664
De scriptis medicis, libri duo. Amstelredami, *J. Blaeu*, 1637.
Van der Linden's book was at the time of its appearance the most complete medical bibliography yet produced. He issued corrected editions in 1651 and 1662, and G. A. Mercklin published a considerably expanded version in 1686.

6744.1 LIPEN, Martin. 1630–1692
Bibliotheca realis medica, omnium materiarum, rerum, et titulorum, in universa medicina occurrentium. Francofurti ad Moenum, *Johannis Friderici*, 1679.
An elaborate subject analysis, with entries arranged alphabetically by subjects, with numerous cross-references and an author index. This formed part of a six-volume work covering various sectors of learning from the beginning of printing.

6745 DOUGLAS, James. 1675–1742
Bibliographiae anatomicae specimen, sive catalogus omnium penè auctorum qui ab Hippocrate ad Harveum rem anatomicam ex professo, vel obiter, scriptis illustrârunt. Londini, *G. Sayes*, 1715.

First attempt at a systematic medical bibliography.

6746 BOERHAAVE, Herman. 1668–1738
Methodus discendi medicinam. London, 1726.

An introduction to medical literature. The edition of 1751, containing the additions of Haller, is the best.

6747 HALLER, Albrecht von. 1708–1777
Bibliotheca medicinae practicae. 4 vols. Basle, *J. Schweighauser*; Berne, *E. Haller*, 1776–88.

Haller compiled four great bibliographies dealing respectively with botany, anatomy, surgery, and medicine. They formed the most complete reference work of the time, consisting of a classified analysis of over 52,000 publications of all countries. Additions and corrections to Haller's *Bibliothecae* were published by C. G. Murr, *Adnotationes ad bibliothecas Hallerianas*, Erlangen, 1805.

6748 BLUMENBACH, Johann Friedrich. 1752–1840
Medicinische Bibliothek. 3 vols. Göttingen, *J. C. Dieterich*, 1783–88.

Includes detailed abstracts of periodical literature.

6749 ——. Introductio in historiam medicinae litterarium. Gottingae, *J. C. Dieterich*, 1786.

6750 PLOUCQUET, Wilhelm Gottfried. 1744–1813
Initia bibliothecae medico-practicae et chirurgicae realis sive repertorii medicinae practicae et chirurgiae. 8 vols. Tubingae, *J. G. Cotta*, 1793–97.

The first important classified bibliography of medical literature covering both monographic material and current periodicals. Continuation and supplement, 4 vols., 1799–1803. Revision, with added material, published as *Literatura medica digesta sive repertorium medicinae practicae, chirurgiae atque rei obstetriciae*, 4 vols. and supplement, 1808–14.

6751 YOUNG, Thomas. 1773–1829
An introduction to medical literature, including a system of practical nosology. Intended as a guide to students, and an assistant to practitioners. London, *B. R. Howlett*, 1813.

The remarkable Thomas Young compiled this bibliography which he considered necessary to a complete medical library. Second edition, 1823.

6752 HAIN, Ludwig Friedrich Theodor. 1781–1836
Repertorium bibliographicum. 2 vols. [in 4]. Stuttgartiae et Tubingae, *J. G. Cottae*, 1826–38.

Alphabetical author-index of 16,299 incunabula. Originally based on the contents of the Munich Hofbibliothek, it was made more useful when W. Copinger published a 3-volume supplement, 1895–1902, which added 6,619 items and corrected 7,000 of the original entries. In 1914 D. Reichling completed a further supplement containing 1,921 items. Until the great *Gesamtkatalog der Wiegendrucke* is completed, "Hain" will remain the greatest bibliography of early printed books.

6753 CHOULANT, JOHANN LUDWIG. 1791–1861
Handbuch der Bücherkunde für die aeltere Medicin zur Kenntniss der griechischen, lateinischen und arabischen Schriften im ärztlichen Fache und zur bibliographischen Unterscheidung ihrer verschiedenen Ausgaben, Uebersetzungen und Erläuterungen. Leipzig, *L. Voss*, 1828.

This is one of the best check lists of the printed works of the older medical writers. It achieved a second edition in 1841, which was reprinted in 1911, 1926 and 1956.

6754 CALLISEN, ADOLPH CARL PETER. 1787–1866
Medicinisches Schriftsteller-Lexicon der jetzt lebenden Aerzte, Wundärzte, Geburtshelfer, Apotheker, und Naturforscher aller gebildeten Völker. 33 vols. Copenhagen & Altona, 1830–45.

Callisen's great medical bibliography gives a complete view of the literature of the period from about 1780 to about 1830. It is, as Garrison points out, one of the greatest achievements of a single man. Reprinted, 1962–65.

6755 FORBES, *Sir* JOHN. 1787–1861
A manual of select medical bibliography. London, *Sherwood, Gilbert, and Piper*, 1835.

"First serious attempt by anyone in the English-speaking world to give a subject classification for medical literature" (Fulton).

6756 CHOULANT, JOHANN LUDWIG. 1791–1861
Bibliotheca medico-historica: sive, catalogus librorum historicorum de re medica et scientia naturali systematicus. Lipsiae, *W. Engelmann*, 1842.

Additamenta, by Julius Rosenbaum, 2 parts, 1842–47. Reprinted (without *Additamenta*), 1960.

6757 ——. Graphische Incunabeln für Naturgeschichte und Medicin. Enthaltend Geschichte und Bibliographie des ersten naturhistorischen und medicinischen Drucke des XV. und XVI. Jahrhunderts, welche mit illustrirenden Abbildungen versehen sind. Leipzig, *R. Weigel*, 1858.

Reprint, Munich, 1924, Hildesheim, 1963.

6758 BRUNET, JACQUES CHARLES. 1780–1867
Manuel du libraire et de l'amateur des livres. 5me. éd. 8 vols. Paris 1860–80.

A useful source for French medical works.

6759 POGGENDORFF, JOHANN CHRISTIAN. 1796–1877
Biographisch-litterarisches Handwörterbuch zur Geschichte der exacten Wissenschaften. 6 vols. Leipzig, *J. A. Barth*, 1863–1940.

Brief biographies, fuller bibliographies. Facsimile reprint (10 vols.), Ann Arbor, 1945.

6760 ROYAL SOCIETY OF LONDON.
Catalogue of scientific papers, compiled and published by the Royal Society of London. 19 vols. London, *Eyre & Spottiswoode*, 1867–1925.

An author-catalogue of all important scientific papers published during the 19th century.

6761 GROSS, Samuel David. 1805–1884
History of American medical literature from 1776 to the present time. Philadelphia, *Collins*, 1876.

6762 INDEX MEDICUS.
A monthly classified record of the current medical literature of the world. Compiled under the supervision of John S. Billings and Robert Fletcher. Vol. 1–21. New York, 1879–99.

A second series, edited by Fletcher and F. H. Garrison, vols. 1–18, appeared between 1903 and 1920; a third series, edited by Garrison, vol. 1–6, 1921–27. In 1927 the *Quarterly Cumulative Index to Current Medical Literature* (12 vols., 1916–26) was amalgamated with the *Index Medicus* to form *Quarterly Cumulative Index Medicus* (1927–56) which, with No. 6777, was superseded in 1960 by a new monthly *Index Medicus* with an annual *Cumulated Index Medicus.* The gap 1900–02 was filled by *Bibliographia medica,* 3 vols., edited by C. Potain and C. Richet.

6763 UNITED STATES. War Dept. Surgeon General's Office. Index-catalogue of the library of the Surgeon-General's Office. Vol. 1–16; 2nd ser., vol. 1–21; 3rd ser., vol. 1–10; 4th ser., vol. 1–11 (A–Mn); 5th ser., vol. 1–3. Washington, *Govt. Printing Office,* 1880–1961.

In 1836 Surgeon-General Lovell established a small collection of medical books for the use of his staff. From it grew the "Surgeon-General's Library", one of the greatest medical libraries in the world. J. S. Billings did much to develop the library; he planned and started the *Index-Catalogue,* probably the finest achievement of medical bibliography. Series 1–4 index about 3,000,000 books, journal articles, and pamphlets. In the 5th series only monographs and theses are included. For continuation see Nos. 6784, 6786.7. The name of the library was changed to Armed Forces Medical Library in 1952; it became the National Library of Medicine in 1956.

6765 STEINSCHNEIDER, Moritz. 1816–1907
Die hebräischen Uebersetzungen des Mittelalters. 2 vols. Berlin, 1893.

Reprinted, 1956.

6766 GYÖRY, Tibor 1869–1938
Bibliographia medica Hungariae, 1472–1899, Budapestini, *sumpt. Athenaei,* 1900.

6767 DIELS, Hermann. 1848–1922
Die Handschriften der antiken Aerzte. *Abhandl. k. preuss. Akad. Wiss.* (*Berl.*), Phil.-hist. Cl., 1905, 1–158; 1906, 1–115; 1907, 1–72.

A catalogue of manuscripts of texts and translations of classical Greek physicians. Republished in book form, 1905–08.

6768 SUDHOFF, Karl Friedrich Jakob. 1853–1938
Deutsche medizinische Inkunabeln. Leipzig, *J. A. Barth,* 1908.

6769 OSLER, *Sir* William, *Bart.* 1849–1919
Incunabula medica. A study of the earliest printed medical books, 1467–1480. Oxford, *Univ. Press,* 1923.

Bibliographical Society Publication. Based on Osler's presidential address to the Bibliographical Society in 1914, the work opens with an essay showing the influence of printing upon the development of modern medicine. Next follows a descriptive list of 217 medical books printed to 1480. This list is edited by V. Scholderer.

6770 GESAMTKATALOG DER WIEGENDRUCKE.
Vol. 1- . Leipzig, *K. W. Hiersemann*, 1925- .

The most exhaustive catalogue of incunabula yet published.

6771 POLLARD, ALFRED WILLIAM. 1859–1944, & REDGRAVE, GILBERT R.
A short-title catalogue of books printed in England, Scotland, and Ireland and of English books printed abroad, 1475–1640. London, *Biographical Society*, 1926.

6772 OSLER, *Sir* WILLIAM, *Bart.* 1849–1919
Bibliotheca Osleriana. A catalogue of books illustrating the history of medicine and science, collected, arranged, and annotated by Sir WILLIAM OSLER, Bt. and bequeathed to McGill University. Oxford, *Clarendon Press*, 1929.

This enormous bibliography of over 7,500 titles is the catalogue of Osler's magnificent library. It is probably the most complete well-annotated bibliography in the history of medicine. It reveals Osler's character better than any of his writings and stands as a monument to him. Reprinted 1969.

6773 GARRISON, FIELDING HUDSON. 1870–1935
Revised students' check-list of texts illustrating the history of medicine, with references for collateral reading. *Bull. Inst. Hist. Med.*, 1933, **1**, 333–434.

An expansion of the list which appeared in the *Index-Catalogue of the Library of the Surgeon-General's Office, Washington*, 1912, 2 ser. **17**, 89–178, also compiled by Garrison.

6774 ——. The medical and scientific periodicals of the 17th and 18th centuries, with revised catalogue and check-list. *Bull. Inst. His. Med.*, 1934, **2**, 285–343.

Addenda and corrigenda by D. A. Kronick, *Bull. Hist. Med.* 1958, **32**, 456–74.

6775 LEFANU, WILLIAM RICHARD. 1904–
British periodicals of medicine. A chronological list. *Bull. Inst. Hist. Med.*, 1937, **5**, 735–61, 827–55; 1938, **6**, 614–48.

Republished in book form, Baltimore, 1938. Supplement, 1938–61, by A. M. Shadrake, *Bull. med. Libr. Ass.*, 1963, **51**, 181–96.

6776 KLEBS, ARNOLD CARL. 1870–1943
Incunabula scientifica et medica. Short title list. Bruges, *St. Catherine Press*, 1938.

Reprinted, Hildesheim, 1963.

6777 CURRENT LIST OF MEDICAL LITERATURE.
Vol. 1–36. Washington, 1941–59.

Published weekly until June 1950, then monthly, with author and subject indexes. Cumulated indexes semi-anually. Superseded 1960 by *Index Medicus*.

6778 POSTELL, WILLIAM DOSITE. 1908–
The development of medical literature. New Orleans, *Louisiana State University*, 1942.

6779 CUSHING, HARVEY WILLIAMS. 1869–1939
The Harvey Cushing collection of books and manuscripts. New York, *Schuman's*, 1943.

Catalogue of the books and manuscripts bequeathed by Harvey Cushing to Yale University. Publication No. 1 of the Historical Library, Yale Medical Library.

6780 WING, DONALD GODDARD. 1904–1972
Short-title catalogue of books printed in England, Scotland, Ireland, Wales, and British America and of English books printed in other countries, 1641–1700. 3 vols. New York, *Columbia University Press*, 1945–51.

Supplements the *Short-title catalogue* of Pollard and Redgrave (No. 6771).

6781 RUSSELL, KENNETH FITZPATRICK. 1911–
A check list of medical books published in English before 1600. *Bull. Hist. Med.*, 1947, **21**, 922–58.

6782 KELLY, EMERSON CROSBY. 1899–
Encyclopedia of medical sources. Baltimore, *Williams & Wilkins*, 1948.

A valuable list of medical eponyms and original sources, arranged alphabetically by authors' names.

6783 SCHULLIAN, DOROTHY MAY. 1906– , & SOMMER, FRANCIS ERICH. 1890–
A catalogue of incunabula and manuscripts in the Army Medical Library. New York, *Henry Schuman*, 1950.

6784 UNITED STATES. National Library of Medicine Catalog. 18 vols. Ann Arbor, Washington, New York, 1950–66.

Two quinquennial and one sexennial cumulations of annual volumes. 6 vols., 1950–54; 6 vols., 1955–59; 6 vols., 1960–65. Author and subject indexes. First series under title "U.S. Armed Forces Medical Library". See also No. 6763; continued by No. 6786.7.

6785 FULTON, JOHN FARQUHAR. 1899–1960
The great medical bibliographers. A study in humanism. Philadelphia, *University of Pennsylvania Press*, 1951.

Gives details of the life and work of all the outstanding contributors to medical bibliography.

6785.1 BRODMAN, ESTELLE. 1914–
The development of medical bibliography. Baltimore, *Medical Library Association*, 1954.

A historical study; includes a list of 255 medical bibliographies published since 1500.

6786 WORLD LIST.
World list of scientific periodicals published in the years 1900–1960. 4th edition. 3 vols. London, *Butterworth*, 1963–65.

Includes standard abbreviations of titles of medical and scientific periodicals and gives their location in British libraries. A historical note on the *World List* appears in *Libr. Ass. Rec.*, 1953, **55**, 245–47.

6786.1 POYNTER, FREDERICK NOEL LAWRENCE. 1908–
A catalogue of incunabula in the Wellcome Historical Medical Library, compiled by F. N. L. POYNTER. London, *Oxford Univ. Press*, 1954.

Gives full bibliographical descriptions of 632 incunabula.

6786.2 SALLANDER, Hans.
Bibliotheca Walleriana. The books illustrating the history of medicine and science collected by Dr. Erik Waller and bequeathed to the library of the Royal University of Uppsala. A catalogue compiled by Hans Sallander. 2 vols. Stockholm, *Almqvist & Wiksell*, 1955.
Contains 23,000 printed items, including 150 incunabula.

6786.3 AUSTIN, Robert B.
Early American medical imprints. A guide to works printed in the United States 1668–1820. Washington, *U.S. Dept. of Health, Education and Welfare*, 1961.

6786.4 GUERRA, Francisco. 1916–
American medical bibliography 1639–1783. New York, *Lathrop C. Harper*, 1962.
Lists and describes 719 books, pamphlets, and broadsides, 506 almanacs, 25 magazines, and 224 newspapers published in the area now forming the U.S.A.

6786.5 WELLCOME HISTORICAL MEDICAL LIBRARY.
A catalogue of printed books in the Wellcome Historical Medical Library. Vol. 1– . London, *Wellcome Historical Medical Library*, 1962– .
Vol. 1: books printed before 1641; vol. 2: books printed from 1641 to 1850, A–E. Under general editorship of F. N. L. Poynter.

6786.6 EMMERSON, Joan Stuart.
Translations of medical classics. A list. Newcastle upon Tyne, 1965.
University Library Publication No. 3. Lists translations of medical works of classical interest and importance published before 1900.

6786.7 UNITED STATES. National Library of Medicine current catalog. Washington, 1966– .
Fortnightly, with quarterly and annual cumulations. Covers all material currently received. Author and subject entries.

6786.8 BLAKE, John Ballard. 1922– , & ROOS, Charles.
Medical reference works 1679–1966; a selected bibliography. Chicago, *Medical Library Association*, 1967.
Contains over 2,700 items, with annotations. Probably the most authoritative list of medical reference books available. Edited by J. B. Blake and C. Roos. Previous editions were published in the *Handbook of medical library practice*, edited by Janet Doe and Eileen R. Cunningham (1943 and 1956).

6786.9 DURLING, Richard Jasper. 1932–
A catalogue of sixteenth century printed books in the National Library of Medicine. Compiled by Richard J. Durling. Bethesda, Maryland, 1967.

6787–6804 MEDICAL LEXICOGRAPHY

6787 ISIDORE, *Bishop of Seville* [Isidorus Hispalensis]. 570–636
Etymologiarum libri xx. Augsburg, *G. Zainer*, 1472.
The principal work of Isidore of Seville, one of the greatest educationists of the Middle Ages. The *Etymologiae*, an encyclopaedic work, presents the sum of contemporary knowledge on all branches of science; Book IV affords a survey of the entire range of medicine. An English translation of the medical and anatomical sections of the *Etymologiae* is in *Trans. Amer. philos. Soc.*, 1964, **54**, pt. 2.

6788 CORDO, Simone [Simon *Januensis* or *Genuensis*]. 1270–1303
Synonyma medicinae, seu clavis sanationis. Mediolani, *Antonio Zarothus*, 1473.

First printed medical dictionary. It was originally published at Ferrara, 1471–2?, of which edition no complete copy is known.

6789 DONDI, Giacomo [Jacobus de Dondis]. 1298–1359
Aggregator, sive de medicinis simplicibus. Strassburg, *Adolph Rusch*, [*circa* 1470].

6790 FRIES, Lorenz [Frisius; Phryesen]. –?1532
Synonima und gerecht Uszlegung der Wörter so man dan in der Artzny, allen Krütern, Wurtzlen, Blůmen, Somen, Gesteinen, Safften unnd anderen Dingen zu schreiben ist. [Strassburg, *J. Grieninger*, 1519.]

6791 ESTIENNE, Henri [Stephanus]. 1528–1598
Dictionarium medicum. [Paris], *H. Fugger*, 1564.

This valuable Greek-Latin dictionary for the ancient medical writers defined and fixed a large number of anatomical terms, and exercised considerable influence on modern anatomical terminology. It was thus an important aid to the full understanding of the ancient texts.

6792 GORRIS, Jean de [Gorraeus]. 1505–1577
Definitionum medicarum libri xxiiii. Lutetiae Parisiorum, *apud A. Wechelum*, 1564.

This dictionary arranges in order of the Greek alphabet all Greek medical terms and carefully explains them in Latin. It was widely used and exerted much influence on modern medical terminology.

6793 FOES, Anuce [Foesius]. 1528–1595
Oeconomia Hippocratis, alphabeti serie distincta. In qua dictionum apud Hippocratem omnium, praesertim obscuriorum, usus explicatur, etc. Francofurdi, *apud A. Wecheli heredes*, 1588.

Foesius spent 40 years in the preparation of this concordance to Hippocrates. It was unsurpassed until Littré's great work appeared 250 years later.

6794 CASTELLI, Bartolommeo. ?–1607
Lexicon medicum Graeco-Latinum ex Hippocrate, et Galeno desumptum. Messanae, *typ. P. Breae*, 1598.

The earlier lexicon of Gorraeus formed the basis of this work, which was reprinted in several editions, the last in 1792.

6795 NAUDÉ, Gabriel. 1600–1653
Quaestio iatrophilologica. Romae, *G. Facciotti*, 1632.

Learned bibliophile and at one period librarian of the Vatican, Gabriel Naudé eventually became Mazarin's librarian and built up for his master a famous collection of books. He wrote an important medical dictionary. Four further parts of the above, with varying titles and places of publication, 1634–47.

6796 BAILLOU, Guillaume de [Ballonius]. 1538–1616
Definitionum medicinarum liber. Parisiis, *J. Quesnel*, 1639.

A glossary of Hippocratic terms.

6797 BLANKAART, Stephan [Blancard]. 1650–1702
A physical dictionary; in which all the terms relating either to anatomy, chirurgery, pharmacy, or chemistry, are very accurately explain'd. London, *J. D. Crouch*, 1684.

The English translation of Blankaart's dictionary was the first medical dictionary to be printed in the British Isles. The original Greek-Latin text was published in Amsterdam, 1679.

6798 CALLARD DE LA DUCQUERIE, Jean Baptiste. 1630–1718
Lexicon medicum etymologicum. Cadomi, *J. Briard*, 1691.

Contains 11,000 definitions.

6799 JAMES, Robert. 1705–1776
A medicinal dictionary. 3 vols. London, *T. Osborne*, 1743–45.

The largest, most exhaustive and most learned medical dictionary written in English prior to the scientific age of medicine which arose in the early 19th century. Dr. Johnson wrote the preface. For an interesting account of the dictionary, see *Ann. med. Hist.*, 1929, n.s. **1**, 180–90.

6800 COPLAND, James. 1791–1870
A dictionary of practical medicine. 3 vols. London, *Longman, etc.*, [1832]–58.

6801 DICTIONNAIRE ENCYCLOPÉDIQUE DES SCIENCES MÉDICALES.
100 vols. Paris, *Asselin et Masson*, 1864–89.

Includes a great number of articles written by the best-known French medical men of the period. A. Dechambre directed it until 1885 when he was succeeded by L. Lereboullet.

6802 LITTRÉ, Maximilien Paul Emile. 1801–1881, & ROBIN, Charles Philippe. 1821–1885
Dictionnaire de médecine. Paris, *J. B. Baillière*, 1865.

This is the twelfth edition of a dictionary first published in 1810, compiled by P. H. Nysten.

6803 POWER, Henry. 1829–1911, & SEDGWICK, Leonard W.
New Sydenham's Society's lexicon of terms used in medicine and the allied sciences. Edited by Henry Power and Leonard W. Sedgwick. 5 vols. London, *New Sydenham Soc.*, 1881–99.

6804 FISCHER, Isidor. 1868–1943
Die Eigennamen in der Krankheitsterminologie. Wien, Leipzig, *M. Perles*, 1931.

The best dictionary of medical eponyms so far produced. It gives references to the original papers and books concerned, and records wherever possible the first use of the eponym.

INDEX OF PERSONAL NAMES

References are to entry numbers; page numbers are not used in the index. References to original works are given in roman type; other references are given in *italic* type.

INDEX OF PERSONAL NAMES

INDEX OF SUBJECTS

References are to entry numbers; page numbers are not used in the index